320
1

AMPHIBIAN MEDICINE
AND
CAPTIVE HUSBANDRY

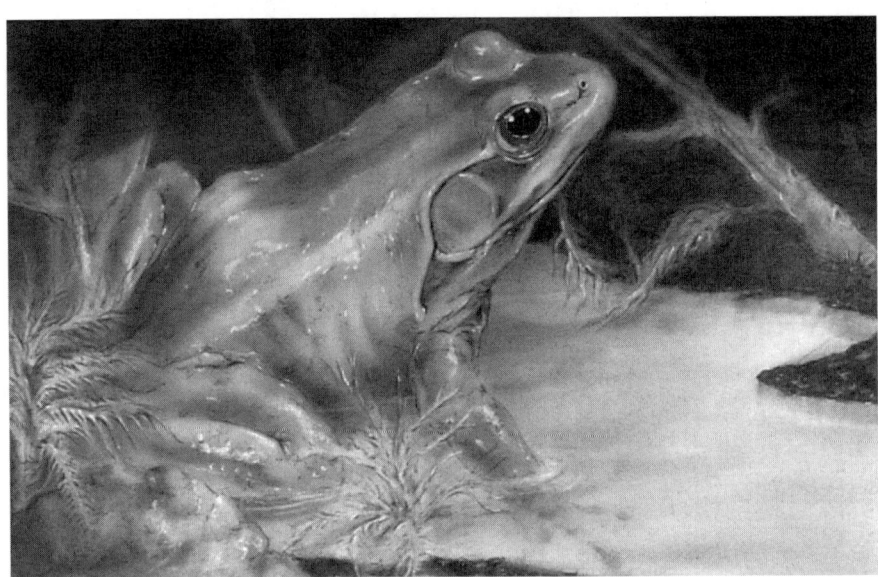
Drawing by Quade Paul

AMPHIBIAN MEDICINE AND CAPTIVE HUSBANDRY

Edited by
Kevin M. Wright, DVM and
Brent R. Whitaker, MS, DVM

KRIEGER PUBLISHING COMPANY

MALABAR, FLORIDA
2001

> **Notice**
>
> The authors and editors of this book are not responsible for any misuse or misapplication of the information provided within this work. Amphibian medicine and husbandry is an evolving field; therefore, new developments ultimately alter the practice. It should be noted that the authors and editors of this work have carefully and extensively researched all of its contents so that it contains the current standards or appropriate applications at the time of writing. Normal safety precautions should be followed. Due to new discoveries and experiences, changes in treatment and therapy may become necessary. To be certain that changes have not been made in the recommended dose or in the contraindications for administration, we advise readers to review product information provided by the manufacturer on all utilized drugs prior to administration. It is the responsibility of those administering a drug to determine the dosages, the best treatment, and the justification for any possible risk to the animal.
>
> The Publisher

Cover illustration: Tim Phelps

Original Edition 2001

Printed and Published by
KRIEGER PUBLISHING COMPANY
KRIEGER DRIVE
MALABAR, FLORIDA 32950

Copyright © 2001 by Krieger Publishing Company

All rights reserved. No part of this book may be reproduced in any form or by any means, electronic or mechanical, including information storage and retrieval systems without permission in writing from the publisher.
No liability is assumed with respect to the use of the information contained herein.
Printed in the United States of America.

> FROM A DECLARATION OF PRINCIPLES JOINTLY ADOPTED BY
> A COMMITTEE OF THE AMERICAN BAR ASSOCIATION AND A
> COMMITTEE OF PUBLISHERS:
> This publication is designed to provide accurate and authoritative information in regard to the subject matter covered. It is sold with the understanding that the publisher is not engaged in rendering legal, accounting, or other professional service. If legal advice or other expert assistance is required, the services of a competent professional person should be sought.

Library of Congress Cataloging-in-Publication Data

Amphibian medicine and captive husbandry / Kevin M. Wright and Brent R. Whitaker,
    editors.—Original ed.
        p.   cm.
        Includes bibliographical references (p.) and index.
        ISBN 0-89464-917-5 (hc : alk. paper)
    1. Amphibians—Diseases. 2. Captive amphibians—Diseases. 3. Veterinary medicine.
    I. Wright, Kevin M., 1962- II. Whitaker, Brent R., 1958- III. Title.

SF997.5A45 A46 2000
639.3'78—dc21   99-086774

DEDICATION

Dedicated to my lovely wife, Marlene, who has lived through the ancient curse of "interesting times" ever since linking up with me. Marlene has cared for the hundreds of beating hearts that are our unusual family, and supported me through the various twists and turns of my professional life. Recognition is also due my parents, Don and Jean, who were the most incredible parents a young herpetologist could have. Even the occasional loose snake popping up in their bathroom was met with considerable aplomb. They gave me the freedom and support to follow my dreams. Thanks also to my grandmother, Grace, who gave me my first redfoot tortoise when I was six. I've met few other people that rival her love of creatures and zest for life. And finally, the parade of lives that have shared their time with me: Spotty, Heidi, Hyla, Svetlana, Chichirivichi, Barnaby, the Imp, Rana, Wally, Charlie, Mr. Smartypants, Apollo, Bubbles, Chani, Apaula, Bob, Butthead, Thing 1 and Thing 2, Rana, Lola, Mbongo, Dongo, Zongo, Peaches, Succubus, Incubus, Corey, Schloemoe, Popeye, Tippie, Rascal, Flower, Spotty, Herman, George, Altair, Scooter, Chet, Abercromby, Suri, Sassy, Sweet-ums, Cleo, Gorgo, and a thousand others.

Kevin M. Wright, DVM

Dedicated lovingly to my wife, Rebecca Ann, who has encouraged me through the years, and our children, whose relentless curiosity must never cease. To my parents who tolerated without question all creatures found in field and stream, and to Tommy V, who taught me that there is a lot to be learned about these wonderful creatures if one is willing to carry the bucket.

Brent R. Whitaker, MS, DVM

CONTRIBUTING AUTHORS

Sandra L. Barnett, MA, Senior Herpetologist, National Aquarium in Baltimore, Baltimore, MD

Val B. Beasely, DVM, PhD, Diplomate ABVT, Professor of Veterinary and Ecological Toxicology, Department of Veterinary Biosciences, College of Veterinary Medicine, University of Illinois at Urbana-Champaign, Urbana, IL

John F. Cover, Jr., BS, Curator of the Rainforest Exhibits, National Aquarium in Baltimore, Baltimore, MD

Stephen G. Diana, MS, DVM, Clinical Research Investigator, Animal Health/Clinical Affairs, Pfizer, Inc., Groton, CT

D. Earl Green, DVM, Diplomate ACVP, Veterinary Pathologist, National Wildlife Health Center, U.S. Geological Survey, U.S. Department of the Interior, Madison, WI

John C. Harshbarger, PhD, Professor of Pathology and Director of Registry of Tumors in Lower Animals, George Washington University Medical Center, Washington, DC

Sandy McCampbell, CAHT, Veterinary Technician, Department of Animal Health, Philadelphia Zoological Garden, Philadelphia, PA

Donald K. Nichols, DVM, Diplomate ACVP, Associate Pathologist, Department of Pathology, National Zoological Park, Washington, DC

Sarah L. Poynton, PhD, Lecturer, Division of Comparative Medicine, The Johns Hopkins University School of Medicine; Research Associate, National Aquarium in Baltimore, Baltimore, MD

Mark D. Stetter, DVM, Diplomate ACZM, Veterinary Operations Manager, Disney Animal Programs, Walt Disney World, Orlando, FL

Sharon K. Taylor, DVM, PhD, Wildlife Manager, Diagnostic Veterinarian Manager, Florida Fish and Wildlife Conservation Commission, Gainesville, FL

Brent R. Whitaker, MS, DVM, Director of Animal Health, National Aquarium in Baltimore, Baltimore, MD

Kevin M. Wright, DVM, Curator/Veterinarian of Amphibians and Reptiles, Philadelphia Zoological Garden, Philadelphia, PA (1993–1999). Currently Curator of Ectotherms, The Phoenix Zoo, Phoenix, AZ

ACKNOWLEDGMENTS

Authors:
We wish to thank our authors for their generous contribution to *Amphibian Medicine and Captive Husbandry*. Each has drawn upon years of study and experience, and searched the literature to provide valuable information that has practical applications.

Reviewers:
Chris Andrews: The Amphibian Eye, Clinical Techniques; Sandy Barnett: Clinical Techniques, Reproduction; Michael Bodri: Protozoa and Metazoa Infecting Amphibians; Kelley Corcoran: The Amphibian Eye; Jack Cover: Water Quality, Clinical Techniques, The Amphibian Eye; Mike Cranfield: Clinical Toxicology, Idiopathic Syndrome, Trauma; Graham Crawshaw: Pharmacotherapeutics, Reproduction, Surgical Techniques; Susan Donoghue: Diets for Captive Amphibians, Nutritional Disorders; John Scott Foster: Applied Physiology; Jack Gaskin: Microbiological Techniques for the Exotic Practice; Greg Lewbart: Hematology; Kelly Myers: Water Quality; R. Andrew Odum: Anatomy for the Clinician, Evolution of the Amphibia, Taxonomy of Amphibians Kept in Captivity; Mark Stetter: Bacterial Diseases, Mycoses, Restraint Techniques; Liz Watson: Diagnostic Imaging of Amphibians; Additional anonymous reviewers who greatly enhanced the presentation of the material.

Literature:
Our sincere appreciation is extended to Susie Ridenour, Librarian at the National Aquarium in Baltimore, who provided us with a substantial portion of the literature needed to complete this text. Her genuine enthusiasm and unfailing ability to acquire even the most obscure of references simplified our task and added to its completeness.

Artwork:
Johns Hopkins School of Medical Illustration: The majority of the artwork presented in this text represents a collaborative effort between graduate students from the Department of Art as Applied to Medicine at Johns Hopkins University and members from the scientific community at the National Aquarium in Baltimore. Over the past six years, graduate students, studying medical and biological illustration, have worked with veterinarians, animal care staff and researchers in developing illustrative plates that explain anatomical and physiological concepts current to amphibian medicine and captive husbandry. Each illustrator's final artwork is based on direct observation and original research as well as on-site sketches. Our deepest gratitude is extended to those who met the challenge, and to their teachers, Brent Bauer, Tim Phelps, and Gary Lees, as well as Juan Garcia, who was instrumental in acquiring the original drawings and preparing them for publication. A listing of contributing individual artists follows: Brent Bauer, Rachel Bedno-Robinson, Reneé Cannon, Wen-Min Chao, Emiko-Rose Koike, Michael Linkinhoker, Quade Paul, Tim Phelps, Bradley Duncan Powell, John Gibb, and Michael Tirenin.

Founded in 1911, the Department of Art as Applied to Medicine was the first of its kind in the world. Johns Hopkins University has trained medical illustrators to advance medical and scientific education internationally for over eighty years. Its graduates continue the Hopkins' tradition of excellence into the 21st century.

Others:
Wilbur Amand, Sandy Barnett, George Grall, Geoff Hall, Keith Hinshaw, Mike Langel, Karl Kranz, Sandy McCampbell, Joyce Parker, and Virginia Pierce are due

thanks for their support that resulted in this book. This work would not have been possible without the support of our institutions, the Philadelphia Zoological Garden and the National Aquarium in Baltimore.

We are also grateful to the following individuals and institutions for their contributions to the photography and art in the book:

Steve Walker, Philadelphia Zoological Garden
Robert Dougan
Florence Robin, Philadelphia Zoological Garden
Tom Dewey, Philadelphia Zoological Garden
Caitlin Hughes
Jenni Jenkins, National Aquarium Baltimore
Christine Steinert, National Aquarium Baltimore
Steve Barten
Lisa Tell, U.S. Government
Scott Citino, Philadelphia Zoological Garden
Heino Möller, Institut für Meereskunde, Kiel, Germany
Philip Rutledge, University of Maryland at Baltimore County
Tracy Barker, Vida Preciosa
Tracey McNamara
Mike Lynn
Jim Walberg
Jay Stefanacci
Barbara Mangold
Ron Conti, Philadelphia Zoological Garden
David Wood
Don Gillespie
F.L. Rose
W.R. Duryee
R. Andrew Odum, Toledo Zoological Society
Scott Highton
Fredric L. Frye

B.J. Cohen
D.H. Ringler, University of Michigan
V.V. Khudoley
C.L. Counts
L.E. DeLanney
C.E. Smith
M.D. McGavin
W. Janisch and T. Schmidt
E. Elkan
G.E. Cosgrove
D.L. Graham
F. Hissom
J.S. Waterhouse
D.J. Mulcare
R.E. Miller
R.L. Snyder
Donald K. Nichols, National Zoological Park
A.J. Herron
R. Verhoeff-DeFremery
J.D. Hardy
J.C. Streett
A.A. Cunningham, The Zoological Society of London
Scott Highton
A. Klembau
K. Wolf and R.L. Herman, National Fish Health Research Laboratory
R. Clapp
C.S. Patton, Armed Forces Institute of Pathobiology
M.M. El-Mofty
G.R. Zug
J. Carney
Wilmer Photography, Johns Hopkins University

Lastly we would like to thank Patty Wolf, Joseph A. Sisneros and Carla L. Fisher at Krieger Publishing Co. for their editorial work on this book. Originally, the book was to be no more than 280 pages. As we prepared our manuscripts and received chapters from contributing authors, it became clear that we had underestimated the wealth of available information on amphibians. We, therefore, wish to thank Elaine Harland and Mr. Krieger for their ever-present patience and support in the creation of this tome. It is our hope that the editors derived as much joy out of managing our text as we did assembling it.

FOREWORD

Rarely do we stop to consider how important amphibians are in our lives. For many of us, our first contact with an amphibian was that frog or toad we encountered during our youth in the back yard or in the park, or we might have seen a redback salamander underneath a log. Our next encounter with amphibians was most likely in high school or in undergraduate school where we dissected a frog in a biology or comparative anatomy class. In veterinary school we may have used the frog muscle in the study of muscle physiology. The point is that amphibians were not high profile animals, not charismatic megavertebrates such as many mammals, and they certainly were not the primary subject in any veterinary text on animal health. Indeed until now there has been no text fully devoted to the health and diseases of these oftentimes colorful and always fascinating creatures.

Although our experience with amphibians has been limited, they have been used as laboratory research animals for more than a century. In addition to their more classic role in developmental biology, amphibians have also been used in the study of comparative, developmental and transplantation immunology, susceptibility to toxicants, teratogen screening, limb regeneration, osmoregulation, physiology and endocrinology of metamorphosis, and embryology and hormone assays. Yet our understanding of amphibian health and disease has been meager. Hence, our ability to provide proper veterinary care for amphibians under captive conditions has been limited.

For more than 50 years, many amphibian species have markedly declined in numbers. Many of these declines have been attributed to adverse human influences acting on local populations of amphibians. However, by the late 1980s herpetologists from many parts of the world were seeing declines in amphibian populations in what appeared to be pristine habitats. With these observations came the suggestion that there may be one or more global factors that are adversely affecting amphibians. By 1991 the concern became so great that the Declining Amphibian Populations Task Force was established by the Species Survival Commission of the World Conservation Union. The Task Force, operating through a network of Working Groups worldwide, collect geographical data on amphibian declines and their causes, and distribute small grants to initiate research projects in key areas.

Recently amphibians have "enjoyed" more public attention. In the summer of 1995, a large number of frogs were discovered in Minnesota with misshapen, extra, or missing limbs. Since then and continuing on to the present time, scientists have been seeking the causes for this phenomenon. Hypotheses abound with many pointing to xenobiotic chemicals as at least one of the reasons for this apparent large increase in amphibian malformations. What drives the interest in and research into the causes of malformed frogs is not purely because of the amphibian itself but rather because of the potential for effects on human health. It would appear that the amphibian is becoming the "canary of the miner" in our modern time as the amphibian is sensitive to numerous stressors in the aquatic environment and may forecast serious threats to our own species.

As noted above, veterinarians have very few sources of information on the health and disease of amphibians. What we have had in the past were single chapters in texts on reptiles or laboratory animal medicine. This text fills a great void in our knowledge of amphibians. Drs. Kevin Wright and Brent Whitaker, along with the individual chapter authors, are to be congratulated for their foresight and dedication to producing a text that provides us with the necessary information to care for amphibians, whether they be private pets, laboratory animals, zoo and aquarium exhibits, or found in the wild. Thanks for a job well done!

Wilbur B. Amand, VMD
Executive Director
American Association of Zoo Veterinarians and
Association of Reptilian and Amphibian Veterinarians
Adjunct Professor, University of Pennsylvania School of Veterinary Medicine

PREFACE

Amphibian Medicine and Captive Husbandry began back in the late 1980's when I suggested to my classmate, Brent, that we should write a book on amphibian medicine. I don't remember his exact response at the time, but considering his tolerance (and even enjoyment) of the *non sequiturs* I spout on a minute by minute basis, I imagine that I received the answer, "Yes, we should do that." Amphibians were a class of animals that were sadly neglected by the professors who taught at my school. This state of affairs was not restricted to the University of Florida (which indeed put more effort into exotic animal medicine than any other school at the time except, perhaps, the University of California at Davis). Somehow, despite being linked to a rather eccentric and offbeat human being who, at times, sported half a beard and wore boxer shorts below cut-off shorts way before it became hip, Brent managed to become staff veterinarian at the National Aquarium in Baltimore, an institution that houses a vast collection of neotropical frogs. With a few more stops, I ended up curator for a smaller but still respectable collection of amphibians that included frogs, salamanders and caecilians. And, after all those years, I once again had the audacity to suggest that we knew enough to put together a book on amphibian medicine.

Elaine Harland took the time to listen to me at the International Herpetological Symposium in Miami, Florida. Several months later, Brent and I started living a life of strange disquiet right after the ink dried on the contract with Krieger Publishing Company.

This book focuses on the literature published in the English language, and is biased heavily toward American publications. It is intended as a good starting point for the clinician interested in amphibians, as well as the most complete reference currently available for those with a strong interest in amphibian medicine.

Undoubtedly this text contains information that will be obsolete or proven erroneous within a few years. Amphibian medicine is in its infancy and needs to develop quickly to catch up with other fields in medicine. Take the time to document your experience, positive or negative, and get that information into print, preferably in a peer-reviewed journal. The field is wide open, and with the appropriate effort anyone can make a contribution. Some people may strongly disagree with the interpretation of the material presented herein, and it is our hope that those with such material to refute our presentation take the time to publish their experience through a peer-reviewed journal. Such information should be disseminated widely, not locked inside their heads.

The information contained within this text has few absolutes. The techniques and drug dosages are ones that have proven effective in many species or, at worst, done no harm. Extra-label use applies to the entire field of amphibian medicine, and the client should be so advised with each and every treatment administered. The risk of treatment failures and the possibility of adverse reactions should be explained carefully to the client before initiating any treatment or procedure with an amphibian. Above all, don't forget the basic tenets of practicing medicine just because your patient is green, coated with mucus and hops. The information contained herein is intended as a guide only, and no responsibility for treatment success or failure is assumed or implied. New information is constantly becoming available, and the clinician must make the effort to keep current with theories and practices involved in all aspects of veterinary medicine.

Enough said. Enjoy.

Kevin M. Wright, DVM

CONTENTS IN BRIEF

Chapter 1	Evolution of the Amphibia
Chapter 2	Taxonomy of Amphibians Kept in Captivity
Chapter 3	Anatomy for the Clinician
Chapter 4	Applied Physiology
Chapter 5	Amphibian Husbandry and Housing
Chapter 6	Diets for Captive Amphibians
Chapter 7	Nutritional Disorders
Chapter 8	Clinical Techniques
Chapter 9	Restraint Techniques and Euthanasia
Chapter 10	Clinical Microbiology of Amphibians for the Exotic Practice
Chapter 11	Amphibian Hematology
Chapter 12	Water Quality
Chapter 13	Bacterial Diseases
Chapter 14	Mycoses
Chapter 15	Protozoa and Metazoa Infecting Amphibians
Chapter 16	Clinical Toxicology
Chapter 17	Trauma
	Color Plates
Chapter 18	Idiopathic Syndromes
Chapter 19	The Amphibian Eye
Chapter 20	Diagnostic Imaging of Amphibians
Chapter 21	Surgical Techniques
Chapter 22	Reproduction
Chapter 23	Quarantine
Chapter 24	Pharmacotherapeutics
Chapter 25	Necropsy
Chapter 26	Spontaneous Neoplasia in Amphibia
Chapter 27	Pathology of Amphibia
Appendix	
Index	

CONTENTS

CHAPTER 1
Evolution of the Amphibia
Kevin M. Wright, DVM
The Phoenix Zoo

Further Reading 1

CHAPTER 2
Taxonomy of Amphibians Kept in Captivity
Kevin M. Wright, DVM
The Phoenix Zoo

Introduction 3	Pelodytidae 9
Order Gymnophiona 3	Myobatrachidae 9
Order Caudata 5	Heleophrynidae 9
Sirenidae 5	Sooglossidae 9
Hynobiidae 6	Leptodactylidae 10
Cryptobranchidae 6	Bufonidae 10
Proteidae 6	Brachycephalidae 11
Dicamptodontidae 6	Rhinodermatidae 11
Amphiumidae 6	Pseudidae 11
Salamandridae 6	Hylidae 11
Ambystomatidae 7	Centrolenidae 11
Plethodontidae 7	Dendrobatidae 12
Order Anura 8	Ranidae 12
Leiopelmatidae 8	Hyperolidae 12
Discoglossidae 8	Rhacophoridae 13
Rhinophrynidae 8	Microhylidae 13
Pipidae 9	Helpful Guides for Identification ... 13
Pelobatidae 9	

CHAPTER 3
Anatomy for the Clinician
Kevin M. Wright, DVM
The Phoenix Zoo

Comprehensive Anatomic Texts 15	Integumentary System 19
Larval Amphibians 15	Alimentary System 21
The Larval Caecilian 15	Urinary System 23
The Larval Salamander 16	Respiratory System 24
The Larval Anuran 16	Cardiovascular System 27
Adult Amphibians 16	Hematolymphopoietic System 28
External Anatomy 16	Endocrine System 28
Musculoskeletal System 17	Reproductive System 29
Nervous System 19	

CHAPTER 4
Applied Physiology
Kevin M. Wright, DVM
The Phoenix Zoo

Thermal Homeostasis	31	Energy Metabolism	33
Water Homeostasis	31	Calcium Metabolism	33

CHAPTER 5
Amphibian Husbandry and Housing
Sandra L. Barnett, MA
National Aquarium in Baltimore
John F. Cover, Jr., BS
National Aquarium in Baltimore
Kevin M. Wright, DVM
The Phoenix Zoo

Introduction	35	Aquatic Stream Enclosures	47
Planning for an Acquisition	35	Stream-Side Enclosure	49
Handling and Transporting a New Acquisition	36	Terrestrial Forest Floor Enclosures	49
Quarantine	37	Terrestrial Fossorial Enclosure	51
Housing	38	Arboreal Enclosures	53
Overview	38	Environmental Control	54
The Basic Amphibian Enclosure	39	Temperature	55
General Guidelines for Enclosure Setup and Maintenance	41	Humidity	57
		Precipitation	57
Enclosure Location	45	Lighting	58
Aquatic Pond Enclosures	45	Nutrition	59

CHAPTER 6
Diets for Captive Amphibians
Kevin M. Wright, DVM
The Phoenix Zoo

Introduction	63	Culturing Food Items	69
Larval Amphibians	63	Introduction	69
Adult Aquatic Amphibians	65	White worms	69
Terrestrial Amphibians	66	Red worms	70
Rodents as a Food Source	67	Springtails	70
Feeding Patterns	67	Flour beetles	70
Vitamin and Mineral Supplementation	67	Mealworms	70
Recording the Diet	69	Fruit flies	71
Dermatophagy	69	Sources of Live Invertebrates	71

CHAPTER 7
Nutritional Disorders
Kevin M. Wright, DVM
The Phoenix Zoo
Brent R. Whitaker, MS, DVM
National Aquarium in Baltimore

Metabolic Bone Disease	73	Gastric Overload and Impaction	79
Hypervitaminosis D_3	76	Scoliosis	80
Thiamine Deficiency	76	Spindly Leg	80
Steatitis	76	Paralysis	80
Renal Calculi	77	Corneal Lipidosis (Lipid Keratopathy)	81
Obesity	77	Cachexia	81

Nutritional Support for the Ill and
Inappetent Amphibian 82

Assist-Feeding 82
Choosing a Formula 83

CHAPTER 8
Clinical Techniques
Brent R. Whitaker, MS, DVM
National Aquarium in Baltimore
Kevin M. Wright, DVM
The Phoenix Zoo

Introduction 89
Transportation of the Amphibian Patient 90
Obtaining a History 91
    Species 91
    Presenting Sign or Complaint 92
    Origin 92
    Husbandry 92
    Diet 95
    Preventive Medicine 95
    Miscellaneous 96
The Examination Room 96
Conducting the Physical Examination 98
    Clinical Examination 98

Clinical Techniques 101
    Celiocentesis 101
    Blood Collection 102
    Cloacal Wash 102
    Culture Collection 103
    Electrocardiography 103
    Endoscopy 105
    Fecal Evaluation 105
    Medication and Nutrient Administration .. 106
    Skin Scrape 107
    Gastric Wash 108
    Touch Preparations 108
    Tracheal Wash 109
    Urine Collection and Analysis 109

CHAPTER 9
Restraint Techniques and Euthanasia
Kevin M. Wright, DVM
The Phoenix Zoo

Manual Restraint 111
Chemical Restraint 114
    Patient Preparation 114
    Anesthetic Monitoring 115

Topical Anesthetics 115
Inhalant Anesthetics 119
Miscellaneous Anesthetics 120
Euthanasia 121

CHAPTER 10
Clinical Microbiology of Amphibians for the Exotic Practice
Sandy McCampbell, CAHT
Philadelphia Zoological Garden

Culture Media for Bacteria 123
    Trypticase Soy Agar with 5% Sheep's Blood
    (Blood Agar Plate) 123
    MacConkey Agar 123
    Columbia Colistin and Nalidixic Acid
    Agar with 5% Sheep's Blood 123
    Thioglycollate Broth 123
Other Media 124
    Salmonella-Shigella Agar 124
    GN Broth 124
    Salmonella Isolation Media 124
Culture Media for Fungi 124
Handling Specimens 124
    Liquid Specimens 124
    Swab Specimens 124

Solid Specimens 125
Antibiotic Sensitivity Testing
    and Bacterial Identification 125
    Gram-Positive Cocci 125
    Gram-Negative Rods 125
    Pathogenic Fungi 126
    Mycobacterium spp. 126
Suggested Samples 126
    Systemic Infections 126
    Skin Infections 126
    Respiratory Infections 126
    Culture for "Normal Microflora" 126
    Necropsies 126
Suppliers of Products Mentioned in Text 128

CHAPTER 11
Amphibian Hematology
Kevin M. Wright, DVM
The Phoenix Zoo

Blood Volume 129	Complete Blood Count 133
An Algorithm for Sample Processing 129	Chemistry 134
Anticoagulants 130	Cytology 134
Blood Collection 130	Interpreting the Hemogram 139
Sample Analysis 132	Interpreting Plasma Biochemistries 140
Stains 132	

CHAPTER 12
Water Quality
Brent R. Whitaker, MS, DVM
National Aquarium in Baltimore

Introduction 147	Hardness 151
Water Temperature 147	Alkalinity 151
Oxygen 148	Total Ammonia Nitrogen 151
Carbon Dioxide 150	Filtration 154
pH, Hardness, and Alkalinity 150	Water Changes 156
pH 150	Water Source 156

CHAPTER 13
Bacterial Diseases
Sharon K. Taylor, DVM, PhD
Florida Fish and Wildlife Conservation Commission
D. Earl Green, DVM, Diplomate ACVP
National Wildlife Health Center
Kevin M. Wright, DVM
The Phoenix Zoo
Brent R. Whitaker, MS, DVM
National Aquarium in Baltimore

Predisposing Factors 159	*Leptospira* 170
Localized Infections 159	*Listeria* 170
Introduction 159	*Salmonella* 170
Superficial Wounds, Ulcers and Abscesses .. 159	*Edwardsiella* 171
Epidermal Discoloration 160	*Yersinia* 171
Rostral Injuries 160	Germ-Free Strains of Amphibians 171
Neurological Infections 160	Bacteriologic Techniques for the
Ocular Infections 161	Diagnostic Laboratory 171
Systemic Infections 161	Specimen Samples 172
Bacterial Dermatosepticemia 161	Culture Media 172
Mycobacterium spp. 167	Bacterial Identification 173
Chlamydia 169	Bacterial Isolate Preservation 175
Rickettsia 170	Antibiotic Sensitivities 175
Nonpathogenic Isolates with Zoonotic Potential 170	

CHAPTER 14
Mycoses
Sharon K. Taylor, DVM, PhD
Florida Fish and Wildlife Conservation Commission

Introduction 181	Egg Mass and Larval Mycoses 186
Localized Mycoses 181	Chromomycosis 187
Mycotic Dermatitis 181	Zygomycoses 188
Mycotic Myositis 185	Candidiasis 188
Mycotic Hepatitis 186	Specimen Samples 189
Mycotic Pneumonia 186	Media and Incubation 189
Intestinal Mycoses 186	Identification of Fungi 189
Systemic Mycoses 186	Culture Preservation 189

CHAPTER 15
Protozoa and Metazoa Infecting Amphibians
Sarah L. Poynton, PhD
Johns Hopkins University School of Medicine
National Aquarium in Baltimore
Brent R. Whitaker, MS, DVM
National Aquarium in Baltimore

Introduction 193	Myxosporea 207
Considerations for Management and Treatment 196	Monogenea 207
Ciliates 196	Digenean Trematodes 208
Ciliates in the Gastrointestinal Tract 196	Cestodes 209
External Ciliates, and Those in	Nematodes 210
the Urinary Bladder 197	Acanthocephala 212
Opalinids 198	Leeches 212
Flagellates 199	Arthropods: Crustaceans, Arachnids, and Insects 213
Ectoparasitic Flagellates 199	Branchiurans 213
Flagellates in the Blood 200	Pentastomids 213
Intestinal Flagellates 200	Mites 214
Amoebae 203	Ticks 214
Apicomplexa 204	Insects 214
Apicomplexa in the Blood 204	Mollusca 215
Apicomplexa in the Tissues 205	Identification of Protozoa and
Microsporidia 205	Metazoa from Amphibians 215
Dermocystidium, the Protozoan-like Fungi . . . 206	

CHAPTER 16
Clinical Toxicology
Stephen G. Diana, MS, DVM
Animal Health Clinical Affairs, Pfizer, Inc.
Val B. Beasely, DVM, PhD, Diplomate ABVT
University of Illinois at Urbana-Champaign
Kevin M. Wright, DVM
The Phoenix Zoo

Introduction 223	Herbicides 226
Principles of Diagnosis 223	Halogens 227
Principles of Treatment 224	Metals 227
Organophosphorus and Carbamate Insecticides 224	Salt 228
Pyrethrin and Pyrethroid Insecticides 226	Dissolved Gas Supersaturation 228
Rotenone 226	Polyvinyl Chloride Glues 229

Nicotine 230	Frog Embryo Teratogenesis Assay
Ammonia, Nitrite and Nitrate 230	Using *Xenopus* (FETAX) 231
	Summary 231

CHAPTER 17
Trauma
Kevin M. Wright, DVM
The Phoenix Zoo

Abrasions 233	Hypothermia 236
Lacerations 234	Dehydration and Desiccation 236
Traumatic Amputations 234	Drowning 237
Skeletal Fractures 235	Electrical Shock 237
Hyperthermia 236	Radiation 237

CHAPTER 18
Idiopathic Syndromes
Kevin M. Wright, DVM
The Phoenix Zoo

Spindly Leg 239	Molchpest 242
Postmetamorphic Death Syndrome 241	Edema Syndrome 242
Gout 241	Rectal, Cloacal, and Gastric Prolapse 243

CHAPTER 19
The Amphibian Eye
Brent R. Whitaker, MS, DVM
National Aquarium in Baltimore

Introduction 245	Cataracts 250
Anatomy 245	Parasites 250
Clinical Evaluation 247	Neoplasia 250
Ocular Disease 248	Glaucoma 250
Panophthalmitis and Uveitis 248	Therapeutic Considerations 250
Corneal Lipidosis 249	Conclusion 251
Keratitis 249	

CHAPTER 20
Diagnostic Imaging of Amphibians
Mark D. Stetter, DVM, Diplomate ACZM
Disney Animal Programs, Walt Disney World

Introduction 253	Colorado River Toad, *Bufo*
Radiography 253	*alvarius*, Ulcerative Dermatitis 264
Radiographic Techniques 254	New Guinea Giant Treefrog, *Litoria*
Amphibian Ultrasonography 258	*infrafrenata*, Anorexia 264
Equipment 260	Tschudi's African Bullfrog, *Pyxicephalus*
Patient Examination 260	*adspersus*, Routine Examination 264
Amphibian CT Scan and MR Imaging 263	Bullfrog, *Rana catesbeiana*, Hydrocoelom
Case Studies 264	and Edema 264
Tiger Salamander, *Ambystoma*	Surinam Toad, *Pipa pipa*, Abdominal
tigrinum, Abdominal Distension 264	Distension 264

CHAPTER 21
Surgical Techniques
Kevin M. Wright, DVM
The Phoenix Zoo

Introduction 273	Major Surgeries 277
Presurgical Preparation of the	Amputation 277
Amphibian Patient 273	Other Orthopedic Procedures 278
Surgical Procedures 274	Laparoscopy and Endoscopy 278
Incision 274	Celiotomy 279
Skin Closure 275	Gonadectomy, Gonadal Biopsy 281
Minor Surgeries 275	Cloacal and Rectal Prolapse 281
Identification Techniques 275	Enucleation 281
Biopsy 276	Postoperative Analgesia 282
Cyrosurgery (Debulking) 277	

CHAPTER 22
Reproduction
Brent R. Whitaker, MS, DVM
National Aquarium in Baltimore

Introduction 285	Oogenesis 288
Reproductive Strategies 285	Spermatogenesis 288
Sexual Dimorphism 286	Hormonal Manipulation 289
Parental Care 287	Artificial Fertilization 294
Reproductive Cycle 287	Reproductive Disorders 296

CHAPTER 23
Quarantine
Kevin M. Wright, DVM
The Phoenix Zoo
Brent R. Whitaker, MS, DVM
National Aquarium in Baltimore

Suggested Quarantine Protocols 301	The Established Collection 306
Acclimation and Maladaptation Syndrome 304	The Quarantined Collection 307
Suggested Disinfection Procedures 306	

CHAPTER 24
Pharmacotherapeutics
Kevin M. Wright, DVM
The Phoenix Zoo
Brent R. Whitaker, MS, DVM
National Aquarium in Baltimore

Introduction 309	Anthelmintics 316
Antiviral Agents 309	Eliminating Other Parasites 318
Antibacterial Agents 309	Maintaining the Electrolyte Balance
Antifungal Agents 313	of the Ill Amphibian 318
Emergency Treatment for the Septic Amphibian 314	Miscellaneous Drugs and Products
Antiprotozoal Agents 315	Used in Amphibians 319

CHAPTER 25
Necropsy
Donald K. Nichols, DVM, Diplomate ACVP
National Zoological Park

Anamnesis 331	Cytology 331
Equipment 331	Necropsy Procedures 332
Culture 331	

CHAPTER 26
Spontaneous Neoplasia in Amphibia
D. Earl Green, DVM, Diplomate ACVP
National Wildlife Health Center
John C. Harshbarger, PhD
George Washington University Medical Center

Introduction 335
    Tumors vs. Neoplasms 335
    Experimental Carcinogenesis 335
Integument 336
    Epithelial Cell Neoplasms 337
    Dermal Gland Neoplasms 343
    Neoplasms of Chromatophores 347
    Neoplasms of Epidermal Neurosensory
        Cells (Lateral Line and Ampullary
        Organ Cells) 350
Neoplasms of the Mesenchymal Tissues 352
    Neoplasms of Fibrous Tissue 352
    Neoplasms of Fat Tissue 353
    Neoplasms of Muscle Tissue 353
    Neoplasms of Blood and Lymph Vessels ... 355
    Miscellaneous, Undifferentiated,
        and Mesenchymal Cell Neoplasms 355
Neoplasms of Hematopoietic and
    Lymphoid Cells and Organs 356
    Lymphoproliferative Diseases 356
    Neoplasms of Granulocytic Cells 360
    Neoplasms of Suspected
        Histiocytic Cells 361
    Neoplasms of Mast Cells 361
    Neoplasms of the Thymus 364
Neoplasms of the Kidneys and Urinary Bladder 364
    Neoplasms of the Kidney 364
    Neoplasms of the Urinary Bladder 369
Neoplasms of the Liver, Biliary System,
    and Pancreas 370
    Hepatic Neoplasms 370
    Bile Duct Neoplasms 372
    Pancreatic Neoplasms 373
Neoplasms of the Alimentary Tract 374
    Neuroepithelioma of the Mouth 374
    Hyperkeratosis of the Tongue 374
    Adenocarcinoma of the Stomach 374
    Intestinal Neoplasms 374
Neoplasms of the Reproductive Systems 377
    Neoplasms of the Male
        Reproductive Tract 377
    Neoplasms of the Female
        Reproductive Tract 379
    Neoplasms of the Female Nongonadal
        Reproductive Organs 381
Neoplasms of the Endocrine Organs 381
    Thyroid Neoplasms 381
    Interrenal Neoplasms 381
    Neoplasms of the Islets of Langerhans
        (Endocrine Pancreas) 381
    Pituitary and Pineal Neoplasms 381
Neoplasms of the Respiratory System 381
Neoplasms of the Central and Peripheral
    Nervous Systems 381
Neoplasms of the Eye and Adnexa 382
Neoplasms of the Bones, Joints, and
    Notochord 382
    Tumorlike Osteochondrous Dysplasia 382
    Chondromyxoma (Myxochondroma,
        Fibromyxochondroma) 383
    Osteosarcoma (Osteogenic Sarcoma) 383
    Chordoma 384
Miscellaneous Neoplasms 384
    Mesothelioma 384
    Teratoma 384
    Hamartoma 384

CHAPTER 27
Pathology of Amphibia
D. Earl Green, DVM, Diplomate ACVP
National Wildlife Health Center

Diseases and Pathology of Eggs and Embryos .. 401
    Genetically Based Egg Pathology 401
    Egg—Toxicological Etiologies 402
    Infectious Diseases of Eggs 406
    Metamorphosis 407
Diseases and Pathology of Larvae, Metamorphs, and Adults 408
    Musculoskeletal System 408
    Integumentary System 415
    Alimentary Tract 438

Urinary System 447
Respiratory System 449
Cardiovascular System 451
Hematolymphopoietic System 453
Endocrine System 458
Reproductive System 459
Central, Peripheral, and Autonomic Nervous Systems 461
Eyes, Ears, and Special Sensory Organs ... 467

Appendix
List of Tables 487

Index 489

Note:
Color Plates follow Chapter 17 ...... C1–C44

CHAPTER 1
EVOLUTION OF THE AMPHIBIA

Kevin M. Wright, DVM

Amphibian fossils have been found in sedimentary rock formations that date back 350 million years. It seems probable that amphibians evolved from rhipidistian crossopterygian fishes, the only known surviving form of this group being the coelacanth, *Latimeria chalumnae*. The rhipidistian ancestors of the amphibians had functional lungs, which freed them of the gilled fish dependence on water for respiration. They also had bony lobed fins that supported the body in a manner sufficient for directed terrestrial locomotion. Amphibians were the first vertebrates to disperse widely into terrestrial habitats. They dominated the Mississippian, Pennsylvanian, and Permian eras, a span of 100 million years. Amphibian fossils are known from the Triassic era, about 200 million years ago, the time in which dinosaurs first came to dominance. Jurassic and Cretaceous era fossils are known, and the modern day orders Anura (frogs) and Caudata (salamanders) are well represented in the Tertiary era, 63 million years ago. A single vertebra represents the earliest known fossil of the Gymnophiona (caecilians) from the late Cretaceous era, while the majority of caecilian fossils are dated to the Pleistocene era, around 1 million years ago. Despite the extensive number of amphibian fossils that have been discovered and analyzed, there are significant gaps in the fossil record, such that the lineages of the three surviving amphibian orders are obscure. Currently all modern amphibians are classified within the subclass Lissamphibia (Haeckel 1866), with the two remaining subclasses, Lepospondylia and Labyrinthodontia, having no known surviving members. Vertebral morphology has been the basis of the division of amphibian subclasses, but this has been met with argument and many taxonomists dispute a monophyletic origin for the Lissamphibia. Barring the uncovering of substantial fossil evidence and concomitant genetic research on modern species, there is little hope that the origins of the Lissamphibia will be unequivocally resolved either way.

The origin of the Lissamphibia is of concern to the veterinary clinician because it serves as a reminder that the modern amphibians are a diverse group of poorly known vertebrates with correspondingly distinct needs. Although extrapolations are made throughout this text on assumed similarities among amphibians with regard to diagnostics and treatment, the very lack of knowledge about the relationships of the three orders of amphibians emphasizes that fact that there is no standard "modern amphibian," therefore many of the assumptions made herein may be proven erroneous by advances in the realms of amphibian biology and medicine.

In order to have the clinical acumen necessary to diagnose and treat the diseases of amphibians, the veterinary clinician must fully appreciate the unique characteristics and biology of modern amphibians and understand the biology of the various species seen in practice.

FURTHER READING

Colbert, E. and M. Morales. 1991. Evolution of Vertebrates: A History of Backboned Animals Through Time. Wily-Liss, New York, NY.
Duellman, W.E. and L. Trueb. 1986. Evolution, *in* Duellman, W.E., and L. Trueb: Biology of the Amphibia. McGraw-Hill Book Company, New York, NY, pp. 415–553.
Goin, C.J., O.B. Goin, and G.R. Zug. 1978. Origin and evolution of amphibians, *in* Goin, C.J., O.B. Goin, and G.R. Zug: Introduction to Herpetology. W.H. Freeman and Co., San Francisco, CA, pp. 56–71.
McFarland, W.N. and J.B. Heiser. 1979. The geology and ecology of tetrapod origin, *in* McFarland, W.N., F.H. Pough, T.J. Cade, and J.B. Heiser: Vertebrate Life. Macmillan Publishing Co., Inc., New York, NY, pp. 285–290.
Porter, K.R. 1972. The origin and phylogenetic relationships of Amphibia, *in* Porter, K.R.: Herpetology. W.B. Saunders Co., Philadelphia, PA, pp. 88–114.
Pough, F.H. 1979a. Origin and radiation of amphibians, *in* McFarland, W.N., F.H. Pough, T.J. Cade, and J.B. Heiser (Eds). Vertebrate Life. Macmillan Publishing Co., Inc., New York, NY, pp. 291–322.
Pough, F.H. 1979b. Modern amphibians, *in* McFarland, W.N., F.H. Pough, T.J. Cade, and J.B. Heiser (Eds): Vertebrate Life. Macmillan Publishing Co., Inc., New York, NY, pp. 323–362.
Stebbins, R.C. and N. Cohen. 1995. A Natural History of Amphibians. Princeton University Press, Princeton, NJ.
Zug, G.R. 1993. Origin and evolution of amphibians, *in* Zug, G.R.: Herpetology: An Introductory Biology of Amphibians and Reptiles. Academic Press, Inc., San Diego, CA, pp. 43–59.

CHAPTER 2

TAXONOMY OF AMPHIBIANS KEPT IN CAPTIVITY

Kevin M. Wright, DVM

2.1 INTRODUCTION

Over 4000 extant species have been described within the class Amphibia belonging to three orders—Anura (Salientia), the frogs and toads; Caudata (Urodela), the salamanders, newts, and sirens; and the Gymnophiona (Apoda), the caecilians. Comparatively few species are represented in zoos or other living collections. Less than one-tenth of the living species are routinely held in captivity, and only within the last decade has broad attention been focused on the husbandry, propagation, and conservation of captive amphibians. The taxonomic scheme used within this text may not account for changes in recent years as it follows the scheme laid out in 1985 (Frost, 1985). The distinguishing taxomonic characters for the families of modern amphibians are beyond the scope of this text, but several texts provide excellent concise reviews (e.g., Duellman & Trueb, 1986a, 1986b; Goin et al., 1978a, 1978b; Mattison, 1987; Porter, 1972; Zug, 1993a, 1993b). These works utilized the taxonomy that was current at the time they were written, hence there are discrepancies between these references. A recent work attempts to standardize the common names given to amphibian species worldwide (Frank & Ramus, 1995). Although the widespread acceptance of this work is yet to be seen, in general, its proposed common names are used in this text. Alternative common names for some species are listed in Table 2.1. This taxonomic review will focus only on those species listed in published inventories of amphibians held in captivity in North America (International Species Information System, 1995; Slavens & Slavens, 1994). The captive amphibian collections in other countries may be quite different from North American collections as a result of various international agreements that control the exportation and importation of amphibian species (e.g., CITES, the Convention on the International Trade in Endangered Species). Many of the species that are common in European collections are virtually unknown in the United States of America. Additional species may be held in North America but are not listed in readily available inventories. Local amphibians that are not part of the commercial trade may be captured and held as pets, so the clinician is advised to become familiar with indigenous species. New species are described and recorded every year, some finding their way into the pet trade before being formally described, which further complicates the picture.

A list of several texts that are available for assisting in the identification of the species of the amphibian patient may be found at the end of this chapter.

Husbandry guidelines are included for some species following the taxonomic review. They include the mode of reproduction, suggested vivarium design, temperature range, and suggested diet.

The summary format is as follows:

Common name, *Scientific name*
Mode of reproduction
Vivarium design:
Temperature range:
Suggested diet:

Mode of reproduction is either oviparous (egg-laying) or viviparous (live-bearing). Further explanations of vivarium design and amphibian husbandry may be found in Chapter 5, while a more complete overview of diets may be found in Chapter 6.

2.2 ORDER GYMNOPHIONA

Very few species of caecilians are reported in captive collections. The Caecilidae (common caecilians) are found throughout the tropical regions of sub-Saharan Africa, India, the Seychelle Islands, and Central and South America. There are around 88 described species of common caecilians, of which the two species best known in captivity are the Mexican caecilian, *Dermophis mexicanus* (Plate 2.1), and the

Varagua caecilian, *Gymnopis multiplicata*. Although many adult caeciliids are between 10 cm (4 inches) and 100 cm (39 inches) in length, this family also includes one of the longest amphibians, Thompson's caecilian, *Caecilia thompsoni*, which reaches lengths in excess of 150 cm (60 inches). Oviparity and viviparity are found in various species, with the majority of the known oviparous caeciliids occurring in the Old World. Ichthyophiidae (fish caecilians) occur throughout southern India, Sri Lanka, Southeast Asia, Indonesia, and the Philippines. There are around 35 species of fish caecilians, of which only the Koh Tao Island caecilian, *Ichthyophis kohtaoensis*, could be considered a regular occurrence in captive collections. Most adult ichthyophiids are around 50 cm (20 inches) in length. Ichthyophiids are oviparous and at least one species, the Ceylon sticky caecilian, *Ichthyophis glutinosus*, is known to guards its eggs in a nest in the mud. Typhlonectidae (aquatic caecilians) occur in the river drainages of northern and southeastern South America. There are around 19 species of aquatic caecilians, of which the Cayenne caecilian, *Typhlonectes compressicauda*, and the Rio Cauca caecilian, *T. natans* (Plate 2.2), are common in captive collections. Typhlonectiids are viviparous. The other families of caecilians are rarely if ever seen outside of museums and research facilities. These families are Rhinatrematidae (beaked caecilians, northern South America, 9 species), Scolecomorphidae (tropical caecilians, tropical sub-Saharan Africa, 7 species), and Uraeotyphlidae (Indian caecilians, southern India, 4 species). The identification of caecilians is problematic in living specimens since many of the species keys are geographically based and utilize skeletal characters not discernible without dissection. Unless the collecting locality for an individual caecilian is known, the task of identifying the caecilian can be quite difficult for anyone but a specialist.

Table 2.1. Common names of amphibians.

Common names	Scientific names
LIMBLESS AMPHIBIANS	**Order GYMNOPHIONA**
Aquatic caecilian	*Typhlonectes* spp.
Flat-tailed caecilian	*Typhlonectes compressicauda*
Rubber eel	*Typhlonectes* spp. although sometimes used for *Amphiuma* spp.
Yellow-striped caecilian	*Ichthyophis kohtaoensis*
SALAMANDERS & NEWTS	**Order CAUDATA**
Arboreal salamander	*Bolitoglossa* spp.
Climbing salamander	*Batrachoseps* spp. or *Bolitoglossa* spp.
European newt	*Triturus* spp. or *Pleurodeles* spp.
Halloween newt	*Tylototriton (verrucosus) shanjing*
Mandarin newt	*Tylototriton (verrucosus) shanjing*
Mushroom tongue salamander	*Bolitoglossa* spp.
Paddle tail newt	*Pachytriton* spp. or *Paramesotriton* spp.
Palm salamander	*Bolitoglossa* spp.
Redbelly newt	*Cynops pyrroghaster* or *Taricha* spp.
Tree salamander	*Bolitoglossa* spp.
Warty newt	*Taricha* spp., *Pleurodeles* spp., or *Paramesotriton* spp.
Waterdog	In the pet trade this is usually the larval form of *Ambystoma tigrinum*, not a true *Necturus* spp.
FROGS AND TOADS	**Order ANURA**
African mouse-eating bullfrog	*Pyxicephalus adspersus*
Argentine horned frog	*Ceratophrys ornata*
Asian horned frog	*Megophrys montana*
Australian green treefrog	*Pelodryas caerulea*
Bell's horned frog	*Ceratophrys ornata*
Budgett's frog	*Lepidobatrachus asper*
Cane toad	*Bufo marinus*
Dumpy treefrog	*Pelodryas caerulea*
Dyeing poison frog	*Dendrobates tinctorius*
Foam-nest frog	*Leptodactylus* spp.
Foam-nest treefrog	*Rhacophorus* spp., *Chiromantis* spp., other rhacophorids
Giant leaf frog	*Phyllomedusa bicolor*
Golden tomato frog	*Dyscophus guineti*

Table 2.1. Common names of amphibians. *(Continued)*

Common names	Scientific names
Golden frog	*Mantella aurantiaca*
Horn frog	*Ceratophrys* spp., *Ceratobatrachus guentheri*, or *Megophrys* spp.
Madagascan treefrog	Usually either a *Mantidactylus* spp. or *Boophis* spp.
Marine toad	*Bufo marinus*
Monkey treefrog	*Phyllomedusa* spp.
Mouse-eating frog	*Bufo marinus, Ceratophrys* spp., *Pyxicephalus adspersus, Rana catesbeiana*
Neotropical giant toad	*Bufo marinus*
Pac-man frog	*Ceratophrys ornata*
Painted frog	In the pet trade this is usually *Kaolula pulchra*, not *Discoglossus* spp.
Painted toad	*Atelopus* spp.
Paradox frog	*Pseudis paradoxa*
Phantasmal dart frog	*Epipedobates* spp.
Pixie frog	*Pyxicephalus delalandii* but also used for *P. adspersus*
Puerto Rican crested toad	*Peltophryne lemur*
Smokey jungle frog	*Leptodactylus pentadactylus*
Smooth-sided toad	*Bufo guttatus*
Solomon Island eyelash frog	*Ceratobatrachus guentheri*
Solomon Island leaf frog	*Ceratobatrachus guentheri*
Waxy treefrog	*Phyllomedusa sauvagii*
White-lipped treefrog	*Litoria infrafrenata*

Husbandry Summary

Mexican caecilian, *Dermophis mexicanus*,
Viviparous
Vivarium design: terrestrial fossorial
Temperature range: tropical lowland
Suggested diet: earthworms

Varagua caecilian, *Gymnopis multiplicata*,
Viviparous
Vivarium design: terrestrial fossorial
Temperature range: tropical lowland
Suggested diet: earthworms

Koh Tao island caecilian, *Ichthyophis kohtaoensis*,
Oviparous
Vivarium design: terrestrial fossorial
Temperature range: tropical lowland
Suggested diet: earthworms

Cayenne caecilian, *Typhlonectes compressicauda*,
Viviparous
Vivarium design: aquatic pond
Temperature range: tropical lowland
Suggested diet: earthworms

Rio Cauca caecilian, *T. natans*,
Viviparous
Vivarium design: aquatic pond
Temperature range: tropical lowland
Suggested diet: earthworms

2.3 ORDER CAUDATA

Caudata contains nine families with a total of around 375 species. Members of this order are referred to as salamanders while certain aquatic forms are also called newts. "Caudates" is an acceptable term for any salamander or newt although it is rarely used. The term "newt" will be restricted primarily to those forms of the Salamandridae that possess a pre-reproductive terrestrial stage and are usually aquatic upon sexual maturity. Salamanders are restricted to the New World and parts of Europe and Asia, with North America containing the greatest diversity of living species.

2.3.1 Sirenidae

Sirenidae (sirens) contains at least four species restricted to southeastern North America. The dwarf sirens, *Pseudobranchus axanthus* and *P. striatus* (Moler & Kezer, 1993), lesser siren, *Siren intermedia*, and the greater siren, *Siren lacertina*, all lack hindlimbs and have external gill plumes (Plate 2.3). Dwarf sirens *Pseudobranchus* spp., are generally under 12 cm (6 inches) in length while the greater siren, *Siren lacertina*, may attain lengths of 100 cm (39 inches). They are occasionally found in collections.

Husbandry Summary

Dwarf siren, *Pseudobranchus* spp.,
Oviparous
Vivarium design: aquatic pond
Temperature range: subtropical

Suggested diet: small red worms, white worms, bloodworms, glass shrimp, other small invertebrates

Lesser siren, *Siren intermedia*,
Oviparous
Vivarium design: aquatic pond
Temperature range: subtropical
Suggested diet: earthworms, other invertebrates, small fish

Greater siren, *Siren lacertina*,
Oviparous
Vivarium design: aquatic pond
Temperature range: subtropical
Suggested diet: earthworms, crayfish, other invertebrates, small fish

2.3.2 Hynobiidae

Hynobiidae (Asian salamanders) contains around 35 species, all of which are uncommon in collections. Hynobiids are generally under 10 cm (4 inches) in length. Although most species are terrestrial, clawed salamanders, *Onychodactylus* spp., are stream-dwellers and are unique among hynobiids since they are lungless.

2.3.3 Cryptobranchidae

Cryptobranchidae (giant salamanders) have a disjunct distribution with the hellbender, *Cryptobranchus alleganiensis*, found in North America, while the Japanese giant salamander, *Andrias japonicus*, and the Chinese giant salamander, *Andrias davidianus* occur in Asia (Plates 2.4, 2.5). Giant salamanders are popular zoo exhibits due to their ugly countenance and large size. The Asian giant salamanders may approach 1.6 meters (5 feet) in length and weigh over 45 kg (100 pounds). All cryptobranchiids are aquatic but lack gills, relying instead on skin folds and lungs as their primary respiratory organs.

Husbandry Summary

All cryptobranchiids
Oviparous
Vivarium design: Aquatic stream
Temperature range: temperate
Suggested diet: fish, crayfish

2.3.4 Proteidae

Proteidae (neotenic salamanders) includes five North American and one European species. The mudpuppy, *Necturus maculosus*, is a common laboratory species (Plate 2.6). Waterdogs, *Necturus* spp., are sometimes sold in pet stores, but most waterdogs in the pet trade are actually larval ambystomids. The cave-dwelling European olm, *Proteus anguinis*, is rare in captive collections. All proteids are aquatic and have external gill plumes.

Husbandry Summary

Mudpuppy, *Necturus maculosus*,
Vivarium design: aquatic stream
Temperature range: temperate
Suggested diet: fish, crayfish, earthworms

2.3.5 Dicamptodontidae

Dicamptodontidae (American giant salamanders) contains seven species found in the northwestern United States. The Pacific giant salamander, *Dicamptodon ensatus*, is the largest terrestrial salamander, reaching lengths of 35 cm (14 inches). It is found in a few collections. The Olympic salamanders, *Rhyacotriton* spp., are small stream-dwelling salamanders sometimes classified in their own family, Rhyacotritonidae. They are uncommon in captive collections.

Husbandry Summary

Pacific giant salamander, *Dicamptodon ensatus*,
Oviparous
Vivarium design: streamside
Temperature range: temperate
Suggested diet: earthworms

2.3.6 Amphiumidae

Amphiumidae (amphiumas) is restricted to southeastern North America. There are at least three species within the genera *Amphiuma*. These large salamanders may exceed 100 cm (39 inches) in length, and although aquatic, they lack gills. Amphiumas are occasionally found in captivity, and are often referred to as "conger eels" due to their elongate body and tiny limbs.

Husbandry Summary

Amphiuma, *Amphiuma* spp.,
Oviparous
Vivarium design: aquatic pond
Temperature range: subtropical
Suggested diet: earthworms, crayfish, small fish

2.3.7 Salamandridae

Salamandridae (true salamanders) has disjunct distribution with species found in eastern and western North America, Europe, and eastern Asia. There are around 55 species of true salamanders, of which around 40 are common in captive collections. The commonly kept species include the Japanese firebelly newt, *Cynops pyrrhogaster* (Plate 2.7), red-spotted newt, *Notophthalmus viridescens viridescens* (Plate 2.8), Tsitou newt, *Pachytriton brevipes,* Spanish ribbed newt, *Pleurodeles waltl,* European fire salamander, *Salamandra salamandra,* roughskin newts, *Taricha* spp. (Plate 2.9), alpine newts, *Triturus* spp., and the crocodile newt, *Tylototriton shanjing* (formerly *T. verrucosus*). Several species have toxins in their mucous that can be irritating or dangerous to humans, and the fire salamander, *Salamandra salamandra,* can actually spray poison from glands along its back.

Husbandry Summary

Japanese firebelly newt, *Cynops pyrrhogaster,*
Oviparous
Vivarium design: aquatic pond
Temperature range: temperate
Suggested diet: small red worms, white worms, other invertebrates

Red-spotted newt, *Notophthalmus viridescens,*
Oviparous
Vivarium design: aquatic pond as adults
Temperature range: subtropical to temperate
Suggested diet: small red worms, white worms, other invertebrates

Tsitou newt, *Pachytriton brevipes,*
Oviparous
Vivarium design: aquatic pond
Temperature range: temperate
Suggested diet: small red worms, white worms, other invertebrates

Spanish ribbed newt, *Pleurodeles waltl,*
Oviparous
Vivarium design: aquatic pond
Temperature range: temperate
Suggested diet: small red worms, white worms, other invertebrates

European fire salamander, *Salamandra salamandra,*
Oviparous or viviparous depending on subspecies
Vivarium design: terrestrial forest floor or streamside
Temperature range: temperate
Suggested diet: small red worms, white worms, small crickets, wax worms, other invertebrates

Roughskin newt, *Taricha* spp.,
Oviparous
Vivarium design: aquatic pond or streamside
Temperature range: temperate
Suggested diet: small red worms, white worms, small crickets, other invertebrates

Alpine newts, *Triturus* spp.,
Oviparous
Vivarium design: aquatic pond
Temperature range: temperate
Suggested diet: small red worms, white worms, other invertebrates

Crocodile newt, *Tylototriton shanjing,* (formerly *T. verrucosus*),
Oviparous
Vivarium design: terrestrial forest floor or streamside
Temperature range: temperate
Suggested diet: small red worms, white worms, small crickets, wax worms, other invertebrates

2.3.8 Ambystomatidae

Ambystomatidae (mole salamanders) is a North American family that contains around 30 species. The axolotl, *Ambystoma mexicanum,* is by far the most common aquatic neotenic species in captivity, and has long been used in biomedical research. A number of color phases exist and are commonly sold through the tropical fish trade. Other neotenic species, such as the Anderson's axolotl, *A. andersoni* (Plate 2.10), may be seen in zoological institutions. The majority of neotenic Mexican salamanders are considered endangered as a result of habitat loss, pollution, and introduced game fish that prey upon larval axolotls. Commonly kept terrestrial ambystomids include the spotted salamander, *A. maculatum,* marbled salamander, *A. opacum,* and the tiger salamander, *A. tigrinum.* (For representative ambystomids, see Plates 2.11, 2.12, 2.13, 2.14).

Husbandry Summary

Axolotl, *Ambystoma mexicanum,*
Oviparous
Vivarium design: aquatic pond
Temperature range: tropical
Suggested diet: earthworms, fish

Tiger salamander, *Ambystoma tigrinum,*
Oviparous
Vivarium design: terrestrial forest floor
Temperature range: subtropical or temperate
Suggested diet: earthworms, wax worms, crickets

2.3.9 Plethodontidae

Plethodontidae (lungless salamanders) contains around 230 species, of which approximately 25 species are in captive collections. The tropical lungless salamanders, *Bolitoglossa* spp. (Plates 2.15, 2.16), dusky salamanders, *Desmognathus* spp. (Plate 2.17), American brook salamanders, *Eurycea* spp., woodland salamanders, *Plethodon* spp. (Plate 2.18), and red salamanders, *Pseudotriton* spp. (Plate 2.19) are commonly kept in captivity. The Texas blind salamander, *Typhlomolge rathbuni*, is a target species for captive propagation in North American zoos.

Husbandry Summary

Tropical lungless salamanders, *Bolitoglossa* spp.,
Oviparous
Vivarium design: arboreal
Temperature range: subtropical to tropical montane
Suggested diet: small crickets, wax worms, earthworms, fruit flies, other invertebrates

Dusky salamanders, *Desmognathus* spp.,
Oviparous
Vivarium design: streamside or terrestrial forest floor
Temperature range: temperate
Suggested diet: small crickets, small red worms, white worms, fruit flies

American brook salamanders, *Eurycea* spp.,
Oviparous
Vivarium design: streamside
Temperature range: temperate
Suggested diet: small crickets, small red worms, white worms, fruit flies

Woodland salamanders, *Plethodon* spp.,
Oviparous
Vivarium design: streamside or terrestrial forest floor
Temperature range: temperate
Suggested diet: small crickets, small red worms, white worms, fruit flies

Red salamanders, *Pseudotriton* spp.,
Oviparous
Vivarium design: aquatic pond or streamside
Temperature range: temperate
Suggested diet: small crickets, small red worms, white worms, fruit flies

2.4 ORDER ANURA

Anura is the most species rich order of amphibians, with over 3500 living species belonging to at least 20 families. Properly termed anurans, members of this order are also called frogs or toads. Although the term "frog" tends to be used for those species found in and around water whereas the term "toad" is used for those terrestrial species, it is not that simple. Some species, such as *Xenopus laevis,* may be called either the African clawed frog or African clawed toad. Regional differences abound, with members of the Hylidae named treefrogs or treetoads in different dialects. In this text "toad" will be used primarily for those anurans of the Bufonidae (true toads), whereas "frog" will apply to all other anurans. Modern anurans are found on every continent except Antarctica. Many of the Australian and Asian frogs are virtually unknown in captive collections outside of their native lands.

2.4.1 Leiopelmatidae

The oldest surviving family is the Leiopelmatidae (tailed frogs) which contains four living species. These are the North American tailed frog, *Ascaphis truei,* and the New Zealand tailed frogs, *Leiopelma* spp. These are uncommon in captive collections. The tail is restricted to male frogs and is actually an outpocketing of the cloaca which serves as an intromittent organ.

Husbandry Summary

North American tailed frog, *Ascaphis truei*,
Oviparous
Vivarium design: streamside
Temperature range: temperate
Suggested diet: crickets, other invertebrates

2.4.2 Discoglossidae

Discoglossidae (painted frogs) contains around 14 species. Three genera are common in captive collections: firebelly toads, *Bombina* spp., from Asia; midwife toads, *Alytes* spp., from Europe and northwestern Africa; and painted frogs, *Discoglossus* spp., also from Europe and northwestern Africa. Firebelly toads, *Bombina* spp., are entirely aquatic. Midwife toads, *Alytes* spp., are interesting since mating occurs on land. The male midwife toad wraps the eggs around its legs and carries the eggs until hatching.

Husbandry Summary

Firebelly toads, *Bombina* spp.,
Oviparous
Vivarium design: shallow aquatic pond with substantial land area
Temperature range: temperate
Suggested diet: small crickets, wax worms, fruit flies

2.4.3 Rhinophrynidae

Rhinophrynidae contains a single species, the Mexican burrowing toad, *Rhinophrynus dorsalis,* and few specimens are reported in captive collections.

> **Husbandry Summary**
>
> **Mexican burrowing toad, *Rhinophrynus dorsalis*,**
> Oviparous
> Vivarium design: terrestrial fossorial
> Temperature range: tropical lowland
> Suggested diet: termites, ants

2.4.4 Pipidae

Pipidae (clawed frogs) has a disjunct distribution with aquatic toads *Pipa* occurring in South America and all other genera found in Africa. There are around 26 species of pipids, and all are aquatic. This family includes the laboratory frog that is also a popular aquarium pet, the African clawed frog, *Xenopus laevis*. Other members of this genus are rarely kept in captivity. The dwarf clawed frogs, *Hymenochirus* spp., are frequently available through tropical fish dealers (Plate 2.20), as is the Surinam toad, *Pipa pipa*. All female clawed toads, *Pipa* spp., deposit their eggs into their dorsal skin, but while tadpoles hatch from other species, tiny froglets emerge from the eggs of the Surinam toad, *P. pipa*.

> **Husbandry Summary**
>
> **African clawed frog, *Xenopus laevis*,**
> Oviparous
> Vivarium design: aquatic pond
> Temperature range: tropical lowland to subtropical
> Suggested diet: earthworms, other invertebrates, small fish
>
> **Dwarf clawed frogs, *Hymenochirus spp.*,**
> Oviparous
> Vivarium design: aquatic pond
> Temperature range: tropical lowland to subtropical
> Suggested diet: white worms, black worms, bloodworms, washed brine shrimp
>
> **Surinam toad, *Pipa pipa*,**
> Oviparous, no tadpole stage
> Vivarium design: aquatic pond
> Temperature range: tropical lowland
> Suggested diet: earthworms

2.4.5 Pelobatidae

Pelobatidae (spadefoot toads) have a worldwide distribution, throughout North America, Europe, and southeastern Asia and Indonesia. There are around 83 species of spadefoot toads, but very few of these are kept in captivity, perhaps because many are secretive or fossorial and therefore are poor displays. The Asian spadefoot toad, *Megophrys montana*, is a large spectacular species that is sometimes available (Plates 2.21, 2.22).

> **Husbandry Summary**
>
> **Asian spadefoot toad, *Megophrys montana*,**
> Oviparous
> Vivarium design: terrestrial forest floor
> Temperature range: temperate to subtropical
> Suggested diet: crickets, earthworms

2.4.6 Pelodytidae

Pelodytidae contains two species commonly called parsley frogs, *Pelodytes* spp. They are found in western Europe and southwestern Asia. Although similar in external appearance to many pelobatids, the parsley frogs are unique among anurans due to a fusion of two "ankle" bones, the calcaneum and astragalus.

> **Husbandry Summary**
>
> **Parsley frogs, *Pelodytes* spp.,**
> Oviparous
> Vivarium design: shallow aquatic pond with land area or streamside
> Temperature range: temperate
> Suggested diet: crickets

2.4.7 Myobatrachidae

Myobatrachidae (Australian froglets) contains around 100 species, but few of these have been reported in captive collections (Plate 2.23). Although the majority of the Australian froglets lead typical anuran lives, the gastric-brooding frog, *Rheobatrachus* spp., is an unusual aquatic frog that incubates its eggs in its stomach. The pathways involved in shutting down the production of stomach acid during the egg incubation promised advances in managing gastric ulcers in humans. Unfortunately this species appears to have become extinct in less than 2 decades after being described and before many of its biochemical mysteries were unraveled.

2.4.8 Heleophrynidae

Heleophrynidae (ghost frogs) contains five species, all of which are uncommon in captivity. Ghost frogs are stream-side dwellers restricted to the highlands of South Africa. They are extremely difficult to locate even when their calls are heard, hence the name "ghost" frogs.

2.4.9 Sooglossidae

Sooglossidae (Seychelles frogs) contains three species, all of which are uncommon in captivity. These small frogs, under 4 cm (1.4 inches) in length, are restricted to the Seychelle Islands. Eggs undergo direct development to froglets in Gardiner's Seychelles frog, *Sooglossus gardineri*, while nonfeeding tadpoles hatch and are tended by the adults in the Seychelles frog, *S. seychellensis*.

2.4.10 Leptodactylidae

Leptodactylidae (tropical frogs) is a New World family that includes some of the more popular pet anurans. There are over 700 species of tropical frogs, but the most common pets belong to the subfamily Ceratophrynae. The ornate horned frog, *Ceratophrys ornata* (Plate 2.24), Cranwell's horned frog, *Ceratophrys cranwelli*, and Paraguay horned frogs, *Lepidobatrachus* spp., are commonly bred in captive collections and are popular pets, in part because of their relatively large size and bizarre appearance. The Surinam horned frog, *Ceratophrys cornuta*, is sporadically available as wild-caught adults, which tend to be difficult to acclimate to captivity (Plates 2.25, 2.26). The genus *Eleuthrodactylus* (robber frogs) contains over 400 species, of which several small species are in captive collections. The genus *Leptodactylus* includes the commonly available South American bullfrog, *Leptodactylus pentadactylus* (Plate 2.27). Some species, such as the Lake Titicaca water frog, *Telmatobius culeus*, are rarely seen in captivity (Plate 2.28).

Husbandry Summary

Ornate horned frog, *Ceratophrys ornata*,
Oviparous
Vivarium design: terrestrial forest floor
Temperature range: tropical lowland
Suggested diet: crickets, earthworms, fish, young mice (sparingly with added vitamin D_3)

Surinam horned frog, *Ceratophrys cornuta*,
Oviparous
Vivarium design: terrestrial forest floor
Temperature range: tropical lowland
Suggested diet: often fixated on other frogs, but may also try crickets, earthworms, fish, young mice (sparingly with added vitamin D_3)

Cranwell's horned frog, *Ceratophrys cranwelli*,
Oviparous
Vivarium design: terrestrial forest floor
Temperature range: tropical lowland
Suggested diet: crickets, earthworms, fish, young mice (sparingly, with added vitamin D_3)

Paraguay horned frogs, *Lepidobatrachus* spp.,
Oviparous
Vivarium design: aquatic pond
Temperature range: subtropical
Suggested diet: earthworms, fish, crickets

South American bullfrog,
Leptodactylus pentadactylus
Oviparous
Vivarium design: terrestrial forest floor or shallow aquatic pond with large land area
Temperature range: tropical lowland
Suggested diet: crickets, earthworms

2.4.11 Bufonidae

Bufonids are the true toads, and are distinguished from all living anurans on the basis of the presence of the Bidder's organ in males, a rudimentary ovary lying on the anterior edge of the testis. There are around 350 species, of which one-tenth are in captive collections. One of the more spectacular species, the golden Alajuela toad, *Bufo periglenes*, of Costa Rica has not been sighted since the late 1980s and is presumed extinct. Considerable effort has been expended to preserve several highly endangered species (e.g., lowland Caribbean toad, *Peltophryne lemur*, Houston toad, *Bufo houstonensis*, Wyoming toad, *Bufo hemiophrys baxteri*; Plates 2.29, 2.30, 2.31) while other bufonids (e.g., European green toad, *Bufo viridis*, spotted toad, *Bufo guttatus*) are among the more popular amphibian pets. The American toad, *Bufo americanus* (Plates 2.32, 2.33), and many other North American bufonids are still quite plentiful in many areas and are often captured and brought home by children for short-term pets. This practice should not be encouraged unless an effort is made to provide appropriate housing and food for the toad. Often the toad is released after being improperly treated for several weeks, thereafter suffering from malnutrition and infections. This ill toad then poses a threat to the toads living at the site of its release. The giant toad, *Bufo marinus*, is a pest species in many parts of the world where it was introduced in an ill-conceived plan to biologically control pests of sugar cane. Efforts in Australia are focused on extirpating this species, as it is responsible for the decline of native wildlife. It is also a serious pest in Florida, Hawaii, the Solomon Islands, and several other tropical locations. Stubfoot toads, *Atelopus* spp., are small, brilliantly colored toads. They are highly valued among herpetoculturists, but are relatively rare in collections and difficult to acclimate (Plate 2.34). Asian tree toads, *Pedostibes* spp., are occasionally found in captive collections (Plate 2.35), but can prove difficult to acclimate since they feed primarily on ants in the wild. One Asian tree toad that fared poorly on 14-day-old and adult crickets began to thrive and gain weight when offered a diet of pinhead crickets (personal communication, D. Harris, 1997).

> **Husbandry Summary**

American toad, *Bufo americanus*,
Oviparous
Vivarium design: terrestrial forest floor
Temperature range: temperate to subtropical
Suggested diet: crickets, earthworms (NOTE—most Bufo spp. can be accommodated in this manner, although some may need tropical lowland temperatures.)

Stubfoot toads, *Atelopus* spp.,
Oviparous
Vivarium design: streamside
Temperature range: subtropical to tropical montane
Suggested diet: small crickets, fruit flies, springtails

Asian tree toads, *Pedostibes* spp.,
Oviparous
Vivarium design: terrestrial forest floor with arboreal furnishings
Temperature range: subtropical to tropical
Suggested diet: pinhead crickets, fruit flies, ants

2.4.12 Brachycephalidae

Brachycephalidae (saddleback toads) is a Brazilian endemic family that contains at least two species that are uncommon in captivity. Originally classified as true toads, these small (1.6 cm or 0.5 inches in length) anurans were removed from Bufonidae due to the lack of a Bidder's organ. Spix's saddleback toad, *Brachycephalus ehippium*, is bright orange to golden yellow in appearance, suggesting a reliance on skin toxins as an anti-predator mechanism.

2.4.13 Rhinodermatidae

Rhinodermatidae (Darwin's frogs) contains two species of mouth-brooding frogs restricted to the temperate forests of southwestern South America. The males of these species carry tadpoles in their mouth and vocal sacs for a variable period of time. Both species are uncommon in captive collections.

2.4.14 Pseudidae

Pseudidae (harlequin frogs) contains around four species and is primarily found throughout eastern South America. The swimming frog, *Pseudis paradoxa*, also known as the paradox frog, is occasionally seen in captivity (Plate 2.36). The tadpole of this frog grows to a much larger size than the adult frog to which it eventually transforms.

2.4.15 Hylidae

Hylidae (treefrogs) is a diverse group of over 650 species, but the relationships within this family are unclear. This may be an artificial grouping of only distantly related species. Treefrogs are found throughout the New World, Europe, Australia, and Asia. Treefrogs have an extremely limited distribution in northwest Africa and are absent from India. Hylid frogs are popular pets, and over 50 species are reported in captive collections. The White's treefrog, *Pelodryas (Litoria) caerulea*, is a candidate for the most popular pet anuran (Plates 2.37A, 2.37B). Other members of this genus such as the New Guinea giant treefrog, *Litoria infrafrenata*, are also held in large numbers. Phyllomedusine frogs such as the red-eyed treefrog, *Agalychnis callidryas*, and leaf or monkey frogs, *Phyllomedusa* spp., (Plates 2.38, 2.39) are also quite popular. The common treefrogs, *Hyla* spp., are well represented in captive collection (Plates 2.40, 2.41) but some species such as the Pine Barrens treefrog, *Hyla andersoni*, are endangered (Plate 2.42). The Cuban treefrog, *Osteopilus septentrionalis*, is a common item in the pet trade, perhaps in part because of its ready availability in Florida. This frog is an introduced species in southern Florida that has become a problem by outcompeting native frogs. Marsupial frogs, *Gastrotheca* spp., are occasionally kept, as are horned treefrogs, *Hemiphractys* spp., chorus frogs, *Pseudacris* spp., and cross-banded treefrogs, *Smilisca* spp.

> **Husbandry Summary**

Most hylid frogs
Oviparous
Vivarium design: arboreal
Temperature range: temperate to tropical lowland
Suggested diet: crickets, other insects

2.4.16 Centrolenidae

Centrolenids (glass frogs) are found from southern Mexico to northern South America. There are around 70 species of centrolenids, which superficially resemble hylid frogs. Many centrolenids have transparent abdominal skin, hence the common name, "glass" frogs. Giant glass frogs, *Centrolene* spp., and glass frogs, *Centrolenella (Cochranella)* spp. (Plate 2.43), are occasionally imported for the pet trade, but identification of these frogs is difficult without supporting data such as the collecting locality.

> **Husbandry Summary**

Most glass frogs
Oviparous
Vivarium design: arboreal
Temperature range: temperate to tropical lowland
Suggested diet: crickets, other insects

2.4.17 Dendrobatidae

Dendrobatidae (poison frogs) contains around 125 species, about 30 of which are held in captive collections. Commonly known as either poison, dart-poison, poison-dart, or poison-arrow frogs, these Central and South American frogs are very popular with the non-herpetoculturist, due in part to their brilliant colorful patterns, small size, and diurnal habits. *Dendrobates* (Plates 2.44, 2.45, 2.46, 2.47), *Epipedobates* (Plate 2.48), and *Phyllobates* (Plate 2.49), are the genera that have been repeatedly bred in captivity over several generations. Rocket frogs, *Colestethus* spp. (Plate 2.50) are unprepossessing dendrobatids that are uncommon in captivity.

Husbandry Summary

Green and black poison frog, *Dendrobates auratus*,
Oviparous
Vivarium design: terrestrial forest floor
Temperature range: tropical lowland
Suggested diet: pinhead crickets, fruit flies, springtails
(NOTE—most of the commonly available *Dendrobates* spp. can be accommodated in this manner.)

Phantasmal poison frog, *Epipedobates tricolor*,
Oviparous
Vivarium design: terrestrial forest floor
Temperature range: tropical montane
Suggested diet: fruit flies, springtails

2.4.18 Ranidae

Ranidae (true frogs) contains around 700 species, but the relationships within the family are unclear. The distribution is worldwide except for southern South America and Australia. Six subfamilies are accepted in this text, only two of which are reported in captive collections—Mantellinae and Raninae. Mantellinae includes a dozen or so mantellas (Madagascan dart-poison frogs), *Mantella* spp. (Plate 2.51), as well as around 20 species of Madagascan frogs, *Mantidactylus*. Around 30 species of Raninae are kept in captive collections, including two common laboratory species, the northern leopard frog, *Rana pipiens* (Plate 2.52), and the bullfrog, *Rana catesbeiana* (Plates 2.53, 2.54). One of the more commonly worked upon "species," the European edible frog, *Rana esculenta*, is not a true species but rather illustrates the klepton concept (Polls Pelaz, 1990). The edible frog is actually the fertile hybrid of the marsh frog *R. ridibunda* and the pool frog *R. lessonae* (Berger, 1973), but the European edible frog is often still referred to as a species rather than as a klepton, e.g., *Rana kl. esculenta*. The wood frog, *Rana sylvatica*, is a species that produces a cryoprotectant allowing acclimated specimens to be frozen for brief periods of time without harm (Plate 2.55). Tschudi's African bullfrog, *Pyxicephalus adspersus*, is another popular pet species that is commonly bred (Plate 2.56). Gunther's triangle frog, *Ceratobatrachus guentheri*, is increasingly common in captive collections (Plate 2.57). This family also includes the largest living anuran, the goliath frog, *Conraua goliath*, which can weigh in excess of 7 kg (15 lbs). This species is currently protected by CITES and the United States Endangered Species Act.

Husbandry Summary

Golden mantella, *Mantella aurantiaca*,
Oviparous
Vivarium design: terrestrial forest floor
Temperature range: subtropical to tropical lowland
Suggested diet: pinhead crickets, fruit flies, springtails
(NOTE: Many *Mantella* spp. may require cooler temperatures than this.)

Northern leopard frog, *Rana pipiens*,
Oviparous
Vivarium design: streamside
Temperature range: temperate
Suggested diet: crickets, earthworms

Bullfrog, *Rana catesbeiana*,
Oviparous
Vivarium design: streamside
Temperature range: temperate to subtropical
Suggested diet: crickets, earthworms, fish

Tschudi's African bullfrog, *Pyxicephalus adspersus*,
Oviparous
Vivarium design: terrestrial forest floor or shallow aquatic pond with large land area
Temperature range: tropical lowland
Suggested diet: crickets, earthworms, fish, small mice (with added vitamin D_3)

Gunther's triangle frog, *Ceratobatrachus guentheri*,
Oviparous, direct development to froglet stage
Vivarium design: terrestrial forest floor
Temperature range: tropical lowland
Suggested diet: crickets

2.4.19 Hyperolidae

Hyperolidae (African reed frogs) contains around 210 species. Hyperolids are restricted to sub-Saharan Africa, Madagascar, and the Seychelle Islands. A few reed frogs, such as the common reed frog, *Hyperolius viridiflavus*, are unique among higher vertebrates due to their ability to change sexes (Grafe & Linsemair,

1989). A few species of African reed frogs, *Hyperolius* spp. (Plate 2.58), and two species of running frogs, *Kassina* spp., are represented in captive collections.

Husbandry Summary

Marbled reed frog, *Hyperolius marmoratus*,
Oviparous
Vivarium design: arboreal
Temperature range: tropical lowland
Suggested diet: small crickets, fruit flies

Running frogs, *Kassina* spp.,
Oviparous
Vivarium design: terrestrial forest floor
Temperature range: tropical lowland
Suggested diet: small crickets, fruit flies

2.4.20 Rhacophoridae

Rhacophorids (flying frogs) are found throughout the tropical areas of the Old World. There are approximately 200 species of rhacophorids, but less than 20 species are common in captive collections. Madagascan bright-eyed frogs, *Boophis* spp., and some flying frogs, *Rhacophorus* spp., are found in captive collections. Despite the common name, few species of the Rhacophoridae actually have adaptations for gliding (e.g., Abah river flying frog, *Rhacophorus nigropalmatus*).

Husbandry Summary

Most rhacophorids can be accommodated as follows
Oviparous
Vivarium design: arboreal
Temperature range: temperate to tropical lowland
Suggested diet: crickets, other insects

2.4.21 Microhylidae

Microhylidae (narrowmouth toads) contains around 290 species (Plate 2.59). Microhylids are found throughout temperate and tropical North America, South America, Africa, Madagascar, and Southeast Asia. The Malaysian narrowmouth toad, *Kaloula pulchra*, is an inexpensive species common in captivity (Plate 2.60). The Sambava tomato frog, *Dyscophus guineti*, is a popular pet and has been captive bred in commercial numbers in recent years. *Dyscophus guineti* is generally yellow to orange in color with a pattern of dark reticulation over its smooth dorsal skin. In contrast, the endangered tomato frog, *D. antongilli*, is generally bright red to reddish-orange, lacks reticulation, and has granular appearing skin on its dorsum. The origin of *Dyscophus antongilli* in the pet trade is legally questionable as many of these were exported from Madagascar without proper permits or were imported bearing the erroneous identification of *D. guineti*.

Husbandry Summary

Sambava tomato frog, *Dyscophus guineti*,
Oviparous
Vivarium design: terrestrial forest floor or shallow aquatic pond with large land area
Temperature range: tropical lowland
Suggested diet: crickets, earthworms

2.5 HELPFUL GUIDES FOR IDENTIFICATION

This should not be considered a comprehensive list of identification guides for amphibians but rather a starting point of texts available to assist in the identification of an amphibian patient.

Altig, R. 1970. A key to the tadpoles of continental United States and Canada. Herpetologica 26:180–207.

Arnold, E.N. and J.A. Burton. 1978. A Field Guide to the Reptiles and Amphibians of Britain and Europe. Collins, London, Great Britain, UK.

Ashton Jr., R.E. and P.S. Ashton. 1988. Handbook of Reptiles and Amphibians of Florida. Part Three. The Amphibians. Windward Publishing, Inc., Miami, FL.

Auerbach, R.D. 1987. The Amphibians and Reptiles of Botswana. Mokwepa Consultants (Pty) Ltd., Gaborone, Botswana.

Bechtel, H.B. 1995. Reptile and Amphibian Variants: Colors, Patterns, and Scales. Krieger Publishing Company, Malabar, FL.

Behler, J.L. and F.W. King. 1979. The Audobon Society Field Guide to North American Reptiles and Amphibians. Alfred A. Knopf, Inc., New York, NY.

Berry, P.Y. 1975. The Amphibian Fauna of Peninsular Malaysia. Tropical Press, Kuala Lumpur.

Bishop, S.C. 1994. Handbook of Salamanders. Comstock Publishing Associates, Cornell University Press, Ithaca, NY.

Cochran, D.M. 1970. Frogs of Colombia. Bulletin of the United States Natl. Museum 288:1–655.

Cochran, D.M. 1961. Living Amphibians of the World. Doubleday & Company, Inc. Garden City, NY.

Cochran, D.M. 1955. Frogs of Southeastern Brazil. Bull. U.S. Natl. Mus. 206:1–423.

Cogger, H.G. 1992. Reptiles and Amphibians of Australia. Cornell University Press, Ithaca, NY.

Collins, J.T. 1993. Amphibians and Reptiles in Kansas, 3rd Edition. University Press of Kansas, Lawrence, KS.

Conant R. and J.T. Collins. 1991. Field Guide to Amphibians and Reptiles of Eastern and Central North America. Houghton Mifflin Co., New York, NY.

Dickerson, M.C. 1969. The Frog Book (North American Toads and Frogs, With a Study of the Habits and Life Histories of those of the Northeastern United States). Dover Publications, Inc., New York, NY.

Duellman, W.E. 1970. The Hylid Frogs of Middle America (two volumes). Monograph of the Museum of Natural History, University of Kansas.

Freytag, G.E., B. Grzimek, O. Kuhn, and E. Thenius (Eds.). 1968. Amphibians, in Grzimek, B (Ed.): Grzimek's Animal Life Encyclopedia, Vol. 5, Fishes II/Amphibian. Van Nostrand Reinhold Co., New York, NY, pp. 269–456.

Glaw, F. and M. Vences. 1994. A Field Guide to the Amphibians and Reptiles of Madagascar, 2nd Edition. Moos-Druck, Leverkusen.

Griffiths, R.A. 1996. Newts and Salamanders of Europe. Academic Press, San Diego, CA.

Green, N.B. and T.K. Pauley. 1987. Amphibians and Reptiles in West Virginia. University of Pittsburgh Press, Pittsburgh, PA.

Hedges, N.G. 1983. Reptiles and Amphibians of East Africa. Kenya Literature Bureau, Nairobi, Kenya.

Henderson, R.W. and A. Schwartz. 1984. A Guide to the Identification of the Amphibians and Reptiles of Hispaniola. Milwaukee Public Museum Special Publications in Biology & Geology Number 4.

Kuzmin, S.L. 1995. The Clawed Salamanders of Asia. Westarp Wissenschaften, Magdeburg.

Leonard, W.P., H.A. Brown, L.L.C. Jones, K.R. McAllister, and R.M. Storm. 1993. Amphibians of Washington and Oregon. Seattle Audubon Society, Seattle, WA.

Leviton, A.E., S.C. Anderson, K. Adler, and S.A. Minton. 1992. Handbook to Middle East Amphibians and Reptiles. Society for the Study of Amphibians and Reptiles, Contributions to Herpetology, Number 8.

Lutz, B. 1973. Brazilian Species of *Hyla*. University of Texas Press, Austin, TX.

Martof, B.S., W.M. Palmer, J.R. Bailey, J.R. Harrison III, and J. Dermid. 1980. Amphibians and Reptiles of the Carolinas and Virginia. The University of North Carolina Press, Chapel Hill, NC.

Menzies, J.I. 1976. Handbook of Common New Guinea Frogs. Wau Ecology Institute Handbook No. 1, Port Moresby, Papua New Guinea.

Meyer, J.R. and C.F. Foster. 1996. A Guide to the Frogs and Toads of Belize. Krieger Publishing Company, Malabar, FL.

Murphy, J.C. (in press). Amphibians and Reptiles of Trinidad and Tobago. Krieger Publishing Company, Malabar, FL.

Norman, D.R. and L. Naylor. 1994. Amphibians and Reptiles of the Paraguayan Chaco, Volume 1. San Jose, Costa Rica.

Obst, F.J., K. Richter, and U. Jacob (Eds.). 1988. The Completely Illustrated Atlas of Reptiles and Amphibians for the Terrarium. TFH Publications, Inc., Neptune City, NJ.

Passmore, N.I. and V.C. Carruthers. 1995. South African Frogs, 2nd Edition. Witwatersrand University Press, Johannesburg.

Petranka, J. W. 1998. Salamanders of the United States and Canada. Smithsonian Institution Press. Washington, DC.

Pfingsten, R.A. and F.L. Downs. 1989. Salamanders of Ohio. Bulletin of the Ohio Biological Survey Vol. 7, #2.

Pickwell, G. 1947. Amphibians and Reptiles of the Pacific States. Stanford University Press, Stanford, CA.

Robb, J. 1980. New Zealand Reptiles and Amphibians in Colour. Collins, Auckland, New Zealand.

Rodriguez, L.O. and W.E. Duellman. 1994. Guide to the Frogs of the Iquitos Region, Amazon, Peru. Natural History Museum, University of Kansas, Lawrence, KS.

Schwartz, A. and R.W. Henderson. 1985. A Guide to the Identification of the Amphibians and Reptiles of the West Indies Exclusive of Hispaniola. Milwaukee Public Museum, Milwaukee, WI.

Stebbins, R.C. 1985. A Field Guide to Western Reptiles and Amphibians, 2nd Edition. Houghton Mifflin Co., Boston, MA.

Stebbins, R.C. and N. Cohen. 1995. A Natural History of Amphibians. Princeton University Press, Princeton, NJ.

Steward, J.W. 1969. The Tailed Amphibians of Europe. David & Charles, Newton Abbot, Great Britain, UK

Stewart, M.M. 1967. Amphibians of Malawi. State University of New York Press, Albany, NY.

Taylor, E.H. 1962. The amphibian fauna of Thailand. University of Kansas Science Bulletin 36:265–599.

Taylor, E.H. 1968. The Caecilians of the World, a Taxonomic Review. University of Kansas Press, Lawrence, KS.

Villa, J., L.D. Wilson, and J.D. Johnson. 1988. Middle American Herpetology. University of Missouri Press, Columbia, MO.

Waite, E.R. 1993 (Orig. Ed. 1929). The Reptiles and Amphibians of South Australia. Krieger Publishing Company, Malabar, FL.

Walls, J.G. 1994. Jewels of the Rainforest. TFH Publications, Inc., Neptune City, NJ.

Wright, A.H. and A.A. Wright. 1949. Handbook of Frogs and Toads of the United States and Canada, 3rd Edition. Cornell University Press, Ithaca, NY.

Zhao, E. and K. Adler. 1993. Herpetology of China. Society for the Study of Amphibians and Reptiles.

REFERENCES

Berger, L. 1973. Systematics and hybridisation in European green frogs of *Rana esculenta* complex. Journal of Herpetology 7:1–10.

Duellman, W.E. and L. Trueb. 1986a. Phylogeny, *in* Duellman, W.E. and L. Trueb: Biology of the Amphibia. McGraw-Hill Book Co., New York, pp. 465–475.

Duellman, W.E. and L. Trueb. 1986b. Classification, *in* Duellman, W.E. and L. Trueb: Biology of the Amphibia. McGraw-Hill Book Co., New York, pp. 493–553.

Frank, N. and E. Ramus. 1995. A Complete Guide to the Scientific and Common Names of Reptiles and Amphibians of the World. Ramus Publishing, Inc., Pottsville, PA.

Frost D. 1985. Amphibian Species of the World. Allen Press, Inc., and The Association of Systematics Collections, Lawrence, KS.

Goin, C.J., O.B. Goin, and G.R. Zug. 1978a. Caecilians, sirens, salamanders, *in* Goin, C.J., O.B. Goin, and G.R. Zug: Introduction to Herpetology. W.H. Freeman and Co., San Francisco, CA, pp. 200–220.

Goin, C.J., O.B. Goin, and G.R. Zug. 1978b. Frogs and toads, *in* Goin, C.J., O.B. Goin, and G.R. Zug: Introduction to Herpetology. W.H. Freeman and Co., San Francisco, CA, pp. 221–251.

Grafe, T.U. and K.E. Linsemair. 1989. Protogynous sex reversal in the reed frog, *Hyperolius viridiflavus*. Copeia 1989 (4): 1024–1030.

International Species Information System. 1995. ISIS Amphibian Abstract as of 30 June 1995. ISIS, Apple Valley, MN.

Mattison, C. 1987. The families of frogs, *in* Mattison, C.: Frogs and Toads of the World. Facts on File, Inc., New York, pp. 150–180.

Moler, P. E. and J. Kezer. 1993. Karyology and systematics of the salamander genus *Pseudobranchus* (Sirenidae). Copeia 1993: 39–47.

Polls Pelaz, M. 1990. The biological klepton concept (BKC). Alytes 8:78–89.

Porter, K.R. 1972. The origin and phylogenetic relationships of Amphibia, *in* Porter, K.R.: Herpetology. W.B. Saunders Co., Philadelphia, PA, pp. 88–114.

Slavens, F.L. and K. Slavens. 1994. Reptiles and Amphibians in Captivity. Breeding, Longevity, Inventory, Current January 1, 1994. Slavewear, Seattle, WA.

Zug, G.R. 1993a. Caecilians and salamanders, *in* Herpetology: An Introductory Biology of Amphibians and Reptiles. Academic Press, Inc., San Diego, CA, pp. 335–355.

Zug, G.R. 1993b. Frogs, *in* Herpetology: An Introductory Biology of Amphibians and Reptiles. Academic Press, Inc., San Diego, CA, pp. 357–385.

CHAPTER 3
ANATOMY FOR THE CLINICIAN

Kevin M. Wright, DVM

3.1 COMPREHENSIVE ANATOMIC TEXTS

The anatomy of the amphibians will be presented with emphasis on clinically salient features. There are several excellent texts that have been published on the anatomy of amphibians, but their availability is limited. The interested clinician is advised to use book search services and inquire with used book dealers with an interest in herpetological texts. An excellent comprehensive text of the anatomy of the European fire salamander, *Salamandra salamandra,* has been published, but it is rare and somewhat expensive (Francis, 1934). There exists a similar comprehensive text of the anatomy of two European ranid frogs, the edible frog, *Rana esculenta,* and European common frog, *R. temporaria* (Haslam, 1971). These two texts are highly recommended and should be consulted for anatomic details not found in this chapter or in the chapters on pathology. The more easily obtainable texts concern the anatomy of the mudpuppy, *Necturus maculosus* (Gilbert, 1973) and the European common frog, *Rana temporaria* (Wells, 1968). An exhaustive text concerning the amphibian ear exists (Wever, 1985). Standard herpetological references also contain anatomic information of use to the clinician (Duellman & Trueb, 1986a, 1986b; Goin et al., 1978; Porter, 1972; Stebbins & Cohen, 1995; Zug, 1993a, 1993b, 1993c), as do some of the popular works on amphibians (e.g., Obst et al., 1988). The clinician is advised to continually review herpetological journals, including, but not limited to, *Copeia, Journal of Herpetology, Herpetological Review,* and *Amphibia-Reptilia,* to build a reprint library of relevant anatomic and physiologic information.

3.2 LARVAL AMPHIBIANS

Reviews of amphibian larval anatomy and metamorphosis are available (Duellman & Trueb, 1986a; White & Nicoll, 1981; Zug, 1993c). Metamorphosis is a complex and metabolically demanding process, and the clinician with a particular interest in amphibian propagation and pediatrics is encouraged to seek out additional sources of information.

3.2.1 The Larval Caecilian

Late stage larval caecilians strongly resemble adult caecilians except for the presence of gills for a few hours after birth (Plate 3.1). The posthatching metamorphosis that is typical of salamanders and anurans is relatively undocumented in caecilians, and all neonates thus studied appear to resemble the adults. Branchial respiration occurs in larval oviparous caecilians within the egg and within the oviduct of viviparous species. Prior to hatching or birth, or within a few hours of birth, the gills are lost. Gill slits disappear during these final stages, as does the larval fins of the terrestrial forms.

The kidney of the larval caecilian functions to excrete nitrogenous waste in the form of ammonia and maintain water balance by excreting excess body water. Paired pronephric kidneys are present in the larva, and the pronephric tubules occur in a metameric (segmental) fashion along the dorsal aspect of the coelom. Depending on the species, 8–12 tubules may be present, which is more than the number of tubules found in species in the other two orders of amphibians. The pronephric kidney filters coelomic fluid via the nephrostome that accesses the coelomic cavity. Glomeruli in the form of outpocketings of the dorsal aorta also serve as an access to the pronephric kidney. The nephrostome drains into a short tubule, which in turn is serviced by the renal portal vein. The short tubule empties into the common (pronephric) duct whereupon the wastes may be excreted into the external environment. This system only allows for filtration, not reabsorption (and thus concentration of the solute level), so the osmolality of the urine of a larval caecilian is equal to the osmolality of its plasma.

During metamorphosis, the pronephros degenerates and is phagocytized while the mesonephros is beginning to function. This transition is to a large degree controlled by fluctuations in the circulating levels of the thyroid hormones triiodothyronine (T_3) and tetraiodothyronine (T_4).

3.2.2 The Larval Salamander

A staging system for the larval development of the spotted salamander, *Ambystoma maculatum*, has been described (Rugh, 1962). Immediately after hatching the larva possesses no external processes except for gills. The larva begins life with a large head bearing three pairs of plumate gills and a streamlined body and tail. Forelimbs erupt a variable length of time later, followed by hind limbs. In species with a terrestrial stage, and in some aquatic species, the gills start to recede shortly before metamorphosis is complete. Salamanders are carnivorous throughout life, and the digestive system changes little with metamorphosis. There may be morphological differences between larvae which suggest either habitat adaptations (a small morph of the tiger salamander, *Ambystoma tigrinum*, adapted to ephemeral ponds and a large morph adapted to permanent ponds) or cannibalism (a morph of the tiger salamander, *A. tigrinum*, with an enlarged head and proportionately larger gape) (Rose & Armentrout, 1976). Some salamander species, such as the axolotl, *Ambystoma mexicanum*, and the mudpuppy, *Necturus maculosus*, continue to mature internally and become reproductive despite the retention of the external appearance of the larva, a process known as neoteny.

Not all salamanders undergo metamorphosis. Some races of the European fire salamander (e.g., *Salamandra salamandra bernardezi*, *S. salamandra fastuosa*) and the alpine salamander, *Salamandra atra*, give birth to fully metamorphosed young that resemble the adults (Griffiths, 1996). Some plethodontids, such as the green salamander, *Aneides aeneus*, develop directly into the adult form from the egg and thereby bypass the free-living larval stages.

The pronephric kidney of the larval salamander is similar to that of the caecilian, however the number of tubules is much reduced. In certain primitive salamanders (e.g., Cryptobranchidae), there is a total of five paired tubules. The number of tubules is reduced to two pairs in more advanced families of salamanders.

3.2.3 The Larval Anuran

Anuran larvae are commonly referred to as tadpoles. Tadpoles are distinctively shaped with a round to oval body and a laterally compressed tail (Plate 3.2). The structure of the tadpole changes dramatically throughout its growth, and various staging systems have been described in an effort to standardize the approach to anuran developmental anatomy. One of the better known staging systems describes the development of the Gulf Coast toad, *Bufo valliceps* (Limbaugh & Volpe, 1957). The oral groove is variably shaped. The shape and structure of the mouth are tailored to the diet of the tadpole and may be taxonomically significant. Anuran tadpoles have a varied diet, and there is considerable variation in diet. The tadpoles within some species may vary in morphology, as some individuals may be programmed for cannibalism. The digestive tract is typically long and coiled in the filter feeding and herbivorous tadpoles and much shorter in carnivorous tadpoles. Paired external nares are present. Gills are visible upon hatching, but eventually are covered by an operculum until a pair of branchial spiracles are present. The cloaca may be located subjugular or more terminally located toward the tail base. There are no known neotenic anurans.

3.3 ADULT AMPHIBIANS

See Figures 3.1A, B and 3.2A, B within this chapter for generalized anatomic drawings of the skeleton of salamanders and anurans. See Figures 3.3, 3.4, 3.5, 3.6, and 3.7 for generalized anatomic drawings of adult specimens of the three orders of amphibians. See Plates 3.3, 3.4, 3.5, and 3.6 within the color section for photographs of the visceral anatomy of a caecilian, salamander, and frog.

3.3.1 External Anatomy

The Adult Caecilian. The body form of caecilians strongly resembles that of annelid worms (e.g., earthworm, *Lumbricus terrestris*) due to the presence of cutaneous folds (primary and secondary annuli) in the skin, suggestive of a segmented body plan, and the absence of limbs. Coloration is variable, from slate grey to bright blue to yellow depending on the species. The eyes are small and covered with skin in many species. The tentacle, a small olfactory and tactile sensory structure, is found in the nasolabial groove immediately ventral or rostral to either eye (Plate 3.7). Small external nares are present. Primary and secondary annuli create the ribbed appearance of the caecilian. Some aquatic species may have a dorsal fin along the caudal third of the body. The cloaca is found at the terminus of the body, and there is usually little if any tail caudal to the cloaca. It has been reported that the sexes of some typhlonectiids and perhaps other caecilians may be externally distinguished by the shape of the cloacal opening, which has been modified in the male so as to enhance its grasping ability during mating. At this point in time, external sexing of caecilians by cloacal morphology is not reliable, for while it was reported that in the Rio Cauca caecilian, *Typhlonectes natans*, the male's cloaca is round and the female's is a longitudinal slit (O'Reilly et al., 1995), this dimorphism has not held true in individuals necropsied at the Philadelphia Zoo.

The Adult Salamander. The adult newt and salamander generally have four limbs, although the sirens only have forelimbs. Many species exhibit the derived trait of less than five toes per limb, and the one-toed amphiuma, *Amphiuma pholeter,* bears only a single digit per limb. Some salamanders, such as the hellbender, *Cryptobranchus alleganiensis,* have light colored soles that should not be mistaken for scar tissue or other lesions (Plate 3.8). Paired external nares and eyes are usually present, although cave-dwelling forms may lack eyes. Tympanic membranes are lacking in salamanders. Aquatic specimens may or may not bear external plumate gills. Axolotls, *Ambystoma* spp., sirens, *Siren* spp., dwarf sirens, *Pseudobranchus* spp., mudpuppies and waterdogs, *Necturus* spp., the olm, *Proteus anguinis,* and blind salamanders, *Typhlomolge* spp., are aquatic species that possess external gills, while hellbenders, *Cryptobranchus* spp., Asian giant salamanders, *Andrias* spp., amphiumas, *Amphiuma* spp., and newts (family Salamandridae) lack these external structures. A tail is present, and in some forms the tail has cleavage planes to allow autotomy as an antipredator defense. In some plethodontid salamanders an obvious constriction ring is present at the tail base immediately caudal to the cloacal slit, and this serves as the site of tail breakage. Many male salamanders may have swollen cloacal lips during times of reproductive activity, whereas female salamanders will show little or no increase in size of the cloacal lips at any time of the year (Plate 3.9). During the breeding season nuptial pads may be present on the forelimbs of some salamanders, such as the Spanish ribbed newt, *Pleurodeles waltl,* and the hindlimbs of others, such as the Eastern red-spotted newt, *Notophthalmus viridescens.* Dorsal crests develop in males of *Triturus* spp. during breeding season. (See also Section 22.3, Sexual Dimorphism.) Costal grooves lend a ribbed appearance to many species and are an important trait needed to identify many species. In some species (e.g., crocodile newt, *Tylototriton shanjing*) sharp points of the actual ribs may break through the skin as a defensive reaction to handling. Large toxin-containing parotid glands are visible caudal to the eye in some species. (These are not to be confused with the parotid gland of mammals, which is a salivary gland. Parotid refers to a location "near the ear." To avoid confusion, the amphibian gland is sometimes called the "parotoid" gland.) Mental glands may be visible underneath the chin of males in some species during the reproductive season.

The Adult Anuran. The adult anuran has four limbs. In anurans that depend on saltatory locomotion, such as ranid frogs, the hindlimbs are much longer and more obviously muscled than the forelimbs, whereas in anurans that tend to walk rather than jump, such as dendrobatids, the leg proportions are more equal. Five digits are present on the hind limbs and four or five are present on the forelimbs. Male anurans may develop nuptial pads on the forelimbs during breeding season. (See Table 3.1 and also see Section 22.3, Sexual Dimorphism.) Paired external nares and eyes are present. Tympanic membranes are present except in a few species. Gills are not present, but modifications of the skin, such as the filaments of the hairy frog, *Trichobatrachus robustus,* and the loose folds of skin of the Titicaca water frog, *Telmatobius culeus,* are functional equivalents. A postmetamorphic tail, actually an outpocketing of the cloacal tissue rather than a true tail, is present only in a few species of Leiopelmatidae and serves as an intromittent organ. The cloaca is found at the tip of the urostyle and may be somewhat dorsally oriented. The cloaca is easier to see when the anuran is in ventral rather than dorsal recumbency. Large parotid glands are visible caudomedial to the eye in some species and are particularly prominent in bufonids. Vocal slits containing the vocal sacs may be visible in the vicinity of the maxillary hinge.

Some of the external characters that may be dimorphic in anurans include skin color (e.g., golden Alajuela toad, *Bufo periglenes*), tympanic membrane size (e.g., bullfrog, *Rana catesbeiana*), presence/absence of nuptial pads (e.g., White's treefrog, *Pelodryas caerulea*), toe shape (e.g., dyeing poison frog, *Dendrobates tinctorius*), adult body size (red-eyed treefrog, *Agalychnis callidryas*), size of certain anatomic structures (e.g., the cranium of the lowland Caribbean toad, *Peltophryne lemur*), presence/absence of modified skin structures (e.g., papillae of the male hairy frog, *Trichobatrachus robustus,* marsupium of the female marsupial treefrog, *Gastrotheca* spp., heavily granulated skin of the male warty toad, *Bufo spinulosus*), presence/absence of vocal sacs (e.g., oak toad, *Bufo quercicus*), presence/absence of "spines" on the forelimbs (e.g., Rosenberg's treefrog, *Hyla rosenbergi*) or lips (e.g., Taosze spiny toad, *Vibrissaphora boringii*), presence/absence of tusks or mandibular odontids (e.g., tusked frog, *Adelotus brevis*), and the presence/absence of a tail (e.g., tailed frog, *Ascaphis truei*).

3.3.2 Musculoskeletal System

The musculoskeletal system of the amphibian has received the most attention of any organ system probably because it is the most common organ system to survive in fossil form. All other organ systems are fairly similar in appearance within an order, but the musculoskeletal system may vary dramatically between members of the same order, and it is often the characteristic used to define relationships among modern amphibians. The elucidation of the particulars of the musculoskeletal anatomy is beyond the scope of this text. Rather, the approach is to familiarize the clinician with basic elements of the amphibian's musculoskeletal system.

Table 3.1. Examples of sexually dimorphic characters in some representative anuran species.

Dimorphic character(s)	Representative species
Skin color	Golden Alajuela toad (*Bufo periglenes*); males are golden, females are brown
Modified skin structures	Hairy frog (*Trichobatrachus robustus*); males develop long papillae on the side during breeding season, females lack these Warty toad (*Bufo spinulosus*); males develop extremely granular skin during breeding season, females remain unchanged Rosenberg's treefrog (*Hyla rosenbergi*); males have "spines" on forelimbs, females have smooth forelimbs Marsupial frogs (*Gastrotheca* spp.); females develop a dorsal marsupium, males have no such opening on their back Taosze spiny toad (*Vibrissaphora boringii*); males have "spines" on lips, females lack these
Tympanic membrane size	Bullfrog (*Rana catesbeiana*); males larger than females
Nuptial pads	White's treefrog (*Pelodryas caerulea*); males have them on forearms during breeding season, females lack them at all times
Toe shape	Dyeing poison frog (*Dendrobates tinctorius*); males have large triangular toe tips, females have smaller more rounded toe tips
Adult body size	Red-eyed treefrog (*Agalychnis callidryas*); mature males are smaller than females
Size of other anatomic structures	Lowland Caribbean toad structures (*Peltophryne lemur*); cranium shape
Vocal sacs	Oak toad (*Bufo quericus*); males have distinct grey pigmented vocal sacs, females sacs are reduced in size and unpigmented
Tusks or mandibular odontids	Tusked frog (*Adelotus brevis*); males have tusks but females lack them
Tail	Tailed frog (*Ascaphis truei*); males have a tail, females lack them

The Adult Caecilian. The majority of the cranial components of a caecilian are fused. Caecilians lack pectoral and pelvic girdles as well as a sacrum. Except for the atlas and terminal vertebrae, the ribs of caecilians are double-headed.

The Adult Salamander. The cranium of the salamander is intermediate between the solid structure of a caecilian and the markedly reduced bone structure of an anuran. The hyoid may be modified to allow for suction feeding or the ejection of the tongue to capture prey items, as in tropical salamanders, *Bolitoglossa* spp. The vertebral column is poorly differentiated into cervical, trunk, sacral, caudal sacral, and caudal regions. Cleavage planes may be present in the caudal region. Pelvic girdles are lacking in sirens, *Siren* spp., and the dwarf siren, *Pseudobranchus* spp. Digits may be lacking in some species.

The Adult Anuran. The musculoskeletal system of the anuran is highly modified from that of other amphibians. Most of the modifications allow for saltatory locomotion, while features for other lifestyles may be secondarily derived from these original modifications. The nomenclature of some of the bones of the anuran skeleton is different from many other vertebrates and should be used appropriately. The cranium bears two large orbits with no bony separation between the ocular globe and the oropharynx. The cranial elements are reduced when compared to the other amphibian orders. The vertebrae are fused, and three regions of the vertebral column are described: the presacral, sacral, and postsacral. A sacrum is lacking, and the pelvic girdle is highly modified. The limbs are highly modified. The distal long bones consist of a fused radioulna in the forelimbs and a fused tibiofibula in the hind limb. The pectoral girdle varies in shape among different genera of anurans, as does the amount of cartilaginous and bony elements making up the pectoral girdle. The pelvic girdle is fused and intimate with the last presacral vertebra. The coccyx or urostyle is a single fused element in most anurans, and forms a point above the dorsocaudal aspect of the pelvic girdle. In many genera the hyoid bones

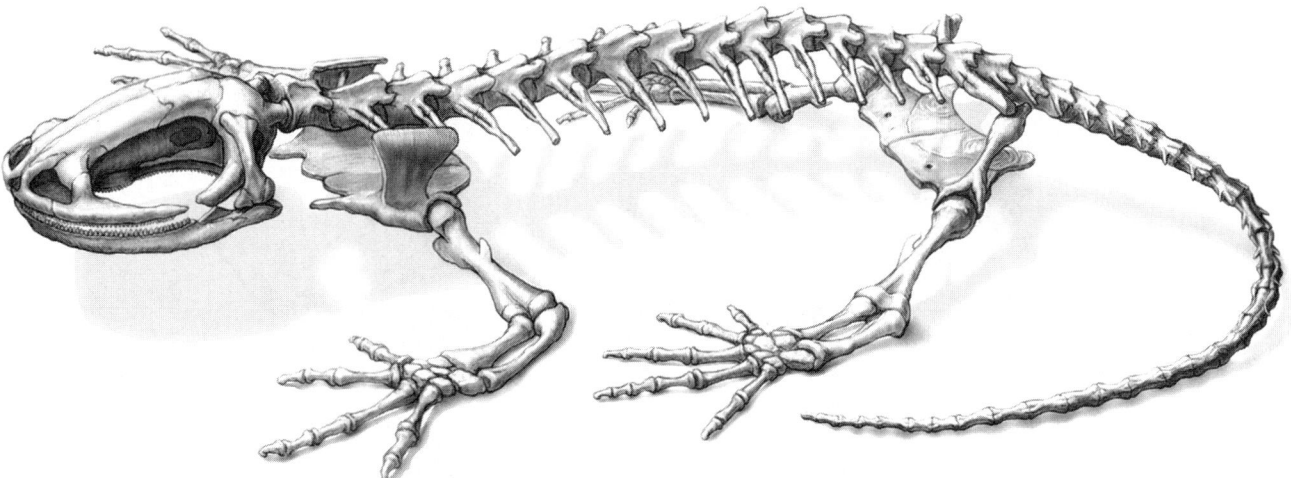

Figure 3.1A. The skeleton of a typical salamander. Not all salamanders have all the skeletal elements depicted here, and the shape and arrangements of some skeletal elements may vary considerably. (John Gibb, Johns Hopkins University Department of Art as Applied to Medicine)

are adapted for ejecting the tongue to capture prey items.

3.3.3 Nervous System

The anatomy of the brain of a caecilian (Kuhlenbeck, 1973), a salamander (Herrick, 1948), and an anuran (Haslam, 1971) have been studied in great detail and compared (Noble, 1931). There is some debate as to the number of cranial nerves. One textbook (Duellman & Trueb, 1986b) lists the cranial nerves as follows: CN I Olfactory (also innervates the tentacle of caecilians); CN II Optic (absent or reduced in many caecilians and cave salamanders); CN III Oculomotor (does not connect with CN V in caecilians); CN IV Trochlear (also innervates an eye muscle); CN V Trigeminal (also innervates the tentacular sheath of caecilians); CN VI Abducens (innervates the retractor of the caecilian tentacle); CN VII Facial; CN VIII Auditory; CN IX Glossopharyngeal; CN X Vagus; CN XI Accessory; CN XII Hypoglossal, which may be considered a spinal nerve and not a true cranial nerve; Lateral-line nerves are innervated by branches of the cranial nerves. As is expected for limbless animals, the brachial and inguinal neural plexi are absent in caecilians, and reduced in salamanders with vestigial limbs (e.g., amphiumas, *Amphiuma* spp., dwarf siren, *Pseudobranchus striatus*, and sirens, *Siren* spp).

3.3.4 Integumentary System

A review of the amphibian integument was recently published (Heatwole & Barthalmus, 1994).

The Adult Caecilian. Caecilians demonstrate the typical amphibian integument that consists of very few cell layers. As a rule the stratum corneum consists of a single layer of keratinized cells. The basal epidermal cell layer is often less than eight cells thick and is underlayed by a basement membrane. The dermis lies immediately beneath this and contains capillaries, nerves, and smooth muscle throughout its two layers. The dermis consists of an outer spongy layer and inner compact layer. Chromatophores and glands are present within the spongy layer, while the compact layer possesses collagen fibers that intimately adhere it to the underlying muscles and bones. Unlike anurans and salamanders, some caecilians possess tiny dermal scales.

Many of the glandular secretions of caecilians can prove irritating if introduced into a human's ocular membranes (O'Reilly et al., 1995). Annuli serve to increase the surface area of the caecilian and may facilitate gas and water exchange.

Shedding of the stratum corneum occurs on a regular basis. Many caecilians eat their shed skin (Weldon et al., 1993).

The Adult Salamander. Salamanders have the typical amphibian integument, but the stratum corneum of some aquatic species is not keratinized. The dermis is firmly attached to the underlying muscles and bones.

The glandular secretions of some salamanders possess toxic compounds. Modifications such as costal grooves, granular skin, and skin folds increase the surface area of the integument and may facilitate gas and water exchange.

Shedding of the stratum corneum occurs on a regular basis. Many salamanders eat their shed skin (Weldon et al., 1993).

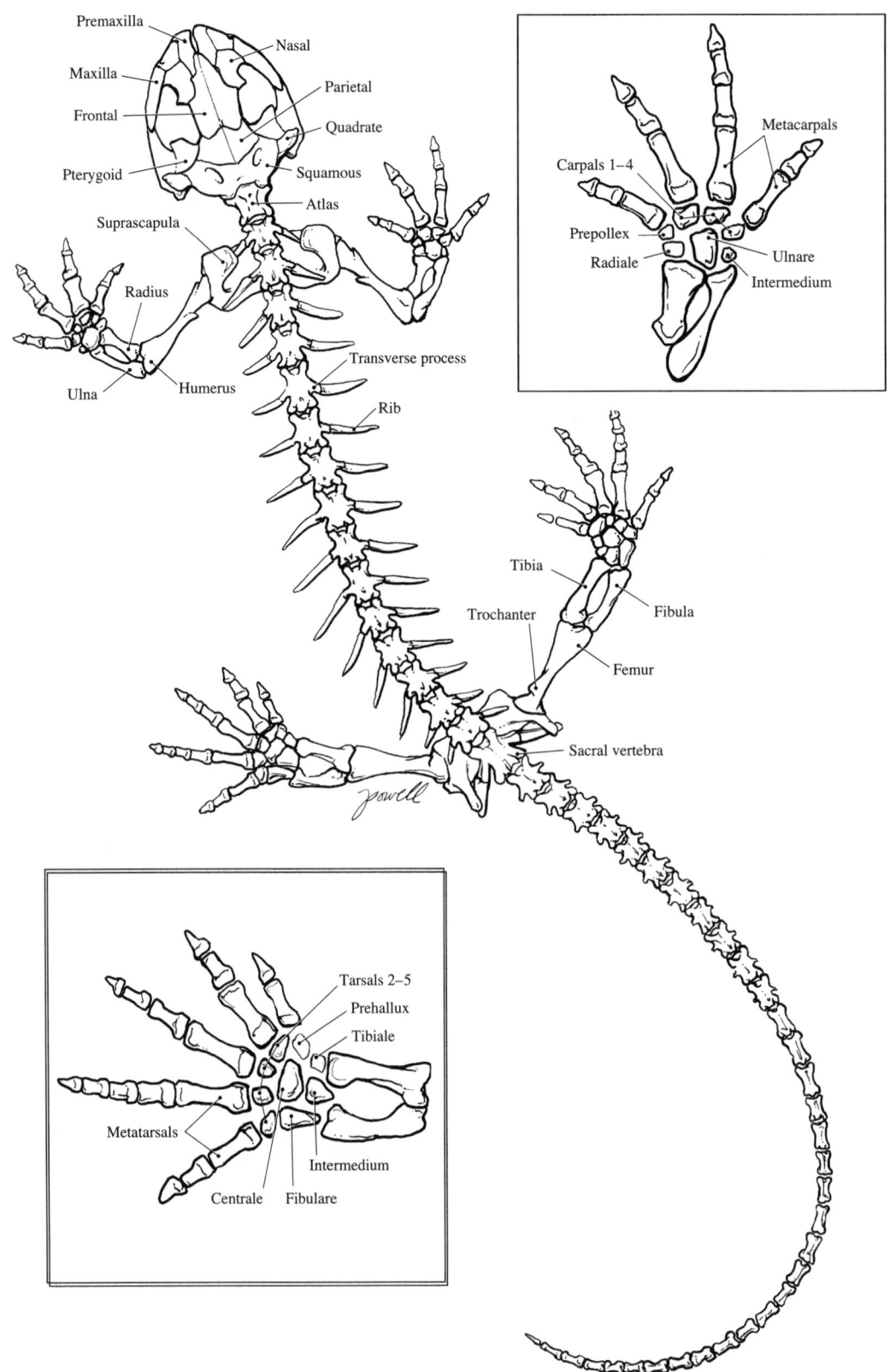

Figure 3.1B. Skeletal nomenclature of a typical salamander. (Bradley Duncan Powell, Johns Hopkins University Department of Art as Applied to Medicine)

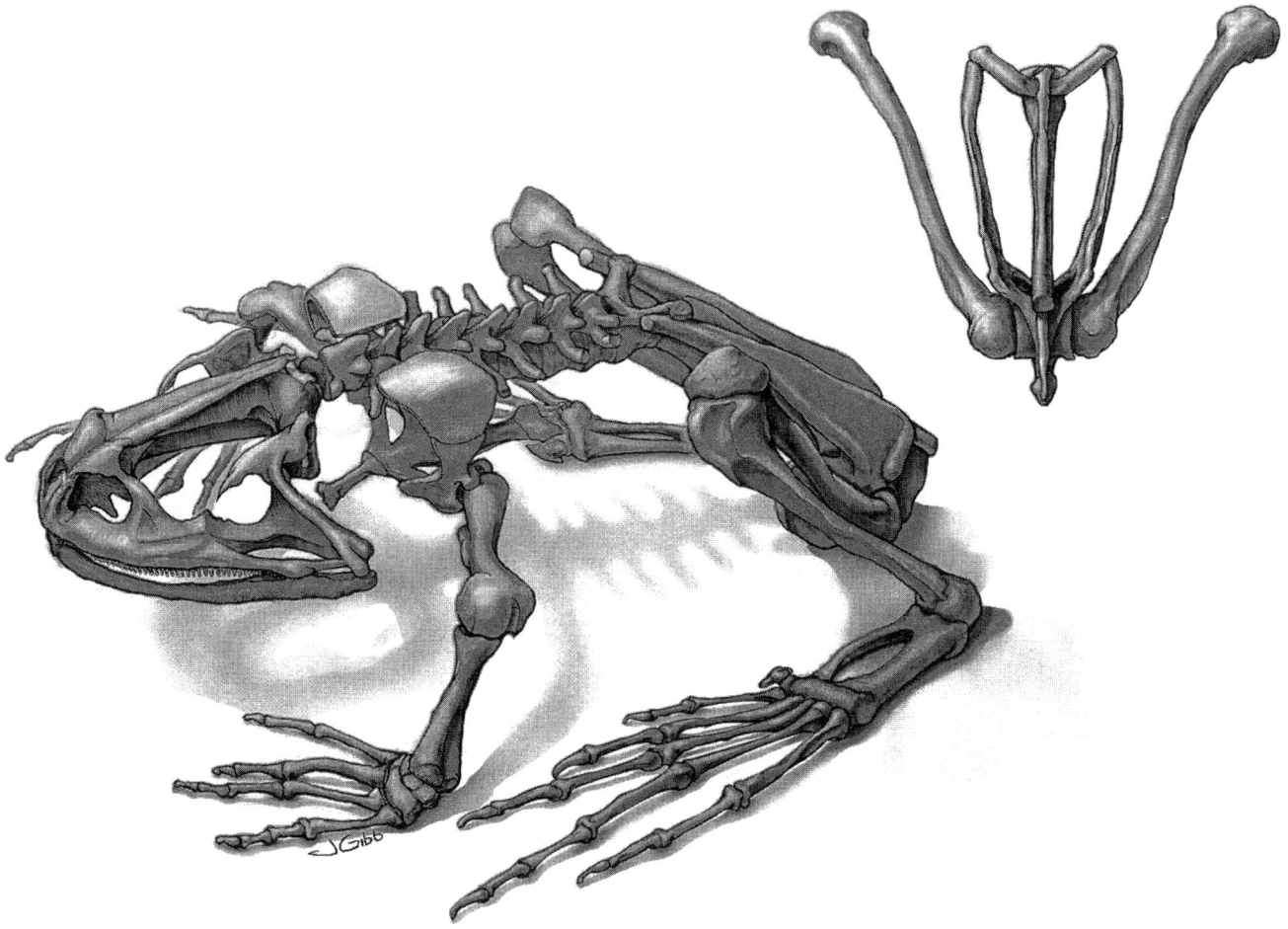

Figure 3.2A. The skeleton of a typical anuran. Not all anurans have all the skeletal elements depicted here, and the shape and arrangements of some skeletal elements may vary considerably. (John Gibb, Johns Hopkins University Department of Art as Applied to Medicine)

The Adult Anuran. Most anurans have the typical amphibian integument, but modifications of the typical plan are numerous. The skin is not as tightly adhered to the underlying structures as it is in caecilians and salamanders, and this potential subcutaneous space can fill with fluid. Thus anurans may appear edematous, a condition not described for caecilians or salamanders. Subcutaneous fluid accumulation in the anuran can be normal, functioning as a reserve of water, or it may be the result of a pathologic process. Anurans generally have a greater range of color changing ability than other amphibians.

The skin over the skull of certain anurans (e.g., bufonids) is co-ossified with the underlying dermal bones, while other frogs (e.g., giant monkey frog, *Phyllomedusa bicolor*) have small bones within the dermis.

Similar to other amphibians, shedding of the stratum corneum occurs on a regular basis and many anurans are keratophagous (Weldon et al., 1993).

3.3.5 Alimentary System

All adult amphibians are primarily carnivorous and have a relatively short and simple gastrointestinal tract. Comprehensive descriptions and reviews of the digestive tract have been published (Olsen, 1977; Reeder, 1964).

Some mastication occurs in the oral cavity, but prey is usually swallowed whole. The oral cavity is separated from the esophagus by a strong sphincter, and the esophagus is separated from the stomach by a sphincter. Cilia lines the esophagus to transport ingesta and secreted material to the stomach. Mucous and some digestive enzymes (e.g., pepsinogen) are secreted by glandular cells lining the esophagus. The stomach is separated from the intestine by a pyloric sphincter, and generally lies to the left of midline within the coelom. The sections of the intestine are not as grossly obvious as in other vertebrates. Gastric emptying is controlled by the duodenum. The liver and gall bladder are intimately connected, and a pancreas is present. The liver has a minimal role in processing nitrogen for excretion

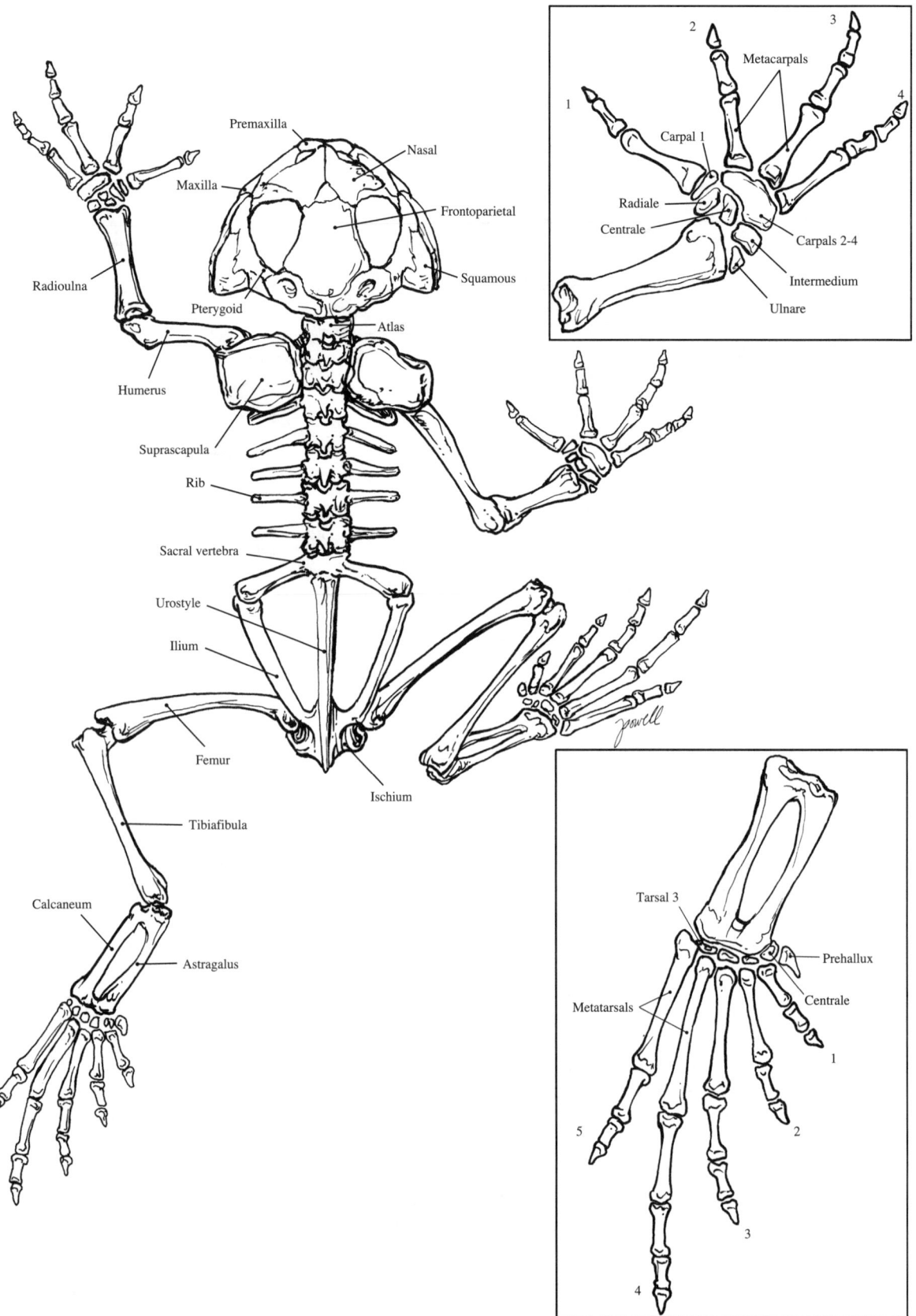

Figure 3.2B. Skeletal nomenclature of a typical anuran. (Bradley Duncan Powell, Johns Hopkins University Department of Art as Applied to Medicine)

in aquatic amphibians, as ammonia is freely diffused into the surrounding environment through the skin and via excretion via the kidneys. In terrestrial amphibians, the liver converts ammonia to the less toxic water-soluble nitrogenous compound urea, and in a few species urea is converted to uric acid as a further method of water conservation. (See Section 4.2, Water Homeostasis.) The pancreas is found in the hepato-gastric ligament between the stomach and anterior intestine. Bile and pancreatic enzymes enter the intestine through ducts that empty into the anterior part of the small intestine (duodenum). The small intestine is the site of enzymatic digestion and carbohydrate, fat, and protein absorption. The large intestine is the site of water and salt absorption and mucous secretion to aid in the passage of fecal boluses. Fecal matter is voided through the cloaca. Amphibian feces will contain undigested parts of the ingesta, including chitin, keratin, cellulose, and the bones that were not decalcified by the acid secretions of the stomach.

The Adult Caecilian. The arrangement and distribution of teeth are diagnostic characters in the identification of many caecilians (Taylor, 1968). Multiple rows of teeth are a common feature of many caecilians. Multiple pancreatic ducts are present, while there is no valve separating the small intestine from the large intestine.

The Adult Salamander. Certain oral glands are lacking in some species of aquatic salamanders (e.g., amphiumas, *Amphiuma* spp., sirens, *Siren* spp.). Pepsinogen secreting cells are absent in some salamandrids (*Salamandra* spp.). Pancreatic ducts range in number from 2–47 depending on the species. There is no valve separating the small intestine from the large intestine.

The Adult Anuran. Teeth are absent in some anurans. Pipid frogs lack tongues and certain oral glands, features that are unnecessary for their mode of aquatic suction feeding. Pepsinogen secreting cells are absent in some pipids. The liver is bilobate. Some anurans can evert their stomach and use their hands to wipe ingesta from the mucosal surface, an apparent adaptation allowing removal of indigestible or toxic substances. There is a single pancreatic duct, but the pancreatic and bile ducts may merge prior to entrance in the intestine in ranids. There is no valve separating the small intestine from the large intestine in many species of primitive anurans.

3.3.6 Urinary System

The Adult Caecilian. The adult caecilian may have different excretory needs than the larva. In aquatic caecilians the role of the kidney is essentially unchanged (i.e., excretion of ammonia and water), whereas in the terrestrial caecilians the kidney may undertake the physiologically more demanding process of urea or uric acid excretion and water reabsorption. (See Section 4.2, Water Homeostasis.)

The excretory system of the caecilian has been described (Wake, 1970a, b, 1972). The mesonephric kidney extends the length of the caecilian's coelomic cavity and retains the metameric arrangement of the larval pronephros (Plate 3.10). Caecilians lack the secondary tubules that arise in anurans and caudates. The mesonephros forms caudal to the pronephros but also functions by filtering both the coelomic and vascular fluids. The excretory route is similar to that described for the larval pronephros, however there are several changes. The nephrostome still connects with the coelomic cavity, but empties into a convoluted tubule. Vascular filtration is achieved by a Malpighian body, consisting of an internal glomerulus and Bowman's capsule, and this structure also empties into the convoluted tubule, which in turn empties into the mesonephric (common) duct. Many species of caecilians are known to have bladders that are bilobate. As with all amphibians, the mesonephric kidney cannot concentrate urine above the solute concentration of the plasma.

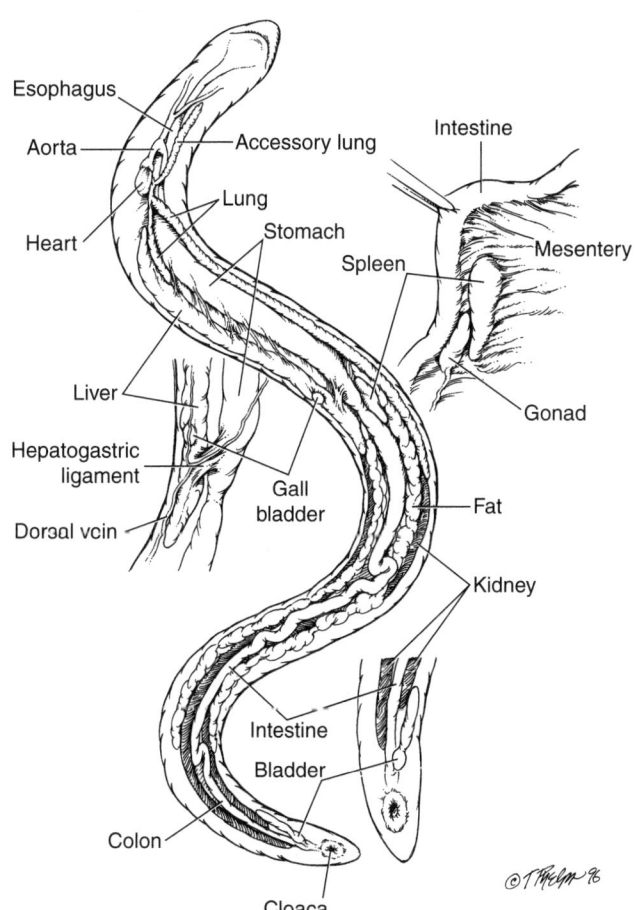

Figure 3.3. General anatomy of a caecilian. Inset view of cloaca and internal anatomy. (Tim Phelps)

The dual filtration of coelomic and vascular fluid by the amphibian's mesonephric kidney may affect the distribution and clearance of intracoelomically administered drugs. Without specific studies documenting the pharmacokinetics of a given drug on a particular species, the clinician must rely on personal clinical judgment when administering intracoelomic drugs.

The Adult Salamander. The mesonephric kidney of the adult salamander arises posterior to the pronephros. The excretory route described for caecilians is similar to one family of caudates, the Amphiumidae, but secondary tubules are found in all other caudates. The secondary tubules arise at branch points of the primary tubules and may have glomeruli. Many tubules lack a nephrostome and are not connected to the coelomic cavity. Thus in many salamanders there is an emphasis on vascular filtration for excretion of nitrogenous wastes. However, as mentioned with caecilians, the role of the kidney is dependent on the Salamander's mode of life—most terrestrial salamanders will conserve water through the excretion of urea and reabsorption of water. The bladder is bilobate, bicornate or cylindrical in salamanders.

The Adult Anuran. The primary nitrogen waste of an anuran is either ammonia, urea, or uric acid, de-

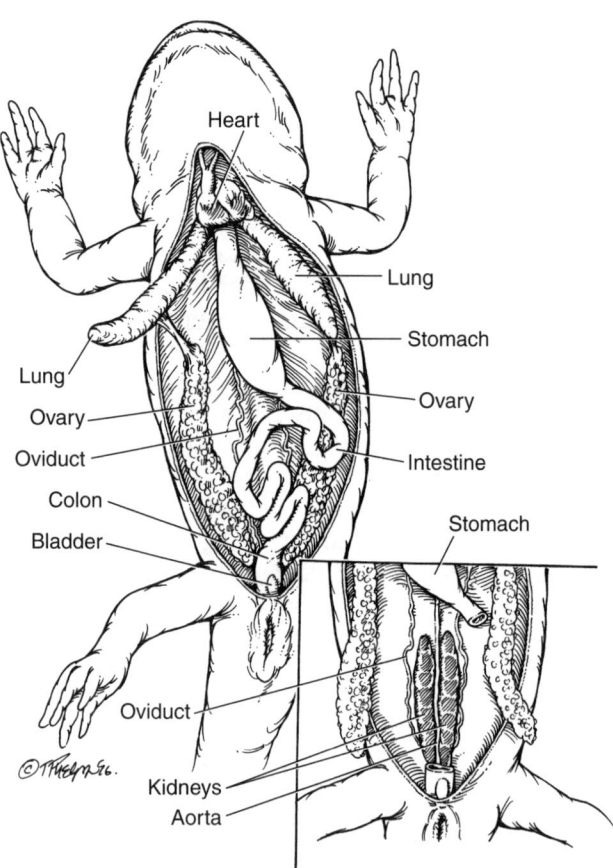

Figure 3.5. Visceral anatomy of a female salamander. Liver and gall bladder removed and right lung reflected. Inset view of retroperitoneal space. (Tim Phelps)

pending on its environment. Aquatic anurans excrete the majority of their nitrogenous waste as ammonia, since water conservation is not an issue. Many terrestrial species, such as bufonids, are not in constant contact with a water-rich environment and excrete a large portion of their nitrogenous waste as urea. Some anurans (e.g., African gray treefrog, *Chiromantis xerampelina,* waxy treefrog, *Phyllomedusa sauvagii*) exploit relatively dry conditions by converting nitrogen wastes to uric acid. (See Section 4.2, Water Homeostasis.) Many of these uricotelic species possess cilia in the urinary bladder (Bolton & Beuchat, 1991).

3.3.7 Respiratory System

The Adult Caecilian. There are three modes of adult respiration within the order Gymnophiona—pulmonic, buccopharyngeal, and cutaneous. The importance of each method undoubtedly varies based on the activity of the caecilian and the dissolved oxygen content of the water in which it lives. Little is known about the respiratory physiology of caecilians, and generalizations are impossible given the disparities in oxygen consumption under differing environmental conditions that have been documented for various species of salamanders and frogs.

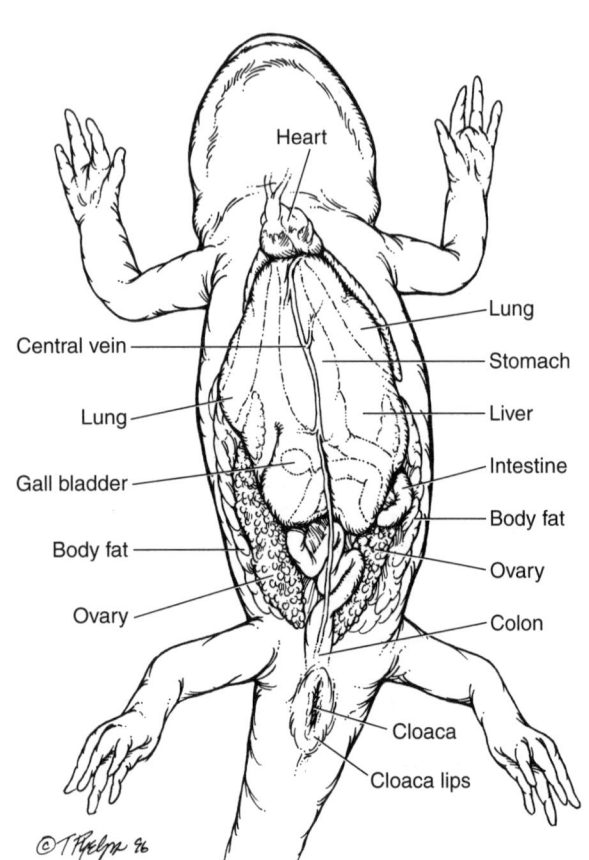

Figure 3.4. Visceral anatomy of a salamander. (Tim Phelps)

The lung of the caecilian is the most important respiratory structure (Bennet & Wake, 1974). Most caecilians have paired elongate lung lobes, with the left lobe reduced in size or absent. In some species (e.g., typhlonectid caecilians), the right and left lobe are of approximately equal size. The alveoli of the caecilian lung is comprised of a mix of smooth muscle, cartilage and other connective tissue, blood vessels, and respiratory epithelium. In the aquatic typhlonectids, it is hypothesized that the lungs serve an additional role as an organ to maintain buoyancy as is noted for some aquatic salamanders (e.g., amphiumas, *Amphiuma* spp.).

Based on a study of a terrestrial caeciliid, the buccopharyngeal structures are the primary mechanical source for the inspiratory and expiratory effort (Mendes, 1945).

The diameter of the external nares and the choana of a caecilian are controlled by smooth muscle. This musculature thereby limits the passage of air through the nasal duct into the buccopharyngeal cavity, and to some extent mediates olfaction by controlling access to the olfactory system. The glottis is at the base of the tongue on the ventral aspect of the buccopharyngeal cavity, and in aquatic amphibians the glottis may be much smaller than expected for a similar sized terrestrial amphibian's glottis. The larynx leads immediately to the trachea. The trachea is well supported through its length with cartilaginous rings. The elongated trachea is lined with ciliated epithelium, and bifurcates into pulmonary bronchi. A tracheal lung has been described in some ichthyophiids and typhlonectids, and this structure actually serves as a structure for gaseous exchange, complete with respiratory epithelium.

The Adult Salamander. There are four modes of adult respiration within the order Urodela: branchial, cutaneous, buccopharyngeal, and pulmonic. The relative importance of any of these is dependent on the species in question.

Neotenic species (e.g., sirens, *Siren* sp., mudpuppies, *Necturus* spp., axolotls, *Ambystoma mexicanum*, olm, *Proteus anguinis*, Texas blind salamanders, *Typhlomolge rathbuni*, etc.), as well as the aquatic larvae of many species, possess external gills and rely heavily on branchial respiration. Some aquatic species (e.g., sirens, *Siren* spp.) possess lungs in addition to their gills. The structure of the gill is dependent on the environment of the species, and the shape and resultant surface area is, to a degree, mutable within a species, dependent on physical parameters. Aquatic environments with a high dissolved oxygen content allow salamanders to have short gills, whereas in areas of low dissolved oxygen content the gills tend to become long and elaborate. Stream-dwelling species tend to have small gills to reduce the drag of the current. The concomitantly high dissolved oxygen content of this environment permits this necessarily small surface area of the gill structure.

Cutaneous respiration is present to a variable degree in all species. This mode of respiration is feasible in salamanders as a result of several anatomic factors: high surface area to volume ratio resultant from the small body size and cylindrical shape, a thin epidermis, and a highly vascularized dermis. All of these features promote the exchange of gases across the skin. Coupled with a salamander's low metabolic rate and its ability to incur an oxygen debt through anaerobic glycolysis, these anatomic features permit cutaneous respiration. In fact, this mode of respiration is so successful that the plethodontids, one of the most species-rich families of salamanders, are lungless. The surface area to volume ratio is enhanced by the presence of lateral folds of skin in the aquatic cryptobranchid salamanders (e.g., hellbender, *Cryptobranchus alleganiensis,* Asian giant salamanders, *Andrias* spp.), and a rocking motion helps increase the diffusion rate across the skin by keeping a current of low dissolved carbon dioxide content water running across the skin. Costal grooves also serve to enhance the surface area of a salamander. The same characteristics that allow cutaneous respiration also play a role in the distribution of topically applied drugs.

The buccal cavity and pharynx serve as a site of gaseous exchange in many species of salamanders. This gaseous exchange is to some extent an extension of the cutaneous respiration, but the muscular pumping action to ventilate this region, as well as peculiarities of the vascular supply of these regions, support buccopharyngeal respiration as a distinct entity. The pumping action is the main source of both buccopharyngeal and pulmonic ventilation for the salamander, both inspiratory and expiratory.

Some salamanders are able to make noises using different anatomic features. The Pacific giant salamander, *Dicamptodon ensatus,* has vocal folds (Maslin, 1950), but the voice of salamanders is derived by forcing air through gill slits or nares or forming a vacuum during inspiration and then opening the mouth.

The lungs of salamanders vary in size and degree of partitioning among species. As a rule, the right and left lung are of approximately equal size, although the right side is slightly smaller than the left. The lungs are generally simple structures with no partitioning or infolding in some aquatic salamanders (e.g., mudpuppies and waterdogs, *Necturus* spp.), while terrestrial salamanders tend to have sacculations and even alveoli in the anterior portion of each lung. Many pond-dwelling species have alveoli too. Although plethodontid salamanders lack lungs, in other families such as the hynobiid clawed salamanders, *Onychodactylus* spp., lungs are reduced in size, or even absent.

The trachea leads to a short bifurcation into the lungs. Cartilaginous rings are present in the trachea, and in some species, the bronchi. The trachea is relatively short in most salamanders, a fact which must be borne in mind when intubating for tracheal washes or intratracheal administration of drugs, and during gaseous anesthesia, or else the intubating device could be inserted too far and damage the pulmonic epithelium. Surprisingly the trachea of many aquatic salamanders, notably the amphiumas, *Amphiuma* spp., is greatly elongated as a result of the position of the lungs, due to the dual functions of gaseous exchange and hydrostasis.

taneous respiration. This option is not available in the warmer waters in which the clawed frog, *Xenopus laevis*, is found.

The buccal cavity and pharynx serve as a site of gaseous exchange in many species of anurans. As in salamanders, buccopharyngeal respiration is a distinct mode of respiration in anurans. The pumping action is the main source of both buccopharyngeal and pulmonic ventilation for the anuran, both inspiratory and expiratory.

Anurans are the most vocal amphibians, with almost every species having a voice. The voice of anurans is derived by forcing air from the lungs across the vocal slits and into the vocal sacs by a combination of buccopharyngeal pumping and pulmonic pumping.

The trachea is extremely short and bifurcates in the lungs. Cartilaginous rings are present in the trachea. The shortness of the trachea must be considered when the clinician is intubating for tracheal washes or intratracheal administration of drugs, and during gaseous anesthesia, or else the intubating device could be inserted too far and damage the pulmonic epithelium.

The lungs of anurans vary in size and degree of partitioning among species. As a rule, the right and left lung are of approximately equal size. The lungs are generally simple structures with no partitioning or infolding.

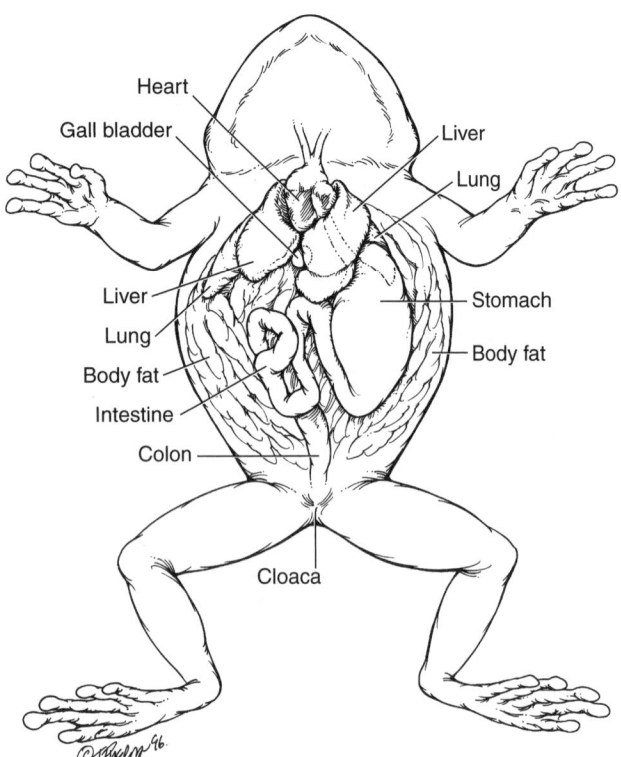

Figure 3.6. Visceral anatomy of a frog. (Tim Phelps)

The Adult Anuran. There are three modes of adult respiration within the order Anura—cutaneous, buccopharyngeal, and pulmonic. The relative importance of any of these is dependent on the species in question.

The aquatic Titicaca water frog, *Telmatobius culeus*, has prominent folds of skin to increase its surface area, and relies heavily on cutaneous respiration, whereas the African clawed frog, *Xenopus laevis*, lacks folds and is primarily a lung breather. This is probably reflective of the dissolved oxygen content of the water in which these species evolved, with the cold well-oxygenated water of the mountain lake allowing the Titicaca water frog, *Telmatobius culeus*, to obtain adequate oxygen saturation of the blood through cu-

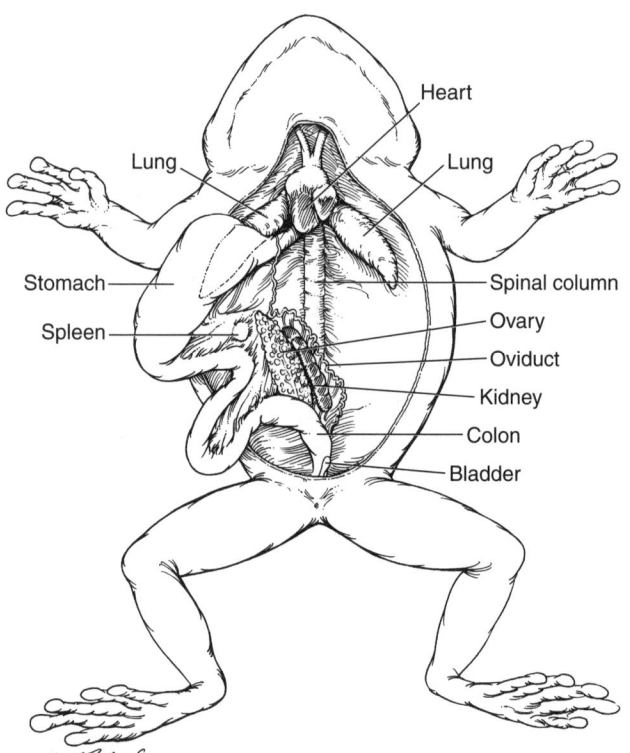

Figure 3.7. Visceral anatomy of a female frog. Liver and gall bladder removed and stomach reflected to reveal urogenital system. (Tim Phelps)

3.3.8 Cardiovascular System

The cardiovascular system includes the arterial, venous, and lymphatic systems. The lymphatic system has unique structures, variously termed lymph sacs, lymph hearts, or lymph vesicles, which serve to restrict flow of lymph unidirectionally so that it returns to the heart. The lymph hearts beat in synchrony at 50–60 beats per minute, independent of the cardiac rate (Conklin, 1930). Given the rapidity of the lymph heart rate, it is sometimes difficult to obtain lymph from these sites. Illness should be expected whenever large volumes of lymph accumulate in any lymph sac. The volume of lymph moved by this system is astounding. One study determined that fluid leakage from the plasma was over 50 times the total plasma volume in a 24-hour period, and this leakage was recovered and circulated by these lymphatics (Isayama, 1924 as cited in Boutilier et al., 1992; Churchill et al., 1927). Well hydrated terrestrial amphibians may be able to route fluid absorbed through the skin directly into the lymphatics (Boutilier et al., 1992), bypassing the arterial blood. Since this fluid is then eliminated by the kidneys, this could have a profound effect on the absorption and distribution of pharmacological agents administered cutaneously. The lymph consists of the components of blood, except for erythrocytes. Variation between the components of plasma versus lymph appears to be poorly documented.

The Adult Caecilian. Caecilians possess the typical amphibian heart, consisting of the right and left atria and one ventricle. The left atrium is usually smaller than the right, and the atrial septum is fenestrated. Due to the lack of limbs, the circulatory system of the caecilian lacks many of the major peripheral arteries and veins found in other amphibians. The routing of blood through the caecilian is largely undocumented, but extrapolating from the patterns established in salamanders and anurans, it is reasonable to assume that the renal and hepatic portal vein systems receive blood from the caudal half of the caecilian (Simons, 1959). Until pharmacokinetics studies document otherwise, it is best to avoid administering drugs that are metabolized or excreted either renally or hepatically in the caudal half of a caecilian.

Caecilians may have over 200 lymph hearts subcutaneously which deliver lymph into the intersegmental veins.

The Adult Salamander. The three-chambered heart is generally found beneath the confluence of the pectoral girdle and sternum. A ventricular septum is present in the lesser siren, *Siren intermedia,* and mudpuppy, *Necturus maculosus* (Putnam, 1975; Putnam & Dunn, 1978). The left atrium is usually smaller than the right. The interatrial septum is fenestrated except in sirens, *Siren* spp., and the hellbender, *Cryptobranchus alleganiensis* (Putnam, 1977; Putnam & Parkerson, 1985). Lungless salamanders (Plethodontidae) have a modified interatrial septum that allows both atria to receive blood from the sinoatrial aperture and prevent stagnation of the flow through the left atria (Putnam & Kelly, 1978). If gills are present, the branchial vasculature is prominent. In darkly pigmented salamanders the superficial vasculature is difficult to discern unless there is obvious hyperemia. However, many salamanders possess white-colored or translucent abdominal skin which may allow direct visualization of the midline abdominal vein. The caudal tail vein runs immediately ventral to the caudal vertebrae, and again may be visible if the skin is translucent.

Both renal and hepatic portal vein systems are present in the caudal half of the salamander. Blood passing through the renal portal vein system passes through the kidneys before entering the postcaval vein, whereas blood passing through the hepatic portal vein system passes through the liver prior to entering the vena cava. It appears that the renal portal system receives a major portion of the blood drainage from the tail, but the factors that determine the routing of blood in the caudal half of the body are largely undocumented. Until pharmacokinetic studies document otherwise, it is best to avoid administering drugs that are metabolized or excreted either renally or hepatically in the hind limbs or tail of salamanders.

The lymphatic system of the European fire salamander, *Salamandra salamandra,* has been extensively described (Francis, 1934). Intestinal lymphatics empty into the subclavian veins, whereas the other lymphatics may empty into the cutaneous, cardinal, subvertebral, or lingual veins. The number of lymph hearts varies with species, but in this medium-sized salamander there are around 11 lymph hearts located in the head and coelom, and four lymph hearts that occur caudal to the sacrum.

The Adult Anuran. The heart of the anuran has been extensively studied (Kumar, 1975). The three-chambered heart is generally found beneath the confluence of the pectoral girdle and sternum. The left atrium is usually smaller than the right, and the interatrial septum is complete, unlike that of the other two orders of amphibians. In some anurans, the ventricular trabeculae are numerous and thick (Plate 3.11). In darkly pigmented anurans the superficial vasculature is difficult to discern unless there is obvious hyperemia. However, many anurans possess white-colored or translucent abdominal skin which may allow direct visualization of the midline abdominal vein. The vasculature of the hindlimb webs and hind limbs are readily identified upon a cursory examination. An extensive lingual venous plexus is present on the underside of the tongue in most species of anurans.

Both renal and hepatic portal vein systems are present in the caudal half of the anuran. Blood passing through the renal portal vein system passes through the kidneys before entering the postcaval vein, whereas blood passing through the hepatic portal vein system passes through the liver prior to entering the vena cava. The factors that determine the routing of blood in the caudal half of the anuran body are largely undocumented. Until pharmacokinetic studies document otherwise, it is best to avoid administering drugs that are metabolized or excreted either renally or hepatically in the hind limbs of anurans.

The lymphatic system of two European ranids has been extensively described (Haslam, 1971), and the structure and function of the lymph hearts of anurans has been reviewed (Carter, 1979). Anurans have few lymph hearts when compared to other amphibians. There may be from 1–5 or more lymph hearts located along the coccyx, and one pair located subscapularly. Enlarged subcutaneous lymphatic spaces occur in varying places on anurans. A prominent pair may be found dorsally on either side of the urostyle in many terrestrial anurans, and this is a convenient site to obtain samples of lymph fluid. Collection of lymph is enhanced in frogs paralyzed with curare (Conklin, 1930).

3.3.9 Hematolymphopoietic System

The hematolymphopoietic system of amphibians has been reviewed (Plyzycz et al., 1995). All amphibians possess a thymus, which is one source of T-lymphocytes in amphibians. The thymus is present throughout life in amphibians, although malnutrition and stress may elicit involution and atrophy of the thymus in captive amphibians (Plyzycz et al., 1995). Hibernation may also cause a reduction in the size of the thymus. The spleen has both red and white pulps in amphibians, which act as the respective centers of erythropoiesis and myelopoiesis. Seasonal variation has been noted in the size of the spleen (Plyzycz et al., 1995). Gut-associated lymphoid tissue (GALT) is present in amphibians. In general, aquatic amphibians lack functional bone marrow, but sites that serve as functional equivalents are found in the liver and kidneys.

The Adult Caecilian. Caecilians lack functional bone marrow, but lymphopoiesis occurs in various sites such as the liver, kidneys, thymus, and spleen.

The Adult Salamander. The bone marrow of terrestrial salamanders has sites of lymphomyelocytopoiesis which are lacking in aquatic salamanders. The ventral meninges of some species of primitive aquatic salamanders also act as hematolymphopoietic tissue. Lymphomyeloid organs are lacking in all caudates.

The Adult Anuran. Terrestrial anurans possess functional bone marrow, but it does not serve as a site for erythropoiesis, only lymphocytopoiesis and myelothrombocytopoiesis. Lymphomyeloid organs are sentinels that process antigens to produce a strong humoral response. The lymphomyeloid organs are not connected with the lymphatic system, rather the afferents of lymphomyeloid organs are either arteries or veins or both.

3.3.10 Endocrine System

The endocrine system of the amphibian is similar to that of other vertebrates, and the function of the various organs is similar, although the actual secretions produced may have significant structural differences from their analogues in other vertebrates (e.g., calcitonin). A review of the endocrine system has been published (Gorbman, 1964). Due to the long use of amphibians as models for study in the fields of embryology and endocrinology, detailed information concerning the amphibian endocrine system may be found in many endocrinology texts. The endocrine glands (and associated secretions) include the following: adrenals (epinephrine, norepinephrine, corticosteroids), gonads (testosterone, estrogen, progesterone), pancreatic islets (insulin), parathyroids (calcitonin, parathyroid hormone), pineal body (melatonin), pituitary (adrenocorticotropin or ACTH, antidiuretic hormone or ADH, arginine vasotocin, follicle-stimulating hormone or FSH, luteinizing hormone or LH, melanophore-stimulating hormone or MSH, oxytocin, prolactin), thymus (thymosin), thyroid (tri-iodothyronine or T_3, tetraiodothyronine or T_4), and ultimobranchial bodies (calcitonin). The locations of the endocrine glands in amphibians are similar to the locations in reptiles, with a few exceptions as noted below.

The Adult Caecilian. The adrenal glands of the caecilian are located on the ventrimesal surface of the kidneys.

The Adult Salamander. The adrenal glands of the salamander are located on the ventrimesal surface of the kidneys. Parathyroid glands are lacking in mudpuppies, *Necturus* spp. The ultimobranchial gland is singular in most species of salamanders but is paired in amphiumas, *Amphiuma* spp., and mudpuppies, *Necturus* spp.

The Adult Anuran. The adrenal glands vary in location depending on the species of anuran, but remain in close association to the kidneys. The adrenals lie lateral to the kidneys in advanced anurans, but are ventrimesal or medial in primitive anurans. It has been documented that the corpora lutea secrete progesterone in some viviparous species (e.g., African tree toads, *Nectophrynoides* spp.). Parathyroid glands regress during the winter in some species and may not be detectable. The ultimobranchial glands are found adjacent to the larynx in most anurans but are lacking in clawed frogs, *Xenopus* spp.

3.3.11 Reproductive System

The reproductive system of the amphibian is fairly standardized considering the diversity of reproductive modes utilized by this class of vertebrates. The gonads are paired, and gametes travel to the cloaca through ducts. The cloaca also receives waste from the digestive tract and the bladder.

The Adult Caecilian. The paired testes of the caecilian are intimately connected to the kidneys by the mesorchium. Seasonal fluctuation in testicular size occurs. The testes are elongated and lobed. Depending on the species, either the anterior lobes or the posterior lobes may be larger, or all lobes may be approximately equal in size (Wake, 1968). Spermatogenesis occurs within locules of the lobe of the testis, and sperm is transported from the testis through vas efferentia to nephric collecting tubules which empty into the Wolffian duct. The Wolffian duct empties sperm into the cloaca. An intromittent organ, the phallodeum, is present, which allows for internal fertilization. Mullerian ducts are present in caecilians. The paired ovaries are intimately connected to the kidneys by the mesovarium. The follicles are surrounded by a thin membranous ovisac. The ovisac must rupture for ovulation to occur, and the ova are released into the coelom. Cilia within the coelom direct the ova to the infundibulum, which lies near the lungs. The oviducts are straight and elongate. In viviparous caecilians the oviductal lining may be consumed by the embryos as a food source (Plate 3.12). Fat bodies are associated with the gonads and probably serve as a nutrient source for the gonads as their size changes in relation to gonadal activity.

The Adult Salamander. The testes of the salamander are lobed, and additional lobes may be added with each breeding season. Sperm transport to the cloaca is similar to that described for caecilians, but in some species of salamanders the nephric collecting tubules empty sperm or ova directly into the cloaca. In female salamanders the dorsal aspect of the cloaca is modified into a spermatheca. Glandular material lines the walls of the cloaca in male salamanders, which engorge during the breeding season. No intromittent organ is present, but internal fertilization is achieved by transfer of a spermatophore. The spermatophore is a gelatinous structure produced by the male that encapsulates the sperm to protect it from the environment before it is taken up by the female's cloaca. External fertilization occurs in two families, Hynobiidae and Cryptobranchidae. The oviducts are minimally convoluted. Ovulation is as described for caecilians. Fat bodies are associated with the gonads.

The Adult Anuran. The testes of the anuran are not lobed, and in some species of anurans the testes are pigmented. Sperm transport to the cloaca is similar to that described for caecilians. A seminal vesicle may be present. The Bidder's organ is a remnant of ovarian tissue that is found on the testes of adult bufonids. Members of the Leiopelmatidae possess an intromittent organ, but this structure is not described for any other frogs. Fertilization is external for most species, but internal fertilization is known or suspected for some species (e.g., the viviparous toads, *Nectophrynoides* spp. and some species of robber frogs, *Eleuthrodactylus* spp.). Mullerian ducts are present in some species of anurans. The oviducts are convoluted. Ovulation is as described for caecilians. Corpora lutea develop in some viviparous species. Fat bodies are associated with the gonads.

REFERENCES

Bennet, A.F. and H.M. Wake. 1974. Metabolic correlates of activity in the caecilian *Geotryptes seraphini*. Copeia 1974(4):764–769.

Bolton, P.M. and C.A. Beuchat. 1991. Cilia in the urinary bladder of reptiles and amphibians: a correlate of urate production? Copeia 1991(3):711–717.

Boutilier, R.G., D.F. Stiffler, and D.P. Toews. 1992. Exchange of respiratory gases, ions, and water in amphibious and aquatic amphibians, *in* Feder, M.E. and W.W. Burggren (Eds.): Environmental Physiology of the Amphibians. University of Chicago Press, Chicago, pp. 81–124.

Carter, D.B. 1979. Structure and function of the subcutaneous lymph sacs in the anura (Amphibia). Journal of Herpetology 13:321–327.

Churchill, E.D., F. Nakazawa, and C.K. Drinker. 1927. The circulation of body fluids in the frog. Journal of Physiology (London) 63:304–308.

Conklin, A.E. 1930. The formation and circulation of lymph in the frog: 1. The rate of lymph production. American Journal of Physiology 1:79–110.

Duellman, W.E. and L. Trueb. 1986a. Eggs and development, larvae, metamorphosis, *in* Duellman, W.E. and L. Trueb, Biology of the Amphibia, McGraw-Hill Book Co., New York, pp. 109–194.

Duellman, W.E. and L. Trueb. 1986b. Morphology: musculoskeletal, integumentary, sensory, and visceral systems, *in* Duellman, W.E. and L. Trueb, Biology of Amphibians. McGraw-Hill Book Co., New York, pp. 287–414.

Francis, Eric T. B. 1934. The anatomy of the salamander. Oxford University Press, London. 381 pp, 25 plates.

Gilbert, S.G. 1973. Pictorial anatomy of the *Necturus*. University of Washington Press, Seattle, WA.

Goin, C.J., O.B. Goin, and G.R. Zug. 1978. Structure of amphibians, *in* Goin, C.J., O.B. Goin, and G.R. Zug: Introduction to Herpetology. W.H. Freeman and Co., San Francisco, CA.

Gorbman, A. 1964. Endocrinology of the Amphibia, *in* Moore, J.A. (Ed.): Physiology of the Amphibia. Academic Press, New York, pp. 371–425.

Griffiths, R.A. 1996. Species Accounts, *in* Newts and Salamanders of Europe. Academic Press, San Diego, CA.

Haslam, G. 1971. Translated, with numerous annotations and additions "Ecker, A. 1889. The anatomy of the frog. Oxford at the Clarendon Press, London." A. Asher and Co. N.V., Amsterdam. 449 pp., 261 figures, and 2 color plates.

Heatwole, H. and G.T. Barthalmus. 1994. Amphibian Biology, Vol. 1. The Integument. Surrey Beatty and Sons Party Limited, Chipping Norton, New South Wales, Australia.

Herrick, C.J. 1948. The Brain of the Tiger Salamander, *Ambystoma tigrinum*. University of Chicago Press, Chicago.

Isayama, S. 1924. Uber die Strimun der Lymph bei den Amphibien. Zeitschrift fur Biologie 82:90–100 as cited in Boutilier et al, 1992.

Kuhlenbeck, H. 1973. The Central Nervous System of Vertebrates, Vol. III, Part 2. S. Karger, Basel.

Kumar, S. 1975. The Amphibian Heart. S. Chand and Company, New Delhi.

Limbaugh, B.A. and E.P. Volpe. 1957. Early development of the Gulf Coast toad *Bufo valliceps* Weigmann. American Mus. Nov. 1842:1–32. Illustrations reprinted in "Reproductive adaptations in amphibians" *in* Porter, K.R. 1972. Herpetology. W.B. Saunders Co., Philadelphia, PA, pp. 352–358.

Maslin, T.P. 1950. The production of sound in caudate amphibia. University of Colorado Studies, Series in Biology 1:29–45.

Mendes, E.G. 1945. Contribucao para a fisiologicca dos sistemas respiratorio e circulatorio de *Siphonops annulatus* (Amphibia-Gymnophiona). Bol. Fac. Filos. Cienc. Letras Univ. Sao Paulo, Zool. 9:25–64. as quoted in Duellman and Trueb, 1986, pp. 405.

Noble, G.K. 1931. The Biology of the Amphibia. McGraw-Hill Book Co., New York.

O'Reilly, Fenolio, D., and M. Ready. 1995. Limbless amphibians: Caecilians. The Vivarium 7(1):26.

Obst, F.J., K. Richter, U. Jacob (Eds.). 1988. The Completely Illustrated Atlas of Reptiles and Amphibians for the Terrarium. TFH Publications, Inc., Neptune City, NJ.

Olsen, I.D. 1977. Digestion and nutrition, *in* A.G. Kluge (Ed.), Chordate Structure and Function. Macmillan Publishing Co., New York, pp. 270–305.

Plyzycz, B., J. Bigaj, and A. Midonski. 1995. Amphibian lymphoid organs and immunocompetent cells. Herpetopathologia (Proceedings of the Fifth International Colloquium on the Pathology of Reptiles and Amphibians), pp. 115–127.

Porter, K.R. 1972. Structural and functional characteristics of living amphibians, *in* Porter, K.R.: Herpetology. W.B. Saunders Co., Philadelphia, PA, 524 pp., numerous figures.

Putnam, J.L. 1975. Septation in the ventricle of the heart of *Siren intermedia*. Copeia 1975(4):773–774.

Putnam, J.L. 1977. Anatomy of the heart of the Amphibia I. *Siren lacertina*. Copeia 1977(3):476–488.

Putnam, J.L. and J.F. Dunn. 1978. Septation in the ventricle of the heart of *Necturus maculosus*. Herpetologica 34:292–297.

Putnam, J.L. and D.L. Kelly. 1978. A new interpretation of interatrial septation in the lungless salamander, *Plethodon glutinosus*. Copeia 1978(2):251–254.

Putnam, J.L. and J.B. Parkerson, Jr. 1985. Anatomy of the heart of the Amphibia II. *Cryptobranchus alleganiensis*. Herpetologica 41(3):287–298.

Reeder, W.G. 1964. The digestive system *in* J.A. Moore (Ed.), Physiology of the Amphibia. Academic Press, New York, pp. 99–149.

Rose, F.L. and D. Armentrout. 1976. Adaptive strategies of *Ambystoma tigrinum* (Green) inhabiting the Llana Estacado of west Texas. Journal of Animal Ecology 45:713–729.

Rugh, R. 1962. Experimental Embryology Techniques and Procedures, 3rd Edition. Burgess, Minneapolis. Illustrations reprinted in "Reproductive adaptations in amphibians" *in* Porter, K.R. 1972. Herpetology. W.B. Saunders Co., Philadelphia, PA, pp. 360–365.

Simons, J.R. 1959. The distribution of the blood from the heart in some amphibians. Proc. Zool. Soc. London 132:51–64.

Stebbins, R.C. and N.W. Cohen. 1995. A Natural History of Amphibians. Princeton University Press, Princeton, NJ.

Taylor, E.H. 1968. The Caecilians of the World, a Taxonomic Review. University of Kansas Press, Lawrence, KS.

Wake, M.H. 1968. Evolutionary morphology of the caecilian urogenital system, Part I. The gonad and fat bodies. Journal of Morphology 126:291–332.

Wake, M.H. 1970a. Evolutionary morphology of the caecilian urogenital system, Part II. The kidneys and urogenital ducts. Acta Anat. 75:321–358.

Wake, M.H. 1970b. Evolutionary morphology of the caecilian urogenital system, Part III. The bladder. Herpetologica 26:120–128.

Wake, M.H. 1972. Evolutionary morphology of the caecilian urogenital system, IV. The cloaca. Journal of Morphology 136:353–366.

Weldon, P.J., B.J. Demeter, and R. Rosscoe. 1993. A survey of shed skin-eating (dermatophagy) in amphibians and reptiles. Journal of Herpetology 27(2):219–228.

Wells, T.A.G. 1968. The frog, a practical guide. Dover Publications, Inc., New York, 44 pp., 49 figures.

Wever, E.G. 1985. The amphibian ear. Princeton University Press, Princeton, NJ, 488 pp., numerous figures.

White, B.A. and C.S. Nicoll. 1981. Hormonal control of amphibian metamorphosis, *in* Gilbert, L.I. and E. Frieden (Eds.). Metamorphosis, a Problem in Developmental Biology. Plenum Press, New York, pp. 363–396.

Zug, G.R. 1993a. Modern groups of amphibians, *in* Herpetology: An Introductory Biology of Amphibians and Reptiles. Academic Press, Inc., San Diego, CA, pp. 4–10.

Zug, G.R. 1993b. General anatomy, *in* Herpetology: An Introductory Biology of Amphibians and Reptiles. Academic Press, Inc., San Diego, CA, pp. 11–38.

Zug, G.R. 1993c. Aspects of larval anatomy, *in* Herpetology: An Introductory Biology of Amphibians and Reptiles. Academic Press, Inc., San Diego, CA, pp. 39–41.

CHAPTER 4
APPLIED PHYSIOLOGY

Kevin M. Wright, DVM

Feder and Burggren's (1992) text *Environmental Physiology of the Amphibians* is essential reading for the veterinary clinician, as it provides unparalleled in-depth coverage of the physiology of amphibians. Brief reviews of amphibian physiology may be found in other texts (Duellman & Trueb, 1986; Goin et al., 1978; Porter, 1972a, 1972b; Stebbins & Cohen, 1995; Zug, 1993). The focus of this chapter will be those aspects of amphibian physiology with immediate clinical relevance.

4.1 THERMAL HOMEOSTASIS

The thermal requirements of amphibians vary tremendously between species and even between geographic variants of the same species. An understanding of a species's thermal preferences and tolerances is essential for guiding vivarium design and husbandry efforts, for many of an amphibian's metabolic processes are impacted by the temperature at which they occur (Hutchison & Dupré, 1992; Rome et al., 1992). (See Chapter 5, Amphibian Husbandry and Housing.) If an amphibian cannot maintain its body temperature appropriately it will fail to thrive in captivity. If an amphibian is maintained at temperatures below its preferred body temperature, it may show signs such as inappetence, lethargy, abdominal bloating from decomposition of ingesta, poor growth rate, and immunosuppression. When maintained at temperatures above its preferred body temperature, an amphibian may show signs such as agitation, excessive movement, changes in skin color, inappetence, weight loss despite good appetite, and immunosuppression. An appropriately constructed vivarium should provide a mosaic of temperatures above and below the preferred body temperature for the species housed so that the inhabitants can thermoregulate.

Some species, such as the White's treefrog, *Pelodryas caerulea*, show a tremendous ability to withstand elevated body temperatures, an adaptation which may serve to conserve water. Individual White's treefrogs, *Pelodryas caerulea*, may bask to achieve a body temperature in excess of 38°C (100°F). Metamorphosing amphibians may seek out temperatures different from the larvae or adults, as may ill amphibians. Behavioral fever in amphibians has been demonstrated (Stebbins & Cohen, 1995), but the fever's potential impact on successful treatment of disease in amphibians has been ignored. Given the limitations of current understanding of the thermal requirements of amphibians, it is important for the enclosures used to provide a mosaic of thermal environments above, below, and including the known or presumed preferred body temperature for the species in question.

4.2 WATER HOMEOSTASIS

Amphibians have developed a wide variety of behavioral and physiological adaptations to cope with the challenges of existing in either an aquatic (Boutilier et al., 1992) or terrestrial (Shoemaker et al. 1992) environment.

The skin of most amphibians, with the exception of a few species of treefrog (e.g., leaf frogs, *Phyllomedusa* spp., reedfrogs, *Hyperolius* spp., foam-nest treefrogs, *Chiromantis* spp.), is a negligible barrier to water loss. The rates of water loss by evaporation are much higher for amphibians than other terrestrial vertebrates, a fact that serves as a limiting factor to the range and activity pattern of amphibian species. Many terrestrial amphibians, especially those lungless forms (e.g., plethodontid salamanders), must remain moist in order for gas exchange to be effective. Thus many amphibians limit their activity patterns to exploit periods of elevated humidity (e.g., during or immediately following rain, during fog, or at night).

Several treefrog species possess a skin that is extremely resistant to evaporative water loss. The underlying etiology of this phenomenon is only well documented in the genera *Phyllomedusa* (Blaylock et al., 1976). Members of this genus have lipid glands in their skin that secrete a waterproof substance composed of waxy esters and other fatty acid compounds (McClanahan et al., 1978). The secretions of these glands are smeared over the surface of the frog with stereotyped movements of its feet. This lipid coating imparts a surface resistant to cutaneous water loss that is comparable to that of many reptiles.

The lipid glands possessed by phyllomedusine frogs are lacking in other species of hylid frogs thus far studied. In other amphibians a combination of several features of the dermis and epidermis may contribute to the waterproofing of the skin. Structures that have been described that may reduce evaporative water loss through the skin include stacked iridophores, a band of undetermined material immediately beneath the stratum corneum, or dried mucus on the surface of the skin. Doubtless other water reduction mechanisms await elucidation.

It is notable that the above described anatomic and physiologic adaptations to reduce evaporative water loss are lacking on the ventral surface of many amphibians. The ventral surface is an important route for the uptake of water from the environment, and in anurans a modified area of the pelvic ventrum is sometimes known as a "drinking patch" (Parsons, 1994). The more adapted an amphibian is to a xeric environment, the more effective it is at extracting moisture from the soil. The drinking patch accounts for up to 80% of the water uptake of an anuran. Little water uptake occurs through the gastrointestinal tract except in some species such as the waxy treefrog, *Phyllomedusa sauvagii* (McClanahan & Shoemaker, 1987). Most amphibians cannot be said to drink in the manner of other terrestrial vertebrates, thus oral fluids are of little help in combatting dehydration in the amphibian. Soaking the dehydrated amphibian in shallow water and, on occasion, subcutaneous or intracoelomic administration of appropriately dilute dextrose/electrolyte solutions are the suggested methods of combatting dehydration.

Certain behaviors minimize water loss to the environment. Hylid treefrogs have a water conserving posture which reduces the surface area exposed to evaporative effects of the environment. The limbs are adducted and the head is pressed against the surface. The ventrum is well protected by the rest of the anuran's body. If a treefrog is consistently in this posture, it suggests that the humidity of the enclosure is too low, and appropriate corrective measures should be undertaken.

The osmolality of a well hydrated amphibian is over 200 mOsm (Bentley, 1971). To increase the water absorbability, some amphibians may selectively retain additional solutes so that it can extract water from much drier soils. Since the amphibian kidney cannot concentrate urine above the osmolality of plasma, one of the main methods of water conservation is the ability to tolerate a wide fluctuation in the osmolality and composition of its plasma. This physiological adaptation can confound the interpretation of a single plasma biochemistry in the amphibian, thus multiple biochemistries, sufficient to assess plasma osmolality, are recommended as part of the amphibian diagnostic evaluation.

Aquatic amphibians are under a different water flux than terrestrial species, as they are immersed in a hyposmotic environment. Aquatic amphibians are adapted to excreting excess water while conserving plasma solutes. Water is continually being absorbed through the skin and gills, if present. If the excretory function of the kidneys fail, or the cutaneous exchange functions fail, the plasma will rapidly dilute with absorbed water while ions and other solutes are lost. This is problematic, for it is difficult to initiate any corrective action (i.e., reestablishing "normal" plasma osmolality via parenteral dextrose/electrolyte solutions or colloid solutions) that does not exacerbate the problem. (See Section 24.9, Maintaining the Electrolyte Balance of the Ill Amphibian.) Volume overload through expansion of the blood (plasma) volume eventually places undue stress on the heart and quickly incapacitates the amphibian.

Aquatic amphibians generally excrete ammonia as their main nitrogenous waste, and this is excreted not only through the kidney but also by the skin and gills, if present. Since ammonia is so toxic, this is not an option for amphibians that aren't surrounded by water at all times. Terrestrial amphibians convert a large portion of their nitrogenous wastes to urea via ornithine cycle enzymes located within hepatocytes. Urea is less cytotoxic than ammonia and can be stored inside the bladder without consequence. When the amphibian has access to water, it will void its urea-laden urine. Some species can actually switch back and forth between ammonia as the main nitrogenous waste and the production of urea, depending on the availability of water (Balinsky et al., 1961). A few species of anurans (e.g., phyllomedusine frogs, rhacophorid foam-nest frogs) are known to produce uric acid as a further water conservation method (Loveridge, 1970, Shoemaker et al., 1972). A common pet anuran, waxy treefrog, *Phyllomedusa sauvagii,* is uricotelic. Amphibians appear to have a different localization of their purine cycle enzymes within the hepatocyte than occurs in other uricotelic vertebrates (i.e., nonavian and avian reptiles), and the level of activity appears slightly lower in amphibians (Smith & Campbell, 1988). A final alternative to nitrogen storage prior to elimination is the incorporation of nitrogen into purines within iridiophores, which occurs in some reed frogs, *Hyperolius* spp., when experiencing dehydration (Geise & Linsenmair, 1986).

Some terrestrial amphibians can tolerate a loss of body water up to 40% of their body weight, and can maintain constant plasma solute concentration until the reservoir of water in the bladder is expended (Shoemaker et al., 1992). Under conditions of restricted water, amphibians cease to produce urine as conservation of body water takes precedence over excretion of nitrogenous wastes. Thus, dehydrated amphibians are often suffering from varying levels of ammonia or even urea intoxication following rehydration. Systemic gout as a result of dehydration is possible although undocumented. Urate bladder stones are a more common sequelae to dehydration and have been discovered in several waxy treefrogs, *Phyllomedusa sauvagii*.

Given the permeability of amphibian skin, many exogenous compounds are freely absorbed. This absorption is useful since it allows many beneficial substances such as antibiotics and anthelmintics to be administered topically. Toxic substances, such as chlorine from chlorinated water, may also readily be absorbed by an amphibian, making them potentially more sensitive to many environmental contaminants.

4.3 ENERGY METABOLISM

Under normal activity levels, energy production in the amphibian is produced primarily by aerobic metabolic pathways, while outbursts of unusual activity are sustained by anaerobic metabolic pathways (Gatten et al., 1992; Pough et al., 1992). Amphibians that make explosive escape attempts, such as ranids, utilize anaerobiosis for this activity and quickly fatigue with the buildup of lactate (any salt derived from lactic acid) in the muscle tissues. Thus those amphibians with a low aerobic scope may suddenly collapse during physical restraint or during capture attempts. The sustainability of this anaerobic activity is brief, often lasting less than 2 minutes. Other amphibians, such as bufonids, have a high aerobic scope and can put up a continuing struggle with minimal signs of fatigue. There is a strong correlation between an amphibian's hunting techniques and its aerobic scope. Sit and wait predators (e.g., ranids, ceratophryne leptodactylids) have a low aerobic scope while active foragers (e.g., bufonids) have a high aerobic scope. There may be marked differences in the aerobic scope between age classes of a given species, with young specimens having a lower aerobic scope (Taigen & Pough, 1981).

Recovery from fatigue varies among species, but the rate of oxygen consumption appears to be one of the main limiting factors (Gatten et al., 1992). The clinician should avoid exhausting the critically ill amphibian patient through excessive handling. Slightly elevated levels of atmospheric oxygen for several minutes prior to and immediately following handling is recommended for the critical patient. Bubbling oxygen through water used to moisten the amphibian patient may help speed recovery. Typically, amphibians return to resting values of oxygen consumption within an hour of exercise-induced exhaustion (Gatten et al., 1992).

The majority of the energy for nonsustainable exercise in amphibians occurs via glycolysis. As glycogen is metabolized, the concentration of lactate in the muscles rises whereas succinate, pyruvate, and other metabolites are relatively unaffected. Total-body lactate can take several hours to clear from an amphibian's system. The metabolism of lactate has been poorly studied in amphibians, but what little is known indicates that it is very different from lactate metabolism in mammals. In one experiment to determine the fate of lactate, specimens of the American toad, *Bufo americanus*, were exercised and treated with radioactively labeled lactate and glucose (Withers et al. 1988). Whereas mammals subjected to similar experiments oxidized the majority of the lactate (up to 95%), the toads oxidized less than 10% of the labeled lactate. Excretion of lactate is limited in amphibians. The lactate level in the urine of amphibians is extremely low, if present at all, and the gills or skin play seemingly insignificant roles in eliminating lactate from the aquatic amphibians studied.

Although increased levels of blood lactate do not appear to directly correlate with muscle fatigue in amphibians, it is known that lactate plays a role in the development of fatigue in amphibians, probably due to its contribution to the level of free hydrogen ions in the muscle. The hydrogen ions contribute to the development of acidified inorganic phosphorus ions, such as H_2PO_4, and appear to be the proximate cause of fatigue in amphibians and mammals (Gatten et al., 1992).

The scarce amount of information on lactate and acid-base metabolism in amphibians has been scarcely addressed compared to the volume of material devoted to mammals. The pH of amphibian blood can vary widely in normal specimens, and although compensatory mechanisms appear similar in amphibians and mammals, the exact nature and contribution of the different mechanisms are not well understood in amphibians (Boutilier et. al, 1992; Shoemaker et. al, 1992). Given that the fate of endogenous lactates is poorly understood in amphibians, as are the compensatory mechanisms for dealing with metabolic acidosis or alkalosis, the clinical use of sodium lactate (found in lactated Ringer's solution) is not advisable in amphibians.

4.4 CALCIUM METABOLISM

Calcium homeostasis is regulated through the interplay of four hormones. The activity of calcitonin and parathormone has been documented in anurans and salamanders, yet vitamin D activity has only been documented in anurans and prolactin activity has only been documented in salamanders. Calcitonin is the hypocalcemic hormone that increases bone calcium deposition. Amphibian calcitonin appears to be significantly different from bovine calcitonin (Boschwitz & Bern, 1971) and salmon calcitonin (Bentley, 1983), and calcitonin may even vary between species, since the black-spotted frog, *Rana nigromaculata*, did not respond to one source of frog-derived calcitonin (Oguro & Sasayama, 1985). Parathormone elevates blood calcium by mobilizing calcium from the bones. Vitamin D elevates plasma calcium levels in adult anurans and increases calcium uptake in larval anurans, while prolactin promotes hypercalcemia in adult salamanders. Calcium is an important regulatory ion, for it is involved in many metabolic pathways throughout the body including activity of muscles and nerves.

Calcium is absorbed from the environment either across the skin or through the gastrointestinal tract, while it is lost to the environment through urine, feces, and the skin. In addition to bone and the endolymphatic sacs, the skin can be a significant storage site of calcium, with up to 30% of the total body calcium stored in the skin of some anurans (Baldwin & Bentley, 1980).

Hypocalcemia is a serious metabolic derangement and can affect the striated and smooth musculature of the amphibian. Tetany may develop in hypocalcemic striated muscle while smooth muscle dysfunction may result in lack of peristalsis and associate gastrointestinal bloating. The permeability of the skin to calcium allows treatment of hypocalcemia via baths of calcium ion solutions such as calcium gluconate. Effects of hypercalcemia are not clinically defined at present.

REFERENCES

Baldwin, G.F. and P.J. Bentley. 1980. Calcium metabolism in bullfrog tadpoles (*Rana catesbeiana*). Journal of Experimental Biology 88:357–365.

Balinsky, J.B., M.M. Cragg, and E. Baldwin. 1961. The adaptation of amphibian nitrogen excretion to dehydration. Comparative Biochemistry and Physiology 3:236–244.

Bentley, P.J. 1971. Endocrines and Osmoregulation: A Comparative Account of the Regulation of Salt and Water in Vertebrates. Springer-Verlag, New York.

Bentley, P.J. 1983. Urinary loss of calcium in an anuran amphibian (*Bufo marinus*) with a note on the effects of calcemic hormones. Comparative Biochemistry and Physiology 79A:1–5.

Blaylock, L.A., R. Ruibal, and K. Platt-Aloia. 1976. Skin structure and wiping behavior of phyllomedusine frogs. Copeia 1976(1):283–295.

Boschwitz, D. and H.A. Bern. 1971. Prolactin, calcitonin, and blood calcium in the toads *Bufo boreas* and *Bufo marinus*. General and Comparative Endocrinology 17:586–588.

Boutilier, R.G., D.F. Stiffler, and D.P. Toews. 1992. Exchange of respiratory gases, ions, and water in amphibious and aquatic amphibians, *in* Feder, M.E. and W.W. Burggren: Environmental Physiology of the Amphibians. University of Chicago Press, Chicago, pp. 81–124.

Duellman, W.E. and L. Trueb. 1986. Relationships with the environment, *in* Duellman, W.E. and L. Trueb: Biology of the Amphibia. McGraw-Hill Book Co., New York, pp. 197–228.

Feder, M.E. and W.W. Burggren (Eds.). 1992. Environmental Physiology of the Amphibians. University of Chicago Press, Chicago.

Gatten, R.E., K. Miller, and R.J. Full. 1992. Energetics at rest and during locomotion, *in* Feder, M.E. and W.W. Burggren (Eds.): Environmental Physiology of the Amphibians. University of Chicago Press, Chicago, pp. 314–377.

Geise, W. and K.E. Linsenmair. 1986. Adaptations of the reed frog *Hyperolius viridiflavus* (Amphibia, Anura, Hyperolidae) to its arid environment: 2. Some aspects of the water economy of *Hyperolius viridiflavus nitidulus* under wet and dry season conditions. Oecologia 68:542–548.

Goin, C.J., O.B. Goin, and G.R. Zug. 1978. Homeostasis, *in* Goin, C.J., O.B. Goin, and G.R. Zug: Introduction to Herpetology. W.H. Freeman and Co., San Francisco, CA, pp. 126–143.

Hutchison, V.H., and R.K. Dupré. 1992. Thermoregulation, *in* Feder, M.E. and W.W. Burggren (Eds.): Environmental Physiology of the Amphibians. University of Chicago Press, Chicago, pp. 206–249.

Loveridge, J.P. 1970. Observations on nitrogenous excretion and water relations of *Chiromantis xerampelina* (Amphibia, Anura). Arnoldia 5:1–6.

McClanahan, L.L. and V.H. Shoemaker. 1987. Behavioral and thermal relations of the arboreal frog, *Phyllomedusa sauvagii*. National Geographic Research 3:11–21.

McClanahan, L.L., J.N. Stinner, and V.H. Shoemaker. 1978. Skin lipids, water loss, and energy metabolism in a South American treefrog (*Phyllomedusa sauvagii*). Physiological Zoology 51:179–187.

Oguro, C. and Y. Sasayama. 1985. Endocrinology of hypocalcemic regulation in anuran amphibians, *in* Lofts, B. and W.N. Holmes (Eds.): Current Trends in Comparative Endocrinology. Hong Kong University Press, Hong Kong, pp. 839–841.

Parsons, R.H. 1994. Effects of skin circulation on water exchange, *in* Heatwhole, H. and G.T. Barthalmus (Eds.): Amphibian Biology, Volume 1, The Integument. Surrey Beatty and Sons, Chipping Norton, New South Wales, Australia, pp. 132–146.

Porter, K.R. 1972a. Amphibian water relations, *in* Porter, K.R.: Herpetology. W.B. Saunders Co., Philadelphia, PA, pp. 275–280.

Porter, K.R. 1972b. Amphibian temperature relations, *in* Porter, K.R.: Herpetology. W.B. Saunders Co., Philadelphia, PA, pp. 288–292.

Pough, F.H., W. Magnusson, M.J. Ryan, K.D. Wells, and T.L. Taigen. 1992. Behavioral energetics, *in* Feder, M.E. and W.W. Burggren (Eds.): Environmental Physiology of the Amphibians. University of Chicago Press, Chicago, pp. 395–436.

Rome, L.C., E.D. Stevens, and H.B. John Alder. 1992. The influence of temperature and thermal acclimation on physiological function, *in* Feder, M.E. and W.W. Burggren (Eds.): Environmental Physiology of the Amphibians. University of Chicago Press, Chicago, pp. 183–205.

Shoemaker, V.H., D. Balding, R. Ruibal, and L.L. McClanahan. 1972. Uricotelism and low evaporative water loss in a South American frog. Science 175:1018–1020.

Shoemaker, V.H., S.S. Hillman, S.D. Hillyard, D.C. Jackson, L.L. McClanahan, P.C. Withers, and M.L. Wygoda. 1992. Exchange of water, ions, and respiratory gases in terrestrial amphibians, *in* Feder, M.E. and W.W. Burggren (Eds.): Environmental Physiology of the Amphibians. University of Chicago Press, Chicago, pp. 125–150.

Smith, D.D., Jr. and J.W. Campbell. 1988. Distribution of glutamine synthetase and carbamyl-phosphate synthetase I in vertebrate liver. Proceedings of the National Academy of Science 85:160–164.

Stebbins, R.C. and N.W. Cohen. 1995. A Natural History of Amphibians. Princeton University Press, Princeton, NJ.

Taigen, T.L. and F.H. Pough. 1981. Activity metabolism of the toad (*Bufo americanus*): ecological consequences of ontogenetic change. Journal of Comparative Physiology 144(A):247–252.

Withers, P.C., M. Lea, T.C. Solberg, M. Baustian, and M. Hedrick. 1988. Metabolic fates of lactate during recovery from activity in an anuran amphibian, *Bufo americanus*. Journal of Experimental Zoology 246(12):236–243.

Zug, G.R. 1993. Herpetology: An Introductory Biology of Amphibians and Reptiles. Academic Press, Inc., San Diego, CA.

CHAPTER 5

AMPHIBIAN HUSBANDRY AND HOUSING

Sandra L. Barnett, MA, John F. Cover, Jr., BS, and Kevin M. Wright, DVM

5.1 INTRODUCTION

Much of the morbidity and mortality in captive amphibians is the result of poor husbandry practices. By developing and utilizing good husbandry skills, keepers of amphibians can minimize or avoid many of the medical problems described in this book, as well as their potentially expensive and time-consuming treatments.

Most amphibians will thrive in captivity, given proper care, correct environment, and a balanced diet. Some species, such as the ornate horned frog, *Ceratophrys ornata*, the African clawed frog, *Xenopus laevis*, and the tiger salamander, *Ambystoma tigrinum*, are remarkably adaptable and can be maintained under a variety of conditions, ranging from spartan to complex. Other species, such as the stubfoot toads *Atelopus* spp. and Darwin's frog, *Rhinoderma darwinii*, remain problematic to maintain for the long term and to breed.

Success in keeping amphibians comes from paying attention to the dozens of small details discussed in this chapter concerning handling, housing, and nutrition. Adherence to these guidelines can make the difference between a captive amphibian that does poorly and dies prematurely, and one that positively thrives.

5.2 PLANNING FOR AN ACQUISITION

The first step toward responsible amphibian ownership is to review the available literature on the desired species, prior to acquiring the animal. Some comprehensive descriptions on the captive care of amphibians have been published (Coburn, 1992; Mattison, 1993a, b; Murphy et al., 1994; National Research Council, 1974; Schulte, 1980; Staniszewski, 1995; Stettler, 1981; Zimmerman, 1986). Advanced Vivarium Systems publishes an open-ended series of booklets (*The Herpetocultural Library*) on the husbandry of commonly kept species of reptiles and amphibians (e.g., de Vosjoli et al., 1996). These inexpensive booklets are available in pet and aquarium stores.

Another source of natural history and husbandry information on amphibians are hobbyist magazines, available in pet and aquarium centers, as well as some book stores and news centers. A wide variety of book sellers advertise in the hobbyist magazines, and are a good starting point for many of the newer books as well as the obscure or out of print texts.

The animal care staff at zoos and aquaria, or members of one's local herpetological society can often provide detailed advice on the husbandry of a particular species. Slavens and Slavens (1998) publishes an annually updated inventory of reptiles and amphibians in zoos and private collections. The Internet offers access to numerous Web sites with information on amphibian husbandry and housing. Not all information is edited and reviewed by experts; use caution.

Sound husbandry practices are based on a thorough understanding of a species's natural history. Valuable information relating to habitat requirements, temperature preferences, behavior, breeding, diet in the wild and the like may be found in scientific journals (Table 5.1) available at the local public or university library, or through direct subscription.

There are several excellent reference books (Duellman & Trueb, 1986; Stebbins & Cohen, 1995; Zug, 1993) that cover the biology and natural history of the amphibians. Mattison (1987) provides an excellent popular account on the natural history of the anurans.

If one is planning to collect amphibians directly from the wild (assuming there are no laws prohibiting it), one has an invaluable opportunity to make firsthand observations on the species's behavior and habitat. These may vary on a daily or seasonal basis, so long-term observations are best.

If a wild-caught amphibian is obtained from someone else, every effort should be made to find out as much as possible about the animal's place of origin, since the natural habitat of the species may vary geographically. It also is useful to find out how long a new purchase has been in captivity, how it has been housed and fed, and what, if any, medications have

Table 5.1. Addresses and publications of scientific herpetological organizations.

Organization	Publications
Society For the Study of Amphibians and Reptiles Dept. of Zoology Ohio University Athens, OH 45701	*Journal of Herpetology* *Herpetological Review* *Contributions to Herpetology* *Catalogue of American Amphibians and Reptiles*
Herpetologists' League, Inc. Dept. of Biological Sciences East Tennessee State University Johnson City, TN 37614	*Herpetologica* *Herpetological Monographs*
American Society of Icthyologists and Herpetologists Florida State Museum University of Florida Gainesville, FL 32611	*Copeia*

been administered. This information is useful in evaluating the amphibian's current physical condition, and may help in determining its food preferences.

It is important to realize that the hardiness of a specimen and suitability for capture may vary seasonally. Thus the northern leopard frog, *Rana pipiens*, that has just completed spring spawning may not be as robust and tolerant of environmental change as an animal collected in the fall following a summer of heavy feeding (National Research Council, 1974).

5.3 HANDLING AND TRANSPORTING A NEW ACQUISITION

After gathering information on the natural history and captive husbandry of the desired species, it is time to make physical preparations for the soon-to-be-acquired amphibian. This includes preparing an appropriate quarantine enclosure as well as permanent housing for the amphibian (see Section 5.5, Housing), making arrangements for a steady food supply (available from the first day the animal arrives), and preparing for the animal's transport to its new home. Only after these steps have been completed should the actual acquisition of the amphibian be undertaken.

In the case of a wild-caught amphibian, captive care begins the moment the animal is collected. The animal should be handled with clean disposable plastic or latex gloves or hands wetted with water to minimize damage to the amphibian's delicate skin and protective mucus coating.

It is convenient to use a pump spray bottle filled with fresh water for wetting one's hands. The sprayer can also be used to gently wash debris off the amphibian. In general, it is advisable not to wipe amphibian skin, and it should only be attempted with a swab or soft cloth premoistened with fresh water. It is very easy to compromise the mucus coating and irritate the skin.

Ideally, the collector should change gloves or wash hands thoroughly between handling different amphibians. This is important not only for hygienic reasons, but to avoid the unintentional transfer of any noxious secretions or pheromone-containing substances from one animal to another. The skin and glandular secretions of one species may be deleterious to another.

Amphibians have a well developed olfactory sense, and pheromones are an important mode of communication in many species (for a review, see Stebbins & Cohen, 1995). Territorial salamanders, for example, communicate their dominance partly via chemical cues. It is possible to transfer these pheromones from one individual to another during handling, thus spreading stressful pheromonal cues among the animals.

Another consideration in the handling of amphibians concerns heat transfer from the collector's hands to the animal. This can be significant with extended handling of small amphibians, and can thermally stress them. Also, amphibians may struggle hard against their captor, leading to skin damage and other injuries, such as dislocated joints.

The newly captured amphibian should be put in a plastic transport container or water-tight plastic bag as soon as possible (see Chapter 8, Clinical Techniques). Each container or bag should hold only a single species, since the defensive skin and glandular secretions of some species are toxic to other species. Sensitive amphibians may not only be poisoned by direct contact with a noxious specimen, but indirectly, by contact with a container contaminated from an earlier use.

Whenever possible, amphibians should be placed in individual containers or bags, to prevent animals from inadvertently or intentionally injuring one another. If a transport container is overcrowded with amphibians, there is a greater risk of dangerous levels of ammonia or urea levels arising from their urination. At a minimum, only same-size specimens should be housed together during transport, and each amphibian should have enough space so that it is not forced to sit on (or under) another animal.

Plastic bags are especially good for transporting large or hyperactive specimens that may injure themselves in hard containers. It is best to use the sturdy plastic bags used in the pet fish trade, as the plastic bags sold for food storage in the supermarket are not reliably watertight. A tiny amount of water should be added to bags holding terrestrial or semiaquatic amphibians. Bags can be one-third filled with water for holding totally aquatic species and larvae. It is preferable to transport an amphibian in the same water in which it has been living, to minimize physiological stress on it. No plant material should be added to the bag, for some plants produce noxious substances, and decaying plant material may foul the water. The bag can be inflated with fresh air and closed with a knot or tightly wound rubber band (a wayward specimen may become injured working its way up under a loose rubber band). The water in the bag must be changed at least once daily to remove dangerous wastes. Amphibians are especially vulnerable to unsanitary conditions because their thin, permeable skin readily absorbs toxins from organic waste.

Plastic food containers with snap-on lids work well for transporting terrestrial amphibians. Some manufacturers treat food containers with antifungal agents which may be toxic to some amphibians, therefore new containers should be soaked and rinsed thoroughly before use.

A few small ventilation holes can be drilled in the upper wall or lid of the plastic containers. The holes should be carefully sanded smooth on the inside surface. Several layers of paper toweling, foam rubber, all-natural sponge, or moss should be added to the container after moistening with fresh water, and then wrung out so it is not heavy enough to injure the amphibian if the material shifts during transport. Also, transport containers should be shielded from direct sunlight at all times to prevent its interior from attaining temperatures lethal to amphibians.

Amphibians should be kept at their preferred temperature during transport. Fossorial species, in particular, are not adapted to dealing with rapid temperature changes and may tolerate only a very narrow thermal range. High altitude species can be kept cool in styrofoam coolers with ice packs, or in climate-controlled food coolers that operate off a battery pack or the cigarette lighter outlet in automobiles. Heat packs can be used in styrofoam boxes to keep warm-adapted species at optimal temperatures when transporting them through cooler climates. Thermal packs should never come in direct contact with an animal or its container. The packs can be secured to the floor of the cooler with duct tape and separated from the animal's container by at least 13 cm (5 in) of crumpled or shredded newspaper. The transport container should be well cushioned and immobilized in the cooler by newspaper. "Popcorn" or styrofoam "peanut" packing material is not recommended for shipping animals, because objects can shift too much in the box during transit. Holes should not be drilled into the cooler. The goal is to isolate the contents of the cooler from outside thermal conditions. Even with a closed lid, most containers allow sufficient gas exchange with the outside to provide ample oxygen in the "closed" environment for an amphibian. However, a transport container crowded with animals may require better ventilation, as may a container subjected to prolonged transport times.

When transporting an amphibian to its new home, do it as quickly as possible to minimize stress. Soon after an animal settles into its quarantine housing, the amphibian should be offered a small meal. This is especially true for very young amphibians and species with a high metabolism, such as mantellas, *Mantella* spp., and poison frogs (family Dendrobatidae).

If a newly acquired amphibian is thin, beware of feeding it heavily at any one meal. It is possible that the animal has not eaten for some time, and consequently the villous lining of its intestinal tract may have atrophied. Without the absorptive surface of the intestine operating, ingested food cannot not be utilized by the animal, and may result in serious digestive distress, even death. Frequent feedings of small amounts is recommended to slowly condition the gastrointestinal tract.

If a newly acquired amphibian is not underweight, it is still advisable to feed small meals. This will safeguard against possible gastrointestinal distress from any abrupt change between its former and current diet.

5.4 QUARANTINE

Newly acquired amphibians should be quarantined away from the established collection to lessen the chance of introducing disease or parasites to the resident animals. The new arrivals may appear healthy and robust, but they could be harboring pathogens to which others animals may be sensitive. Also, the new animals may themselves become ill after arrival, due to the stress experienced in transit and during adjustment to a new environment and diet. Detailed aspects of housing appropriate for quarantine are discussed elsewhere (Chapter 23, Quarantine), as are medical protocols for processing amphibians through quarantine.

It is stressful for an animal to move into a new and unfamiliar environment. Depending on the source, the amphibian may have been subjected to a variety of additional stressors before reaching its final destination. Among these stressors are inadequate hydration, inappropriate temperature and rapid temperature fluctuations, food deprivation, physical jostling and mishandling, unsanitary conditions, crowding, and housing with inappropriate cagemates. Furthermore, the amphibian may have abraded or cut its delicate skin in transport, creating avenues for pathogens to enter the body. The situation is compounded by the effect of stress, which depresses the animal's immune function, thereby making it more vulnerable to infection.

At the National Aquarium in Baltimore (NAIB), stress on newly acquired amphibians is minimized by housing the animals in well enriched enclosures that include the essential elements of the species's natural habitat. At NAIB, small nonaquatic amphibians are moved temporarily into plastic containers (e.g., Small Pal Pens®, Rolf C. Hagen USA Corporation, Mansfield, MA; Smallworld®, Penn Plax, Garden City, NY) just long enough to collect uncontaminated fecal samples for laboratory analysis. Large frogs are put in grey plastic trash cans with a fiberglass screened lid. A moist paper towel substrate and a plastic hut (retreat) are put in the temporary quarters to reduce the amphibian's stress level. Upright strands of plastic leaves may be added for treefrogs to perch on.

The containers and trash cans used for fecal collection are rinsed with fresh water and the paper toweling is changed daily. Usually, however, amphibians are kept in these containers no longer than a couple of hours for a diurnal species, or overnight for a nocturnal one. Comparable spartan caging has been successfully used at the Philadelphia Zoo for the full quarantine period and even for long-term maintenance of some adaptable species of amphibians. However, the more conservative route of using an enriched enclosure is advisable when there is doubt about the hardiness of a specimen.

During quarantine, handling of animals and human activity in the area should be kept to a minimum. Rostral abrasions can occur when amphibians spook and jump at the transparent walls of their enclosure. These abrasions provide avenues for pathogens to enter the body, and they can take months to heal. Even when the lesions have healed, there can be unattractive, permanent loss of pigmentation and scarring.

One aid in preventing wild jumping at the tank walls is to tape multicolored paper to the outside walls to provide a visual barrier. Solid color barriers may not be as easily perceived by some amphibians. Black barriers can actually make a clean glass or plastic surface act like a mirror. The mirror images of the animal, its live food, and the cage interior may actually encourage striking behavior.

One option for minimizing striking trauma is to tape, glue, or use plastic suction cups to adhere plastic bubble wrap to the inside wall of the enclosure as a cushion. The translucent bubble wrap may also make the wall more obvious to the amphibian and prevent striking behavior in the first place. Another alternative is to place plants near the wall, to discourage jumping and to cushion against any strikes.

In the case of aquatic enclosures with a barren, transparent floor, it is best to place the tank on an opaque surface to discourage the amphibian from trying to swim through the bottom of the tank. This behavior can also result in rostral abrasions.

Provision of adequate refugia prevents or reduces restless behavior. If an amphibian appears ill at ease with its surroundings, the enclosure should be reexamined to eliminate stressful conditions.

5.5 HOUSING

5.5.1 Overview

Enclosures for captive amphibians can range from spartan to highly complex systems. The initial cost of spartan enclosures is quite low and the setup time is minimal when compared to naturalistic enclosures. However, spartan enclosures lack the natural biological filtration of the complex systems, and thus require more manual cleaning and servicing. This intervention disrupts the amphibians' daily life and, for some species, may be quite stressful.

Spartan enclosures are not aesthetically pleasing, and in some cases they may not accommodate the full range of behavior for a species. In order to achieve breeding success with many amphibians, and to simply keep many of the more delicate species alive, a more naturalistic enclosure may be needed.

Amphibians are ectotherms. They have little metabolic control of their body temperature and derive their temperature from the ambient environment—air, water, substrate, and, in some species, through basking in the sun. Like all other animals, amphibians prefer temperatures at which their body functions optimally for a given activity. Temperatures above and below the preferred temperature may be stressful and impair the animal's ability to function normally. Thermal stress may lead to illness or even death.

Given a thermal gradient, amphibians are able to exercise some thermal control, often within rather broad limits, by behavioral and physiological adjustments. A thermal gradient allows an amphibian to develop a behavioral fever when combatting infection.

Amphibians have glandular skin through which they passively absorb and lose water, as well as respire (marginally so in caecilians); they do not drink water. Amphibians are subject to desiccation if put in a totally dry environment, and most species require frequent contact with a moist substrate and relatively humid air to maintain a positive water balance. However, some amphibians have difficulty with excessive water retention if put in an environment that is too wet. Given a moisture gradient, amphibians are able to osmoregulate by moving in and out of different moisture regimes, and by making postural adjustments.

Most amphibians have small body size, or at least "stand short." Their microhabitat is the interface of the leaf litter, the surface of a leaf, the top layer of the soil or stream bottom, or the subsurface environment of rocks and burrows. Care must be taken to look beyond the larger, macroenvironment where temperature, humidity, and light levels may be strikingly different than they are in the world occupied by these small animals.

Most amphibians are secretive. In their natural habitat, they are often preyed upon by other animals. Cryptic behavior, often augmented by camouflage, is an integral part of their life. Even bold species with bright aposematic (warning) coloration usually flee or hide if sufficiently threatened.

The olfactory sense is well developed in most amphibians, especially in burrowing toads, newts, salamanders, and in caecilians (see Duellman & Trueb, 1986 for a review). Pheromones are important elements in the behavior of many species. The spatial pattern of pheromonal signals can strongly define an amphibian's world.

When selecting housing for an amphibian, it is important to consider not only the lifestyle of the desired species, but how the enclosure will be maintained over the long term. Ideally, an enclosure and its life support system should require little servicing, and can be tended with a minimum of disturbance to the cage inhabitants. A stable environment, with minimal interference by human hands, can be critical to success with delicate species of amphibians.

It is wise to plan ahead and have an emergency setup available, should a sick or injured amphibian suddenly need to be separated from the group. When possible, compromised animals should be treated in their home enclosure. This is the familiar environment in which they will feel the least stressed, and presumably, their immune systems will function at their best. If the problem is social in origin, it may be necessary to temporarily or permanently remove cagemates. In any event, it may be less stressful for the sick or injured animal to be isolated in its normal vivarium and allowed to recover without interference or possible stress from cagemates. If there is an adequate second enclosure, it may be best to remove the healthy animals from the home cage, since they are in better condition to cope with the stress of a move than their sick or injured cagemate. However, residual pheromone contamination from the former cagemates may continue to be a source of stress to an ill amphibian left in its original housing. If pheromone contamination or any other chemical contamination is suspected, the ill amphibian should be moved into a previously unoccupied vivarium.

5.5.2 The Basic Amphibian Enclosure

The most commonly used materials for amphibian enclosures are glass and plastic. Plastic has the advantage that it can be easily cut and drilled, such as is done to install plumbing and create ventilation holes. A major disadvantage of plastic is that it scratches easily. In time, this may obscure viewing into the tank. Scratching also roughens the wall surfaces, making it easier for small climbing food insects to escape. Plastics also are more absorbent than glass, and may pick up and later leach out disinfectants or other contaminants deleterious to the cage inhabitants. Many plastics become yellow and brittle after prolonged exposure to UV light yet such light is commonly used over amphibian cages for its possible health benefits to the animals (see Section 5.6.4, Lighting).

Glass is not as easily drilled as plastic, but glass companies and some aquarium stores will drill holes in the walls and floor of untempered glass tanks for a small fee.

At NAIB, plumbed glass aquariums and plumbed plastic containers (e.g., Small Pal Pens®, Rolf C. Hagen USA Corp., Mansfield, MA) are used to house most of the amphibian collection (approximately 50 species of anurans, 1800 specimens). The tank dimensions and enrichment vary with the particular habitat requirements of the housed specimens, but the same basic tank design is used throughout the collection (Figure 5.1). It is applicable to a wide range of amphibians, as described below.

NAIB uses custom-made hinged lids fashioned from vinyl window screen framing over all amphibian cages (see Figure 5.1), except for the plastic "Pal Pens," which come with snap-on plastic lids. The vinyl framing is relatively weather-resistant and nonabrasive. The frames are inset with removable panels of fiberglass window screening. The panels allow fresh air to enter the cage and allow the transmission of potentially beneficial ultraviolet (UV) radiation from overhead sources. By using hinged lids,

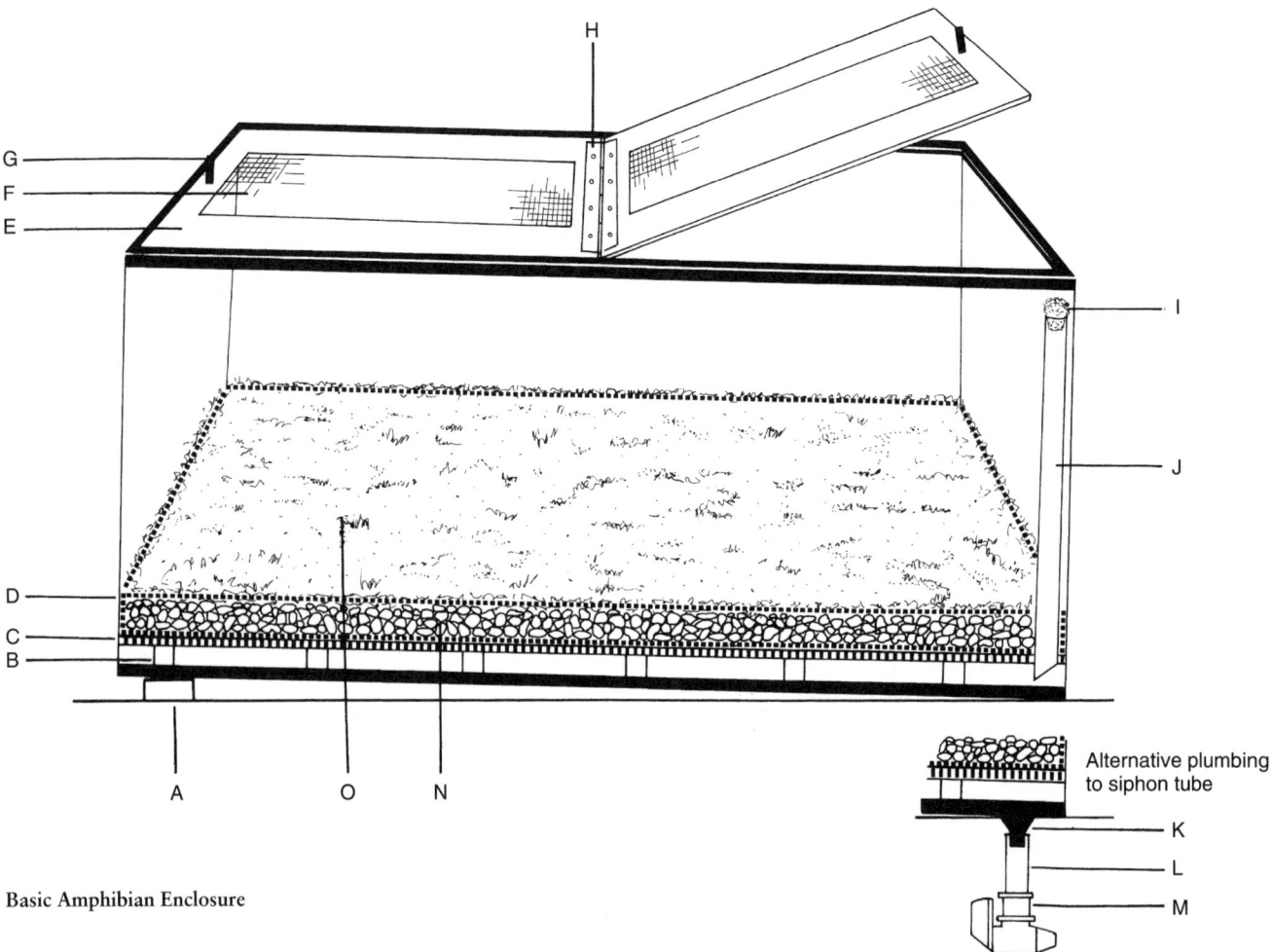

Basic Amphibian Enclosure

Figure 5.1. Lateral view of the unfurnished basic amphibian enclosure used at the National Aquarium in Baltimore. **A.** cross section of nominal 2.5 × 5 cm (1" × 2") board supporting the rim of the tank, tipping it toward the drain. **B.** plastic biofilter rings 2.5 cm outer diameter (1" OD) used as pilings for the false floor, sections of PVC pipe can be substituted as pilings. **C.** false floor made from a sheet of plastic "egg-crate" or light-diffusing panels. **D.** single layer of fiberglass window screening with 2.5 cm (1") border turned up and pressed against the tank wall by overlying gravel, or sealed to the tank wall with silicone rubber. **E.** two-panel lid made from 2.5 cm (1") wide vinyl window screen framing. **F.** removeable fiberglass window screen panel. **G.** nylon nut and bolt lid handle; other plastic or stainless steel hardware can be substituted. **H.** all plastic piano hinge attached with nylon nuts and bolts; stainless steel hardware may be substituted. **I.** aquarium filter floss used as a stopper in the siphon well, to keep animals and debris out. **J.** clear plastic siphon well permanently sealed in place with silicone rubber; the well extends below the false floor, to allow debris and dirty water to be siphoned out of the subfloor zone using a removeable soft plastic hose fed down the well. **N.** layer of pea gravel. **O.** moist cover of rehydrated dried sheet moss or sphagnum moss. (Inset) As an alternative to using a siphon well, the bottom of the tank may be plumbed using a bulkhead system (**K, L, M**). A hole must be drilled in the bottom glass of the aquarium to use this system. **K.** A removable bulkhead system can be installed and connected to a drain hose. Alternatively, a nylon or polyethylene male connector/reducer tube fitting with a 2.5 cm (1.0") outer diameter threaded end can be epoxied into the drain hole and cut flush with the inside floor of the tank; the tapered end press-fits into the flexible drain hose; a plastic garden hose connector can be substituted for the male connector/reducer tube fitting. **L.** flexible vinyl tubing 1.7 cm (11/16") outer diameter; 1.3 cm (0.5") inner diameter. **M.** plastic stopcock. (Sandy Barnett)

rather than one-piece construction, only part of the cage needs to be uncovered during servicing which helps to minimize the chances of escape by amphibians and food insects.

All-aluminum window screen framing may be substituted for vinyl framing, which is not readily available in stores, but any metal should be used with caution in an amphibian enclosure due to the risks of metal toxicoses. Standard fiberglass window screening will pass small insects (e.g., fruit flies), but screening that is fine enough to hold back very tiny insects is prohibitively expensive. Galvanized hardware cloth lids and lids made with aluminum window screening are not recommended since they can easily abrade the delicate skin of amphibians. There is also the possibility that galvanized metal screens will leach harmful levels of zinc.

Custom-cut sheets of clear thermoplastic (e.g., Plexiglas®, Lexsan®) can also serve as lids. Numerous small holes should be drilled in the plastic for ventilation. Care should be taken that the holes are perfectly smooth on the inside surface of the lid for the animals' safety. The major disadvantages of solid plastic or glass lids is that they significantly reduce ventilation (see Section 5.6.2, Humidity), and they screen out potentially beneficial UV light (see Section 5.6.4, Lighting). Also, some plastics tend to warp over time, which may create gaps of sufficient size to allow the inhabitants to escape.

There are some commercially available plastic vivarium tops that are designed to tightly fit onto the top of all glass aquariums (e.g., "Pal Pen Tank Lids," distributed by Hagen). These lids fit well and, in general, provide good ventilation and illumination. However fruit flies and small insects may be able to crawl through the ventilation slits.

5.5.3 General Guidelines for Enclosure Setup and Maintenance

Glues and Sealants. Only glues approved for aquarium applications should be used in amphibian enclosures. New constructions should be thoroughly cured, and then soaked for several days in repeated baths of clean water to reduce harmful levels of contaminants. Whitaker (1993) describes hyperactivity in a large number of poison frogs (family Dendrobatidae) exposed to PVC pipes that had been freshly glued with PVC cement.

At NAIB, the two-part epoxy paste "PC-7" (Protective Coating Co., Allentown, PA) is used to repair crack lines in plastic aquariums, to attach bulkheads to glass and plastic tanks, and to glue various porous and nonporous amphibian cage furnishings together. This epoxy is easy to work with, has a long setup period, and bonds well even when rather imprecisely measured and mixed. A similar product by the same company, "PC-11," can be used on wet surfaces. Aquastick™ (Two Little Fishies, Inc., Coconut Grove, FL) is another safe epoxy paste that comes premeasured for use. It has the advantage of attaching to damp surfaces and curing underwater. Any time an epoxy is used it should be allowed to completely cure for at least 24 hours, and the cured epoxy should be flushed with clean water several times before placing the item in contact with a living amphibian.

Water Quality. The water used in an amphibian enclosure should be free of harmful substances such as chlorine, chloramine, ammonia, and heavy metals.

Although most adult amphibians are tolerant of fairly high levels of chlorine, eggs and larvae may be extremely sensitive. It is recommended that tap water intended for use with amphibians be run through an activated charcoal filter or aged for at least 24 hours in an open container to outgas the chlorine. The addition of an air stone will greatly speed up the aging process. Caution should be used following the addition of a water filtration system, as the mineral content of the water may be altered in addition to removing chlorine. As an example, tadpoles of the dyeing poison frog, *Dendrobates tinctorius,* were raised successfully in aged tapwater at the Philadelphia Zoo, but tadpoles from the same parents who were offered the same food developed spindly leg when raised in carbon-filtered water. Switching back to aged tapwater eliminated the spindly leg problem in subsequent batches of tadpoles. Although spindly leg has been noted in various dendrobatids at the National Aquarium in Baltimore, a clear link to the use of carbon-filtered water has not been demonstrated.

It is recommended that water conditioners sold for use with tropical fish not be used for preparing water for amphibians. O'Reilly et al. (1995) report that tap water treated with conventional chemicals used for tropical fish is often fatal to the Rio Cauca caecilian, *Typhlonectes natans,* the most commonly sold caecilian in the United States. Also, some water conditioners reduce or remove medication dyes such as malachite green, methylene blue, and potassium permanganate, and thus could interfere with a medical treatment.

Completely deionized water is harmful to aquatic amphibians, as the effort needed to maintain the osmotic balance of their body tissues cannot be sustained long against such a gradient. Artificial pond water consisting of distilled or reverse osmosis water and mineral additives has been used with much success with aquatic amphibians (see Table 24.1.). Bottled spring water is also commonly used with amphibians. Any new water added to an amphibian enclosure should be the same temperature as that in the home tank to avoid thermal shock to the animals. (See Chapter 12, Water Quality.)

If water is offered in a bowl to amphibians, it is imperative that the water be clean. Bacteria can colonize water bowls quickly, and at an even faster rate when the water is contaminated with feces, food, or shed skin. This mandates that the bowl be cleaned daily and disinfected several times weekly to reduce the chance that the bowl will be a source of pathogenic organisms (see Wright, 1993, for information on disinfectants). Keeping an emergent rock in the water bowl will allow any food insects that fall in to escape. Drowned insects quickly pollute the water.

Substrate. A medium-grade gravel substrate can serve as an excellent biological filter in an amphibian enclosure. The gravel should either be too large for the amphibian to ingest or so small and smooth that it can be passed through the digestive tract. Otherwise, the amphibian may suffer complications arising from a gastrointestinal foreign body impaction. It is wise to use smooth gravel to minimize the possibility of damage to the amphibian's delicate skin, especially if the animal tends to dig. Smooth gravel will also minimize internal damage and facilitate passage, should the amphibian ingest some of it. The gravel should be of a color typical of the animal's natural habitat. For many ground- and rock-dwelling amphibians, this means that the animal will blend in with the substrate. This camouflage is not only interesting to observe, but presumably helps to make the amphibian feel less vulnerable and less stressed.

If sand is to be used to overlay the gravel, it is better to use horticultural silver sand rather than builder's sand. The latter tends to form a crust after it has been dampened and dries.

It is recommended that soil or potting mixes be used sparingly, unless essential to the lifestyle of the amphibians being kept (e.g., fossorial or woodland species). A soil substrate is more work to service and drains less well than a simple gravel substrate covered with moss or leaf litter. With proper planning, it is possible to create a lush planted enclosure using soil just around plant roots, or using epiphytic plants (which require no soil) and rehydrated dried mosses and leaf litter (Plate 5.1).

If soil is used over gravel, a layer of fiberglass window screening can be sandwiched in between to prevent the soil from clogging up the gravel layer. Weed guard fabric, available in hardware and garden stores, can also be used for this purpose, but tends to clog up with tiny soil particles over a period of months.

Many commercially sold topsoil and potting mixes are unsuitable for amphibian enclosures because they contain potentially dangerous chemical additives. These include surfactants for moistening the soil, antifungal agents, fertilizers, and aerating agents that are potentially dangerous if ingested (e.g., perlite, styrofoam). Manure-containing compost should be avoided altogether, because it is too acidic and there are often undesirable chemicals present. Peat moss and potting mixes containing peat moss should be avoided. They are too acidic for many amphibians and will irritate their skin. Caecilians, in particular, are very sensitive to contact with peat (O'Reilly et al., 1995).

When soil is used, the composition should match that of the amphibian's natural habitat. For example, the spadefoot toads, *Scaphiopus* spp. and *Spea* spp., do best in sandy, loamy soil, whereas lungless salamanders (family Plethodontidae) prefer rich, organic soil that is pH neutral.

Soil of appropriate composition can be collected in the field, so long as it is free of contaminants (e.g., motor oil, gasoline, pavement salt, paint). Generally, there are few negative health implications of using clean but not sterile soil. Some of the organisms present in the soil, in fact, may help to keep the vivarium healthy, breaking down waste products from the amphibians and dead plant material. However, if one wants to be absolutely safe against possibly exposing a captive amphibian to undesirable organisms, such as trombiculid mites, the soil should be heat- or cold-treated. Heat treatment is often effective in killing arthropod parasites, and may also destroy the ova of helminth parasites. The soil being treated should be arranged in a layer no more than 2.5 cm (1 in) deep, and baked at a temperature of at least 95°C (200°F) for 30 minutes or more. Alternatively, exposing the soil to temperatures well below the freezing point of water (0°C, 32°F) for several weeks may kill soil arthropods. Another option is to place the soil in a dark plastic bag and place it in strong direct sunlight for several hours.

Wood rot (crumbled wood from decaying logs) is an excellent substrate for many woodland amphibians. Fresh material may even contain invertebrate species that are nutritious food for the captive amphibian. Again, however, one must weigh the benefits of using a living substrate against the possibility of introducing undesirable invertebrates and disease into the captive environment. If wood rot is desired to be pest free it can be treated by freezing or by placing it in a dark plastic bag in direct sunlight. Oven treating may cause the wood to char or otherwise alter its composition.

The soil in a vivarium should drain readily, so that pools of water do not form in it. Also, the soil should have a moisture gradient, so that the amphibian can carry out normal osmoregulatory functions (see Section 5.6.2, Humidity). The range of the moisture gradient that should be provided will depend on the particular requirements of the species being housed.

If an amphibian appears to avoid the soil in its enclosure (e.g., if a fossorial species stays on the surface), or shows signs of contact irritation (i.e., erythema of the ventral surface, inappetence), the moisture content or soil composition may be inappropriate and the soil should be replaced.

Ground Cover. Common ground covers include live moss, rehydrated sheet and sphagnum moss, hardwood mulch and nuggets, and leaf litter. All of these materials, except for the leaf litter, can be purchased at garden centers.

Properly maintained, these substrates will develop a complex community of beneficial microorganisms that will help to keep the substrate "healthy," breaking down waste products from the amphibians and dead plant material. Of course, this living system will fail if the vivarium is overcrowded and the bio-load is too high. A balance must be found. Prompt removal of large droppings by hand is recommended, with spot replacement of heavily soiled or decomposed substrate at least every few months.

Living mosses often do poorly in vivariums because

the light levels tend to be inadequate and moisture levels too high or too low. Some amphibians (e.g., some specimens of terrestrial caecilians) appear to be irritated by prolonged contact with sphagnum moss or sheet moss (O'Reilly et al., 1995).

Sphagnum moss is considerably less expensive than sheet moss. Moist sphagnum is an affordable solution when a substrate is needed for temporarily housing a terrestrial or fossorial anuran or salamander, as, for example, during a medical procedure or quarantine. The major disadvantages of sphagnum are that it crumbles easily (small pieces stick to amphibians and are easily ingested with prey items), and it is easily tracked into the water. As the sphagnum decomposes and packs down (over a period of many weeks), water and wastes do not pass through it readily, and it may become a breeding ground for undesirable anaerobic bacteria. However, when kept moist and changed regularly, it can be used over a long period of time to house many species of amphibians.

Sheet moss is expensive but attractive. It can be arranged to form a smooth, carpetlike substrate which gives food insects few places to hide and facilitates their capture by surface-feeding amphibians. Moreover, the structural integrity of sheet moss reduces the chances that the amphibian will accidentally ingest moss during food capture.

A tight carpet of sheet moss is useful for stabilizing the bank along a stream or pond, and for preventing an amphibian from tracking debris into the water.

Cedar and pine mulches and nuggets should be avoided, as they contain natural compounds that are potentially toxic to amphibians. Only untreated hardwood mulches should be used. Care should be taken to remove from mulch any shards of wood that could injure the amphibian. Mulch retains moisture well and aids in humidifying the vivarium. The mulch should be replaced at least every few months.

Freezing or sunlight sterilization are the best options for treating moss, leaves, and bark to rid them of undesirable organisms.

A heterogenous substrate may be needed to accomodate different aspects of an amphibian's behavior from tunneling in soil to foraging underneath dry leaves. The natural world is rarely a homogeneous environment, and neither is the healthy vivarium.

In some instances, it may be desirable to house amphibians on a substrate of moist paper toweling (see Section 5.5.8, Terrestrial Forest Floor Enclosures). Unbleached paper toweling is a very hygienic substrate when fresh, but it degrades rapidly and organic wastes accumulate on the surface. Many amphibians are restless and seemingly stressed on a paper towel substrate, although others (e.g., many species of terrestrial salamanders) do fine on it (see Section 5.5.8). Providing hiding spots in the form of crumpled balls of paper or folds in the towel substrate may relieve the stress experienced by some individuals.

Plants. Plants, whether artificial or living, serve many functions in the vivarium. They provide cover and rest spots, elevated perches for territorial displays, sites for oviposition in some terrestrial and arboreal species, and they act to filter the overhead light, creating the more subdued lighting at ground level that most amphibians prefer. Live plants provide additional benefits over artificial plants. Some common indoor plants help purify the air and utilize organic wastes in the soil (Raloff, 1989). Live plants also increase the humidity in an enclosure. Aquatic plants help to oxygenate the water and rid it of harmful organic wastes.

Both terrestrial and aquatic plants can be rooted directly into the substrate, or they can be placed in individual pots that are buried in the substrate. Keeping plants in their pots facilitates cage cleaning and replacement of old plant material, with a minimum of disturbance to the cage inhabitants. Also, pots protect plants against amphibians that tend to dig. Plastic pots are preferable to terra cotta for the former are lightweight, nonabrasive, non-absorbent and easily cleaned.

Plants that thrive in low light levels are recommended for amphibian enclosures, where subdued lighting is most appropriate. Hardy terrestrial plants that are especially tolerant of low light include the peace lily, *Spathiphyllum tasson,* the emerald beauty, *Aglaonema commutatus,* the silver queen, *Aglaonema roebelinii,* golden pothos, *Epipremnum aureum,* and the dwarf palm, *Chamaedorea elegans.* An extensive review of plant species appropriate for the vivarium is given in Mattison (1993b).

Many of the common vivarium plants contain oxalates. If consumed by prey insects, there is a potential for these oxalates to create problems in the amphibians consuming the insects. It is preferable to release only as many plant-eating feeder insects into a planted amphibian enclosure as can be eaten within a few hours. When crickets are being offered, a small dish of cricket food can be placed in the enclosure to offer the insects an alternative to eating the vivarium plants. Commercially prepared cricket food, which is fortified, will also boost the nutritional content of the feeder insects (Allen & Oftedal, 1989).

Whatever plants are used in the amphibian enclosure should be free of sharp spines and edges and stiff tips. Many bromeliads have rigid leaves with spines along the edges. Such plants could impale or cut into the delicate skin of an amphibian jumping across the enclosures or tussling with a cagemate. These plants should be avoided.

Plants that are purchased from a nursery will often be contaminated with fertilizer, pesticides, fungicides, and detergents (to enhance the shine of the plants' leaves). The potting soil may be similarly contaminated. As a safeguard against these hazards, all plants should be removed from their original pot and as much soil as possible should be removed from the roots. The entire plant should then be thoroughly rinsed in fresh water and repotted.

Arboreal bromeliads and other epiphytes can be lightly wrapped in *Osmunda* fern fiber or wired to a tree fern plaque. These absorbent natural products provide an anchor for the roots, keeping them moist but not wet. Tree fern boards are derived from the stems of certain wild tropical ferns, and for this reason, one may wish to avoid using this product. Compressed peat logs are not recommended because of their high acid content.

There is a small risk that plants will be contaminated with the ova of nematodes pathogenic to amphibians. A common source of the contamination for store-bought plants is the feces of infected Cuban treefrogs, *Osteopilus septentrionalis,* which thrive in the greenhouses of south Florida. Unfortunately, there is no known treatment that will kill these ova without also killing the plants or contaminating the plant with chemicals deadly to amphibians. To reduce the parasite load, all soil should be removed from the plant and the plant should be rinsed well before repotting.

If aquatic plants are used, it is advisable to treat them with a molluscicide or rinse them thoroughly in fresh water to eliminate aquatic snails. Snails can serve as the intermediate host for many parasites of amphibians, and snails will eat amphibian egg masses. The plants can be soaked in a 0.25 mg/L copper sulfate solution for 48 hrs at 30°C (85°F) to eliminate any adult freshwater snails (Cardeilhac & Whitaker, 1988). The plants should then be rinsed thoroughly in fresh water to remove all dead snails, their egg masses, and any copper residues. As an additional safeguard against copper residues, the plants should be held in copper-free water for several days before being incorporated into the amphibian aquarium. Copper-removing solutions (e.g., NovaAqua®, Novalek, Inc., Hayward, CA), are available at pet and aquarium centers.

Green algae often grows in the undisturbed pools and streams of vivariums. Green algae can be beneficial in cleansing the water, as well as in contributing to the diet of herbivorous and omnivorous larval amphibians.

Branches, Rocks, and Other Heavy Furnishings. Whenever heavy objects (e.g., rocks, branches, ceramic flower pots, large potted plants) are used in an amphibian enclosure, one must always consider the potential for injury to the cage inhabitants if there is a cave-in or the furnishings topple over.

Furnishings should be solidly built so that there is no possibility of collapse. If the amphibian tends to dig, heavy tank furnishings should rest directly on the (false) floor rather than on top of the substrate. Otherwise, the animal may undermine the furnishings and be injured or killed in a cave-in. It is also possible that glass or plastic cage walls could be damaged in such an accident.

If a rock wall or waterfall is desired, the rocks should be securely fixed together with silicon rubber or a waterproof nontoxic epoxy (e.g., Aquastick™, Two Little Fishies, Inc., Coconut Grove, FL). Attach the rocks to a frame (e.g., rigid sheet plastic), and the entire system can be removed, if needed. This can greatly facilitate cage cleaning and maintenance work on the furnishings. It also means that the configuration of the rock structure will not change from cleaning to cleaning. Familiar retreats and perches will be left intact. This constancy in cage furnishings may help to reduce the stress of cage cleaning on the amphibians.

Rocks collected in the field should be thoroughly rinsed in clean, running water before use. Branches can be sun sterilized in a sealed, clear or black plastic bag left in strong direct sunlight for a day. Alternatively, branches can be frozen to eliminate undesirable organisms.

To be safe, only rocks and wood suitable for use in freshwater fish tanks should be used in aquatic enclosures. As in the case of mulches, branches should be hardwood.

Water bowls should be shallow, preferably with sloping sides. They should be tip-proof and flat-rimmed for comfortable perching. Heavy (shatter-proof) unleaded glass, glazed ceramic bowls, or plastic dishes are recommended because they can be easily cleaned and disinfected. If a ceramic bowl cracks or chips, it should be discarded, because of the possibility of lead leaching out. Cracked containers also may have dangerous sharp edges, and they may harbor pathogens that are not easily removed during cleaning.

Retreats. Amphibians are secretive animals, and most spend a considerable amount of time hiding. It is essential to provide them with adequate options for such retreat or camouflage to prevent undue stress. Appropriate hiding spots should be provided at different points in the thermal and moisture gradient, so that the amphibians are not forced to choose between meeting physiological needs and security.

The type of refuge that is most appropriate depends on the species of amphibian involved. The Surinam horned frog, *Ceratophrys cornuta,* will camouflage itself in a layer of moss or leaf litter to avoid detection by potential predators and prey, while an arboreal red-eyed treefrog, *Agalychnis callidryas,* will seek refuge in lush green foliage.

Cork bark, hollow coconut shells, hardwood

branches, and smooth rocks can be used to provide refuges as well as visual barriers within the enclosure. There should be a minimum of one retreat per amphibian, more if the species in question is territorial. The retreats should be scattered throughout the enclosure in areas of different temperature and humidity, so that an amphibian is able to hide in a spot with an appropriate microclimate. Cave-style retreats should not be used with species of amphibians that will not use them (e.g., the giant monkey treefrog, *Phyllomedusa bicolor*). For many of these amphibians, caves are havens for live prey that go uneaten.

Cork bark can serve double duty as a retreat and as a feeding platform for many species of small frogs, such as the mantellas, *Mantella* spp., the stubfoot toads, *Atelopus* spp., and the poison frogs (family Dendrobatidae). Small insects (fruit flies, hatchling crickets, springtails) can be sprinkled onto the bark, where they are easy prey for the frogs. Even if the enclosure is freshly misted, insects will not stick to the bark, because it absorbs and passes moisture quickly. Cork bark can be autoclaved for sterilization without altering its appearance.

Amphibian retreats can be fashioned from darkly colored plastic containers. Examples include plastic bowls, storage containers, plant pots, and the reinforcement cup on the bottom of many soda bottles. The chosen container is simply turned upside down, and an access hole slightly taller and wider than the amphibian is cut into the wall. The edge of the access hole and the interior surface of the retreat should be smooth, so that the amphibian cannot injure itself. The size of the retreat will depend on the number, size, and species of amphibian being housed. The retreat should be deep enough to enable the amphibian to fully hide its body inside in a relatively dark environment. Most amphibians that use hideaways prefer one with a low ceiling, so that they can wedge their body beneath it with their dorsum touching or nearly touching the ceiling. Among the possible explanations for this preference are water conservation, thermoregulation, and predator avoidance.

Similar to other amphibian habitats, aquatic enclosures should include multiple dark retreats. A subordinate amphibian should not be forced to share a retreat with a more dominant animal, and animals should not need to venture far to seek cover. Furnishings should be arranged so that when food is offered, it is relatively near a refuge, such as a submerged rock or wood cave, or section of PVC pipe.

5.5.4 Enclosure Location

Surrounding Activity. It is important to place an amphibian enclosure in an appropriate location. Locate animals away from areas of high traffic and loud noises (salamanders and caecilians have poorly developed auditory sensitivity, but at least some species can detect substratum vibration which traffic and loud sounds may generate). Some amphibians are shy and easily spooked. If one hopes to witness their complex array of behaviors, it is helpful to be still or move slowly and be quiet!

Vibration. Locate animals away from sources of vibration. Research has shown that some amphibians are stressed by exposure to constant vibrations (National Research Council, 1974). When possible, do not put canister filters, air pumps, and other motorized apparatus that vibrate on the same surface as an amphibian enclosure. If this must be done, put a pad under the apparatus to absorb as much of the vibration as possible.

Controlled Environment. Locate animals where they can be provided with the temperature, humidity, and lighting that they would experience in the wild. This is probably best accomplished in a dedicated animal room where human activity and the ambient environment can be carefully controlled. Avoid rooms with strong daily temperature fluctuations or strong drafts.

Avoid Direct Sunlight. Do not locate amphibian enclosures in direct sunlight. Lethal temperatures can be reached quickly in glass or plastic vivariums exposed to direct sunlight. Moreover, even if lethal temperatures are not reached, the rapid change in temperature may put thermal stress on the amphibians.

Escapes. Plan for escapes! If an amphibian escapes into a dry room, it can quickly succumb to desiccation. One solution is to set up one or more moist "oases" for the amphibian on the floor of the room. These can be as simple as a lidless plastic container turned on its side, and padded with moist moss and a dark hide box. It is recommended that the oases be set along the wall, since amphibians often travel along the perimeter of an enclosure (in this case, the room).

5.5.5 Aquatic Pond Enclosures

Complex Pond Enclosure. The pond enclosure is appropriate for aquatic amphibians adapted to living in relatively still or low-flow bodies of water. These amphibians include pond-dwelling larvae, neotenic pond-dwelling salamanders, aquatic newts, and aquatic frogs (*Xenopus* spp. and *Pipa* spp.). These species are often restless in an aquarium with significant water movement.

The amphibian pond enclosure requires only a slight modification of the standard fish aquarium to accommodate the need of many amphibians to breathe air.

The basic, low-maintenance pond enclosure (Figure 5.2, Plate 5.2) utilizes an undergravel filter with a gravel substrate about 5 cm thick. The filter can be operated by air lift. Alternatively, an external canister filter can be used to create a reverse flow undergravel filter. Outflow water from the canister is sent into the lift tube, to move under the false floor and up through the gravel bed. This diffuses the water current for still water inhabitants. The return water is suctioned from the water column above the gravel, on the opposite side of the tank from the tank inflow. It is important to screen the tank outflow so that the amphibians cannot be trapped by the force of its suction. A filter screen with a wide surface area is recommended to disperse the force of the uptake.

The enclosure should include shallow areas where amphibians can rest and gulp air. Many aquatic amphibians rely to some degree on pulmonary respiration and may drown if not provided with the opportunity to surface without strenuous effort. Shallow rest areas can be created by sturdy floating or emergent vegetation, smooth rocks or wood projecting at a low angle out of the water, or floating bark. For some semiaquatic species, such as the South American bullfrog, *Leptodactylus pentadactylus*, it is necessary to provide a large land area bordering the water to accommodate their full range of behaviors.

Similar to other amphibian habitats, aquatic enclosures should include multiple dark retreats. These refuges can be made from piled rocks, submerged wood, or sections of PVC pipe. A minimum of one retreat per amphibian is recommended, although additional retreats may be placed throughout the vivarium to allow access to a range of temperatures.

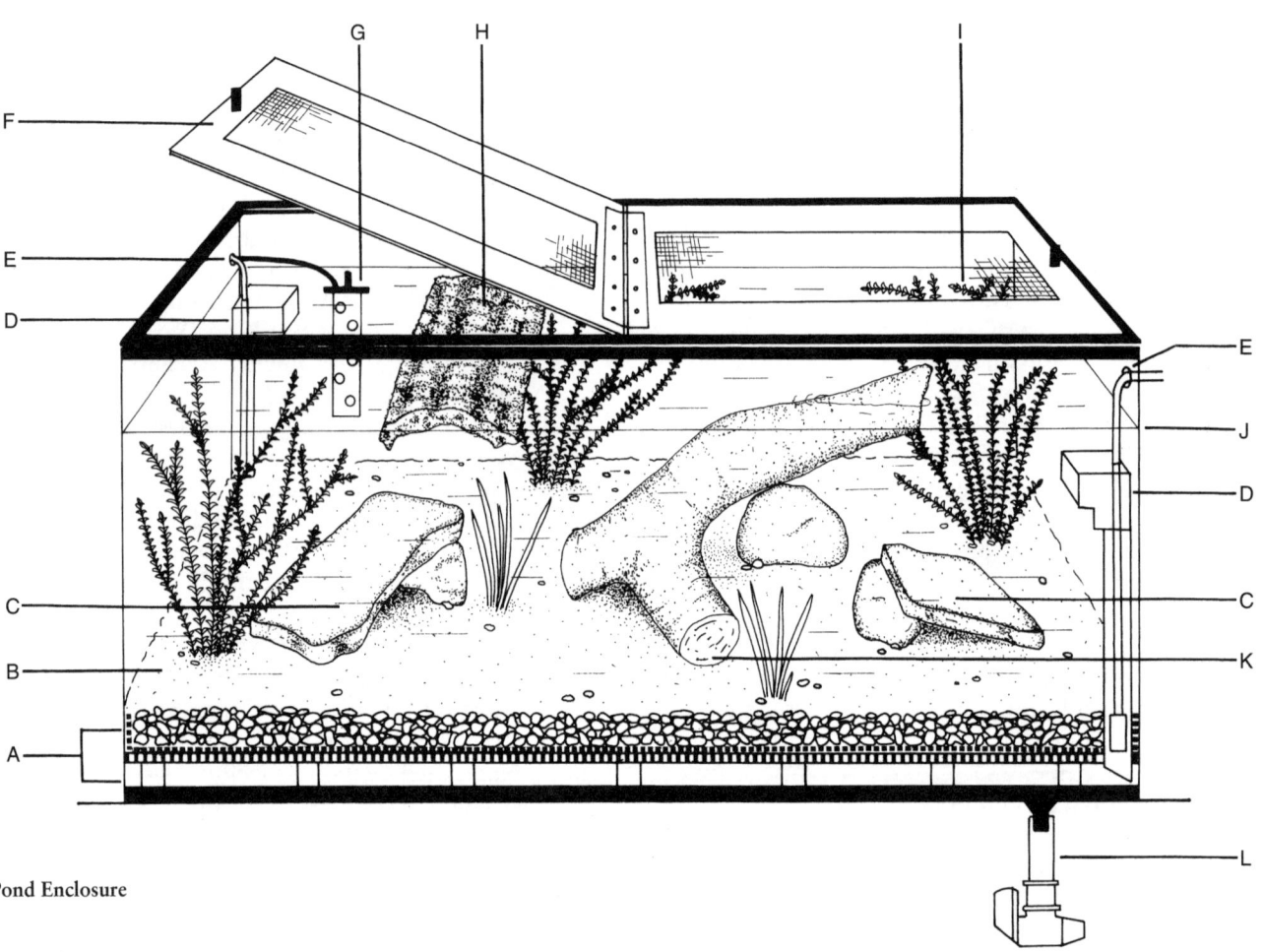

Pond Enclosure

Figure 5.2. Lateral view of pond enclosure for amphibians. **A.** false floor assembly (see Figure 5.1 B—D). **B.** pea gravel layer approximately 2" (5 cm) thick. **C.** underwater rock cave. **D.** air lift tube sealed to the tank wall and false floor with silicone rubber (also serves as access port to subfloor for siphoning up debris). **E.** hole in the tank wall for the air line and heater cord; alternatively, a hole could be cut into the lid. **F.** lid (see Figure 5.1 E—H). **G.** aquarium heater (for additional protection, this may be sheathed in a perforated PVC pipe). **H.** anchored cork bark island. **I.** aquatic plant tall and strong enough to provide a perch close to the water surface for the tank inhabitants. **J.** water line. **K.** emergent hardwood log providing an underwater retreat and shallow water rest area. **L.** drain assembly (see Figure 5.1 K—M). (Sandy Barnett)

Spartan Pond Enclosure. It may be necessary to isolate an amphibian in a simple tank where the contents can be regularly replaced or disinfected. Such spartan enclosures may have no substrate, and only plastic plants and perhaps PVC piping for underwater enrichment. Floating pieces of styrofoam, plastic shelves, or plastic plants can be placed in the enclosure to create shallow water or exposed rest areas.

The dump and fill system can be used for water maintenance in the spartan tank. A siphon or water vacuum should be used to remove all uneaten food and other debris daily, and regular partial water changes are recommended to prevent buildup of ammonia and urea. The frequency of the water changes and amount of water that should be exchanged will depend on the volume of water in the enclosure and on the number, size, and species of amphibians being kept. As a starting point, a 10% water change should be made every 2 days. Change water should be aged and brought to the same temperature as the home tank water to avoid chemical and thermal shock to the amphibians.

An airstone can be added to the spartan tank to prevent scum buildup on the water's surface and to oxygenate the water. A sponge filter can be used for biological filtration, but it should be augmented by regular partial water changes and prompt removal of gross debris, such as feces or uneaten food. Sponge filters cannot handle high levels of ammonia and are best suited to small groups of small amphibians, such as anuran and salamander larvae adapted to living in ponds. If an amphibian harbors or is suspected of harboring an infectious disease, it will be necessary to periodically discard the sponge filter, since it cannot be completely disinfected. However, sponge filters are relatively inexpensive and easily replaced. Keep in mind that the sponge filter takes time to reach peak efficiency in biological filtration, and frequent replacements will prevent this from happening. Also, the beneficial organisms in the filter may be eliminated by some medications in the water.

Another filtration option in the spartan tank is a small in-tank box filter that provides biological, mechanical, and chemical filtration, but is not strong enough to create a significant current. Such a filter can easily be disinfected, and the filtering material can be replaced at the same time. However, box filters, like sponge filters, need time to reach peak efficiency, and frequent replacement of all filter material will prevent this from happening. Also, activated charcoal eliminates certain medications from the water.

Natural porous materials are not recommended in the spartan hospital tank, as they are more difficult to clean and disinfect. If an amphibian is undergoing treatment for an infectious disease that is difficult to eliminate, the enclosure and all furnishings should be cleaned and disinfected after each treatment.

There are some exceptionally hardy species of amphibians, such as the axolotl, *Ambystoma mexicanum,* and the African clawed frog, *Xenopus laevis,* that are often successfully maintained for a long time in relatively spartan aquatic enclosures.

Spartan pond enclosures are often used for rearing pond-dwelling larval frogs to metamorphosis. Plastic plants or hardy live aquatic plants that do not require rooting in the substrate (such as *Elodea canadensis*) can be added to provide cover and rest areas. Living plants will also help to rid the water of harmful organic wastes. Some tadpoles will eat the vegetation, or the algae that grows on it. Cork bark, styrofoam, plastic shelves, or a sloping shore can serve as a landing for new metamorphs, as well as provide cover and a surface for algae growth.

These spartan nursery tanks require more daily maintenance than an enclosure set up with undergravel filtration, but the barren floor in the spartan enclosure can greatly facilitate the retrieval of small tadpoles. In gravel-bottom tanks, small tadpoles can be very difficult to catch, as they seek cover in between the rocks when alarmed.

5.5.6 Aquatic Stream Enclosures

Complex Aquatic Stream Enclosure. The aquatic stream enclosure is suitable for amphibians adapted to living in well oxygenated, usually cool streams with a significant current. Typical species include the stubfoot toads, *Atelopus* spp., the tailed frog, *Ascaphus truei,* the hellbender, *Cryptobranchus alleganiensis,* and the larvae of many stream-dwelling and riparian salamanders, such as the American brook salamanders, *Eurycea* spp., the spring salamanders, *Gyrinophilus* spp., and the Pacific giant salamander, *Dicampton ensatus.*

The basic stream enclosure (Figure 5.3) has a false floor overlayed by gravel, similar to the pond enclosure. The deep area of the stream should have underwater caves and crevices where the tank occupants can seek refuge, as well as shallow water areas where the amphibian can rest and gulp air. Depending on the species, the water may be shallow throughout, allowing the amphibian at any point to reach its head up to gulp air while keeping its feet on the stream floor. There may also be exposed land areas, if appropriate for the species.

Unlike the pond tank, the stream enclosure has a moderate to strong power filter for rapid water turnover. It is set up so that it provides undergravel filtration, in addition to cycling the water through an outside canister filter or powerhead.

Outside canister style filters are preferable to in-tank models on amphibian enclosures. Outside filters are less work to remove and clean, and a shut-off valve on the supply hose allows the filter media to be changed with a minimum of disturbance to the

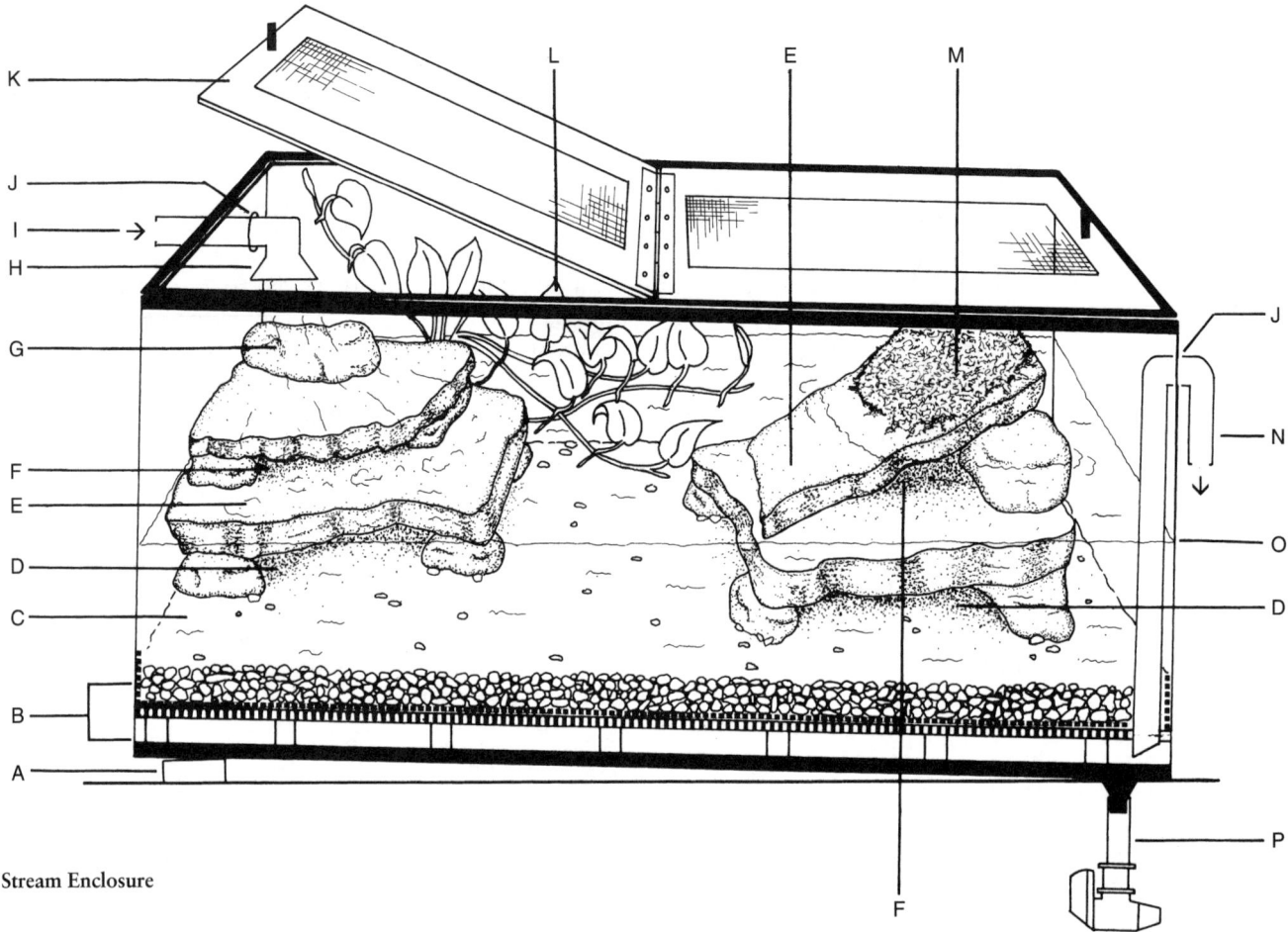

Figure 5.3. Lateral view of stream enclosure for amphibians. **A.** cross-section of board supporting the rim of the tank, tipping it toward the water outflow end. **B.** false floor assembly (see Figure 5.1 B—D). **C.** pea gravel layer approximately 5 cm (2") thick. **D.** underwater rock cave. **E.** shallow water rest area. **F.** partially flooded rock cave. **G.** waterfall. **H.** hose fitting to spread the water flow. **I.** water outflow from the canister filter. **J.** hole in the tank wall just large enough to pass the canister filter tubing. **K.** lid (see Figure 5.1 E—H). **L.** golden pothos, *Epipremnum aureum,* a hardy vine able to live "rooted" in water and tolerant of considerable root disturbance. **M.** emergent rockwork covered with moist sheet moss. **N.** water inflow to the canister filter. **O.** water line. **P.** drain assembly (see Figure 5.1 K—M). (Sandy Barnett)

animals. A trickle filter addition on the return water can further increase filtration and dissolved oxygen levels.

The outflow from the canister filter can be used to create a waterfall. A waterfall adds aesthetic appeal, can provide additional underwater and terrestrial habitat for the animals, and helps oxygenate and biologically filter the water. A waterfall can also serve to channel or disperse the force of the water current, depending on the configuration of the rockwork. Many stream-dwelling amphibians fare better in enclosures with a current. The hellbender, *Cryptobranchus alleganiensis,* seems to prefer an enclosure that provides a current strong enough to ripple its skin folds. The animal will rock from side to side if a current is not provided, presumably to better oxygenate its skin for respiration. If a current is provided in an enclosure, some of the underwater shelters should be arranged perpendicular to the current so that areas of calm water are available to the animals.

If the water intake for the canister filter is located above the substrate, care should be taken to screen the opening so that the amphibians cannot be trapped by the force of the filter's suction. If feces need to be collected for parasite examination, the canister filter may be temporarily removed, and the dump and fill method used to maintain water quality. A strong air pump can be temporarily added to the setup, similar to how it is used in the aquatic pond tank, to keep the undergravel filter operating and healthy during the down-time for the canister filter. An airstone can also be placed in the main water body to further oxygenate the water. If the canister filter is left off for more than a few hours, it should be broken down and cleaned before reuse, as anaerobic bacteria will grow and render the filter media unfit for use.

It may be difficult to find aquatic plants that will thrive in a stream enclosure, due to the strong water current and uprooting by the tank occupants. Golden pothos, *Epipremnum aureum,* a very hardy creeping vine, can be anchored without soil to emergent rockwork or a dead branch, and trailed into the water. It will not only filter the overhead light and provide cover for the tank occupants, but it will also help to clean the water, removing harmful wastes.

Amphibians adapted for living in a stream habitat generally require water that is highly saturated with dissolved oxygen and contains undetectable levels of ammonia or nitrite. Stream dwellers are extremely sensitive to toxins and pH fluctuations. It is recommended that ammonia-absorbing resins be used in combination with activated charcoal in the filter. Also, partial water changes (10–20% weekly) are highly recommended. Large debris should be siphoned out daily.

Spartan Stream Enclosure. A much simplified version of the stream enclosure may be advisable. Such a spartan enclosure has no substrate. It has simple rock or PVC pipe retreats, and a land area made from piled rocks, sheet plastic, or styrofoam. Water quality is maintained with a canister filter. Such an enclosure is easily disassembled for cleaning and disinfection.

There are many species of stream-dwelling amphibians that do poorly in a spartan setup, even on a temporary basis. Larvae of the Pyrenees Mountain salamander, *Euproctus asper,* do better when maintained on a gravel substrate than on a barren floor (Wisniewski, 1986). Possibly the substrate allows the larvae to rest in more ergonomic positions than those larvae deprived of the substrate.

5.5.7 Stream-Side Enclosure

The stream-side enclosure is appropriate for amphibians that live on the margins of streams or ponds. These amphibians are generally good swimmers, and some spend considerable amounts of time in the water. Others stay on land or near the water's edge, entering the water only to breed or travel to another bank. Stream-side dwellers include the stubfoot toads, *Atelopus* spp., the green frog, *Rana clamitans,* the bullfrog, *Rana catesbeiana* (also adapted to living in a pond habitat), the hairy frog, *Trichobatrachus robustus,* the tailed frog, *Ascaphus truei,* the American brook salamanders, *Eurycea* spp., the dusky salamanders, *Desmognathus* spp., the spring salamanders, *Gyrinophilus* spp., and the Pacific giant salamander, *Dicamptodon ensatus.*

The basic stream-side enclosure (Plate 5.3, Figure 5.4) includes a stream and a land area covered with moss and/or leaf litter over a gravel substrate. The enclosure should be as long as possible to accommodate different aspects of the stream. The size of the stream should be tailored to the lifestyle of the species of amphibian being housed. It should have areas of faster and slower moving water, including riffles and relatively quiet eddies. If an amphibian has to struggle against a current for extended periods of time, it may become exhausted. The depth of the water should at no point exceed the shoulder height of the amphibian, unless the particular species is known to be a strong swimmer.

At the head of the stream there may be a waterfall formed from stacked rocks. Nooks and crannies in the rockwork may provide cool, wet retreats for the amphibians. A grooved piece of cork bark can be used as a stream base. The outflow from the canister filter can be directed to the high end of the cork, and water can spill down the cork into the pool at the far end. Alternatively, "egg crate" and plastic screening can be fastened together to form a channel for the stream bed. A combination of large river rock and pea gravel can be used to fill in the stream bed. The gravel can be bonded to the egg crate with silicon rubber to provide a secure framework for the stream, and loose gravel and rocks can be added to create the desired water movement. Large pieces of rock or wood can be oriented at an angle to the current to form eddies where water movement is minimal. A split section of PVC pipe can be used for the same purpose. The water in the stream-side enclosure needs to be well oxygenated at all times, which it will be if the current and stream contours are appropriate.

Ideally, the land area in the stream-side enclosure includes a moisture gradient ranging from saturated near the water's edge and the waterfall, to fully drained but still slightly moist farthest from the stream. Small areas with dry, but not dusty leaf litter, dry rocks or fallen branches, and live plants will further diversify the moisture options available to the amphibian.

Living vegetation, rocks, branches, flower pots, and cork bark can be used to create terrestrial retreats, as well as refuges in shallow water. The latter refuges should allow the amphibian to rest in water no deeper than shoulder height, so that the animal can gulp air without treading water.

Some vegetation should be planted near and overhanging the streamway to provide cover and perches, as well as oviposition sites for some species of terrestrial and arboreal amphibians.

5.5.8 Terrestrial Forest Floor Enclosures

Terrestrial Forest Floor Complex Enclosure. The terrestrial forest floor enclosure is appropriate for

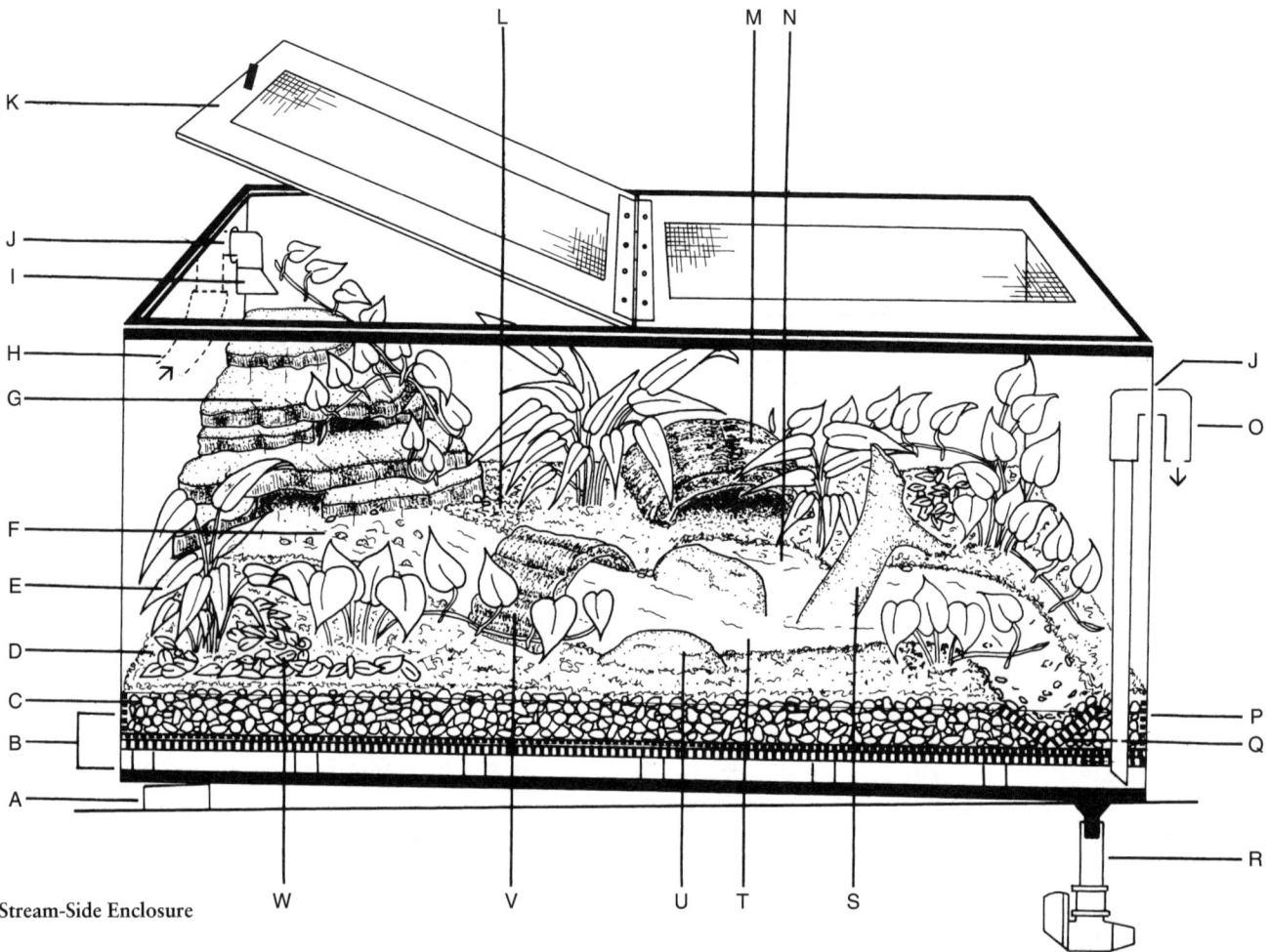

Figure 5.4. Lateral view of stream-side enclosure for amphibians. **A.** cross-section of board supporting the rim of the tank, tipping it toward the water outflow end. **B.** false floor assembly (see Figure 5.1 B—D). **C.** pea gravel layer approximately 5 cm (2") thick. **D.** moist sheet moss. **E.** live, potted plant with the base of the pot resting on the fiberglass screen. **F.** riffle. **G.** waterfall running over rocks stacked to create moist crevice retreats. **H.** water outflow from the canister filter. **I.** hose fitting to spread the water flow. **J.** hole in tank wall just large enough to pass the canister filter tubing. **K.** lid (see Figure 5.1 E—H). **L.** mucky area. **M.** cork bark cave/feeding platform. **N.** eddy. **O.** water inflow to the canister filter. **P.** water line. **Q.** gravel siliconed to egg crate screening to form the streambed. **R.** drain assembly (see Figure 5.1 K—M). **S.** hardwood branch. **T.** streamway. **U.** rock perch. **V.** cork bridge over shallow water, providing a semi-aquatic retreat. **W.** leaf litter over moist sheet moss. (Sandy Barnett)

many species of ground-dwelling and semiarboreal anurans. Also, many species of lungless salamander (Plethodontidae) and mole salamander (Ambystomatidae) will do well in a terrestrial environment.

The terrestrial forest floor enclosure (Plate 5.4, Figures 5.5, 5.6) has a gravel substrate, with the land area covered by a layer of moist moss, leaf litter, hardwood mulch, wood rot, and/or soil. There may be a shallow pond or water bowl for species that utilize standing water, but many terrestrial caecilians and salamanders tend to avoid standing water and may drown if they become trapped in water deeper than they are tall.

The terrestrial forest floor enclosure is enriched similarly to the land area of the stream-side vivarium (see Section 5.5.7, Stream-Side Enclosure). Care must be taken not to overplant the terrestrial enclosure. While amphibians require some cover, it is possible to plant the foliage so densely that the animals have difficulty finding and catching prey, or they expend too much energy in the hunt. The end result is underweight amphibians, a vivarium full of uneaten live food and their droppings, and in the case of some food insects, a lot of insect-damaged plants! On the other hand, an enclosure that is too sparsely vegetated may leave the amphibians feeling exposed and excessively stressed.

Terrestrial Spartan Enclosure. There are some terrestrial amphibians that can be maintained for a long term in spartan enclosures. Most salamanders are somewhat sedentary in the wild, and many terrestrial species thrive in such simple setups as plastic shoe or sweater boxes enriched with moist, crumpled paper toweling (Maruska, 1994) or petri dishes containing several layers of moist filter paper (Jaeger, 1992).

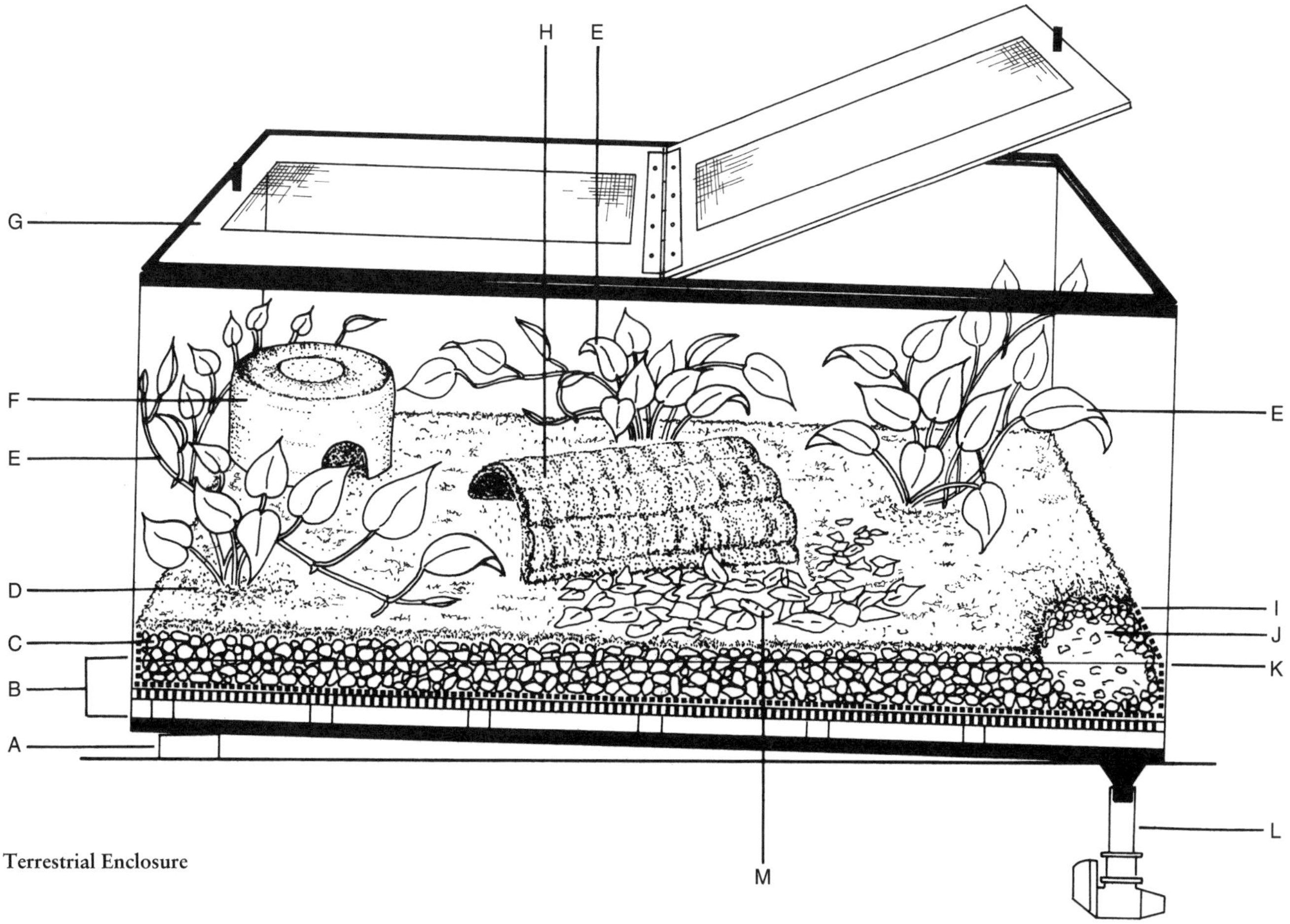

Figure 5.5. Lateral view of terrestrial enclosure for amphibians. **A.** cross-section of board supporting the rim of the tank, tipping it toward the drain. **B.** false floor assembly (see Figure 5.1 B—D). **C.** pea gravel layer approximately 2.5–5 cm (1–2") thick. **D.** moist sheet moss. **E.** live, potted plant with the base of the pot resting on the fiberglass screen. **F.** dark plastic hut. **G.** lid (see Figure 5.1 E—H). **H.** cork bark cave/feeding platform. **I.** upturned edge of fiberglass floor screen; it provides an escape route for food insects that fall into the pool and swim or drift to the glass wall. **J.** shallow pool. **K.** water line. **L.** drain assembly (see Figure 5.1 K—M). **M.** leaf litter over moist sheet moss. (Sandy Barnett)

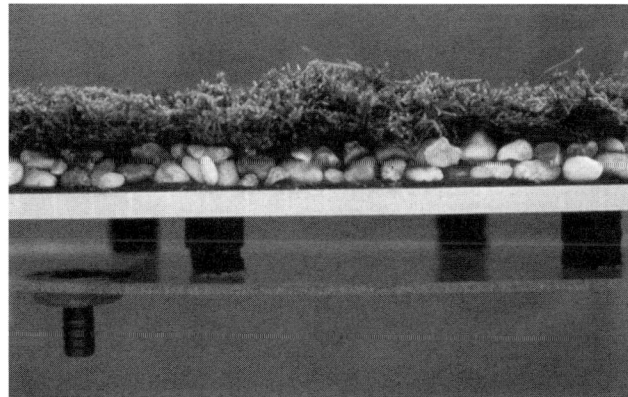

Figure 5.6. Cross-sectional view of substrate layers in a terrestrial enclosure. (George Grall, National Aquarium in Baltimore)

5.5.9 Terrestrial Fossorial Enclosure

The terrestrial fossorial enclosure is appropriate for terrestrial caecilians, many of the mole salamanders, *Ambystoma* spp., some of the lungless salamanders (family Plethodontidae), the tomato frogs, *Dyscophus* spp., and the spadefoot toads (family Pelobatidae).

The basic design for a terrestrial vivarium is appropriate for fossorial amphibians, although the latter animals need a deep soil base of at least 10 cm (4 in) for burrowing (Figure 5.7). The pool area can be quite small or eliminated altogether, unless the species needs a large pool for breeding.

It is best to use an enclosure that maximizes floor space. The height of the fossorial vivarium needs to be only a little taller than the depth of the soil. A 76 L (20 gal) long aquarium works well for a breeding group of medium sized species, such as the marbled salamander, *Ambystoma opacum,* while larger species such as the Mexican caecilian, *Dermophis mexicanus*, should be housed in a 114 L (30 gal) breeder aquarium.

It is essential that a moisture gradient exists throughout the fossorial enclosure, with one end of the tank having drier soil than the other, and the bottom soil being more moist than the surface soil. This will allow the amphibian to seek out an appropriate microenvironment. The easiest way to set up this environment is to use a long aquarium, and tilt it lengthwise with a brick or board under the high end. Always rest the weight of a glass vivarium on the framed rim and not on the glass itself to prevent cracking of the glass or loosening of the seals. Water is then added only at the lower end of the enclosure. This creates a gradient of wet to dry soil from the lower to the higher end.

It is essential to have well-drained soil and an unclogged drain, so that water does not back up into the burrows. To keep the gravel bed from clogging with dirt, a layer of window screening can be laid between the gravel and the soil layer.

Many fossorial amphibians are quite strong for their size and can easily push open a poorly secured cage lid. It is recommended that the lid have a locking mechanism, or be weighted down with a brick or comparably heavy object.

Fossorial species, by their nature, spend much of their time underground, out of view. One strategy for increasing their display value, while still allowing them to exhibit normal burrowing behavior, is to stack pea gravel in a high mound in the center of the tank and place a moat of deep soil around the perimeter, filling in the space between the gravel mound and the walls of the vivarium. This setup allows the amphibian to construct burrows that are visible in cross section. Black plastic or dark paper should be placed

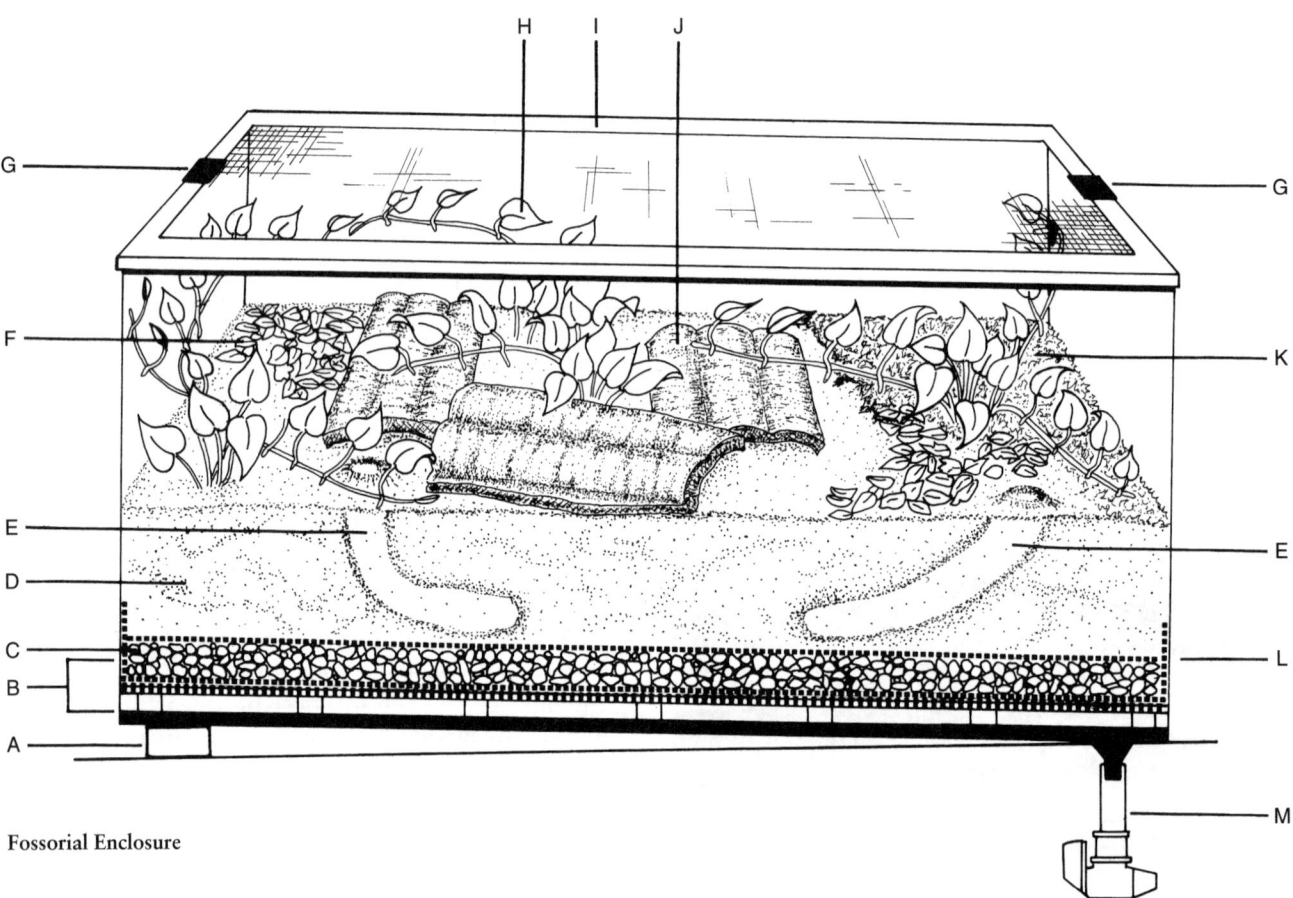

Fossorial Enclosure

Figure 5.7. Lateral view of fossorial enclosure for amphibians. **A.** cross-section of board supporting the rim of the tank, tipping it toward the drain. **B.** false floor assembly (see Figure 5.1 B—D). **C.** pea gravel layer approximately 2.5–5 cm (1–2") thick. **D.** soil at least 10 cm (4 in) deep. **E.** burrow made by a fossorial amphibian. **F.** leaf litter. **G.** clip to secure the lid against escapes. **H.** live, potted plant with the base of the pot resting on the fiberglass screen. **I.** standard one-piece screened aquarium/vivarium lid. **J.** hardwood bark or cork bark. **K.** moist sheet moss. **L.** single layer of fiberglass window screening to keep the overlying soil from clogging the gravel layer beneath. **M.** drain assembly (see Figure 5.1 K—M) (Sandy Barnett)

over the wall of the burrow to maintain a dark environment whenever the vivarium is not being observed.

Plenty of ground cover in the form of dead leaves, flat rocks, bark, clumps of sphagnum moss, or sheet moss is recommended so that fossorial amphibians can forage on the surface of the soil but remain under cover. Small sections of thermoplastic (e.g., Plexiglas) may be placed on the surface of the soil, which an amphibian may use for cover when on the surface. Dark-tinted thermoplastic is needed for many salamanders to feel secure, but caecilians have such poor eyesight that clear plastic can be used for these burrowers.

PVC pipes with rounded edges can be sunk at an angle in the soil to provide ready-made burrows. A see-through burrow can be made by cutting the pipe lengthwise and placing the open side up against the glass. Many ambystomid salamanders will readily use these structures.

Live plants generally fare poorly with fossorial amphibians; the burrowing activity constantly disrupts the root system. Golden pothos, *Epipremnum aureum,* and Cordatum philodendron, *Philodendron oxycardium,* are among the hardy plants that handle such disturbances well. If other plants are going to be used, it is best to keep them in their pots. A layer of gravel can be put in the top of each pot to discourage digging.

Another way to add greenery to a fossorial cage is to use an epiphyte log. Its construction is described by de Vosjoli (1995). Basically, the epiphyte log is a roll of cork or a suitable hardwood branch covered with epiphytes of different sizes and shapes.

The fossorial enclosure can be used to estivate certain amphibians, such as sirens, *Siren* spp., and spadefoot toads (family Pelobatidae). The soil layer should be deep, in excess of 30 cm (12 in), and should be wetted thoroughly. The enclosure can be left to dry out so that the surface of the soil develops cracks from the dryness. Healthy amphibians of cocoon-forming species will create a nest chamber and estivate through this period of dryness. Moistening the soil again will bring the amphibians out of estivation. After the soil has been moistened a few days, buried terrestrial amphibians can be dug up and allowed to rehydrate in a shallow bath. Aquatic amphibians can be returned to their normal aquatic enclosure.

5.5.10 Arboreal Enclosures

Complex Arboreal Enclosure. The basic design for a terrestrial forest floor vivarium is appropriate for arboreal amphibians, although the arboreal enclosure should be as tall as possible and provided with tall plants and branches. Hexagonal aquariums that are especially suitable for this purpose are available in a variety of sizes.

Arboreal enclosures can be very complex, taking on the appearance of a richly stratified forest, with branches covered with mosses and epiphytic plants, terrestrial vegetation, and a pool. The back and side walls may be covered with sheets of cork bark or tropical fern fiber and planted with more epiphytic vegetation, or climbing vines. Wall growth is encouraged by trickling water down the wall with a recirculating pump, powerhead, or canister filter.

A much simpler enclosure that still satisfies the needs of arboreal anurans has been successfully used for years at the National Aquarium in Baltimore (Plate 5.5, Figures 5.8, 5.9). It consists of a gravel substrate overlaid by moist sheet moss. One or two large potted plants, usually a broad-leaved species of *Agleonema,* are partially buried in the gravel. The plants fill out most of the open vertical space in the enclosure. One or two hardwood branches, with a strong horizontal inclination, provide arboreal perches for the amphibians, but some vertically inclined branches should be also available. On the floor of the cage, there is a pool or shallow water bowl. A small golden pothos, *Epipremnum aureum,* or peace lily, *Spathiphyllum* sp., may be planted next to the water to provide cover for the animals. The water section of the arboreal vivarium is not deep. A water depth of 2.5 cm (1 in) is adequate.

Broad-leaved plants should be used if leaf-spawning anurans are to be housed in the enclosure. Since some anurans oviposit on leaves that overhang water, care must be taken to locate plants near the water's edge.

Some arboreal anurans (e.g. the hourglass treefrog, *Hyla ebraccata,* and the orange-sided leaf treefrog, *Phyllomedusa hypochondrialis*) readily sleep on the smooth inside wall of retreats made from dark plastic containers. While such refuges are not particularly attractive, they make it quick and easy to inventory and monitor frogs that might otherwise be difficult to find during their sleep period.

Cliffside Arboreal Enclosure. Many crevice dwelling amphibians, such as the green salamander, *Aneides aeneus,* and some of the slender salamanders, *Batrachoseps* spp., are not arboreal, and do best in a tall enclosure with high rock faces rather than cork or other plant material. The rocks should be securely fixed together with silicon rubber or a waterproof nontoxic epoxy, and stacked in such a way that there are a variety of crevices to serve as retreats. A slight trickle down one face of the rock surface will create a moisture gradient that may encourage breeding in those areas (similar to conditions in the wild).

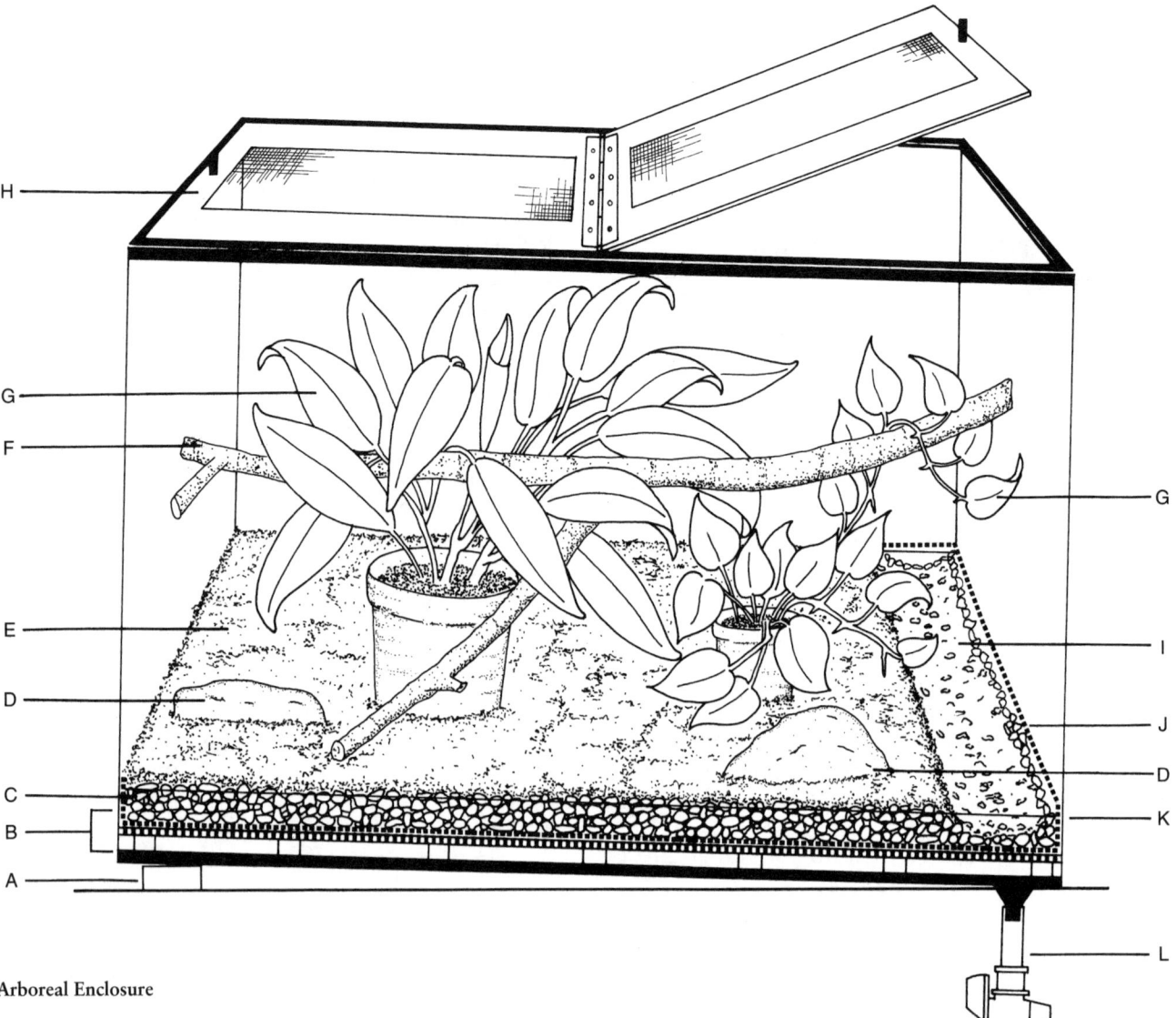

Arboreal Enclosure

Figure 5.8. Lateral view of arboreal enclosure for amphibians. **A.** cross-section of board supporting the rim of the tank, tipping it toward the drain. **B.** false floor assembly (see Figure 5.1 B—D). **C.** pea gravel layer approximately 2.5–5 cm (1 to 2") thick. **D.** rock perch. **E.** moist sheet moss. **F.** cut hardwood branch or sturdy vine with no sharp edges or points. **G.** live, potted plant with the base of the pot resting on the fiberglass screen. **H.** lid (see Figure 5.1 E—H). **I.** shallow pool. **J.** upturned edge of fiberglass floor screen; it provides an escape route for food insects that fall into the pool and swim or drift to the glass wall. **K.** water level. **L.** drain assembly (see Figure 5.1 K—M). (Sandy Barnett)

Spartan Arboreal Enclosure. A spartan version of the arboreal terrarium has been used successfully at the Philadelphia Zoo to house some species of amphibians during quarantine and for the duration of certain medical treatments. The tank floor is covered with moist paper toweling. Enrichment is limited to a water bowl and strips of mylar plastic or plastic plants draped down the walls. The amphibians can hide behind the plastic strips or plastic plants, clinging to the walls or plastic. A dark strip of plastic is hung on the outside of one wall of the enclosure to block the light. Breeding of the New Granada cross-banded frog, *Smilisca phaeota,* occurred in such an enclosure.

5.6 ENVIRONMENTAL CONTROL

Temperature, humidity, precipitation, and lighting are environmental parameters that profoundly affect the health of an amphibian, as well as its behavior and reproductive success. Successful husbandry depends on controlling these parameters to produce the functional equivalent of the amphibian's natural microhabitat in captivity. The captive environment should include any daily fluctuations of these parameters encountered by the amphibian in the wild.

For many species of amphibians, it may be necessary to simulate the seasonal fluctuations in certain

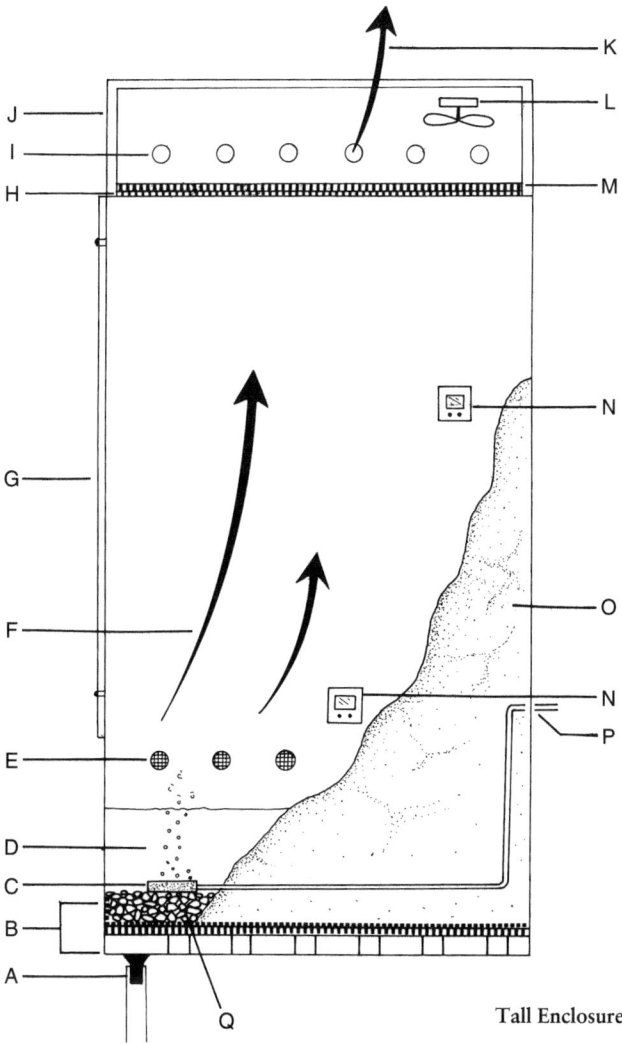

Figure 5.9. Lateral view of a tall enclosure for arboreal amphibians showing appropriate air circulation patterns (after Stettler, 1981). Even tall vivariums can ventilate well with proper placement of ventilation holes/panels to create cross air currents. A. drain. B. false floor assembly (see Figure 5.1 B—D). C. air stone connected to an outside aquarium air pump. D. pool. E. screened ventilation holes in one wall of enclosure, at a low level (alternatively, an aquarium air pump can be used to add fresh air low in the enclosure). F. warm, moist air rising from the heated water or land mass (e.g. heated by a submersible aquarium heater, undertank heating pad or tape, or buried heating cable). G. front of the enclosure with a sliding or hinged access door. H. screened ceiling. I. ventilation holes in the vivarium hood for warm air to escape. J. vivarium hood holding fluorescent and spot lights. K. vented air. L. small venting fan inside hood. M. white egg-crate screening to reduce glare from overhead lights. N. hygrometer/thermometer. O. land mass. P. hole in wall for electrical and air lines. Q. pea gravel. (Sandy Barnett)

environmental variables to stimulate reproductive cycles. This includes conditions appropriate for hibernation or estivation in many temperate species. However, eliminating these cycles of dormancy will not harm the amphibians themselves. In fact, creating appropriate conditions for hibernation or estivation and making sure that the amphibians are physically prepared to handle it can be difficult, and these arrangements are best left in the hands of experienced herpetoculturists.

Information on climatic conditions around the world (temperature, humidity, wind, precipitation) is available on computer disc (WeatherDisc Associates, 1995). The library of the National Oceanic and Atmospheric Administration in Silver Springs, MD (301/713-2600 ext. 124) will fax a limited amount of this climatological data to any caller at no charge. Many public and university libraries also have access to this material. This data can be useful in setting up appropriate conditions in the captive environment.

5.6.1 Temperature

The optimal air temperature in an amphibian enclosure will depend on the species being housed and on the specimen's place of origin. Approximate temporal-spatial temperature gradients suggested for keeping postlarval terrestrial amphibians are presented according to broad habitat type: tropical lowland species 24–30°C (75–85°F); tropical montane forms 18–24°C (65–75°F); subtropical forms 21–27°C (70–80°F); and temperate forms, summer 18–24°C (65–75°F), winter hibernation 10–16°C (50–60°F). These ranges are only rough guidelines, and temperatures may need to be adjusted higher or lower depending on a particular amphibian's response to the temperatures provided.

The optimal water temperature in an aquatic amphibian enclosure will depend on the species being housed and on the specimen's place of origin. Approximate temporal-spatial temperature gradients suggested for keeping aquatic larval and adult amphibians are presented according to broad habitat type: tropical lowland species 24–30°C (75–85°F), tropical montane species 18–24°C (65–75°F), subtropical species 21–27°C (70–80°F), temperate stream species in summer 16–21°C (60–70°F), and temperate pond species in summer 18–24°C (65–75°F). Most temperate species of aquatic amphibians experience a drop of 9°C (15°F) or more in the winter, so a chilling unit may be needed. Alternatively, the entire room can be cooled with an air conditioner. These ranges are only rough guidelines, and temperatures may need to be adjusted higher or lower depending on a particular amphibian's response to the temperatures provided.

Some amphibians undergo a daily shift in thermal preference. Diurnal species may seek lower temperatures at night while nocturnal species may seek such temperatures in the daytime. When placed in a thermal gradient in the laboratory, the mudpuppy, *Necturus maculosus,* a completely aquatic, nocturnally active species, selects considerably higher temperatures at night than it does during the day (Hutchison & Spriestersbach, 1986).

A maximum-minimum thermometer should be maintained at the warmest and coolest points in the enclosure at all times to make sure that the daily temperature range (temporal and spatial) is appropriate. Digital maximum-minimum thermometers, with a remote sensor for a second location, are available at some electronics/appliance stores (e.g., Dual Display In/Outdoor Thermometer, Cat. No. 63–1020, Radio Shack, Ft. Worth, TX) as well as through laboratory and herpetological supply companies. Some models also include a hygrometer for measuring relative humidity.

Tropical lowland and subtropical species of amphibians can normally be kept and bred at a fairly constant temperature year-round. However, many temperate species of amphibians are stimulated to reproduce only after a period of hibernation at cooler temperatures. Seasonal drops of 6–8°C (10–15°F) or more may be necessary to induce the cycle of gonad atrophy and recrudescence needed for breeding.

Amphibians control their body temperature by both behavioral and physiological mechanisms (for a review, see Duellman & Trueb, 1986; Stebbins & Cohen, 1995). Behavioral control involves movement from place to place within the temperature mosaic of the environment and postural adjustments that increase or decrease contact with environmental temperature sources. Physiological control includes changing the rate and amount of evaporative water loss from the skin, changing skin color to affect the absorption and reflectance of solar radiation, and possibly peripheral vasodilation and constriction.

For many species of amphibians, a thermal gradient within the enclosure is desirable throughout most of the year to enable the animals to thermoregulate. In most cases the warmest area should be no more than 5–8°C (10–15°F) above the coolest area in the enclosure. Substrate heating can be accomplished by using a low wattage undertank heating pad, or flexible heating tape or cable (see Fogel, 1993 for a review of heating equipment). Electrical "hot rocks" are too hot for amphibians and should never be used. For temperate amphibians, the thermal gradient in the enclosure can be reduced in magnitude or eliminated during the winter hibernation.

Basking appears to be important in body temperature regulation in some species of amphibians (for a review, see Stebbins & Cohen, 1995). Basking may take place in direct sunlight, or under rocks or other material warmed by the sun. Many newly metamorphosed anurans seem especially prone to sitting in the sun when there is adequate substrate moisture or the opportunity to move quickly into water to compensate for evaporative water loss. Juveniles of the green toad, *Bufo debilis,* accelerate feeding, digestion, and growth by elevating their body temperature through basking (Seymour, 1972).

A basking spot can be provided by a low wattage ceramic heating lamp or an incandescent spotlight. The former type of lamp produces no visible light and is preferable where nighttime heating is needed, or where the basking amphibian is photophobic. Incandescent lights are preferable for daytime use with species of amphibians that normally bask in sunlight. Heliophilic lizards can be confused by unnatural combinations of light and temperature (e.g., bright light with low temperatures) and fail to thermoregulate properly (Sievert & Hutchison, 1991). It is possible that basking amphibians could experience the same difficulty.

Care must be taken that any heat-generating light does not overly dry the air. Also, it is important that amphibians do not come into direct contact with the heat source, which could cause desiccation and thermal burns; however, fluorescent tubes emit only small amounts of heat (unlike the starter unit, which can become quite warm). Agile treefrogs will often rest on lit tubes, presumably for the warmth. This is not known to be deleterious to these amphibians. It is best to shield the starter unit with screening, or to use a remote ballast located outside the cage. Used inside the enclosure, however, the starter unit can serve as a source of ambient heat.

Heating requirements for aquatic species and the larvae of terrestrial species are easily met using standard aquarium heaters. A simple way to prevent the amphibian from directly contacting the heater is to sheath it in a section of PVC pipe. Holes should be drilled in the pipe to improve water flow through it. The pipe should be small enough in diameter to keep the amphibian out, but large enough so that the heating element does not touch the interior wall of the pipe. Clear plastic tubes are also available, albeit more expensive than PVC pipe, and have the advantage that the heater's indicator light can be seen without obstruction. These clear tubes must be ordered from plastic specialty supply companies.

Aquarium heaters can also be used to add heat to terrestrial enclosures that have a pond or stream. Again, the heater should be sheathed in a piece of highly perforated PVC pipe or clear plastic, or otherwise located so that the cage inhabitants cannot directly contact the heating element.

5.6.2 Humidity

The humidity in an amphibian enclosure should match that of the species's natural microhabitat. Humidity is generally controlled by adjusting the amount of ventilation, and by varying the amount of water that is added to the cage and released into the air.

A pump spray bottle can be used several times daily to increase humidity, but the effect each time is temporary. Reducing the amount of ventilation in an enclosure, by draping a sheet of plastic over the top, for example, will increase the humidity. But it may also create a stagnant atmosphere, reducing thermal and moisture gradients, and increasing the amphibian's susceptibility to disease (Baetjer, 1968). Also, many species of plants fail to thrive in poorly ventilated environments.

An effective way to raise the humidity without reducing ventilation is to create areas of moving water—install a waterfall or stream, or put an airstone in a pool or bowl of water. Live plants will also help to increase the humidity.

Tall vivariums are especially prone to the accumulation of stagnant air near the bottom. Such enclosures often have very poor thermal and humidity gradients, due to a lack of air circulation. Small cooling fans, such as the ones used for cooling computers, can be put at the top of the tank to turn over the air. The fans should be directed downward, toward an inside wall of the enclosure, with the goal of minimizing any strong air flow onto the amphibians themselves. Alternatively, ventilation holes can be drilled in a lower wall of the tank to create a cross current (see Figure 5.9). The strength of the air current can be increased by installing a small fan facing upward at the top of the enclosure, so that it pulls air up through the vivarium.

Most species of nonaquatic amphibians spend large portions of their time in sheltered microhabitats where the relative humidity is high. Even species found in xeric macrohabitats may spend much of their time in burrows or under rocks where humidity levels are high. Activity patterns can be affected by humidity levels. For example, rain forest dendrobatid frogs will exhibit high levels of activity on a wet substrate in high humidity, but will seek refugia as humidity levels drop. A relative humidity above 70% suits most species of amphibians. However, it is best to provide a humidity gradient within the enclosure, so an amphibian can seek its preferred microenvironment. Some amphibians (e.g., the waxy treefrog, *Phyllomedusa sauvagii,* the giant monkey frog, *Phyllomedusa bicolor*) will develop skin problems if continuously exposed to high humidity and are, in fact, adapted to spending at least part of their daily cycle in a low humidity environment. An area of lower humidity can be established using low wattage spotlights over part of the enclosure during the daytime. Refuges should be available throughout the humidity gradient in an enclosure, so an amphibian is not forced to select between security and meeting physiological needs.

If a room can be dedicated for housing amphibians, an area humidifier can be installed. Care must be taken to clean and disinfect the unit weekly, since it can harbor and spread potentially pathogenic bacteria and fungi (Hunter, 1989). A solution of 120 ml (4 fl oz) of white vinegar and 946 ml (1 qt) of water can be used to dissolve any mineral deposits and clean the humidifier (Pinkham & Higgenbotham, 1976).

This should be followed by a disinfecting bath or spray of sodium hypochlorite (bleach) at a dilution of 30 ml (1 fl oz) of bleach to each quart (946 ml) of water. The solution should be left on the humidifier parts for at least 15 minutes, then rinsed well with fresh water (Wright, 1993).

With regard to ventilation in the room, 1–2 air changes per hour should provide a satisfactory level of ventilation while still maintaining adequate humidity levels for amphibians (Pough, 1992).

5.6.3 Precipitation

Precipitation is an essential trigger for breeding behavior in many species of amphibians (for a review, see Duellman & Trueb, 1986; Stebbins & Cohen, 1995; Zug, 1993). For tropical terrestrial amphibians, it is often the onset of the rainy season following the dry season that stimulates reproductive behavior. Flooding (associated with rain) and a drop in water temperature elicits breeding behavior in many tropical aquatic and stream-breeding terrestrial species. And among many temperate species, hibernation followed by spring rains is often the stimulus for reproduction.

Simulating these environmental cues in a captive setting is essential to successfully propagate many species of amphibians. Wright (1994) discusses various options for constructing "rain chambers" for breeding amphibians.

The basic NAIB amphibian enclosure can be modified to provide rain showers. The outflow of a canister filter is diverted into a perforated tray positioned over the cage top. The intensity of the rain shower is controlled by the number of holes in the tray, and the rate of water flow. The goal is to have a gentle rain over a portion of the tank, allowing the amphibians to avoid it if they choose to. (This pattern of rain also provides a drier area where live food insects can congregate, which minimizes insect losses due to drowning.)

If the filtration material in the canister is removed, and the unit is used strictly to move water, it can be set on a timer to automatically rain on the enclosure, as needed. A timer should not be used with a filter-loaded canister, since the system will become anaerobic if the water flow is shut down for more than a few hours, and the nitrifying bacteria will die.

5.6.4 Lighting

The proper illumination for health and reproductive success in captive amphibians is a subject of much debate. A conservative approach, and the one that is recommended here, is to provide lighting that mimics, as closely as possible, the spectral characteristics, intensity, and duration of light found in the amphibian's natural habitat.

There are numerous brands of fluorescent lights on the market purporting to be "full-spectrum," i.e., to duplicate the spectrum of natural sunlight. Of particular concern to the herpetoculturist is the emission of light in the ultraviolet-B portion of the spectrum (285–320 nm). It is well known that ultraviolet-B radiation plays a key role in the biogenesis of vitamin D_3 in the exposed skin of endothermic vertebrates (Holick, 1989). There is evidence that this is also true for at least some species of reptiles (Allen, 1989) and amphibians (St. Lezin, 1983). As a precaution against vitamin D_3 deficiency and its complications, most herpetoculturists use full-spectrum lighting (which emits ultraviolet-B radiation) over amphibians, in addition to fortifying the diet with this vitamin as part of a multivitamin, multimineral supplementation program.

Unfortunately, the amount of ultraviolet-B radiation emitted from many of the full-spectrum fluorescent lights, especially over an extended period of time, is suspect. It is recommended that whatever full-spectrum lights are chosen, they be replaced every 6–12 months. Also, the lights should be positioned no more than 46 cm (18 in) from the cage floor, since the intensity of the emissions falls off rapidly with increasing distance from the source. At NAIB, at least two 4-ft (122 cm) "Instant Sun" fluorescent tubes (Verilux, Stamford, CT) are placed over all amphibian enclosures approximately 8 cm (3 in) above the screened lids. Some other bulbs have been manufactured and distributed recently that emit a higher proportion of their output as ultraviolet-B radiation (e.g., ReptiSun 310®, ZooMed, San Luis Obispo, CA; Reptile D-Light, 8% Type, Ultraviolet Resources International, Cleveland, OH) (Gehrmann, 1996), but there is no long-term track record for their use with amphibians at this time.

It should be noted that many of the "full-spectrum" and "wide-spectrum" tungsten filament incandescent lamps currently on the market produce no ultraviolet-B radiation (Gehrmann, 1992) or very low levels of ultraviolet-B radiation (Gehrmann, 1996). These lights are useful for providing visible light and heat, but their modest output of ultraviolet light, either ultraviolet-A or ultraviolet-B radiation, makes their role in vitamin D biogenesis questionable. A radiometer that measures ultraviolet-B emission and one that measures ultraviolet-A emission is currently available in the pet trade, but is somewhat expensive (ZooMed, San Luis Obispo, CA). These radiometers may not separate out the biologically relevant wavelengths within the categories, and are different from those used to report ultraviolet emission of commercially available bulbs (Gehrmann, 1996). Other radiometers are commercially available that can help identify the suitability of bulbs (biological activity) as well as their useful lifespan.

Ultraviolet radiation does not transmit well through standard glass or plastic. There now are specialty plastics on the market that are designed specifically for ultraviolet light transmission, but they are expensive and not commonly available. This means that when lights are placed above an enclosure lid made from glass or plastic (including thin pliable sheet plastic), ultraviolet-B radiation is screened out. For this reason, lights should not be encased in a plastic shield, and they should only be located above a screened lid that allows direct penetration of light. Alternatively, uncovered fluorescent lights can be located inside the enclosure.

Recently, a low-lead glass aquarium cover was introduced into the marketplace that purports to allow ultraviolet light transmission. In fact, small amounts of ultraviolet-A radiation are transmitted through the glass, but little or no ultraviolet-B radiation (Messonnier, 1995).

The lighting needs of nocturnal amphibians are poorly known, but low-level lighting to replicate the cycle of the moon should be provided. At NAIB, light-emitting diode (LED) night-lights, placed directly above a cage lid, appear to produce adequate light for nocturnal anurans to hunt, and yet do not appear to interfere with other nighttime activity (e.g., male calling, breeding, feeding). Red light (15-watt incandescent lights behind a red filter), and "bright" (4- watt) white night-lights placed within several feet (less than 1 m) of an enclosure, appear to interfere with normal nocturnal behavior. The moonlight bulbs designed for marine aquariums may have some utility in the herpetoculture of nocturnal amphibians, but this remains to be studied.

In general, amphibians appear to prefer subdued lighting (basking in sunlight is a notable exception). The glare from lights over an amphibian enclosure can be reduced by putting a sheet of plastic egg-crate screening directly underneath the light fixture. This screening is sold in many hardware and lighting stores for use with fluorescent ceiling lights. It has a large, open square pattern that permits direct transmission of overhead light.

Although the enclosure lighting should first and foremost meet the needs of the amphibians, a secondary consideration must be the lighting requirements of the enclosed plants. By selecting plants that thrive in moderate to low light levels, planting the most light-demanding ones closest to the lights, and arranging plants to shade at least some of the areas frequented by the amphibians, it is possible to have a vivarium that meets the needs of both plants and animals. It should be noted that the incandescent and fluorescent lights sold specifically for growing indoor plants (e.g., Gro-Lux® and Gro-Lux/ws®, Sylvania Corporation, Danvers, MA) do not produce ultraviolet-B radiation (Gehrmann, 1994) and should not be used in place of full-spectrum fluorescent lighting in animal enclosures.

The photoperiod in the vivarium should be maintained in a cycle that mimics that found within the amphibian's natural range. The United States Naval Observatory Web site (http://aa.usno.navy.mil/AA/data/docs/RS_OneYear.html) provides a calculator to determine the time of sunrise and sunset anywhere in the world. Day length data is also available in the printed serial, *Astronomical Almanac* (Nautical Almanac Office, 1999).

It is recommended that the lights over an amphibian enclosure be arranged to turn on and off in sequence, to simulate dawn and dusk. Twilight transitions have been shown to have a significant effect in normalizing activity patterns of laboratory animals (Greenberg, 1992). While this research did not include amphibians, it is reasonable to assume that sighted amphibians may benefit from gradual rather than abrupt lighting changes, just as they occur in the wild.

5.7 NUTRITION

Prior to metamorphosis, anurans may be herbivorous, omnivorous, or carnivorous, depending on the species. After metamorphosis, diets typically shift to being completely carnivorous, although there are a few exceptions. Larval and adult salamanders and caecilians are strictly carnivorous. (See also Chapter 6, Diets for Captive Amphibians.)

Prey type and size vary, depending on the life stage, size, and species of amphibian. The adult stage of some species specialize on tiny leaf litter insects. Larger species of amphibians tend to be opportunistic and prey on a variety of species ranging from arthropods to small vertebrates.

It is a misconception that wild animals are nutritionally wise and will always select a balanced diet if given a choice (Allen, 1989). A captive diet should not be based simply on what items an amphibian eats most readily. Keep in mind that selection of food in the wild depends on a number of factors, including seasonal shifts in composition and abundance of prey, the amphibian's prior experience with a particular prey species, as well as prey attributes of size, movement (orientation and speed), palatability and nutritive value (Stebbins & Cohen, 1995). It is the responsibility of herpetoculturists to devise varied and balanced diets for their captive amphibians.

Captive weights and body outline should mimic wild weights and body appearance. It is especially important that amphibians be in good weight prior to any breeding attempt, as this is an energetically expensive undertaking, and in some species, a period of little or no food intake.

Overfeeding and obesity can be a problem for some species of amphibians in captivity (e.g., White's treefrog, *Pelodryas caerulea,* ornate horned frog, *Ceratophrys ornata,* tiger salamander, *Ambystoma tigrinum*). The recommended frequency of feeding varies with the species, age, and activity level (which may be influenced by cage enrichment and environmental variables) of the amphibian. Young, growing animals, and active foragers thrive on daily feeding. Mature sit-and-wait predators (e.g., the horned frogs, *Ceratophrys* spp.) will usually maintain good body weight with a large meal every 2 weeks.

In general, larval amphibians should be fed small amounts daily, rather than several large meals weekly. For species prone to cannibalism, it is important to provide food *ad libitum* if the tadpoles are to be raised communally. It is recommended that feeding, as well as cleaning, be done on a variable time schedule. Larvae of the bullfrog, *Rana catesbeiana,* respond to a fixed schedule of disturbance (feeding and tank cleaning) by accumulation of coelomic fat and delayed metamorphosis (Culley, 1991; Horseman et al., 1976). The excess fat restricts the mobility of some froglets, leading to starvation and death in some instances. The studies concluded that the larvae must be disturbed on an irregular time schedule, from hatching through to metamorphosis, to prevent these problems.

Common invertebrate foods for postlarval terrestrial amphibians include red worms, earthworms, white worms, crickets, fly maggots and adults, fruit flies, springtails, mealworm larvae, waxmoth larvae, and *Zophobas* beetle larvae. Aquatic amphibians also accept invertebrates such as bloodworms, black worms, washed brine shrimp, *Artemia* spp., glass shrimp, and crayfish. Techniques for culturing live food are covered in Chapter 6, Diets for Captive Amphibians, as well as the following sources: Axelrod &

Schultz, 1990; Brown, 1995; Culley, 1991; Frye 1991, 1992; Masters, 1975; National Research Council, 1974. Additional sources with information on diets and care of some of the more commonly kept amphibians are: anurans (Cover et al., 1994; de Vosjoli, 1990a, 1990b; de Vosjoli et al. 1996; Fenolio & Ready, 1995; Le Berre, 1993) salamanders (Balsai, 1994; Fenolio & Ready, 1996; Harkavy, 1993; Jaeger, 1992; Maruska, 1994; Staniszewski, 1996; Webb, 1994), caecilians (O'Reilly et al., 1995; Wake, 1994).

Field sweepings and leaf litter invertebrates from areas where pesticides and herbicides have not been used are excellent food sources for amphibians. As a precaution, though, brightly colored insects should be avoided unless they are positively known not to be toxic. Mosquito larvae are a good food for many larval salamanders as well as for some tadpoles. A bucket of water left outside in warm weather will often be seeded within a few days. Equipment for catching and keeping insects is available from Bio-Quip Products (17803 La Salle Ave, Gardena, CA).

The National Research Council (1974) notes that cooked spinach, a food commonly fed to many herbivorous tadpoles, should be avoided because it can cause kidney stones. Cooked romaine and escarole lettuces do not cause this problem, though their nutritional adequacy remains uncertain. At NAIB, the tadpoles of nearly all species of anurans are fed dried fish food. (Sera Micron: Stage 1 Powdered Food for Newborn Fry, Sera, Heinsburg, Germany). At NAIB, stream-dwelling larvae of the harlequin stubfoot toad, *Atelopus v. varius,* feed on Sera Micron, as well as algae that is cultured in-house on PVC pipe fittings and on rocks.

REFERENCES

Allen, M.E. 1989. Nutritional Aspects of Insectivory. Ph.D. Dissertation, Michigan State University, East Lansing, MI, 205 pp.

Allen, M.E. and O.T. Oftedal. 1989. Dietary manipulation of the calcium content of feed crickets. Journal of Zoo and Wildlife Medicine 20(1):26–33.

Axelrod, H.R. and L.P. Schultz. 1990. Handbook of Tropical Aquarium Fishes. TFH Publications, Inc., Neptune City, NJ, 718 pp.

Baetjer, A.M. 1968. Role of Environmental Temperature and Humidity in Susceptibility to Disease. Arch Environ Health 16:565-570.

Balsai, M.J. 1994. Axolotls. Reptile and Amphibian Magazine (March/April):41–51.

Brown, L.E. 1995. Successful mealworm raising. Reptile & Amphibian Magazine (March/April):74–79.

Cardeilhac, P.T. and B.R. Whitaker. 1988. Copper treatments, uses and precautions. Veterinary Clinics of North America: Small Animal Practice 18(2):435–448.

Coburn, J. 1992. The Proper Care of Amphibians. TFH Publications, Inc., Neptune City, NJ, 256 pp.

Cover, J.F. Jr., S.L. Barnett, and R.L. Saunders. 1994. Captive management and breeding of dendrobatid and neotropical hylid frogs at the National Aquarium in Baltimore, *in* J.B. Murphy, K. Adler, and J.T. Collins (Eds.): Captive Management and Conservation of Amphibians and Reptiles. Society for the Study of Amphibians and Reptiles, St. Louis, MO, pp. 267–273.

Culley, D.D. 1991. Bufo culture, *in* C.E. Nash (Ed.): Production of Aquatic Animals, World Animal Science C4. Elsevier Science Publishers, British Vancouver, Canada, pp. 185–205.

de Vosjoli, P. 1990a. The General Care and Maintenance of Horned Frogs. Advanced Vivarium Systems, Lakeside, CA, 32 pp.

de Vosjoli, P. 1990b. The General Care and Maintenance of White's Tree Frogs and White-lipped Tree Frogs. Advanced Vivarium Systems, Lakeside, CA, 28 pp.

de Vosjoli, P. 1995. Vivarium design. A tropical rainforest vivarium. The Vivarium 7(2):14–16.

de Vosjoli, P., R. Mailloux, and D. Ready. 1996. Care and Breeding of Popular Tree Frogs. Advanced Vivarium Systems, Santee, CA.

Duellman, W.E. and L. Trueb. 1986. Biology of Amphibians. McGraw-Hill Book Co., New York, 670 pp.

Fenolio, D. and M. Ready. 1995. Phyllomedusine frogs of Latin America in the wild and in captivity. The Vivarium 5(6):26–37.

Fenolio, D. and M. Ready. 1996. California: the *Ensatina* State. The Vivarium 7(4):32–60.

Fogel, D. 1993. Heating Herps in the 1990s. The Vivarium 4(6):8–11.

Frye, F.L. 1991. A Practical Guide for Feeding Captive Reptiles. Krieger Publishing Co., Malabar, FL, 171 pp.

Frye, F.L. 1992. Captive Invertebrates: A Guide to Their Biology and Husbandry. Krieger Publishing Co., Malabar, FL, 160 pp.

Gehrmann, W.H. 1992. No UV B from Tungsten Filament Incandescent Lamps. Bulletin of the Association of Reptilian and Amphibian Veterinarians 2(2):5.

Gehrmann, W.H. 1994. Spectral characteristics of lamps commonly used in herpetoculture. The Vivarium 5(5):16–29.

Gehrmann, W.H. 1996. Reptile lighting: a current perspective. The Vivarium 8(2):44–45, 62.

Greenberg, N. 1992. The saurian psyche revisited: lizards in research, *in* D.O. Schaeffer, K.M. Kleinow, and L. Krulisch (Eds.): The Care and Use of Amphibians, Reptiles and Fish in Research. The Scientists Center for Animal Welfare, Bethesda, MD, pp. 75–86.

Harkavy, R. 1993. Mole salamanders — genus *Ambystoma*. Reptile & Amphibian Magazine (Sept/Oct):6–17.

Holick, M.F. 1989. Phylogenetic and evolutionary aspects of vitamin D from phyto-plankton to humans, *in* P.K.T. Pang and M.P. Schreibman (Eds.): Vertebrate Endocrinology: Fundamentals and Biomedical Implications. Vol. 3, Regulation of Calcium and Phosphate. Academic Press, New York, pp. 7–43.

Horseman, N.D., A.H. Meier, and D.D. Culley, Jr. 1976. Daily variations in the effects of disturbance on growth, fattening and metamorphosis in the bullfrog (*Rana catesbeiana*) tadpole. J. Exp. Zool. 198:353–357.

Hunter, L.M. 1989. The Healthy Home. Rodale Press, Emmaus, PA, 313 pp.

Hutchison, V.H. and K.K. Spriestersbach. 1986. Diel and seasonal cycles of activity and behavioral thermoregulation in the salamander *Necturus maculosus*. Copeia 1986(3):612–618.

Jaeger, R.G. 1992. Housing, handling, and nutrition of salamanders, *in* D.O. Schaeffer, K.M. Kleinow, and L. Krulisch (Eds.): The Care and Use of Amphibians, Reptiles and Fish in Research. The Scientists Center for Animal Welfare, Bethesda, MD, pp. 25–29.

Le Berre, F. 1993. Notes on three species of frogs of the genus *Mantella*. The Vivarium 4(6):19–22.

Maruska, E.J. 1994. Procedures for setting up and maintaining a salamander colony, *in* J.B. Murphy, K. Adler, and J.T. Collins (Eds.): Captive Management and Conservation of Amphibians and Reptiles. Society for the Study of Amphibians and Reptiles, St. Louis, MO, pp. 229–242.

Masters, C.O. 1975. Encyclopedia of Live Foods. TFH Publications, Inc., Neptune City, NJ.

Mattison, C. 1987. Frogs and Toads of the World. Facts on File, Inc., New York, 191 pp.

Mattison, C. 1993a. The Care of Reptiles and Amphibians in Captivity. Sterling Publishing Co., Inc., New York, 317 pp.

Mattison, C. 1993b. Keeping and Breeding Amphibians: Caecilians, Newts, Salamanders, Frogs and Toads. Blandford, London, UK, 222 pp.

Messonnier, S.P. 1995. Incorrect ultraviolet light usage. Bulletin of the Association of Reptilian and Amphibian Veterinarians 5(3):4.

Murphy, J.B., K. Adler, and J.T. Collins (Eds.). 1994. Captive Management and Conservation of Amphibians and Reptiles. Society for the Study of Amphibians and Reptiles, St. Louis, MO, 408 pp.

National Research Council. 1974. Amphibians: Guidelines for the Breeding, Care, and Management of Laboratory Animals. National Academy of Sciences, Washington, DC, 153 pp.

Nautical Almanac Office, US Naval Observatory. 1999. Astronomical Almanac 2000. Government Printing Office, Washington, DC.

O'Reilly, J., D. Fenolio and M. Ready. 1995. Limbless amphibians: Caecilians. The Vivarium 7(1):26–54.

Pinkham, M.E. and P. Higgenbotham. 1976. The Best of Helpful Hints. Mary Ellen Enterprises, Minneapolis, MN, 95 pp.

Pough, F.H. 1992. Setting Guidelines for the Care of Reptiles, Amphibians and Fishes, in D.O. Schaeffer, K.M. Kleinow, and L. Krulisch (Eds.): The Care and Use of Amphibians, Reptiles and Fish in Research. The Scientists Center for Animal Welfare, Bethesda, MD. pp. 7–17.

Raloff, J. 1989. Greenery filters out indoor air pollution. Science News 136(14):212.

Schulte, R. 1980. Froesche und Kroeten. Eugen Ulmer GmbH, Stuttgart, Germany, 240 pp.

Seymour, R.S. 1972. Behavioral thermoregulation by juvenile green toads, *Bufo debilis*. Copeia 1972(2):572–575.

Sievert, L.M. and V.H. Hutchison. 1991. The influence of photoperiod and position of a light source on behavioral thermoregulation in *Crotaphytus collaris* (Squamata: Iguanidae). Copeia 1991(1):105–110.

Slavens, F.L. and K. Slavens. 1998. Reptiles and Amphibians in Captivity: Breeding - Longevity and Inventory Current January 1, 1998. Woodland Park Zoological Gardens, Seattle, WA, 423 pp.

St. Lezin, M.A. 1983. Phylogenetic Occurrence of Vitamin D and Provitamin D Sterols. M.S. Dissertation, MIT Press, Cambridge, MA.

Staniszewski, M. 1995. Amphibians in Captivity. TFH Publications, Inc., Neptune City, NJ, 544 pp.

Staniszewski, M. 1996. The maintenance and breeding of Banded Newts in captivity. Reptile & Amphibian Magazine (May–June):46–54.

Stebbins, R.C. and N.W. Cohen. 1995. A Natural History of Amphibians. Princeton University Press, Princeton, NJ, 316 pp.

Stettler, P.H. 1981. Handbuch der Terrarienkunde: Terrarientypen, Tiere, Pflanzen, Futter. Franckh'sche Verlagshandlung, Stuttgart, Germany, 228pp.

Wake, M.H. 1994. Caecilians (Amphibia: Gymnophiona) in captivity, in J.B. Murphy, K. Adler, and J.T. Collins (Eds.): Captive Management and Conservation of Amphibians and Reptiles. Society for the Study of Amphibians and Reptiles, St. Louis, MO, pp. 223–228.

WeatherDisc Associates. 1995. The World WeatherDisc. Computer disc produced biannually by WeathDisc Associates, Seattle, WA.

Webb, G.R. 1994. The Mole Salamander, *Ambystoma talpoideum*: An Ideal Aquarium Species. Reptile & Amphibian Magazine (Jan/Feb):71–79.

Whitaker, B.R. 1993. The use of polyvinyl chloride glues and their potential toxicity to amphibians. 1993 Proceedings of the American Association of Zoo Veterinarians, pp. 16–18.

Wisniewski, P.J. 1986. Substrate and tadpole survival in *Euproctus a. asper*. British Herpetological Society Bulletin 18:19.

Wright, K. 1993. Disinfection for the herpetoculturist. The Vivarium 5(1):31–33.

Wright, K. 1994. The importance of rain chambers in herpetoculture. The Vivarium 6(1):38–40.

Zimmerman, E. 1986. Breeding Terrarium Animals: Amphibians and Reptiles. Care, Behavior, Reproduction. TFH Publications, Inc., Neptune City, NJ, 384 pp.

Zug, G.R. 1993. Herpetology: An Introductory Biology of Amphibians and Reptiles. Academic Press, Inc., San Diego, CA, 527 pp.

CHAPTER 6
DIETS FOR CAPTIVE AMPHIBIANS

Kevin M. Wright, DVM

6.1 INTRODUCTION

Larval and adult amphibians consume very different diets in the wild than offered in captivity, and undoubtedly that is the etiology of many of the nutritional diseases known in captive amphibians. The prey species consumed in the wild is known for few species of amphibians, and from very small sample sizes of those species studied (e.g., Cornish et al., 1995; DeBruyn et al., 1996; Duellman & Lizana, 1994; Evans & Lampo, 1996; Tocque et al., 1995). The nutrient composition of many actual or potential prey species are either incompletely studied (e.g., Reichle et al., 1969) or virtually unknown—it is not feasible to scientifically formulate diets for captive amphibians based on the fieldwork done thus far. Analyses of species of some of the invertebrates and vertebrates used as food items have been compiled and reported (e.g., Dierenfeld & Barker, 1995), however these analyses are incomplete with regard to the levels of vitamin D_3 and other nutrients. When one considers the controversies that exist in the well-documented field of human nutrition, the long term suitability of a diet described for captive amphibians is difficult to assess. Fortunately many of the species commonly held in captivity adapt well to readily available food items, which may indeed be the reason why these species are common in captivity. Multigenerational breeding by more than one captive population is one of the few objective measures of success for a diet, and has occurred in only a few species (e.g., White's treefrog, *Pelodryas caerulea*, the green and black poison dart frog, *Dendrobates auratus*, the dyeing poison frog, *D. tinctorius*, the African clawed frog, *Xenopus laevis*, the Cayenne caecilian, *Typhlonectes compressicauda*, and the axolotl, *Ambystoma mexicanum*). Extensive field research and analysis of the nutrient composition of prey items and gastrointestinal contents is needed if the discipline of captive amphibian nutrition is ever to become a hard science.

6.2 LARVAL AMPHIBIANS

The diets fed to larval salamanders and neonatal caecilians are generally similar to those fed adults, although the items must be smaller in size. Tadpoles, however, may have diets radically different from adult anurans, for while adults are carnivorous many anuran species have tadpoles that are herbivorous or filter feeders. The tadpoles of some dendrobatids (e.g., strawberry poison dart frog, *Dendrobates pumilio*) are obligatorily oophagous and consume infertile eggs laid by their mother (Figure 6.1). According to one classification system based on the arrangement of the mouth and opercula, there are at least five types of anuran tadpoles (Duellman & Trueb, 1986; Orton, 1953; Sokol, 1975), and this oral structure is linked to the dietary preference. Some larval amphibians may have different morphologies depending on food availability, and may become cannibalistic in times of food shortages. This has been noted in the Plains spadefoot toad, *Spea bombifrons*, where some tadpoles have the typical scraping mouthpart while others develop an enlarged beak and jaw muscles and become predatory feeding on tadpoles (Bragg, 1965; Orton, 1954). A similar morphological range is noted in some populations of the tiger salamander, *Ambystoma tigrinum*. Some larvae develop much larger heads (and consequent mouth gape) and longer teeth than others and become cannibalistic (Rose & Armentrout, 1976). It is essential that one understand the life cycle of an anuran species when choosing a diet to feed the tadpole, or else malnutrition will result.

Carnivorous tadpoles, larval salamanders, and neonatal caecilians can be reared using a variety of whole and chopped invertebrates and vertebrates. Newly hatched larvae may be so small that fresh zooplankton netted from an unpolluted natural water source may be needed to establish feeding (e.g., Baker, 1988), although once they have reached a larger size other items can be used. Cultured protozoa (e.g., *Paramecium* spp.) and small crustaceans (e.g., *Cy-*

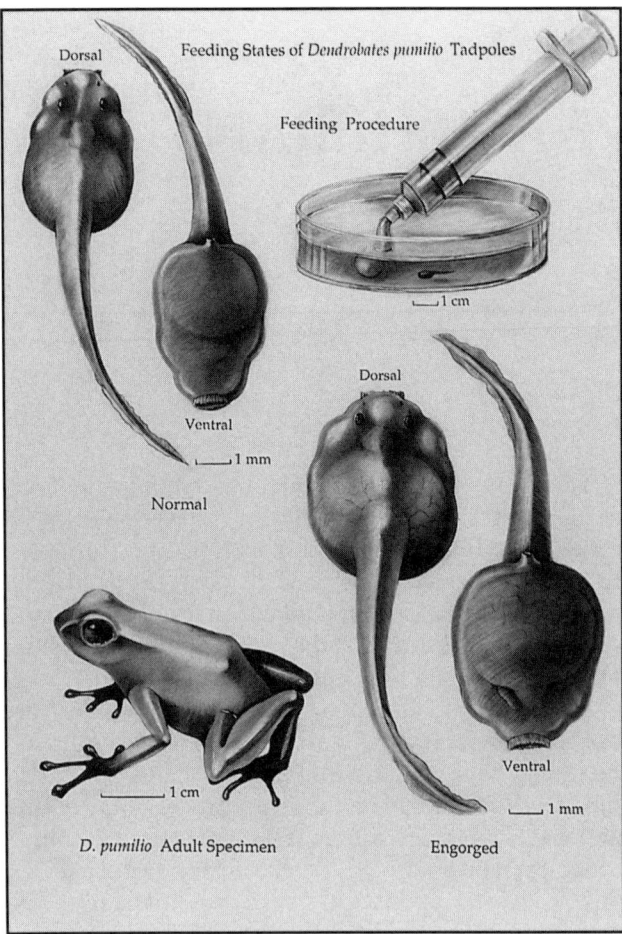

Figure 6.1. Obligatory oophagous tadpoles, such as the strawberry poison frog, *Dendrobates pumilio*, engorge themselves during feeding. Unfortunately attempts to rear these tadpoles on artificial diets as depicted here have met with minimal success (Heselhaus, 1992). (Caitlin Hughes)

clops spp.) have been used as a food source for small larvae (Wisniewski & Paull, 1983). Cultured rotifers are used extensively in raising fish fry and can be used as a food for larval salamanders. Other small crustaceans (e.g., *Daphnia* spp., newly hatched brine shrimp, *Artemia salina*) can be cultured as food sources. Once the larvae have reached an appropriate size, generally over 10 mm (0.4 in) in length, larger food items may be offered. Some larvae have large enough mouths upon hatching to immediately take these larger food items. Small earthworms or chopped adult earthworms, bloodworms, glassworms, white worms, black worms, tubifex worms, mosquito larvae, small live freshwater fish, and chopped whole freshwater fish can be offered. Some larvae may learn to accept extruded, pelleted, or flake food designed for fish or reptiles (Baker, 1988). It is suggested that several different items are offered in the course of a week so that a varied diet can be consumed by the larvae. It should be noted that frozen zooplankton and other invertebrate food items are packaged and sold as fish food and are readily available at most pet stores that sell fish and fish supplies. The clinician is advised to determine local sources for these food items so that the client can quickly acquire food when the need arises.

Omnivorous tadpoles can be fed brands of flaked or pelleted food designed for omnivorous fish. The problem with many fish foods is that as the food particle size gets smaller, it has an increasing surface area-to-volume ratio which in turn increases the rate of leaching of water soluble nutrients. At least one study has documented that there is significant leaching of the water soluble vitamins from flaked foods, with up to a 90% reduction in cyanocobalamin (B_{12}) within 30 seconds of immersion in water (Pannevis & Earle, 1994). This loss of B vitamins appears responsible, at least in part, for the development of scoliosis, spindly leg, and paralysis of developing anurans. (See also Sections 7.8, Scoliosis; 7.9, Spindly Leg; 7.10, Paralysis; 18.1, Spindly Leg.) To minimize the loss of important nutrients, feed schedules should occur so that food is consumed immediately. Tadpoles that feed at the surface may be offered floating foods, while bottom feeding tadpoles may be offered sinking foods. It is often helpful to have live aquatic vegetation and (green) algae present in the water of omnivorous (and herbivorous) tadpoles as an alternate food source. One study documented the faster growth rate of tadpoles raised in a tank containing live algae, diatoms, and commercial food and supports the important role of good algal growth in tadpole growth (Kupferberg et al., 1994). Food items suggested for carnivorous larvae may be offered sparingly to omnivores.

Herbivorous tadpoles can be fed flaked fish foods designed for herbivorous fish. Spirulina tablets are often used as a supplement to this diet with herbivorous tadpoles. As already mentioned, the presence of live aquatic vegetation and algae is suggested for good tadpole growth (Kupferberg et al., 1994). Blanched or microwaved romaine lettuce or other heat-treated greens can be offered in addition to the aquatic vegetation, but the produce should be replaced daily. Proper heat treatment of produce does not degrade the vitamins while it breaks down the structure so the tadpoles can easily graze upon it. Oxalate-containing vegetables such as kale and spinach are to be avoided as a food source to prevent renal disease from oxalate accumulation (National Research Council, 1974). Decorative plants such as the silver queen, *Aglaonema roebelinii*, may also contain calcium oxalate. Oxalate-containing plants should be considered a potential hazard due to the development of renal disease in some frogs at the National Aquarium in Baltimore held in enclosures containing silver queen, *A. roebelinii* (see Section 7.5, Renal Calculi).

Microencapsulated foods designed for filter-feeding invertebrates and fish fry have been used with some detritivorous tadpoles. However, better growth rates may be achieved by rearing the tadpoles in a tank containing a combination of algae, diatoms, and artificial food (Kupferberg, 1994).

There have been some studies documenting the effect of diet on growth of larvae and metamorphosis into normal adults (reviewed by Kaltenbach & Hagedorn, 1981), but a formula for success for a given species is still elusive. The efficacy of any diet is determined solely by trial and error, and evaluating the efficacy is incumbent upon standardization of other parameters such as water quality and temperature. Water quality should always be evaluated if growth rates of larvae are not optimal or if abnormalities of growth (i.e., delayed development) are noted. Furthermore, there may exist significant differences between the morphology, development, and behavior of the larvae of subspecies and geographic races within a single species (Wisniewski, 1992), and these differences may be erroneously interpreted as nutritionally related rather than having a genetic basis. The effects of crowding or isolation, wherein the population density of the larvae within a tank is less than optimal, can also influence growth rates (Woodward, 1987), as can lack of appropriate cage furnishings (Wisniewski & Paull, 1983). Inappropriate lighting may influence growth rates (Rugh, 1935), although this has received little attention since early studies. The frequency and predictability of cage servicing and feeding may delay metamorphosis and have other physiological effects, as was noted with the bullfrog, *Rana catesbeiana*, (Horseman et al., 1976). Some researchers have suggested that there are other growth inhibition agents that affect tadpole development, and the existence and exact nature of these agents have been debated (Beebee, 1995; Petranka, 1995). All these items must be considered whenever there appears to be a failure in development of larvae in order to determine if there is indeed a nutritional link.

Scoliosis and 100% mortality occurred in captive bred tadpoles of a phyllomedusine frog, *Phyllomedusa* cf *tarsius*, at the National Aquarium in Baltimore (B. Whitaker, personal communication, 1996), and high mortality from spindly leg was noted in the tadpoles of several species of dendrobatid frog (*Epipedobates* spp., *Dendrobates* spp., *Phyllobates* spp.). Successful rearing was achieved when vitamin B complex (Vitamin B Complex, VEDCO, Inc., St. Joseph, MO) was added to the tank water at a dose of 0.5 to 1 ml per gallon of tank water. One ml of this product contains 12.5 mg thiamine, 2 mg riboflavin, 5 mg pyridoxine hydrochloride, 12.5 mg niacinamide, 10 mg d-panthenol, and 5 µg cyanocobalamin. New water used for water changes was supplemented at this level, and water changes occurred twice weekly. However, there was greater growth of algae in the supplemented tank than unsupplemented tanks, so the mechanism by which normal maturation occurred is unclear. Young specimens of the phantasmal poison frog, *Epipedobates tricolor*, were especially prone to spindly leg unless this rearing regimen was used. However, adding this vitamin complex to the water used at the Philadelphia Zoo did not prevent spindly leg in this species. The uncertainties associated with the B vitamin complex supplementation emphasizes the difficulty in evaluating larval diets for amphibians.

6.3 ADULT AQUATIC AMPHIBIANS

Invertebrates make up the bulk of the natural diet of most species of aquatic amphibians, whether they are frogs, salamanders, or caecilians, and generally they accept very similar diets in captivity. There are some species of aquatic amphibians that are specialists and feed on only one or a few types of prey in the wild, but many of these adapt to a different diet in captivity. Some species of aquatic caecilians, such as the Cayenne caecilian, *Typhlonectes compressicauda*, have been kept and bred over multiple generations on a diet consisting primarily of earthworms. Aquatic salamanders such as the axolotl, *Ambystoma mexicanum*, and the red-spotted newt, *Notophthalmus viridescens*, generally accept whole or chopped annelid worms as well as other whole or chopped invertebrates. Earthworms, *Lumbricus* spp., bloodworms (midge larvae, family Chironomidae), black worms, *Lumbriculus variegatus*, tubifex worms, *Tubifex tubifex*, white worms, *Enchytraeus* spp., glassworms, washed brine shrimp, *Artemia salina*, water fleas, *Daphnia* spp. and *Cyclops* spp., grass shrimp, *Palaemonetes* spp., crayfish, springtails, *Collembola* spp., flour beetles and larvae, *Tribolium confusum*, newly molted mealworm larvae, *Tenebrio molitor*, crickets, wax worms (larvae of either *Galleria mellonella* or *Achroia grisella*) and fly larvae and wingless adult flies (*Musca* spp. or *Drosophila* spp.) are commercially available invertebrates that can be used as elements of the diet for captive salamanders. Feeder fish (e.g., guppy, platy, goldfish, and loach) can be offered to the larger aquatic amphibians, as can many of the smaller freshwater fish, such as whole smelt.

Live moving prey is accepted more eagerly than dead stationary prey, but most aquatic amphibians will learn to accept dead prey. Many caecilians, salamanders, and frogs will learn to accept food offered on forceps or impaled on the tip of a broom straw, while others remain timid and reluctant to feed in the presence of humans. An amphibian that learns to accept dead prey is easily fed, since frozen invertebrates and vertebrates are packaged and sold as fish food and are readily available at most pet stores that sell fish and fish supplies. A change in appetite, either gradual or sudden, is often the first clue to an amphibian's health, so hand feeding is encouraged for it allows the caregiver to keep track of the amphibian's appetite.

Live food is also available through most pet and bait stores, but may only be available seasonally. The clinician is advised to determine local sources for these food items so that the client can quickly acquire food when the need arises. These commercially available prey items can be supplemented with invertebrates that can be collected in the field. Small insects, sometimes referred to as meadow plankton, can be harvested with a sweep net brushed through tall grasses and light shrubs. Slugs, small grasshoppers, mosquito larvae, and other invertebrates are relished by many aquatic amphibians. Wild-collected food items are not without hazards however, for these items may be contaminated with pesticides and other harmful compounds and may be an intermediate host for parasites affecting amphibians. Mosquito larvae and other aquatic invertebrates can be collected from natural water sources, but may serve as a vector for infectious diseases.

Care should be taken to screen aquatic prey items to avoid introducing pathogens such as ectoparasitic protozoa. A 10- or 20-gallon glass tank can be used for quarantine holding of live food items, and a program to remove parasites instituted. A safe and simple treatment to reduce the numbers of ectoparasites on aquatic invertebrates is immersion in a saltwater bath (25 g sea salt/L water). Different species of invertebrates can tolerate different lengths of time immersed in a salt bath, and should be monitored for signs of distress to a maximum time of 60 minutes. Fish can be treated similarly using either sea salts or a formaldehyde treatment (0.4 ml 37% formaldehyde/L water) can be used. All prey items should be thoroughly rinsed with fresh water following treatment, and allowed several hours in the quarantine tank before being used as amphibian food. Prophylaxis of bacterial disease may lead to the development of resistant strains of pathogenic bacteria and is not recommended for food items. If the items were collected from an unsanitary area or raised in an unsanitary manner, they should not be used as a food source for amphibians. Equal care should be given to screening frozen fish offered to amphibians, for *Aeromonas salmonicida* was introduced into a colony of the African clawed frog, *Xenopus laevis*, through contaminated food fish (Frye, 1989).

Some aquatic frogs and salamanders may learn to eat pelleted foods, displaying an individual preference for either floating or sinking pellets. It is important to remember that many of the fish foods are geared toward omnivorous fish and are not designed to be used as a diet for carnivorous vertebrates. Even the pelleted turtle diets are geared toward an omnivore rather than a strict carnivore. These omnivore diets may not meet the protein, fat, and fat-soluble vitamin needs of the carnivorous adult salamander or frog. Amphibians that receive a large portion of their calories from artificial diets may develop a variety of health problems, such as hydrocoelom from protein deficiency and skin lesions from fat deficiencies. Depending on the levels of fat and fat soluble vitamins in the food, disease from either vitamin D deficiency or toxicity might develop.

6.4 TERRESTRIAL AMPHIBIANS

The majority of terrestrial amphibians prey primarily on invertebrates. The prey items suggested for aquatic amphibians can also be offered to terrestrial amphibians, although as a rule most terrestrial amphibians are reluctant to accept any pelleted diets. There are some specialist feeders that are extremely reluctant to feed on the prey items commonly offered in captivity, and some species (e.g., Surinam horned frog, *Ceratophrys cornuta*) must be given assistance in feeding for prolonged periods of time (de Vosjoli & Mailloux, 1987).

One study documented improved growth in newly metamorphosed bullfrogs, *Rana catesbeiana*, that were fed a diet of mosquito fish, *Gambusia affinis*, over those frogs fed either crickets, *Acheta domestica*, or earthworms, *Lumbricus* spp. (Modzelewski & Culley, 1974). In addition, the frogs that were fed mosquito fish had no rickets. The study suggested that fish were a superior food source due to their higher calcium content over the nonsupplemented invertebrates. Four other fish species were mentioned in the study as being used to successfully rear bullfrogs, *R. catesbeiana*, including the molly, *Molliensia latipinna*, golden shiner, *Notemigonus crysoleucas*, and two species of sunfish, *Lepomis* spp. Inclusion of fish in a diet consisting of crickets and earthworms showed growth rates similar to that achieved by feeding fish alone. Vitamin D_3 levels of the prey items were undocumented in that study but vitamin D_3 levels have been reported for some fish species consumed by humans (Ensminger et al., 1994; Souci et al., 1989) and are generally adequate to prevent hypovitaminosis D in other vertebrates. A similar study was performed on the Woodhouse toad, *Bufo woodhousei* (Claussen & Layne 1983), and that study concluded that mealworms alone were a better diet than crickets, cabbage loopers, or a combination of the three items.

6.5 RODENTS AS A FOOD SOURCE

Neonatal mice and neonatal rats (pinkies) can be offered on occasion to aquatic and terrestrial amphibians, however one study reported that the levels of vitamin A in these domestic rodents are high (Douglas et al., 1994). If this study is valid, hypervitaminosis A could contribute to the development of metabolic bone disease if mice or rats are used on a regular basis without vitamin D_3 supplementation. (See also Section 7.1, Metabolic Bone Disease, and Toxicological Etiologies—Hypervitaminosis A in Section 27.2.1, Musculoskeletal System.) Given a whole body content of about 27 iu vitamin A/g body weight for rat pinkies (Douglas et al., 1994), a supplement of at least 2.7 iu vitamin D_3/g body weight may be needed to offset the high levels of vitamin A in rat pinkies. However, this supplementation rate has yet to be tested for long-term safety and efficacy in amphibians and may well result in toxicities from the fat-soluble vitamins. To avoid this risk the feeding of rodents to amphibians should be minimized.

6.6 FEEDING PATTERNS

It is important to offer food items at a time that is cued to the activity pattern of the species as well as the individual specimen. Establishment of a regular photoperiod in an enclosure allows the inhabitants to develop appropriate activity patterns. Avoid sudden shifts in the photoperiod as these may disrupt the amphibian's biorhythms and alter its feeding behavior. Diurnally active amphibians, such as dendrobatid frogs, should be offered food in the morning and early afternoon, while nocturnally active amphibians will feed most readily if offered food in the early evening. The lighting of an enclosure may influence an amphibian's activity pattern (Jaeger & Hailman, 1981); thus the illumination should be appropriate to the species. Some nocturnally active snakes show a cycle in foraging activity that corresponds to the phase of the moon and associated illumination intensity (Personal communication, P. Andreadis, 1997), thus a regular fluctuation of the nighttime illumination may prove beneficial to some amphibians. The radiation wavelength of the light source used in an enclosure may also influence the behavior of animals (White et al., 1994), and the light source should be chosen to meet the known needs of the species. Species that are diurnally active but live on the forest floor may not be accustomed to intense lighting and may hide rather than eat if kept under inappropriately high light levels, possibly giving the caretaker the erroneous impression that the species is crepuscular or nocturnal. Erratic behavior is often noted when the light levels or photoperiod is inappropriate.

If food items are offered at inappropriate times (e.g., first thing in the morning for a nocturnally active species), the vitamin and mineral supplementation may not be effective, as the amount dusted onto the prey may be groomed or wiped off, and the contents of the gut may be excreted.

If an amphibian is not hungry, the uneaten prey may in turn consume the amphibian. Crickets are notorious for eating small amphibians or eating wounds on larger amphibians. An amphibian may be hungry and willing to eat, but if too many prey items are present an amphibian may be reluctant to feed due to tactile stimulation of prey items crawling on its body.

The amount of food offered and frequency of feeding depends on the energy budget of the species in question. Small, actively foraging amphibians may need to be fed twice a day to maintain good body weight, whereas large ambush predators may gain excess weight if fed to satiation more often than once or twice a month.

Environmental cues such as temperature and humidity can influence feeding behavior. Body temperatures far below or above the preferred body temperature for a species can make an amphibian reluctant to feed, as can a decrease in total body water such as may be brought about by inappropriately low humidity within an enclosure. Poor water quality caused by an elevated pH or low levels of dissolved oxygen can put an amphibian off feed, and should be evaluated whenever there is a problem feeder.

6.7 VITAMIN AND MINERAL SUPPLEMENTATION

Vitamin and mineral supplementation of captive amphibian diets is done on an empirical basis. There are a tremendous number of supplements marketed for the herpetocultural hobbyist, but the bioavailability of the contents of these supplements as well as the need for the contents in any given species's diet is undocumented.

Most supplementation programs are designed to ensure adequate levels of calcium (i.e., from 0.5% to 1.5% total diet dry matter) and vitamin D_3, as well as a balanced ratio of calcium to phosphorus (i.e., 1.5:1.0). This can be difficult given the inverse calcium-to-phosphorus ratio of many invertebrate species. The earthworm is a notable exception with a positive calcium-to-phosphorus ratio and adequate total levels of calcium (Dierenfeld & Barker, 1995). There are "gut-loading" diets that can be fed to crickets and other insects to increase their total calcium content, a concept that can be traced back to a study that documented the increased calcium content of the mealworm, *Tenebrio molitor*, fed solely vitamin-mineral preparations for 24 hours prior to use as a food for insectivorous animals (Zwart & Rulkens, 1979). When fed solely a diet that contained 11.65% calcium and 0.55% phosphorus (Carnicon®, Trouw Company, Putten, Netherlands), the calcium-to-phosphorus values of mealworms increased from 1:3.7 to 1.38:1 and yielded a final calcium content of 0.84% calcium. Subsequent studies document the differing tolerances of insect species to high-calcium diets, and along the way the term "gut-loading" came into common usage in herpetoculture.

The ideal gut-loading diet for an invertebrate species should result in an active live prey item that has a nutritional composition no lower than 0.5% and no higher than 2% total calcium content (dry matter basis) and a calcium-to-phosphorus ratio of 1.5:1. The wax worm, *Galleria mellonella*, when maintained on a diet of 5.7% calcium, survived over 72 hours, and achieved a calcium content of 0.31% with a calcium-to-phosphorus ratio of 1.29:1 at 72 hours (Strzelewicz et al., 1985) whereas one species of cricket, *Acheta domestica*, could not tolerate a diet in excess of 0.14% calcium for prolonged periods of time (McFarlane, 1991). Commercial gut-loading diets for crickets have calcium levels of up to 8% and cause significant mortality if fed for more than 48 hours.

Gut-loading diets are not balanced diets due to the high levels of calcium present, and are not intended for optimal growth and development of the insects. The gut-loading diets should be placed within the cricket cage no sooner than 48 hours prior to use as an amphibian food source. Either water or slices of fruit (e.g., apple or orange) can be used as a water source concurrent with the gut-loading diet, as the calcium content of the crickets were the same for either source in one study (Trusk & Crissey, 1987). Crickets given no access to moisture die within hours if fed the gut-loading diet. Given a diet containing 8% calcium, crickets achieved a dry matter calcium content of 1.3% (Allen, 1983; Allen & Oftedal, 1989; Allen et al., 1993). The crickets will begin to excrete their high-calcium ingesta almost immediately, so only as many insects as will be consumed by the amphibian within 2–4 hours should be offered.

It is noted that adults of the Cuban treefrog, *Osteopilus septentrionalis*, maintained adequate total body calcium levels while on either a high-calcium diet (i.e., crickets containing 1.26% Ca and 0.89% P) or a low-calcium diet (i.e., 0.23% Ca and 0.82% P) (Allen, 1983; Allen et al., 1993). No significant differences were noted in total body calcium, phosphorus, or in radiographic appearance between frogs raised on either diet. The frogs' overall body calcium declined by 25% during the 7-month study, although it is possible that this decline was due to the frogs' maintenance in deionized water and other factors, such as lack of ultraviolet-B irradiation, inappropriate levels of vitamin D_3, or a normal seasonal fluctuation in calcium. Whether the calcium levels would have been adequate in the face of growth, reproduction, or unusual activity is unknown.

A 5.7% calcium gut-loading diet for the wax worm, *Galleria mellonella*, has been reported (Strzelewicz et al., 1985). It consisted of 12.0 ml honey, 18.9 g high-protein baby cereal (Gerber High Protein Baby Cereal, Gerber Products Company, Remont, MI; this product may no longer be available), 5.7 g calcium carbonate, 10.0 ml glycerol (Glycerine USP 99.5%), and 4.0 ml distilled water. Wax worm larvae should be maintained on this diet for a minimum of 72 hours at 30°C (86°F) in order to achieve a calcium content of 0.31% and a calcium-to-phosphorus ratio of 1.29:1.

An alternative diet for gut-loading crickets and mealworms consists of 20% calcium carbonate powder and 80% nutritionally complete layer chicken mash (Dierenfeld & Barker, 1995). This diet has a final calcium content of 8%.

Crickets may eat less in the final weeks of their life, so gut-loading may be less effective for older crickets. This may hold true for other insects as well.

A small amount of powdered supplement can be placed into a container, and prey items can be shaken in the container to become thoroughly coated with the supplement. This technique is known as dusting and is based on the assumption that finely ground vitamin-mineral powders adhere to prey items, which in turn bolsters the prey's intrinsic nutritional value. Dusting is usually used with small prey items such as fruit flies and pinhead crickets for which gut-loading diets are lethal or impractical. Dusting does itself significantly decrease the life span of very small insects and should only be done immediately prior to feeding out the insects. It is generally assumed that these smaller insects have inverse calcium-to-phosphorus ratios and thus require dusting; however, one study suggests that this may not be a valid assumption as pinhead crickets had an average dry matter calcium of 2.1% (Dierenfeld & Barker, 1995). If this analysis of pinhead cricket calcium content holds true (i.e., pinhead crickets are truly a high-calcium food), then dusting pinhead crickets may have had little to do with the successes of rearing small amphibians.

One study failed to achieve a positive calcium-to-phosphorus ratio in adult crickets (unknown species) using a dust that contained 11% calcium and 3.2% phosphorus (Trusk & Crissey, 1987). The highest calcium-to-phosphorus ratio achieved was 0.18:1 within

5 minutes of dusting, and this tapered off to 0.15:1 within 3 hours. As with gut-loading, it is suggested that no more insects be offered than can be consumed within a few hours to maximize the calcium gain achieved by dusting. Pure calcium carbonate or other nonphosphorus forms of calcium should be the calcium source for any mineral supplement to offset the inverse calcium-to-phosphorus ratio of most prey species.

The benefits of dusting with regard to improving the vitamin content of prey species appears to be undocumented. There are a variety of vitamin-mineral supplements marketed for amphibians and reptiles; however, full-spectrum human vitamin-mineral supplements are cheap, readily available products that can be used for dusting if one is willing to grind the tablets into a fine powder. The bioavailability of the human products may actually be better than those marketed specifically for amphibians and reptiles (Donoghue & Langenberg, 1996). One is cautioned to review the label of any vitamin, pet or human, prior to purchase, as substitutions and reformulations frequently occur. As an example, in many human formulations vitamin D_3 has been replaced recently with vitamin D_2.

It is noted that further studies are needed to validate the conclusions of one dusting study (Trusk & Crissey, 1987). If dusting achieves much lower levels of supplementation than does gut-loading, then the recommendations for supplementation of invertebrate prey may change. Currently it is recommended that small insects, such as fruit flies, pinhead crickets, and houseflies, should be dusted with a vitamin-mineral mix prior to being fed to young growing amphibians. Adult amphibians may do well on a schedule with prey insects dusted from 1 to 3 feedings a week.

Vertebrate prey rarely need additional supplementation in this manner (but see Section 6.5, Rodents as a Food Source), although frozen whole fish may need additional thiamine to offset thiaminase activity. (See Section 7.3, Thiamine Deficiency.) If only muscle portions of fish are used, supplementation is recommended to offset calcium, vitamin A, vitamin D, and iodine imbalance of the muscle meat.

6.8 RECORDING THE DIET

It is extremely important to keep accurate records of the diet fed to captive amphibians, as many disorders seen in captivity are first revealed by changes in their appetite or may have an underlying nutritional etiology. The actual design of the record depends on both the caregiver and the amphibians in the collection. Ideally the records should be easy to maintain, concise, and accurate. At a minimum the date and time of feeding and the amount of each type of food item offered should be recorded, along with the exact brand name and amounts of any vitamin-mineral supplements that are used. If gut-loading diets are used for invertebrates, the brand name of the diet and lot number should be recorded on the feed record. If commercially prepared foods such as flaked fish food or pelleted feeds are offered to amphibians, the brand name and lot number should be recorded. Weight records should be a part of the feed record so that any apparent weight gain or loss in an amphibian can be objectively evaluated.

6.9 DERMATOPHAGY

Dermatophagy, the act of consuming shed skin, occurs in all three orders of Amphibia (Weldon et al., 1993) (Plates 6.1, 6.2). The reason for this process is unknown, but recapture of critical nutrients and predator avoidance have been proposed.

6.10 CULTURING FOOD ITEMS

6.10.1 Introduction

Although rodents and many invertebrates can be purchased from commercial suppliers, shortfalls in distribution can occur during inclement weather, thus many herpetoculturists maintain small colonies of insects and rodents to ensure a steady supply of food for their amphibians. Further details of cultivation of food items are available elsewhere (e.g., Andrews, 1986; Frye, 1991; Jaycox, 1971; Martin et al., 1976; Mason, 1994; Masters, 1975; Mattison, 1982; Obst et al., 1988; Zimmerman, 1986). In addition to the amphibian and reptile literature, tropical fish magazines and other newsletters often have detailed articles about culturing live food items that are suitable for amphibians. Following is brief overview of the culturing of some of the invertebrate species readily maintained in the average home.

It is difficult to estimate how many food item colonies are needed to maintain a collection, but most shortages occur when attempting to rear amphibian metamorphs. In order to avoid shortages, as a general rule one sweaterbox-sized thriving colony of springtails should be available for each newly metamorphosed small anuran or salamander. A similar sized colony of white worms should be maintained for slightly larger salamanders.

6.10.2 White worms

The white worm, *Enchytraeus albidus*, is an annelid worm of the family Enchytraeidae. White worms can be raised in a lidded dark plastic container (e.g., shoebox). Ventilation holes are not required, but if present should be covered with foam or fine mesh screen to prevent infestation with parasitic mites or flies. Moist potting soil and peat moss should fill the container to within a few inches of the top. A quantity of white worms can be introduced to this container. White worms should be cultured at temperatures between 7 and 20°C (45° and 68°F), but do best at the lower end of this range. Oatmeal, white bread that has been soaked in milk or aged tap water, tropical fish food flakes, and vegetables should be placed on top of the soil on a regular basis. Water should be sprayed into the culture as needed to keep soil moist. Feed sparingly and remove food before it spoils.

6.10.3 Red worms

The annelid red worm, *Lumbricus rubellus,* can be cultured in the manner of the white worm, *Enchytraeus albidus,* but requires warmer temperatures in the range of 16–20°C (60°–68°F). Burlap or cardboard should be laid on top of the soil to provide hiding spaces. Cricket chow, trout chow, cornmeal, oatmeal, and vegetables should be placed underneath the burlap or cardboard but on top of the soil on a regular basis. Water should be sprayed into the culture as needed to keep soil moist. Feed sparingly and remove food before it spoils.

6.10.4 Springtails

Springtails are tiny primitive insects of the order Collembola that are natural prey items of many amphibians throughout the world. Springtails are easy to culture and the adults rarely exceed 3 mm in length. Springtails can be raised in a lidded, clear plastic container (e.g., shoebox or sweaterbox). Ventilation holes are not required, but if present should be covered with foam or fine mesh screen to prevent infestation with parasitic mites or flies. Moist potting soil free of surfactants, antifungal agents, and fertilizers should fill the container to within 2 inches of the top. A quantity of springtails can be introduced to this container. Springtails can be cultured at temperatures between 20 and 27°C (68° and 80°F). Flaked fish food can be fed on a regular basis and water sprayed into the culture as needed to keep soil moist. It generally takes a month or more for a new colony to produce enough for harvesting. A minimum of one sweaterbox-sized colony of springtails should be maintained for each small salamander or anuran. Colonies of springtails have also been maintained on damp gravel with a small amount of moist potting soil at one end of the container.

6.10.5 Flour beetles

Flour beetles, *Tribolium* spp., are small insects that are relatives of the common mealworm, *Tenebrio molitor.* Flour beetles are available from many biological supply houses or can be obtained from infested grain items. The generation time and number of eggs produced varies between species of flour beetles, but generally a colony of the confused flour beetle, *Tribolium confusum,* is thriving within 60 days of founding if maintained at temperatures between 24 and 28°C (75 and 82°F). Flour beetles can be maintained in a lidded, clear plastic container (e.g., shoebox) that is well aerated. Ventilation holes should be plugged with cotton or foam or otherwise screened to prevent invasion by pests such as mites. Excess humidity can quickly kill a flour beetle colony. The substrate can be just the food items used. Commercial cricket diets (not gut-loading diets) can be used to maintain colonies of flour beetles, as can pelleted trout chow, dog food, monkey biscuit, and rodent blocks. The substrate should be kept dry and free of mold. Small wedges of apples or oranges or a moist cotton ball need to be placed within the colony on a daily basis to provide water for the beetles. The fruit or cotton should be placed on a small plastic bottle cap to prevent molding of the substrate. Either adult or larval beetles can be offered as food. New colonies should be started from colonies less than 60 days old.

6.10.6 Mealworms

The common mealworm, *Tenebrio molitor,* is easily maintained in the average household. The chitinous exoskeleton of mealworm larvae limits its use as a food item. Many amphibians swallow their prey whole, and mealworms may appear nearly whole in feces if the exoskeleton was not sufficiently crushed and pierced by the mouth of the amphibian. This problem is not apparent when using newly moulted mealworm larvae, which appear pale white beside the hardened exoskeleton of other larvae. If hard-shelled larvae are to be used, the exoskeleton should be slit with a razor prior to feeding to ensure the penetration of stomach acid and digestive enzymes. The head of the mealworm larvae may also be crushed prior to feeding to minimize the risk of injury to the amphibian's stomach caused by the mealworm's escape attempts after ingestion.

There are many possible methods of rearing mealworms, but this author has used the following simple system with great success. Mealworms can be maintained in a lidded, clear plastic container (e.g., sweaterbox) that is well aerated. Ventilation holes should be plugged with cotton or foam or otherwise screened to prevent invasion by pests, such as mites. Excess humidity can quickly kill a mealworm colony. Dry sphagnum moss works well as a substrate, and will become finely powdered by the action of the mealworms. Low-fat monkey biscuits (e.g., Zupreem® monkey biscuits) are used as a food source and are constantly available on the surface of the moss. Slices of apple or potato are placed on the surface of the moss and replaced as needed to provide moisture. Additional moss is added as needed. New colonies should be started from colonies that are less than 60 days old.

6.10.7 Fruit flies

Fruit flies (*Drosophila melanogaster, D. hiedii*) are easily maintained using either commercially available media (Carolina Biological Supply, Burlington, NC) or on homemade media. One formula consists of a volume of 1 part brewer's yeast to 10 parts instant potato flakes, which is then mixed with an equal volume of dechlorinated water (Waddle, 1996). A mold inhibitor (e.g., tegosept at 4 g/gal water) can be added to the water used for the mix. Wadded paper towels or cotton gauze can be placed into the mix to prevent the media from getting too liquid (from the growth of the fruit fly larvae). Colonies do best if maintained between 24 and 25°C (75 and 77°F), and new colonies are best started from cultures less than 30 days old.

6.11 SOURCES OF LIVE INVERTEBRATES

The advertising section of many of the national herpetoculturally oriented magazines and newsletters of regional herpetological societies list the commercial suppliers of invertebrates and vertebrates for food. Some of the larger established companies are listed below. Inclusion in this list is not to be considered an endorsement of any establishment over any not listed, but is solely provided as a convenience to the reader. These companies were all commercially active providing invertebrates as of 2001.

Armstrong's Cricket Farm, POB 125, West Monroe, LA 71294. (318) 387-6000.
Bassett's Cricket Ranch, Inc. 365 S. Mariposa, Visalia, CA 93292. (800) 634-2445.
Carolina Biological Supply Company, Burlington, NC 27215. (800) 334-5551.
Fluker Farms, Baton Rouge, LA (800) 735-8537.
Grubco, Inc., POB 15001, Hamilton, OH 45015. (800) 222-3563.
Rainbow Mealworms and Crickets, POB 4525, Compton, CA 90220. (310) 635-1494.
Top Hat Cricket Farm, Inc. 1919 Forest Drive, Kalamazoo, MI 49002. (800) 638-2555.
Ward's Natural Science Establishment, 5100 W. Henrietta Road, Rochester, NY 14692. (716) 359-2502.

REFERENCES

Allen, M.E. 1983. Geckos, treefrogs, crickets and calcium. 1983 Proceedings of the American Association of Zoo Veterinarians Annual Conference, pp. 189–191.
Allen, M.E. and O.T. Oftedal. 1989. Dietary manipulation of the calcium content of feed crickets. Journal of Zoo and Wildlife Medicine 20(1):26–33.
Allen, M.E., O.T. Oftedal, and D.E. Ullrey. 1993. Effect of dietary calcium on mineral composition of fox geckos (*Hemidactylus garnoti*) and Cuban treefrogs (*Osteopilus septentrionalis*). Journal of Zoo and Wildlife Medicine 24:118–128.
Andrews, C. 1986. Fish breeding. Salamander Books, London, UK.
Baker, J. 1988. Maintenance and breeding of *Triturus karelini*. British Herpetological Society Bulletin 25:14–15.
Beebee, T.J.C. 1995. Tadpole growth: Is there an interference effect in nature? Herpetological Journal 5:204–205.
Bragg, A.N. 1965. Gnomes of the Night: The Spadefoot Toads. University of Pennsylvania Press, Philadelphia, PA.
Claussen, D.L. and J.R. Layne. 1983. Growth and survival of juvenile toads *Bufo woodhousei*. Journal of Herpetology 17:107–112.
Cornish, C.A., R.S. Oldham, D.J. Bullock, and J.A. Bullock. 1995. Comparison of the diet of adult toads (*Bufo bufo*) with pitfall trap catches. Herpetological Journal 5:236–238.
De Bruyn, L., M. Kazadi, and J. Hulselmans. 1996. Diet of *Xenopus fraseri* (Anura, Pipidae). Journal of Herpetology 30(1):82–85.
de Vosjoli, P. and R. Mailloux. 1987. The husbandry and captive propagation of the Surinam horned frog (*Ceratophrys cornuta*). Northern California Herpetological Society Special Publication #4, pp. 1–10.
Dierenfeld, E.S. and D. Barker. 1995. Nutrient composition of whole prey commonly fed to reptiles and amphibians. 1995 Proceedings of the Association of Reptilian and Amphibian Veterinarians, pp. 3–15.
Donoghue, S. and J. Langenberg. 1996. Nutrition, *in* Mader, D.R. (Ed.): Reptile Medicine and Surgery. W.B. Saunders Co., Philadelphia, PA, pp. 148–174.
Douglas, T.C., M. Pennino, and E.S. Dierenfeld. 1994. Vitamins E and A, and proximate composition of whole mice and rats used as feed. Comp. Biochem. Physiol. 107A (2):419–424.
Duellman, W.E. and M. Lizana. 1994. Biology of a sit-and-wait predator, the leptodactylid frog *Ceratophrys cornuta*. Herpetologica 50(1):51–64.
Duellman, W.E. and L. Trueb. 1986. Larvae, *in* Duellman, W.E., and L. Trueb: Biology of Amphibians. McGraw-Hill Book Co., New York, pp. 141–171.
Ensminger, H.H., M.E. Ensminger, J.E. Konlande, and J.R.K. Robson. 1994. Foods and Nutrition Encyclopedia. 2nd Edition. CRC Press, Boca Raton, FL, 2264 pp.
Evans, M. and M. Lampo. 1996. Diet of *Bufo marinus* in Venezuela. Journal of Herpetology 30(1):73–76.
Frye, F.L. 1989. *Aeromonas* and *Citrobacter* epizootics in an institutional amphibian collection [Abstr.] 3rd International Colloquium on Pathology of Reptiles & Amphibians, 13–15 January 1989, Orlando, FL, pp. 31–32.
Frye, F.L. 1991. Culture of prey species, *in* Frye, F.L.: Captive Invertebrates: A Guide to Their Biology and Husbandry. Krieger Publishing Co., Malabar, FL, pp. 83–97.
Heselhaus, R. 1992. "The genus *Dendrobates*," *in*: Poison-arrow Frogs—Their natural history and captive care. Ralph Curtis Books, Sanibel Island, FL, pp. 56–80.
Horseman, N.D., A.H. Meier, and D.D. Culley, Jr. 1976. Daily variations in the effects of disturbance on growth, fattening and metamorphosis in the bullfrog (*Rana catesbeiana*) tadpole. J. Exp. Zool. 198:353–357.
Jaeger, R.G. and J.P. Hailman. 1981. Activity of neotropical frogs in relation to ambient light. Biotropica 13(1):59–65.
Jaycox, E.R. 1971. Rearing wax moth larvae. Cooperative Extension Service, University of Illinois, Urbana-Champaign. #H-671.
Kaltenbach, J.C. and H.H. Hagedorn. 1981. Effects of nutrition in metamorphosis, *in* Rechcigl, M. (Ed.): CRC Handbook of Nutritional Requirements in a Functional Context. Vol. 1. Development and Conditions of Physiologic Stress. CRC Press, Boca Raton, FL.
Kupferberg, S.J., J.C. Marks, and M.E. Power. 1994. Effects of variation in natural algal and detrital diets on larval anuran (*Hyla regilla*) life-history traits. Copeia 1994(2):446–457.
McFarlane, J.E. 1991. Dietary sodium, potassium and calcium requirements of the house cricket, *Acheta domesticus* (L.). Comp. Biochem. Physiol. 100A:217.
Martin, R.D., J.P.W. Rivers, and U.M. Cowgill. 1976. Culturing mealworms as food for animals in captivity. International Zoo Yearbook 16:63–70.
Mason, W.T. 1994. A review of life histories and culture methods for five common species of Oligochaeta (Annelida). World Aquaculture 25(1):67–75.
Masters, C.O. 1975. Encyclopedia of Live Foods. TFH Publications, Inc., Neptune City, NJ.
Mattison, C. 1982. Foods and feeding, *in* Mattison, C.: The Care of Rep-

tiles and Amphibians in Captivity. Blandford Press, Poole, Great Britain, UK, pp. 50–66.

Modzelewski, E.H. and D.D. Culley, Jr. 1974. Growth responses of the bullfrog *Rana catesbeiana* fed various live foods. Herpetologica 30(4):396–405.

National Research Council. 1974. Amphibians: Guidelines for the Breeding, Care, and Management of Laboratory Animals. National Academy of Sciences, Washington, DC. 153 pp.

Obst, F.J., K. Richter and U. Jacob (Eds.). 1988. The Completely Illustrated Atlas of Reptiles and Amphibians for the Terrarium. TFH Publications, Inc., Neptune City, NJ.

Orton, G.L. 1953. The systematics of vertebrate larvae. Syst. Zool. 2:63–75.

Orton, G.L. 1954. Dimorphism in larval mouthparts in spadefoot toads of the *Scaphiophus hammondi* group. Copeia 1954(1):97–100.

Pannevis, M.C. and K.E. Earle. 1994. Nutrition of ornamental fish: water soluble vitamin leaching and growth of *Paracheirodon innesi*. Journal of Nutrition 124:2633S–2635S.

Petranka, J.W. 1995. Interference competition in tadpoles: Are multiple agents involved? Herpetological Journal 5:206–207.

Reichle, D.E., M.H. Shanks, and D.A. Crossley, Jr. 1969. Calcium, potassium, and sodium content of forest floor arthropods. Ann. Entomol. Soc. Am. 65:57.

Rose, F.L. and D. Armentrout. 1976. Adaptive strategies of *Ambystoma tigrinum* (Green) inhabiting the Llana Estacado of West Texas. Journal of Animal Ecology 45:713–729.

Rugh, R. 1935. The spectral effect on the growth rate of tadpoles. Physiological Zoology 8:186–195.

Souci, S.W., W. Fachman, and H. Kraut. 1989. Food Composition and Nutrition Tables. 3rd Edition. Wissenschaftliche.

Sokol, O.M. 1975. The phylogeny of anuran larvae: a new look. Copeia 1975(1):1–23.

Strzelewicz, M.A., D.E. Ullrey, S.F. Schafer, and J.P. Bacon. 1985. Feeding insectivores: Increasing the calcium content of wax moth (*Galleria mellonella*) larvae. Journal of Zoo Animal Medicine 16:25–27.

Tocque, K., R. Tinsley, and T. Lamb. 1995. Ecological constraints on feeding and growth of *Scaphiopus couchii*. Herpetological Journal 5:257–265.

Trusk, A.M. and S. Crissey. 1987. Comparison of calcium and phosphorus levels in crickets fed a high calcium diet versus those dusted with supplement. Proceedings of the Sixth and Seventh Dr. Scholl's Conferences on the Nutrition of Captive Wild Animals, Seventh Annual Conference, pp. 93–99.

Waddle, F. 1996. Raising fruit flies (letter). Reptiles 4(2):29–30.

Weldon, P.J., B.J. Demeter, and R. Rosscoe. 1993. A survey of shed skin-eating (dermatophagy) in amphibians and reptiles. Journal of Herpetology 27(2):219–228.

White, R.H., R.D. Stevenson, R.R. Bennett, and D.E. Cutler. 1994. Wavelength discrimination and the role of ultraviolet vision in the feeding behavior of hawkmoths. Biotropica 26(4):427–435.

Wisniewski, P.J. 1992. Morphological and behavioral differences between larvae of various races of *Salamandra salamandra*. British Herpetological Society Bulletin 39:26–27.

Wisniewski, P.J. and L.M. Paull. 1983. A note on the captive maintenance of the Pyrenean Mountain salamander (*Euproctus asper asper*) [Duges]. British Herpetological Society Bulletin 6:21.

Woodward, B.D. 1987. Interactions between Woodhouse's toad tadpoles (*Bufo woodhousei*) of mixed sizes. Copeia 1987(2):380–386.

Zimmerman, E. 1986. Keeping and breeding important food animals, *in* Zimmerman, E: Breeding Terrarium Animals. TFH Publications, Inc., Neptune City, NJ, pp. 44–47.

Zwart, P. and R.J. Rulkens. 1979. Improving the calcium content of mealworms. Intl. Zoo Yearbook 19:254–255.

CHAPTER 7
NUTRITIONAL DISORDERS

Kevin M. Wright, DVM and Brent R. Whitaker, MS, DVM

A variety of nutritional problems have been seen in captive amphibians. Zoo curators, veterinarians and nutritionists typically focus on the analysis of nutrients in the diet offered, but the impact of water quality upon the development of these disorders needs to be addressed in the future.

7.1 METABOLIC BONE DISEASE

In our experience, metabolic bone disease is the most commonly recognized nutritionally related disorder of captive amphibians, and was reported as a problem associated with hypervitaminosis A in the African clawed frog, *Xenopus laevis*, 50 years ago (Bruce & Parkes, 1950). Metabolic bone disease is a broad term that does not specify a particular etiology, although common etiologies in amphibians are an imbalance in the ingested dietary levels of calcium, phosphorus, and vitamin D_3, or ingestion of other substances (e.g., fat-soluble vitamins, various minerals, oxalates) that interfere with the absorption, excretion, or utilization of any of these three compounds.

Unlike bony fishes, reptiles, birds, and mammals, amphibians utilize lipoproteins as the transport mechanism for the active vitamin D metabolite 25-hydroxycholecalciferol (Hay & Watson, 1976). This difference in transport mechanisms may have untoward consequences for amphibians consuming diets that contain inappropriate levels and balances of fatty acids and fats, but adequate dietary levels of calcium, phosphorus, and vitamin D_3. This may be a contributing factor in the development of metabolic bone disease in those amphibians fed rodents and other items that are not typically a part of their natural diet.

Recent reviews have demonstrated the comparative paucity of knowledge regarding amphibian calcium metabolism (Bentley, 1984; Boutilier et al., 1992; Larsen, 1992; Shoemaker et al., 1992; Stiffler, 1993). This is a physiological process that has a profound impact on the development and maintenance of normal mineralized skeletons, and the obscurity of this basic process makes treatment of metabolic bone disease less scientific than desirable.

Many of the arthropods and other invertebrates that are cultured for the diets of amphibians have an inverse calcium-to-phosphorus ratio and are considered a calcium deficient food source for vertebrates (Dierenfeld & Barker, 1995). Two methods of offsetting this imbalance are gut-loading and dusting. (See Section 6.7, Vitamin and Mineral Supplementation.) Some of the salient points are worth reiterating here. It is important to feed the insects a properly designed maintenance diet, for a malnourished cricket will result in a malnourished amphibian. The readily available species of domesticated cricket (e.g., *Acheta domestica*) that are used as a staple for many amphibian diets must be carefully managed on a gut-loading diet containing around 8% calcium for 48 h prior to feeding in an attempt to maintain a positive balance of calcium to phosphorus. However, even frogs fed a gut-loaded cricket may continue to lose calcium (Allen & Oftedal, 1989), suggesting that a variety of other factors may influence calcium uptake, distribution, and excretion in the amphibian.

There are commercially available and home-made diets specifically designed to increase the calcium content of insects through a process termed "gut-loading" whereby the gastrointestinal tract of the insect is filled with a high-calcium (5% to 8%) diet. The prey item should have access to the gut-loading diet for up to 48 h prior to its presentation to the amphibian. A significant disadvantage of gut-loading is that many insects cannot survive on a diet containing such high levels of calcium and will die if this diet is the sole source of nutrients beyond a 48-h period. A further problem is that the insect must be eaten soon after ingesting the high-calcium diet or else the ingesta will be voided and the insect will no longer have a positive calcium balance.

Another option to enhance the calcium and vitamin content of ingested prey is to dust the prey item with a mineral-vitamin mix immediately prior to feeding out the item. Pinhead crickets, fruit flies, *Drosophila* spp., and flour beetles, *Triboleum* spp., are commonly fed to small amphibians such as dendrobatid frogs and newly metamorphosed froglets of many species. Unfortunately gut-loading with high-calcium diets seems to kill an insect with a small body mass in a matter of a few hours after ingestion so the method used to enhance the calcium and vitamin D_3 level is to dust the insect with a vitamin-mineral mix. If too many of the insect prey are offered, the mineral-vitamin powder may be groomed off or otherwise lost prior to consumption by the targeted amphibian, and one study suggests that dusting does little to improve the calcium content of the insects (Trusk & Crissey, 1987). Consumption of the undusted insects may promote hypocalcemic conditions. Pinhead crickets may actually have adequate levels of calcium (Dierenfeld & Barker, 1995), but this awaits confirmation. A review of the feeding regimen should resolve the question of how many items are offered at one time, when the food is offered, how many feedings are made in the course of one day, and how quickly all of the items are consumed.

The high levels of vitamin A found in domestic mice and rats (Douglas et al., 1994) may interfere with the absorption and utilization of vitamin D_3. Hypervitaminosis A is a possible etiology of metabolic bone disease in large amphibians (Bruce & Parkes, 1950), and has been suspected as the underlying etiology of metabolic bone disease in several specimens of the ornate horned frog, *Ceratophrys ornata*, maintained on a rodent-based diet at the Philadelphia Zoo. Supplementation of domestic rodents with calcium (e.g., calcium glubionate, Neo-Calglucon syrup, Sandoz Pharmaceuticals, East Hanover, NJ) and vitamin D_3 immediately prior to feeding out is recommended to offset the probable hypervitaminosis A that results from the feeding of commercially available rodent diets. A supplement of 2.7 iu vitamin D_3/g body weight may be needed to offset the high levels of vitamin A in rodents. However, this supplementation rate has yet to be tested for long-term safety and efficacy in amphibians and may well result in toxicities from the fat-soluble vitamins. To avoid this risk the feeding of rodents to amphibians should be restricted.

Metabolic bone disease has been reported in the African clawed frog, *Xenopus laevis,* (Bruce & Parkes, 1950) and the bullfrog, *Rana catesbeiana,* (Modzelewski & Culley, 1974), and has been observed by the authors in many other species, including, but not limited to, Tschudi's African bullfrog, *Pyxicephalus adspersus,* ornate horned frog, *Ceratophrys ornata,* South American bullfrog, *Leptodactylus pentadactylus,* Australian giant frog, *Litoria infrafrenata,* Pine Barren treefrog, *Hyla andersoni,* various bufonids, the axolotl, *Ambystoma mexicanum,* and the mexican caecilian, *Dermophis mexicanus.* Signs suggestive of metabolic bone disease or hypocalcemia include mandibular deformity, abnormal posture with one or more limb splayed, scoliosis, reluctance to move, long bone fracture, tetany, bloating (gastrointestinal gas), hydrops, subcutaneous edema, and gastric, rectal or cloacal prolapse (Plates 7.1, 7.2; Figures 7.1, 7.2, 7.3, 7.4). Confirmation of metabolic bone disease requires radiographic studies. Radiographic features suggestive of metabolic bone disease include abnormally shaped and radiolucent mandibles, thin cortices of long bones, expansion of the marrow cavity, overall loss of bone density, angular limb deformities, and the presence of pathologic fractures (see Figure 7.3). In addition to pathological fractures of the femur and humerus, pelvic luxation, spinal fractures, and coracoid fractures are commonly noted in anurans with metabolic bone disease. In addition to gross mandibular deformity, the one caecilian diagnosed with metabolic bone disease had less radiodense lateral vertebral processes than healthy

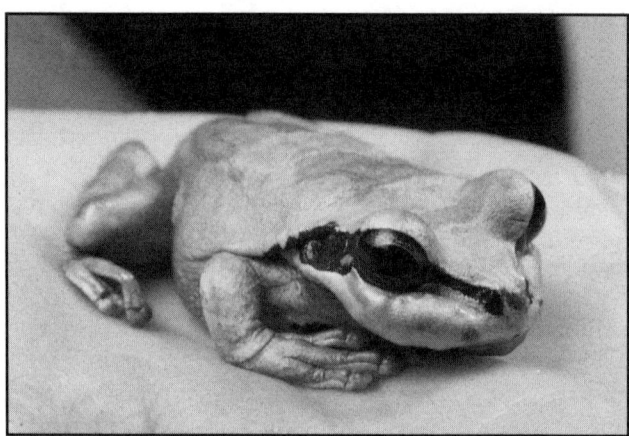

Figure 7.1. New Granada cross-banded frog, *Smiliscus phaeota*, with deformities of the mandible, maxilla, and premaxilla caused by metabolic bone disease. (George Grall, National Aquarium in Baltimore)

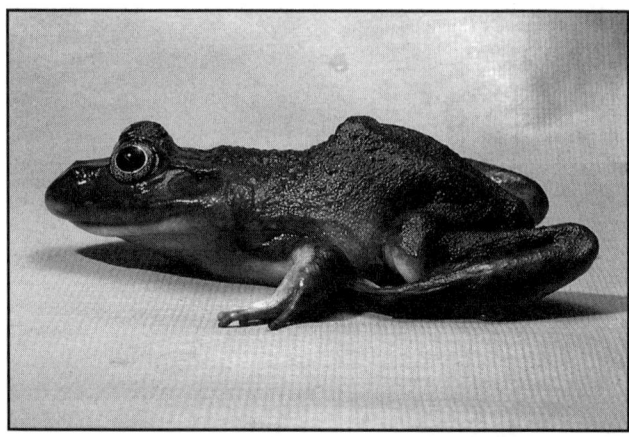

Figure 7.2. Bullfrog, *Rana catesbeiana*, with metabolic bone disease. Due to multiple pathologic fractures, the frog cannot elevate its head and the sacrum is abnormally positioned. (George Grall, National Aquarium in Baltimore)

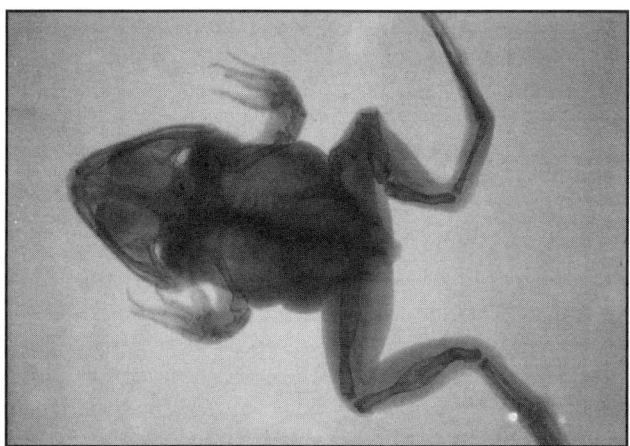

Figure 7.3. Radiograph of the bullfrog, *Rana catesbeiana*, in Figure 7.2. Multiple pathological fractures of the long bones are evident. (George Grall, National Aquarium in Baltimore)

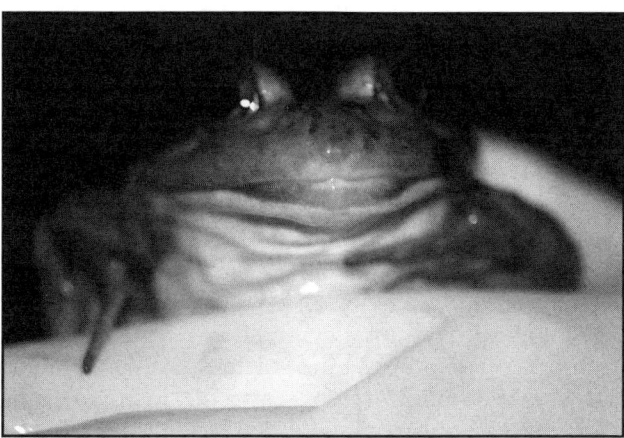

Figure 7.4. Bullfrog, *Rana catesbeiana* with a slight mandibular deformity that may be the first obvious sign of metabolic bone disease. (Kevin Wright, Philadelphia Zoological Garden)

specimens. In young caecilians, it is typical for the caudal vertebrae to be less radiodense than cranial vertebrae since growth occurs by addition of vertebrae caudally. The affected caecilian had markedly less radiodense caudal vertebraes than healthy caecilians. Hypocalcemia and/or hyperphosphatemia may support the diagnosis of metabolic bone disease, especially in adult amphibians, but given the flux typical in amphibian plasma these two ions are often within parameters assumed to be normal for a species.

Treatment of the amphibian with metabolic bone disease can be frustrating. Supplementation with oral calcium and vitamin D_3 is recommended. Calcium glubionate in the form of Neo-Calglucon can be given at 1 ml/kg PO daily, and should be administered for a minimum of 30 days or until bones resume normal density on radiographs. Alternatively, 1- to 2-hour daily baths in 2.3% calcium gluconate may be considered as a treatment for amphibians that are difficult to dose orally. Parenteral calcium (100 mg/kg of 10% calcium gluconate IM, IV, or intracoelomically) is recommended for amphibians showing tetany or gastrointestinal bloating, and may be administered every 4–6 h for up to 24 h. After 24 h of initiating calcium therapy, if tetany has subsided, the amphibian may be given parenteral vitamin D_3 (1000 iu/kg IM). Oral supplementation of vitamin D_3 (High-D 2X Vitamin D_3 Liquid Concentrate, 4,000,000 iu/oz., I.D. Russell Company, Laboratories, Longmount, CO) is suggested at a lower dose (e.g., 100–400 iu/kg) concomitant with oral calcium supplementation. The elucidation of calcitonin's role in amphibians has been problematic (Herman, 1992) and therapeutic regimes modified from those described for the green iguana, *Iguana iguana*, (Mader, 1993) have proven unrewarding in amphibians. Increased dosages of calcitonin (i.e., over 50 iu/kg IM) or a more frequent dosing schedule (i.e., more frequently than every 7 days) may be productive. It is extremely important to continue calcium and vitamin D_3 supplementation until the skeleton structures are radiographically normal, a process which may take 6 weeks or longer. Discontinuing the oral supplements too early will result in continued problems, such as pathologic fractures.

An adjustment of the dietary management of the amphibian should occur concomitant with calcium and vitamin D_3 supplemental therapy. Anamnesis of the feeding regimen is mandated, and instructions regarding the proper care of the feed items as well as proper preparation and presentation of the diet should be distributed. As an example, the contributing factor to the development of metabolic bone disease in a juvenile Mexican caecilian, *Dermophis mexicanus*, appears to have been failure to feed the earthworm colony used as its food source.

The link between ultraviolet radiation and the active metabolites of vitamin D_3 has not been well-documented for amphibians, but is likely to play a role in the development of metabolic bone disease in some species of amphibians. Exposure to ultraviolet-emitting fluorescent bulbs should be considered as adjunct therapy in the treatment of metabolic bone disease in amphibians, unless it has been demonstrated that a particular species of amphibian does not have a need for ultraviolet radiation. The amphibian patient should be provided access to illumination which provides unfiltered ultraviolet-B in the range of 280–310 nm. Several brands of fluorescent bulbs are known to be weak emitters of ultraviolet in these frequencies (Ball, 1995; Bernard, 1995; Gehrmann, 1987, 1992, 1994, 1996). As of this writing, there is a plethora of brand name bulbs that claim to be ultraviolet emitters, and some of the brands have been redesigned to improve their output of ultraviolet radiation. This makes it impossible for us to recommend any particular brand at this time. The clinician is advised to become familiar with the claims of one or more brands and to obtain spectral graphs and irradiance claims from the manufacturer, as well as any independent investigations of the product. Radiometers can be used to quantify the output of either ultraviolet-A (long wave) or ultraviolet-B (short wave) radiation from a bulb (See Gehrmann, 1987, 1992, 1994, 1996). If independent test results are available, that data can be compared to the manufacturer's claims, and the usefulness of that brand of bulb can be better evaluated. It is known that there is a significant decline in the output of some of these bulbs within the first week of use, and a later decline again several months later. Thus the bulbs should be replaced at a minimum of every 6–12 months unless there is evidence to suggest otherwise. The date that a bulb is first used (or date for replacement) should be marked directly on the bulb with an indelible marker to allow rapid assessment of the bulb's lifespan. Incandescent sunlamps are not recommended, nor are any lamps that produce high levels of ultraviolet-A. Many of the metal halide lamps used in maintaining marine invertebrates may prove beneficial with amphibians, but the intensity of the light may be too high for amphibians. If the amphibian shows signs of stress or radiation damage (e.g., corneal opacities, erythema, excess mucus production, etc.), then the ultraviolet light source should be discontinued.

The kidney is the site of the final step in the activation of vitamin D_3 into 1,25-dihydroxycholecalciferol (Baksi et al., 1977), thus renal disease may contribute to the development of metabolic bone disease despite adequate intake of vitamin D_3. Additionally, large amounts of calcium ions filtered from the plasma are reabsorbed from the renal tubules (Stiffler, 1993), and could result in a significant loss of ingested calcium if the transport mechanism is damaged. Renal disease should be suspected whenever there is an apparent failure for an amphibian with metabolic bone disease to respond to appropriate therapy.

7.2 HYPERVITAMINOSIS D_3

There has been one report of a syndrome suggestive of hypervitaminosis D_3 in an anuran (Frye, 1992). Progressive lethargy, anorexia, weakness, hydrops (ascites or anasarca), and edema of the thighs were noted in a young male ornate horned frog, *Ceratophrys ornata*. An acellular coelomic transudate was strongly positive for urea nitrogen suggestive of renal disease. This frog had been fed goldfish that were themselves fed a diet that allowed accumulation of potentially high levels of vitamin D_3. Soft tissue mineralization was noted in the heart and kidneys, and the histopathology was suggestive of hypervitaminosis D_3.

7.3 THIAMINE DEFICIENCY

Aquatic salamanders and frogs, as well as the horned frogs, *Ceratophrys* spp., the bullfrog, *Rana catesbeiana*, and Tschudi's African bullfrog, *Pyxicephalus adspersus*, can be easily trained to accept thawed frozen fish. Thiamine deficiency may be expected in amphibians that are fed a diet consisting primarily of frozen fish containing thiaminase, an enzyme that rapidly inactivates any thiamine present. Thiaminase is commonly found in freshwater and marine fish species, as well as some mollusks and crustaceans (National Research Council Committee on Animal Nutrition, 1993; National Research Council Subcommittee on Warmwater Fish Nutrition, 1983).

Although there has not been a definitive study of thiamine deficiency in amphibians, given the universality of signs described for this disease in mammals (Ullrey & Allen, 1986), birds (Ward, 1971), and reptiles (Donoghue & Langenberg, 1996), thiamine deficiency should be suspected in amphibians exhibiting neurological dysfunction including fasciculations, tremors, opisthotonos, and seizures. Any amphibian showing these clinical signs with a diet history that includes fish should immediately receive thiamine at a dosage of 25–100 mg/kg body weight either intramuscularly or intracoelomically. Supplemental parenteral thiamine should be given until muscular contractions or seizures cease. Thereafter oral thiamine can be given as a dietary supplement at 25 mg/kg body weight with each meal for several weeks after the resolution of clinical signs, or a maintenance dose may be allometrically derived from the known thiamine requirement of a primate (i.e., 0.03 mg/kg/day) (Waisman & McCall, 1944). Thiamine is relatively nontoxic, so even higher levels of thiamine may be given without fear of adverse effects.

The diet should be adjusted to include fresh whole animals such as insects, earthworms, or mice. If this is not possible, vary the fish species offered. If thawed frozen fish are used, a regular supplement containing up to 250 mg thiamine per kilogram fish is recommended (Snyder & Terry, 1986).

7.4 STEATITIS

Steatitis is likely to occur in those amphibians that have been fed improperly stored and handled frozen fish or dead rodents that have become rancid. Vitamin E by itself or in combination with selenium may be administered but the successful elimination of steatitic nodules using this approach is unlikely. Surgery to remove these nodules from the fat bodies may be warranted if the amphibian appears to have discomfort upon abdominal palpation. A combination of 1 mg/kg body weight vitamin E and 0.1 mg/kg body weight selenium may be administered once IM, followed by weekly administration of 100–400 iu/kg body weight vitamin E orally.

7.5 RENAL CALCULI

Oxalate-containing plants such as spinach have been linked to the development of oxalate-containing renal calculi in the tadpoles of some ranid frogs. However, other frogs have been raised on spinach with no ill effects. It seems likely that the herbivorous larvae of anurans have coevolved with the plants in their environment and are adapted to processing the toxins of the plants and algae upon which they normally feed. Problems arise in captivity, and presumably in the wild, when a tadpole ingests an unfamiliar compound and lacks the metabolic pathway for efficient detoxification and/or elimination. This information is usually attained by trial and error, and it is imperative that a thorough literature review precedes development of a rearing diet for a species. Commercially available tropical fish food products are reasonable alternative diets, and as yet there have been no reports of renal calculi linked with these products.

Individuals of the waxy frog, *Phyllomedusa sauvagii*, developed hydrocoelom, subcutaneous edema and lethargy (Figure 7.5). These frogs were housed in an enclosure containing an oxalate-producing plant, the silver queen, *Aglaonema roebelinii*. Crickets fed to the frogs were suspected of eating this plant, and this was the presumed manner of oxalate ingestion by the frogs. As this species is uricotelic and excretes little urinary water, it is presumed that this caused the oxalates to become concentrated to pathologic levels. This disease may not occur in ammonitelic or ureotelic species of amphibians. Saline diuresis was attempted but all severely affected frogs died. Histopathology of the affected frogs revealed oxalate crystals in the kidneys suggesting that renal failure was responsible for the clinical signs of fluid accumulation and lethargy. Once the plant was replaced with a peace lily, *Spathophyllium* spp., no further incidence was noted, but the link between species of plants within an enclosure and the development of presumptive oxalate toxicosis is speculative.

7.6 OBESITY

Obesity is caused by consumption of a diet in excess of the amphibian's energy needs. Many species of amphibians are conditioned to gorge on prey when it is available, thus building up fat reserves for when prey is not available. This feeding cycle is valuable in preparing the body for estivation, hibernation, and reproductive activity, but may not be linked with this appropriate physiological outlet in captivity. Obesity is most often seen in captive specimens of the White's treefrog, *Pelodryas caerulea* (Plates 7.3, 7.4, 7.5), horned frogs, *Ceratophrys* spp., and Tschudi's African bullfrog, *Pyxicephalus adspersus*. The axolotl, *Ambystoma mexicanum*, and tiger salamander, *Ambystoma tigrinum*, are the most common pet salamanders seen with this condition. Fat deposition typically occurs in the fat bodies, causing an enlarged abdomen in the obese amphibian that must be differentiated from egg production (Plates 7.6, 7.7). The fat bodies may be palpable, and may obscure the organs normally visible through the abdominal wall. Some obese specimens of the White's treefrog, *Pelodryas caerulea*, may develop enlarged crests over the eyes that can impede vision.

Treatment of obesity requires counseling the client on the estimated energetic needs of the amphibian. (The formulas to determine the basal metabolic rate of an amphibian are presented in Section 7.13.2 Choosing a Formula; and Tables 7.1, 7.2, and 7.3.) All other variables being equal, larger animals require proportionately fewer calories than smaller ones. For example, a 50 g White's treefrog, *Pelodryas caerulea*, held at 25°C (77°F) is calculated to require approximately 0.54 kcal/day to maintain its basal metabolic rate, while a

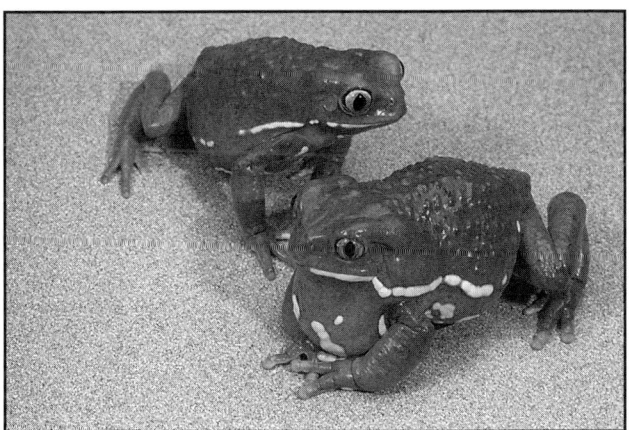

Figure 7.5. Oxalate toxicosis in the waxy frog, *Phyllomedusa sauvagii*. Note fluid accumulation in the ventral throat and abdomen. (George Grall, National Aquarium in Baltimore)

500 g ornate horned frog, *Ceratophrys ornata*, is calculated to need 3.7 kcal/day (see Table 7.4). Thus although there is a 10-fold increase in body size between the two frogs, there is less than a 7-fold increase in overall caloric needs. A 5000-g goliath frog, *Conraua goliath*, held at 25°C is calculated to need 25 kcal/day, reflecting less than a 48-fold increase in overall caloric needs despite a 100-fold increase in body mass.

With activity, the metabolic demands increase and a corresponding increase in caloric intake is required. With strenuous exercise the metabolic rate may be 9 times that of a resting amphibian (Gatten et al., 1992). If the obese amphibian is an active forager, such as is the case for dendrobatid frogs, increasing the enclosure size or adding new cage furnishings may stimulate increased activity and increase its metabolic demand.

With many sit-and-wait foragers, such as horned frogs, *Ceratophrys* spp., it is difficult to manipulate their environment so as to increase their activity level for weight reduction. With these amphibians, weight reduction is best achieved by dietary manipulation to reduce the amount of food offered over a weekly period until the amphibian is eating slightly less than is needed for maintenance. A mild elevation in environmental temperature may increase the amphibian's metabolism after acclimation, but prolonged exposure to temperatures above the preferred body temperature may have adverse physiological effects. At the clinician's discretion, a period of fasting is in order, but this may shift the animal's metabolism to a conserva-

Table 7.1. Equations for calculating resting metabolism of anurans. To convert oxygen consumption to caloric needs, assume standard conversion of 4.8 kcal/1000 ml O_2 or 0.0048 kcal/ml O_2. (Adapted from Table 12.2 found in Gatten et al., 1992.)

Temperature °C (°F)	Oxygen Consumption (ml/hr)
5 (40)	$0.049 \, (BW \text{ in } g)^{0.81}$
10 (50)	—
15 (60)	$0.104 \, (BW \text{ in } g)^{0.79}$
20 (68)	$0.103 \, (BW \text{ in } g)^{0.82}$
25 (77)	$0.174 \, (BW \text{ in } g)^{0.84}$

Table 7.2. Equations for calculating resting metabolism of salamanders. To convert oxygen consumption to caloric needs, assume standard conversion of 4.8 kcal/1000 ml O_2 or 0.0048 kcal/ml O_2. (Adapted from Table 12.2 found in Gatten et al., 1992.)

Temperature °C (°F)	Oxygen Consumption (ml/hr)
5 (40)	$0.02 \, (BW \text{ in } g)^{0.81}$
10 (50)	—
15 (60)	$0.045 \, (BW \text{ in } g)^{0.81}$
20 (68)	$0.068 \, (BW \text{ in } g)^{0.80}$
25 (77)	$0.095 \, (BW \text{ in } g)^{0.80}$

Table 7.3. Equations for calculating resting metabolism of caecilians. To convert oxygen consumption to caloric needs, assume standard conversion of 4.8 kcal/1000 ml O_2 or 0.0048 kcal/ml O_2. (Adapted from Figure 2 found in Smits & Flanagin, 1994.)

Temperature °C (°F)	Oxygen Consumption (ml/hr)
5 (40)	—
10 (50)	—
15 (60)	—
20 (68)	$0.023 \, (BW \text{ in } g)^{1.05}$
25 (77)	$0.067 \, (BW \text{ in } g)^{1.06}$

Table 7.4. Standard Metabolic Rate of anurans by body mass and body temperature. During injury or illness, the caloric needs should be increased by a minimum of 50%.

Bodyweight in grams	kcal/day @ 5°C	kcal/day @ 15°C	kcal/day @ 20°C	kcal/day @ 25°C
1	0.006	0.01	0.01	0.02
5	0.02	0.04	0.04	0.08
10	0.04	0.07	0.08	0.14
20	0.06	0.13	0.14	0.25
30	0.09	0.18	0.19	0.35
40	0.11	0.22	0.24	0.45
50	0.13	0.26	0.29	0.54
60	0.16	0.30	0.34	0.63
70	0.18	0.34	0.39	0.71
80	0.20	0.38	0.43	0.80
90	0.22	0.42	0.47	0.88
100	0.24	0.46	0.52	0.97
500	0.87	1.6	1.9	3.7

tion mode and actually reduce the calories used each day. A weekly weight chart and feed diary should be maintained by the client and evaluated every 4–6 weeks until the amphibian has returned to an appropriate weight.

If the client desires to breed the obese amphibian, the clinician may advise inducing estivation or hibernation as a means to reducing excess fat. The goal of this effort is to convert the body fat to egg masses in the female and to stimulate courtship activity that is energetically demanding in the male. For example, the male marbled reed frog, *Hyperolius viridiflavus*, uses ten times more energy during calling than does a resting frog (Grafe, 1988). This is only advised for those clients that have the skill and available equipment to monitor the amphibian during this period of environmental extremes. For estivating species known to form cocoons as a response to drying conditions, the obese amphibian can be placed in a bucket of river mud which is allowed to slowly dry. Food should be withheld for 14 days prior to estivation, and the amphibian should be soaked in water for several hours immediately prior to allow defecation and micturition. The specimen may be estivated for 2–6 months after the mud has dried. Moistening the dried mud will bring the amphibian out of estivation. Estivation can also be achieved using a deep bed of moist sphagnum moss; the top layer is allowed to dry out, but the bottom layers must remain slightly moist. If the bottom layers of moss dry out, the amphibian may desiccate. If a species is known to hibernate, it can be hibernated with a similar precondition as described for estivation. The temperature of the hibernaculum can be lowered 2°C every day until the desired temperature is reached. Hibernation temperatures should be appropriate for the species and should last no longer than 4 months. These cycles may induce ovulation in female frogs. If oviposition does not occur, it may be assisted with hormones or manual stripping (see Chapter 22, Reproduction). Failure to oviposit can create additional medical problems, so again the clinician is cautioned that these techniques are not recommended for the average client.

7.7 GASTRIC OVERLOAD AND IMPACTION

Many species of amphibians exhibit a strong feeding response which can result in the ingestion of an overly large food item or an excessive number of smaller food items. This is an especially common phenomenon in horned frogs, *Ceratophrys* spp., and Tschudi's African bullfrog, *Pyxicephalus adspersus*, although it has been noted in many species of smaller frogs and salamanders (Plates 7.8, 7.9, Figure 7.6). The distended stomach decreases the inspiratory volume of an amphibian, leading to hypoxia and hypercarbia. The circulation becomes compromised as the distended stomach compresses the major veins, leading to hypovolemic shock within a few hours. Amphibians that die at this stage will have stomach contents showing little or no digestion or decomposition. If the amphibian can survive these physiologic stresses, it eventually succumbs to toxins associated with putrefying ingesta.

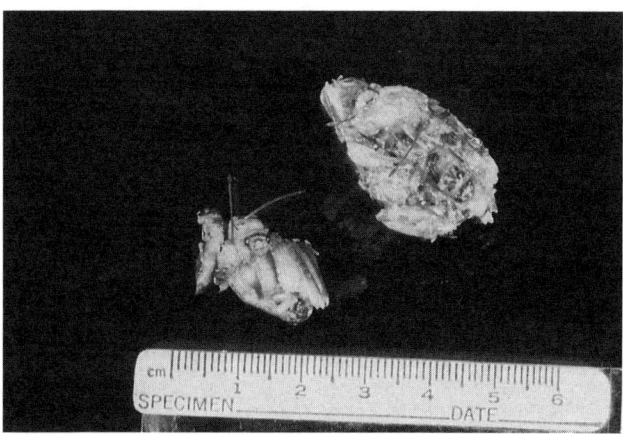

Figure 7.6. Although the stomach was only mildly distended by this meal, the ovipositor of one cricket had caused numerous punctures in the stomach of a spotted toad, *Bufo guttatus*, contributing to its death. (Virginia Pierce, Philadelphia Zoological Garden)

Gastric overload is a medical emergency. Attempts can be made to retrieve items through the oropharynx using thumb forceps or alligator forceps, but objects should not be forced out, as sharp edges and points on the prey item (e.g., cricket legs, mouse toenails) may rupture the strained wall of the stomach. On occasion it is possible to dislodge material by passing a small gauge red rubber feeding catheter into the stomach and performing a gentle gavage with small amounts of warmed saline. Endoscopic retrieval of foreign bodies has been successful on many patients. This is generally considered a surgical emergency, and a celiotomy and gastrotomy is warranted if the objects can not be removed otherwise. Preoperative corticosteroids are recommended, as are postoperative fluids.

Impaction may result when foreign objects are ingested. Stones, mulch, and other debris may be consumed along with the food item. These items may be large enough to cause a gastric impaction, or may be passed into the intestine, causing intestinal obstruction and concomitant fecal impact. Lethargy and abdominal bloating are suggestive of an obstruction or impaction. Palpation may reveal a firm intra-abdominal mass. Radiographic examination and ultrasound examination can confirm the presence of a foreign object. Contrast studies are not usually needed for diagnosis, but may allow differentiation from other internal masses. Medical therapy in the form of oral fluids and gentle gavage may be attempted, but generally a gastrotomy or enterotomy is warranted.

7.8 SCOLIOSIS

Mild to severe scoliosis and 100% mortality occurred in captive bred tadpoles of the giant monkey frog, *Phyllomedusa* cf *tarsius,* at the National Aquarium in Baltimore (Figures 7.7, 7.8). Successful rearing was achieved when vitamin B complex (Vitamin B Complex, VEDCO, Inc., St. Joseph, MO) was added to the tank water at a dose of 1 ml per gallon of tank water (each ml of B complex provided 12.5 mg thiamine, 2 mg riboflavin, 5 mg pyridoxine hydrochloride, 12.5 mg niacinamide, 10 mg d-panthenol, 5 µg cyanocobalamin). This supplementation may have offset leaching of B vitamins from the fish food offered, however there was greater growth of algae in the supplemented tank than in unsupplemented tanks, so the mechanism by which normal maturation occurred is unclear. Subsequent use of vitamin B supplementation in this manner with other hylid and dendrobatid frogs has met with similar success.

7.9 SPINDLY LEG

Spindly leg (i.e., skeletomuscular underdevelopment) has long been recognized as a developmental disease affecting tadpoles and recently metamorphosed dendrobatid frogs (e.g., Espinosa poison frog, *Epipedobates espinosai, E. antoni,* black-legged poison frog, *Phyllobates bicolor*) and hylid frogs (e.g. Phyllomedusine frog, *Phyllomedusa* cf *tarsius,* New Granada cross-banded frog, *Smilisca phaeota*). Most of these amphibians do not survive. This syndrome has been linked with flaked fish foods as a sole diet, perhaps due to leaching of B vitamins. Feeding tadpoles a quality fish flake food (e.g. Aquarian®, Wardley Corporation, Secaucus, NJ) that contains significant levels of vitamins and minerals (including B vitamins) or the addition of vitamin B complex to the water (described in Section 7.8, Scoliosis) has drastically reduced spindly leg among the species mentioned, suggesting the importance of a proper diet in preventing this disease. The provision of living aquatic vegetation and algae as a food source also seems to decrease the incidence of spindly leg (See also Section 18.1, Spindly Leg).

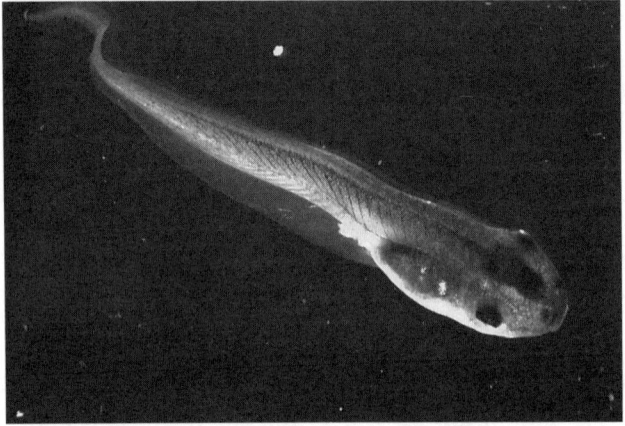

Figure 7.7. Mild scoliosis of the tail in a young tadpole of an undescribed *Phyllomedusa* sp. (George Grall, National Aquarium in Baltimore)

7.10 PARALYSIS

Hindlimb and forelimb paralysis has been observed in numerous anurans maintained in captive populations. Dendrobatid frogs and atelopid toads have shown a progressive paralysis of the hindlimbs, and less frequently the forelimbs, that can culminate in the death of the affected amphibian in a matter of days to weeks. We have observed atelopids with a rigid paralysis, whereas other frogs have typically shown a flaccid paralysis. Pathological examination of several affected dendrobatids from the National Aquarium in Baltimore demonstrated a demyelination of the peripheral nerves consistent with thiamine and other B-vitamin deficiencies. A suspected *Clostridium botulinum* was isolated from one atelopid enclosure, but was lost during attempts to confirm the identification. Affected individuals were

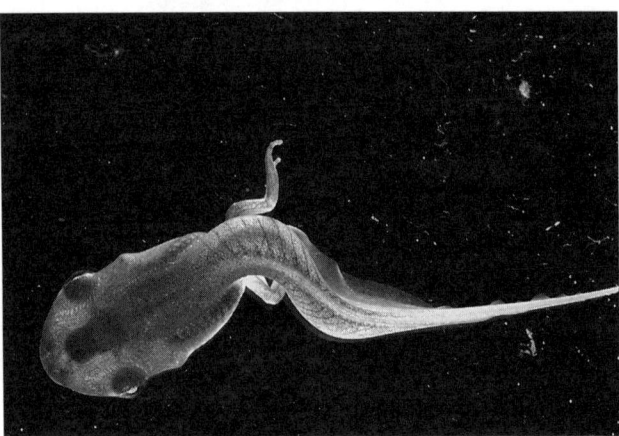

Figure 7.8. Severe scoliosis in a late stage tadpole of an undescribed *Phyllomedusa* sp. This condition is progressive and terminal. (George Grall, National Aquarium in Baltimore)

treated with vitamin B complex at 0.1 ml/300 g body weight PO every 24 h for 7 days, then every 48 h (B Complex, VEDCO Inc. St. Joseph, MO); corticosteroids; antibiotics (penicillin-G 40,000 iu/kg every 24 h for 7 days); botulism antitoxoid (1:1000 dilution of 300 mg/ml standard antitoxoid); and parenteral calcium. The treatments were effective, although a full recovery took longer than 1 month. To date, similar treatment regimes have effectively been used to treat cases of paralysis in the green and black poison frog, *Dendrobates auratus,* harlequin poison frog, *D. histrionicus,* yellow-banded poison frog, *D. leocomelas,* dyeing poison frog, *D. tinctorius,* pleasing poison frog, *Epipedobates bassleri,* three-striped poison frog, *E. trivittatus,* black-legged poison frog, *Phyllobates bicolor,* lovely poison frog, *P. lugubris,* and the Veragoa stubfoot toad, *Atelopus varius.* The effectiveness of any one of the pharmaceuticals used in this "shotgun" approach is unknown and obscures the underlying etiology of the paralysis. Thiamine deficiency, other B-vitamin deficiencies, hypocalcemia, botulism, and infection are possible etiologies for this syndrome.

7.11 CORNEAL LIPIDOSIS (LIPID KERATOPATHY)

One of the theories explaining corneal lipidosis is related to the compositional differences between the prey items fed in captivity and the prey items consumed in the wild, particularly in regard to the balance of fatty acids and fats.

There is ample evidence that different orders of insects have different essential fatty acids (i.e., fatty acids that they cannot synthesize). For example, *Ephestia* moths fail to develop wings when fed a diet lacking linoleic acid, but *Tenebrio* mealworms will undergo normal development and metamorphosis (Fraenkel & Blewett, 1947, as cited in Prosser, 1950). The linoleic acid content of the fat of the two insects was compared after one insect was fed a linoleic acid-free diet and the other was fed a linoleic acid-supplemented diet. *Tenebrio* had a linoleic acid content of 10% when fed a deficient diet, and a 20% content when on a supplemented diet. *Ephestia* has a linoleic content of 1% when fed the deficient diet, and a 15% content on the supplemented diet. If an insect prey, such as the domestic mealworm, *Tenebrio molitor,* has a particular fatty acid in amounts far in excess of an amphibian's needs, this could result in derangement of the amphibian's metabolism, resulting in a disorder such as corneal lipidosis.

Cholesterol is required in the diets of *Drosophila, Tribolium, Tenebrio, Blatella* (cockroaches), and most other insects, but vertebrates such as amphibians can synthesize the cholesterol they need (Prosser, 1950). It is possible that the cholesterol content in a diet composed of domestic insects is too high for amphibians to metabolize properly, and that corneal lipidosis is analagous to hypercholesterolemia-related diseases in man.

The incidence of this disease in wild amphibians is unreported. Given the compositional differences known for some insects, it is likely that the amphibian metabolism is adapted to the fluctuating nutrient levels associated with the variety of invertebrate species consumed by free-ranging amphibians. Constant exposure to inappropriate levels of a compound, such as excessive ingestion of cholesterol, may overwhelm the metabolic pathway, leading to a storage disorder, in this case, corneal lipidosis.

Although corneal lipidosis likely is a primary nutritional disorder, a multifactorial etiology may be likely. For example, many amphibians with corneal lipidosis are captive females that have failed to oviposit in one or more seasons. When the ova is absorbed instead of deposited to the environment, the nutrients in the ova must be metabolized or stored. Since this is not a normal result of follicle development in the wild, the mechanisms for efficient reabsorption of the nutrients may be lacking. A possible consequence of improper transport and storage of fatty acids is corneal lipidosis (see also Chapter 19, The Amphibian Eye).

7.12 CACHEXIA

Amphibians are often presented in a cachectic state (Plates 7.10, 7.11, Figure 7.9). The effects of starvation are consistent with that described in other vertebrates, including utilization of fat stores (fat bodies), muscle loss through protein catabolism, and gluconeogenesis from hepatic and muscular glycogen stores (Merkle & Hanke, 1988). Long-term starvation in the African clawed frog, *Xenopus laevis,* has two distinct phases (Merkle, 1990). Phase I, which lasts for the first 4–6 weeks (or longer in obese frogs), is marked by reduced activity, reduced oxygen consumption, depletion of glycogen reserves, atrophy of the fat body, and atrophy of the gonads (with concomitant mobilization of lipids from any ova that are present). Phase II begins when the fat body is completely atrophied and catabolism of tissue proteins accelerates as the glycogen and fat stores are depleted. Marked skeletal muscle atrophy follows. The cardiac and renal mass remain unchanged throughout prolonged periods of starvation, from 6–12 months in duration, but the hepatic mass may decrease by more than 20%. Ovarian mass may decrease by 70%, while the mass of the fat bodies may decrease by 99%. As the muscle protein

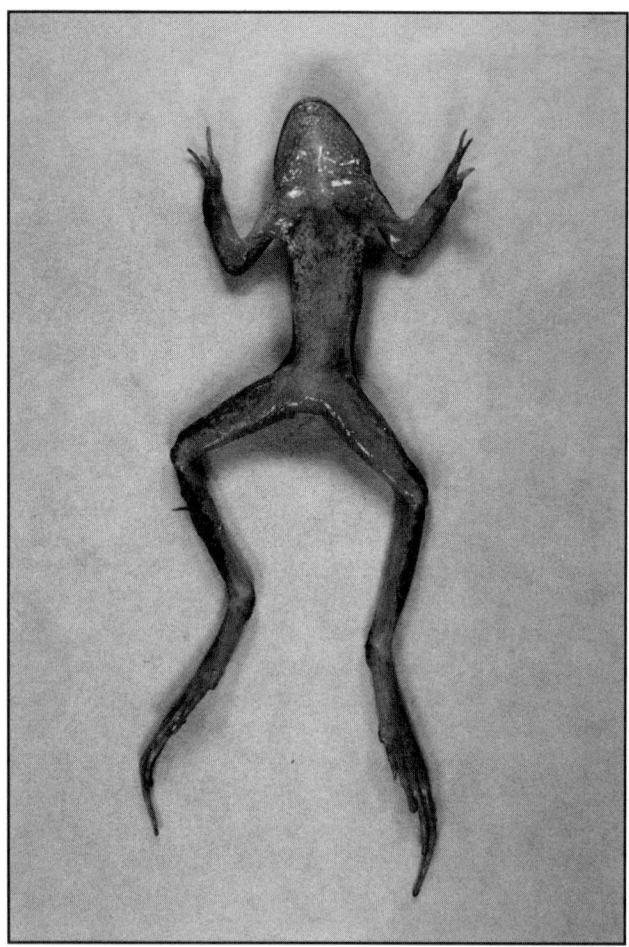

Figure 7.9. Severe starvation of a northern leopard frog, *Rana pipiens*, used by a university biology class. Amphibians are excluded from the animal care and use guidelines of many institutions. (Sharon K. Taylor)

decreases, the water content of the muscles rises similarly to the protein-water line reported in starving fish (Love, 1980).

Physiologic changes similar to those described for the edible frog, *Rana kl. esculenta,* are expected in terrestrial amphibians that are starving (Grably & Peiry, 1981). Terrestrial amphibians are likely to become dehydrated if they are away from standing water or a humid environment, due to the conflicting demands of energy conservation and the movement required for water homeostasis. The Puerto Rican coqui, *Eleutherodactylus coqui,* will conserve body water by reducing movement and foraging, staying in a humid microclimate and opting for starvation over dehydration (Stewart, 1995). A starving terrestrial amphibian may develop increased body water if in a suitably wet environment (Grably & Peiry, 1981).

Clinical signs of starvation vary between aquatic and terrestrial amphibians. Fat bodies may be undetectable by palpation or transillumination, and the female amphibian may lack developed ova (however, both of these signs occur in female amphibians after spawning). The gall bladder may be markedly distended. The limbs and abdomen may appear thin in terrestrial amphibians, and the pelvis or urostyle can appear prominent. Aquatic amphibians may appear bloated and edematous due to the gain in body water associated with protein catabolism. Terrestrial amphibians may appear dehydrated and have marked weight loss (in excess of 20%), especially if they are dehydrated. The globes of the eyes may be sunken in the orbits of terrestrial amphibians. The skin may become thinner (Grably & Peiry, 1981) and may be more easily torn when the amphibian is manually restrained.

Often there are underlying problems that are the cause of cachexia, but sometimes it is solely the result of the client's failure to understand the amphibian's energy needs (i.e., underfeeding) or to present the food in an appropriate fashion.

Treatment of cachexia should include supplemental feeding with a high-calorie formula until the amphibian is gaining weight (see Section 7.13, Nutritional Support for the Ill and Inappetent Amphibian). Once this has been achieved, weaning the amphibian onto a program of self-feeding follows. The client should be counseled on any husbandry problems that are contributing to the amphibian's inappetence. Common husbandry issues include feeding diurnal animals in the afternoon or evening, feeding nocturnal animals in the morning, feeding inappropriately sized food items (e.g., small crickets to a full grown ornate horned frog, *Ceratophrys ornata,* feeding adult crickets to Boulenger's tree toad, *Pedostibes hosei*), and feeding inappropriate food items.

7.13 NUTRITIONAL SUPPORT FOR THE ILL AND INAPPETENT AMPHIBIAN

7.13.1 Assist-Feeding

Assist-feeding (hand-feeding) is a preferred route of nutritional support for some debilitated amphibians. Many amphibians will swallow a piece of food (e.g., an earthworm, a headless cricket, or neonatal mouse) that is placed in their mouth. The mouth may need to be opened by a speculum, but some specimens will engulf the food if it is touched lightly to the mouth. To increase the speed of enzymatic breakdown of the prey, the skin of the mouse should be incised, and the head of the cricket should be removed. The food item may be predigested by an injection of a solution of water and pancreatic enzyme (e.g., Prozyme®, The Prozyme Company, Elk Grove Village, IL) immediately prior to feeding. Frozen and thawed prey items may be subject to faster digestion and assimilation than freshly killed items.

Objects that may be used as oral speculums include a plastic credit card, developed radiograph film, a thin plastic wedge (e.g., a piece of the lid of a yogurt container), a metal flat spatula (chemical scoop), waterproof paper, an index card or business card, an eyelid speculum, an IV catheter slip cover, a teaspoon, a rubber-coated baby spoon, or a rubber spatula (Figure 7.10). The speculum is pressed into the filtrum (divot at the rostral edge of the mouth), upon which many amphibians will open their mouths. The speculum should be inserted further until a suitable gap is present. At this point, food items may be inserted and placed in the back of the mouth. Remove the speculum and allow the amphibian a chance to swallow. If the item is rejected, a smaller item should be used. If the item is again spat out, it should be lubricated with a water-soluble gel and gently pushed into the esophagus before allowing the amphibian a chance to swallow on its own.

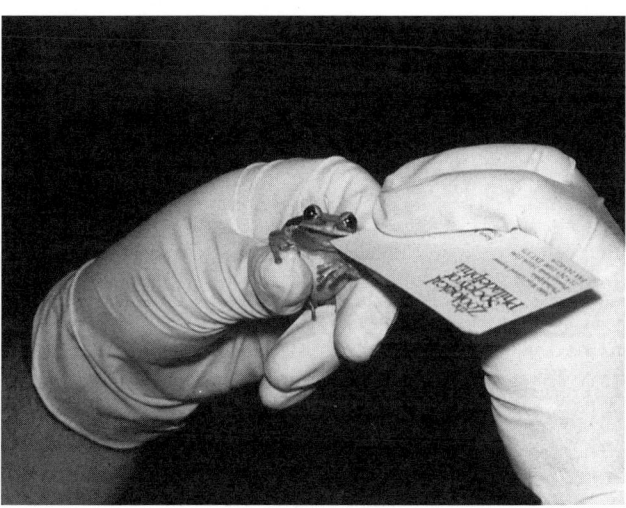

Figure 7.10. A business card can be used as a speculum to open the mouth of a New Granada cross-banded treefrog, *Smiliscus phaeota*. (Philadelphia Zoological Garden)

In many instances it is less stressful and more practical to tube feed the amphibian. A rodent gavage tube, an intravenous catheter, a polypropylene urinary catheter (e.g., tomcat urinary catheter), or a red rubber feeding tube may be used as a gavage tube (Figure 7.11). In the event of tube feeding, the tube should be measured and marked so that the length of tube inserted into the amphibian's gastrointestinal tract is no more than one-third to one-half the body length. Given the fact that adult amphibians have a short esophagus, the clinician must take care not to damage the stomach with too long a tube.

Weight should be recorded after defecation/urination to determine the patient's true body mass. Every effort should be made to provide an enclosure that meets the needs of the species in question, and appropriate prey items should be provided between the assisted feedings. Avoid unnecessary intrusions into the amphibian's enclosure to allow the animal to feel secure.

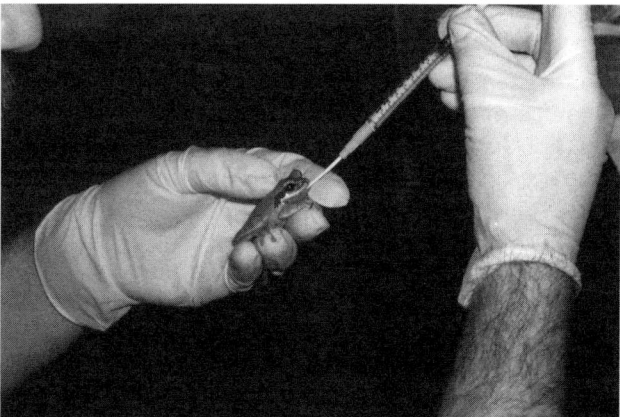

Figure 7.11. Tube-feeding a New Granada cross-banded treefrog, *Smiliscus phaeota*. (Philadelphia Zoological Garden)

7.13.2 Choosing a Formula

Feeding regimens vary with species and should be tailored to the amphibian's body condition. The standard metabolic rate (SMR), sometimes known as resting or basal metabolic rate, for the three orders of amphibians is approximated by the oxygen consumption formulas noted in Tables 7.1, 7.2, and 7.3 (Gatten et al., 1992; Smits & Flanagin, 1994). This rate can be converted to a daily caloric need by using the standard assumption of 4.8 kcal/l oxygen consumed (or 0.0048 kcal/ml O_2) and multiplying this by 24 h. Oxygen consumption rates for various types of physical exertion have been recorded and can be over nine times the rate determined for an amphibian at rest (Gatten et al., 1992).

Although we are unaware of reports concerning the SMR of ill amphibians, it is reasonable to assume that the metabolic demands of an ill or recovering amphibian are in excess of the basal metabolic rates determined for apparently healthy inactive amphibians. The metabolic rate of ectotherms varies with temperature, and if an amphibian is inducing a behavioral fever, this will also increase its energy needs. Pending reports otherwise, nutritional support for the ill amphibian should exceed the energy demands of basal metabolism by a minimum of 50%. (See Tables 7.4, 7.5, and 7.6 for daily caloric needs of amphibians by weight and body temperature.) The values in these tables reflect values obtained for temperatures up to 25°C (77°F), and the caloric needs at higher temperatures are doubled for each 10°C (16 to 18°F) increase (Gatten et al., 1992).

If the amphibian has undergone surgery, is severely underweight, or fails to maintain weight at this lower level, increase the offered calories to 2 times or greater than that of the calculated SMR. If the amphibian continues to lose weight, does not gain weight, or in any way appears to have a prolonged recovery, the offered calories can be increased up to 10 times the calculated standard metabolic rate. We prefer to work in 7-day time periods so that while every feeding may not be in excess, the planned excess (e.g., 50% or more) should be provided in that time span. Working in the 7-day framework decreases the handling necessary, as assist feeding need not be attempted daily. If the pharmacotherapeutic regimen warrants daily handling, then daily assist-feeding can be undertaken without undue additional stress.

On an as-fed basis, the majority of prey items fed to amphibians are between 1 and 2 kcal/gm (Table 7.7). This allows the clinician to calculate the ability of a diet to meet an amphibian patient's energy needs based on the prey items available. Although the domestic cricket, *Acheta domestica*, has a reported caloric value of 1.9 kcal/g and the house cricket, *Gryllus domesticus*, has a reported value of 1.0 kcal/g (Donoghue, 1995), this data is based on limited studies and may not be reflective of the true biological energy. In most instances it is practical to use an estimated caloric value of 1.5 kcal/g for live feed items when calculating energetic needs of the amphibian patient. Well fed and hydrated adult crickets maintained in colonies at the Philadelphia Zoo weigh approximately 0.3 to 0.4 g each.

As a general rule, additional protein and fat supplements are not needed if well-nourished whole prey items are fed. However, protein and amino acid pow-

Table 7.6. Standard Metabolic Rate of caecilians by body mass and body temperature. During injury or illness, the caloric needs should be increased by a minimum of 50%.

Bodyweight in grams	kcal/day @ 20°C	kcal/day @ 25°C
1	0.003	0.008
5	0.01	0.04
10	0.03	0.09
20	0.06	0.19
30	0.09	0.27
40	0.13	0.38
50	0.16	0.47
60	0.19	0.59
70	0.23	0.70
80	0.26	0.80
90	0.29	0.91
100	0.33	1.0
500	1.8	5.6

Table 7.5. Standard Metabolic Rate of salamanders by body mass and body temperature. During injury or illness, the caloric needs should be increased by a minimum of 50%.

Bodyweight in grams	kcal/day @ 5°C	kcal/day @ 15°C	kcal/day @ 20°C	kcal/day @ 25°C
1	0.002	0.005	0.008	0.01
5	0.008	0.02	0.03	0.04
10	0.015	0.03	0.04	0.07
20	0.03	0.06	0.09	0.12
30	0.04	0.08	0.12	0.17
40	0.05	0.10	0.15	0.21
50	0.055	0.12	0.18	0.25
60	0.06	0.14	0.21	0.29
70	0.07	0.16	0.23	0.33
80	0.08	0.18	0.26	0.36
90	0.09	0.20	0.29	0.40
100	0.10	0.21	0.31	0.44
500	0.35	0.80	1.1	1.6

Table 7.7. Estimated caloric content of some prey items fed to amphibians. Adapted from Donoghue, 1995.

Prey item	Energy as fed (kcal/g)
Cricket *Acheta domesticus* House cricket	1.9
Gryllus domesticus Mealworm larvae	1.0
Tenebrio molitor Earthworm	2.1
Lumbricus terrestris Mouse pinkie, 1 g Mouse pinkie, 4 g Mouse adult, 27 g	0.5 0.8 (has not nursed) 1.7 (after nursing) 1.7

ders can be added to the formula of severely cachectic individuals to help regain muscle mass. The diet of "poor-doers" should be evaluated to rule out fat excess/protein deficiency as a cause.

Example 7.1. The patient is an inappetent 50-g White's treefrog, *Pelodryas caerulea,* held at 25°C with an ulcerative rostral lesion. Assume a metabolic demand 50% over standard metabolic rate.

Standard Metabolic Rate (see Table 7.1).

$$\text{ml O}_2 \text{ consumed/hr} = 0.174 \, (50 \text{ g})^{0.84} = 4.68 \text{ ml O}_2/\text{hr}$$

Convert to caloric need (or refer to Table 7.4).

$$(4.68 \text{ ml O}_2/\text{hr}) \, (0.0048 \text{ kcal/ml O}_2)$$
$$(24 \text{ hr/day}) = 0.54 \text{ kcal/day}$$

Grams of cricket *Acheta domestica* needed for SMR

$$(0.54 \text{ kcal/day}) \, (1 \text{ g cricket}/1.5 \text{ kcal}) = 0.36 \text{ g crickets/day}$$

Grams of crickets/day needed during illness

$$0.36 \text{ g crickets/day} + 0.5 \, (0.36 \text{ g crickets/day}) = 0.54 \text{ g crickets/day}$$

Grams of crickets/week needed during illness

$$7(0.54 \text{ g crickets}) = 3.8 \text{ g crickets/week}$$

Number of adult crickets needed during illness assuming a weight range of 0.3 to 0.4 g/adult cricket

$$(3.8 \text{ g crickets/week})(1 \text{ adult cricket}/0.3 \text{ to } 0.4 \text{ g}) = 10 \text{ to } 12 \text{ adult crickets/week}$$

Amphibians are obligate carnivores with rare exceptions. Extrapolating from other animals, carnivores are adapted for a diet consisting of 50% protein, 45% fat, and 5% carbohydrates. The domestic cricket, *Acheta domestica,* is 50% protein, 44% fat, and 6% carbohydrates on a % kcal basis, whereas a 1.5 g mouse pinkie is 57% protein, 40% fat, and 3% carbohydrates on the same basis. Any tube-feeding formula based on whole animal products such as crickets or 1- to 2-day-old mice should have the calcium content adjusted to create a positive calcium-to-phosphorus balance. As a general rule, 1 level tsp of ground calcium carbonate provides approximately 6.5 g of calcium.

Any commercial reptile and amphibian diet should be evaluated with regard to its carbohydrate content before being used as diet for the amphibian patient. If the major ingredients of the diet are grain products rather than animal protein, that diet is probably inappropriate for adult amphibians. Inordinate levels of simple and complex sugars may induce an osmotic diarrhea and provide little if any sustenance to the patient.

Meat baby food can serve as the base for a temporary diet. A multivitamin-mineral supplement should be added to the baby food to make the formula as nutritionally complete as possible. Products marketed for human consumption may be more complete and have a more appropriate balance of vitamins and minerals than any of the products targeted for amphibians and reptiles (Donoghue, 1995). Even with human-targeted products, the formula may change, as happened with Centrum® (Lederle, American Cyanamid Corporation, Pearl River, NY 10965), which changed from vitamin D_3 to vitamin D_2. The label should be reviewed with each new purchase to ensure consistency in the formulation. The calcium-to-phosphorus ratio of meat can be adjusted by adding 0.5 to 1.0 g calcium carbonate (40% calcium by weight) to each 100 g meat to yield a formula adequate for dogs and cats, and presumably this formula is adequate for amphibians. This formula yields a caloric value of approximately 1 kcal/ml. A multivitamin-mineral supplement can be added to the formula to yield a vitamin D_3 level of 20–100 iu/100 g diet. Prozyme® may be added to the formula to liquefy it, but the formula may need to be thinned with water in order to pass through the small-bore feeding tubes, and the dilution of as-fed calories in the formula may necessitate an increased number of feedings to meet the amphibian's needs. Thus the clinician needs to monitor the amount of water used to thin the formula for accurate assessment of energy intake of the amphibian patient.

Certain enteral products designed for humans or domestic mammals have been used with success in carnivorous reptiles (Donoghue & Langenberg, 1996) and are applicable to amphibians. Clinical Care Feline Liquid® (Pet-Ag, Elgin, IL) provides 0.92 kcal/ml with a caloric distribution of 30% protein, 45% fat, and 25% carbohydrates, and is a common product in most small animal clinics. This formula and other similar enteral products may be used for tubefeeding in the event a prey-based formula is not available. These products are, in fact, often preferable due to the ease of administration through narrow-bore feeding tubes and consistency of nutritional levels. If other products are used, their caloric distribution should approach that eaten by carnivores, and the caloric concentration should be noted and included in any calculations. With small amphibians (body mass under 5 g) it is helpful to dilute the enteral formula with water to more accurately meet the caloric needs of the patient.

In many instances it is reasonable to predigest the tube-feeding formula, whether it is prey-based (e.g., crickets) or baby food–based, with powdered pancreatic enzyme (e.g., Prozyme®) to ease passage of the formula through the feeding tube without diluting the amount of energy per ml. This is also a recommended procedure if the patient is being treated for any gastrointestinal disorders, such as a frog recovering from a gastrotomy to remove a foreign body.

Regardless of the formula used, it is important to make the mixture fresh daily or as needed. This serves to minimize the risk of bacterial contamination of the product. Refrigerate the formula at or just below 3°C (45°F) until needed, and warm to the amphibian's preferred body temperature immediately prior to feeding.

As a general rule, the volume of formula fed should not exceed 10% of the amphibian's weight per 24-h period. Amphibians can and do often exceed this volume when eating on their own, but animals in need of force-feeding may not be able to assimilate large meals.

Although a mathematical basis has been laid out for determining the nutrient needs of a patient, the clinician is reminded to treat the patient, not the formula. These formulas are approximations of data collected from many different species of amphibians, and there may be significant deviations from these calculated values among species and individuals. Nutrition is not an exact science, and in many instances a range of values should be worked from rather than trying to meet the exact caloric values obtained by metabolic rate formulas. For example, a 54-g healthy frog at rest held at 25°C (77°F) is considered to have an approximate caloric need between 0.54 kcal/day (value for a 50-g frog) and 0.63 kcal/day (value for a 60-g frog) (see Table 7.4). Rather than calculating a formula for a 54-g frog, it is practical to provide nutritional support somewhere between those two values, and to increase the amount fed if the patient is losing weight and to decrease the amount fed if the patient is becoming clinically obese.

Example 7.2. The patient is an inappetent 50-g White's treefrog, *Pelodryas caerulea*, held at 25°C with an ulcerative rostral lesion. Assume a metabolic demand 50% over standard metabolic rate.

Standard Metabolic Rate (See Table 7.1).

$$\text{ml } O_2 \text{ consumed/hr} = 0.174 \, (50 \text{ g})^{0.84} = 4.68 \text{ ml } O_2/\text{hr}$$

Convert to caloric need (or refer to Table 7.4).

$$4.68 \text{ ml } O_2/\text{hr} \times 0.0048 \text{ kcal/ml } O_2 \times 24 \text{ hr/day} = 0.54 \text{ kcal/day}$$

ml Clinical Care Feline Liquid® needed for SMR

$$(0.54 \text{ kcal/day})(1 \text{ ml}/.92 \text{ kcal}) = 0.6 \text{ ml/day}$$

ml Clinical Care Feline Liquid® needed per day during illness

$$0.6 \text{ ml} + 0.5 \, (0.6 \text{ ml}) = 0.9 \text{ ml /day}$$

Note: This volume of Clinical Care Feline Liquid® is approximately 2% of the entire body mass of the patient.

Example 7.3. The patient is an inappetent 50-g White's treefrog, *Pelodryas caerulea*, held at 30°C following foreleg amputation. Assume a metabolic demand 250% over standard metabolic rate. Since 30°C is not a value in the equations or on a chart, refer to 20°C values and double them since the metabolic rate approximately doubles for each 10°C rise in temperature.

Standard Metabolic Rate at 20°C (see Table 7.1).

$$\text{ml } O_2 \text{ consumed/hr at } 20°C = 0.103 \, (50 \text{ g})^{0.82} = 2.55 \text{ ml } O_2/\text{hr}$$

Standard Metabolic Rate at 30°C

$$\text{ml } O_2 \text{ consumed/hr at } 30°C = 2.55 \text{ ml } O_2/\text{hr} \times 2 = 5.1 \text{ ml/hr}$$

Convert to caloric need (or refer to Table 7.4).

$$5.1 \text{ ml } O_2/\text{hr} \times 0.0048 \text{ kcal/ml } O_2 \times 24 \text{ hr/day} = 0.59 \text{ kcal/day}$$

ml Clinical Care Feline Liquid® needed for SMR

$$(0.59 \text{ kcal/day})(1 \text{ ml}/.92 \text{ kcal}) = 0.64 \text{ ml/day}$$

ml Clinical Care Feline Liquid® needed per day during illness

$$0.64 \text{ ml} + 2.5 \, (0.64 \text{ ml}) = 2.24 \text{ ml /day}$$

Note: This volume of Clinical Care Feline Liquid® is approximately 5% of the entire body mass of the patient.

REFERENCES

Allen, M.E. and O.T. Oftedal. 1989. Dietary manipulation of the calcium content of feed crickets. Journal of Zoo and Wildlife Medicine 20(1):26–33.

Baksi, S.N., S.M. Galli-Gallardo, and P.K.T. Pang. 1977. Vitamin D metabolism in amphibia and fish. Fedn. Am. Socs. Exp. Biol. 36:1097.

Ball, J.C. 1995. A comparison of the uv-b irradiance of low-intensity, full-spectrum lamps with natural sunlight. Bulletin of the Chicago Herpetological Society 30(4):69–72.

Bentley, P.J. 1984. Calcium metabolism in the Amphibia. Comp. Biochem. Physiol. 79A:1–5.

Bernard, J.B. 1995. Spectral Irradiance of Fluorescent Lamps and their Efficacy for Promoting Vitamin D Synthesis in Herbivorous Reptiles. Doctoral dissertation, Michigan State University, East Lansing, MI.

Boutilier, R.G., D.F. Stiffler, and D.P. Toews. 1992. Exchange of respiratory gases, ions, and water in amphibious and aquatic amphibians, in Feder, M.E. and W.W. Burggren (Eds.): Environmental Physiology of Amphibians. University of Chicago Press, Chicago, pp. 81–124.

Bruce, H.M. and A.S. Parkes. 1950. Rickets and osteoporosis in *Xenopus laevis*. Journal of Endocrinology 7:64–81.

Dierenfeld, E.S. and D. Barker. 1995. Nutrient composition of whole prey commonly fed to reptiles and amphibians. 1995 Proceedings of the Association of Reptilian and Amphibian Veterinarians, pp. 3–15.

Donoghue, S. 1995. Clinical nutrition of reptiles and amphibians. 1995 Proceedings of the Association of Reptilian and Amphibian Veterinarians, pp. 16–37.

Donoghue, S. and J. Langenberg. 1996. Nutrition, in Mader, D.R. (Ed.): Reptile Medicine and Surgery. W.B. Saunders Co., Philadelphia, PA, pp. 148–174.

Douglas, T.C., M. Pennino, and E.S. Dierenfeld. 1994. Vitamins E and A, and proximate composition of whole mice and rats used as feed. Comp. Biochem. Physiol. 107A(2):419–424.

Fraenkel, G. and M. Blewett. 1947. Linoleic acid in nutrition of *Ephestia* and *Tenebrio*. Biochem. J. 41:475–478.

Frye, F.L. 1992. Anasarca in an Argentine horned frog *Ceratophrys ornata*. Journal of Small Exotics Animal Medicine 1(4):148–149.

Gatten, R.E., Jr., K. Miller, and R.J. Full. 1992. Energetics at rest and during locomotion, in Feder, M.E. and W.W. Burggren (Eds.): Environmental Physiology of the Amphibians. University of Chicago Press, Chicago, pp. 314–377.

Gehrmann, W.H. 1987. Ultraviolet irradiances of various lamps used in animal husbandry. Zoo Biology 6:117–127.

Gehrmann, W.H. 1992. No UV B from Tungsten Filament Incandescent Lamps. Bulletin of the Association of Reptilian and Amphibian Veterinarians 2(2):5.

Gehrmann, W.H. 1994. Spectral characteristics of lamps commonly used in herpetoculture. The Vivarium 5(5):16–29.

Gehrmann, W.H. 1996. Reptile lighting: a current perspective. The Vivarium 8(2):44–45, 62.

Grably, S. and Y. Peiry. 1981. Weight and tissues changes in long term starved frogs, *Rana esculenta*. Comparative Biochemistry and Physiology 69A:683–688.

Grafe, T.U. 1988. Untersuchungen zur Fortpflanzungs biologie und Zu Lebensstrategien von *Hyperiolius viridiflavus* (Amphibia, Anura, Hyperoludae). Master's thesis, Bayerische Julius-Maximillans Universisität, Würzburg, Germany.

Hay, A.W.M. and G. Watson. 1976. The plasma transport proteins of 25-hydroxycholecalciferol in fish, amphibians, reptiles, and birds. Comp. Biochem. Physiol. 53B:167–172.

Herman, C.A. 1992. Endocrinology, in Feder, M.E. and W.W. Burggren (Eds.): Environmental Physiology of Amphibians. University of Chicago Press, Chicago, pp. 40–54.

Larsen, L.O. 1992. Feeding and digestion, in Feder, M.E. and W.W. Burggren (Eds.): Environmental Physiology of Amphibians. University of Chicago Press, Chicago, pp. 378–394.

Love, R.M. 1980. The Chemical Biology of Fishes. Academic Press, London, UK.

Mader, D.R. 1993. Use of calcitonin in green iguanas (*Iguana iguana*). Bulletin of the Association of Reptilian and Amphibian Veterinarians 3(1):5.

Merkle, S. 1990. Effects of starvation in *Xenopus*. Fortschritte der Zoologie 38:311–320.

Merkle S. and W. Hanke. 1988. Long-term starvation in *Xenopus laevis* Daudin: 1. Effects on general metabolism. Comparative Biochemistry and Physiology 89B:719–739.

Modzelewski, E.H. and D.D. Culley, Jr. 1974. Growth responses of the bullfrog, *Rana catesbeiana*, fed various live foods. Herpetologica 30 (4):396–405.

National Research Council. Committee on Animal Nutrition. Board on Agriculture. 1993. Requirements of Fish. National Academy Press, Washington, DC.

National Research Council. Subcommittee on Warmwater Fish Nutrition. 1983. Nutrient Requirements of Warmwater Fishes and Shellfishes. National Academy Press, Washington, DC.

Prosser, C.L. 1950. Chapter 5, Nutrition, in Prosser, C.L. (Ed.): Comparative Animal Physiology. W.B. Saunders Co., Philadelphia, PA, pp. 112–143.

Shoemaker, V.H., S.S. Hillman, S.D. Hillyard, D.C. Jackson, L.L. McClanahan, P.C. Withers, and M.L. Wygoda. 1992. Exchange of water, ions, and respiratory gases in terrestrial amphibians, in Feder, M.E. and W.W. Burggren (Eds.): Environmental Physiology of Amphibians. University of Chicago Press, Chicago, pp. 125–150.

Smits, A.W. and J.I. Flanagin. 1994. Bimodal respiration in aquatic and terrestrial apodan amphibians. American Zoologist 34:247–263.

Snyder, R.L. and J. Terry. 1986. Avian nutrition, in Fowler, M.E. (Ed.): Zoo and Wild Animal Medicine. W.B. Saunders Co., Philadelphia, PA, pp. 190–200.

Stewart, M.M. 1995. Climate driven population fluctuations in rain forest frogs. Journal of Herpetology 29:437–446.

Stiffler, D.F. 1993. Amphibian calcium metabolism. J. Exp. Biol. 184:47–61.

Trusk, A.M. and S. Crissey. 1987. Comparison of calcium and phosphorus levels in crickets fed a high calcium diet versus those dusted with supplement. Proceedings of the Sixth and Seventh Dr. Scholl Conferences on the Nutrition of Captive Wild Animals, Seventh Annual Conference, pp. 93–99.

Ullrey, D.E. and M.E. Allen. 1986. Principles of zoo mammal nutrition, in Fowler, M.E. (Ed.): Zoo and Wild Animal Medicine. W.B. Saunders Co., Philadelphia, PA, pp. 516–532.

Waisman, H.A. and K.B. McCall 1944. A study of thiamine deficiency in the monkey *Macaca mulatta*. Arch. Bioch. 4:265.

Ward, F.P. 1971. Thiamine deficiency in a peregrine falcon. Journal of the American Veterinary Medical Association 159:599.

CHAPTER 8
CLINICAL TECHNIQUES

Brent R. Whitaker, MS, DVM and Kevin M. Wright, DVM

8.1 INTRODUCTION

Amphibians become ill or fail to thrive for a variety of reasons. When presented with an amphibian patient, the clinician is tasked with determining a course of action based upon clinical findings and subsequent conclusions. Anurans, salamanders, and caecilians present a unique challenge to the veterinary practitioner, as great diversity exists within and between each order. A library of herpetological texts is, therefore, a valuable investment for those practicing amphibian medicine.

Receiving an amphibian patient requires preparation and client education. Special considerations must be given to the transport of animals to and from the veterinary hospital. Several modifications should also be made to the examination room in order to make it "amphibian-friendly." Most well-equipped veterinary hospitals will have the equipment needed to examine amphibians, especially those prepared to see reptiles and birds. Useful information on many of the commercially available products mentioned in the text is found in Table 8.1.

A systematic problem-oriented approach should be taken when working with the amphibian patient. First, a complete history of the animal must be obtained including a description of the animal's nutritional plan and appetite; recent and current environmental parameters, such as humidity, temperature, water quality, and lighting; social structure and reproductive status; the recent introduction or loss of animals; and the administration of medications or other chemicals within the past few months. Any problems noted by the client should be described in detail at this time. Clients should be asked to bring any husbandry records, such as food and water quality logs, as they are very useful in identifying important trends that have developed over time. In addition, a water sample from the amphibian's home vivarium should accompany the patient so that water quality parameters may be assessed. A physical examination is then performed. Based upon the clinician's initial findings, a list of differential diagnoses is prepared. Further clinical tests are often necessary in order to determine a final diagnosis and formulate a therapeutic plan.

This chapter will present special considerations and techniques that are useful when working with amphibian patients. It is hoped that creativity in combination with an understanding of fundamental concepts will allow the clinician to develop new and innovative approaches to diagnosing the diseases of amphibians.

Table 8.1. Commercially available products for amphibian veterinary care.

Equipment	Product Name	Manufacturer
Blood culture tubes containing tryptic soy broth	Bacto® Tryptic Soy Broth w/ SPS & CO_2	DIFCO Laboratories, Detroit, MI
Clay for capillary tubes	Critoseal®	Manufactured for Monoject Scientific, Division of Sherwood Medical, St. Louis, MO
Culture swabs with transport media	Mini-tip Culturette® Collection and Transport System	Becton Dickinson Microbiology Systems, Cockeysville, MD
Disinfectants 1). 2% chlorhexidine 2). iodine-based	1). Chlorhexidine Solution 2). Betadine®	1). Distributor: VEDCO, St. Joseph, MO 2). The Purdue Frederick Co. Norwalk, CT

Table 8.1. Commercially available products for amphibian veterinary care. *(Continued)*

Equipment	Product Name	Manufacturer
Fecal float solution	Fecasol®	EVSCO Pharmaceuticals, Buena, NJ
Flexible red-rubber tubes	Sovereign® Feeding Tube and Urethral Catheter;	Sherwood Medical, St. Louis, MO
Lithium heparin blood tubes	Microtainer® Brand Tube with Lithium Heparin Reorder Number 36-5971	Becton Dickinson and Company, Franklin Lakes, NJ
Microhematocrit tubes	Standard®	Clay Adams Division of Becton-Dickinson Parsippany, NJ
Microliter pipette	Eppendorf Autoclavable Pipetter 0.5–10 µl 2–20 µl	Distributor: Brinkman, Westbury, NY
Portable doppler	Ultrascope Doppler Arterial and Venous Blood Flow Detector, Model 8, 8 MHz	EMS Products, Inc., Kirkland, WA
Stain: cytological evaluation 1). Wright-Geimsa 2). Gram 3). Acid-fast	1). Protocol™ 2). Bacto® Gram 3). Bacto® Acid-fast	1). Biochemical Sciences, Inc., Swedesboro, NJ 2). DIFCO Laboratories, Detroit, MI 3). DIFCO Laboratories, Detroit, MI
Temporary/transport containers	Pal Pens®	Hagen Corp., Mansfield, MA
Tomcat catheter	Sovereign® 3.5 Fr Tomcat Catheter	Sherwood Medical, St. Louis, MO
Tricaine methane sulfonate	MS-222	Argent Chemical Laboratories, Redman, WA
Water test kits	Various kits available: 1). Hach aquaculture test kits 2). LaMotte test kits 3). Tetra kits	1). Hach Co., P.O. Box 608 Loveland, CO 2). LaMotte, Chestertown, MD 3). Tetra Werke Dr. rer. nat. Ulrich Baensch Gmblt, D-4520 Melle 1. Germany

8.2 TRANSPORTATION OF THE AMPHIBIAN PATIENT

Transportation of the amphibian patient for examination can be safely achieved using a container that has a moist substrate, such as a wetted, nonbleached paper towel or sphagnum moss. Aquatic species and tadpoles will require a water-tight container that can be sealed. Plastic bags, either moistened for terrestrial animals or partially filled with water for aquatic species and larvae, can be inflated with air and closed using rubber bands. Small plastic containers (e.g., Small Pal Pens®, Rolf C. Hagen USA Corporation, Mansfield, MA.) or deli cups with lids having small ventilation holes (made from the inside out to prevent the amphibian from contacting an abrasive surface) work well for smaller terrestrial amphibians (Figures 8.1, 8.2). A plastic trash

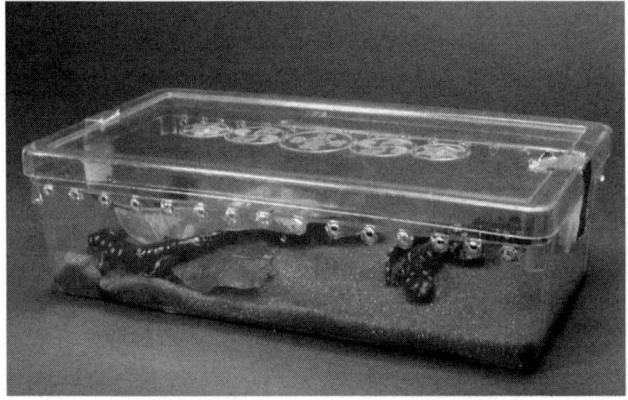

Figure 8.1. Small plastic containers are excellent for transporting amphibians short distances. A moistened sponge is an excellent temporary substrate for amphibians such as the spotted salamander, *Ambystoma maculatum*. (George Grall, National Aquarium in Baltimore)

can with a snug-fitting lid is useful for larger species of anurans (e.g., the giant toad, *Bufo marinus*) that will traumatize themselves in smaller enclosures (Figure 8.3). Care must be taken not to expose the animals rapidly to dramatically different temperatures. This can be avoided by placing the animal's transport bag or box into a pillow case or a cooler filled with newspaper strips. Although unnecessary for short trips in a climate-controlled car, some coolers now offer temperature control by merely plugging them into the vehicle's cigarette lighter.

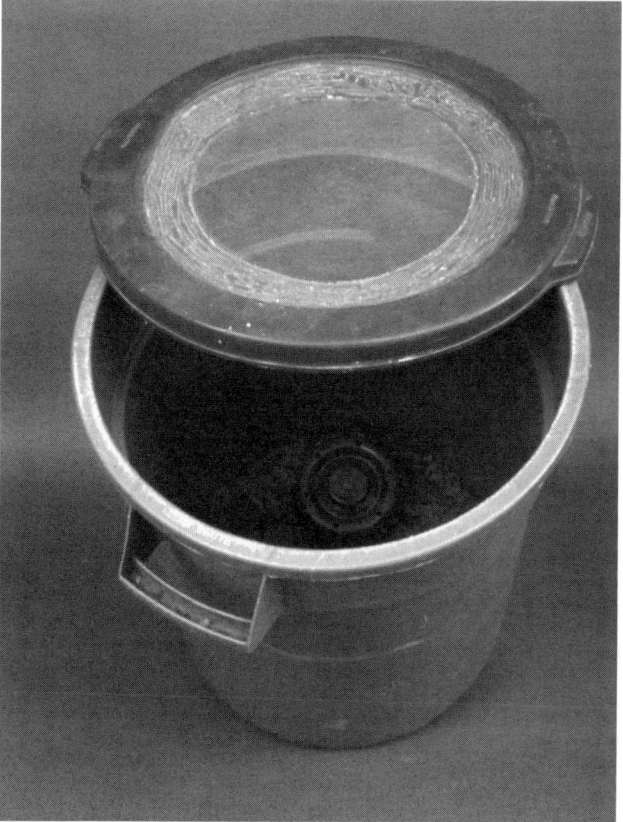

Figure 8.3. Clean plastic garbage cans can be used as transport containers for large amphibians. (George Grall, National Aquarium in Baltimore)

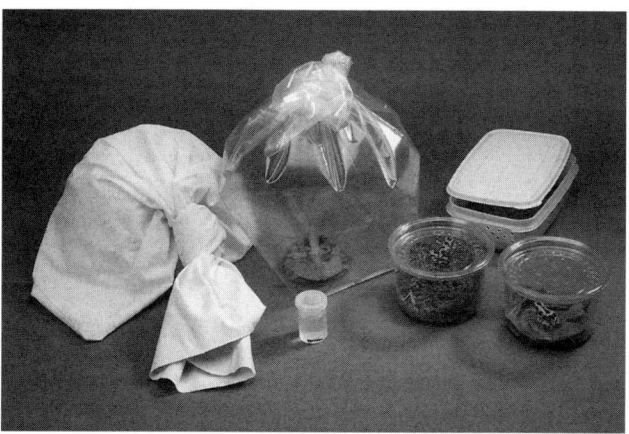

Figure 8.2. A variety of containers can be used to safely transport the amphibian to the veterinarian. Shown here are deli cups with a moistened paper towel, a plastic container filled with sphagnum moss, a moistened plastic bag, and a film container for tadpoles. Placing these containers in a pillowcase will minimize heat loss or gain when transporting short distances. (George Grall, National Aquarium in Baltimore)

Motion sickness leading to emesis has been reported in larval and adult salamanders and postmetamorphic frogs (Naitoh & Wassersug, 1994; Wassersug et al., 1993) however, it is rare. If regurgitation or emesis occurs, a sample should be collected for laboratory analysis.

After the journey is completed, the transport container should be disinfected by filling it with diluted household bleach (e.g., 50 ml bleach per liter of water) for 20 minutes. Always be sure to rinse the vessel thoroughly and allow it to dry. Iodine-based products are best avoided due to their potential toxicity in amphibians (Stoskopf et al., 1985).

8.3 OBTAINING A HISTORY

A thorough medical history is an essential part of the evaluation of an amphibian patient. This is especially important since husbandry requirements vary so widely between species, and even within a species at different times of the year. Obtaining a complete history is facilitated by the use of standardized forms. The receptionist and veterinary technician can obtain most of the history through the use of these forms which can be filled out by the client while in the waiting or exam room. The information is then reviewed by the veterinarian, who should attempt to obtain any missing information. Investigating the following topics is helpful in determining a diagnostic plan for the amphibian patient.

8.3.1 Species

The common name and scientific name should be recorded for each patient, but the medical record is best kept under the scientific name to avoid confusion. Common names are often pet store names designed to make a species more desirable to the impulse buyer, and do little to reveal the actual identification of the animal. The ornate horned frog, *Ceratophrys ornata*, and Cranwell's horned frog, *C. cranwelli*, are often sold under the name "pac-man frog." Likewise Tschudi's African bullfrog, *Pyxicephalus adspersus*, is sometimes sold as a "pixie frog," an obvious reference to its scientific name, although it may also reflect an attempt to disguise the fact that this frog gets as large as it does. Accurate species identification facilitates literature acquisition and communication with colleagues about the case. A quick perusal through the indices of several herpetocultural texts may allow the clinician to glean general husbandry information about an unfamiliar species prior to the physical examination (Freytag et al., 1968; Mattison, 1987; Obst et al., 1988; Staniszewski, 1995; Zimmerman, 1986). Unfortunately, many excellent texts on amphibian husbandry are not available in English as yet (Herrmann, 1993a, 1993b, 1994). An inventory of captive amphibians and reptiles is published annually, and people experienced with that species may be contacted through their listing in this book (Slavens, 1995). If presented with an unfamiliar species on which little information is readily available, extrapolation from similar animals within the same family may be useful. A general synopsis of amphibian families can be found in many herpetological texts (Duellman & Trueb, 1994; Mattison, 1987; Porter, 1972).

8.3.2 Presenting Sign or Complaint

A clear and detailed description of the reason (i.e., the presenting sign or complaint) that the amphibian has been brought for veterinary evaluation should be recorded. The duration of the problem should be noted as well as a detailed description of its progression. Skilled questioning may be required to obtain objective information as many clients are reluctant to admit that the animal's problem was not promptly brought in for evaluation. Any additional signs or complaints should be noted.

8.3.3 Origin

The previous owner(s) and origin of the amphibian, whether it came from a pet store, a mail order dealer, a swap meet, or was captured by the owner, can provide clues to the underlying etiology of the presenting complaint. Amphibians recently acquired by the client may have had multiple owners in a short time with little chance to acclimate and feed well along the way. Thus a pet store amphibian is more likely to exhibit consequences of stress-related immunosuppression (e.g. septicemia, overt parasitism) and malnutrition than an amphibian purchased directly from a breeder. The date obtained allows the problem to be put into perspective. Many problems commonly observed by new owners shortly after acquisition include rostral and other skin abrasions, skin discoloration, unusual lumps, corneal opacity, emaciation, lethargy, unresponsiveness, bloat, missing digits, and anorexia.

These problems are often the result of rough handling, suboptimal husbandry conditions, prior medical ailments, or extreme shipping conditions (i.e., package was exposed to temperatures that were too hot or too cold).

In developing a diagnostic algorithm it is helpful to distinguish whether the amphibian was captive-bred or wild-caught, for many of the common problems in wild-caught amphibians (e.g., heavy parasitism, malacclimation/maladaptation syndrome, rostral abrasions) are less common in captive-bred amphibians. For captive-bred amphibians, the egg hatch date (or date of birth for live-bearers), and date of metamorphosis should be obtained. Adult amphibians are less likely to suffer from certain nutritional diseases (e.g., metabolic bone disease) than young amphibians, and certain idiopathic syndromes (e.g., spindly leg) can be conclusively dismissed from the differential diagnosis of adults. It is rare for captive-bred adults to be available as many herpetoculturists prefer to transfer newly metamorphosed animals, thus avoiding the laborious and costly task of raising small amphibians. If the length of time between either the lay date and hatch date *or* the hatch date and date of metamorphosis is prolonged compared to information known for this species, it suggests husbandry problems (e.g., incubation temperature is too low, malnutrition of the larvae, exposure to toxins such as low levels of ammonia), congenital problems (e.g., genetic defects), or perhaps erroneous information. Questioning of the previous owner, if available, may provide further clues to the underlying cause of the presenting complaint. Sex, if known, should be obtained. Abdominal swelling may be normal as an adult female in breeding season undergoes follicular growth, but is abnormal in an adult male amphibian. Dark colored egg masses may be visible through the ventrum of reproductively active adult female amphibians. The veterinarian who is able to identify the gender of an amphibian often helps to strengthen the bond that a client feels with their companion amphibian. Sexually dimorphic traits to look for include, but are not limited to, nuptial pads, cloacal swellings, dorsal crests, size of tympanum, and coloration (see Chapter 22, Reproduction).

8.3.4 Husbandry

The quality of the husbandry afforded a captive amphibian has a major impact on its health. Although some amphibians are seemingly resistant to the poor husbandry of neglectful owners (e.g., Tschudi's African bullfrog, *Pyxicephalus adspersus*), their life span is probably shortened when compared to their well-attended cohorts. Some owners even pride themselves on neglect—"I only change the water once a month!"—but may not reveal this attitude without careful questioning. Cagemates can influence the health of each other. The number, sex, and species of the cagemates are important factors to consider. Males may live quite compatibly with each other only to erupt in agonistic behavior upon the introduction of a female, as happens with the seal salamander, *Desmognathus monticola*. Too many of one species may result in territorial behaviors and dominance hierarchies with untoward effects (e.g., starvation) for the least dominant individuals. In social species such as the golden mantella, *Mantella aurantiaca*, too few animals may result in poor propagation. Some species produce skin secretions that are deadly to other species. The secretions of a pickerel frog *Rana palustris*, will incapacitate and kill many other amphibians. If there is a major size difference between cagemates, the smaller individual may be ingested by the larger individual. Some species are best kept alone. The proclivity of Tschudi's African bullfrog, *Pyxicephalus adspersus*, is to eat anything that moves, including the limbs and digits of any cagemates. Asking about the health status of cagemates often provides valuable information and an indication of chronicity. Persistent parasitism in an amphibian colony for example, can be problematic due to direct life cycles and resistance to treatment. Rectal prolapse is often linked to intestinal nematodiasis, and several inhabitants of a cage may prolapse a few weeks or months after an infected cagemate is introduced. Sudden die-offs of cagemates may suggest outbreaks of bacterial septicemia or intoxication, yet the client may not mention these events unless directly asked. The health status of the rest of the collection (i.e., other amphibians and reptiles that do not share the same cage but are in the same room or cared for by the same person) should be reviewed. Clients often fail to wash their hands or properly disinfect tools between cages thus potentiating the spread of contagious diseases.

Cage design should be documented, with emphasis on the materials used to build and furnish the enclosure. Various paints and treated woods contain substances that are toxic to amphibians, and outgassing from uncured fiberglass and polyurethane can prove deadly. Improperly maintained fiberglass may shed small particles into the enclosure, resulting in skin irritation and perhaps chronic dermatitis. The use of metals in construction of the cage should not be overlooked, as oxidation of metal screening and galvanized metals can be deleterious to amphibians. The dimensions of the enclosure are also noted to determine if the volume of space is adequate for the species housed.

The method of illumination should be documented. The actual brand name and wattage of any bulbs used should be obtained, as well as the type of fixture used to hold the bulb. The age of the bulb may be important for certain broad spectrum fluorescent bulbs, and the client is encouraged to use an indelible ink pen to write on the bulb the date of first use. A regular yearly rotation of the broad-spectrum and ultraviolet-emitting bulbs is encouraged so that the spectrum of illumination does not skew away from the desired output. It is important to know whether the illumination is direct or filtered. If a pane of glass or fine screen mesh is between the emitting bulb and the amphibian, then many of the benefits of the ultraviolet-emitting (i.e, broad-spectrum) bulbs are lost, for these radiation frequencies are absorbed by the intervening material. There has been little work to elucidate the importance of ultraviolet light in the activation of vitamin D in amphibians, but the lack of appropriate illumination may underlie some cases of metabolic bone disease, as well as less obvious problems, such as maladaptation. The photoperiod and its seasonal cycle should be documented. Many amphibian species may have their reproductive cycle cued by seasonal changes in day length. Failure to feed during parts of the breeding season is not uncommon for many amphibians, so inappetence at certain times of the year may be normal if the light cycle is appropriate. Recent power outages should be documented, as they can disrupt environmental conditions including temperature and lighting regimens. Electrical timers, for example, should be checked, as they are often relied upon to create a photoperiod.

The substrate used is important, as is the treatment of the substrate prior to its use in the cage. Certain materials are not recommended due to the presence of potentially toxic compounds (e.g., cedar mulch, pine shavings) and chemical additives (e.g., potting soil with fertilizer enhancement). Sphagnum moss and peat moss are rich in tannins and acidify an enclosure, which may prove detrimental to alkaline-adapted amphibians such as cave-adapted plethodontid salamanders. Coral rock and limestone alkalinize the water of an enclosure, and are a better choice for these alkaline-adapted amphibians. Pretreatment of the substrate should be investigated. Mulch, soil, and sand may be heat-treated, frozen, or sun-sterilized prior to incorporation in an enclosure to reduce the risk of introducing mites and other parasites (see Section 5.5.3, General Guidelines for Enclosure Setup and Maintenance). Potted plants should be rinsed free of their original soil and replanted with the clean materials. The frequency of cleaning is important as a new substrate may be irritating to some amphibians shortly after it has been placed in the vivarium. Alternatively, substrate heavily soiled with fecal material may also lead to the development of health problems. In some instances it is important to vary servicing frequency for optimal health (Horseman et al., 1976).

The types of plants present can have an impact on the amphibian's health. Oxalate-containing plants may be linked to renal disease (see Section 7.5, Renal Calculi). Overplanting of an enclosure may allow prey insects to escape capture, resulting in a amphibian starving in the midst of plenty.

Other cage furnishings may introduce toxins or pathogens into the system. Avoid items such as resin-containing branches and metals. The use of glues and epoxies should be documented, especially in suspected cases of intoxication.

The method of water presentation should be documented, whether it is provided by daily misting, an unfiltered closed system (e.g., water bowl or other dump-and-fill system), a filtered closed system (e.g., aquarium with an undergravel or canister filter), or an open (flow-through) system. If the water isn't offered in an appropriate manner, the amphibian may fail to access it, dehydrate, and eventually desiccate. Arboreal frogs and salamanders rarely come down to soak in pools on the floor of a cage, so it is best to use a misting system to provide water. Deep water bowls can drown nonaquatic amphibians and should be avoided if an amphibian's swimming and climbing abilities are limited. Standing pools are likely to become fouled with animal waste and can quickly develop toxic levels of ammonia and urea, as well as unsanitary levels of coliform bacteria. Filtered pools can lull the herpetoculturist into a false sense of complacency, for the water may look clear yet have dangerous levels of ammonia or nitrites if the biological or chemical filter isn't fully functional. Regular water testing is essential to prevent problems with filtered closed systems. The date that the biological filter was established should be documented, as new systems (i.e., systems <30 days old) are more likely to have dangerous levels of ammonia or nitrites than well-established systems. Water additives such as medications and conditioners (dechlorinizers, ammonia removers) should be documented. Antibiotics can decimate the bacteria responsible for denitrification, leading to the rapid death of multiple animals in well-established systems. Influxes of poor quality water (e.g., municipal water with high levels of chloramines) can also destroy the biological filter.

It is important to document the source of the water used in the vivarium. Chloramine and chlorine are often added to municipal water supplies, while the pipes that carry tap water may leach heavy metals (e.g., copper and zinc). Distinguish between aged tapwater, and filtered tapwater as there may be a difference in the dissolved solutes in these two sources. If activated carbon is used to remove various impurities and potential toxins, be sure to ask the client when it was last changed. Distilled water lacks any solutes and can create osmotic stress in amphibians exposed to it for extended periods of time.

The presence of a marine aquarium in the household should be investigated. Accidental introduction of seawater or sea salt into an amphibian's enclosure can result in salt intoxication or milder forms of osmotic stress. If the marine aquarium is in close proximity to the amphibian's enclosure, the two systems should be moved as far apart as possible.

The enclosure's daily high and low humidity should be documented, as well as any seasonal cycling of humidity. The client should be encouraged to record this information. A hygrometer put at the driest end of the cage gives the lowest possible humidity to which the animal may be exposed. Excessively high humidity can promote the development of infectious lesions of the skin, whereas excessively low humidity can cause chronic dehydration, renal failure, and desiccation. The method of ventilation should also be investigated, as good air flow is essential to prevent stagnation in a high-humidity enclosure.

The enclosure's daily high and low air temperatures should be documented, as well as any seasonal cycling of temperature. If the client does not record this information, they should be encouraged to do so. The warmest microenvironment of the cage can be measured by using a maximum-minimum thermometer. In general a 6–8°C (10–15°F) temperature gradient should be found when comparing the coolest point in the enclosure to the warmest point (see Section 5.6.1, Temperature). Even a brief exposure to above or below optimal temperatures can cause immunosuppression and derangement of other metabolic processes, thus it is important that each enclosure has a range of temperatures so that the amphibian can thermoregulate. Temperatures above that to which an animal is adapted can cause regurgitation, whereas exposure to cold environments may cause ingested food to putrefy, resulting in gastric or intestinal bloating prior to regurgitation. Inappropriate temperatures may be the cause of lethargy, agitation, skin discoloration, or refusal or inability to feed. Many problems can result from inappropriate hibernation or estivation techniques (e.g., corneal coagulopathies following hibernation), so the history should detail any attempts at seasonal cycling of the temperatures.

The heating and cooling devices used to maintain temperatures in the vivarium should be documented. Resistance-method heat devices (e.g., under-the-tank heaters) can develop hot spots which, if undetected, can be the source of thermal burns. Thermostats with automatic shut-offs are recommended to prevent overheating of an enclosure, while a secondary heating device, set at a lower temperature, will prevent the chilling of animals if the primary system fails. A redundant system with two thermostats for each heating device will minimize the risk of overheating or chilling in the event of the failure of the primary thermostat. The design and placement of the heating and cooling devices should allow a thermocline within the cage so that its inhabitants have the opportunity to thermoregulate. The temperature within a new vivarium should always be stabilized for a minimum of 24 hours before any amphibians are introduced. Recent fluctuations in room temperature (e.g., broken window, loss of air conditioning, loss of heating, etc.) should be investigated, as the vivarium's individual devices may have been unable to maintain appropriate parameters.

People unfamiliar with the needs of amphibians can unknowingly create an unhealthy environment. The use of the following products should be avoided or strictly controlled in a room containing amphibians: pesticides (e.g., aerosols, powders, foggers), room deodorizers, air fresheners, tobacco products, flea powders, paints, epoxies, petroleum products, resins, varnishes, and volatile cleaning agents and disinfectants. The location of the amphibian room in the dwelling should be investigated. If a garage, a hobby room (e.g., building scale models using volatile glues and paints), or a kitchen is adjacent to the amphibian room, fumes emanating from these rooms may contribute to the amphibian's ill health. Free-ranging pets such as cats, dogs, ferrets, parrots, and iguanas, may cause problems by intimidating the amphibians. Even the most harmless of domestic pets may seem like a predator to an amphibian. Small children attempting to "play" with their amphibian pet in the absence of adult supervision may cause injury. On occasion, caretakers may change (e.g., vacation), sometimes causing inadequate care of the animals. Written instructions and a phone number of a veterinarian may prevent developing medical problems from going unrecognized until the owners return. The clinician should be careful not to lay blame upon the other caretaker, nor ask questions in an accusatory tone about the care given.

The disinfectants that are used in or around the vivarium and on food and water bowls should be documented, as well as the concentrations used, the actual cleaning procedures, and the rinsing procedure if any. Chlorine bleach and ammonia are the least problematic disinfectants if used appropriately and rinsed thoroughly. Iodine-containing disinfectants (e.g., Wescodyne®) and other disinfectants may penetrate into wood and plastics, and can later leach into the amphibian's enclosure, intoxicating its inhabitants. Soap and detergents should be avoided, as they can be especially difficult to rinse away. Soapy residues can cause skin discoloration, severe chemical dermatitis, and possibly death.

8.3.5 Diet

The complete diet should be documented, including items fed and quantity, and the actual presentation of the food. If too many insects are put into the enclosure at one time, they may attempt to feed upon the amphibian, causing skin lesions. Excessive amounts of prey items may intimidate an amphibian, causing it to refuse feed. Inadequate amounts of prey may cause cagemate aggression. Some amphibians will learn to eat unmoving (dead) prey, whereas others are stimulated to feed by movement. If the food items are not presented in a recognizable form, they may be refused. The pretreatment of prey items to boost diet quality should be investigated. Only high-quality foods should be fed to prey items. Most vertebrate prey items do not need additional calcium, but "gut-loading diets" are suggested for many insects and other invertebrates. The frequency of feeding (e.g., daily, twice daily, every 48 hrs, 2 times a week, 3 times a week, every 7 days, every 14 days, every 30 days) and time of day that the amphibians are fed should be documented. The vitamin and mineral supplements given should be evaluated. Clients should be asked to bring the actual bottles used so that the label can be reviewed with regard to the nutritional analysis/report and expiration date. If there is no expiration date on the label, the date that the client purchased the supplement can serve as a guide. Opening the supplements quickly reveals their status. If clumps are present it suggests that the supplement has been kept too moist and may not offer optimal bioavailability. The method of storage of the supplements should be documented, as excessive heat can also degrade the potency of certain vitamins. The exact method and frequency of use should be documented. Are the insects dusted immediately before being put into the enclosure? Are the items put in the enclosure at an appropriate time, or do the insects have time to groom off the vitamin dust prior to being eaten? For example, gut-loaded or dusted crickets fed to treefrogs in the morning but not eaten until night may no longer be of top nutritional value.

8.3.6 Preventive Medicine

Knowledgeable clients are likely to have implemented a preventative medicine program. These practices should be elucidated when collecting the history as they often provide the clinician with valuable information that is useful in the diagnosis and management of health problems. The quarantine procedure should be discussed and documented, as it is the single most important step to preventing health problems in a collection of captive amphibians. At minimum, all amphibians should enter a 30-day quarantine upon arrival, although a 60-day quarantine period is not an unreasonable length of time for anurans of wild-caught or uncertain origin (see Chapter 23, Quarantine).

A collection that undergoes a rigorous quarantine and has regular fecal parasite examinations and anthelmintic treatments is likely to have different problems than a poorly managed collection. The date of last fecal parasite exam and its results, the date of last veterinary exam and its results, and previous medical treatments should be documented.

If there were any deaths in the collection in the last 30 days this should be documented, along with the cause if known. Outbreaks of bacterial septicemia can quickly ravage a collection, and sometimes the first clue to an impending epizootic is the recent occurrence of one or two sudden deaths.

8.3.7 Miscellaneous

It does take practice to become skillful at anamnesis of the amphibian patient. It is difficult to remember all the questions that should be asked for a given patient unless a written guide is followed. Inaccurate information may be relayed by the client either through forgetfulness, evasiveness, or deliberate misinformation. Clients are often reluctant to admit their husbandry practices, and they may not be forthcoming about previous medical treatments. The client may be unaware of activities by other members of the household. It is sometimes helpful to review questions and ask the questions in slightly different ways throughout the examination in order to obtain a more accurate picture of the amphibian's background. Nevertheless, the effort that goes into obtaining the medical history is worthwhile, for it can help the clinician build a holistic view of the amphibian, which in turn may avoid fruitless diagnostic tests. An accurate diagnosis obtained quickly not only benefits the amphibian patient, but will also result in a highly appreciative client.

8.4 THE EXAMINATION ROOM

The examination room for amphibians should be designed to allow a safe and thorough physical examination of the amphibian patient. A list of suggested supplies for the examination room is given in Table 8.2. Because most amphibians are susceptible to desiccation, a relative humidity of at least 60% should be maintained. This can be accomplished with a small room humidifier. The room temperature should also be in the low to mid 70s °F. A heated table or water pad should be available on which to set the amphibian's traveling enclosure. This is especially important for tropical amphibians requiring warmer temperatures. Care should be taken to avoid having items with sharp edges in the room that may cause injury to escapees. Quite often the underside of exam room tables are a maze of sharp edges, grease, and other elements that are potentially dangerous for the escaped amphibian.

Many of the precautions that should be used for reptiles and small mammals are also recommended when working with amphibians. Although these animals are less likely to escape during the examination than other patients, some anurans can make explosive jumps. Seeing a red-eyed treefrog, *Agalychnis callidryas*, climbing into the air conditioning ductwork after jumping out of a weigh basket does little to inspire a client's confidence. Escape routes should be blocked—the ventilation grid should have a fine screen mesh in place, and the drain in the sink should have a suitable screen in place. Cabinetry should be flush with the floor, and modifications made to enclose the underside of draw-

Table 8.2. Suggested supplies for the examination room.

Small room humidifier
Heated table or water pad
Penlight
Cool light source such as a small (1.7–2.7 mm) arthroscope
Ophthalmoscope and/or slit lamp
Latex gloves
Water quality test kit
Dechlorinated water
Tricaine methanesulfonate
Unbleached paper towels
Clean deli cups with clear lids
Milligram balance
Disinfectants:
Chlorine bleach, 2% chlorhexidine, 5–10% ammonia, quaternary ammonium compounds
Oral Speculums:
Plastic cards of varied thicknesses, waterproof paper, weigh spatula, plastic or rubber spatula
Cotton tipped swabs
Fine tipped sterile culture swabs
Tryptic soy broth tubes for blood culture
Tomcat catheters
Flexible feeding/urethral tubes
Needles—20 to 30 gauge
Syringes—1 to 3 cc; several 12–35 cc syringes
Scalpel blades no. 15
0.9% saline
Lithium heparin tubes
Liquid heparin
Serum collection tubes
Microhematocrit tubes
Clay
Microslides and coverslips
8 MHz doppler
Water soluble lubricant gel
Microliter syringe or pipette
Assortment of commonly used drugs

ers and doors, thus limiting access to the other areas of the building. Weather stripping can be easily added to the doors so that they are flush with the floor preventing unwanted egress from the room.

Room lights should be on a dimmer switch. A dim room may quiet the patient in between handling, and it is also essential for a good ophthalmic examination and transillumination of the amphibian. A light source for transillumination should also be readily available. A cool light source, such as that which emanates from the tip of most high quality endoscopes, is recommended. Many of the inexpensive fiberoptic light sources produce a light that can burn amphibian skin within seconds. An illuminated magnifying loupe is very useful when examining the smaller amphibian patient, as it provides greater detail than can be appreciated without it.

A reservoir of dechlorinated water (e.g., artificial pond water reconstituted from distilled water, carbon filtered tap water, aged tap water, or bottled spring water) should be readily available in the room. This can be used to rinse off the disposable vinyl or latex gloves used to handle an amphibian, to moisten the amphibian as needed, and to prepare the proper dilution of any pharmaceutical baths that may be necessary. A small spray bottle filled with water is useful in wetting gloves prior to handling and occasionally misting the amphibian during the examination.

A water quality test kit should be part of the in-house diagnostic laboratory. The client should be instructed to bring approximately one liter of water from their amphibian's enclosure. A small amount of the sample will be analyzed as part of the anamnesis. The levels of ammonia, nitrite, and chlorine, as well as the pH and general hardness of the water should be obtained prior to physical examination. An inexpensive copper test kit is useful in cases where heavy metal toxicity is suspected. The rest of the sample may be needed to dilute the tricaine methanesulfonate solution if anesthesia is needed.

Only unbleached paper towels should be used in the room. This limits the exposure of the amphibian patient to some of the toxic chemicals that have been used in the dyeing process.

Accurate weights need to be obtained for all amphibian patients. This usually requires placing smaller animals into a clean lightweight container, such as a deli cup or a clear plastic bag, and larger ones into plastic shoe boxes or buckets (Figure 8.4). Given the small body size of many amphibians, a milligram balance is recommended in addition to the commonly available centigram balance. A small mass of known weight should be used to periodically check the accuracy of the milligram balance. The weight should be recorded in the context of the examination—if the amphibian voids cloacal water or defecates immediately after being weighed, a follow-up weight should be obtained and the physiological activity noted. This allows the clinician to assess the reserve water capacity and/or the colonic capacity of the amphibian, facts that will guide the choice of fluid therapy and nutritional support if deemed necessary. The lowest body weight obtained is used to develop the therapeutic regime.

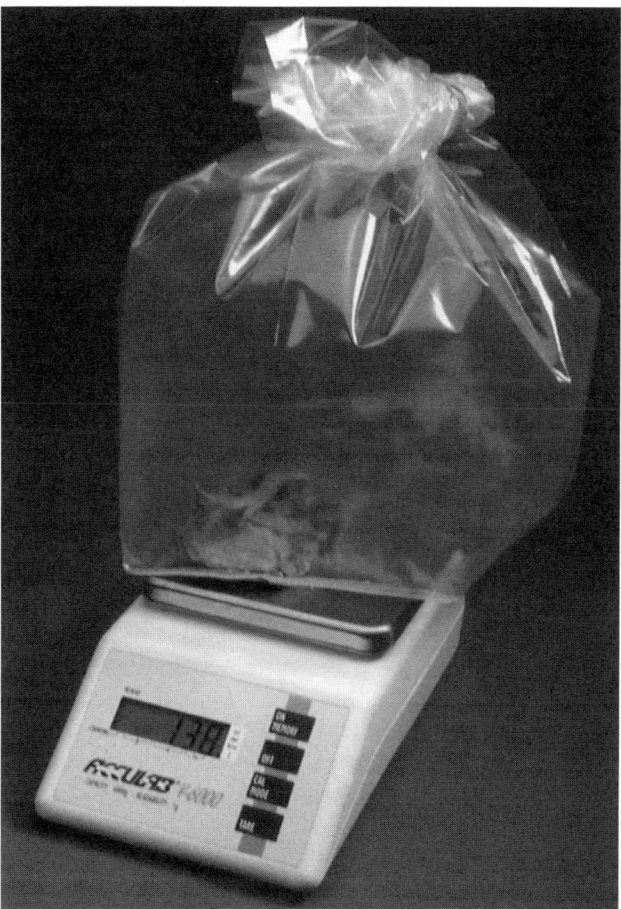

Figure 8.4. This Surinam horned frog, *Ceratophrys cornuta*, is easily restrained in a plastic bag while being weighed. (George Grall, National Aquarium in Baltimore)

All reusable items that come into contact with the amphibian patient should be thoroughly cleaned, disinfected, and rinsed before being used on the next patient. Chlorine bleach, 2% chlorhexidene, or 5–10% ammonia (full-strength household ammonia), are useful disinfectants (Wright, 1993). After an item has been disinfected, it should be wiped down with a damp unbleached paper towel or rinsed with water to remove any disinfectant residue. Failure to do this can result in contact irritation and other clinical signs of toxicosis. Under no circumstances should povidone iodine compounds be used on organic items (e.g., plastics, wood) as the iodine may leach out and cause iodine toxicity (Stoskopf et al. 1985).

In addition to cotton tip applicators and swabs for culture (e.g., Mini-tip Culturette Collection and Transport System®, Becton, Dickinson and Company, Cockeysville, MD) should be readily available in the exam room. Blood culture tubes (e.g., thioglycollate broth) should also be accessible. The choice of microbial sampling devices is dependent on the preference of the laboratory that will actually be culturing the samples obtained.

A variety of items may be used as oral speculums, the choice depending on the size of the patient. Stiff waterproof paper, a business card, a plastic credit card, a metal weigh spatula, a thin plastic or rubber spatula are readily available tools that can be used as speculums. Tomcat catheters and flexible feeding/urethral tubes should be kept handy. The latter can be trimmed to size and attached to a syringe using a large gauge needle. These have many uses including tube feeding, collecting stomach or tracheal wash samples, and administering medications.

Lithium heparin microcontainers (e.g., Microtainers®, Becton, Dickinson and Company, Cockeysville, MD), and microhematocrit tubes (e.g., Standard®, Monoject Scientific, St. Louis, MO) and clay (e.g., Critoseal®, Monoject Scientific, St. Louis, MO) should be accessible for blood collection. An assortment of needles (20–30 gauge) and volume syringes suitable for blood collection should be stocked in the room. A bottle of liquid heparin should be on hand so that the collection needle and syringe can be primed to avoid coagulation of samples not destined for blood culture.

It is helpful to have premeasured amounts and concentrations of commonly used drugs readily available. Given the small body size of most amphibians, the stock concentrations of many drugs are too concentrated for use without dilution. It is helpful to maintain compounded forms of commonly used drugs (e.g., levamisole, ivermectin, fenbendazole, praziquantel, amikacin, and oxytetracycline) so that they can be dispensed at a volume of 0.02 ml per 10 g body weight. This serves to minimize the time spent calculating dosages and diluting drugs to meet the needs of the amphibian patient. Various sized graduated cylinders and designated water syringes should be available for preparing pharmaceutical solutions. A microliter syringe is handy to accurately administer small amounts of drug.

An 8 MHz doppler probe suitable for detecting cardiovascular sounds should be available within the room. As most amphibians are fairly small, it is important to use a doppler with a small patient contact surface. One probe that has been used is an 8.0 MHz unit with a 9-mm patient contact surface diameter (Ultrascope Doppler Arterial and Venous Blood Flow Detector, Model 8, 8 MHz; EMS Products, Inc., Kirkland, WA). The doppler also readily locates the heart for cardiac puncture.

8.5 CONDUCTING THE PHYSICAL EXAMINATION

In general, amphibians make great patients. Most are easily restrained allowing a complete physical examination with minimal stress to both animal and handler. Smaller amphibians, some of which weigh only grams, require the use of magnification for proper evaluation. By modifying techniques used commonly in other animals, diagnostic samples and administration of treatments can easily be accomplished.

With a complete history in hand, a physical examination is then performed. When possible, blood is collected for a routine complete blood count (CBC) and serum chemistry analysis. Unfortunately, many amphibians are simply too small to provide a significant sample size. Because some anurans release a significant stream of urine when first restrained, the clinician should be prepared to catch a sample for laboratory analysis. Radiographs should also be considered on a periodic basis to survey for the presence of metabolic bone disease. Stool samples are easily collected and may provide valuable information if examined in a timely fashion. Equipped with new information, problems identified during the clinical examination are considered and a differential diagnosis is formed. Additional clinical tests are then performed to provide the data needed to eliminate or confirm the clinician's hypothesis. Once the necessary tests have been performed, all of the information is considered and a final diagnosis is made. Lastly, an appropriate treatment regime is formulated including a plan to monitor the amphibian's progress.

8.5.1 Clinical Examination

Evaluation of the amphibian should begin with a hands-off observation of behavior and overall body condition. Posture of the animal should be appropriate for the species. Anurans typically rest with their heads up and legs held flexed beside their body. The head, eyes, and limbs should be symmetrical. Malformation, nutritional deficiencies, parasitic, and microbial infections may all result in a grossly abnormal animal. The amphibian should be well fleshed, showing little of the underlying skeleton. Evidence of bloat, hydrocoelom or emaciation is easily observed and often a first sign that the animal is in trouble (Figure 8.5). Gas bubbles in the skin or eyes of aquatic species indicate that the water in their environment is supersaturated with air. Further observation of the animal attempting to feed may provide information about its vision and neuromuscular capabilities.

Amphibians should be handled gently using wetted powder-free gloves. Examination then proceeds in a

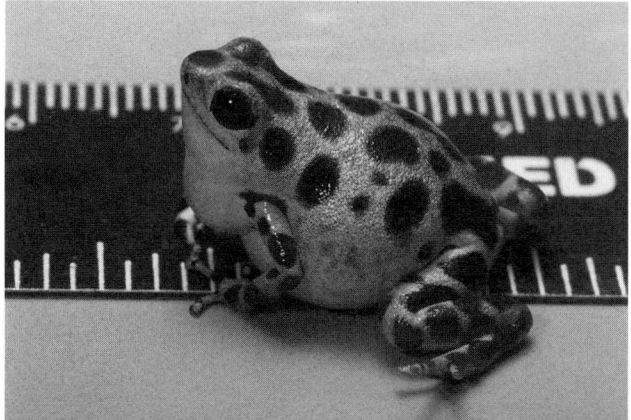

Figure 8.5. The rapid accumulation of fluid (hydrocoelom) in this strawberry poison frog, *Dendrobates pumilio,* was associated with sudden cessation of egg laying and subsequent illness. (George Grall, National Aquarium in Baltimore)

consistent and orderly fashion that minimizes the amount of handling time. Many amphibians resist restraint by kicking with their rear legs and pulling with their forelegs. A withdrawal reflex can easily be elicited by grasping each limb distally and extending it. When placed upside down, most amphibians will quickly exhibit a righting reflex, although patience may be required for those species that play dead. The blink reflex is elicited by gently touching the eyes, which, in response, should close and withdraw. Loss of one or more of these reflexes is indicative of a seriously ill patient.

A bright focal light source, such as a high-quality penlight, and magnification are useful during the physical examination. A binocular dissecting microscope is ideal for examining small amphibians, such as aquatic larvae. During the exam, care must be taken to prevent the animal from dehydrating or overheating. A supply of fresh, chemical-free, clean water should be kept on hand and used to keep the patient moist. A spray bottle works well for this purpose. Weight, although extremely variable due to hydration status, food in the stomach, and the presence of urine, should be recorded for every animal. The skin of amphibians is moist, except in toads and some species of frogs. The giant monkey frog, *Phyllomedusa bicolor,* for example, lives high within the rain forest canopy and waxes its skin to retain body fluids. Some anurans will periodically slough their superficial epidermis and then consume it unless they are ill. Pigment loss, erythema, hemorrhage, and ulceration of the integument (Figure 8.6) are commonly associated with microbial or parasitic infections.

Erosions and ulcerations on the feet are seen in animals housed on dirty or inappropriate substrates. Rostral abrasions are commonly found in animals attempting to escape their vivarium, although myiasis should be considered. Impression smears or biopsies are recommended for all skin lesions in order to determine etiology and develop a successful clinical plan. The heart rate may be determined in some animals by watching the surface of the skin in the area of the xiphoid. The ultrasonic doppler probe has been used on amphibians the size of a dendrobatid frog, and with practice the clinician can differentiate and characterize the cardiovascular sounds (e.g., atrial and ventricular contractions, atrioventricular and aortic valvular, aortic, brachiocephalic artery, and vena caval sounds) (Frye, 1994). It is helpful to move the probe along the transverse and longitudinal axis of the ventral thorax to locate these sounds. As a general rule, sounds originating from high pressure structures (e.g., ventricle, arteries) are louder and less sibilant than those from low pressure structures (atria, venous system). Evidence of respiration is readily seen as rapid movements at the intermandibular space. Both heart and respiratory rate vary with environmental temperature, as well as the activity level and condition of the animal. Auscultation is practical with larger amphibians only. The nares should be clean. Respiratory disease is suspected if excessive mucous or bubbles are noted.

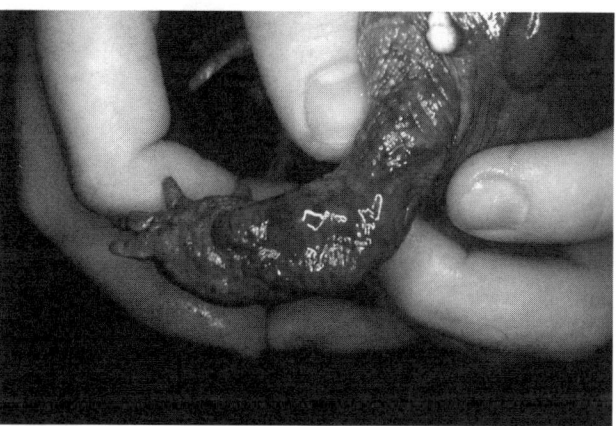

Figure 8.6. Ulceration of the skin may result from trauma or be associated with bacterial, fungal, or parasitic agents, or neoplasia. Failure to wear gloves puts the handler at risk of contracting zoonotic infections. (Kevin Wright, Philadelphia Zoological Garden)

Muscle wasting is indicative of starvation or chronic disease. Inadequate caloric intake eventually forces the animal to break down its muscle mass in an effort to derive the energy needed for survival. Improper nutrition, social structure, restricted vision, and illness may prevent the animal from feeding normally. Chronic infections with microsporidia and mycobacteria must be considered. Other diseases, such as a protein-losing enteropathy, prevent the animal from assimilating nutrients into the body. The long bones are easily palpated on large anurans. Deformities may be the result of prior trauma or metabolic bone disease.

The eyes are examined using a penlight, ophthalmoscope or slit-lamp (Figure 8.7). A slit-lamp is optimal, as it provides both illumination and magnification, allowing the viewer to inspect the cornea, iris, lens, retina, and anterior and posterior chambers. Aquatic and all larval frogs lack eyelids, while terrestrial adults have short lids and a translucent conjunctival fold. Most salamanders have well-developed lids. Like fish, the iris of many amphibians species have a vertical inferior stripe. Corneal and lenticular lesions are common. Special stains, such as fluorescein, can be used to further define corneal damage. (See Chapter 19, The Amphibian Eye.) Uveitis and panophthalmitis may be associated with the presence of infectious organisms. Topical ophthalmic medicated drops may easily be used, however, the size of drop (dose), and placement of the drug should be considered, as these animals have semipermeable skin allowing systemic assimilation.

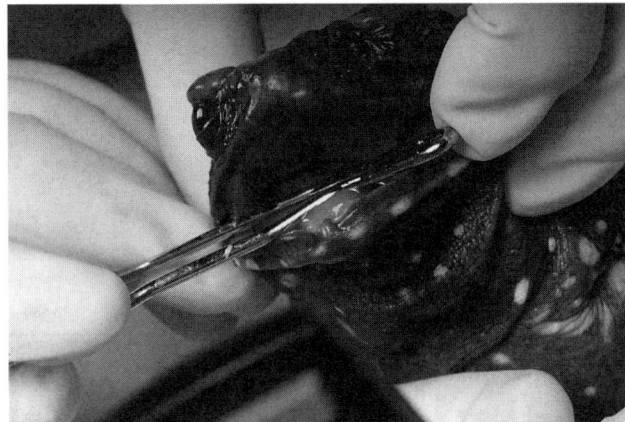

Figure 8.8. An oral speculum may be necessary to keep the mouth open for a thorough exam in larger species of amphibian such as this spotted toad, *Bufo guttatus*. (George Grall, National Aquarium in Baltimore)

Twisting the wrong way can result in mandibular fractures. Mucous membranes are then examined for appropriate color and the presence of lesions. The eye is separated from the buccal cavity by only a thin membrane, which should be carefully inspected, especially if an ocular problem has been noted. A tongue is present in most species (Figure 8.9). The lingual plexus can be evaluated by drawing the tongue forward using a cotton tip applicator. Occasionally ectoparasites may be found in the oral cavity and should be removed using a cotton tip applicator or eyelid forceps for identification. Gastric intussusception into the mouth has been seen in terminally ill and ascitic amphibian. However, some anurans can evert their stomach through the mouth as a normal behavior and use their forelegs to wipe toxic or otherwise undigestible materials off the stomach's mucosa.

Medications and blended foods are easily given orally. A blunted, flexible tube may be used in larger patients, while the accurate dosing of smaller amphibians

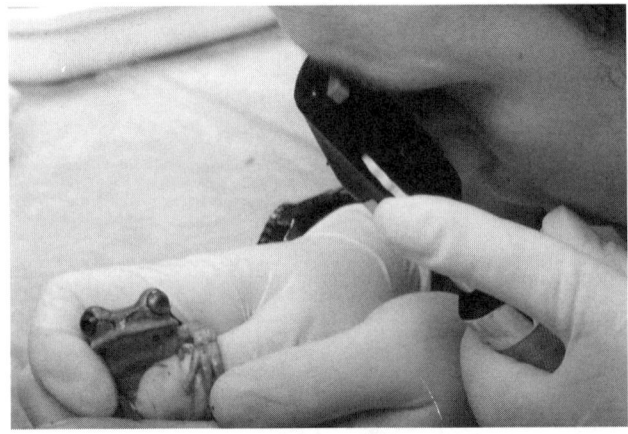

Figure 8.7. An ophthalmoscope can be used to assess the eye and surrounding tissues. (George Grall, National Aquarium in Baltimore)

The oral cavity is examined by gently opening the animal's mouth using either a small piece of waterproof paper, plastic card, oral speculum, or rubber spatula (Figure 8.8). Some amphibians, such as the commonly kept ornate horned frog, *Ceratophrys ornata*, are capable of inflicting a forceful bite, requiring that proper precautions be taken. As the mandibular and hyoid bones are generally quite fragile, a thorough oral exam may require chemical restraint in some animals to decrease the chance of severe iatrogenic trauma. The clinician is also advised that certain salamanders move the upper part of the jaw rather than the mandible, so the opening of the jaw should be attempted by gentle lifting of the maxillary region rather than forcing the mandible down.

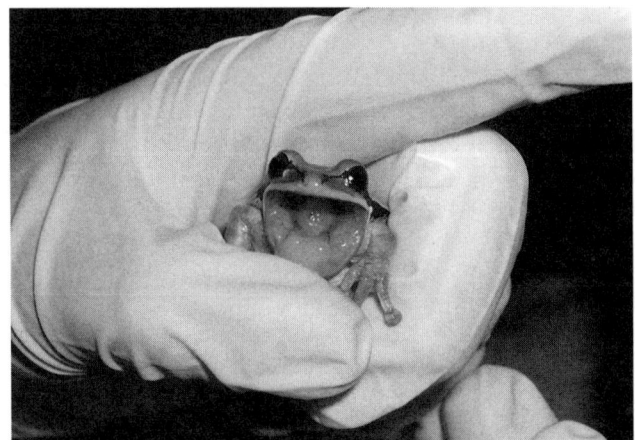

Figure 8.9. The tongue, glottis, lingual plexus, and mucous membranes are easily examined in this New Granada cross-banded treefrog, *Smilisca phaeota*. (Kevin Wright, Philadelphia Zoological Garden)

requires the use of a microliter syringe or pipette (Figures 8.10, 8.11). The Eppendorf® pipette (Brinkman Distributor, Westbury, NY) provides efficient and exact administration of very small quantities. The amount to be administered is simply set, and the disposable tip enables expedient placement of the drug in the animal's mouth. Most of the drugs used will be swallowed by the animal with little resistance.

Some amphibians defensively inflate themselves when handled, making abdominal palpation a challenge. Others are easily examined, allowing palpation of the stomach, liver, and egg masses if prominent (Figure 8.12). Abdominal masses including gastrointestinal obstruction and bladder stones may also be identified. Radiographs or ultrasound may provide additional information. Rectal, cloacal, and urinary bladder prolapse is not uncommon. This may be associated with heavy par-

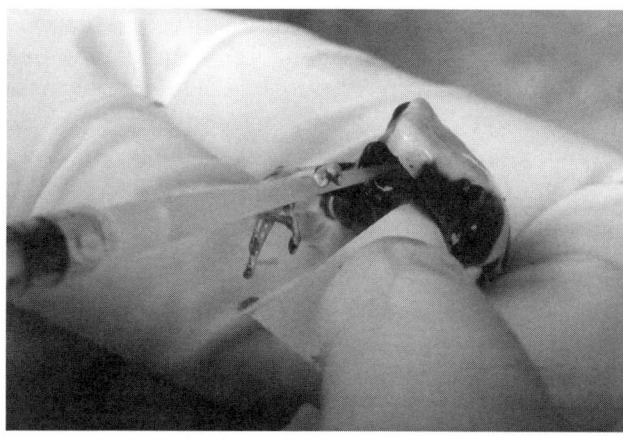

Figure 8.11. Oral administration of medication to a dyeing poison frog, *Dendrobates tinctorius*, using a microliter pipette. (George Grall, National Aquarium in Baltimore)

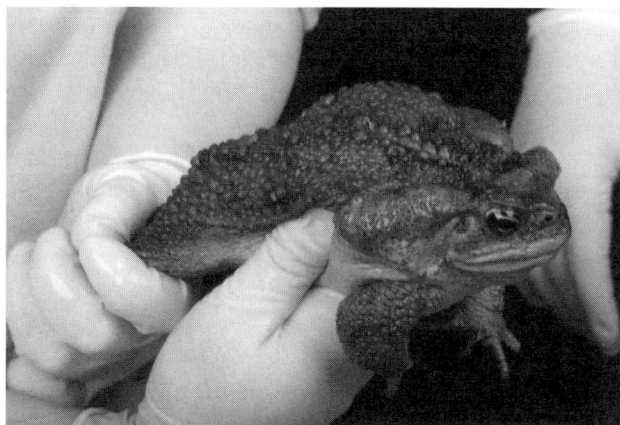

Figure 8.12. Abdominal palpation of the giant toad, *Bufo marinus*. (George Grall, National Aquarium in Baltimore)

asitism or traumatic injury. Animals with evidence of a possible prolapse must be palpated very gently.

8.6 CLINICAL TECHNIQUES

To make a diagnosis or monitor an amphibian's progress, the clinician may need to perform one or more clinical tests. The value of the potential knowledge must be always be weighed against the inherent risk in the procedure. Proper restraint combined with skilled collection, however, minimizes stress and the likelihood of injury to either handler or animal.

The size of the amphibian patient, its condition, and the skills of the clinician must always be considered when determining if a clinical technique can be safely accomplished.

8.6.1 Celiocentesis

Celiocentesis is the process of aspirating fluid from the coelom of bloated amphibians. Fluid commonly

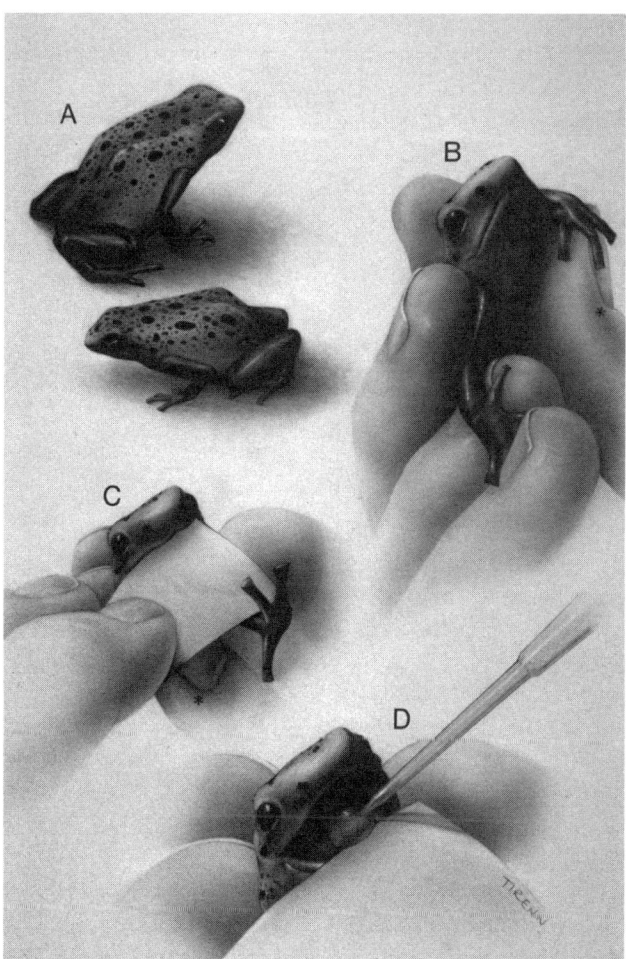

Figure 8.10. **A.** A healthy dendrobatid frog sits erect compared to an unhealthy animal. **B.** The thumb and forefingers should be used to grasp the subject firmly. Failure to wear gloves may damage the amphibian's skin and put handler at risk of intoxication from the animal's defensive secretions. **C.** A thin piece of waterproof paper or stiff plastic may be used to open the mouth gently. **D.** A microtip pipette is used to deliver oral medications. (Mike Tirenin, Johns Hopkins University Department of Art as Applied to Medicine)

accumulates as a result of cardiovascular failure, hepatic, or renal disease resulting in hydrocoelom (fluid within the coelom) or anasarca (generalized edema). Failure of the lymph hearts may result in abnormal fluid accumulation. In anurans, the lymph hearts located under the scapula and adjacent to the urostyle nay become especially prominent in addition to the excess fluid in the coelom. Samples are collected using a small-gauge needle and syringe. The animal should be palpated just prior to sample collection. With an amphibian in dorsal recumbency, dilute chlorhexidene (1 ml of 2% chlorhexidene solution, e.g., Novalsan®, mixed into 40 ml water) may be used to gently clean the selected site, generally in the paralumbar region or just off midline (Figure 8.13). When using the latter site, care should be taken to avoid the midabdominal vein. Samples should be submitted for fluid analysis including specific gravity, total protein, cytology, culture, and chemistry analysis. In several cases, clinicians have reported the collection of a clear, blue, or green fluid. Its clinical significance is presently unknown.

8.6.2 Blood Collection

Even small amounts of blood can yield important information, such as white blood cell count, red blood cell count, hematocrit, leukocyte differential, total protein, and the presence of parasites. Blood may be collected from frogs and toads using cardiac puncture, the femoral vein, the ventral abdominal vein, or the lingual vein (Figure 8.14). The ventral tail vein is the easiest site to collect blood from most salamanders. Lithium heparin is the anticoagulant of choice. A dilute chlorhexidene solution (1:40) may be used to prepare the puncture site. Because amphibians have an extensive lymphatic system, samples may become diluted with lymph. Hemostasis is achieved by applying direct pressure to the puncture site. Cotton tipped swabs are excellent for this purpose, as they concentrate the pressure directly to the vessel, especially in smaller patients (see also Chapter 11, Amphibian Hematology).

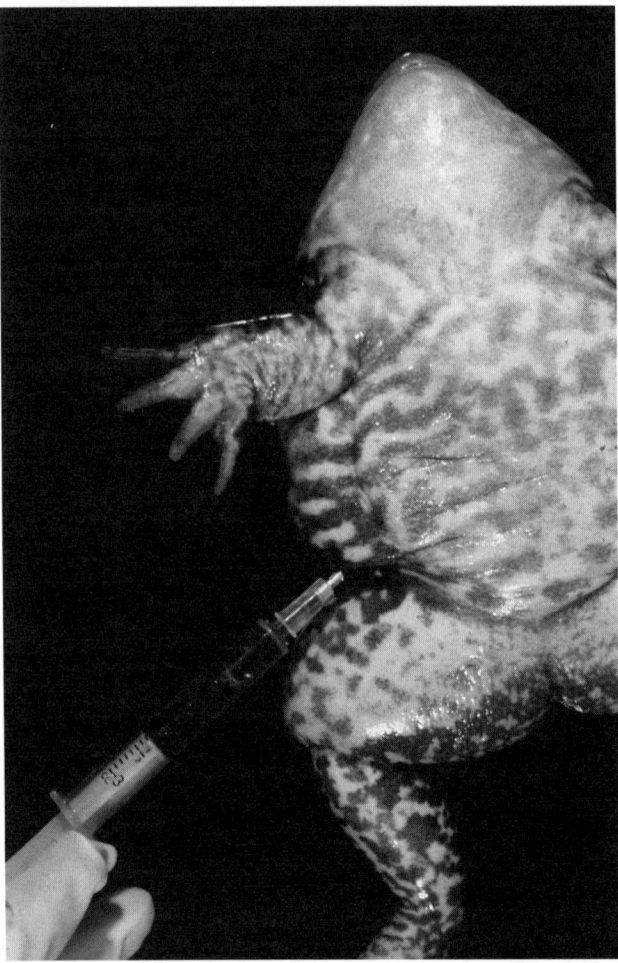

Figure 8.13. Celiocentesis is easily performed in amphibians using a small gauge needle placed paramedially or in the paralumbar region. (Kevin Wright, Philadelphia Zoological Garden)

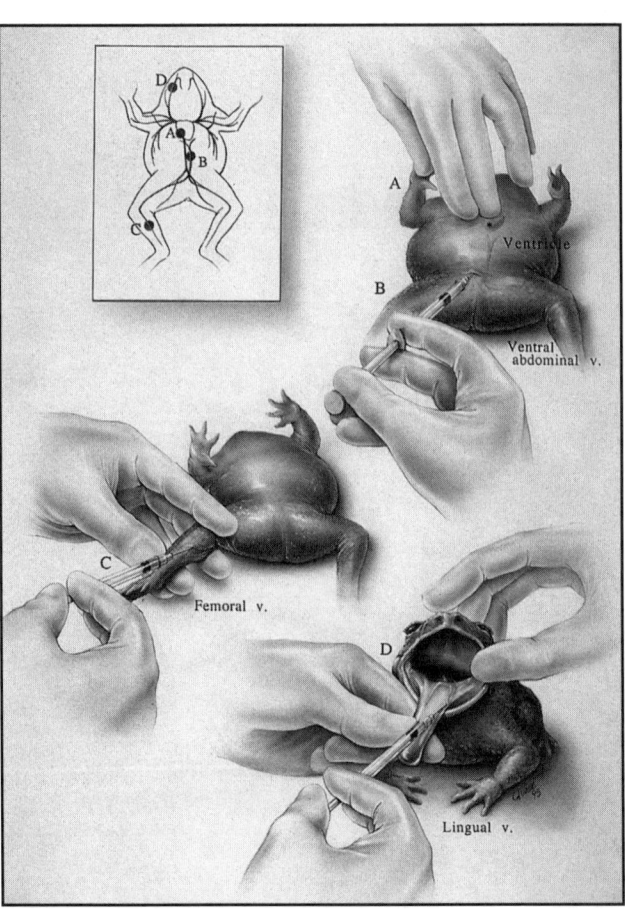

Figure 8.14. Commonly used phlebotomy sites in the anuran: **A**—Heart, **B**—Ventral Abdominal vein, **C**—Femoral Vein, **D**—Lingual Vein. (Quade Paul, Johns Hopkins University Department of Art as Applied to Medicine)

8.6.3 Cloacal Wash

A cloacal wash is easily performed using a tomcat catheter, an appropriately sized red rubber catheter, or a polypropylene intravenous catheter and 3-ml syringe (Figure 8.15). This technique is especially useful if repeated attempts to collect fresh stool have been unsuccessful. Protozoans, metazoans, bacteria, fungi, as well as inflammatory and neoplastic cells may be identified. The catheter is lubricated with a water-soluble sterile gel and gently inserted into the cloaca. A small amount (0.05–1 ml) of saline is then gently instilled and aspirated back into the syringe. Once collected, the sample must be immediately examined using light microscopy. Smears are then allowed to dry and stained for detailed cytological evaluation.

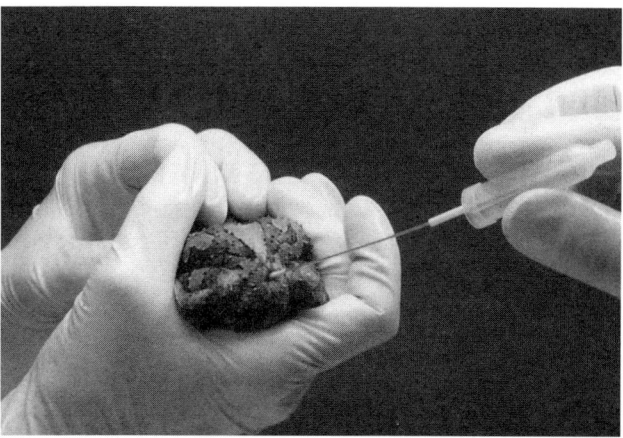

Figure 8.16. A moistened sterile swab can be inserted into the cloaca to obtain a culture. (George Grall, National Aquarium in Baltimore)

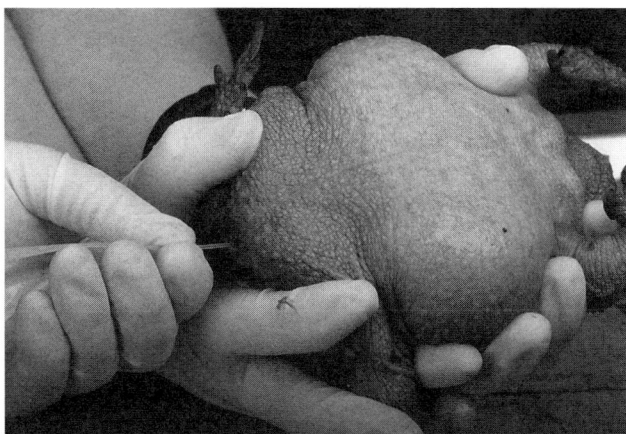

Figure 8.15. A cloacal wash is accomplished in this giant toad, *Bufo marinus*, using a tomcat catheter and 0.5 cc of 0.9% NaCl (Saline). (George Grall, National Aquarium in Baltimore)

8.6.4 Culture Collection

Bacterial and fungal cultures are readily collected from amphibians. Sites commonly sampled include dermal, oral, and ocular lesions; and the cloaca (Figure 8.16). Complete analysis of diagnostic specimens such as coelomic fluid, blood, urine, and feces may include microbial assessment. Postmortem tissues routinely collected for culture are liver, spleen, kidney, and heart. Samples are taken using fine-tipped sterile swabs which are placed immediately into transport media (e.g., Mini-tip Culturette® Collection and Transport System Becton Dickinson Microbiology Systems, Cockeysville, MD). Tissue damage and irritation is minimized by first wetting the swab with transport media or sterile saline. Anaerobic, aerobic, and/or fungal cultures are then made by plating samples onto appropriate media and incubating as required (see Chapter 10, Clinical Microbiology of Amphibians for the Exotic Practice, and Section 13.6, Bacteriologic Techniques for the Diagnostic Laboratory). Pediatric blood culture tubes (Figure 8.17) containing tryptic soy broth (DIFCO Laboratories, Detroit, MI) may be successfully used for the culture of very small blood samples (>0.05 ml) and may also enable the isolation of difficult-to-grow

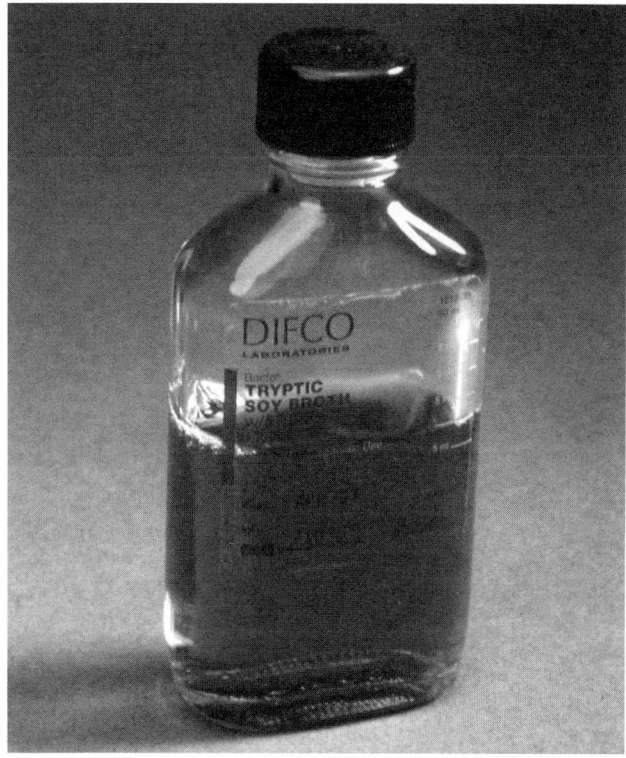

Figure 8.17. Tryptic soy broth works well for aerobic and anaerobic culture of the blood or other samples. Several drops of fluid or merely the tip of the culture swab are sufficient to inoculate the medium. (George Grall, National Aquarium in Baltimore)

microorganisms from other sites. A thioglycollate broth tube can be used for a blood culture too.

8.6.5 Electrocardiography

Amphibians have rarely been subjected to electrocardiographic studies and analysis, and one published electrocardiographic study of amphibians did not correlate electrocardiogram (ECG) changes with a specific pathology (Mullen, 1974). The amphibian patient has been excluded from cardiac cycle analysis for a variety of reasons, including, but not limited to, small body size, uncooperative patients necessitating anesthesia, failure to recognize disease, and the variation of the ectotherm metabolism associated with temperature. The small body size of most amphibians has made it difficult to attach the probes. Furthermore, small body size can influence the shape of the ECG, as the placement of the leads can affect the recording of the electrical impulses, a fact amply demonstrated in reptiles (Valentinuzzi et al., 1969). The amphibian must be anesthetized for an accurate ECG recording. The type of anesthetic used may influence the shape of the ECG. The practicality of using an ECG to diagnose disease in amphibians is limited, as there are few normal values to serve as an interpretive base (Table 8.3). In ectotherms such as reptiles it has been shown that the environmental temperature has an exponential relationship with heart rate within physiological limits (Francaz & Aupy, 1969; Jacobson & Whitford, 1970; Jacobson & Whitford, 1971), thus the ECG will have a different morphology at small temperature increments. The amplitude of the R wave also increases proportionately with temperature (Francaz & Aupy, 1969).

The morphology of the amphibian heart causes unique waves in the ECG. Amphibians can produce a low magnitude SV wave during depolarization of the bulbus cordis (Mullen, 1974) which may occur before the P wave. The B wave is another low magnitude wave that occurs after ventricular depolarization. Neither wave may be distinguishable from the other components (i.e., P, QRS, and T waves) due to their low amplitude.

The excitation sequence of the amphibian heart is species-dependent and not correlated with habitat type. Two terrestrial bufonids, the giant toad, *Bufo marinus*, and leaf toad, *Bufo* cf *typhonius*, had a base-to-apex

Table 8.3. Electrocardiogram information on four anurans maintained under sodium pentobarbital anesthesia (.025–.03mg/gm). Adapted from Mullen, 1974.

Common name	South American common toad	Giant toad	Buerger's robber frog *Eleuthrodactylus buergeri*	Mountain water frog
Scientific name	*Bufo cf typhonius*	*Bufo marinus*		*Telmatobius montanus*
Sample size	4	3	5	5
Body weight (g)	7 (2–23)	10 (3–17)	9 (6–13)	53 (46–59)
Temp. (°C)	19	19	13	12–14
Intervals				
RR	0.906s (0.094–1.31)	0.97s (0.86–1.10)	1.89s (1.46–2.34)	1.83s (1.72–1.90)
PR	0.225s (0.20–.24)	0.23s (0.20–.26)	0.34s (0.31–.41)	0.44s (0.39–.51)
QRS	0.075s (0.06–.08)	0.04s (0.04)	0.14s (0.10–.20)	0.10s (0.06–.12)
QT	0.72s (0.66–.82)	0.62s (0.52–.74)	0.93s (0.76–1.06)	1.18s (1.02–1.36)
PR:RR	0.208 (0.17–.82)	0.24 (0.18–.30)	0.186 (0.14–.23)	0.24 (0.22–.27)
QT:RR	0.65 (0.63–.70)	0.65 (0.63–.67)	0.51 (0.32–.64).64	0.64 (0.59–.72)
Wave forms				
QRS	131° (+75° to −160°)	105° (+75° to +165°)	−73° (−150° to −25°)	+73° (−20° to +165°)
T	−77° (−120° to −30°)	−62° (−140° to +20°)	−142° (+170° to −110°)	−165° (+160° to −100°)

sequence of ventricular depolarization and repolarization, which is the same cycle described for the aquatic leptodactylid frog, *Telmatobius montanus* (Mullen, 1974). The terrestrial leptodactylid, *Eleuthrodactylus buergeri* had an apex-to-base sequence of ventricular depolarization and repolarization (Mullen, 1974). Given the lack of guidelines for this basic physiological function, the clinician is advised to determine "normal" values by analyzing a clinically healthy amphibian of the same species as the clinically ill amphibian. The interpretation of the ill amphibian's ECG can then be predicated on the assumed normal ECG in combination with the results of ultrasonic doppler examination and, if possible, ultrasonographic examination (see Chapter 20, Diagnostic Imaging of Amphibians).

Analysis of the amphibian ECG is further complicated by the low surface electrical potential of amphibians. Low surface electrical potential can make identification of isoelectric leads difficult if not impossible with standard ECG equipment. A lack of isoelectric leads eliminates the possibility of determining the mean electrical axis.

Despite the difficulties encountered in electrocardiographic analysis of the amphibian patient, it does merit further attention. The following suggested techniques are used to obtain a standardized ECG:

1) Acclimate the amphibian(s) for a minimum of 4 h to the temperature of the room where the ECG will be made. Longer acclimation times may be necessary for amphibians over 500 g.
2) Note the date, time, and temperature at which the ECG was obtained directly on the ECG. The ambient temperature should be at 21°C (70°F) unless this is stressful to the species.
3) Perform an ECG on a healthy amphibian in addition to the ill amphibian.
4) The patient should be at a surgical level of anesthesia induced by tricaine methanesulfonate (see Chapter 9, Restraint Techniques and Euthanasia) with supplemental oxygen bubbled through anesthetic solution.
5) The patient should have needle electrodes placed intramuscularly if size allows, otherwise electrodes can be placed subcutaneously.
6) The electrodes for the right arm (RA) and left arm (LA) should be placed ventrally at the distal third of the humerus. The electrode for the left leg (LL) is placed midventrally and that for the right leg (RL) is placed ventrally in the right gastrocnemius.

The field of electrocardiography is largely unexplored. It would be helpful to compile an ECG table that records the different values obtained in healthy individuals of different species acclimated to different temperatures so that temperature acclimation would not be a necessary part of the process needed to obtain an ECG in amphibians.

8.6.6 Endoscopy

Valuable information may be gained by passing a small rigid scope through the oropharynx and into the stomach of larger sedated amphibians. Examination of the cloaca may also be carried out. Depending on the size of the amphibian, a 1.7-mm needle endoscope, a 1.9-mm arthroscope, or a 2.7-mm arthroscope, may be selected. As a general rule, larger scopes will provide better optics and field of view. Insufflation may improve images substantially. This is best accomplished using a red rubber tube and 12–35-ml syringe to inflate the stomach or cloaca with air. Foreign bodies can be removed or small biopsies taken using a pair of biopsy forceps.

8.6.7 Fecal Evaluation

Analysis of fresh fecal samples can provide valuable information, even in the smallest of amphibians. Fresh samples are best as some protozoans will encyst with environmental change escaping detection. Furthermore, with time cellular degradation and the increased presence of free ranging organisms complicates assessment. To avoid these problems, many amphibians can be force-fed and placed on a moist, nonbleached paper towel in a clean container (Figure 8.18). A slurry of ReptoMin® (distributed by Tetra Sales, Blacksburg, VA) works well for this purpose as it is rapidly passed through the animal. Routine evaluation of the sample includes form and color, a wet mount using 0.9% saline, and a float using a sodium nitrate solution with a specific gravity of 1.200 (e.g., Fecasol®). Samples should not be stored in the refrigerator, as this may cause many protozoans to encyst, hindering identification. Commonly found organisms include flagellates, opalinids, ciliates, nematode eggs and larvae. Cytological evaluation is performed

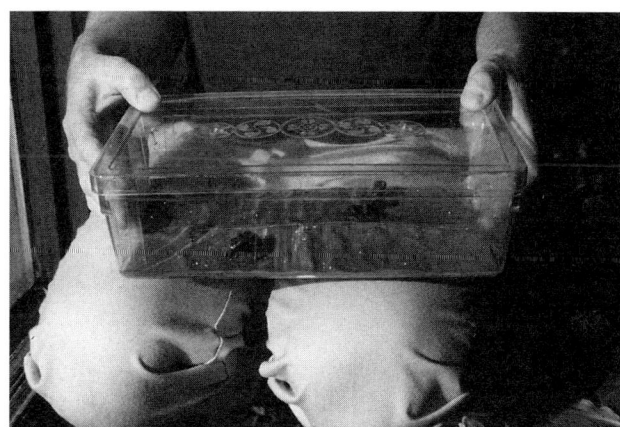

Figure 8.18. Collecting a group fecal sample from recently fed blue poison frogs, *Dendrobates azureus*. (Brent Whitaker, National Aquarium in Baltimore)

where suspicion of coccidiosis, or other gastrointestinal disease exists. Wright-Giemsa stain and Gram stain work well for this purpose. The presence of red blood cells and inflammatory cells is indicative of active infection requiring immediate therapy. An acid-fast stain is useful if *Cryptosporidium*-like agents are suspected. Many of the metazoa and protozoa are considered normal flora in small to moderate numbers. Culture of the stool in most cases is often unrewarding. Salmonella, aeromonads, and other bacteria can be found and most often appear to be of little clinical significance, although their zoonotic potential must be considered. On rare occasions a fecal culture may reveal a single species of bacteria. A sole isolate may in fact represent the primary etiological agent.

8.6.8 Medication and Nutrient Administration

Administration of Injectable Medications. Injectable medications may be given intracoelomically, intravenously, intramuscularly, or subcutaneously. Injections into the anuran's dorsal lymph sac is also an excellent option that results in extremely rapid assimilation of drug. The puncture site is first cleaned with dilute chlorhexidine (1:40). Intracoelomic injections are best accomplished with the animal in dorsal recumbency with its head tipped slightly downward. A small (23–30 gauge) needle is slowly inserted just off midline or in the paralumbar region. Because of the potential danger to impale other organs, proper restraint is mandatory. Intravenous administration is difficult in small amphibians, but can be achieved in larger animals through the midabdominal vein, lingual vein, or heart (see Figure 8.14). Intramuscular injections can be given to amphibians large enough to provide an adequate muscle mass (Figure 8.19). Insulin syringes with fixed needles work well for this purpose. Subcutaneous injections may also be used in anurans, but in salamanders and caecilians this is problematic, due to the adherence of the skin to the underlying muscle. Lymph sac injections are readily accomplished by locating one of the many lymph sacs that lie just below the skin. The dorsal lymph sac of anurans, which extends from the tip of the urostyle to the tip of the snout, is easily found for injection just lateral and anterior to the urostyle. Because there is rapid assimilation of drugs, such as ketamine, the dorsal lymph sac is the preferred site for injection of anurans.

Administration of Oral Medications and Nutrients. Medications and prepared foods may be given to amphibians orally (see Chapter 24, Pharmacotherapeutics, and Section 7.12, Cachexia). The mouth is opened gently using piece of waterproof paper, plastic card, rubber spatula, or other nontraumatic speculum. Excessive force will cause mandibular fractures and must be avoided. In resistant animals, such as the Surinam horned frog, *Ceratophrys cornuta*, two smooth plastic cards stacked upon one another, may be inserted into the mouth allowing a tube or instrument to be passed between them (Figure 8.20). A microliter syringe, tomcat catheter or other blunted tube may be used to administer the desired material into the mouth (Figure 8.21; see also Figure 8.10). If necessary to tube feed the animal, a blunted, flexible tube (e.g., Sovereign® Feeding Tube and Urethral Catheter) may be advanced carefully down the esophagus and into the stomach of larger amphibians, allowing greater quantities of fluid, food, or medication to be administered.

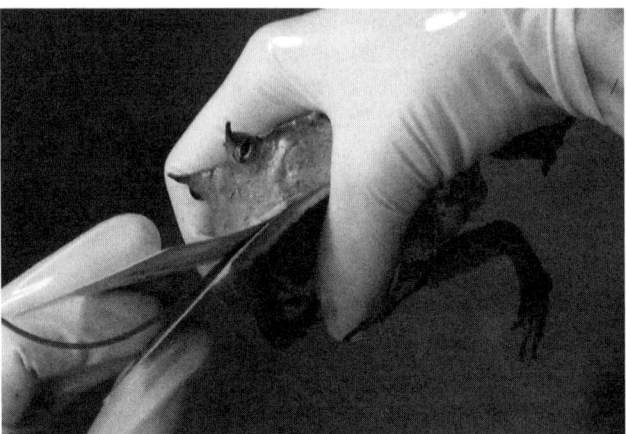

Figure 8.20. Giving oral medication to this Surinam horned frog, *Ceratophrys cornuta*, is facilitated using two smooth plastic cards to open the mouth. (George Grall, National Aquarium in Baltimore)

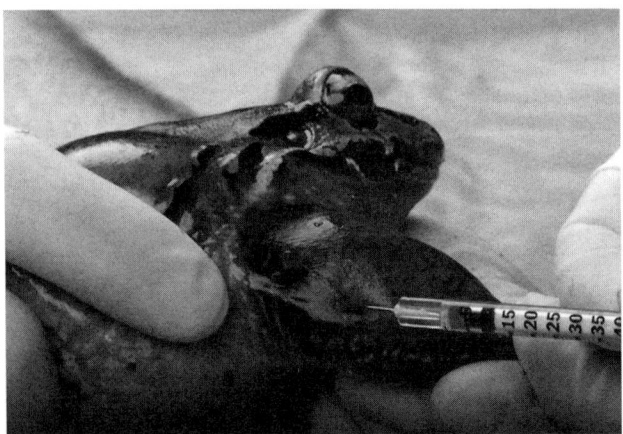

Figure 8.19. An intramuscular injection is given in the forelimb of this South American bullfrog, *Leptodactylus pentadactylus*, using an insulin syringe. (Brent Whitaker, National Aquarium in Baltimore)

CLINICAL TECHNIQUES —— 107

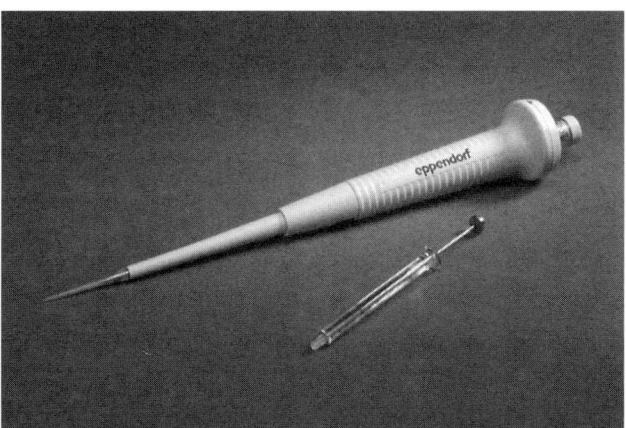

Figure 8.21. The Eppendorf pipette system can be used to deliver minute volumes of medications to amphibians. (George Grall, National Aquarium in Baltimore)

Topical Administration of Medications. Many amphibians have semipermeable skin that allows the systemic uptake of medications applied percutaneously (Figure 8.22). This rapid route of administration can be advantageous where small quantities are required, especially in animals that are easily stressed when handled. Some drugs, however, contain carriers that are irritating to amphibians, minimizing their usefulness topically. Injectable enrofloxacin, for example, contains benzyl alcohol which in some species appears to cause discomfort for a short time following its administration. Caution must also be taken when treating ocular lesions frequently throughout the day, as most medicated drops contain relatively high concentrations of drug. Overdosing small amphibians can be avoided by diluting ophthalmic drops and calculating the total possible dose an animal of a given size may tolerate.

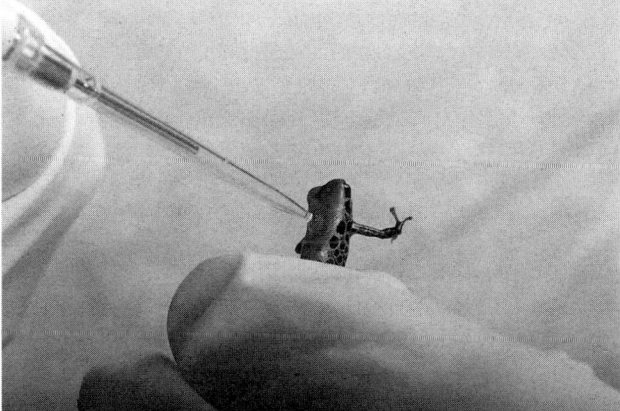

Figure 8.22. The topical administration of small quantities of medication is accomplished using a microliter pipette. (George Grall, National Aquarium in Baltimore)

Medicated Baths. Medicated baths have long been used to treat the ailments of fishes and amphibians. It is an especially useful technique when treating a large number of amphibians, especially those that are aquatic. Because amphibians possess a semipermeable skin, medications mixed into a physiological solution are readily absorbed. Care must be taken to ensure that the resulting solution is pH-balanced and that the chemicals used are not irritating to the amphibian.

Terrestrial amphibians may be given short-term baths by placing them into a container filled so that their ventrum is immersed in the solution. Deli cups lined with a paper towel wetted with the medicated solution can be used for smaller amphibians. A second moistened paper towel can be placed gently on top, trapping the amphibians in small medicated caves. Larger animals may be put into tubs containing medicated solution. Escape of climbing amphibians from the container is prevented by placing a lid or wad of nonabrasive bubble wrap approximately 2 cm (1 in) above the solution's surface. Amphibians should be closely monitored to ensure that they do not abrade their rostrum during this process.

In some cases, medicated baths may be performed directly in the tanks that house aquatic amphibians. A large water change should be carried out just prior to adding the chemical in an effort to reduce the concentration of the pathogen. Biological filtration should be removed from the tank if possible, as many chemicals such as antibiotics may injure or kill the nitrifying bacteria responsible for converting toxic ammonia and nitrite to relatively nontoxic nitrate. Activated carbon must also be removed as it will bind many of the drugs commonly used. Additional aeration may be necessary, especially when using chemicals such as formalin. Once the bath is completed, 75–90% of the water should be changed with aged water, and filtration with activated carbon should be initiated. If filtration with activated carbon is not possible, then a minimum of three 100% water changes should be made to ensure that only negligible quantities of the chemical are left in the system. Biological filtration can then be returned to the tank.

8.6.9 Skin Scrape

Successful treatment of integument disease requires proper classification of the offending organism(s). Many metazoans, protozoans, fungi, and bacteria that infect the skin may be readily identified in minutes after making an inspection of cells obtained from active lesions. Samples are collected by gently pulling the edge of a glass slide, coverslip, or the blunted edge of a scalpel blade over the surface of the skin (Figures 8.23, 8.24, 8.25, 8.26). The material collected is smeared onto a glass slide and a cover slip is placed gently on top. Saline (0.9% NaCl) is used to wet the smear if needed. If a microscope is not immediately

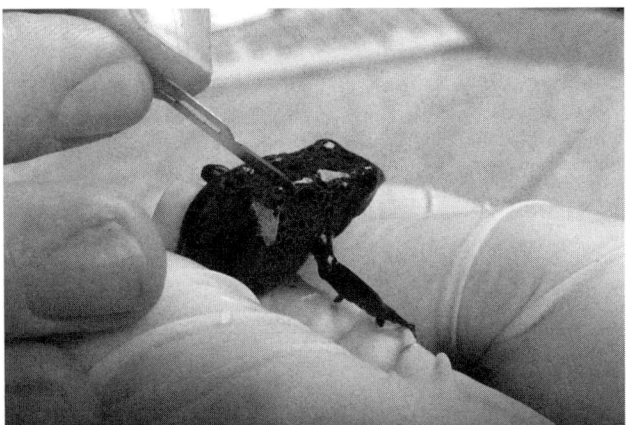

Figure 8.23. A skin scraping is taken from a blue poison frog, *Dendrobates azureus*, using the blunted edge of a #15 scalpel blade. (George Grall, National Aquarium in Baltimore)

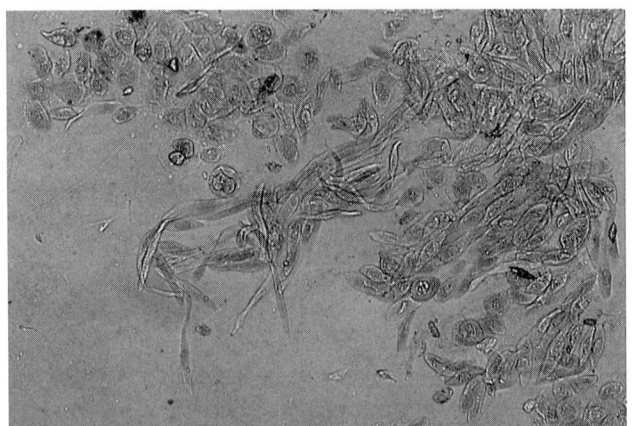

Figure 8.24. Normal epithelial cells of an Anderson's axolotl. *Ambystoma andersoni*, obtained by skin scrape and examined unstained in a wet mount. (Sandy McCampbell, Philadelphia Zoological Garden)

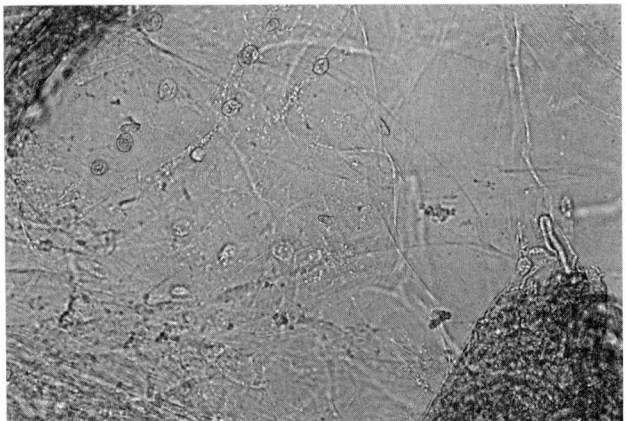

Figure 8.25. Fungal elements obtained by skin scrape and examined unstained in a wet mount confirming saprolegniasis in a Rio Cauca caecilian, *Typhlonectes natans*. (Sandy McCampbell, Philadelphia Zoological Garden)

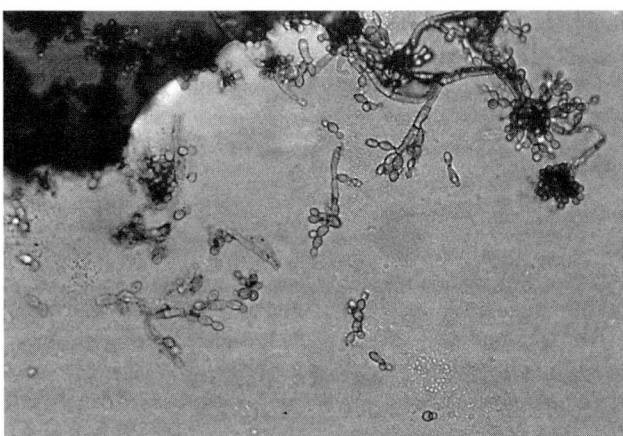

Figure 8.26. *Phialophora*-like fungal elements obtained by skin scrape and examined unstained in a wet mount. (Sandy McCampbell, Philadelphia Zoological Garden)

available, desiccation can be prevented by placing the slide on a moist paper towel in a covered petri dish. Once examined, the smear can be dried and stained as needed to enhance diagnostic value.

8.6.10 Gastric Wash

In larger animals, a small pliable tube (e.g., 5–8 French catheter) lightly coated with sterile water-soluble gel may be gently advanced into the amphibian's stomach. Up to 1–2 ml of saline (0.9%) is then slowly administered using a 6-ml syringe. After approximately 30 seconds the fluid is gently aspirated back into the catheter. A portion of the sample is examined immediately using a light microscope and slides are prepared for cytological examination using Wright-Giemsa and Gram stains. Cultures are often unrewarding, however, this should be considered by the clinician.

8.6.11 Touch Preparations

A touch preparation complements the skin scrape or may be used where there is concern that a scraping may cause further trauma to the affected tissue. Rostral abrasions and cloacal prolapses, which are commonly seen in anurans, are easily sampled by lightly touching the lesion one or more times with a clean glass slide (Figure 8.27). Several slides are prepared and allowed to air dry. Samples are stained using Wright-Giemsa to provide cellular definition. Gram stain is applied to a second slide. Bacteria, fungi, parasites, and inflammatory cells may be detected on the stained slides allowing the clinician to determine an appropriate course of action.

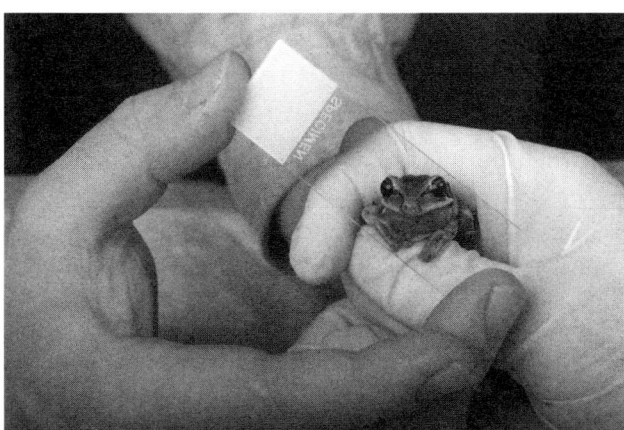

Figure 8.27. A touch preparation is made using a clean glass slide from the rostral abrasion on a New Granada cross-banded treefrog, *Smilisca phaeota*. (George Grall, National Aquarium in Baltimore)

8.6.12 Tracheal Wash

A tracheal wash may provide the clinician with evidence of parasitic, bacterial, or fungal pneumonia. Samples are best collected in anesthetized animals using a sterile tomcat catheter which is inserted *very gently* through the glottis and into the trachea (Figure 8.28). A small amount of sterile saline is instilled and then aspirated back into the syringe. A wet mount performed immediately may provide guidance in choosing therapeutics which can be administered before the patient recovers from anesthesia. Further analysis of the sample should include culture and cytology.

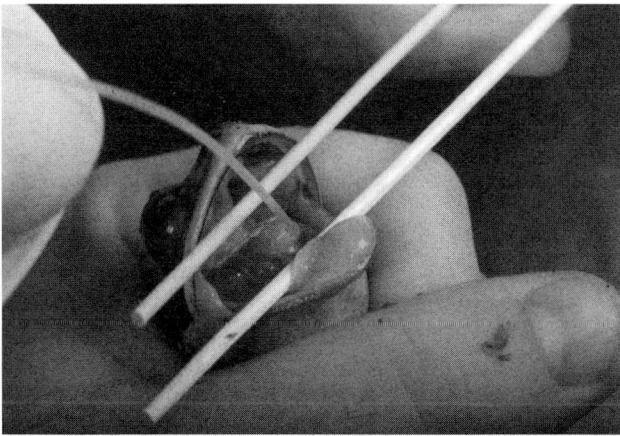

Figure 8.28. A tomcat catheter is inserted into the glottis in preparation for a tracheal wash. Note the thin membrane that separates the eye from the oral cavity. (George Grall, National Aquarium in Baltimore)

8.6.13 Urine Collection and Analysis

Urine may be collected from anurans with frequent success. Aquatic frogs, such as the African clawed frog, *Xenopus laevis*, have small urinary bladders capable of holding relatively little urine in comparison to anurans that inhabit arid environments (Duellman & Trueb, 1994; Prosser, 1973). When first handled, many anurans will release a significant stream of urine that can be caught in a sterile cup. Those that do not may be encouraged to produce a urine sample by stimulating the cloaca with a small rubber tube (Figure 8.29). A complete urinalysis is performed, including a wet mount which is scrutinized for the presence of cells and parasites. Slides are prepared for staining at a later time with Wright-Giemsa and Gram stains.

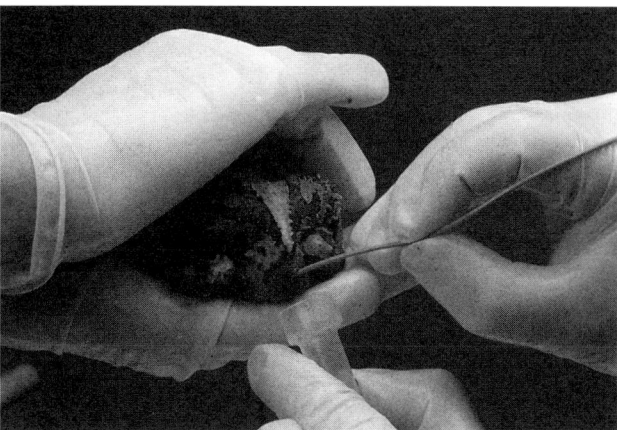

Figure 8.29. Many anurans can be stimulated to urinate by the insertion of a small red rubber catheter. (George Grall, National Aquarium in Baltimore)

Interpretation of results should be based upon comparison to urine collected from clinically healthy members of the same species. Environmental conditions, diet, and the physiological state of the amphibian may influence urine composition. Glucosuria for instance, may be more prominent in winter-adapted frogs, such as the wood frog, *Rana sylvatica*, that produce a massive hyperglycemia in order to prevent cryoinjury (Layne et al., 1996). Under normal circumstances, filtration rates of 30 ml/kg/h have been determined in frogs. Functional glomeruli produce a filtrate void of protein, but with concentrations of chloride and glucose similar to that of blood plasma. Sodium, chloride, and glucose are absorbed by the tubule. Although the proximal and distal tubule absorb both sodium and water, the distal tubule has low water permeability, causing urine to be hyposmotic (Prosser, 1973).

Active transport may also occur in the urinary bladder of amphibians. The giant toad, *Bufo marinus*, adapted to brackish water produces cloacal urine with 10–12 times the sodium content compared to ureteral urine as fresh water is absorbed. Dehydration and reduced blood volume stimulate the absorption of water from the bladder while amphibians that are well hydrated reabsorb sodium (Prosser, 1973).

REFERENCES

Duellman, W.E. and L. Trueb. 1994. Biology of Amphibians. Johns Hopkins University Press, Baltimore, MD, 670 pp.

Francaz, J.M. and M. Aupy. 1969. Action de la temperature sur la forme de l'electrocardiogramme chez quelques amphibiens et reptiles. Comptes Rendus des Seances de la Societe de Biologie. Extrait du Tome 163(1):48–50.

Freytag, G.E., B. Grzimek, O. Kuhn, and E. Thenius. 1968. Amphibians, *in* Grzimek B., (Ed): Animal Life Encyclopedia, Vol. 5 Fishes II and Amphibians. Van Nostrand Reinhold Co., New York.

Frye, F.L. 1994. Ultrasonic doppler blood flow detection in small exotic animal medicine. Seminars in Avian and Exotic Pet Medicine 3(3): 133–139.

Herrmann, Hans-Joachim. 1993a. Laubfroesche. Tetra, Germany. ISBN 3-89356-161-7. (emphasizes Hylidae)

Herrmann, Hans-Joachim. 1993b. Ruder and Riedfroesche. Tetra, Germany. ISBN 3-89356-160-9. (emphasizes Rhacophoridae and Hyperolidae)

Herrmann, Hans-Joachim. 1994. Amphibien im Aquarium. Tetra, Stuttgart, Germany. ISBN 3-8001-7287-9.

Horseman, N.D., A.H. Meier, and D.D. Culley. 1976. Daily variations in the effects of disturbances on growth, fattening and metamorphosis in the bullfrog (*Rana catesbeiana*). Journal of Experimental Zoology 198:353–357.

Jacobson, E. and W.G. Whitford. 1970. The effect of acclimation on physiological responses to temperature in the snakes *Thamnophis proximus* and *Natrix rhombifer*. Comp. Biochem. Physiol. 35:439–449.

Jacobson, E. and W.G. Whitford. 1971. Physiological responses to temperature in the patch-nosed snake *Salvadora lexalepis*. Herpetologica 27(3):289–295.

Layne, J.R., R.E. Lee, and M.M. Cutwa 1996. Post-hibernation excretion of glucose in urine of the freeze tolerant frog *Rana sylvatica*. Journal of Herpetology 30:1:85–87.

Mattison, C. 1987. Frogs and Toads of the World. Facts on File, Inc., New York.

Mullen, R.K. 1974. Electrocardiographic characteristics of four anuran Amphibia. Comp. Biochem. Physiol. 49A:647–654.

Naitoh, T. and R.J. Wassersug. 1994. Emesis in larval salamanders, *Hynobius nebulosus* (Hynobiidae). J. of Herpetology 28:2:245–247.

Obst, F.J., K. Richter, and U. Jacob. 1988. The Completely Illustrated Atlas of Reptiles and Amphibian for the Terrarium. TFH Publications, Inc., Neptune City, NJ.

Porter, K.R. 1972. Herpetology. W.B. Saunders Co., Philadelphia, PA.

Prosser, C.L. 1973. Water: Osmotic balance; hormonal regulation, *in* Prosser, C.L., (Ed.): Comparative Animal Physiology. W.B. Saunders Co., Philadelphia, PA, pp. 1–78.

Slavens, F.L. 1995. Reptiles and amphibians in captivity: breeding, longevity, and inventory. Published annually by Frank L. Slavens, POB 30744, Seattle, WA 98103.

Staniszewski, M. 1995. Amphibians in Captivity. TFH Publications, Inc., Neptune City, NJ.

Stoskopf, M.K., A. Wisneski, and L. Pieper. 1985. Iodine toxicity in poison arrow frogs. Proc. Amer. Assoc. Zoo Vet. pp. 86–88.

Valentinuzzi, M.E., H.E. Hoff, and L.A. Geddes. 1969. Electrocardiogram of the snake: Effect of the location of the electrodes and cardiac vectors. Journal of Electrocardiology 2(3):245–252.

Wassersug, R.J., A.Izumi-Kurotani, M. Yamashita, and T. Naitoh. 1993. Motion sickness in amphibians. Behavioral and Neural Biology 60:42–51.

Wright, K.M. 1993. Disinfection for the herpetoculturist. Vivarium 5(1):31–33.

Zimmerman, E. 1986. Breeding Terrarium Animals. TFH Publications, Inc., Neptune City, NJ.

CHAPTER 9
RESTRAINT TECHNIQUES AND EUTHANASIA

Kevin M. Wright, DVM

9.1 MANUAL RESTRAINT

When restraining amphibians, the safety of the veterinarian and veterinary assistant and the comfort and safety of the patient must be taken into account. The skin of many species of anurans and salamanders are known to produce secretions which contain potentially toxic compounds and are the focus of intensive research (Erspamer, 1994; Habermehl, 1974), while the skin secretions of caecilians have been the subject of little, if any, investigation. Many of the compounds that have been isolated and described from amphibian skin secretions are toxic to man and probably evolved as antipredator defenses, although other purposes have also been delineated (Barthalmus, 1994). Most of these toxins must come into direct contact with mucous membranes in order to be absorbed into the human body, however transdermal absorption, inoculation into abrasions or lacerations, inhalation, and ingestion are other possible routes of human exposure to amphibian secretions.

Many species of amphibians produce skin secretions that cause mild to severe inflammation of mucous membranes (e.g., Cuban treefrog, *Osteopilus septentrionalis*, members of the Bufonidae) (Chen & Chen, 1933). Alvarobufotoxin and other digitalis-like substances have been isolated from the Colorado river toad, *Bufo alvarius* (Hanson & Vial, 1956). If ingested, the secretions of the Colorado river toad and the giant toad, *Bufo marinus*, cause salivation, regurgitation, dyspnea, convulsions, and even death. Both species are well known for producing hallucinogenic substances similar to bufotenine. Bufotenine was placed under restriction by the U.S. Drug Enforcement Administration in the late 1960's (Horgan, 1990). The abuse potential of the toads has been overemphasized in the press with tales of people licking toads to ingest these mind-altering substances. This media blitz in turn has led to legislation that prohibits possession of these toads in certain areas. The truth of the matter is that the other toxic compounds present in the secretions of these toads will cause sickness and possibly death in anyone foolhardy enough to attempt "toad-licking." Lethal toxins are also present in the skin secretions of many poison frog species (e.g., golden poison frog, *Phyllobates terribilis*) (Grenard, 1994). The toxins in some species are especially dangerous, and even a minute amount of the skin secretion produced by some dendrobatid frogs can cause human death.

Some amphibians lack compounds that are noticeably toxic to humans, but their skin secretions are still an effective means of defense against predation by other creatures. Members of the slimy salamander complex, *Plethodon glutinosus*, produce mucilaginous secretions, as does the Sambava tomato frog, *Dyscophus guineti*. The average tensile strength of the tomato frog's secretion is five times stronger than rubber cement and can effectively glue a clinician's fingers together (Evans & Brodie, 1994). These gluey secretions are difficult to remove even with soap and warm water, as are the secretions of many other amphibians (e.g. South American bullfrog, *Leptodactylus pentadactylus*, Japanese giant salamander, *Andrias japonicus*). Some handlers may find these residues irritating, especially if introduced to a mucous membrane. Some species produce foul-smelling secretions when frightened (e.g., mink frog, *Rana septentrionalis*), and this odor may linger on the handler despite vigorous washing with soap and warm water.

Recent research suggests that many pharmacologically valuable compounds are present in the skin secretions of some amphibians. A variety of amphibian produced antimicrobial compounds and analgesics are being investigated by pharmaceutical companies. Extracts from the splendid treefrog, *Pelodryas (Litoria) splendida*, showed significant activity against two human pathogens—*Staphylococcus aureus* and *Herpes simplex* (Tyler, 1994, 1995). Interest in harvesting the secretions of frogs for pharmacological investigations has led to the development of a nonlethal "milking" process using electric probes to stimulate the release of material from the glands (Tyler et al., 1992).

The amount of toxin produced may vary with the physical state of the amphibian, a fact that has been exploited by native Americans to produce various artifacts such as immobilizing blowdarts and hallucinogenic substances used in tribal rituals (Bainbridge, 1993; Meadows, 1993; Milton, 1994). An injured or otherwise agitated amphibian is more likely to exude toxic substances than a calm specimen. In certain instances, the toxic secretions may be expelled with considerable force. The European fire salamander, *Salamandra salamandra*, and various toads, *Bufo* spp., are notorious for eruptions of their parotid glands. This author once handled a spotted toad, *Bufo guttatus*, that squirted parotid gland contents over a distance of 6 feet. A Colorado river toad, *Bufo alvarius*, ejected parotid gland contents a distance over 12 feet (Hanson & Vial, 1956). The concentration of toxins present in an amphibian's secretion may vary with time spent in captivity as many long-term captive specimens and captive-produced specimens of dendrobatid frogs are less toxic than their wild or recently imported cohorts (Meadows, 1993). Information about toxin decline in other families of amphibians is lacking, so it is prudent to treat all specimens as potentially dangerous.

Moistened talc-free latex gloves should be worn whenever an amphibian is handled to minimize contact with these defensive secretions (Figure 9.1). After use, the glove should removed and turned inside out, tied shut, and discarded directly into the biohazardous waste receptacle so as to avoid the possibility of intoxicating other staff members. One anecdote recounts that a researcher became intoxicated when he wiped his forehead with his handkerchief—a handkerchief that had been used to bag a dendrobatid frog and that still contained the dried secretions of that dendrobatid frog. If in doubt, protective eyewear should be worn by all present in the room whenever there is a question about the glandular ejection capability of a species. Eyewash stations should be present in or near any room where amphibians are restrained for examination and treatment. If an amphibian's secretions contact the eyes, one should immediately flush the eyes and face with eyewash or fresh water. If any symptoms of intoxication develop (e.g., epiphora, erythema, edema, paralysis of the ocular muscles, nausea, vomiting, dyspnea, hallucination, etc.) a qualified physician should evaluate the affected person.

Latex gloves are also important for the protection of the skin of the amphibian patient. An amphibian will struggle when manually restrained, and the thin epidermis may be abraded by the ridges and callosities of the restrainer's hand. A covering of moistened latex or vinyl will smooth over these irregularities and lessen the damage to the amphibian resulting from the examination. The gloves should be rinsed off with distilled water prior to handling the amphibian to remove talc or other lubricating powders. A thin coating of a water-soluble nontoxic gel or an artificial slime (e.g., Shield-X®, Aquatronics, Malibu, CA, or Polyaqua®, Kordon Division of Novalek, Hayward, CA), should be applied to the gloves prior to handling specimens. This is especially important for species with delicate skin, such as glass frogs (Centrolenidae), small dendrobatids, cave salamanders (*Eurycea* sp.), among others. The clinician must be aware that any restraint in amphibians may damage the epidermis. Cells injured during the restraint procedure are probably phagocytized by the amphibian's macrophages (Kollias, 1984). If the damage is extensive, it is likely that the monocyte count on subsequent hemograms may be depressed if monocytes are sequestered in the tissue or elevated if they are still circulating.

A shallow container of oxygenated toxin-free water at room temperature or a water sample from the amphibian's enclosure, if it has been evaluated and deemed appropriate, should be readily available for moistening the patient throughout the examination.

Amphibians may struggle during capture and restraint. While some become resigned to restraint and cease to struggle, other specimens may exhibit various antipredator behaviors. Death feigning may occur in species like the big-eyed forest treefrog, *Leptopelis macrotis* (Kofron & Schmitt, 1992), and an incautious handler's grip may loosen. The amphibian may then show an explosive burst of activity such as either leaping or biting to escape. This behavior must be differentiated from signs of true distress, an analysis that may be difficult to make when restraining an unfamiliar species. The handler must remain on guard to prevent escape. Proceed with caution if any amphibian appears unduly stressed by the restraint. Other defensive reactions include inflation (ceratophryne frogs), micturition (bufonids), biting (ceratophryne frogs, amphiumas), release calls (various anurans), writhing (salamanders and caecilians), rolling (salamanders [Garcia-Paris &

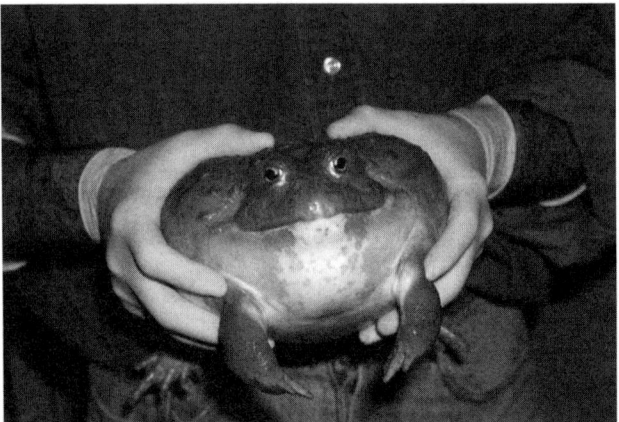

Figure 9.1. Moistened powder-free disposable gloves should be worn whenever amphibians, such as this Tschudi's African bullfrog, *Pyxicephalus adpsersus*, are handled. (Kevin Wright, Philadelphia Zoological Garden)

Deban, 1995]), and tail autotomy (salamandrid [Arntzen, 1994] and plethodontid salamanders).

Examination of small amphibians is facilitated by the use of a clear glass jar, a deli cup with a transparent lid, or a clear plastic bag (Figure 9.2). Detailed observations can be made. Special attention should be given to the ventrum. Capillary blush (dermal erythema) may be suggestive of a serious underlying illness or simply reflect an agitated patient. Erythema is most easily noted on pale skin such as on the ventral surface of a frog. Ventral erythema due to excitement alone will usually dissipate if the patient is left undisturbed in a quiet, dimly lit room for several minutes, but erythema due to illness will still be noted. Some species (e.g., glass frogs, Centrolenidae) have transparent abdominal skin, and evaluation of the internal organs is possible as they sit on a transparent surface. The visual examination may be enhanced by transillumination. Normal structures such as the heart, lungs, liver, midline abdominal vein, intestine, and ova are readily detected by transillumination. Transillumination can reveal otherwise overlooked details, such as visceral parasites or masses in muscle and organ parenchyma. A cool light source should be used for transillumination to prevent thermal burns to the patient. Best results are achieved from transillumination when the light source is in direct contact with the amphibian's body. Additional information can be obtained by internal transillumination. The tip of the light source can be passed into the amphibian's stomach to highlight some of the internal organs more sharply than is achieved by whole body transillumination. Internal transillumination may also help define the heart's location for cardiocentesis attempts. Chemical restraint may be necessary for internal transillumination, thus it may be part of a follow-up examination rather than a part of the initial physical examination.

Larger anurans and salamanders may be manually restrained without difficulty. Anurans should be grasped immediately anterior to the hindlimbs, and a second grip secured around the forelegs. Due to their more flexible body, salamanders should be grasped in the opposite fashion to control the head. Grasp a salamander immediately behind the forelegs first, and then secure a grip in front of the hind legs. Two handlers may be needed to secure large specimens (e.g., Asian giant salamanders, *Andrias* spp.). Care should be taken to avoid gripping the tail in many salamander species since the tail may break, a trait known as tail autotomy.

Medium-sized anurans and salamanders can be handled as above, or they may be gripped in a fist for access to the oral cavity and cloaca (Figures 9.3, 9.4).

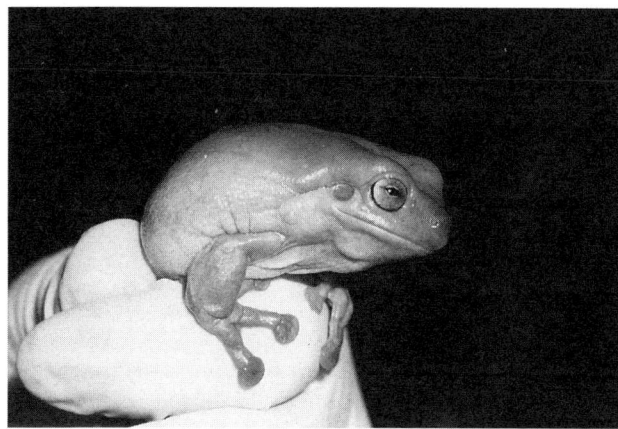

Figure 9.3. A fist grip encircling the hind limbs can be used to firmly restrain medium-sized anurans such as this White's treefrog, *Pelodryas caerulea*. (Kevin Wright, Philadelphia Zoological Garden)

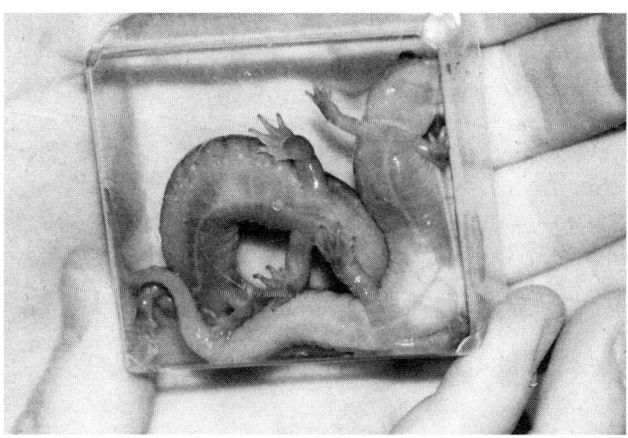

Figure 9.2. A male and female seal salamander, *Desmognathus monticola*, are restrained in a clear plastic box for examination. The large white objects visible through the ventrum of the female salamander are ova. (Philadelphia Zoological Garden)

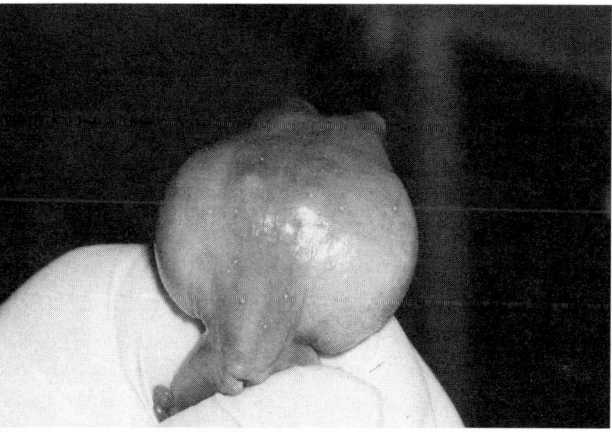

Figure 9.4. Many anurans will inflate as a defensive behavior when restrained. The fist grip allows the handler to safely control the patient as demonstrated with this White's treefrog, *Pelodryas caerulea*. (Kevin Wright, Philadelphia Zoological Garden)

The small amphibian may be restrained with a loose grip (Figure 9.5), but chemical restraint is recommended instead to minimize the risk of traumatic injuries. Some species react very poorly to manual restraint, and the spot-legged poison frog, *Epipedobates pictus*, has been known to die after only a few minutes of handling (Buchanan & Jaeger, 1995). A small anuran can have its hindlimbs secured between the handler's thumb and forefinger so that the anuran lies across the palm of the hand facing the handler's little finger. This restraint technique works well for anurans that have a tendency to climb or walk rather than jump (e.g., many arboreal frogs). This technique is not recommended for ranid frogs as they can injure their hindlegs attempting to jump free of the handler's grip.

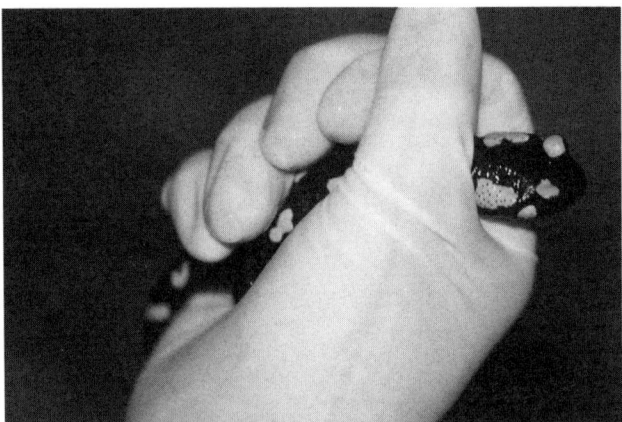

Figure 9.5. Small amphibians, such as this young fire salamander, *Salamandra salamandra*, are best restrained with a loose grip that encircles the whole body. (Kevin Wright, Philadelphia Zoological Garden)

Caecilians, sirens, *Siren* spp., dwarf sirens, *Pseudobranchus* spp., and amphiumas, *Amphiuma* spp., can be difficult to restrain without chemical sedation. A clear plexiglass tube, such as is used for restraining venomous snakes, may be used for visual examination of the patient. Smaller individuals of these amphibians can be pressed between two pieces of foam rubber, and portions of the foam moved to access sections of the body. This type of restraint can be used with certain other salamanders (e.g., mudpuppy, *Necturus maculosus*, hellbender, *Cryptobranchus alleganiensis*). Larger specimens may require a squeeze box lined with damp foam rubber to press the animal into immobility. The exposure allowed by the squeeze box is minimal, but will restrain the patient sufficiently for injections. Chemical restraint is recommended if a prolonged exam or extensive diagnostic sampling is required of large specimens.

Large amphibians may bite when provoked. Sirens and amphiumas can produce deep lacerations that bleed copiously. Horned frogs, *Ceratophrys* spp., can also produce severe bites. Other amphibian species that are known to have inflicted painful bite wounds include Tschudi's African bullfrog, *Pyxicephalus adspersus*, the hellbender, *Cryptobranchus alleganiensis*, the Asian giant salamanders, *Andrias* spp., and the mudpuppy, *Necturus* spp. If a bite breaks through the latex glove and skin of the handler, the wound should be rinsed and washed thoroughly with antibacterial soap. Given the prevalence of Gram-negative bacteria in the oropharynx of amphibians, a physician should be consulted if red streaks radiate from the wound within 48 hours, as this could be a sign of serious infection.

Larval amphibians should be handled sparingly, and careful attention given to keeping their skin moist. If the skin changes texture and becomes wrinkled, or if the tail tip begins to curl, the larva is too dry and must be immediately moistened or returned to its aquatic environment.

9.2 CHEMICAL RESTRAINT

Some amphibian patients may be difficult to fully evaluate when they are completely awake. Different planes of anesthesia are routinely used in the evaluation and treatment of the amphibian patient. Several anesthetics that have been used in amphibians will not be discussed, as they are either not readily available, have adverse side effects, or produce equivocal results. For one or more of the above reasons the author does not recommend the clinical application of the following anesthetic agents that appear in the literature: urethane, chloretone, ether, phencyclidine, acepromazine, and procaine hydrochloride (Buchanan & Jaeger, 1995; Moore, 1964; Noble, 1931; Rie, 1973; Subcommittee on Amphibian Standards, 1974). Cooling of the amphibian for hypothermic restraint is not recommended due to its probable lack of analgesia as well as potential long-term immunosuppressive effects (Green & Cohen, 1977). In addition, the slower response time of the hypothermic animal may mask pain reflexes, thus obscuring the true plane of analgesia achieved. Many of the more familiar anesthetic agents (e.g., ketamine hydrochloride, halothane, isoflurane) can be used in amphibians. However, the anesthetic agent of choice in amphibians is tricaine methanesulfonate.

9.2.1 Patient Preparation

Aspiration of regurgitated stomach contents is an extremely rare event in amphibians, as the larynx is usually closed when an amphibian patient is anesthetized. Aspiration pneumonia subsequent to anesthesia has not been noted in the amphibian collections of the Philadelphia Zoo or the National Aquarium in

Baltimore, or in the amphibian collection of the Wildlife Conservation Society (personal communication, M. Stetter, 1997), despite the lack of a prolonged fast in the majority of cases. However, it is prudent to minimize the risk of anesthetic emesis as this can be a physiologically demanding event due to the loss of ingesta and associated gastric secretions such as chloride ions. If at all possible, the stomach should be empty of ingesta in the amphibian that is to be anesthetized. Based on a study of the Eastern red-spotted newt, *Notophthalmus viridescens* (Jiang & Claussen, 1993), a fasting time of 48 hours allows adequate time for gastric emptying of most insectivorous salamanders and medium-sized anurans (i.e., anurans with a body weight of 20 g or more). If the environmental temperature is lower than the amphibian's preferred body temperature, the fasting time may be extended up to a period of 10 days to ensure gastric emptying (Jiang & Claussen, 1993). Amphibians that eat vertebrates such as rodents may have significantly prolonged gastric emptying, and a minimum fast of 7 days is recommended. Many small anurans (i.e., anurans with a body weight under 20 g) may be safely anesthetized with only a brief fast of 4 hours or less with minimal risk of emesis. The length of fasting recommended is dependent on the patient's condition. An elective procedure on a healthy specimen, such as laparoscopy for sexing, should minimize the risk of adverse effects such as emesis, while a clinically ill amphibian with a surgical condition, such as gastrointestinal obstruction, should not have treatment delayed for a fasting period.

9.2.2 Anesthetic Monitoring

Monitoring of the heart rate, buccopharyngeal or pulmonic respiratory rate if present, and blood (hemoglobin) oxygen saturation are recommended during an anesthetic procedure.

The cardiac impulse may be visualized in some specimens and heart rate determined simply by counting the heart beats. Small doppler probes have been used to monitor heart rates. As most amphibians are fairly small, it is important to use a doppler with a small patient contact surface. An 8.0 mHz unit with a 9-mm patient contact surface diameter is recommended (Ultrascope Doppler Arterial and Venous Blood Flow Detector, Model 8, 8 MHz; EMS Products, Inc.) (Frye, 1994). This probe has been used to detect cardiovascular sounds in amphibians weighing 2 g, and the sounds may be differentiated and characterized (e.g., atrial and ventricular contractions, atrioventricular and aortic valvular, aortic, brachiocephalic artery, and vena caval sounds) (Frye, 1994). The probe should be moved laterally and longitudinally across the ventral thorax to help differentiate the sounds. As a general rule, sounds originating from high pressure structures (e.g., ventricle, artery) are louder and less sibilant than those from low pressure structures (e.g., atria, venous system). ECG monitoring has not been used as a general rule by this author, but it can be used to monitor heart rate (personal communication, M. Stetter, 1997). Advances in the electrode clip systems and sensitivity of the ECG machine may well make this a more viable option in the near future. Oxygen flow should be increased (either via increased bubbling through the anesthetic solution, endotracheal tube, or oxygen flow across the skin of the patient) and the anesthesia discontinued or lightened, if possible, whenever a patient shows a significant decrease in cardiac rate, hemoglobin oxygen saturation, or any other sign of metabolic derangement.

Many amphibians have both a hypoxic and a hypercapnic respiratory drive, but the magnitude of change needed to activate respiration varies considerably (West & Van Vliet, 1992). Buccopharyngeal and pulmonic respiratory movements usually cease if an amphibian is maintained under hyperoxic conditions during surgery. Normal respiratory movements may not return if an amphibian is maintained under pure oxygen, thus room air should be used for ventilation during recovery to help elicit respirations in the patient.

Many of the new pulse oximetry devices now have small clips that can be placed on the toes or tails of amphibians, probes that can be laid directly on the ventrum over the heart, or esophageal probes. Pulse oximetry allows the clinician to directly assess the hemoglobin oxygen saturation in the face of inapparent pulmonary ventilation. As a general rule amphibians have a lower hemoglobin oxygen saturation than may be expected for mammals, but no values have been published from clinical cases. Under normoxic conditions (Partial Pressure of Oxygen, PO_2, 150 mm Hg), the oxygen saturation of the blood (hemoglobin) of the tiger salamander, *Ambystoma tigrinum*, ranges upwards from 95% (Burggren & Just, 1992). As a general rule, a decrease of the oxygen saturation of 5% or more should elicit a reevaluation of the patient and possible adjustment of the anesthetic regimen.

The amphibian should have normal respiratory movements and appear alert and responsive before recovery from anesthesia can be considered complete.

9.2.3 Topical Anesthetics

Tricaine Methanesulfonate. Tricaine methanesulfonate (FINQUEL® or MS-222, Argent Chemical Laboratories, Redmond, WA) is the water-soluble white salt of the insoluble tricaine (3-amino benzoic acid ethyl ester), that is an isomer of another useful anesthetic agent in amphibians, benzocaine (4-amino benzoic acid ethyl ester). Tricaine methanesulfonate is known also as ethyl *m*-amino benzoate. When present in solution in the un-ionized form, tricaine methanesulfonate is a practical immobilizing agent at extremely low concentrations (as low as 0.05%), yet it is safe at much higher levels. A common problem stems from the fact that methanesulfonate is an acidic salt. When the water-soluble tricaine salt is dissolved in distilled water, the resultant solution is physiologically challenging due to its low pH, which ranges down to a value of 3.0 for the concentrations normally used for amphibian anesthesia (Ohr, 1976). This low-pH environment also causes the majority of the tricaine to be in an un-ionized form, which cannot be absorbed and therefore cannot act as an anesthetic.

A stock solution of buffered tricaine methanesulfonate can be made easily and should be kept readily available. A helpful practice is to have a premeasured amount of 2 g of tricaine methanesulfonate powder in a small container (e.g., Whirlpak®), which is then taped to a container holding 2 liters of well oxygenated distilled water to which has been added 34–50 ml of 0.5 M Na_2HPO_4 (Downes, 1995) (Na_2HPO_4 available from Sigma Scientific Company, St. Louis, MO). When the anesthetic solution is needed, the tricaine methanesulfonate can be added to the water to yield the stock concentration of 1 g/L (0.1%). The sodium phosphate acts as a buffer so that the final pH of the 1 g/L tricaine methanesulfonate solution is within a physiological range between 7.0 and 7.4. The pH of the solution should be checked prior to use to ensure an appropriate level of buffering has been achieved. Another buffering option that has worked is to add sodium bicarbonate ($NaHCO_3$, baking soda) to a solution of pure tricaine methanesulfonate and distilled water to achieve a physiological range between pH 7.0 and 7.4. Several other 1-liter containers of well-oxygenated, toxin-free water at room temperature should also be available for diluent if needed so the 1 g/L stock solution can be diluted further with water to levels appropriate for the individual amphibian.

The anamnesis and initial evaluation should include a water quality analysis of water from the amphibian's enclosure. If the parameters of water quality are acceptable, it is recommended to use this water as the diluent when preparing an anesthetic solution from the stock solution of tricaine methanesulfonate. This will minimize health problems in the anesthetized amphibian that can be associated with sudden changes in various parameters of water quality. If this is not possible, well-oxygenated, toxin-free water should be used as the diluent. The temperature of the amphibian and the anesthetic solution should be allowed to equilibrate before induction to minimize stress associated with thermal shock.

In the past, tricaine methanesulfonate concentrations ranging from 0.5 g/L to 5.0 g/L were recommended as the concentrations needed to induce anesthesia in amphibians. A 0.5 g/L (0.05%) solution of tricaine methanesulfonate was reported to anesthetize tadpoles and other amphibian larvae, while a range of 1 g/L to 2 g/L (0.1% to 0.2%) solution was recommended for induction of surgical level anesthesia in most frogs and urodeles. A 3 g/L (0.3%) solution was often recommended for large bufonids (Anonymous, 1987; Crawshaw, 1989). Higher dosages, such as 3.5 mg/L, have been recommended, in one case to prevent muscular movement in the red-spotted newt, *Notophthalmus viridescens* (Vanable, 1985). It may well be that these recommendations were made because the solutions were not buffered and the tricaine was in the unavailable ionized form.

The author concurs with a recent review that disputes the need for these higher levels of tricaine, and recommends a induction concentrations of 0.2 g/L in buffered solution for larvae, and 1 g/L in buffered solution for adult amphibians (Downes, 1995). In exceptionally large specimens, higher concentrations may be needed for induction, but these should always be buffered back to a physiologically neutral pH (i.e., pH 7.0–7.4). Induction time is generally under 30 minutes at these concentrations. Small deviations from the recommended concentration will affect the time needed to achieve sternal recumbency in an amphibian, and there is a general correlation between lower concentrations and increased length of time for induction. Upon attainment of the desired anesthetic state, the amphibian should be removed from the induction solution and moved to fresh water. In most cases an anesthetized amphibian removed from its tricaine bath will remain anesthetized long enough for most diagnostic or surgical procedures. If the amphibian starts to recover, the clinician may return it to deep anesthesia by bathing it in a solution that has a tricaine methanesulfonate concentration no more than 50% of the induction solution (Figure 9.6). This can be easily achieved by using a 1:1 solution of well-oxygenated, toxin-free water and induction solution.

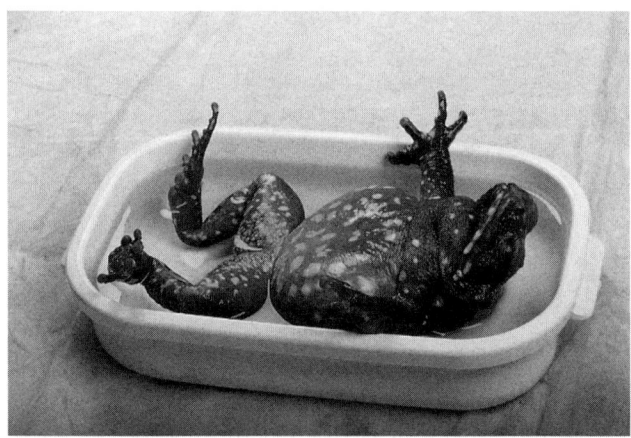

Figure 9.6. A spotted toad, *Bufo guttata*, immobilized in a bath of tricaine methanesulfonate. Note that the nostrils are elevated above the surface of the liquid to prevent aspiration. (George Grall, National Aquarium in Baltimore)

Clear plastic bags (e.g., Whirlpak® or Ziploc® bag) work well as induction chambers for many amphibians. For large amphibians, such as the Asian giant salamanders, *Andrias* spp., sweater boxes, styrofoam coolers, and lock-top plastic tubs (e.g., Rubbermaid®) are durable and easily cleaned and disinfected. Cat induction chambers (generally a modified aquarium) may also be used. Caution should be exercised when choosing an induction chamber, as compounds that leach from some plastics may prove toxic to amphibians. The induction chamber should be designed to ensure that the amphibian can not climb away from the anesthetic solution, yet the design of the chamber should allow sufficient air space so that the patient can breathe readily during induction. In the case of flighty anurans, if an induction chamber other than a plastic bag is used, the chamber should be lined with a plastic bag or bubble wrap. These shock absorbers will minimize damage to the rostrum and eyes that may be inflicted by erratic hopping movements during the excitatory phase of induction. Except in amphibians that rely entirely on branchial respiration, drowning may occur if the nostrils are submerged for any length of time. Amphibians should be watched constantly throughout the induction to prevent accidental drowning. Should anesthetic complications arise, immediately rinse the patient with copious amounts of well-oxygenated clean water until it has fully recovered.

Induction times for amphibians vary, but generally a surgical plane of anesthesia will occur within 30 minutes of immersion into a 1 g/L buffered solution of tricaine methanesulfonate. Respiratory efforts, including ventilation of the gills, will slow down, and may stop, during tricaine methanesulfonate anesthesia, but the cardiac rate is unaffected or even slightly increased, except in very deep levels of anesthesia. As a result of anesthetic-induced apnea, blood gas values of the anesthetized amphibian will change markedly during prolonged anesthesia at normal clinic temperatures (e.g., 22°C [72°F] and above), with hypoxia, hypercarbia, and acidosis the normal manifestations resulting from lack of pulmonary ventilation in amphibians (Downes, 1995; Gottlieb & Jackson, 1976). Provision of 100% oxygen bubbling into the maintenance anesthetic solution is recommended, as it will help insure that cutaneous oxygen diffusion meets the amphibian's respiratory demands (Downes, 1995) In the face of normoxia (PO_2 = 150 mm Hg), the concomitant acidosis and hypercarbia still present in the apneic anesthetized amphibian does not appear to compromise the patient in the time frame of most diagnostic or therapeutic procedures (Downes, 1995). Large amphibians may need to be ventilated with oxygen via an endotracheal tube if undergoing prolonged anesthesia.

Erythema of the ventrum or other light-skinned areas of the amphibian's body is the first sign of anesthetic induction by tricaine methanesulfonate. This is a transient erythema similar to the "emotional" erythema associated with stressful conditions such as manual restraint. The amphibian may appear agitated, and a frenzied exploration of the induction chamber may occur. Anurans often leap in a random manner as they attempt to escape from contact with the anesthetic solution. It is emphasized that inducing an amphibian inside a flexible plastic bag will minimize the trauma associated with these movements. Lining an induction chamber with plastic bubble wrap may also reduce injury.

A light plane of anesthesia from tricaine methanesulfonate is characterized by the loss of the righting reflex and corneal reflex, but the withdrawal reflex (deep pain), spontaneous movement, gular respiration, and the cardiac impulse (visible heartbeat) are retained. A deep plane of anesthesia is the stage when only the cardiac impulse is present (Figure 9.7). The withdrawal reflex (to deep pain) is the last reflex to go (Figure 9.8). The level of anesthesia can be maintained by trickling the maintenance anesthetic solution over the amphibian's body, and a reversal of the effect can be had by rinsing the body with clean, well-oxygenated water (Figure 9.9). An overdose is indicated when the cardiac impulse slows or becomes difficult to detect. A decrease in the cardiac rate of 20% or greater is indication for immediate removal of the amphibian from the anesthetic. The clinician may rinse the body with clean water to increase the amount of excretion of tricaine methanesulfonate that occurs by diffusion instead of relying solely on metabolism of the drug for excretion.

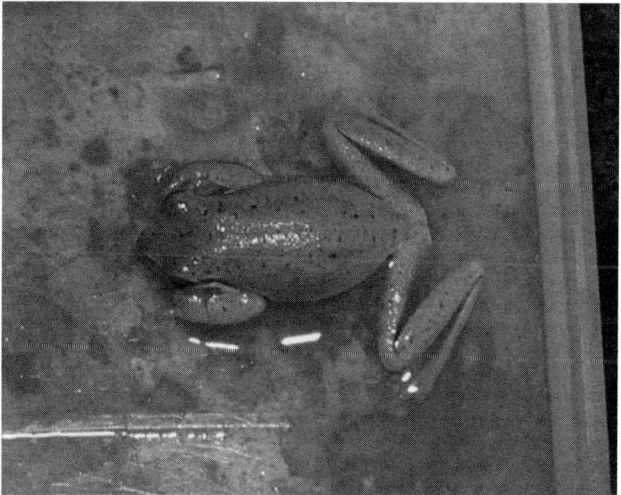

Figure 9.7. A dwarf treefrog, *Litoria fallax*, in a deep plane of anesthesia from tricaine methanesulfonate. At this anesthetic plane there is no voluntary or involuntary movement and the cardiac impulse can be detected through the ventral skin. (Kevin Wright, Philadelphia Zoological Garden)

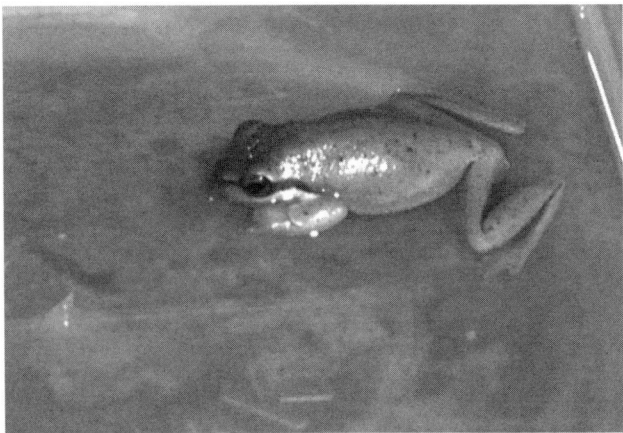

Figure 9.8. Adduction of the limb in response to deep pain is the last reflex to disappear during anesthesia with tricaine methanesulfonate. It is the first reflex to reappear. This dwarf treefrog, *Litoria fallax*, is beginning to adduct its hindlimbs. (Kevin Wright, Philadelphia Zoological Garden)

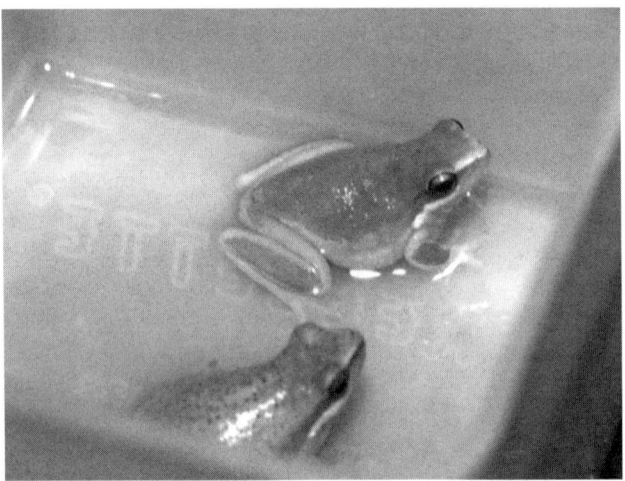

Figure 9.9. A dwarf treefrog, *Litoria fallax*, fully recovered from anesthesia with tricaine methanesulfonate. Note the tightly adducted limbs, elevated head and torso, and overall alert appearance. (Kevin Wright, Philadelphia Zoological Garden)

Renal circulation may become reduced if high concentrations of tricaine methanesulfonate are used, but the impact this has on pharmacokinetics of renal metabolized and excreted compounds is undocumented. Nevertheless, monitoring of the cardiovascular sounds via doppler is recommended during anesthesia, and the patient should be removed from the anesthetic solution if blood flow appears significantly impaired, as indicated by diminishing volume of the sounds of the peripheral circulation (e.g., midline abdominal vein, femoral veins, or iliac arteries).

The methanesulfonate moiety is presumed to remain in the anesthetic solution when the tricaine component is absorbed via the skin and gills. Tricaine's effectiveness as an anesthetic is predicated on the rapidity of the amphibian's metabolism. Tricaine is converted to relatively inactive metabolites via hydrolysis of the ester bond and conjugation of the aromatic amine, and these metabolic pathways appear to be present throughout the amphibian body, although these pathways are reduced or absent in the amphibian liver when compared with the liver of mammals. The apparent lack of hydrolytic pathways in the amphibian liver is the reason that tricaine is a good anesthetic in these animals—if the liver contained significant amounts of tricaine esterases then tricaine would be metabolized too rapidly to maintain systemic levels effective for anesthesia. However, due to the widespread locations of these metabolic pathways in other tissues of amphibians, tricaine is eliminated more rapidly than many other pharmaceuticals and this allows the amphibians to recovery more rapidly from tricaine than any other currently available anesthetic. The metabolic by-products of tricaine are then either eliminated by cutaneous diffusion or via renal excretion. There is some evidence to suggest that cutaneous diffusion is extremely important in smaller amphibians, which have a correspondingly larger surface area–to-volume ratio than larger amphibians (Wayson et al., 1976a, 1976b).

It should be noted that tricaine methanesulfonate can be administered intracoelomically or via the dorsal lymph sac (Downes, 1995; Letcher, 1992). A recent review advocates a tricaine dosage range of 175–200 mg/kg for induction of amphibians, with supplemental dosages of 50–100 mg/kg given as needed (Downes, 1995). A formula was proposed for an injectable solution of tricaine: "200 mg tricaine methanesulfonate neutralized and precipitated in 0.8 ml 1 N aqueous NaOH, redissolved by addition of 0.5 ml dimethyl sulfoxide (DMSO) and 0.5 ml ethanol yielding a final volume of 1.8 ml. All of the diluents can be obtained in sterile solutions and tricaine methanesulfonate can be autoclaved" (Downes, 1995). In order to simplify the creation of an injectable form of tricaine, 200 mg of tricaine methanesulfonate can be placed in a clot tube and the air evacuated by aspiration. This tube is then autoclaved, and the tricaine can be put into solution through the aseptic introduction of the sterile diluents noted above. Several containers of sterile tricaine methanesulfonate can be prepared at one time and stored for use as needed. In this author's opinion, there is little advantage to this technique for most clinical procedures, and the steps needed to prepare an aseptic solution limit the use of this route in most clinical practices.

Benzocaine. Benzocaine (ethyl *p*-aminobenzoate) is related to tricaine methanesulfonate and has been used to achieve surgical levels of anesthesia in many species of amphibians, including ambystomids, plethodontids, salamandrids, a proteid (the mudpuppy, *Necturus maculosus*), ranids, and pipids. A solution of 0.02–0.03% benzocaine can be used to anesthetize many adult amphibians, whereas significantly lower concentrations are effective for larva (e.g., 0.01–0.005%) (Borgens et al., 1984; Vanable et al., 1983). Recovery occurs within 60 minutes of rinsing the amphibians with benzocaine-free water. Since benzocaine is more soluble in ethanol than water, it is expedient to dissolve the benzocaine in a small amount of absolute ethanol, and then add water to achieve the desired benzocaine concentration while not exceeding a final ethanol concentration of 1%. The benzocaine solution is stable for up to 2 weeks at room temperature. Given the availability of tricaine methanesulfonate as an anesthetic, there is little cause to use benzocaine as an anesthetic in clinical practice.

9.2.4 Inhalant Anesthetics

The term "inhalant anesthetic" refers to the usage of these agents in reptiles, birds, and mammals. The distinction between inhaled and topical anesthetics is blurred by the multiple modes of respiration occurring in amphibians. Inhalant anesthetics can be used in amphibians, but there is little cause to use them if tricaine methanesulfonate is available. Apnea, the main side effect of tricaine anesthesia, also occurs when inhalant anesthetics are used (Downes, 1995). A disadvantage of gaseous anesthetics is the potential for exposure of personnel to waste gases, a situation exacerbated by the chamber method of induction. In the author's experience, the scavenging systems in use in most clinics leave noticeable amounts of inhalant anesthetics in the induction chamber. Methoxyflurane (Wass, 1974), halothane (Wright, 1996), and isoflurane (Downes, 1995; Stetter et al., 1996) have been used in amphibians. No comparative studies have been published to guide choice of anesthetic in a given situation, but halothane and isoflurane have been used by the author without ill effect.

Induction of anesthesia using a gaseous agent can be accomplished via a chamber (Olson, 1986), by bubbling the solution through water, intubation, or by direct application of anesthetic to the skin of the amphibian patient with or without a carrier vehicle (Stetter et al., 1996). Anesthetic saturations of 2–5% usually promote a surgical plane of anesthesia within 5–20 minutes. Induction rate is highly variable, as is the length of time an amphibian remains sedated following removal from anesthetic. In one study, two bullfrogs took 61–103 minutes to recover from 5% isoflurane induction, as compared to 43–47 minutes from two bullfrogs induced in 1 g/L tricaine methonesulfonate (Downes, 1995). It has been this author's experience that some amphibians may start struggling within moments of removal from the induction chamber despite the absence of a withdrawal reflex while within the chamber.

Intubation is one method of gaseous anesthetic delivery in the amphibian patient, but its use is limited due to the narrow diameter of the glottis, even in amphibians that are quite large. Cole tubes, uncuffed endotracheal tubes, red rubber catheters, polypropylene intravenous catheters, and open-ended tomcat urinary catheters can all be used for intubation. Given the extremely short trachea of many amphibians, the endotracheal tube should be advanced minimally beyond the epiglottis to avoid damage of the lower respiratory tract structures. The endotracheal tube should be secured in position to minimize advancement of the endotracheal tube during the procedure. This can be accomplished by taping the tube and the patient to the piece of plexiglass functioning as the surgical platform. This plexiglass surgical platform should have a slight lip for water retention to prevent dehydration of the patient during the procedure. The entire platform can then be positioned as needed for the procedure. Maintaining a steady level of anesthesia via this route is difficult due to the additional respiratory surfaces that are not in contact with the anesthetic agent (e.g., skin, buccopharynx).

Methoxyflurane. Methoxyflurane has been reported as a practical anesthetic in laboratory frogs (Wass & Kaplan, 1974). The technique described consists of soaking cotton with 10 ml of methoxyflurane and placing this within a 1-gallon glass jar with ventilation holes in the top. The study was performed at 21°C (70°F) using leopard frogs, *Rana pipiens,* that had been acclimated to 21°C (70°F) for 2 days previously. Frogs placed within this anesthetic chamber went through a 1 minute excitatory phase which included ventral erythema, but were at a deep plane of anesthesia within 2 minutes as indicated by the absence of motion, loss of the pedal reflex, and loss of response to deep pain. A total exposure time of 5 minutes in the chamber resulted in a surgical plane of anesthesia for approximately 40 minutes with a recovery time of approximately 7 hours. Respiratory rate was markedly depressed throughout deep anesthesia and early recovery, but cardiac rate was only minimally depressed.

Isoflurane. Isoflurane can be used in the manner described for methoxyflurane, but a flow-through anesthetic chamber with scavenging capabilities is the preferred method to use given isoflurane's volatility when compared to methoxyflurane. In the authors experience, a 5% isoflurane saturation at a low oxygen flow rate will induce unconsciousness within 5–20 minutes in most amphibians. A small amount of water may be placed in the anesthetic chamber to offset the dehydrating effect of tank oxygen. Recovery time is quicker than for methoxyflurane, and it generally takes less than 100 minutes for an amphibian to recover to a righting phase from a surgical plane of anesthesia.

A comparative study of five methods of application of isoflurane has been published (Stetter et al., 1996). The aquatic clawed frog, *Xenopus laevis,* and terrestrial toads, *Bufo* sp., were used in the study as representatives of diverse ecological and, hence, physiological adaptations. The routes of application were as follows: 1) direct topical application of 100% isoflurane utilized a dose of 0.007 ml/g body weight for the clawed frog, *X. laevis,* and 0.015 ml/g body weight for the toad *Bufo* sp.; 2) a bath of 0.28% isoflurane (i.e., 0.25 ml isoflurane in 125 ml of water); 3) topical administration of isoflurane gel—3 ml isoflurane in a carrier vehicle of 3.5 ml water soluble gel (i.e., KY jelly) and 1.5 ml water administered at a topical dose of 0.025 ml/g for *X. laevis* and .035 ml/g for *Bufo* sp.; 4) 5% isoflurane bubbled through water; 5) 5% isoflurane in an anesthetic chamber.

Direct application of full-strength isoflurane provided lighter levels of sedation than other techniques. The 0.28% isoflurane bath provided consistent levels of surgical anesthesia, but the patient had to be removed from the solution immediately after loss of the righting reflex to avoid excessively deep anesthesia and prolonged recovery. The isoflurane gel also worked well, but had to be wiped off immediately following loss of the righting reflex to avoid deep anesthesia and prolonged recovery. The vaporized isoflurane in water and vaporized isoflurane in a chamber had longer induction times and faster recovery rates, and are more suitable for short procedures.

Halothane. Halothane should be used in the manner described for isoflurane, although no recipes for baths and topical gels have been described.

9.2.5 Miscellaneous Anesthetics.

Ketamine Hydrochloride. Ketamine hydrochloride has been reported as an option for anesthesia of amphibians (Frank, 1976; Vogelnest, 1994a, b; Wright,1994). Dosage ranges of 20–210 mg/kg IM were reported. One report discourages the use of ketamine injected into the dorsal lymph sac at ranges from 55–210 mg/kg, and does not recommend ketamine as an anesthetic. Other reports are more favorable—a surgical plane of anesthesia was obtained within 15 minutes in White's treefrog, *Litoria caerulea,* and the Australian giant treefrog, *L. infrafrenata,* at 70–100 mg/kg (Vogelnest, 1994a, b), and within 20 minutes in a two-toed amphiuma, *Amphiuma means,* at 120 mg/kg (Wright, 1994). Uncoordinated muscle movements were still noted in the amphiuma despite lack of response to painful stimuli. Recovery was unspecified in the frogs, but the amphiuma was fully recovered 18 h postanesthesia. Clinical experience with ketamine hydrochloride in the bullfrog, *Rana catesbeiana,* giant toad, *Bufo marinus,* and tiger salamander, *Ambystoma tigrinum,* indicates that a dosage of 70–100 mg/kg IM is adequate for many surgical procedures, including celiotomy, provided that an allowance is made by the surgeon for the random muscle contraction. Recovery is uneventful and all individuals are completely recovered within 12 hours. Lower dosages are recommended for minor procedures.

Tiletamine HCl and Zolazepam. There is at least one report in the literature concerning the use of tiletamine/zolazepam as an anesthetic agent in anurans (Letcher & Durante, 1995). Due to the wide variation in response to this anesthetic combination in the two species of ranid frogs studied, the investigators reported that the drug was an unsuitable agent in anurans. The only anesthetic alteration that could be reliably induced was modification of locomotor behavior. A dosage of 20 mg/kg IM produced a deep level of anesthesia in the northern leopard frog, *Rana pipiens,* but over 10 hours elapsed between time of injection and loss of deep pain. Recovery took up to 32 hours, a time frame that is not helpful in clinical situations. In contrast this dosage had little effect on several specimens of the bullfrog, *Rana catesbeiana,* that were used in the study. There was variation in the level of anesthetic response tested at each dosage level. This author concurs that tiletamine/zolazepam is not a useful anesthetic agent in these two species, and cautions against its use in other species of amphibians.

Ethanol (Ethyl Alcohol). Ethanol at a 10% solution is an anesthetic that has been used in terminal procedures, such as harvesting internal parasites for ecological studies of amphibians. The use of ethanol as an anesthetic for anurans was documented in 1961 (Kaplan & Kaplan, 1961). Ethanol is not recommended as an anesthetic for the amphibian patient except in nonsurvival studies, due to its marked physiological effects beyond loss of consciousness. In the author's experience, the amphibian patient may undergo respiratory and cardiac arrest with prolonged exposure to 5% ethanol, while this occurs within minutes of immersion in 20% ethanol.

Barbiturates. Pentobarbital and other barbiturates are used in biological labs for euthanasia. Pentobarbital at levels of 30–60 mg/kg intracoelomically has been recommended for anesthesia (Kaplan et al., 1962). Sodium pentobarbital at a dosage of 20 mg/kg either topically or intracoelomically induced anesthesia in the roughskin newt, *Taricha granulosa* (Rie, 1973). Supportive care in the form of flushing the patient with oxygenated fresh water was needed to speed recovery. However pentobarbital at levels of 60–100 mg/kg intracoelomically, intracardially, or via the subcutaneous lymph sacs has been reported as a method to euthanatize an amphibian (Burns, 1995). Given the wide range of dosages reported in the literature, the author cautions against the use of pentobarbital in amphibians, except as a euthanasia agent.

9.3 EUTHANASIA

Most people hope for a peaceful, painless death, and it is this concept that is the basis for defining appropriate methods of euthanasia in animals. Considerable debate has focused on the concept and pathways of pain as well as the nomenclature of nociceptive responses in the various classes of animals (Stevens, 1995), but there is no doubt that living amphibians can feel pain. The method of euthanasia is dependent on the condition of the amphibian patient, the wishes of the client, and the need for postmortem diagnostics or body preservation. The choice of method is best made by the clinician involved with the case.

Tricaine Methanesulfonate Overdose. Prolonged immersion in tricaine methanesulfonate appears to be one of the least stressful forms of euthanasia. Intracoelomic injection of concentrated dosages of tricaine (200 mg/kg) apparently does not alter the appearance of gross or histopathological lesions in amphibians (Wayson et al., 1976b). The body cavity can be opened and the heart removed to ensure death.

Ethanol Overdose. Concentrations of ethanol of 20% or more can be used as a euthanasia solution. Initial sedation in 5% ethanol is recommended followed by exposure to the higher concentration. Ethanol overdose is one of the recommended forms of euthanasia for preserving an amphibian for a museum specimen, as it does not cause the agitation and muscle distortion that contact with 10% buffered formalin may cause in living specimens.

Barbiturates. Pentobarbital administered at a dosage of 100 mg/kg intracoelomically should cause death within 30 minutes. Intracardiac injection will result in rapid death, while injection of pentobarbital into the subcutaneous lymph sacs takes up to 30 minutes for death. Some pathologists dislike pentobarbital because it causes tissue alteration and inhibits some microbiological assays of postmortem tissues. Intracardiac injections may ruin the heart for histopathological investigations.

Pithing. Pithing can be used in unconscious amphibians, and should be done in a rostral direction from the foramen magnum as well as in a caudal direction inside the vertebral canal. This method should be avoided in the face of neurological signs, as it renders the majority of the nervous system unfit for histopathological analysis.

Freezing. Freezing can be used in unconscious amphibians provided it can be done in a rapid manner. Immersion of unconscious small amphibians (<40 g body weight) into liquid nitrogen is an acceptable form of euthanasia (National Research Council Committee on Pain and Distress in Laboratory Animals, 1992). Placing the animal into a regular refrigerator freezer held at −2°C to 0°C (28–32°F) is unacceptable, as it is too slow a process. Furthermore, some species (e.g., wood frog, *Rana sylvatica,* spring peeper, *Pseudacris crucifer*) can tolerate freezing for over 48 h. Freezing is an unacceptable method for many nearctic and montane species.

Traumatic. Striking the amphibian's head against a heavy solid object (traumatic euthanasia) has been described as a method of euthanasia, but accuracy is essential to inflict a quick death (Cooper et al., 1989). Alternatively, the object may be struck against the amphibian's cranium with a point of impact centering on the brain. This renders the central nervous system and other tissues unfit for histopathological analysis.

Unacceptable Methods of Euthanasia. Due to the tolerance of many amphibians to hypercarbic conditions, carbon dioxide administration is not a satisfactory method of euthanasia due to the prolonged time required for death to occur. Other unacceptable methods of euthanasia include decapitation, hyperthermia, electrocution, and exsanguination (except in unconscious amphibians) (Cooper et al., 1989).

REFERENCES

Anonymous. 1987. Argent Finquel® Package Insert, NDC 051212-0001-1, revised October 1987.

Arntzen, J.W. 1994. Allometry and autotomy of the tail in the golden-striped salamander, *Chioglossa lusitanica.* Amphibia-Reptilia 15:267–274.

Bainbridge, J.S. 1993. Frogs that sweat—not bullets, but a poison for darts. Smithsonian (July), pp. 70–76.

Barthalmus, G.T. 1994. Biological roles of amphibian skin secretions, *in* Heatwole, H. and G.T. Barthalmus (Eds.): Amphibian Biology, Vol. 1, The Integument. Surry Beatty and Sons, Chipping Norton, New South Wales, Australia, pp. 382–410.

Borgens R.B., M.E. McGinnis, J.W. Vanable, Jr and E.S. Miles. 1984. Stump currents in regenerating salamanders and newts. Journal of Experimental Zoology 231:249–256.

Buchanan, B.W. and R.G. Jaeger. 1995. Amphibians, *in* Rollins, B.E. (Ed.): The experimental animal in biomedical research. Volume II. Care, husbandry, and well-being, An overview by species. CRC Press, Boca Raton, FL, pp. 32–48.

Burggren, W.E. and J.J. Just. 1992. Developmental changes in physiological systems, *in* Feder, M.E. and W.W. Burggren (Eds.): Environmental Physiology of Amphibians. University of Chicago Press, Chicago, pp. 467–530.

Burns, R. 1995. Considerations in the euthanasia of reptiles, amphibians, and fish. Proceedings of the Joint Conference of the AAZV, WDA, and AAWV, pp. 243–249.

Chen, K.K. and A.L. Chen. 1933. A study of the poisonous secretions of five North American species of toads. Jour. Pharmacol. Exp. Therap. 49:526–542.

Cooper, J.E., R. Ewbank, C. Platt, and C. Warwick 1989. Euthanasia of Amphibians and Reptiles. Universities Federation for Animal Welfare & World Society for the Protection of Animals, London, UK.

Crawshaw, G.J. 1989. Medical care of amphibians. Proceedings of the American Association of Zoo Veterinarians 1989, pp. 166–172.

Downes, H. 1995. Tricaine anesthesia in Amphibia: a review. Bulletin of the Association of Reptile and Amphibian Veterinarians 5(2):11–16.

Erspamer, V. 1994. Bioactive skin secretions of the amphibian integument, in Heatwole, H. and G.T. Barthlamus (Eds.): Amphibian Biology, Vol. 1, The Integument. Surrey Beatty and Sons, Chipping Norton, New South Wales, Australia, pp. 178–350.

Evans, C.M. and E.D. Brodie, Jr. 1994. Adhesive strength of amphibian skins secretions. Journal of Herpetology 28(4):499–502.

Frank W. 1976. (translated 1982 by G. Speckmann. 3.29.2 Amphibia-Reptilia Restraint. in Klos H-G. and E.M. Lang (Eds.): Handbook of Zoo Medicine. Van Nostrand Reinhold Co., New York, pp. 355–356.

Frye, F.L. 1994. Ultrasonic doppler blood flow detection in small exotic animal medicine. Seminars in Avian and Exotic Pet Medicine 3(3): 133–139.

Garcia-Paris, M. and S.M. Deban. 1995. A novel antipredator mechanism in salamanders: rolling escape in *Hydromantes platycephala*. Journal of Herpetology 29(1):149–151.

Gottlieb, G. and D.C. Jackson. 1976. Importance of pulmonary ventilation in respiratory control in the bullfrog. Am. J. Physiol. 230:608–613.

Green, N. and N. Cohen. 1977. Effect of temperature on serum complement levels in the leopard frog *Rana pipiens*. Developmental and Comparative Pathology 1:59–64.

Grenard, S. 1994. Medical Herpetology. NG Publishing, Inc., Pottsville, PA.

Habermehl, G.G. 1974. Venoms of Amphibia, in Florkin, M. and B.T. Scheer (Eds.): Chemical Zoology. Vol. IX, Amphibia and Reptilia. Academic Press, New York, pp.161–183.

Hanson, J.A. and J.L. Vial. 1956. Defensive behavior and effects of toxins in *Bufo alvarius*. Herpetologica 12:141–149.

Horgan, J. 1990. Bufo abuse—a toxic toad gets licked, boiled, teed up, and tanned. Scientific American, August 1990, pp. 26–27.

Jiang, S. and D.L. Claussen. 1993. The effects of temperature on food passage time through the digestive tract in *Notophthalmus viridescens*. Journal of Herpetology 27(4):414–419.

Kaplan, H.M., N.R. Brewer, and M. Kaplan. 1962. Comparative value for some barbiturates in the frog. Proceedings of the Animal Care Panel 12: 141.

Kaplan, H.M. and M. Kaplan. 1961. Anesthesia in frogs with ethyl alcohol. Proceedings Animal Care Panel 11:31–36.

Kofron, C.P. and C.G. Schmitt. 1992. Death-feigning in a West African treefrog. Amphibia-Reptilia 13(1992):405–407.

Kollias, G.V. 1984. Immunologic aspects of infectious disease. in Hoff, G.L., Frye, F.L., and E.R. Jacobson (Eds.): Diseases of Amphibians and Reptiles. Plenum Press, New York.

Letcher, J.L. 1992. Intracoelomic use of tricaine methane sulfonate for anesthesia of bullfrogs (*Rana catesbeiana*) and leopard frogs (*Rana pipiens*). Zoo Biology 11:243–251.

Letcher, J. and R. Durante. 1995. Evaluation of use of tiletamine/zolazepam for anesthesia of bullfrogs and leopard frogs. JAVMA 207(1):80–82.

Meadows, R. 1993. Frogs with a poisonous potential. Zoogoer December 1993, pp. 6–11.

Milton, K. 1994. No pain, no game. Natural History 103(9):44–51.

Moore, J.A. 1964. Physiology of the Amphibia. Academic Press, New York.

National Research Council Committee on Pain and Distress in Laboratory Animals. 1992. Recognition of pain and distress in laboratory animals. National Academy Press. Washington, DC.

Noble, G.K. 1931. The Biology of the Amphibia. McGraw-Hill Book Co., New York.

Ohr, E.A. 1976. Tricaine methanesulfonate—I. pH and its effects on anesthetic potency. Comparative Biochemistry and Physiology 54(C):13–17.

Olson, M.E. 1986. A simple anesthetic chamber. Laboratory Animal Science 36(6):703.

Rie, I.P. 1973. Application of drugs to the skin of salamanders. Herpetologica 29:55–59.

Stevens, C.W. 1995. An amphibian model for pain research. Lab Animal, pp. 32–36.

Stetter, M.D., B. Raphael, F. Indiviglio, and R.A. Cook. 1996. Isoflurane anesthesia in amphibians: Comparison of five application methods. 1996 Proceedings of the American Association of Zoo Veterinarians, pp. 255–257.

Subcommittee on Amphibian Standards. 1974. Committee on Standards, National Research Council, (Eds.): Amphibians: Guidelines for the breeding, care, and management of laboratory animals. National Academy Press Inc., Washington, DC.

Tyler, M.J. 1994. Frog cures herpes. Australian Natural History, 23(4):10–12.

Tyler, M.J. 1995. Frogs and drugs. Australian Natural History 24(12): 46–51.

Tyler, M.J., D.J.M. Stone, and J.H. Bowie. 1992. A novel method for the release and collection of dermal glandular secretions from the skin of frogs. J. Pharmacol. Toxicol. Meth. 28(4):199–200.

Vanable Jr., J.W. 1985. Benzocaine: an excellent amphibian anesthetic. Axolotl Newsletter Spring 1985 14:19–21.

Vanable Jr., J.W., L.L. Hearson, and M.E. McGinnis. 1983. The role of endogenous electrical fields in limb regeneration, In Fallon, J.F. and A.I. Caplan (Eds): Limb Development and Regeneration Part A. A.R. Liss Inc., New York.

Vogelnest, L. 1994a. Transponder implants for frog identification. Bulletin of Association of Reptile and Amphibian Veterinarians 4(1):4.

Vogelnest, L. 1994b. Myiasis in a green treefrog *Litoria caerulea*. Bulletin of the Association of Reptile and Amphibian Veterinarians 4(1):4.

Wass, J.A. and H.M. Kaplan. 1974. Methoxyflurane anesthesia for *Rana pipiens*. Laboratory Animal Science 24(4):669–671.

Wayson, K.A., H. Downes, R.K. Lynn, and N. Gerber. 1976a. Anesthetic effects and elimination of tricaine methane-sulphonate (MS-222) in terrestrial vertebrates. Comparative Biochemical Physiology 55C:37–41.

Wayson, K.A., H. Downes, R.K. Lynn, and N. Gerber. 1976b. Studies on the comparative pharmacology and selective toxicity of tricaine methanesulfonate: metabolism as a basis of selective toxicity in poikilotherms. Journal of Pharmacolo. Exp. Therap. 198:695–708.

West, N.H. and B.N. Van Vliet. 1992. Sensory mechanisms regulating the cardiovascular and respiratory systems, in Feder, M.E. and W.W. Burggren (Eds.): Environmental Physiology of Amphibians. University of Chicago Press, Chicago, pp. 151–182.

Wright, K.M. 1994. Amputation of the tail of a two-toed amphiuma, *Amphiuma means*. Bulletin of Association of Reptile and Amphibian Veterinarians 4(1):5.

Wright, K.M. 1996. Amphibian husbandry and medicine, in Mader, D.R. (Ed.): Reptile Medicine and Surgery. W.B. Saunders Co., Philadelphia, PA, pp. 436–459.

CHAPTER 10

CLINICAL MICROBIOLOGY OF AMPHIBIANS FOR THE EXOTIC PRACTICE

Sandy McCampbell, CAHT

The culturing, isolation, and antibiotic sensitivity testing of amphibian pathogens can be accomplished in most veterinary practices without great expense or complexity. Equipment needs are minimal, and include space in a refrigerator to hold unused media, a medical incubator, and the capability to flame sterilize bacteriological loops and microscope slides. Prepared media and identification systems are readily available. The following is a synopsis of the systems in use at the Philadelphia Zoological Garden.

10.1 CULTURE MEDIA FOR BACTERIA

All samples to be assayed for aerobic activity are plated onto three plates and inoculated into thioglycollate broth. All cultures are incubated at 36–37°C (98–99°F) even though amphibians are ectotherms. Incubating cultures at room temperature or the preferred body temperature of the amphibian patient may more accurately reflect the needs of the microorganisms, however, their growth at these temperatures can be exceedingly slow, delaying the diagnosis for several days. In general, the pathogenic bacteria isolated from amphibians will grow faster at the higher temperature, providing a timely identification of the antibiotic sensitivity spectrum. This is extremely useful to the clinician responsible for developing a therapeutic plan for the amphibian patient.

Using the different plates described below, one can readily distinguish between broad groups of bacteria.

10.1.1 Trypticase Soy Agar with 5% Sheep's Blood (Blood Agar Plate)

Blood agar is an enriched all-purpose medium that grows most microorganisms. Fastidious microorganisms may be overgrown by more aggressive ones, so other plated media may be needed for isolation. The blood present in the agar allows visualization of the hemolytic capacity of colonies. Even though mammalian blood is used as the base, the pathogenicity of an organism isolated from an amphibian is often correlated with its hemolytic ability. Beta hemolysis is complete hemolysis, and the media immediately surrounding a colony of bacteria will become transparent. Alpha hemolysis is partial hemolysis, and a translucent greenish zone may become apparent around the colony. Gamma hemolysis is no hemolysis, and the erythrocytes in the medium will remain unchanged.

All bacterial colonies that grow on the blood agar plate should be Gram stained and examined. Gram-negative organisms should be subcultured to selective media such as MacConkey and eosin-methylene blue agars; however, it is not unusual to find Gram-negative rods that are too fastidious to grow on MacConkey agar.

10.1.2 MacConkey Agar

MacConkey agar is a selective and differential medium that grows Gram-negative organisms and inhibits the growth of most Gram-positive organisms by the inclusion of crystal violet and bile salts. Incorporation of the pH indicator neutral red distinguishes between lactose fermenters and non–lactose fermenters by causing lactose-fermenting colonies to become pink. Non–lactose fermenters are tan or uncolored. As a general rule, the pathogenic bacteria of amphibians are often non–lactose fermenting Gram-negative bacteria.

10.1.3 Columbia Colistin and Nalidixic Acid Agar with 5% Sheep's Blood

The Columbia CNA Agar with 5% Sheep's Blood plate selects for Gram-positive organisms because of the antibiotic activity of colistin and nalidixic acid against many Gram-negative bacteria.

10.1.4 Thioglycollate Broth

All samples are also placed into thioglycollate broth (Thio) to encourage the growth of fastidious or scant bacteria. After a day or so, the broth is subcultured onto the above three plates. Because the techniques for anaerobic culturing are time consuming and represent a significant additional expense, anaerobic cultures are not performed on-site at the Philadelphia Zoo. Including Thio as part of the initial culturing effort enables anaerobes to grow at the bottom of the tube. Their presence is usually indicated by large amounts of bubbles when the tube is moved and the presence of growth in the bottom of the tube (but not on the plates when the broth is subcultured) and is confirmed by Gram-staining growth from the bottom of the tube. If isolation and identification of the anaerobic microflora is desired, cultures are sent to a commercial lab for identification.

10.2 OTHER MEDIA

10.2.1 Salmonella-Shigella Agar

Salmonella-Shigella agar (SS) is selective for Gram-negative bacteria, differentiates between lactose fermenters and nonlactose fermenters, and differentiates hydrogen sulfide producers (such as *Salmonella* spp.) from nonhydrogen sulfide producers. The inclusion of sodium thiosulfate and ferric citrate turns hydrogen sulfide-producing colonies black. Although neither *Salmonella* or *Shigella* are considered pathogens of amphibians at this time, their detection could prove of zoonotic significance.

10.2.2 GN Broth

GN broth is an enrichment medium used to encourage growth of fecal pathogens, especially *Shigella* and *Salmonella*. After a day or two, the broth is subcultured onto an SS plate. This media is often used in mammals to detect enteric pathogens such as *Salmonella* spp. and *Yersinia* spp., although the pathogenicity of many of these organisms for amphibians has not been determined.

10.2.3 *Salmonella* Isolation Media

Specific media are available for the growth *of Salmonella* spp. (e.g, XLT4, DIFCO Laboratories, Detroit, MI). Another agar, Selenite (DIFCO Laboratories, Detroit, MI) is helpful, as it inhibits the growth of other coliforms which typically overgrow and prevent the isolation of *Salmonella* spp.

10.3 CULTURE MEDIA FOR FUNGI

Fungal organisms can be recovered with a variety of special media. Sabouraud Dextrose Agar grows both pathogenic and nonpathogenic fungi. Some Gram-negative organisms can proliferate on this medium, so antibiotics such as chloramphenicol and gentamicin may be incorporated to curb bacterial growth. Dermatophyte Test Medium is designed to isolate and identify dermatophytes that utilize proteins in the medium to cause an alkaline pH change and a resultant red color surrounding the colonies. It can be used to grow amphibian fungal isolates, but it is not a differential medium for them. Mycosel Agar contains cycloheximide and chloramphenicol to permit growth of pathogenic fungi and to discourage growth of Gram-negative bacteria and saprophytic fungi. Fungal cultures are incubated at room temperature. Often, fungi present in clinical specimens will grow on culture media used to isolate bacteria. While *Aspergillus* and other fungi develop typical hyphae-form colonies on culture media, yeast (*Candida* sp.) colonies resemble *Staphylococcus* colonies; thus all cultures should be Gram-stained to permit microscopic interpretation.

10.4 HANDLING SPECIMENS

If a bacterial culture needs to be submitted to an outside lab for analysis, or if a prolonged period of time elapses between collection of the sample and processing, a suitable transport media should be used to ensure survival of the aerobic and anaerobic bacteria (e.g., BBL Port-A-Cul, BBL Media, Cockeysville, MD).

10.4.1 Liquid Specimens

Liquid specimens are usually collected in a syringe, and may include blood, coelomic aspirates, tracheal washes, gastric washes, cloacal washes, urine, or purulent exudate. A drop of specimen is placed on each of the appropriate plates and they are streaked for bacterial isolation. A few drops are placed into thioglycollate broth. The specimen is Gram-stained if enough remains.

If the expected microbial load is light (such as with blood or synovial fluid), the sample can be placed in thioglycollate broth to grow for a few days, then subcultured onto plates.

10.4.2 Swab Specimens

A swab may be used to collect material from purulent exudates, discharges from body orifices, ocular lesions, skin lesions, the trachea, the stomach, the cloaca, the large intestine, and the coelom during a celiotomy. The swab is used to inoculate each agar, which is then streaked for bacterial isolation. The culture swab is then placed into the thioglycollate broth. The swab is either stirred to leave the inoculant in broth, then removed, or broken off to allow the entire swab to be incubated. The metal support wire for the minitip swab can be cut with utility scissors. The cut end of the wire should be flamed before it is allowed to slide into the broth.

A Gram stain can be performed with the swab before placing it in the thioglycollate broth if a flamed (sterile) slide is used. If a fungal culture is also needed, stir the swab through the Thio, then imbed the swab tip in the chosen fungal medium. The swab should be broken off at an appropriate level or the cut-and-flame method can be used so it will fit into the slant tube.

10.4.3 Solid Specimens

Typical solid specimens submitted for culture include caseous exudates, feces, biopsies of skin lesions or internal organs, or organ samples taken at necropsy. The specimen should be collected and treated as aseptically as possible. Using sterile implements (e.g., flamed forceps and a sterile scalpel blade), the specimen can be cut in cross section and the interior swabbed for culture and Gram-staining. Small pieces can be cut from the specimen with sterile implements and used to inoculate other media (e.g., fungal media or *Salmonella-Shigella* medium). It can be difficult to plate pieces of tissue, so more commonly organ pieces are placed into thioglycollate broth and subcultured onto plates.

If the sample was contaminated on the exterior, and if it is large enough, a hot flamed spatula is used to lightly sear the surface before the culture sample is taken. A sterile scalpel is then used to cut into the sample below the seared area.

If the expected bacterial load is light (such as in a fresh organ sample), or if the solid specimen is difficult to plate, a piece can be placed in thioglycollate broth only, allowed to incubate until growth is noticed, then subcultured onto the plates.

10.5 ANTIBIOTIC SENSITIVITY TESTING AND BACTERIAL IDENTIFICATION

Once an organism is isolated, it can be identified and, if bacterial, tested for sensitivity to antibiotics. In some cases the identification of an isolate can be hastened by comparison of its colony morphology to color plates depicting typical growth of common bacteria (for color plates, see Quinn et al., 1994; for identification, see Larone, 1995), but a comprehensive review of the characteristics of pathogenic and nonpathogenic bacteria is beyond the scope of this text. For further details on identification of bacterial isolates, standard microbiological texts should be consulted (Carnahan et al., 1991; Farmer et al., 1985; Finegold & Baron, 1990; Holt, 1989; Holt et al., 1994; Quinn et al., 1994).

10.5.1 Gram-Positive Cocci

Gram-positive cocci, such as *Staphylococcus* spp. and *Streptococcus* spp., are differentiated by the catalase test. The catalase test is performed by placing a drop of 3% hydrogen peroxide onto a clean glass slide. With an applicator stick, a bit of the colony to be tested is added to the drop. Bubbling indicates the colony is catalase-positive, while no reaction means the colony is catalase-negative.

Staphylococcal organisms are catalase-positive. Although they can be speciated with a staphylococcal identification kit, most laboratories simply grade them on the basis of coagulase reactivity. A colony of *Staphylococcus* spp. is inoculated into a small amount of prepared rabbit plasma, which then is incubated overnight. Coagulase-positive *Staphylococcus* spp. will clot (gel) the plasma. This reaction can be easily seen by tilting the tube and observing the tenacity of the solution. There is a strong correlation between pathogenicity and a coagulase-positive reaction in birds and mammals. *Staphylococcus* spp. can also exhibit hemolysis on a blood-containing agar. Hemolysis is not graded as with the streptococci, but should be noted. Sensitivity testing is done using the Kirby-Bauer method.

Streptococcus spp. are catalase-negative. They are graded by their hemolytic reaction on blood agar as alpha, beta, or gamma (non) hemolytic streptococci. The majority of beta-hemolytic streptococci are pathogenic. Enterococcal streptococci (*Enterococcus* spp.) are identified by the ability to split esculin products on Bile Esculin Agar (which turns black if the colony is positive) and growth in 6.5% NaCL trypticase soy broth.

Antibiotic sensitivity testing of Gram-positive bacteria is done by the Kirby-Bauer method on a 150 mm Mueller-Hinton Agar plate. A Mueller-Hinton Agar plate containing 5% sheep blood can be used for the more fastidious bacteria; however, sulfa drugs will not provide accurate zones due to the presence of para-aminobenzoic acid in the blood. Some bacteria including *Streptococcus* spp. will only grow on agar plates containing blood.

Yeast can resemble *Staphylococcus* spp. on an agar plate and they are also catalase-positive. If a sensitivity is mistakenly performed on a yeast, it will be resistant to all antibiotics tested; thus, all types of colonies on a plate should be Gram-stained to assess the morphology of the organisms.

10.5.2 Gram-Negative Rods

Many of the bacteria isolated from ill amphibians are Gram-negative rods. Gram-negative bacteria can be readily broken into two broad groups by the oxidase test. To perform the oxidase test, a pure isolate must be taken from a dye-free agar (e.g., blood agar). The isolate is mixed with oxidase reagent on a piece of white filter paper. Oxidase-positive bacteria form a deep blue to purple color within 30 seconds of mixing with the reagent while oxidase-negative bacteria remain unchanged. Oxidase-positive bacteria which have been isolated from ill amphibians include, but are not limited to, *Alcaligenes, Aeromonas,* and *Pseudomonas* (some species of which are oxidase-negative). Oxidase-negative bacteria infecting amphibians include, but are not limited to, *Acinetobacter, Citrobacter, Enterobacter, Klebsiella, Proteus,* and *Pseudomonas* (some species of which are oxidase-positive). Identification of Gram-negative bacteria may be performed with a variety of integrated test kits such as the API 20E (API 20E Enterobacterial Identification System, BioMerieux Vitek, St. Louis, MO), and the RapID One System and RapID NF Plus System for Gram-negative organisms (Innovative Diagnostics, Inc., Norcross, GA). It is important to note that these systems are intended for use on bacteria of human origin, and may not identify isolates or species recovered from amphibians. Isolates that are not successfully identified by these systems need to be evaluated by conventional microbiological tests (Carnahan et al., 1991; Farmer et al., 1985; Holt, 1989; Holt et al., 1994; Quinn et al., 1994).

Antibiotic sensitivity testing is done using the Kirby-Bauer method. The bacterial saline suspension used in setting up the API 20E can also be used to inoculate the Mueller-Hinton Agar plate with a pure culture for sensitivity testing. In order for the sensitivity testing to be standardized, the final turbidity of the saline suspension should equal a 0.5 McFarland standard, and the Mueller-Hinton agar should be 4 mm in depth.

10.5.3 Pathogenic Fungi

Dermatophytes such as *Microsporum* spp. and *Trichophyton* spp. are uncommon isolates in amphibians, and such an identification should be considered suspect. Saprophytic fungi are commonly recovered, but many species have not been associated with disease in amphibians. *Candida* spp. of yeast also grow on fungal media and may infect amphibians. *Candida* spp. can be identified using a yeast-identification kit but, since these test kits were developed for human medical use, many amphibian pathogens are not included in their profile. Many fungi pathogenic to amphibians require specialized culture techniques, so sample submission to a diagnostic laboratory may be necessary.

Identification of many fungi can be performed in the laboratory by microscopic examination. To conserve colony morphology, a piece of transparent tape is pressed, sticky side down, onto the colony and placed, still sticky side down, onto a microscope slide to which a drop of lacto-phenol cotton blue stain or saline has been added.

10.5.4 *Mycobacterium* spp.

Mycobacterium spp. can be pathogenic in amphibians. Culture and identification of *Mycobacterium* spp. is best accomplished by submission to a diagnostic laboratory.

10.6 SUGGESTED SAMPLES

See Table 10.1 for a list of microbial isolates from ill amphibians.

10.6.1 Systemic Infections

Samples to culture include blood, coelomic fluid, and subcutaneous fluid. Cloacal and oropharyngeal swabs can be difficult to interpret due to high numbers of normal microflora.

10.6.2 Skin Infections

Since many signs of systemic infection appear as skin discoloration or lesions, samples to culture include all those already mentioned for systemic disease. Skin lesions may be cultured directly prior to cytologic sampling. Surface samples may be difficult to interpret due to the high numbers of normal microflora, or, in some cases, bacterial growth may be inhibited by antibacterial compounds present in the amphibian's slime layer that contaminate the swab. Cultures may be taken from exudates, purulent material, debrided material, or deep swab of the lesion, taking care not to contaminate the swab with skin microflora. It can be helpful to run comparisons between samples of surface microflora of the ill amphibian with swabs of the skin from a healthy amphibian from the same enclosure. However, because infectious diseases can spread quickly, it is possible that apparently healthy amphibians may be harboring pathogenic organisms.

10.6.3 Respiratory Infections

Culturing of the trachea may be warranted if an amphibian displays buoyancy problems, nasal exudate, or lethargy. Some clear mucus is normally present in the mouth of most animals, and care should be taken to avoid contaminating the sample with this mucus. A microtip culturette can be used to swab the trachea. A sterile catheter can be placed in the trachea, and sterile saline flushed and aspirated to obtain a tracheal wash.

10.6.4 Culture For "Normal Microflora"

Although it may be cost prohibitive, it is often beneficial to do bacterial cultures on an amphibian while it is healthy. This documents the normal bacterial microflora so that pathogens may be identified more readily when the animal is ill.

10.6.5 Necropsies

Timely necropsies are invaluable, especially in a "herd" disease outbreak (see Chapter 25, Necropsy). Cultures can be taken from organ samples obtained at

Table 10.1. Representative microbial isolates recovered from ill anurans at the National Aquarium in Baltimore over the course of one year. (Compare to Tables 13.1, Some bacteria associated with red leg syndrome, and 13.3, Bacteria generally considered to be nonpathogenic to amphibians.)

Amphibian	Bacterial Isolate	Culture Site
Agalychnis callidryas	*Aeromonas hydrophila*	skin lesion
Agalychnis callidryas	*Citrobacter freundii*	skin lesion
Agalychnis callidryas	*Flavobacterium odoratum*	skin lesion
Agalychnis spurrelli	*Aeromonas hydrophila*	feces
Agalychnis spurrelli	*Citrobacter freundii*	feces
Agalychnis spurrelli	*Morganella morganii*	feces
Agalychnis spurrelli	*Streptococcus viridans*	feces
Bufo guttatus	*Flavobacterium indologenes*	egg mass
Bufo guttatus	*Providencia rettgeri*	egg mass
Bufo guttatus	*Staphylococcus* spp.	egg mass
Bufo guttatus	*Proteus vulgaris*	liver
Bufo guttatus	*Staphylococcus* spp.	liver
Ceratophrys cornuta	*Aeromonas hydrophila*	gastric wash
Ceratophrys cornuta	*Citrobacteri freundii*	gastric wash
Ceratophrys cornuta	*Morganella morganii*	gastric wash
Ceratophrys cornuta	*Streptococcus* spp.	gastric wash
Hyla miliaria	*Pseudomonas* spp.	liver
Hyla miliaria	*Citrobacter freundii*	lung
Hyla miliaria	*Pseudomonas aeruginosa*	lung
Hyla miliaria	*Serratia marcescens*	lung
Hyla miliaria	*Staphylococcus* spp.	lung
Hyla miliaria	*Staphylococcus* spp. hemolytic	lung
Hyla miliaria	*Streptococcus* spp.	lung
Mantella aurantiaca	*Aeromonas hydrophila*	brain
Mantella aurantiaca	*Hafnia alvei*	brain
Phyllobates bicolor	*Aeromonas hydrophila*	coelom
Phyllobates bicolor	*Citrobacter freundii*	coelom
Phyllobates bicolor	*Klebsiella* spp.	coelom
Phyllobates bicolor	*Pseudomonas putrefaciens*	coelom
Phyllobates bicolor	*Aeromonas hydrophila*	coelom
Phyllobates bicolor	*Pseudomonas putrefaciens*	coelom
Phyllobates bicolor	*Flavobacterium indologenes*	liver
Phyllobates bicolor	*Sphingobacterium multivorum*	liver
Phyllobates bicolor	*Vibrio hollisae*	liver
Phyllomedusa bicolor	*Aeromonas hydrophila*	feces
Phyllomedusa bicolor	*Bacillus* spp.	left leg*
Phyllomedusa bicolor	*Flavobacterium meningosepticum*	left leg
Phyllomedusa bicolor	*Providencia rustigianii*	left leg
Phyllomedusa bicolor	*Serratia marcescens*	rostral abrasion
Phyllomedusa celestiae	*Proteus mirabilis*	aspirate of mass
Phyllomedusa celestiae	*Citrobacter amalonaticus*	urolith
Phyllomedusa celestiae	*Proteus mirabilis*	urolith
Phyllomedusa iherengii	*Acinetobacter calcoaceticus*	feces
Phyllomedusa iherengii	*Alcaligenes xylosoxydans xylosoxydans*	feces
Phyllomedusa iherengii	Anaerobic Gram-negative rod	feces
Phyllomedusa iherengii	*Bacillus* spp.	feces*
Phyllomedusa iherengii	*Citrobacter freundii*	feces
Phyllomedusa iherengii	*Proteus vulgaris*	feces
Phyllomedusa iherengii	*Staphylococcus* spp.	feces
Phyllomedusa iherengii	*Streptococcus* spp.	feces
Phyllomedusa iherengii	budding yeast	feces

* indicates probable environmental contaminant

necropsy. The specimen should be collected and treated as aseptically as possible. Culture of heart blood may determine the cause of a septicemia. Flame-searing the surface of an organ will reduce potential contaminants, and a sample can be taken from a stab incision through the seared area. If the necropsy is performed in an aseptic manner, small pieces can be cut from the specimen with sterile implements and used for culture.

10.7 SUPPLIERS OF PRODUCTS MENTIONED IN TEXT

BBL Media, BD Micro Systems, Cockeysville, MD 21030 supplies the following products: Trypticase Soy Agar with 5% sheep blood, MacConkey Agar, Columbia CNA Agar with 5% sheep blood, Mueller-Hinton Agar, Coagulase plasma EDTA, Oxidase reagent, BBL Port-A-Cul.

Innovative Diagnostics, Inc., Norcross, GA supplies the RapID One System for medically important Enterobacteriaceae and oxidase-negative Gram-negative rods and RapID NF Plus System for medically important glucose nonfermenting and selected glucose-fermenting Gram-negative bacteria.

BioMerieux Vitek, St. Louis, MO supplies the API 20E (Enterobacterial Identification System).

REFERENCES

Carnahan, A.M., S. Behram, and S.W. Joseph. 1991. Aerokey II: A flexible key for identifying clinical Aeromonas species. American Society for Microbiology 29(12):2843–2849.

Farmer, J.J., B.R. Davis, F.W. Hickman-Brenner, A. McWhorter, G.P. Huntley-Carter, M.A. Asbury, C. Riddle, H.G. Warthen-Grady, C. Elias, G.R. Fanning, A.G. Steigerwalt, C.M. O'Hara, G.K. Morris, P.B. Smith, and D.J. Brenner. 1985. Biochemical identification of new species and biogroups of Enterobacteriaceae isolated from clinical specimens. Journal of Clinical Microbiology 21:46–76.

Finegold, S.M. and E.J. Baron. 1990. Bailey and Scott's Diagnostic Microbiology. The C.V. Mosby Co., St. Louis, MO.

Holt, J.G. 1989. Bergey's Manual of Systematic Bacteriology, Vol. 1–4. Williams and Wilkins. Baltimore, MD.

Holt, J.G., N.R. Krieg, P.H.A. Sneath, J.T. Staley, and S.T. Williams 1994. Bergey's Manual of Determinative Bacteriology, 9th Edition, Vol. 1. Williams and Wilkins, Baltimore, MD.

Larone, D. 1995. Medically Important Fungi, A guide to Identification, 3rd edition. ASM Press, Washington DC.

Quinn, O.J., M.E. Carter, B. Markey, and G.R. Carter. 1994. Clinical Veterinary Microbiology. Moseby Year Book Europe, Ltd., Wolfe Publishing, Spain.

CHAPTER 11
AMPHIBIAN HEMATOLOGY

Kevin M. Wright, DVM

11.1 BLOOD VOLUME

The small body size of many amphibians often dissuades the veterinary clinician from pursuing a hematological work-up of an amphibian patient. The blood volume of many aquatic species is incredibly high, from 13.4% of the body mass in the African clawed frog, *Xenopus laevis,* to 25% in aquatic caecilians, *Typhlonectes* spp. Terrestrial forms are more in keeping with other terrestrial vertebrates, with blood volume approximately 9.5% in the northern leopard frog, *Rana pipiens,* and 7.4% in the marine toad, *Bufo marinus* (Boutilier et al., 1992; Thorson, 1964). As a general rule, it is safe to take a blood volume of no more than 1% of a healthy amphibian's body weight, and no more than 0.5% should be taken from a seriously ill amphibian. For example, no more than 0.1 ml of blood should be removed from a healthy 10-g frog, and no more than 0.05 ml from an ill 10-g frog. Valuable information can be obtained from even small samples of blood, so the clinician is encouraged to include hematology as a standard part of the diagnostic evaluation of the amphibian.

11.2 AN ALGORITHM FOR SAMPLE PROCESSING

A healthy 7-g frog can provide up to 0.07 ml of blood (i.e., approximately the volume of a single microhematocrit tube), a volume adequate to evaluate for several parameters. A suggested algorithm for analyzing small volumes of blood is to first evaluate a wet mount of whole blood to detect trypanosomes and other extracellular hemoparasites. Movement of the blood cells often facilitates detection of flagellated protozoa, such as trypanosomes. A stained blood film can be evaluated for the presence of parasites, erythrocyte morphology, leukocyte differential, thrombocyte presence, and the number of leukocytes counted per high power field (WBC/HPF). This evaluation should be done before performing the actual total white blood cell count (TWBC/mm^3), as it may determine whether or not performing the TWBC/mm^3 is an appropriate use of the remaining blood sample. An unstained blood film should be set aside for additional staining techniques if needed. If the WBC/HPF seems excessively high, or if toxic granulocytes or phagocytic monocytes are noted, then it is reasonable to use a portion of the blood sample for the TWBC/mm^3. Decant the exact amount of the sample needed for an actual total white blood cell count (TWBC/mm^3) and perform the count. If there are large numbers of parasitized erythrocytes, performing a total erythrocyte count (RBC/mm^3) and hemoglobin concentration may be a productive use of some of the remaining blood sample. After the cellular analysis has been completed, the hematocrit tube can be scanned under a light microscope to determine if microfilaria or protozoa are moving in the blood. Afterwards, the hematocrit tube can be centrifuged. Note that there are calibrated microhematocrit tubes that are of a smaller inner diameter than regular hematocrit tubes, thus requiring a smaller volume of blood for processing. The packed cell volume (PCV), percent buffy coat, and icteric index can be obtained. Some amphibians may have unusually colored plasma. The Japanese giant salamander, *Andrias japonicus,* may have a bluish tint to its plasma, and shades of green and orange have been noted in the plasma of other apparently healthy amphibians on occasion. The hematocrit tube can then be examined under low power on a microscope to screen for microfilaria (Figure 11.1), and then the plasma can be removed to analyze for various chemistries and total solids or total protein until the sample is depleted. With dry film chemistry analyzers usually one or two additional parameters can be measured from a small sample. Amphibians weighing more than 40 g can provide a sufficient volume of blood to run complete blood counts and multiple plasma chemistries.

Unless a blood culture is to be performed on the sample, it is important to heparinize the syringe in venipuncture attempts to avoid coagulation of the sample before it is transferred to the appropriate whole blood tube. If a blood sample is to be obtained for microbial culture, no anticoagulant should be

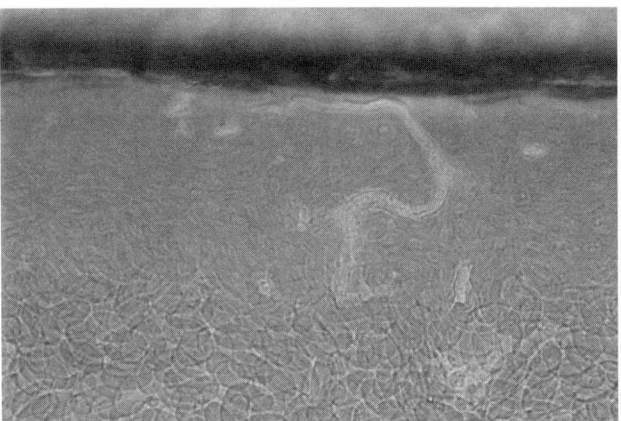

Figure 11.1. Microfilariae can be detected in the hematocrit tube if it is scanned by light microscopy under low power before and after centrifugation for packed cell volume. (Sandy McCampbell, Philadelphia Zoological Garden)

used to pretreat the syringe, needle, or capillary tube, as this might affect the growth of some organisms. However, unheparinized glass (e.g., plain hematocrit tubes) may promote clotting of amphibian blood (Zwemer, 1991), thus transfer of the blood sample to the culture media must be prompt.

11.3 ANTICOAGULANTS

Lithium heparin is the anticoagulant of choice for pretreating the syringe and storage of blood since it does not appear to affect the values of plasma calcium, sodium, or ammonia. A small amount of sterile distilled or reverse osmosis-derived water (i.e., 0.05 ml or less) can be placed into a lithium heparin-containing tube (e.g., Microtainer®, Becton Dickinson and Company, Cockeysville, MD), and this liquid is used to pretreat the syringe. The liquid should be blown out of the syringe by plunging to flush air and liquid out of the syringe chamber. Arterial blood gas kits contain syringes coated with lithium heparin (e.g., BardParker® A-line Kit, Becton Dickinson Acute Care, Franklin Lakes, NJ), but these kits are expensive and only contain 3-ml syringes. Ammonium heparin is a common liquid form of heparin in most practices. It can be used to pretreat the syringe, but it is important to avoid the use of ammonium heparin when obtaining a sample that is to be analyzed for ammonia (NH_3) levels or else a falsely elevated reading will result. Sodium heparin can be used to pretreat a syringe, but it should be avoided when electrolyte values are desired. Ethylenediamine-tetra-acetic acid (EDTA) may lyse the erythrocytes of certain species of amphibians, so this anticoagulant is not recommended for amphibian blood unless its efficacy is known for the species in question. A solution of 3% EDTA in distilled water is an effective anticoagulant for the blood of the axolotl, *Ambystoma mexicanum*, and is preferred by some authors (Zwemer, 1991).

11.4 BLOOD COLLECTION

There are several options available for obtaining blood from a frog. A relatively simple procedure is to bleed from the lingual venous plexus that lies immediately beneath the tongue (Baranowski-Smith & Smith, 1983) (Figure 11.2). This method works well on frogs as small as 25 g although some species (e.g., pipid frogs) do not have tongues with suitable anatomy. Care must be taken to gently pry open the mouth in order to avoid breaking the thin mandibular bones. A small firm rubber spatula works well as a mouth speculum, as does developed x-ray film, a plastic credit card, business card, or even a cotton minitip applicator. In some animals it is easier to work from the lateral edge of the oral commissure, while in other animals it is easiest to insert the speculum into the philtrum, a small divot found just beneath the tip of the nose. Once the mouth is opened, a cotton tip applicator is used to draw the tongue forward, as if the tongue was flipping out to catch a prey item. The lingual venous plexus is then visible on the underside of the tongue and the buccal floor. Most frogs have pale colored tongues, so the purple-to-red network of veins is readily apparent. One large vein can then be punctured with a 26 or 25 gauge needle, and a heparinized microhematocrit tube can be used to collect the blood that oozes from the vein. Once an adequate sample of blood is obtained, release the tongue. In most cases, this serves to put enough pressure on the vein that it stops bleeding. Occasionally it is necessary to put direct

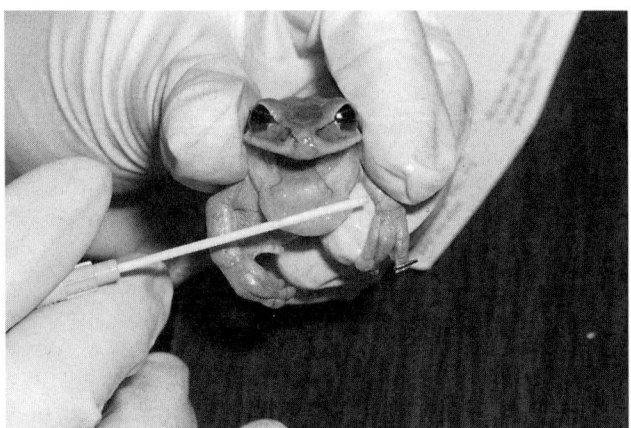

Figure 11.2. Lingual venous plexus in a New Guinea white-lipped treefrog, *Litoria infrafrenata*. (Kevin Wright, Philadelphia Zoological Garden)

pressure on the venipuncture site with a dry cotton tip applicator to achieve hemostasis. The disadvantage to this technique is that the samples can be contaminated with saliva and mucous, but this can be minimized if care is taken to swab clean the surface of the plexus with a dry cotton tip applicator before venipuncture. In the case of a fractious animal, blood collection can be facilitated by sedating or anesthetizing the patient with tricaine methanesulfonate (see Section 9.2.3, Topical Anesthetics).

Large frogs and toads can be bled quite easily from the midline abdominal vein. This relatively large vein runs subcutaneously over the linea alba along the ventrum of the animal (Figure 11.3). A 26 or 27 gauge needle can be carefully inserted in a craniodorsal direction into this vein, and gentle pressure applied to withdraw blood into the syringe. A good insertion site is the point midway between the sternum and the pelvis. Unfortunately, the passage through the bore of these small gauge needles does tend to distort some blood cells, but if a larger gauge needle is used there is a risk of lacerating the midline abdominal vein.

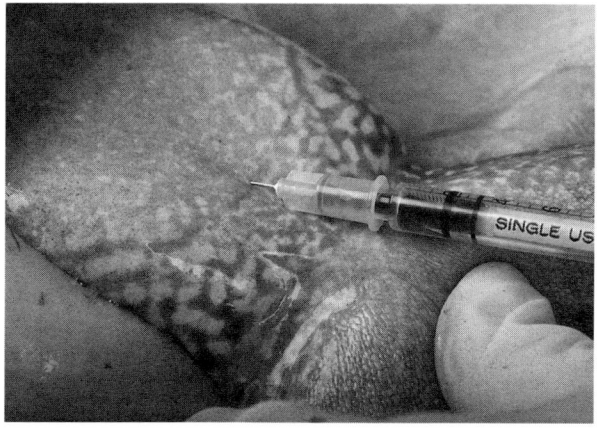

Figure 11.3. Phlebotomy of the midline abdominal vein in a South American bullfrog, *Leptodactylus pentadactylus*. (George Grall, National Aquarium in Baltimore)

Salamanders may be bled from the anterior (midline) abdominal vein in the manner described above, but it is more difficult to identify the venipuncture site in this order of amphibians. A doppler probe may help locate the vein. An additional site for venipuncture is the ventral caudal vein, also called the tail vein, that runs immediately ventral to the vertebral bodies (Figure 11.4). In salamanders less than 80 g, a 27 gauge needle is the most practical choice for venipuncture attempts, but a 26 or 25 gauge needle may be used for larger animals. Some salamanders and newts have tail autotomy, and in these species one should not attempt this method since it could result in the loss of the specimen's tail during the venipuncture endeavor.

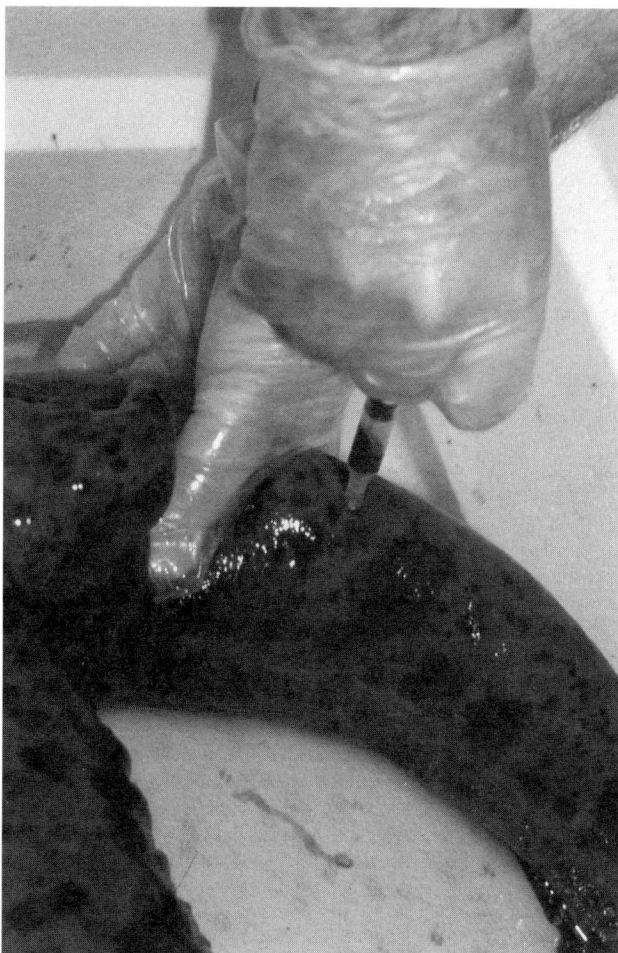

Figure 11.4. Phlebotomy from the ventral tail vein of an anesthetized Japanese giant salamander, *Andrias japonicus*. (Philadelphia Zoological Garden)

Cardiocentesis has worked equally well for anurans, most salamanders, and even caecilians. If the animal is difficult to restrain, it should be sedated or anesthetized with tricaine methanesulfonate to minimize the risk of pericardial, ventricular, or atrial laceration. The animal is placed in dorsal recumbency, and its cardiac impulse is identified visually. A doppler probe may assist in locating the heart (Figure 11.5). An instrument with a cool light source (e.g., an arthroscope) can be advanced down the esophagus into the stomach for internal transillumination of the heart in some amphibians. Once the cardiac impulse is noted or the cardiac image defined, a 25, 26, or 27 gauge needle may be inserted so as to penetrate the apex of the ventricle. Gentle pressure is applied, and the needle slowly advanced or withdrawn until a flash of blood is visible in the hub of the syringe. If a clear or cloudy yellow fluid appears instead, the needle should be withdrawn, as the sample is most likely fluid from the pericardial sac. If sufficient pericardial fluid is obtained, it can

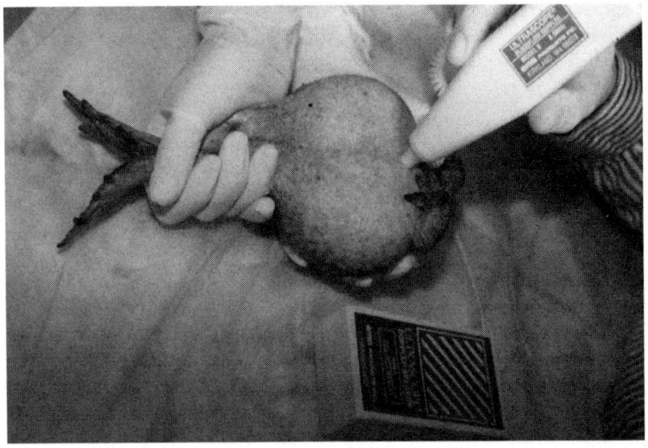

Figure 11.5. Doppler examination of the heart of a giant toad, *Bufo marinus*. (Christine Steinert, National Aquarium in Baltimore)

be analyzed for biochemical parameters. However, usually it is of small quantity and is better examined by light microscopy to determine if inflammatory cells or other abnormal items are present. On occasion it may be more productive to culture the pericardial fluid, but the heparin in the syringe may interfere with bacterial growth. A new needle and syringe should be used for a second attempt. There is an increased risk of a problem arising with each subsequent puncture of pericardial or cardiac tissue. If a blood flash is detected, pressure should be let off the syringe. A cycle of gentle pressure and release will coax blood into the syringe with each heartbeat. Once an adequate sample is obtained, pressure is released and the needle withdrawn from the ventricular chamber.

In very small amphibians, the heart may be punctured with a small gauge needle (i.e., 28 gauge) and blood collected from the hub with a microhematocrit tube. This technique has been proven effective even in amphibians as small as tadpoles of the wood frog, *Rana sylvatica* (R. Boltz, personal communication, 1995).

Digital amputation and tail amputation have been used as the route of collecting blood samples from animals in the field. This method cannot be recommended for the amphibian patient due to the pain and disfigurement associated with these options. However, if toe-clipping is being used as a form of identification, concomitant blood collection may be undertaken.

With any of the methods described for obtaining blood, it is suggested that heparinized microhematocrit tubes be on hand so that any blood that wells up on the surface of the amphibian can be collected for analysis. Sometimes this blood may be the only sample obtained.

11.5 SAMPLE ANALYSIS

11.5.1 Stains

Wright's solution (Camco Quik Stain, American Scientific Products, McGaw Park, Illinois) is the stain of choice for hematological evaluations at the Philadelphia Zoo. When treated with Wright-Giemsa stain, a mature erythrocyte will have an eosinophilic cytoplasm (deep pink to red) with a basophilic staining multilobed nucleus (blue). Thrombocytes will have a pale gray cytoplasm, and may aggregate. Lymphocytes will have small amounts of a gray to deep blue cytoplasm, while monocytes will have large amounts of a gray to light blue cytoplasm. The leukocyte differential count will usually be heavily biased with basophilic-staining granulocytes when using Wright-Giemsa stain. It is important to remember that granulocytes are described on the basis of their staining characteristics, and that the classes of granulocytes have not been proven conclusively to be either homologous or analogous to the mammalian granulocytes with similar staining characteristics. Thus an eosinophilic-staining granulocyte in an amphibian is not proven to be linked with parasitism or allergic conditions as is generally assumed with the mammalian eosinophil. It is important to document collection data (e.g., date and time collected, ambient temperature/animal's body temperature, sex of animal, etc.) as well as the disease accompanying the differential leukogram in order to elucidate the role of the various leukocytes seen in amphibians.

Other staining techniques may be warranted, especially use of stains that document histochemical properties (see Alleman et al., 1996; Mateo et al., 1984; Yam et al., 1971), or the unstained blood film may be sent to a diagnostic lab for further analysis. A Gram-stain of the blood film may reveal bacteria supporting a diagnosis of bacteremia. Rickettsia, protozoa and inclusions (inclusion bodies) caused by viruses may be detected on appropriately stained blood smears (Desser, 1992; Graczyk et al., 1996; Marcus, 1981; Reichenbach-Klinke & Elkan, 1965; Schmittner & McGhee, 1961). Trypanosomes and microfilaria are extraerythrocytic (Plate 11.1). Hemogregarine parasites are common basophilic intraerythrocytic inclusions in amphibians (Plate 11.2). The relative percentage of erythrocytes afflicted with inclusions may be an important clinical prognostic indicator. Due to the movement of trypanosomes and microfilaria, an unstained wet mount of fresh blood may more readily reveal these parasites than air-dried blood smears. Low levels of hemoparasites are probably unimportant (Graczyk et al., 1996; Schmittner & McGhee, 1961), or may only be a minor contributing factor to the amphibian's signs. Moderate to high levels of inclusions may be significant, especially if coupled with signs of anemia such as low PCV or RBC, polychromatic erythrocytes, microcytosis, or hypohemoglobinemia.

11.5.2 Complete Blood Count

Complete blood counts may be performed in the same manner as described for avian and reptilian species (Campbell, 1996, 1988). Natt-Herrick's solution was first used to evaluate chicken blood cells (Natt & Herrick, 1952), but has since been used with success in amphibians (Cathers et al., 1997; Wright, 1996). This technique allows one to make a count of leukocytes, erythrocytes and thrombocytes from the same sample using a hemocytometer and an erythrocyte diluting pipette (e.g., erythrocyte Unopette®, Becton Dickinson, Rutherford, NJ) (Plate 11.3). Furthermore, the leukocyte differential does not need to be determined in order to yield the total leukocyte count. The main disadvantage to this technique is that the Natt-Herrick's solution must be made and manually diluted (see Table 11.1). Parasites such as microfilaria are occasionally encountered in the charged chamber of the hemocytometer (Figure 11.6).

Table 11.1. Natt-Herrick's solution (Natt & Herrick, 1952).

NaCl	3.88 g
Na_2SO_4	2.50 g
$Na_2HPO_4 \cdot 12H_2$	2.91 g
KH_2PO_4	0.25 g
formalin (37%)	7.50 ml
methyl violet 2B	0.10 g
water, distilled	

Dissolve all the chemicals in the order listed in distilled water. Once all chemicals have been dissolved, dilute soltuion with distilled water to a total volume of 1000 ml. Let solution stand overnight, then filter through fine filter paper (Whatman #2). Natt-Herrick's solution is now ready for use. Store in a sealed container to prevent evaporation.

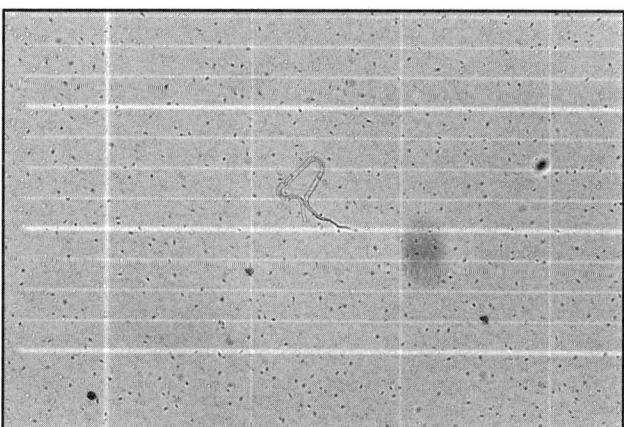

Figure 11.6. Microfilaria and other parasites are occasionally discovered in the charged chamber of the hemocytometer during the white blood cell count. (Sandy McCampbell, Philadelphia Zoological Garden)

Natt-Herrick's Solution. In order to perform a total leukocyte or total white blood cell count per mm^3 (TWBC/mm^3) using the Natt-Herrick's solution, an uncoagulated blood sample is pipetted into an erythrocyte diluting pipette to a level of the 0.5 mark. Natt-Herrick's solution is then drawn into the pipette to provide a 1:200 dilution. The diluting pipette should be thoroughly mixed by repeated inversion, and then some of its contents can be discharged into the hemocytometer counting chamber. The freshly charged hemocytometer should be allowed to sit in a humid chamber for at least 5 minutes or the count will be inaccurate. The count should be confined to the large central square of the Neubauer grid of the hemocytometer. Since many amphibians possess large erythrocytes, a survey of the four corner and center squares should be done at low power to determine if a count can be accurately made of the erythrocytes in these sections. If this can be done, count and record the erythrocyte number. If the cells are not distinct at low power, higher power dry lenses should be used. The total erythrocyte count in these five chambers is multiplied by 10,000 to yield the total erythrocyte count per mm^3 of blood. Once the hemoglobin concentration is determined, the erythrocyte values such as mean corpuscular volume (MCV), mean corpuscular hemoglobin (MCH), and mean corpuscular hemoglobin concentration (MCHC) can be determined in the standard manner. The total leukocyte count (TWBC/mm^3) can be made from the same charged hemocytometer chamber only the count includes all leukocytes in the nine large squares of the Neubauer grid. The total count is increased by 10% and then this new total is multiplied by 200 to yield the total leukocyte count per mm^3 of blood. Total thrombocyte count per mm^3 of blood is performed similarly as the total leukocyte count from the same charged hemocytometer chamber.

Eosinophil Unopette® Method. Another option for determining the total leukocyte count per mm^3 of blood is to use an eosinophil Unopette® #5877 (Becton Dickinson, Rutherford, NJ) to count granulocytes followed by a leukocyte differential count of a stained blood film to determine total white blood cell count. Heterophilic granulocytes and eosinophilic granulocytes accumulate the phloxine B stain in the solution within the eosinophil Unopette® #5877 and appear a brighter red than other cells (Plate 11.4). Basophilic granulocytes are readily distinguished from heterophils and eosinophils during the actual counting process since the basophilic granules refract light brightly and are quite obvious. The eosinophil pipette draws up an aliquotted sample of blood which is discharged into the eosinophil Unopette® #5877. The hemocytometer is charged with this solution and allowed to incubate in a humid chamber for a minimum of 10 minutes to allow the blood cells to settle and the granulocytes to uptake the stain. A count is made of all red staining cells in the nine large squares of the Neubauer grid on both sides of the counting chamber (a total of 18 squares). If the count differs by more than 10% between the two sides, the count should be considered suspect (Dein et al., 1994). If sufficient solution remains, the hemocytometer should be cleaned and recharged. If there is still a discrepancy, and sufficient blood remains, a new solution should be prepared and used. Once the box count is obtained, the total white blood cell count per mm^3 is calculated using the leukocyte differential.

To obtain the count of heterophils and eosinophils per mm^3 (HE/mm^3), multiply the cells counted by 320 and divide this total by 18, the number of squares counted in the Neubauer grid. A leukocyte differential must be performed to determine the total percentage of white blood cells that are heterophils and eosinophils (%HE). The total leukocyte count per mm^3 ($TWBC/mm^3$) is determined by dividing the total eosinophil and heterophil count per mm^3 by the total percentage of eosinophils and heterophils in the leukocyte differential multiplied by 100.

In summary, the total leukocyte count is a two step process when using the eosinophil Unopette® method:

Step 1. Count of heterophils and eosinophils.

$$HE/mm^3 = \{320 \times (\# \text{ granulocytes in box count})\}/18$$

Step 2. Total leukocyte count.

$$TWBC/mm^3 = \{(HE/mm^3)/(\%HE)\} \times 100$$

The eosinophil Unopette® method may not work in all amphibian species. At the Philadelphia Zoo, it has worked well in the giant toad *Bufo marinus,* ornate horned frog, *Ceratophrys ornata,* South American bullfrog, *Leptodactylus pentadactylus,* bullfrog, *Rana catesbeiana,* hellbender, *Cryptobranchus alleganiensis,* Japanese giant salamander, *Andrias japonicus,* Anderson's axolotl, *Ambystoma andersoni,* the lesser siren, *Siren intermedia,* the Mexican caecilian, *Dermophis mexicanus,* among others. The eosinophil Unopette® technique may be applicable to a wide variety of amphibians. For each species encountered, it is recommended that the eosinophil Unopette® technique not be used until it is verified for that species. This may be done by performing simultaneous counts using the Natt-Herrick's solution/Unopette method and the eosinophil Unopette® method (Dein et al., 1994). If the counts are consistently within 5% of each other, then the eosinophil Unopette® method may be used on future hematology specimens of that species. An advantage to the eosinophil Unopette® method is that it is much easier to count the stained granulocytes than it is to distinguish leukocytes from erythrocytes in the Natt-Herrick's solution. Furthermore, in some amphibians the lymphocytes, thrombocytes, and free erythrocyte nuclei may appear very similar when stained with Natt-Herrick's solution. However, with suitable training the Natt-Herrick's solution allows an accurate $TWBC/mm^3$ independent of the granulocyte differential count. This is important since in amphibians the granulocytes have been poorly described and may vary tremendously in staining characteristics and gross morphology between species. It is unknown whether many of the cells that appear basophilic with a Wright-Giemsa stain uptake phloxin B. Considerable expertise is needed for an accurate leukocyte differential count using either method.

11.5.3 Chemistry

With the advent of small inexpensive dry film analyzers (e.g., Kodak Ektachem DT60 Analyzer, Eastman Kodak Co., Rochester, NY), it is practical to obtain plasma chemistries on amphibians. Typically these analyzers can analyze plasma samples for total protein, albumin, aspartate (AST), alanine aminotransferase (ALT), blood urea nitrogen (BUN), calcium, phosphorus, glucose, electrolytes, and various other chemistries. The small volume of sample needed for analysis by these machines (i.e., 10 µl) allows even a 0.5 ml plasma sample to yield the results of up to five different chemistries. Blood samples should be spun down soon after collection and plasma decanted from the cellular component.

11.5.4 Cytology

An excellent review of amphibian hematology (Turner, 1988) and an atlas of the hematology of the African clawed frog, *Xenopus laevis,* (Hadji-Azimi et al., 1987) have been published.

Erythrocyte. The erythrocytes of amphibians include the largest average mean cell volume of any vertebrate. Depending on the species, erythrocyte size varies from 10 to 70 µm in diameter, with an erythrocyte volume (mean cell volume or MCV) that is correspondingly variable (Table 11.2). Immature erythrocytes may be found in the circulating blood, and may herald viral infection in some species (Gruia-Grey & Desser, 1992). Most amphibian erythrocytes are nucleated elliptical cells, and the nucleus probably allows protein synthesis and adjustment of metabolic processes (Boutilier et al., 1992). In some amphibians, especially terrestrial anurans and lungless salamanders, anucleated erythrocytes (also known as erythroplastids or plasmocytes) have been documented at species-specific levels ranging from 2% in the red-backed salamander, *Plethodon cinereus* (Turner, 1988), to 90% in slender salamanders *Batrachoseps* spp. (Cohen, 1982; Emmel, 1924). It is assumed that the loss of the nucleus is associated with an improved ability to absorb and

Table 11.2. Average values for hematocrit, hemoglobin, erythrocyte count, erythrocyte volume, and erythrocyte dimensions for some amphibians. Adapted from Boutilier et al., 1992, Cathers et el., 1997, Duellman and Trueb, 1986a, b, Jerret and Mays, 1973, and Pfeiffer et al., 1990.

Species	Hct %	Hb g/dl	RBC + $10^6/\mu l$	MCV μm^3	Dimensions μm
GYMNIOPHONA					
Boulengerula taitanus	40.0	10.3	0.68	588	22.1 × 15.6
Typhlonectes compressicaudus	37.6	11.3			
CAUDATA					
Ambystoma mexicanum (gilled)	27.7	7.5			
Ambystoma mexicanum (metamorphosed)	29.8	7.6			
Amphiuma tridactylum	23.0	5.7			
Amphiuma means			0.03	13,857	62.5 × 36.3
Cryptobranchus alleganiensis	40.0–43.3	8.32–10.07	0.07	7,425	40.5 × 21.0
Cynops pyrrhogaster	40 ± 1.9		0.023		
Desmognathus fuscus	28.0	7.5			
Dicamptodon ensatus	24.2	4.4	0.05	4,938	51.4 × 29.3
Necturus maculosus	19.0	4.5	0.02	10,070	52.8 × 28.2
Taricha granulosa	36.7	9.5			
ANURA					
Chiromantis petersi	21.1				
Hyla versicolor			0.9		
Rana catesbeiana (larva)	20.9	3.7			
Rana catesbeiana (adult)	22.2–23.5	5.7–6.3	0.44	670	24.8 × 15.3
Rana catesbeiana (adult)	22.1	4.72			
Rana esculenta	27.3	7.8	0.43	659	
Rana pipiens			0.32	768	23.8 × 16.2
Telmatobius culeus	27.9	8.1	0.73	394	17.0 × 12.0
Xenopus laevis	28.3–38.7	8.3–11.3			

transport oxygen. Erythrocyte nuclei may be found free in the blood, but these are unlikely to persist. In the amphibians studied, nucleated erythrocytes tend to live upwards of 100 days (Porter, 1972), a fact perhaps related to the ability to control and alter their metabolism. The longevity of erythrocytes may make blood transfusion a viable therapeutic option for the large amphibians that are anemic, but there have been no clinical investigations published that document transfusion attempts. Providing supplemental oxygen is the currently recommended supportive therapy for the anemic amphibian.

The spleen is the primary site of erythropoiesis in adult amphibians, although the kidney (mesonephroi), bone marrow and liver also have erythropoietic capacity in many adult amphibians (Turner, 1988). Erythropoiesis in larval amphibians occurs in the kidney (pronephroi or mesonephroi) and liver with the spleen playing a minor role.

Maturation stages of erythrocytes have been described from experimentally induced erythropoiesis in the crested newt, *Triturus cristatus* (Grasso, 1973a, b). "Erythroid precursors" may occur in various sizes but typically appear similar to lymphocytes. A first stage erythrocyte or erythroid precursor is rounded, with a high nucleus to cytoplasm ratio, large nucleolus, weakly basophilic chromatin clumps in the nucleus, and a cytoplasm that is either weakly basophilic or clear (Wright-Giemsa stain). Basophilic erythroblasts are the next maturation stage, and are similar in appearance to the erythrocyte precursor but with a more intensely basophilic cytoplasm. Polychromatophilic erythroblasts are next, and have a less basophilic cytoplasm than the previous stage. The rounded nucleus is slightly smaller and more condensed than in the basophilic erythroblast, and the nucleolus is less obvious. The polychromatophilic erythroblast cannot synthesize RNA although it continues to produce hemoglobin. The reticulocyte has a heterochromatic cytoplasm as hemoglobin starts to accumulate. The reticulocyte has an slightly oval shape, and the nucleus is starting to elongate. The nucleolus may or may not be visible at this stage. The reticulocyte is the last stage which can still undergo mitosis (Plate 11.5), and is the last stage for which prominent vacuoles are normal. The mature erythrocyte is elliptical and flattened, with an intensely eosinophilic homogenous cytoplasm and deeply basophilic elongated nucleus. The nucleolus is no longer visible, and the cytoplasm lacks vacuoles or other visible inclusions.

Erythrocyte maturation has also been described in the African clawed frog, *Xenopus laevis* (Chegini et al., 1979; Stearner, 1950), and follows the same scheme outlined for the newt. In the bullfrog, *Rana catesbeiana*, larval erythrocytes originating from the kidney are larger (27 µm) and have a peripheral nucleus while those erythrocytes originating from the liver are smaller (24 µm) and have a centralized nucleus (Broyles et al., 1981). A difference between the cytoplasm of adult erythrocytes and larval erythroctes was noted using dark field microscopy (Tyler et al., 1982). Larval erythrocytes had a granular luminescence that was lacking in adult eryrthocytes.

Several different types of circulating erythrocytes have been described in the Rio Cauca caecilian, *Typhlonectes compressicauda* (Boschini, 1979) and Koh Tao Island caecilian, *Ichthyophis kohtaoensis* (Zapata et al., 1982). Boschini (1979) and Zapata et al. (1982) described at least four types of erythrocytes: 1) a rounded erythrocyte possessing a distinctly visible nucleolus, a high nucleus to cytoplasm ratio and a nucleus filled with flocculent chromatin (erythroid precursor); 2) a large rounded erythrocyte lacking a visible nucleolus, a lower nucleus to cytoplasm ratio, a round nucleus containing more tightly condensed chromatin, and cytoplasm that may contain occasional azurophilic granules (polychromatic erythroblast); 3) a large discoid erythrocyte with a dense oval nucleus, very low nucleus to cytoplasm ratio and abundant small azurophilic granules (reticulocyte); and 4) a mature discoid erythrocyte with an intensely basophilic, dense oval nucleus (Wright-Giemsa stain), a very low nucleus to cytoplasm ratio, and an eosinophilic homogeneous cytoplasm.

Thrombocyte. The amphibian thrombocyte is a nucleated elliptical to spindle-shaped cell. The nucleus may range in shape from round to oval. The variable morphology of the thrombocyte may be influenced by the pressure used in preparing the blood film, although certainly *in vivo* processes may alter its appearance. Fragmentation of a thrombocyte may yield anucleate objects that are analogous to the mammalian platelet (Foxon, 1964). This process is more common among the plethodontid salamanders than any other amphibian family studied to date (Porter, 1972).

Thrombocytes are similar in appearance to lymphocytes by light microscopy. In the Japanese fire-bellied newt, *Cynops pyrrhogaster*, thrombocytes were reported as having a denser appearing cytoplasm than lymphocytes (Pfeiffer et al., 1990). In other species the thrombocytes may have a clear cytoplasm resembling the cytoplasm of the mammalian neutrophil. A cleft nucleus has been described in the northern leopard frog, *Rana pipiens*, (Campbell, 1970) and a sticky caecilian, *Ichthyophis* sp., (Welsch & Storch, 1982); this is most readily distinguished by electron microscopy and is of little help in the clinical evaluation of a blood film.

It is rare to find immature thrombocytes (i.e., thromboblasts) in the circulating blood of an amphibian except in a splenectomized specimen (Fey, 1965, 1966 as cited in Turner, 1988). The thromboblasts also may be confused with lymphocytes. In the clawed frog, *Xenopus laevis*, the thromboblast may be differentiated from the lymphocyte by its eccentrically placed irregularly shaped nucleus, fine chromatin and weakly basophilic cytoplasm (Fey, 1965 as cited in Turner, 1988). Experimentally, the level of circulating thrombocytes in the northern leopard frog, *Rana pipiens*, is affected little by radiation while lymphocytes markedly decline (Stearner, 1950).

Thrombocytes may be found singly or in aggregates (Pfeiffer et al., 1990), and this feature helps distinguish them from lymphocytes since lymphocytes rarely aggregate. Amphibian thrombocytes rarely form into rafts of several cells common for reptilian thrombocytes. The amphibian thrombocyte aggregate most commonly consists of a few cells. It is problematic to obtain an accurate thrombocyte count since the cells aggregate and are nonrandomly distributed throughout the chamber of a hemocytometer or on a stained blood film.

The thrombocytes of several species of amphibians have been analyzed cytochemically and an excellent summary table published (Turner, 1988). As a general rule for anurans, the thrombocytes stain alkaline phosphatase-positive while lymphocytes stain alkaline phosphatase-negative. In two genera of salamanders, *Ambystoma* and *Triturus,* both thrombocytes and lymphocytes are alkaline phosphatase-positive, and share similar cytochemical characteristics for the peroxidase test, acid phosphatase test, esterase test, and periodic acid-Schiff test. The thrombocytes of the aquatic caecilian, *Typhlonectes compressicaudus,* were periodic acid-Schiff-positive while the lymphocytes were not (Boschini, 1980 as cited in Turner, 1988).

The amphibian thrombocyte plays a major role in coagulation as does the mammalian platelet. Fibrin threads may be exuded from the thrombocyte to contribute to clot formation. The thrombocyte rapidly disintegrates once it has produced these threads.

Leukocytes. The ratio of leukocytes to erythrocytes in amphibian blood is generally between 1:20 and 1:70, and the size of the leukocyte is around 30–32 μm in length (Duellman & Trueb, 1986b). Normal leukocyte counts are known for a few species, and few studies have addressed leukogram changes with disease (Cathers et al., 1997; Kaplan 1951; Pfeiffer et al., 1990).

Granulocytic Leukocytes. Although there has been some work elucidating the structure and histochemical properties of reptilian leukocytes (Alleman et al., 1996; Cooper et al., 1985; Frye, 1991; Hawkey & Dennett, 1989; Mateo et al., 1984), comparatively little attention has been given to the granulocytic leukocytes that are found in amphibian blood (Fey, 1962; Fey, 1967b as cited in Turner, 1988). Amphibian granulocytes are named according to their morphological description when prepared using Wright-Giemsa stain, often with little attention given to histochemical properties, yielding the terms eosinophilic granulocyte (large eosinophilic granule leukocyte), heterophilic granulocyte (small eosinophilic granule leukocyte), basophilic granulocyte, neutrophilic granulocyte, and azurophilic granulocyte (Cannon & Cannon, 1979; Cowden et al., 1964; Hawkey & Dennett, 1989; Jerret & Mays, 1973; Pfeiffer et al., 1990; Surbis, 1978). The abbreviated terms eosinophil, heterophil, basophil, neutrophil, and azurophil will be used in this text, however it is implicit that this in no way defines their functional role(s) which await further cytological investigations. Band stages suggestive of immature granulocytes are occasionally noted (Pfeiffer et al., 1990).

Eosinophils commonly contain round or oval eosinophilic granules of variable size. Some amphibians may have two distinguishable types of eosinophilic granules (Surbis, 1978). The eosinophil has a smoother, less lobulated nucleus than the heterophil. Eosinophils are often the same size as circulating heterophils.

Eosinophils are known to be able to disrupt the integument of the trematode, *Gorgoderina vitelliloba* (Mitchell, 1982). There is evidence to suggest that eosinophils are not equally effective for all life stages of an amphibian or for many other metazoan parasites (Elkan, 1976). Eosinophils are poorly phagocytic, and appear to play little or no role in combatting bacterial or fungal disease.

Heterophils have smaller eosinophilic granules than eosinophils, and the granules are typically rod-shaped rather than round or oval (Plates 11.6, 11.10, 11.14, 11.15, 11.18). The eosinophilic granules of the heterophil may be irregularly shaped rather than consistently rod-shaped. Since these granules are smaller than those found in eosinophils, it may be simpler to define these cells as either a small eosinophilic granule leukocyte (heterophil) or a large eosinophilic granule leukocyte (eosinophil). Histochemical descriptions of heterophils vary with species (Turner, 1988), but typically the heterophil is peroxidase-positive while basophils and eosinophils are peroxidase-negative.

Heterophils are able to phagocytize bacteria. The circulating population of heterophils often increases in initial stages of bacterial infection, but may lower as heterophils are depleted. "Band" stages of heterophils, wherein the nucleus is less lobulated, are rarely seen except in chronic infections.

Neutrophils are synonymized with heterophils by some authors (Turner, 1988). However, granulocytes that uptake little Wright-Giemsa stain are sometimes seen in small numbers, often less than 5% of leukocyte differential. Based on this neutral staining these leukocytes may be termed neutrophilic granulocytes or neutrophils (Plate 11.13), and may be considered a distinct population of granulocytes rather than a subpopulation of heterophils. Whether this light microscopy distinction is merited awaits histochemical description of these neutrophils in a species, and subsequent comparison to the characteristics of heterophils of that species.

Basophils are typically less than 1% of the circulating leukocyte population for most amphibian species (Cannon & Cannon, 1979), but may sometimes be the predominant granulocyte in others (Cowden, 1965; Pfeiffer et al., 1990; Takaya, 1968 as cited in Turner, 1988) (Plates 11.7, 11.11, 11.16, 11.18). Basophils are variable in size between species, and may be smaller, the same size or larger than the heterophils and eosinophils. The basophil nucleus is round, and the basophilic granules may be round to oval.

Basophils are commonly noted in the process of

degranulating in blood films of amphibians made at the Philadelphia Zoo, and this has been commented upon in the Japanese fire-bellied newt, *Cynops pyrrhogaster* (Pfeiffer et al., 1990), and other newts (Cowden et al., 1964). Heparin-like substances have been described in the basophils of some amphibians (Turner, 1988). The ready degranulation of basophils noted in ill amphibians may contribute to the development of petechia and ecchymoses independent of bacterial hemolysins. Basophils may play a surveillance role and recruit eosinophils in the event of helminth infection as is known for other vertebrates.

Mast cells may be confused with basophils. Typically the mast cell has an oval to elliptical nucleus, rather than the rounded nucleus of a basophil, and the mast cell has significantly more cytoplasm than the basophil (Csaba et al., 1970, as cited in Turner, 1988; Kapa et al., 1970, as cited in Turner, 1988). In addition, the mast cell often has smaller, finer granules than the basophil (Cowden et al., 1964). Whether the basophil and mast cell are merely different developmental stages has not been resolved, although Cowden et al. (1964) demonstrated similar histochemical properties for the two in the red spotted newt, *Notophthalmus viridescens*.

Azurophils possess light gray-blue cytoplasm within which may be distinguished fine irregularly shaped granules. The azurophil is thought to be the same cell type as the mammalian monocyte (Hawkey & Dennett, 1989: Montali, 1988) or possibly the neutrophil in reptiles (Cooper et al., 1985) (Plates 11.8, 11.14). It is possible that the amphibian neutrophil and azurophil are in fact either immature or senescent granulocytes from the other granulocytic cell lines or immature or senescent monocytes rather than a distinct cell type.

Lymphocytes. Lymphocytes generally are the smallest leukocyte, half the size of or smaller than an erythrocyte or granulocyte, round to ovoid in shape, and with a small amount of cytoplasm (Plates 11.9, 11.12, 11.17, 11.18). The nucleus is generally round (Turner, 1988) but in some species the nucleus may be bilobed or cleft (Herrmann, 1989; Pfeiffer et al., 1990).

The lymphocyte is often confused with the thrombocyte (see *Thrombocyte*). In the fire-bellied newt, *Cynops pyrrhogaster,* the cytoplasm of the lymphocyte is lighter than in the similar appearing thrombocyte (Pfeiffer et al., 1990), but this is not the case in many other species wherein the cytoplasm is intensely basophilic. Lymphocytes are generally found singly, whereas thrombocytes may aggregate. Distinct azurophilic granules occur in the cytoplasm of the lymphocytes of some ranid frogs.

The lymphocytes of several species of amphibians have been analyzed cytochemically and an excellent summary table published (Turner, 1988). A significant difference was found with respect to the cytochemical differences between the lymphocyte of the Colorado River toad, *Bufo alvarius,* and mammalian lymphocytes; the bufonid lymphocyte lacked β-glucuronidase and aryl sulphatase activity (Cannon & Cannon, 1979).

Lymphocytes may also be confused with monocytes (see *Monocyte*), plasma cells and immature erythroid cells. Plasma cells are an extremely uncommon cell in the circulating blood (Fey, 1967b as cited in Turner, 1988), and are therefore unlikely to be encountered in most amphibian patients. Immature erythroid cells possess hemoglobin, and can be distinguished from lymphocytes with hemoglobin-specific stains.

Immunoglobulin production has been studied in amphibians (Balls & Ruben, 1968; Evan & Cooper, 1990; Hadji-Azimi, 1979). Lymphocytes are known to produce three immunoglobulin isotypes—IgM, IgY (also known as IgG-like isotype), and IgX (Haynes et al., 1992). Bacterial infections stimulate lymphocytes to produce only high molecular weight IgM, while viral infections cause initial production of IgM followed by low molecular weight IgY (Turner, 1988). Immunoglobulin analysis deserves exploration to develop its potential as a practical diagnostic tool for the amphibian patient.

Lymphocytes are believed to be involved in many other immunological functions in amphibians such as antibody-dependent cell-mediated cytotoxicity. Additional functional analyses of amphibian lymphocytes will require improved methods of harvesting them from the circulating blood (McKnight et al., 1982).

Monocytes. Most monocytes are only slightly larger than a granulocyte, although they may range in size from much smaller to much larger than the granulocytes. A monocyte generally has a larger proportion of cytoplasm than a mature lymphocyte. A Wright-Giemsa stained monocyte typically has a light blue to grey blue cytoplasm, occassionally with small azurophilic granules visible. The cytoplasm may contain a few or many vacuoles, or the cytoplasm may appear foamy with no obvious vacuoles. Pseudopodia may be detected on monocytes, but it may be difficult to differentiate true pseudopodia from distortions caused by blood sample processing.

The morphology of the monocyte nucleus varies with species, and may be round, kidney-shaped or horseshoe-shaped (Cannon & Cannon, 1979; Fey, 1962 as cited in Turner, 1988; Hildeman & Haas, 1962 as cited in Turner, 1988; Jordan, 1938 as cited in Turner, 1988). Sometimes a vacuolated monocyte may be mistaken for an azurophil, but generally the monocyte has a more rounded nucleus that is never lobulated. Phagocytic monocytes containing bacteria and other debris may sometimes be seen in the circulating blood (Plate 11.19). If a blood sample is allowed to sit a day or more before processing, monocytes may actually phagocytize other blood cells. Phagocytic activity may be determined in the laboratory by uptake of carbon or latex; monocytes, not lymphocytes, will phagocytize those particles.

Monocytes can be difficult to distinguish from lymphocytes. One constant that holds true across the various amphibian species is that monocytes are peroxidase-positive while lymphocytes are peroxidase-negative. May-Grunwald stain may distinguish monocytes from lymphocytes in some amphibians (Schermer, 1967).

Monocytes are phagocytic, and may leave the blood to become macrophages in tissues. In addition to direct killing of ingested pathogens, monocytes and macrophages appear to process certain antigens in a way that stimulates antibody production by lymphocytes. Monocyte counts often become elevated with infectious disease.

Plasma cell. Plasma cells are rarely detected in amphibian circulating blood, or at least remain unidentified at this time (Fey, 1967b as cited in Turner, 1988). However, plasma cells are identified readily in histopathological preparations when present.

Miscellaneous. Cells that do not fit readily into the described categories of blood cells may be found occasionally in the circulating blood of amphibians. Two unusual cell types were noted in the Japanese fire-belly newt, *Cynops pyrrhogaster,* a large macrophagic cell with thin pseudopodia and a giant cell containing granulocytes (Pfeiffer et al., 1990). Multinucleated leukocytes and other unusual morphologies may be noted. These unusual cells may represent immature cells from the hematopoietic cell lines, cells derived from other stem cells yet to be defined, or the result of pathologic processes. Amphibian blood cells tend to be more pleomorphic and with more variation in their staining characteristics than the blood cells of birds and mammals. These characteristics have made advances in amphibian hematology limited as many labs are not equipped for the special stains and harvesting procedures necessary to define cell function.

11.6 INTERPRETING THE HEMOGRAM

The wide range of hematological values published for "healthy" amphibians is undoubtedly influenced by variations in sampling techniques, sampling conditions, limited sample size, analytical techniques, physiological state, gender, season, unrecognized pathologies, and even erroneous identification of the amphibians, which obscures the value of the hemogram. There is little to no clinical value to most published reports on amphibian hematology. There is only one current report of normal values for an amphibian, the bullfrog, *Rana catesbeiana* (Cathers et al., 1997), and this study is of limited value for it is based on a sample size of fourteen anesthetized frogs and a single sampling from each frog.

Drawing assumptions based on conventional wisdom is fraught with pitfalls, for the body of knowledge used in interpreting the mammalian hemogram has not been proven valid in amphibians. The hemogram must be interpreted with the clinical picture of the amphibian, and the clinician is reminded that a hemogram with no apparent abnormalities is still helpful in the diagnostic process. It is beneficial to obtain serial samples from the affected amphibian as well as samples from clinically normal controls in order to more fully evaluate the hemogram. Whenever healthy specimens of the same species are available as the patient, they should be used as a baseline to complement the hemogram of the ill amphibian.

Whenever an amphibian is manually restrained, there is some damage to the thin epidermis. For this reason, moistened latex gloves should be worn by the handler to ameliorate the cutaneous injury to the patient. Although the humoral and cell-mediated immunologic response in amphibians is poorly delineated, monocytes are responsible for phagocytic removal of cellular debris and bacteria (Kollias, 1984; Turner, 1988). Due to the presence of injured epithelial cells after handling, an amphibian's monocyte count may show a relative and absolute increase on subsequent leukocyte profiles.

Glucocorticoids, whether exogenous (e.g., dexamethasone) or endogenous (e.g., restraint-associated stress), result in lymphopenia and "neutrophilia" (Garrido et al., 1987). Neutrophilia is interpreted as an increase in the circulating heterophils and neutrophils rather than the deeply staining eosinophils and basophils. Lymphocytosis and a severe drop in the hematocrit has been associated with tail amputations in the Japanese fire-bellied newt, *Cynops pyrrhogaster* (Pfeiffer et al., 1990). These processes may occur within hours or it may take several days. Serial monitoring of the amphibian hemogram is warranted as single samples may lead to erroneous diagnostic assumptions.

In many instances the morphology of the erythrocytes and leukocytes are the most important facet of the hemogram. Viral inclusions, parasites, and bacteria noted in the blood film may suggest serious illness despite apparently normal parameters in the hematocrit and total white blood cell count. Iridovirus infection of anurans may result in substantial changes in the erythrocyte parameters (Graczyk et al., 1996; Gruia-Gray & Desser, 1992). In the bullfrog, *Rana catesbeiana*, the erythrocyte volume (MCV) may increase up to 20% during iridovirus infection, and there may be an increase in circulating immature erythrocytes (Gruia-Gray & Desser, 1992). The erythrocyte count may drop close to 30% while the hematocrit remains minimally changed. However, in the giant monkey frog, *Phyllomedusa bicolor*, a decrease in the erythrocyte volume was noted in erythrocytes with viral inclusions (Graczyk et al., 1996).

11.7 INTERPRETING PLASMA BIOCHEMISTRIES

The documented sources of plasma glucose level variation within the northern leopard frog, *Rana pipiens*, include the following: collection locality (i.e., geographic origin of a population), season, time of day, handling and shipping, anesthesia, and the assay method (Baranowski-Kish & Smith, 1976; Baranowski-Smith & Smith, 1983; Farrar & Frye, 1979; Hutchison & Turney, 1975; Jungreis, 1970; Jungreis & Hooper, 1970; Mizell, 1965). Sex-related differences have been noted in the plasma protein, calcium, and sodium values in the bullfrog, *Rana catesbeiana* (Cathers et al., 1997). This variation for a single biochemical parameter is indicative of the difficulty engendered in obtaining meaningful insight from a single plasma sample taken from an amphibian patient, a difficulty that is multiplied for the values that have received little attention in the literature (e.g., AST, BUN).

Common sources of hyperglycemia in the amphibian are the handling involved in the transport of the patient from its enclosure to the examination room, as well as the manual restraint and anesthesia needed to obtain the sample. Hyperglycemia must be interpreted within the context of the order Amphibia which has values significantly lower than that seen in birds, mammals, and even reptiles. Plasma glucose values are commonly under 50 mg/dl. In one study the mean plasma glucose was 30.1 ± 1.0 mg/dl prior to handling and the hyperglycemic level was 38.1 mg/dl $\pm$ 1.0 mg/dl after handling (Baranowski-Smith & Smith, 1983). This is almost a 25% increase in circulating glucose, but the low absolute value of the glucose when compared to more familiar animal patients may be overlooked unless the clinician is in the proper mindset. Amphibians with tetany should be evaluated for hypoglycemia as well as hypocalcemia. Blood from amphibians suspected of ammonia intoxication can be tested for ammonia, but the plasma needs to be analyzed immediately. Renal disease may be suspected if BUN is elevated in the face of a well-hydrated amphibian.

The osmolality of a well hydrated amphibian is over 200 mOsm (Bentley, 1971). To increase its water absorbency, an amphibian may selectively retain additional solutes so that it can extract water from much drier soils. Since the amphibian kidney cannot concentrate urine above the osmolality of plasma, one of the main methods of water conservation is the ability to tolerate a wide fluctuation in the osmolality and composition of its plasma. This physiological adaptation can obfuscate the interpretation of a single plasma biochemistry in the amphibian, thus multiple biochemistries (i.e., electrolytes), enough to assess plasma osmolality, may be required for a complete amphibian diagnostic evaluation.

Allozyme variations have been noted in common plasma enzymes (e.g., lactate dehydrogenase or LDH) of anurans (e.g., Prakash, 1995), and diversity of serum albumin and proteins have been noted (e.g., Cei & Bertini, 1961; Hass et al., 1995). Unfortunately for the clinician, the work in this area has focused on taxonomic questions and has not been evaluated as a diagnostic tool.

Unfortunately, given the paucity of clinicopathologic information about amphibians, even with serum chemistry data and hematological values it is still more of an art than a science to interpret clinicopathologic values in the context of the clinical picture of an amphibian (see Tables 11.3A–11.3I). Whenever possible, samples from a control (i.e., unaffected) amphibian should be submitted for analysis concomitant with samples from the ill amphibian in order to better detect and interpret abnormalities as well as to establish baseline values for a species. If a consistent systematic approach is maintained when evaluating an amphibian, then each practitioner will have the potential to contribute to the development of this field of veterinary medicine.

AMPHIBIAN HEMATOLOGY —— 141

Table 11.3A. Hemograms and plasma chemistries of a captive bullfrog, *Rana catesbeiana* (400109), with metabolic bone disease.

Date	Hct %	Hgb g/dl	RBC ×10⁶	WBC ×10³	Het %	Lymp %	Mono %	Eos %	Baso %	Azuro %	T.S. mg/dl	Gluc mg/dl	Ca mg/dl	P mg/dl	AST 1μ/L	ALT 1μ/L	Chol mg/dl	
23 Sep 1994	36	9.4	0.3	1.2	13	54	0	0	1	6	5.7		6.4	5.1			80	
5 Jan 1995	34	8.9	0.3	2.5	9	62	19	0	5	5			5.8	4.6	57		58	uric acid <0.3
20 Jan 1995	30			7.0	2	64	0	0	3	10	4.4		6.4					
14 Apr 1995	24	6.8	0.3	8.8	2	70	0	0	15	8	3.5		6.9	3.5	51			uric acid <0.3

Table 11.3B. Hemograms and plasma chemistries of a captive bullfrog, *Rana catesbeiana* (400157), with metabolic bone disease. The bullfrog was supplemented with calcium glubionate/vitamin D after diagnosis on 6 Sep 1994.

Date	Hct %	Hgb g/dl	RBC ×10⁶	WBC ×10³	Het %	Lymp %	Mono %	Eos %	Baso %	Azuro %	T.S. mg/dl	Gluc mg/dl	Ca mg/dl	P mg/dl	AST 1μ/L	ALT 1μ/L	Chol mg/dl	
06 Sep 1994	20										2.3		<3.0	3.5				
23 Sep 1994	14	4.0	0.2	3.6	7	56	0	0	20	3	2.0		3.5	1.1				
09 Oct 1994	25			3.5	1	64	0	1	22	3	2.9		7.9	1.1				*

* Moderate anisocytosis, poikilocytosis, polychromasia, and marked hypochromasia noted in erythrocytes.

Table 11.3C. Hemograms and plasma chemistries of a free-ranging bullfrog, *Rana catesbeiana*.

Date	Hct %	Hgb g/dl	RBC ×10⁶	WBC ×10³	Het %	Lymp %	Mono %	Eos %	Baso %	Azuro %	T.S. mg/dl	Ca mg/dl	P mg/dl	AST 1μ/L	Chol mg/dl	ALT 1μ/L	
14 Jun 1995	32.5	9.0	0.32	10.6	1 hets 10 neut	60	0	0	20	9	5.7	10.1	4.6	8.0	<35		uric acid <0.3

Table 11.3D. Average values for hemograms of anesthetized captive bullfrogs, *Rana catesbeiana*, maintained at 20–25°C. (Cathers et al., 1997)

Hct %	Hgb g/dl	RBC ×10⁶	WBC ×10³	AST 1µ/L	Het %	Lymp %	Mono %	Eos %	Baso %	Azuro %
22.1	4.72		5.2	44.7	22 defined as segmented neutrophils 0.2% segmented bands noted	62.9 2.8% reactive lymphocytes noted	0.6	9.9	2.5	0

Table 11.3E. Average values for serum chemistries of anesthetized captive bullfrogs, *Rana catesbeiana*, maintained at 20–25°C. (Cathers et al., 1997)

T.P. mg/dl	Ca mg/dl	P mg/dl	AST 1µ/L	LDH 1µ/L	Albumin g/dl	Creatinine mg/dl	Mg mEq/L	Na mEq/L	K mEq/L	Cl mEq/L	Anion Gap	TCO₂	BUN mg/dl	Uric Acid mg/dl
4.0 both sexes	8.0 both sexes	3.2	44.7	33	1.6	1.0	2.0	107.9 both sexes	2.7	77	9.8	24.9	3.2	0.06
4.4 female	8.7 female							110.6 female						
3.7 male	7.4 male							105.1 male						

Table 11.3F. Hemograms and plasma chemistries of two specimens of the Japanese giant salamander, *Andrias japonicus*. The salamanders were immobilized with unbuffered tricaine methanesulfonate for preshipment physical examinations.

ID	Hct %	Hgb g/dl	RBC ×10⁶	WBC ×10³	Het %	Lymp %	Mono %	Eos %	Baso %	Azuro %	T.S. mg/dl	Gluc mg/dl	Ca mg/dl	P mg/dl	AST 1µ/m	ALT 1µ/m	Uric Acid mg/dl	BUN mg/dl	AP 1µ/L	CPK 1µ/L
008	42	10.6	0.05	1.5	6	37	0	0	4	53	3.9*	31	9.0	7.0	192	<3.0	<0.3	12	1243	836
009	50	11.6	0.07	0.7	9	71	0	1	2	12	3.8*	<20					<0.3			

* Plasma was clear blue.

Table 11.3G. Hemograms and plasma chemistries of an adult male South American bullfrog, *Leptodactylus pentadactylus* (400038), with metabolic bone disease.

Date	Hct %	Hgb g/dl	RBC ×10⁶	WBC ×10³	Het %	Lymp %	Mono %	Eos %	Baso %	Azuro %	T.S. mg/dl	Gluc mg/dl	Ca mg/dl	P mg/dl	AST 1µ/L	ALT 1µ/L	Chol mg/dL	AP 1µ/L
22 Sep 1993	20		0.69	2.08	33	41	0	0	5	21	4.6		9.0	5.2			220	
01 Dec 1994	28	9.2	0.5	7.5	14	64	0	0	16	0	5.3		8.9	4.5			290	185

Table 11.3H. Hemograms and plasma chemistries of an adult female South American bullfrog, *Leptodactylus pentadactylus* (400037), with corneal lipidosis. Note that this was fed the identical diet to # 400038 (above).

Date	Hct %	Hgb g/dl	RBC ×10⁶	WBC ×10³	Het %	Lymp %	Mono %	Eos %	Baso %	Azuro %	T.S. mg/dl	Gluc mg/dl	Ca mg/dl	P mg/dl	BUN mg/dl	Uric Acid mg/dl	Chol mg/dl	AP 1µ/L
15 Nov 1991	44			4.12	4	67	0	14	10	5	8.7	40	9.3		1.0	<0.3	628	
27 Mar 1992	40		0.99	7.01	5	74	0	8	8	5	8.0						>850	
22 Sep 1993	33		0.57	2.04	57	37	6	0	6	0	7.3		9.3	6.1		<0.3	1944	
29 Oct 1995	19	6.2									6.9*		7.0	3.3				

* Plasma was clear blue.

Table 11.3l. Hemograms and plasma chemistries of an adult female axolotl, *Ambystoma mexicanum* (400015), with ovarian neoplasia.

Date	Hct %	Hgb g/dl	RBC ×10⁶	WBC ×10³	Het %	Lymp %	Mono %	Eos %	Baso %	Azuro %	T.S. mg/dl	Gluc mg/dl	Ca mg/dl	P mg/dl	AST 1µ/L	ALT 1µ/L	CPK 1µ/L	BUN mg/dl
10 Jul 1992	16	<5.0	0.06	2.5	22	63	0	15	0	0	<2.0	<20			845	92	2578	2.0
11 Aug 1993	44	9.0	0.18	1.12	44	24	2	0	10	20	1.5							
8 Aug 1993	40		0.25	2.8	35	34	24	0	3	4	1.8				1020			
20 Aug 1993	40		0.13	1.71	35	24	53	0	6	2	1.3	29	7.7	2.8	870			2.0*

* Uric Acid <0.3, Cl 77, Na 108, K 1.4

REFERENCES

Alleman, A.R., E.R. Jacobson, and R.E. Raskin. 1996. Morphologic and cytochemical characteristics of blood cells from the desert tortoise (*Gopherus agassizii*). Association of Reptilian and Amphibian Veterinarians 1996 Proceedings, pp. 51–55.

Balls, M. and L.N. Ruben. 1968. Lymphoid tumors in Amphibia: a review. Progressive Experimental Tumor Research 10:238–260.

Baranowski-Kish, L.L. and C.J.V. Smith. 1976. A diurnal study of plasma glucose levels in adult *Rana pipiens*. American Zoologist 16:249.

Baranowski-Smith, L.L. and C.J.V. Smith. 1983. A simple method for obtaining blood samples from mature frogs. Lab Animal Science 33(4):338–339.

Bentley, P.J. 1971. Endocrines and Osmoregulation: A Comparative Account of the Regulation of Salt and Water in Vertebrates. Springer-Verlag, New York.

Boschini Filho, J. 1979. Elementos figurados do sangue periferico de *Typhlonectes compressicaudus*. Descicao das formas eritrocitarias aos niveis optico e electronico. Boletim de Fisiologia Animal, University Sao Paulo 3:33–38.

Boschini Filho, J. 1980. Caracterizacao do trombocito do sangue periferico de *Typhlonectes compressicaudus* (Amphibia-Apoda) pela reacao citoquimica do P.A.S. Boletim de Fisiologia Animal, University Sao Paulo 5:75–80.

Boutilier, R.G., D.F. Stiffler, and D.P. Toews. 1992. Exchange of respiratory gases, ions, and water in amphibious and aquatic amphibians, *in* Feder, M.E. and W.W. Burggren (Eds.): Environmental Physiology of Amphibians. University of Chicago Press, Chicago, pp. 81–124.

Broyles, R.H., A.R. Dorn, P.B. Maples, G.M. Johnson, G.R. Kindell, and A.M. Parkinson. 1981. Choice of hemoglobin type in erythroid cells of *Rana catesbeiana*, *in* Stamatoyannopoulos, G. and A.W. Nienhuis (Eds.): Hemoglobins in Development and Differentiation. A.R. Liss Inc., New York, pp. 179–191.

Campbell, F.R. 1970. Ultrastructure of the bone marrow of the frog. American Journal of Anatomy 129:329–356.

Campbell, T.W. 1988. Avian Hematology and Cytology. Iowa State University Press, Ames, IA, pp. 9–10.

Campbell, T.W. 1996. Clinical pathology, *in* Mader, D.R. (Ed.): Reptile Medicine and Surgery. W.B. Saunders Co., Philadelphia, PA, pp. 248–257.

Cannon, M.S. and A.M. Cannon. 1979. The blood leukocytes of *Bufo alvarius*: a light, phase-contrast, and histochemical study. Canadian Journal of Zoology 57:314–322.

Cathers, T., G.A. Lewbart, M. Correa, and J.B. Stevens. 1997. Serum chemistry and hematology values for anesthetized American bullfrogs (*Rana catesbeiana*). Journal of Zoo and Wildlife Medicine 28(2): 171–174.

Cei, J.M. and F. Bertini. 1961. Serum proteins in allopatric and sympatric populations of *Leptodactylus ocellatus* and *L. chaquensi*. Copeia 1961(3):336–340.

Chegini, N., V. Aleporou, G. Bell, V.A. Hilder, and N. Maclean. 1979. Production and fate of erythroid cells in anaemic *Xenopus laevis*. Journal of Cell Science 35:403–416.

Cohen, W.D. 1982. The cytomorphic system of anucleate nonmammalian erythrocytes. Protoplasma 113:23–32.

Cooper, E.L., A.E. Klempau, and A.G. Zapata. 1985. Reptilian immunity, *in* Gans, C.A., F. Billett, and P.F.A. Maderson (Eds.): Biology of the Reptilia, Vol. 14, Development A. John Wiley and Sons, New York, pp. 599–678.

Cowden, R.R. 1965. Quantitative and qualitative cytochemical studies on the *Amphiuma* basophil leukocyte. Z. Zellforsch. 67:219–233.

Cowden, R.R., A. Narain, and G.C. Beveridge. 1964. Basophil leukocytes and tissue mast cells in the newt *Diemyctylus viridescens*. Acta. Haematol. (Basel) 32:250–255.

Csaba, G., I. Olha, and E. Kapa. 1970. Phylogenesis of mast cells. II. Ultrastructure of the mast cells in the frog. Acta Biologie Academy Science Hungary 21:255–264.

Dein, F.J., A. Wilson, D. Fischer, and P. Langenberg. 1994. Avian leukocyte counting using the hemocytometer. Journal of Zoo and Wildlife Medicine 25(3):432–437.

Desser, S.S. 1992. Ultrastructural observations on an icosahedral cytoplasmic virus in leukocytes of frogs from Algonquin Park, Ontario. Canadian Journal of Zoology 70:833–836.

Duellman, W.E. and L. Trueb. 1986a. Ecology, *in* Duellman, W.E. and L.

Trueb (Eds): Biology of the Amphibia. McGraw-Hill Book Co., New York, pp. 196–287.

Duellman, W.E. and L. Trueb. 1986b. Morphology, *in* (Duellman, W.E. and L. Trueb (Eds): Biology of the Amphibia. McGraw-Hill Book Co., New York, pp. 288–415.

Elkan, E. 1976. Pathology in the Amphibia, *in* Lofts, B. (Ed.): Physiology of the Amphibia, Vol. III. Academic Press, New York, pp. 273–314.

Emmel, V.E. 1924. Studies on the non-nucleated elements of the blood: 2. The occurrence and genesis of non-nucleated erythrocytes or erythroplastids in vertebrates other than mammals. American Journal of Anatomy 30:347–405.

Evan, D.L. and E.L. Cooper. 1990. Natural killer cells in ectothermic vertebrates. Bioscience 40(10):745–749.

Farrar, E.S. and B.E. Frye. 1979. Factors affecting normal carbohydrate levels in *Rana pipiens*. General Comparative Endocrinology 39:358–371.

Fey, F. 1962. Hamatologische Untersuchungen an *Xenopus laevis* Daudin. I. Die morphologie des Blutes mit einigen vergleichenden Betrachtungen bei *Rana esculenta* und *R. temporaria*. Morph. Jb. 103:9–20.

Fey, F. 1965. Hamozytologische Untersuchungen nach Splenektomie an *Xenopus*—Froschen. Acta Biol. Med. Germ. 14:417–422.

Fey, F. 1966. Vergleichende Hamozytologie niederer Verbebraten. II. Thrombozyten. Folia Haematol. 85:205–217.

Fey, F. 1967a. Vergleichende Hamozytologie niederer Verbebraten. III. Granulozyten. Folia Haematol. 86:1–20.

Fey, F. 1967b. Vergleichende Hamozytologie niederer Verbebraten. IV. Monozyten, Plasmozyten, Lumphozyten. Folia Haematol. 86:133–147.

Foxon, G.E.H. 1964. Blood and respiration, *in* Koore, J.A. (Ed.): Physiology of the Amphibia. Academic Press, London, Great Britain, UK, pp. 151–209.

Frye, F.L. 1991. Hematology as applied to clinical reptile medicine, *in* Frye, F.L. (Ed.): Biomedical and Surgical Aspects of Captive Reptile Husbandry. Krieger Publishing Co., Malabar, FL, pp. 209–277.

Garrido, E., R.P. Gomariz, J. Leceta, and A. Zapata. 1987. Effects of dexamethasone on the lymphoid organs of *Rana perezi*. Developmental and Comparative Immunology 11:375–384.

Graczyk, T.K., M.R. Cranfield, E.J. Bicknese, and A.P. Wisnieski. 1996. Progressive ulcerative dermatitis in a captive wild-caught South American giant treefrog (*Phyllomedusa bicolor*) with microsporidial septicemia. Journal of Zoo and Wildlife Medicine 27(4):522–527.

Grasso, J.A. 1973a. Erythropoiesis in the newt, *Triturus cristatus* Laur. I. Identification of the erythroid precursor cell. Journal of Cell Science 12:463–489.

Grasso, J.A. 1973b. Erythropoiesis in the newt, *Triturus cristatus* Laur. II. Characteristics of the erythropoietic process. Journal of Cell Science 12:491–523.

Gruia-Gray, J. and S.S. Desser. 1992. Cytopathological observations and epizootiology of frog erythrocytic virus in bullfrogs (*Rana catesbeiana*). Journal of Wildlife Diseases 28:34–41.

Hadji-Azimi, I. 1979. Anuran immunoglobulins, a review. Devel. and Comparative Immunology 3:223–243.

Hadji-Azimi, I., V. Coosemans and C. Canicatti. 1987. Atlas of adult *Xenopus laevis laevis* hematology. Developmental and Comparative Immunology 11(4):807–874.

Hass, C.A., J.F. Dunski, L.R. Maxson, and M.S. Hoogmoed. 1995. Divergent lineages within the *Bufo margaritifera* complex (Amphibia: Anura; Bufonidae) revealed by albumin immunology. Biotropica 27(2):238–249.

Hawkey, C.M. and T.B. Dennett. 1989. Color Atlas of Comparative Veterinary Hematology. Wolfe Medical Publications, Ltd., London, Great Britain, UK, pp. 9–147.

Haynes, L., F.A. Harding, A.D. Koniski, and N. Cohen. 1992. Immune system activation associated with a naturally occurring infection in *Xenopus laevis*. Developmental and Comparative Immunology 16:453–462.

Herrmann, H.J. 1989. Blutbild und asterelektronenmikroskopische Darstellung der Blutzellen von *Rana temporaria* Linne, 1758. Amphibia-Reptilia 10:85–92.

Hildemann, W.H. and R. Haas. 1962. Developmental changes in leukocytes in relation to immunological maturity, *in* Hasek, M., A. Langerova, and M. Vojitskova (Eds): Mechanisms of Immunological Tolerance. Publishing House of the Czechoslovak Academy of Science, Prague, Czechoslovakia, pp. 35–49.

Hutchison, V.H. and L.D. Turney. 1975. Glucose and lactate concentrations during activity in the leopard frog *Rana pipiens*. Journal of Comparative Physiology 99:278–295.

Jerret, D.P. and C.E. Mays. 1973. Comparative hematology of the hellbender, *Cryptobranchus alleganiensis* in Missouri. Copeia 1973 (2):331–337.

Jordan, H.E. 1938. Comparative hematology, *in* Downey, H. (Ed.): Handbook of Hematology Vol. II. Harper, New York, pp. 704–862.

Jungreis, A.M. 1970. The effects of long-term starvation and acclimation temperature on glucose regulation and nitrogen anabolism in the frog *Rana pipiens*—II. Summer animals. Comparative Biochemical Physiology 32:433–444.

Jungreis A.M. and A.B. Hooper. 1970. The effects of long-term starvation and acclimation temperature on glucose regulation and nitrogen anabolism in the frog *Rana pipiens*—I. Winter animals. Comparative Biochemical Physiology 32:417–432.

Kapa, E., M. Szigeti, A. Juhasz, and G. Csaba. 1970. Phylogenesis of mast cells. I. Mast cells of the frog, *Rana esculenta*. Acta Biology Academy Science Hungary 21:141–147.

Kaplan, H.M. 1951. A study of frog blood in red leg disease. Transactions of Illinois State Academic Sciences. 44:209–215.

Kollias, G.V. 1984. Immunologic aspects of infectious disease, *in* Hoff, G.L., F.L. Frye and E.R. Jacobson (Eds.): Diseases of Amphibians and Reptiles. Plenum Press, New York, pp. 661–691.

Marcus, L.C. 1981. Veterinary Biology and Medicine of Captive Amphibians and Reptiles. Lea & Febiger, Philadelphia, PA.

Mateo, M.R., E.D. Roberts, and F.M. Enright. 1984. Morphological, cytochemical, and functional studies of peripheral blood cells of healthy American alligators (*Alligator mississippiensis*). American Journal of Veterinary Research 45:1046–1053.

McKnight, B.J., T.C. Ford and D. Rickwood. 1982. An improved method for the isolation of leukocytes from *Xenopus laevis* blood. Developmental and Comparative Immunology 6:381–384.

Mitchell, J.B. 1982. The effect of host age on *Rana temporaria* and *Gorgoderina vitelliloba* interactions. International Journal of Parasitology 12:601–604.

Mizell, S. 1965. Seasonal changes in energy reserves in the common frog *Rana pipiens*. Journal of Cellular Comparative Physiology 66:251–258.

Montali, R.J. 1988. Comparative pathology of inflammation in the higher vertebrates (reptiles, birds, mammals). Journal of Comparative Pathology 99:1–26.

Natt, M.P. and C.A. Herrick. 1952. A new blood diluent for counting the erythrocytes and leukocytes of the chicken. Poultry Science 31:735.

Pfeiffer, C.J., H. Pyle, and M. Asashima. 1990. Blood cell morphology and counts in the Japanese newt (*Cynops pyrrhogaster*). Journal of Zoo and Wildlife Medicine 21(1):56–64.

Porter, K.R. 1972. Structural and functional characteristics of living amphibians, *in* Porter, K.R.: Herpetology. W.B. Saunders Co., Philadelphia, PA, pp. 17–87.

Prakash, S. 1995. Allozyme variations in natural populations of *Rana limnocharis* (Anura: Ranidae). Zoos' Print July 1995:17–21.

Reichenbach-Klinke, H. and E. Elkan. 1965. Diseases of Amphibians. TFH Publications, Inc., Neptune City, NJ.

Schermer, S. 1967. The frog, *in*: Schermer, S. (Ed.): Blood Morphology of Laboratory Animals, 3rd Edition. F.A. Davis Co., Philadelphia, PA. pp. 171–187.

Schmittner, S.M. and R.B. McGhee. 1961. The intra-erythrocytic development of *Babesioma stableri* n. sp. in *Rana pipiens pipiens*. Journal of Protozoology 8:381–386.

Stearner, S.P. 1950. The effects of X-irradiation on *Rana pipiens* (leopard frog), with special reference to survival and to the response of the peripheral blood. Journal of Experimental Zoology 115:251–262.

Surbis, A.Y. 1978. Ultrastructural study of granulocytes of *Bufo marinus*. Florida Scientist 41:42–45.

Takaya, K. 1968. Mast cells and histamine in a newt, *Triturus pyrrhogaster* Boie. Experientia 24:1053–1054.

Thorson, T.B. 1964. The partitioning of body water in Amphibia. Physiological Zoology 37:395–399.

Turner, R.J. 1988. Amphibians, *in* Rowley, A.F. and N.A. Ratcliffe (Eds.): Vertebrate Blood Cells. Cambridge University Press, Cambridge, MA, pp. 129–209.

Tyler, L.W., D.C. Piotrowski, and J.C. Kaltenbach. 1982. Tadpole erythrocytes: optical properties with dark field microscopy. American Zoologist 22:946.

Welsch, U. and V. Storch. 1982. Light microscopic and electron microscopic observations on the caecilian spleen: a contribution to the evolution of lymphatic organs. Developmental and Comparative Immunology 6:293–302.

Wright, K.M. 1996. Amphibian husbandry and medicine, in Mader, D.R. (Ed.): Reptile Medicine and Surgery. W.B. Saunders Co., Philadelphia, PA, pp. 437–459.

Yam, L.T., C.Y. Li, and W.H. Crosby. 1971. Cytochemical identification of monocytes and granulocytes. American Journal of Pathology 55:283–290.

Zapata, A., R.P. Gomariz, E. Garrido, and E.L. Cooper. 1982. Lymphoid organs and blood cells of the caecilian *Ichthyophis kohtaoensis*. Acta Zoologie (Stockholm) 63:11–16.

Zwemer, C.F. 1991. An effective acquisition and stable containment technique for *Ambystoma mexicanum* whole blood. Axolotl Newsletter 20:39–40.

CHAPTER 12
WATER QUALITY

Brent R. Whitaker, MS, DVM

12.1 INTRODUCTION

Amphibians are bound to water rich microenvironment, using their moist skin and gills for respiration and osmoregulation. As a result, waterborne toxins including ammonia, nitrite, heavy metals, disinfectants, pesticides, chlorine, and chloramine are of particular concern when keeping amphibians. Due to the tremendous diversity of species and the variable tolerance of individual specimens, some amphibians exposed to water of poor quality may be unaffected while others become ill or die. Clinical signs suggesting poor water quality are often nonspecific and include lethargy, anorexia, color change, increased respiratory effort, loss of coordination, and loss of equilibrium. Due to the rapid dispersal of water-soluble toxins, more than one animal in an enclosure is usually affected by poor water quality.

Water temperature, pH, ammonia, and nitrite should be tested daily in newly created aquatic environments using a reliable kit that can be purchased at most tropical fish stores (Figure 12.1). Dissolved oxygen is also important to monitor, but requires additional equipment such as an oxygen probe or commercial test kit. Unfortunately, the detection of pesticides or other toxins may be more difficult and costly for routine measurement. Once water parameters appear stable and within acceptable limits (Table 12.1), weekly sampling may be sufficient. Nitrates and water hardness should be tested several times a month. Whenever illness or death occurs among amphibians, the water quality should be analyzed immediately and actions taken to correct any abnormal parameters detected.

Vigilant record keeping ensures that proper water quality is maintained and allows potentially dangerous trends to be identified. Keeping a water quality log (Table 12.2) enables rapid detection of developing problems that can often be corrected before the animals are adversely affected. Proper filtration, in combination with regular water changes and the routine removal of uneaten food or other organic debris from the tank, promotes a healthy environment for amphibians.

12.2 WATER TEMPERATURE

Amphibians are unable to maintain body heat beyond that of the surrounding environment. Species-specific tolerance, developmental stage, natural history, seasonal variation, and the reproductive strategy are considered in determining the air and water temperatures appropriate for an enclosure. In most cases, water temperature will parallel that of the air, however, some amphibians in the wild live in microhabitats which differ greatly from that expected of their geographic location. Temperate amphibians usually do well at temperatures ranging from 18 to 24°C (65 to 75°F), although cooler temperatures may be needed seasonally. Recommended winter air temperatures for many temperate salamanders are as low as 10–16°C (50–60°F) or lower. Aquatic caecilians typically thrive at warmer temperatures of 27–30°C (80–85°F). Tropical lowland frogs can be kept at 24–30°C (75–85°F) with 27°C (80°F) an acceptable target temperature for

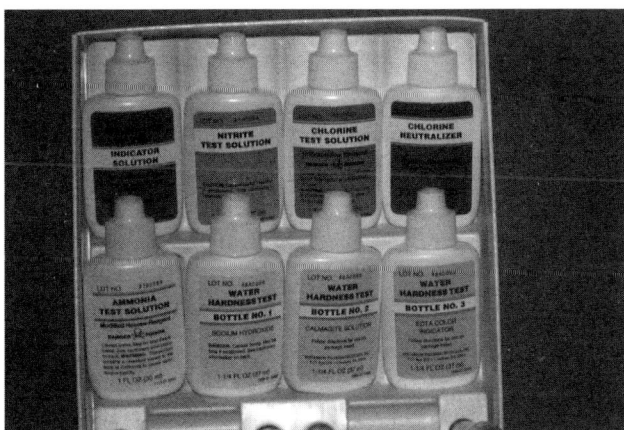

Figure 12.1. Water quality test kits are readily obtained from local pet stores, and should be used by both clinician and herpetologist to assess water parameters. (Kevin Wright, Philadelphia Zoological Garden)

Table 12.1. Suggested water quality parameters for most adult and larval amphibians.

Parameter	Measure	Comments
Temperature 　Caecilians 　Salamanders 　Anurans 　　temperate 　　tropical 　　　lowland 　　　highland	 25–28°C 16–20°C 16–24°C 22–28°C 18–23°C	In most cases water temperature and air temperature are similar; requirements are highly species-specific and may vary with seasonal change in temperate species; increased growth rate in many larval forms occurs at slightly higher temperatures
pH	6.5–8.5*	If species requirements are unknown, a pH of 7.0 is desirable; peat moss may lower pH and hardness
Salinity	0–5 ppt	Most species do not tolerate elevated salinity for long periods of time
Hardness	75–150 mg/L	Measures mineral ions needed by animals; requirements dependent on origin of animals; hard water may cause lesions in some caecilians
Alkalinity	15–50 mg/L	Measures buffering capacity of water; requirements vary greatly with species of animal
Dissolved oxygen	>80% saturation	Low oxygen levels are tolerated well by many amphibians; oxygen is also required by nitrifying bacteria, plants, and heterotrophic organisms
Carbon dioxide	<5 mg/L*	Agitation and aeration minimizes carbon dioxide accumulation; elevated carbon dioxide associated with decreasing pH
Un-ionized-ammonia	<0.02 mg/L	Undetectable levels accomplished with proper filtration and established biofilter; the indiscriminate use of chemicals in the water may result in a sudden increase in ammonia
Nitrite	<1 mg/L	Very low levels maintained with an active biological filter; animals found in fast moving streams typically more sensitive to nitrites/nitrates
Nitrate	<50 mg/L	Control with water changes and removal of organic debris; see nitrites
Chlorine	undetectable	Oxidizing compound easily removed using sodium thiosulfate or agitation of water

*Subcommittee on Amphibian Standards. 1974. Amphibians: Guidelines for the Breeding, Care, and Management of Laboratory Animals. National Academy of Sciences, Washington DC, 153 pp.

most species. Tropical montane frogs generally thrive when maintained at 18–24°C (65–75°F). Most eggs and larvae of neotropical hylids and dendrobatids do best when kept at 25–27°C (77–80°F) (Cover et al., 1994). Gradual changes in temperature allow thermal acclimation to occur in those amphibians capable of it. Temperatures that fall below those for which the animal is adapted hinder metabolic processes such as digestion, immunological function, drug absorption, and drug utilization. Secondary parasitism or microbial infection is seen where potential pathogens are less affected by altered temperatures than the host. For cool adapted species or those requiring seasonal changes, an environmental chamber, room air conditioner, or water chiller can be used to create the desired conditions. Warmer water temperatures are easily achieved using submersible heaters.

12.3 OXYGEN

Aquatic amphibian larvae acquire oxygen by gulping air, using gills, and/or absorbing it through their skin (Duellman & Trueb, 1986). Many adult amphibians breathe air making them less dependent upon dissolved oxygen within the water. The amount of dissolved oxygen required by an amphibian varies with species. Amphibians that have evolved in cas-

Table 12.2. Water quality log.

Date:_____to_____   Page:_____

Species:_____

DATE	TEMP	pH	AMMONIA	NITRITE/ NITRATE	HARDNESS	ALKALINITY	OTHER/ COMMENTS

Enclosure:_____

cading streams typically depend upon higher concentrations of dissolved oxygen than do pond dwellers. A certain minimum concentration of dissolved oxygen is also necessary for nitrifying bacteria, plants, and the heterotrophic organisms that are responsible for the initial breakdown of organic waste. Without a dissolved oxygen concentration over 80%, foul-smelling anaerobic bacteria flourish and the vivarium becomes unsanitary for resident amphibians, as well as offensive to the caretaker.

Aeration and circulation of the water may be accomplished using a standard aquarium air pump and air stone (Figure 12.2), or by using a water pump to cascade water over tank decor. The actual amount of dissolved oxygen present in freshwater is dependent upon two factors: atmospheric pressure and water temperature. Fresh water is said to be "saturated" with oxygen when it holds its theoretical maximum for a given temperature and atmospheric pressure. As temperature increases and/or pressure decreases it becomes increasingly more difficult to maintain oxygen in solution.

Too much air dissolved in water is referred to as su-

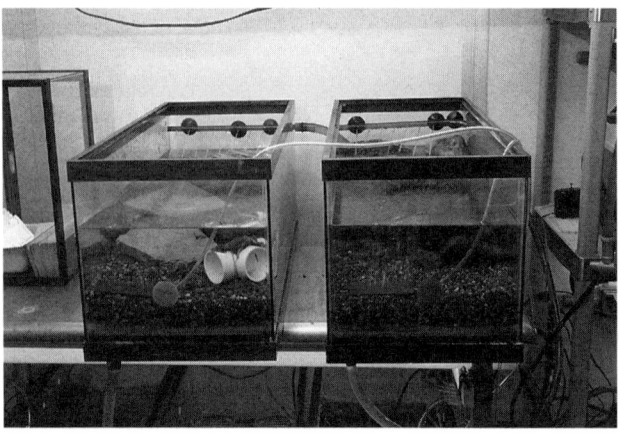

Figure 12.2. Airstones can be used to provide adequate levels of dissolved gases and water circulation in an aquatic system. (George Grall, National Aquarium in Baltimore)

persaturation and can result in gas bubble disease. Careful examination of affected animals may reveal the presence of gas bubbles in their skin, eyes, or gastrointestinal tract. Aquatic frogs, such as the African clawed frog, *Xenopus laevis,* have been observed with gas bubbles in the webs of their feet (Colt et al., 1984). Erythema, hemorrhage and death may occur dependent upon the location of air emboli. Supersaturation is most often seen when loose fittings, cracked pipes, or a low level sump allows air to mix with water prior to undergoing pressurization by pumps or filters. The presence of small air bubbles in the water, on the animals, and covering all surfaces of the aquarium is a warning that should be investigated immediately. Affected amphibians must be removed from their environment and supportive therapy provided. Once the source of the problem has been corrected, dissolved air is easily removed by stirring the water and agitating the substrate (see also Section 16.11, Dissolved Gas Supersaturation).

12.4 CARBON DIOXIDE

There are many sources of carbon dioxide (CO_2) found in water of the home aquarium or vivarium. Aquatic plants consume inorganic carbon, in the form of CO_2, and through photosynthesis reduce it to potentially edible organic carbon. Bacteria living in the environment ultimately oxidize organic carbon found in food, plant, and animal waste thus producing CO_2 once again. Although minimal in comparison to the bacterial contribution, amphibians also contribute to environmental CO_2 which through respiration is released from their blood in exchange for oxygen.

When present in water, a small amount of available CO_2 is hydrated to carbonic acid. In significant concentrations this may cause a noticeable lowering of water pH. In addition to the regular removal of organic debris, proper aeration and agitation of the water should be enough to release CO_2 to the atmosphere before it can become concentrated to the point that it lowers pH. Dissolved CO_2 should be kept to a level below 5 mg/L for a healthy aqueous environment.

If exposed to slightly elevated levels of environmental CO_2, many amphibians such as the giant toad, *Bufo marinus,* the bullfrog, *Rana catesbeiana,* and the African clawed frog, *Xenopus laevis,* are able to eliminate excess gas by simply increasing pulmonary respiration. Alternatively, some aquatic amphibians like the amphiumas, *Amphiuma* spp., do not elevate respiration. In greater concentrations, carbon dioxide can accumulate within amphibians causing blood pH to decline and plasma carbonate to increase. Should acidosis of the animal continue, additional mechanisms work to convert molecular CO_2 to carbonate by nonbicarbonate buffering. Furthermore, the accumulation of carbonate via ion exchange processes help to return blood pH to normal (Boutilier et al., 1992).

12.5 pH, HARDNESS, AND ALKALINITY

12.5.1 pH

The pH of water is determined by the proportion of hydrogen (H^+) and hydroxide ions (OH^-) present.

Each pH unit represents a 10-fold change in the number of hydrogen ions. At a pH of 7, hydrogen ions equal hydroxide ions. Water becomes more acidic with increasing hydrogen ions resulting in a lower pH. While many amphibians are able to tolerate wide swings in pH for short periods of time, this can be stressful. Thus the herpetoculturist should strive to maintain a fairly constant pH value in the vivarium's water system. Newly hatched tadpoles are particularly sensitive to inappropriate pH values. Mortality among tadpoles of the bullfrog, *Rana catesbeiana*, is substantial above a pH of 7.2 which has been associated with an increase in gut bacteria (Culley, 1992). A pH of 7.0 is recommended as a starting point for a species if the optimal pH is unknown. An educated guess can be made for the pH after reviewing what is known about the animal's natural habitat. Salamanders found in limestone aquifers are likely to need a more alkaline environment than those species found in or near sphagnum bogs. It is important to remember that higher pH values favor the more harmful form of some potential toxins, such as ammonia, and should be avoided whenever possible (see Section 16.14). Nitrification also produces acid which, unless buffered, will lower pH. Certain substances found in water (e.g., bicarbonate ions) provide natural buffers preventing sudden changes in pH.

12.5.2 Hardness

Water hardness is a measure of the mineral ions present in water. While copper, zinc, iron, boron, and silicon contribute to hardness, only calcium and magnesium are normally found in substantial amounts. Soft water contains up to 75 mg/L calcium carbonate compared to hard water which typically measures 150–300 mg/L. In general the hardness of the water should be not exceed 150 mg/L unless the species' natural history suggests otherwise. Exposure to elevated hardness may result in skin lesions in some aquatic species such as the typhlonectiid caecilians.

12.5.3 Alkalinity

The alkalinity of water is a measure of its buffering capacity and reflects the combined presence of negatively charged ions, primarily bicarbonate (HCO_3^-), and carbonate (CO_3^{-2}). When total hardness exceeds total alkalinity, calcium and magnesium ions are associated with anions other than HCO_3^- and CO_3^{-2}. Alternatively, when total alkalinity exceeds total hardness, a portion of HCO_3^- and CO_3^{-2} ions are associated with sodium and potassium ions (Beleau, 1988). For these reasons, soft water generally has less buffering capacity than hard water, requiring more frequent replenishment through water changes or the addition of buffers in order to maintain the desired pH. Heavy metals including copper, zinc, and aluminum may form relatively nontoxic precipitates and dissolved carbonate and bicarbonate complexes, decreasing their toxicity in water having a higher alkalinity (Tucker, 1993). In general, an alkalinity range between 15 and 50 mg/L is recommended unless a species natural history suggests otherwise.

12.6 TOTAL AMMONIA NITROGEN

Unlike their terrestrial counterpart, nearly all aquatic amphibians are ammoniotelic, producing ammonia as their primary means of nitrogen excretion. Energetically, this approach is frugal, however, these animals rely on their aquatic environment to rapidly dilute and remove this highly toxic waste. In closed systems, this challenge is met using a biological filter in which beneficial nitrifying bacteria populate the filter media and substrate (Figure 12.3).

Total ammonia nitrogen (TAN) produced by animals and the breakdown of organic matter such as uneaten food, comprises very toxic un-ionized ammonia (NH_3), and less toxic ionized ammonia (NH_4^+). Tadpoles of the bullfrog, *Rana catesbeiana*, eat continuously, producing up to 400 μg of ammonia per gram of tadpole in one day (Culley, 1992). The higher the pH of the water, the greater the portion of dangerous un-ionized ammonia. While most test kits measure only TAN, the actual amount of toxic ammonia varies with temperature and pH of the water. Table 12.3 shows the percent NH_3 present for a given pH and temperature. Fortunately, the presence of ammonia tends to drop the pH of the water favoring the less toxic form while signaling the hobbyist to scrutinize all water quality parameters.

Clinical signs of ammonia intoxication include lethargy, dyspnea, color change, increased mucous production (Plate 12.1A), erythema, and possibly neurological dysfunction. Adult anurans may raise their body off the substrate in an effort to minimize contact with contaminated water (Plate 12.1B). The onset of symptoms is usually acute with more than one animal affected. Death of one or more individuals is frequently reported in the clinical history. Damage of the respiratory epithelium rapidly leads to mortality of larval forms. Other effects occur as levels of ammonia rise within the amphibian. Elevated water pH not only appears to enhance uptake of the un-ionized ammonia from the environment, but may also lead to an increase in blood pH facilitating the movement of ammonia across the blood-brain barrier and into other tissues (Campbell, 1973). As levels build, the ability of the liver to detoxify ammonia is quickly exceeded resulting in the disruption of oxidative metabolism. Chronic exposure to low levels of ammonia can lead to

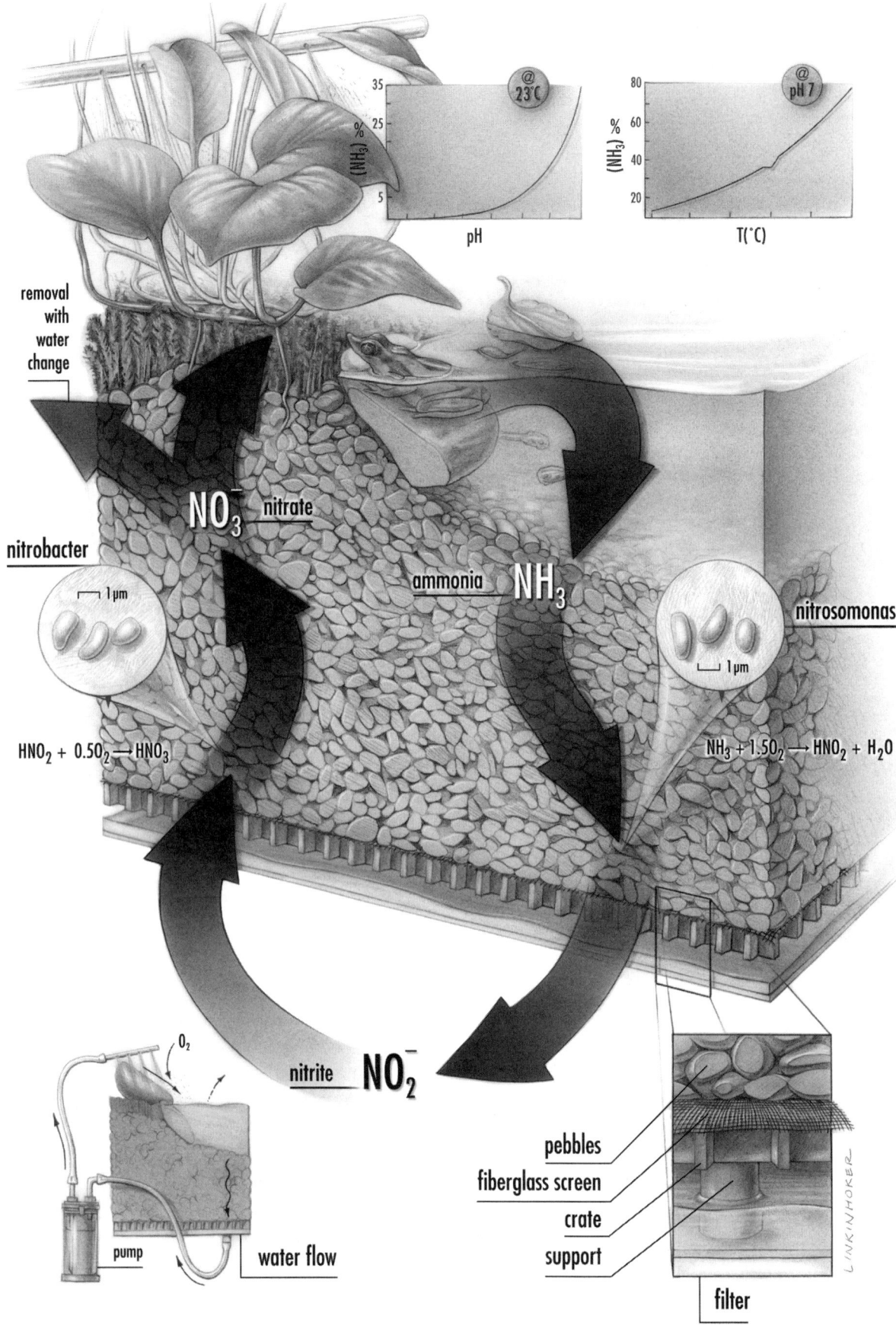

Figure 12.3. Nitrogenous waste resulting from amphibian excretory products, as well as that generated from the bacterial decay of uneaten food, decaying plants debris, and other organic materials, are broken down by heterotrophic and nitrifying bacteria into less toxic products. Recycling the water from the undergravel filter through an aerating system, such as a spray bar, helps provide oxygen (required by the nitrifying bacteria) and stabilizes the pH of the system by outgassing carbon dioxide. The toxic form of ammonia (NH_3) increases with increasing temperature and pH (see also Table 12.3). (Michael Linkinhoker, Johns Hopkins University Department of Art as Applied to Medicine)

Table 12.3. Percent of total ammonia in un-ionized form for 5–30°C and pH 6 to 9.

Temp °C	pH						
	6.0	6.5	7.0	7.5	8.0	8.5	9.0
5	0.0125	0.0395	0.125	0.394	1.23	3.80	11.1
6	0.0136	0.0429	0.135	0.427	1.34	4.11	11.9
7	0.0147	0.0464	0.147	0.462	1.45	4.44	12.8
8	0.0159	0.0503	0.159	0.501	1.57	4.79	13.7
9	0.0172	0.0544	0.172	0.542	1.69	5.16	14.7
10	0.0186	0.0589	0.186	0.586	1.83	5.56	15.7
11	0.0201	0.0637	0.201	0.633	1.97	5.99	16.8
12	0.0218	0.0688	0.217	0.684	2.13	6.44	17.0
13	0.0235	0.0743	0.235	0.738	2.30	6.92	19.0
14	0.0254	0.0802	0.253	0.796	2.48	7.43	20.2
15	0.0274	0.0865	0.273	0.859	2.67	7.97	21.5
16	0.0295	0.0933	0.294	0.925	2.87	8.54	22.8
17	0.0318	0.101	0.317	0.996	3.08	9.14	24.1
18	0.0343	0.108	0.342	1.07	3.31	9.78	25.5
19	0.0369	0.117	0.368	1.15	3.56	10.5	27.0
20	0.0397	0.125	0.369	1.24	3.82	11.2	28.4
21	0.0427	0.135	0.425	1.33	4.10	11.9	29.9
22	0.0459	0.145	0.457	1.43	4.39	12.7	31.5
23	0.0493	0.156	0.491	1.54	4.70	13.5	33.0
24	0.0530	0.167	0.527	1.65	5.03	14.4	34.6
25	0.0569	0.180	0.566	1.77	5.38	15.3	36.3
26	0.0610	0.193	0.607	1.89	5.75	16.2	37.9
27	0.0654	0.207	0.651	2.03	6.15	17.2	39.6
28	0.0701	0.221	0.697	2.17	6.56	18.2	41.2
29	0.0752	0.237	0.747	2.32	7.00	19.2	42.9
30	0.0805	0.254	0.799	2.48	7.46	20.3	44.6

Adapted from Emerson et al., 1975.

immunosuppression and secondary infection. A water sample should always be submitted for complete analysis when illness is suspected. Treatment is supportive and must include the provision of fresh, well oxygenated water. Calcium may be administered if tetany is present, but the prognosis in such cases is poor.

Although flow-through systems may be necessary where a large number of amphibians are kept in a relatively small volume of water, ammonia and nitrite can be kept at undetectable levels by using proper filtration, and removing organic debris on a regular basis. Denitrification is accomplished by two genera of bacteria. The first, *Nitrosomonas* spp., oxidize ammonia to less toxic nitrite. Like other animals exposed to high levels of nitrite, amphibians can develop methemoglobinemia or brown blood disease leading to respiratory compromise. Methylene blue baths (e.g., 2 mg/L) and supplemental oxygen may result in effective treatment, or methylene blue (e.g., methylene blue injection USP 1%, American Regent Laboratories, Inc., Shirley, NY) may be administered intracoelomically or intravenously to effect, not to exceed a total dosage of 9 mg/kg. A second population of nitrifying bacteria, *Nitrobacter* spp., consume nitrite and produce nitrate which is removed via routine water changes and through assimilation by plants.

Because the biological filter is actually a living component of the environment, care must be taken to preserve it. Nitrifying bacteria take 4–6 weeks to grow and require oxygenated water. An established biological filter (biofilter) is one in which the number of nitrifying bacteria present are sufficient to meet the current biological load. A sudden increase in organic matter, such as that which occurs when suddenly adding a large number of amphibians to a system, can overwhelm the capabilities of resident bacteria resulting in an ammonia spike. This is commonly referred to as "New Tank Syndrome." Nitrifying bacteria may also be destroyed or inhibited by adding chemicals such as antibiotics and dyes to the water, which can also result in a sudden increase in ammonia. Whenever using compounds within the aquarium/vivarium, water quality should be monitored daily.

12.7 FILTRATION

Filters that are commercially available for fishes work well for amphibians. The specific filter used is dependent upon the size of the system, organic load expected, flow requirements, and personal preference. A good filter will provide both the physical removal of large organic debris (mechanical filtration), as well as denitrification through biological processes (biological filtration). Ammonia-absorbing clays, activated carbon, and resins may be added to the filter to modify water chemistry (chemical filtration). Filters are powered by air, rotary impeller motors, or water pumps. In all cases, efficiency of the filter will decline as collected debris inhibits the flow of water through the media. When this occurs, a thorough cleaning of the filter is needed during which care must be taken to preserve the nitrifying bacteria. This is done by gently rinsing a generous portion of the media in chlorine-free water which is the same temperature as the tank water, and returning it to the filter. The nitrifying bacteria, which adhere to all surfaces of the filter and substrate, will not be lost unless washed in hot water, vigorously scrubbed, exposed to disinfectants, or allowed to dry.

Undergravel filters provide inexpensive and effective in-tank biological and mechanical filtration. Some are modified for the addition of chemical filtration. Because water flow through this type of filter is accomplished using air-lift tubes, nitrifying bacteria are provided with an abundant supply of oxygen (Figure 12.4). In order to maintain optimal performance, only the top layer of gravel should be cleaned at each water change using a special siphon that is enlarged at one end. Debris that has been trapped is removed leaving the heavier gravel behind.

The air-driven sponge or foam filter, which is also placed directly in the tank, is particularly useful in tanks where young larvae may be drawn into the swift outflow of other units (Figure 12.5). Sponge filters consist of an air-lift tube inserted into a piece of foam and work very well in small systems that have no substrate. Their operation is so gentle that small tadpoles will actually graze over the surface of the foam. The mesh work within the foam provides a great amount of surface area for nitrifying bacteria and works well to trap debris, but it must be rinsed clean relatively frequently in order to maintain effectiveness. Sponge filters are quickly overwhelmed in systems with large numbers of animals. Care must be taken during the cleaning process not to kill the nitrifying bacteria.

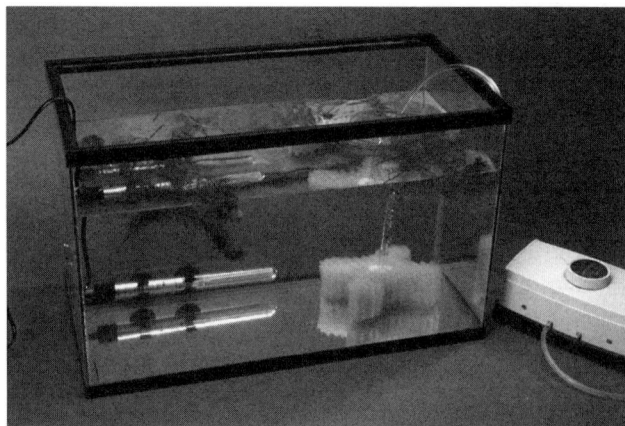

Figure 12.5. Sponge filters are often used with amphibian larvae as the water circulation does not entrap even very small specimens. (George Grall, National Aquarium in Baltimore)

Box or corner filters use air to create water flow through a plastic box in which filter floss, activated carbon, and gravel are layered to provide mechanical, chemical, and biological filtration. As with sponge filters, box filters are inexpensive, but only work well in small systems with relatively low organic load. They are easily removed for cleaning and can be adjusted to provide the flow rate desired.

Outside power and canister filters should be selected for larger systems maintaining amphibians (Figure 12.6). Because water must exit the aquarium via one or more siphon tubes, a noncorrosive guard must be fashioned around the outflow to keep animals away while allowing proper water flow to the unit. Canister filters are advantageous because they are large enough to accommodate many layers of different types of media. Peat moss, for example, may be

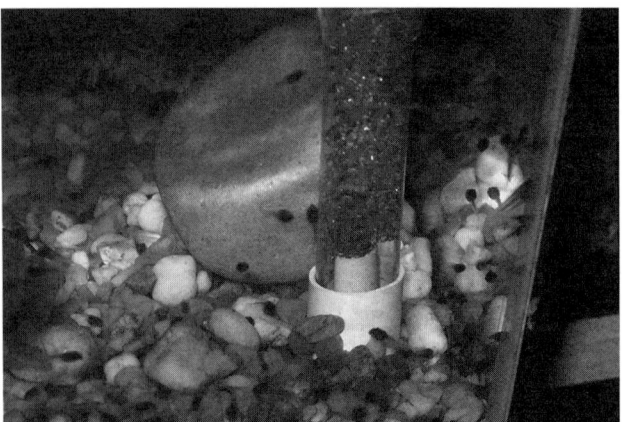

Figure 12.4. Adequate levels of oxygen and water circulation are needed for an undergravel filter bed to act as a biological filter. (Kevin Wright, Philadelphia Zoological Garden)

WATER QUALITY —— 155

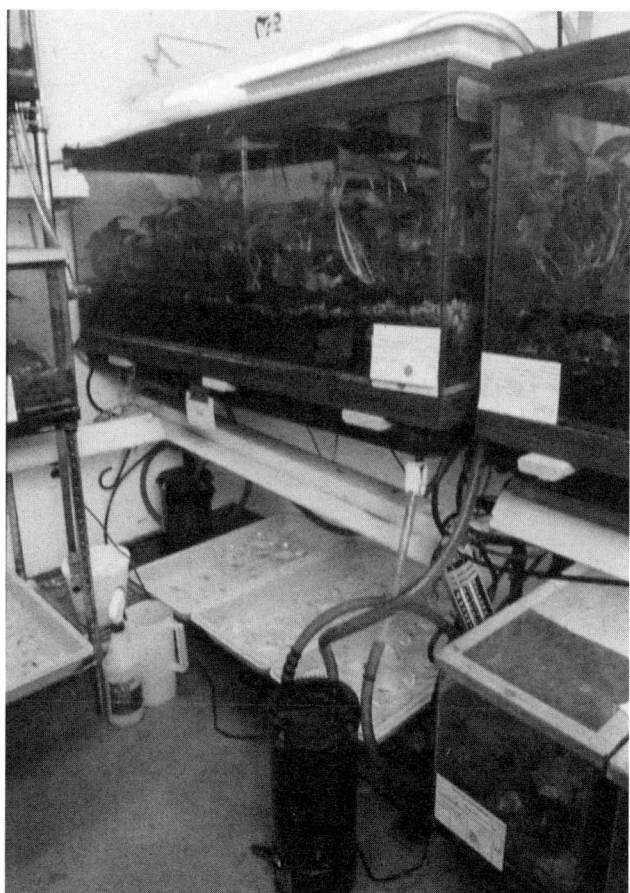

Figure 12.6. A canister filter works well for many systems where high flow of water is desirable, and provides excellent mechanical, chemical, and biological filtration. (George Grall, National Aquarium in Baltimore)

added to acidify and color the water for certain species. A separate source of air may be necessary unless the water is agitated upon return to the tank.

Trickle or wet-dry filters may also be used for larger aquatic systems. Water is sprayed over a column of biological filtration media (e.g., plastic "bioballs" or filter floss) which is active with nitrifying bacteria. As it trickles down, carbon dioxide is lost and oxygen gained. The water then passes through a series of chambers which may contain a variety of media before returning to the aquarium.

Ponds and streams can be created in a vivarium using an undergravel filter plate and a submersible water pump. Alternatively, an external power filter or water pump may be used. In this way, water collects in the pond and is pulled down through biologically active gravel. It is returned, with or without additional filtration, to the pond or the beginning of a stream. Regular water changes and cleaning of the gravel is required.

Larger tanks may also be modified to house many animals, such as carnivorous tadpoles, in separate compartments thus eliminating the laborious task of cleaning individual bowls daily. This is done by using acrylic to make a tray that is divided into individual cells. The length, width and depth of the cells depend on the species being kept. Plastic ice cube trays work well for some species. The bottom of this tray is made of noncorrosive fiberglass screen so that waste material and uneaten food can pass through while retaining the animal. The tray is set into the tank so that the top of the partitions remain above water level (Figure 12.7). As needed, the entire tray is lifted from the tank and gently rinsed to remove debris caught in the screening (Figure 12.8). The opportunity should be taken at this time to also clean the large tank. External or internal filtration is used to provide appropriate water treatment.

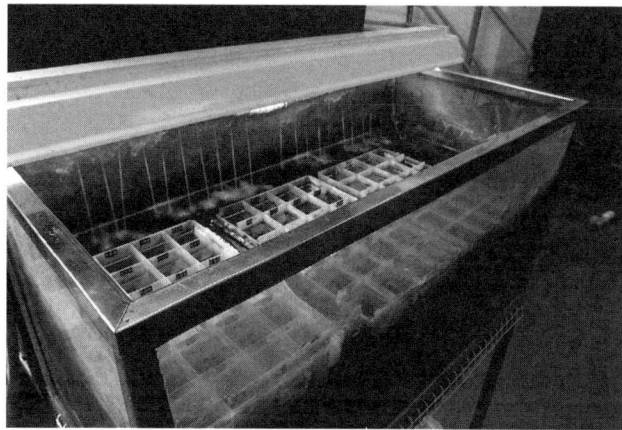

Figure 12.7. A partitioned tray may be used to separate larval amphibians into individual compartments. This is especially useful for raising carnivorous larvae. (George Grall, National Aquarium in Baltimore)

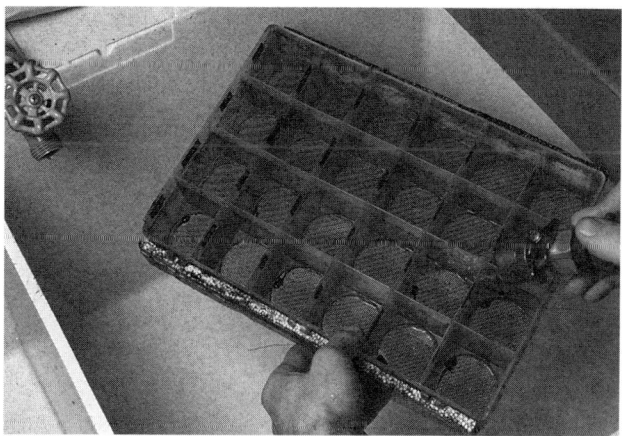

Figure 12.8. A tadpole tray can be rinsed gently with water to remove debris. (George Grall, National Aquarium in Baltimore)

12.8 WATER CHANGES

With proper filtration a 10% water change weekly or a 20% water change every 2 weeks should be sufficient to maintain good water quality. Systems without filtration may require large daily water changes to remove uneaten food and potentially toxic waste. All water changes should be made using only clean and chlorine/chloramine-free water. The temperature, pH, alkalinity, and hardness should match that in which the animals are living. Water may be preconditioned by placing it in a large plastic garbage barrel with submersible heaters and circulating it through a canister filter charged with activated carbon. This process improves water clarity as it removes organic substances. Potential chemical toxins, including any remaining chlorine, are also extracted. Activated carbon must be changed periodically to be effective. Once this is accomplished, further conditioning may be done by replacing the activated carbon with other substrates such as peat moss which imparts a light brown color to the water. This is often used for amphibians that require slightly acidic and soft water. Making the time and effort to ensure proper water quality is a wise investment that is rewarded with healthy amphibians.

12.9 WATER SOURCE

Amphibians rely upon the water in which they live to provide them with many of the constituents needed to carry out metabolic processes. Frogs can absorb sodium through their skin from relatively dilute pond water thus balancing sodium loss (Prosser, 1973). Like many fish, larva of the bullfrog, *Rana catesbeiana,* appear to absorb calcium across their gills (Boutilier et al., 1992) and when reared in water containing less then 4 mg/L calcium developed skeletal deformities akin to spindly leg syndrome (Marshal et al., 1980). In calcium-deficient water amphibians may actually lose this ion through cutaneous diffusion. The Northern leopard frog, *Rana pipiens,* and the North American tiger salamander, *Ambystoma tigrinum,* have been reported to lose up to 0.1% of their total body calcium daily (Bentley, 1984). It becomes clear that a variety of mechanisms have evolved allowing some species to absorb specific ions from their food while others remain dependent upon absorption from the water using their skin and/or gills.

Water used for captive amphibians must be of the highest quality and meet the specific requirements of the animals being kept. Although there are some species that can live in brackish water such as the Philippine frog, *Rana cancrivora* (Duellman & Trueb, 1986), most amphibians require fresh water. Distilled and reverse osmosis water contain none of the elements required by amphibians and should be not be used without modification. Water collected from ponds, springs, streams, or rivers may contain parasites, pesticides, bacteria, and viruses, but a healthy natural water source yields high quality water. Well water varies greatly in composition and may need to be conditioned before use. A variety of chemicals are often added to municipal water supplies. In buildings with copper pipes, water should be tested periodically for this heavy metal. Leaching of copper is exacerbated in standing water of low pH. If detected, allow the pipes to be thoroughly flushed before collecting a sample for retesting. Unfortunately, activated carbon will not effectively remove this form of copper from water. Letting water run through the tap for several minutes prior to collection will eliminate copper-contaminated water.

Water should be free of chlorine and chloramine. These oxidizing agents are added to local water supplies to reduce microbial levels. At lower concentrations these chemicals cause skin, gill, and eye irritation. Higher levels lead to toxicosis as blood cells are destroyed and the iron present in hemoglobin is oxidized to a steady state, thus disrupting oxygen transfer (Smith, 1982). One report suggested that red leg disease was less prevalent in frogs held in chlorine-free water (Scott, 1928). Some species, such as the bullfrog, *Rana catesbeiana,* will tolerate chlorine up to 3 mg/L (Culley, 1992), but despite this tolerance the use of a dechlorinating agent or activated carbon is highly recommended. Most dechlorinators contain sodium thiosulfate and remove chlorine rapidly, allowing the water to be used immediately. Vigorous aeration in an open barrel overnight will also effectively remove chlorine. Chloramine, a combination of chlorine and ammonia, is more toxic and stable than chlorine. The use of water conditioners specifically designed to remove chloramine often results in the release of ammonia (Blasiola, 1992), which activated carbon will not remove. Conditioning chloramine-treated water is best accomplished using a canister filter charged with an ammonia-absorbing material such as clinoptilolite, in addition to activated carbon.

REFERENCES

Beleau, M.H. 1988. Evaluating water problems, *in* Stoskopf, M.K. (Ed.): The Veterinary Clinics of North America: Tropical Fish Medicine. W.B. Saunders Co., Philadelphia, PA, pp. 291–302.

Bentley, P.J. 1984. Calcium metabolism in the amphibia. Comp. Biochem. Physiol. 79A, No. 1:1–5.

Blasiola, G.C. 1992. Diseases of ornamental marine fishes, *in* Gratzek, J.B. and J.R. Matthews (Eds.): Aquariology: The Science of Fish Health Management—Master Volume. Tetra Press, Morris Plains, NJ, pp. 275–300.

Boutilier, R.G., D.F. Stiffler, and D.P. Toews. 1992. Exchange of respiratory gases, ions, and water in amphibious and aquatic amphibians, *in* Feder, M.E. and W.W. Burggren (Eds.): Environmental Physiology of the Amphibians. University of Chicago Press, Chicago, pp. 81–124.

Campbell, J.W. 1973. Nitrogen excretion, *in* Feder, M.E. and W.W. Burggren (Eds.): Environmental Physiology of the Amphibians. University of Chicago Press, Chicago, pp. 279–316.

Colt, J., K. Orwicz and D. Brooks. 1984. Gas bubble disease in the African clawed frog, *Xenopus laevis*. Journal of Herpetology 18:131–137.

Cover, J.F., Jr., S.L. Barnett, and R.L. Saunders. 1994. Captive management and breeding of dendrobatid and neotropical hylid frogs at the National Aquarium in Baltimore, *in* Murphy, J.B., K. Adler, and J.T. Collins (Eds.): Captive Management and Conservation of Amphibians and Reptiles, Society for the Study of Amphibians and Reptiles. Contributions to Herpetology, volume 11, Ithaca, NY, pp. 267–273.

Crawshaw, G.J. 1992. Amphibian medicine, *in* Kirk, R.W. and J.D. Bonagura (Eds.): Current Veterinary Therapy Vol. XI. W.B. Saunders Co., Philadelphia, PA, pp. 1219–1230.

Culley, D.D. 1992. Managing a bullfrog research colony, *in* Schaeffer, D.O., K.M. Kleinow, and L. Krulisch (Eds.): The Care and Use of Amphibians, Reptiles and Fish in Research. Scientists Center for Animal Welfare, Bethesda, MD, pp. 30–40.

Duellman, W.E. and L. Trueb. 1986. Biology of Amphibians. Johns Hopkins University Press, Baltimore, MD, 670 pp.

Emerson, K., R.C. Russo, R.E. Lund, and R.V. Thurston. 1975. Aqueous ammonia equilibrium calculations: Effect of pH and temperature. J. Fish. Res. Board Can. 32(12):2379–2383.

Marshall, G.A., R.L. Amborski, and D.D. Culley. 1980. Calcium and pH requirements in the culture of bullfrog *Rana catesbeiana* larvae. Proc. World Maricul. Soc. 11:445–453.

Prosser, C.L. 1973. Water: Osmotic balance; hormonal regulation, *in* Prosser, C.L.: Comparative Animal Physiology. W.B. Saunders Co., Philadelphia, PA, pp. 1–78.

Scott, J.M.D. 1928. Pink-belly disease in frogs. Am. J. Physiol. 85:405.

Smith, L.S. 1982. Introduction to Fish Physiology. TFH Publications, Inc., Neptune City, NJ.

Subcommittee on Amphibian Standards. 1974. Committee on Standards, National Research Council, (Eds.): Amphibians: Guidelines for the breeding, care, and management of laboratory animals. National Academy Press Inc., Washington DC, 153 pp.

Tucker, C.S. 1993. Water analysis, *in* Stoskopf, M.K. (Ed.): Fish Medicine. W.B. Saunders Co., Philadelphia, PA, pp. 166–197.

CHAPTER 13
BACTERIAL DISEASES

Sharon K. Taylor, DVM, PhD, D. Earl Green, DVM, Diplomate ACVP,
Kevin M. Wright, DVM, and Brent R. Whitaker, MS, DVM

13.1 PREDISPOSING FACTORS

Bacterial infections often are difficult to recognize in a colony of amphibians until disease has progressed to the point that mortality ensues in some or all of the affected specimens. Confirming a diagnosis in living specimens is difficult due to the relative paucity of published clinicopathological evaluations of ill amphibians. The majority of bacterial infections reported in amphibians are caused by Gram-negative organisms for which there are readily available antibiotics. Unfortunately the pharmacokinetics of these agents in most amphibian species are as yet unknown (see Chapter 24, Pharmacotherapeutics). Many bacterial infections are thought to be associated with stress caused by lapses in appropriate husbandry and consequent immunosuppression. Any outbreak of bacterial disease mandates thorough documentation of the captive care with a species-specific review to uncover likely contributing factors.

The two stressors most commonly documented in outbreaks of bacterial disease are shipment and improper husbandry, which may include deficiencies in water quality, humidity, temperature, photoperiod, substrate, population density, social structure, cage furnishings (i.e., hiding cover), and nutrition. Brief exposure to even minor adverse environmental conditions may prove disastrous to amphibians, altering their immune response and metabolism beyond their ability to cope with infectious diseases.

Hibernation affects both the immune system and the gastrointestinal bacterial flora. Studies conducted on the aerobic bacteria in the intestinal tract of the bullfrog, *Rana catesbeiana*, and the northern leopard frog, *R. pipiens*, have shown that hibernation temperatures may provide a selective advantage for potentially pathogenic bacterial species (Banas et al., 1988; Carr et al., 1976). Research has also shown that it is actually the decrease in temperature, not the accompanying state of fasting, which induces this microbial shift during hibernation (Gossling et al., 1982a). This microbial shift may be a transient event. Once hibernation has been established for several weeks or months the numbers and types of bacteria may return to the prehibernation state (Gossling et al., 1982b). There is also evidence to support a seasonal variation in the immune response of amphibians (Zapata et al., 1992). In the European common frog, *R. temporaria*, maximal development of the thymus has been reported to occur in the summer months with marked regression as winter approaches. The thymus regressed even in those frogs which were maintained in an active state in a warm environment and not hibernated. The square-marked toad, *Bufo regularis*, has been noted to have lower humoral responses to heterologous erythrocytes in the autumn as compared to the spring and summer (Zapata et al., 1992). Thus amphibians may be at a microbial disadvantage at the time of hibernation in addition to having a suppressed immune system.

13.2 LOCALIZED INFECTIONS

13.2.1 Introduction

Localized infections in amphibians are rarely reported in the literature. This is due, in part, to the presence of antimicrobial factors in the external mucus coat of the amphibian integument. Antimicrobial peptides, magainins, have been isolated from the skin of the African clawed frog, *Xenopus laevis* (Zasloff, 1987). This previously unidentified defense may explain how amphibians remain healthy in an aquatic environment filled with potential bacterial pathogens. Abrasions, chemical disruptions, and thermal injuries may compromise this first line of defense, and may lead to superficial ulcers (Plates 13.1, 13.2, 13.3) and abscesses, which in turn may progress to septicemia.

13.2.2 Superficial Wounds, Ulcers and Abscesses

Superficial wounds, ulcers and abscesses usually reveal a diversity of Gram-negative bacteria including, but not limited to, *Acinetobacter* spp., *Aeromonas* spp., *Citrobacter* spp., *Flavobacterium* spp., *Providencia* spp., and *Pseudomonas* spp., and, on occasion, a Gram-positive organism (Plate 13.4).

A superficial open wound or ulcer may be treated daily with a variety of topical antibiotics, topical antiseptics or other compounds to prevent development of an abscess. In general, silver sulfadiazine cream is an excellent choice for localized lesions, and has the advantage of antifungal activity in addition to its antibacterial spectrum. Gentamicin ophthalmic ointment or drops applied one to three times a days is a good choice for localized lesions, however caution is advised when treating small amphibians given the potential for toxicity from percutaneous absorption of this drug. Oxytetracycline ointments may be efficacious, however many Gram-negative organisms may be resistant to this. In one report, the product Bactine™ (Miles Laboratories, Ltd.) was used until white scar tissue covered the wound (Martin & Hong, 1991), and it was believed that this regime decreased healing time. Another report recommended that a wound be sprayed with a topical furazolidone (Boyer et al., 1971). The course of treatment was to dry off the amphibian by holding it out of water for five minutes, apply the furazolidone spray, and holding the amphibian out of water for another five minutes to ensure adherence of the drug. Other topical antiseptics and antibiotics have been used, and the choice depends on the severity of the wound and the nature of the amphibian. Plasticized hydrocarbon pastes (e.g., Orabase®, Colgate Oral Pharmaceuticals, Canton, MA) can be applied directly to superficial lesions once every one to two days (Hoogesteyn & Stetter, 1996), but this bandaging should be accompanied by a course of systemic antibiotics. Aquatic amphibians are better treated by maintaining them in a medicated bath. This approach may be stressful for some species of terrestrial amphibians. A serious breach of the integument warrants prophylaxis with systemic antibiotics (see Chapter 24, Pharmacotherapeutics). In many amphibians, the margins of a healing wound will be darker than surrounding normal skin.

Bacterial abscesses should be treated by removing all encapsulated material and flushing the cavity with an antiseptic (e.g., chlorhexidine) or an antibiotic (e.g., gentamicin). Additional therapy may include daily treatment with an appropriate topical antiseptic or antibiotic as well as systemic antibiotics based on the sensitivity patterns of bacteria isolated from the abscess.

13.2.3 Epidermal Discoloration

Some amphibians may develop skin discoloration suggestive of a bacterial dermatitis. The affected skin may become grey, brown or black (Plate 13.5). No organisms have been consistently linked with these lesions as yet, but it is noteworthy that it takes several days to weeks before affected amphibians show signs consistent with generalized infection. Topical and systemic broad spectrum antibiotics, such as enrofloxacin (5–10 mg/kg IM, ICe, SQ, PO, or topically q 24 h), may eliminate the lesion, although a permanent lightening of the skin color may be evident (Plate 13.6).

13.2.4 Rostral Injuries

Rostral abrasions are a common injury in captive anurans and may serve as the site of initial invasion by pathogens (see also Section 17.1, Abrasions). These lesions are often the result of improper housing or exposure to a noxious agent that causes the amphibian to attempt escape (e.g., polyvinyl chloride glues, ammonia). A bullfrog, *Rana catesbeiana*, developed severe ulceration of the rostrum and maxilla exposing underlying bone (Li & Lipman, 1995). *Aeromonas hydrophila, Citrobacter freundii, Pseudomonas* spp., and a group D *Streptococcus* were isolated from the lesion. The frog was euthanized and *Aeromonas hydrophila* was isolated from its heart blood suggesting that septicemia probably originated from the rostral abrasion.

A small captive group of Darwin's frog, *Rhinoderma darwini*, was observed with ulceration and necrosis of the rostrum (Cooper et al., 1978). Clinical signs were grayish discoloration, ulceration, and necrosis of the rostrum, and some frogs' rostral projections were atrophied. The predominant organism isolated and thus implicated was *Aeromonas liquefaciens*, however *Acinetobacter* spp. and *Citrobacter freundii* were also cultured. These Gram-negative organisms are common in aquatic and soil environments (Juni, 1984; Popoff, 1984; Sakazaki, 1984), and it is assumed that physical injury to the projecting rostral fold predisposed the frogs to infection.

Treatment of rostral abrasions should begin immediately as there is little soft tissue overlying the bone in this region (see Section 17.1, Abrasions). Healing is particularly slow and the client should be warned that permanent discoloration of the rostrum is likely. Alternative housing is suggested to prevent further trauma, and topical and systemic antibiotic therapy may be warranted. If alternate housing is not available, foam or bubble wrap should cover the areas where the trauma is occurring (e.g., screen tops).

13.2.5 Neurological Infections

Bacterial meningitis has been identified rarely in amphibians. *Flavobacterium meningosepticum* was isolated from a captive colony of the northern leopard frog, *Rana pipiens*. Clinical signs indicative of neurologic disease include circling, head tilt, and an inability to right themselves (Taylor et al., 1993). Meningitis, panophthalmitis and bilateral suppurative otitis were confirmed histologically. Treatment with chloramphenicol at 250 mg/19 L of water for 10 days was not effective in reducing clinical signs or preventing the development of additional cases. However, assuming that the organisms were sensitive to this drug, this treatment may not have reached therapeutic levels in blood or cerebrospinal fluid. *Flavobacterium meningosepticum* has been reported as the cause of over 100 human cases of meningitis (Holmes et al., 1984), however there has been no known association of zoonotic transmission with amphibians. This Gram-negative aerobic rod is frequently found in soil and water (Holmes et al., 1984).

13.2.6 Ocular Infections

Panophthalmitis and uveitis may be caused by a variety of Gram-negative and Gram-positive bacteria. Specimens of a large colony of the firebelly toad, *Bombina orientalis,* developed anorexia, bloating, and cloudy eyes (hypopyon) 3 weeks after being shipped from Japan to Florida (Brooks et al., 1983). Some toads displayed circling, opisthotonos, head tilt, and poor righting reflexes. Panophthalmitis and otitis interna were found histologically. *Aeromonas hydrophila, Citrobacter freundii,* and *Providencia alcalifaciens* were isolated from internal organs and aqueous humor. All of these organisms are Gram-negative (Penner, 1984; Popoff, 1984; Sakazaki, 1984). Treatment with oxytetracycline at 26 mg/L of water daily did not decrease mortality, however this is well below the concentration of oxytetracycline (100 mg/L) that has been efficacious in treating other amphibian bacterial infections (Wright, 1996). Intracameral, intramuscular, intracoelomic, or subcutaneous routes of administration should be considered in addition to the topical route for the treatment of severe ocular infections.

See Chapter 19, The Amphibian Eye, for further discussion on infectious processes of the ocular system.

13.3 SYSTEMIC INFECTIONS

Multiple bacterial taxa are often isolated from amphibians with red leg syndrome and septicemias. Multiple bacterial genera from one individual may be attributed in part to decompositional bacteria that rapidly invade tissues of aquatic organisms. Despite the volume of literature which supports the concept that mixed bacterial infections are common in amphibians (Brooks et al., 1983; Frye, 1989; Glorioso et al., 1974a; Hubbard, 1981), most bacterial isolates have been from dead amphibians and must be viewed cautiously. All Gram-negative bacteria which have been associated with clinical disease in amphibians are included in the discussion of red leg syndrome below.

There are several reasonable theories on the pathogenesis of bacterial dermatosepticemias or red leg syndrome, but little experimental proof (Glorioso et al., 1974a). It seems likely that red leg syndrome may be attributed to one or more of the major theories:

1) Infections occur as a result of the complex interaction of multiple taxa of bacteria or from the overwhelming presence of a single species of bacterium;
2) Infections occur as a result of immunosuppression from the elevation of endogenous corticosteroids associated with physical stressors such as temperature changes, crowding, water quality, and chemicals, or the immunosuppression is directly caused by other means such as the hormonal and immunological effects of trace levels of organochlorine pesticides (Carey, 1993; Fox, 1992; Gross et al., 1994);
3) Infections occur as a result of other biological agents (such as viruses) which exert physiological (immunological) changes resulting in enhancement of bacterial colonization (Cunningham et al., 1993; Speare et al., 1994);
4) Infections occur as a result of infection of minor skin lesions by environmental bacteria, including flora originating from arthropods used as live food, or intestinal bacteria (Dusi, 1949; Elkan, 1976; Kulp & Borden, 1942; Vander Waaij et al., 1974); and,
5) Infections occur via colonization of the skin damaged by ultraviolet-B radiation (Blaustein et al., 1994) or other physical agents such as gas-supersaturated water (Colt et al., 1984).

The theory of immunosuppressive viral infections has received scant attention in cases of amphibian dermatosepticemias prior to 1996. Although viruses were not detected in the wild-caught tadpoles of the bullfrog, *Rana catesbeiana,* culture attempts were limited to fat-head minnow (fish) cell lines (Glorioso et al., 1974a). This failure to isolate any viruses is in conflict with the widespread distribution of viruses, especially ranaviruses and other iridoviruses, in the bullfrog, *R. catesbeiana* (Gruia-Gray & Desser, 1992; Wolf et al., 1968, 1969). Determining the role of viral infections in red leg epidemics is important to our understanding of the pathogenesis of bacterial infections in captive and wild amphibians.

13.3.1 Bacterial Dermatosepticemia

Red Leg Syndrome. Red leg syndrome in amphibians is so named due to the hyperemia of the ventral skin of the thighs and abdomen of septicemic anurans, and is now synonymous with any generalized bacterial infection in amphibians. Red leg syndrome is better termed bacterial dermatosepticemia, but the common name is firmly entrenched in the literature. Historically, this disease is associated with *Aeromonas* *hydrophila* and other aeromonads, but many other infectious agents produce similar integumentary signs.

A common clinical sign of red leg syndrome is ventral and digital erythema due to dilation of dermal vessels (Plates 13.7, 13.8, 13.9). There may be multiple foci of necrosis or ulceration of the epidermis, hemorrhagic papules, and petechial or ecchymotic hemorrhages in the dermis (Gibbs et al., 1966; Glorioso et al., 1974a; Hubbard, 1981; Kulp & Borden, 1942) (Plate 13.10). Other lesions include edematous, fibrinocellular or sanguinous fluids in the subcutis of the upper limbs and ventral abdomen, hemorrhagic ulceration of the tips of digital skin (which may expose phalangeal bones or cause sloughed digits), ulcerated jaws, pale yellowish or sanguinous coelomic transudates or effusions, and hemoptysis (Gibbs et al., 1966; Kulp & Borden, 1942). Subcutaneous edema may be so severe that it causes the appearance of generalized cutaneous pallor, a lack of erythema or hemorrhage within dermal ulcers, and a bloated appearance (sometimes termed edema syndrome) (Glorioso et al., 1974a) (Plates 13.10, 13.11, 13.12, 13.13). Petechial and ecchymotic hemorrhages in adult amphibians may also be detected in skeletal muscles, kidneys, spleen, coelomic mesothelial surfaces, and nearly any other organ in which vascular thrombi and bacillary emboli develop (Cunningham et al., 1993; Frye, 1989; Kulp & Borden, 1942; Olson et al., 1992). Hypopyon or hyphema may be noted. Mild weight loss to obvious emaciation may be evident in adult amphibians as atrophy of muscles and fat bodies occurs. Many amphibians succumbing peracutely or acutely to bacterial dermatosepticemias may have minimal to no gross lesions (Abrams, 1969; Boyer et al., 1971; Frye, 1989; Gibbs et al., 1966; Kulp & Borden, 1942).

In tadpoles and salamander larvae, erythema and petechia are noted on ventral and lateral body skin, the tail, and legs. Hemorrhages may be present over the eyes in tadpoles of the bullfrog, *Rana catesbeiana* (Glorioso et al., 1974a). Immature amphibians also may have minimal to moderate subcutaneous edema composed of clear, cloudy, or sanguinous fluids, but others in the same group may appear emaciated (Glorioso et al., 1974a; Nyman, 1986).

Red leg syndrome has been attributed to the bacterium *Aeromonas hydrophila* without appropriate diagnostic investigation. Clinical signs of red leg syndrome may be caused by other infectious agents including, but not limited to, ranaviruses (e.g., tadpole edema virus, frog virus-3), other bacteria (Table 13.1), *Chlamydia psittaci* (Newcomer et al., 1982), and *Basidiobolus ranarum* (Taylor et al., 1995). Additionally there are noninfectious causes of ventral erythema that are usually transient, such as may be caused by contact with a heated substrate, chemical irritation or the stress of being handled.

One of the earliest reports attributing mortality in frogs to *Aeromonas hydrophila* occurred within a captive research colony of frogs at Rush Medical College (Russell, 1898). This extensively descriptive manuscript outlines the syndrome, which in 1905 became known as "red leg" (Emerson & Norris, 1905). Red leg syndrome attributed to *A. hydrophila* has occurred in numerous captive amphibian species since those initial reports. The species list from the literature is sparse and should not be considered a comprehensive list of potential host species. Species reported with red leg syndrome include the African clawed frog, *Xenopus laevis*, the northern leopard frog, *Rana pipiens*, the northern cricket frog, *Acris crepitans*, the giant toad, *Bufo marinus*, the Texas salamander, *Eurycea neotenes*, and the axolotl, *Ambystoma mexicanum* (Boyer et al., 1971; Gibbs, 1963; Hubbard, 1981; Hunsaker & Potter, 1960; Paul & Dillehay, 1991; Smith, 1950). The disease in these captive animals was associated with improper husbandry (overcrowding, poor water quality, malnutrition), shipping stress, and surgery.

Reports of naturally occurring red leg epizootics occurring in free-ranging populations are rare. Trends in peak densities of *Aeromonas hydrophila* have been observed to occur during March and June in a South Carolina reservoir (Hazen, 1979), and these trends may influence epizootics. It is likely that underlying stressors have been involved in these outbreaks causing the amphibians to be predisposed to infection by this ubiquitous bacterial genus. In 1948, an outbreak occurred in a population of the American toad, *Bufo americanus*, in West Virginia (Dusi, 1949). Within 48 hours of onset, the majority of the more than 300 individuals of this free-ranging population were dead. *Aeromonas hydrophila* was isolated from heart blood of these toads.

Susceptibility to red leg syndrome varies between species of amphibians. In a vernal-autumnal pond in Rhode Island mass mortality attributed to *Aeromonas hydrophila* occurred in the wood frog, *Rana sylvatica*, and larvae of the spotted salamander, *Ambystoma maculatum*, while at the same time larvae of the gray treefrog, *Hyla versicolor*, and adults of the bullfrog, *R. catesbeiana*, displayed petechiae but suffered no detected mortality (Nyman, 1986). Mass mortality attributed to *A. hydrophila* occurred over a 2-week period in a population of the Texas salamander, *Eurycea neotenes*, the northern leopard frog, *R. pipiens*, and the northern cricket frog, *Acris crepitans*, which inhabited a stream near San Antonio, Texas (Hunsaker & Potter, 1960).

Free-ranging and captive-reared specimens of the Wyoming toad, *Bufo hemiophrys baxteri*, were re-

Table 13.1. Some bacteria associated with red leg syndrome. Clinical disease and mortalities were noted for each bacterial species listed. This list should not be considered a definitive list of species associations. Compare to Table 10.1, Representative microbial isolates recovered from ill anurans at the National Aquarium in Baltimore over the course of one year.

Bacteria	Host	Reference
Aeromonas hydrophila	Various	Various, see text.
Aeromonas salmonicida	*Xenopus laevis*	Frye, 1989
Aeromonas sp.	Various	Various, see text.
Acinetobacter haemolyticus (= *A. calcoaceticus*)	*Ambystoma tigrinum*	Worthylake & Hovingh, 1989
Alcaligenes faecalis	*Rana* sp.	Miles, 1950; Isolated but considered nonpathogenic by Glorioso et al. 1974a
Citrobacter freundii	*Rana pipiens, Ambystoma tridactyla, Bombina orientalis*	Brooks, et al., 1983; Frye, 1989; Gibbs, 1963; Gibbs et al., 1966;
Enterobacter spp.	*Rana mucosa*	Bradford, 1991
Flavobacterium indologenes	*Rana pipiens*	Olson et al. 1992
Flavobacterium sp.	*Rana catesbeiana*	Glorioso et al., 1974a
Klebsiella sp.	*Bufo hemiophrys baxteri*	Taylor et al., 1995
Mima polymorpha	*Rana catesbeiana*	Gibbs et al., 1966; Glorioso et al., 1974a
Proteus mirabilis	*Rana catesbeiana*	Glorioso et al., 1974a
Proteus morganii	*Rana catesbeiana*	Glorioso et al., 1974a
Proteus rettgeri	*Rana catesbeiana*	Glorioso et al., 1974a
Proteus vulgaris	*Rana catesbeiana*	Glorioso et al., 1974a
Pseudomonas aeruginosa	*Rana catesbeiana*	Glorioso et al., 1974a
Pseudomonas fluorescens	*Rana catesbeiana*	Reichenbach-Klinke & Elkan, 1965
Pseudomonas putida	*Rana catesbeiana*	Glorioso et al., 1974a
Staphylococcus epidermis	*Rana* sp.	Gibbs et al., 1966
Streptococcus, Group B	*Rana catesbeiana*	Amborski et al., 1983

ported to have a mycotic dermatitis caused by *Basidiobolus ranarum* with a secondary septicemia which was predominantly caused by *A. hydrophila* (Taylor et al., 1995). The clinical signs of this condition were indistinguishable from red leg syndrome.

Treatment of red leg syndrome has met with varied success. Most of the published regimes are more than 25 years old. Numerous chemicals (chlorhexidine, sodium chloride, potassium permanganate, chloride of lime, copper sulfate, mercuric chloride, formalin, phenol, tricresol) have been evaluated for their *in vitro* and *in vivo* efficacy (Kaplan & Light, 1955). The majority of these compounds have been shown to be lethal to amphibians if used at concentrations necessary to eliminate bacteria. Cold therapy, 9–11 days at 0–5°C, (32–40°F) was the first treatment that met with some success (Emerson & Norris, 1905), perhaps by inhibiting bacterial growth to the point that the amphibian's cytologic and humoral mechanisms could eliminate the bacteria. Wounds or surgical incisions that may predispose amphibians to infections may be treated with a topical antibiotic (e.g., antibiotic ophthalmic drops or ointments) or antiseptic (e.g., sprayed with a topical furazolidone (Boyer et al., 1971), Bactine™ (Martin & Hong, 1991), or Orabase® (Hoogesteyn & Stetter, 1996)). Other topical treatments, such as localized application of hypertonic saline or baths in electrolyte solutions such as Holtfreter's or Steinberg's solutions, have been used to prevent colonization of surface wounds. It is highly recommended that systemic antibiotics be used in addition to topical treatments for deep or extensive wounds (see Section 24.3, Antibacterial Agents).

Several drug regimes have been reported as having efficacy in the treatment of red leg syndrome (Ambrus et al., 1951; Boyer et al., 1971; Gibbs, 1963; Gibbs,

1973; Hunsaker & Potter, 1960; Koivastik, 1950; Miles, 1950; Smith, 1950), but little regard has been paid to the culture and sensitivity of the bacterial isolates thus limiting the value of these reports. The use of saline (0.15 %) as the amphibian's water source in combination with externally applied antibiotic treatments may decrease mortality (Menard, 1984). Maintenance of the amphibian's electrolyte balance is suggested as concomitant therapy (see Section 24.9, Maintaining the Electrolyte Balance of the Ill Amphibian). Parenteral broad spectrum antibiotics are recommended for any amphibian with a suspected septicemia (see Sections 24.3, Antibacterial Agents, and 24.5, Emergency Treatment for the Septic Amphibian).

Edema Syndrome. Edema syndrome refers to the combination of hydrocoelom and subcutaneous edema in amphibians. This syndrome may or may not be associated with bacterial septicemia (see Plate 13.13). There is a marked excess of clear or clear yellowish fluid in the subcutis and coelomic cavity. Edema syndrome in the septic amphibian is assumed to result from the disruption of capillaries and lymphatics compromising the return of interstitial fluid to the circulatory system, as well as a disruption in the integrity of the skin resulting in an increased uptake of water. Renal and hepatic failure, as may occur from bacterial invasion or bacterial toxins, may result in edema syndrome along with other factors which damage or decrease the contractions of the lymph hearts. It is important to evaluate other potential causes of impaired osmoregulation such as a toxic insult or water quality problems (i.e., lack of adequate solutes in the water), to rule out renal, hepatic, and cardiovascular disease, and to confirm the presence of pathogenic bacteria before attributing edema syndrome to a bacterial infection. Edema syndrome has been associated with *Flavobacterium* spp. infections, but it is likely that other bacterial species will be confirmed upon investigation of additional outbreaks.

Aeromonas. Aeromonas hydrophila has been previously called *Aerobacter liquefaciens, Achromobacter punctation, Bacillus hydrophilus, Bacillus hydrophilus fuscus, Bacillus icthyosomium, Bacillus punctatus, Bacillus ranicida, Bacterium hydrophilus fuscus, Bacterium punctatus, Bacterium ranicida, Escherichia icthyosomium, Proteus hydrophilus, Pseudomonas punctata, Proteus icthyosomium, Pseudomonas fermentans,* and *Pseudomonas icthyosomium* (Kulp & Borden, 1942; Shotts, 1984). Organisms within the genus *Aeromonas* are motile Gram-negative polar-flagellated rods (Nygaard et al., 1970). Aeromonads are known to be common in aquatic environments and are found over wide ranges of salinity, conductivity, temperature, pH, and turbidity (Hazen et al., 1978; Palumbo, 1993; Popoff, 1984).

Aeromonas hydrophila is ubiquitous in aquatic environments and may be considered a primary pathogen, but most often is a secondary or opportunistic invader of all classes of vertebrates, especially amphibians and fish (Cahill, 1990; Cartwright et al., 1994). Few reports of *Aeromonas*-related disease in amphibians hold up to careful scrutiny. For example, there are very few studies of virulence determinants of *Aeromonas hydrophila* isolated from amphibians with clinical disease (Cahill, 1990; Kulp & Borden, 1942), and seldom have viral and fungal cultures been attempted on amphibians with red leg syndrome. It is very difficult to assess whether the motile aeromonads associated with clinical disease in amphibians were primary or secondary pathogens, or even incidental environmental or decompositional organisms. When attempts at fulfilling Koch's postulates were reported using isolates from *Aeromonas hydrophila*-related disease, often the challenged amphibians suffered much milder or inapparent infections (Boyer et al., 1971; Dusi, 1949; Hubbard, 1981) or large numbers of organisms had to be administered parenterally (Glorioso et al., 1974a; Kulp & Borden, 1942). Low mortality also occurred in healthy northern leopard frogs inoculated with large numbers of *Pseudomonas aeruginosa* bacilli (Brodkin et al., 1992). Wild-caught clinically healthy firebelly toads, *Bombina* spp., normally have live bacteria in their spleens, and more so when the toads occupy bacteria-rich water (Mika et al., 1995). Bacteria disappear from the spleen in captive toads maintained in bacteria-free water, suggesting anurans experience a constant invasion of bacteria into the circulation with a rapid clearance of these organisms by the spleen and possibly other organs with reticuloendothelial cells (Mika et al., 1995).

The confusion over *Aeromonas hydrophila*-associated disease may be attributed in part to shifting taxonomy. Only recently have the systematics of the genus *Aeromonas* been clarified from that in which *Aeromonas* was considered a monotypic genus (i.e., *A. hydrophila*) (Joseph & Carnahan, 1994) (Table 13.2). The scientific literature, especially those works published prior to 1985, includes unreliable or outdated classifications for identifying aeromonads to the species level (Pazzaglia, 1993). Overlaps among classification schemes and failure of many reports to detail methods of identification have resulted in many scientific and clinical articles which cannot unequivocally identify *Aeromonas* isolates to species levels. Of the more than twelve species of *Aeromonas* now identified (Joseph & Carnahan, 1994), it is unclear how many of these species may participate in clinical disease in amphibians. Many reported isolates of *A. hydrophila* from amphibians may have been one of the other species of aeromonads.

A number of virulence factors have been identified in

Table 13.2. Species of *Aeromonas* isolated from amphibians. (Taxonomy according to Joseph & Carnahan, 1994.)

Aeromonas sp.	Pathogenic to Fish	Isolated from Amphibians	Reference
Allosaccharophila	unknown	no	
Caviae	no	yes	Green, unpublished data
Enteropelogenes	unknown	no	
Eucrenophila	unknown	no	
Hydrophila	yes	yes	many
Ichthiosmia	unknown	no	
Jandaei	unknown	no	
Media	unknown	no	
Salmonicida	yes	yes	Frye, 1989
Schuberti	unknown	yes	Green, unpublished data
Sobria	yes	yes	Paniagua et al., 1990; Green, unpublished data
Trota	unknown	yes	Green, unpublished data
Veronii	unknown	no	

the motile aeromonads including endotoxins such as lipopolysaccharides, extracellular choleralike enterotoxins, cytotoxins, hemolysins (aerolysin), dermonecrotic factor, pili, cell adherence factors, an S-layer surface protein, and other extracellular proteases (Cahill, 1990; Cartwright et al., 1994). The presence and contribution of these virulence determinants to clinical disease in amphibians is very inadequately studied with few exceptions (e.g., Kulp & Borden, 1942), yet such factors as cell adherence, extracellular proteases, cytotoxins, and hemolysins probably play a significant role in the pathogenesis of amphibian mortalities. Many motile aeromonads are psychrotrophic, and capable of producing hemolysins and enterotoxins at the cool temperatures preferred by most amphibians (Cahill, 1990). From fish, 72% of strains of *Aeromonas hydrophila* produced enterotoxins, and 100% of *A. sobria* strains produced it. Again from fish isolates, hemolysin and protease were found to be extracellular products of *A. hydrophila* and *A. sobria,* and may have been the principal lethal factors to experimental fish (reviewed by Cahill, 1990). Hemolysin is released by *Aeromonas* spp. in an inactive form, and is activated by extracellular proteases. It is not clear whether amphibian cellular and serum proteases are capable of activiting hemolysin. The proteases of *Aeromonas* spp. include a thermostable metalloprotease, and a thermolabile serine protease. This array of virulence factors in motile aeromonads gives the bacteria the capability to act as opportunistic pathogens in susceptible hosts, although the virulence mechanisms of these bacteria in ectotherms and endotherms may be different (Cahill, 1990).

The chief microbial toxin believed to be responsible for the pathogenicity is aerolysin (Parker et al., 1994). This water-soluble protein changes form to produce a transmembrane channel that destroys sensitive cells by disrupting their permeability barriers leading to cell death.

The optimum temperature for recovery of the organism varies widely. The fish pathogen, *Aeromonas salmonicida,* grows optimally at a temperature of 35°C (95°F). Thirteen aeromonads (purported strains of *A. hydrophila* under the taxonomic scheme of the time) tested for optimal growth temperature varied from 5°C to 55°C (41°F to 131°F) (Rouf & Rigney, 1971). It was originally reported that strains of *A. hydrophila* obtained from infections in amphibians were indistinguishable by cultural and biochemical reactions from those causing disease in fish (Reed & Toner, 1942), but this sweeping generalization has been invalidated by the current taxonomic scheme (Joseph & Carnahan, 1994).

In experimental studies to determine the pathogenicity of *Aeromonas hydrophila* in the northern leopard frog, *Rana pipiens,* it was determined that extremely high numbers of bacteria (1.5×10^9) were required to induce mortality (Rigney et al., 1978). It was also found that the strain of the organism used was not very virulent and required the influence of endotoxin and hemolysin. This information supports the finding of a survey for *A. hydrophila* in free-ranging populations of the northern leopard frog, *R. pipiens*, conducted in Minnesota in which the bacteria was isolated from 94 (32%) of 294 clinically healthy frogs (Hird et al., 1981). Thus *A. hydrophila* is not always pathogenic. Morbidity and mortality are likely to be the result of other factors including virulence, poor water quality, pre-existing disease, and other stressors. *Aeromonas hydrophila* may be isolated commonly from the feces of amphibians. In one captive-bred group of the giant leaf frog, *Phyllomedusa bicolor*, bred at the National Aquarium in Baltimore, recent metamorphs developed diarrhea, lost weight, and died. *Aeromonas hydrophila* was cultured consistently from many individuals. Oral trimethoprim-sulfa was administered resulting in immediate improvement and subsequent survival of many of the affected frogs. The ease with which most suspected pathogenic bacteria can be isolated from the skin and gastrointestinal tract of clinically healthy free-ranging populations necessitates additional proof of the pathogenicity of bacterial isolates.

Aeromonas salmonicida is the only major non-motile aeromonad. *Aeromonas salmonicida* is principally a pathogen of fish although it has caused disease in a colony of the African clawed frog, *Xenopus laevis* (Frye, 1989). The source of infection was fresh Pacific salmon in the laboratory which presumably contaminated the tank water of the frogs. Clinical signs included reddened skin, dermal hemorrhages, and extensive dermal ulcerations. Necrosis of ulcerated tissues resulted in the loss of digits and exposure of patellae. *Aeromonas salmonicida massucida* was isolated from the internal organs of necropsied frogs.

Pure isolates of *Aeromonas hydrophila* from specimens of the Wyoming toad, *B. hemiophrys baxteri*, have been most susceptible *in vitro* to enrofloxacin, gentamicin, and neomycin. Resistance to ampicillin, amoxicillin, amoxicillin/clavulinic acid, cephalothin, erythromycin, lincomycin, penicillin, and sulfa/trimethoprim has been noted frequently. The sensitivity of these isolates to amikacin and advanced penicillins is unknown. When dealing with endangered species, further testing needs to be conducted on isolates in vitro, and in vivo in a surrogate species, to identify an antibiotic agent, dose, and route of administration that might be more efficacious and safe.

Aeromonas spp. have zoonotic potential and thus basic hygiene precautions should taken. In humans, *A. hydrophila* may cause soft tissue infections which are often a result of water-related trauma or consumption of contaminated water (Seidler et al., 1980; Slotnick, 1970). The organism has been isolated as the sole pathogen in cases of human diarrhea (Palumbo, 1993). Infection may be lethal in compromised individuals (Bulger & Sherris, 1966; Ketover et al., 1973).

Flavobacterium. Bacteria in the genus *Flavobacterium* are Gram-negative, aerobic rods (Holmes et al., 1984). *Flavobacterium indolgenes* has caused infection in a captive colony of the northern leopard frog, *Rana pipiens* (Olson et al., 1992). Affected frogs showed weight loss, swollen abdomens, corneal edema, uveitis, subcutaneous edema, petechial hemorrhage, incoordination, and respiratory distress. Necropsy revealed the coelomic cavity contained serosanguineous fluid and all visceral vessels were congested. In addition, lungs were congested, livers were enlarged and pale, and the myocardia were flaccid and pale. A portal of entry into the body and a high concentration of organisms were necessary to replicate the disease experimentally.

Edema syndrome has been associated with *Flavobacterium indolgenes* infection in both free-ranging and captive populations of the Wyoming toad, *Bufo hemiophrys baxteri*, as well as free-ranging larvae of the tiger salamander, *Ambystoma tigrinum*. In addition to subcutaneous edema or hydrocoelom, affected toads were frequently observed to have edematous tongues. Histologically, the skin showed scattered foci of ballooning degeneration in the epidermis. There was hepatocellular degeneration with variable sized eosinophilic bodies in the cytoplasm of many hepatocytes. The lesions in the liver were noninflammatory suggesting that a toxemia or physiologic change caused the hepatocellular swelling. Renal tubular degeneration and glomerulopathy frequently occurred. Eosinophilic fluid present in the renal tubules suggested that protein was being lost, possibly from endothelial damage within the glomeruli. Bacteria were not observed microscopically.

Pseudomonas. *Pseudomonas aeruginosa* is a Gram-negative rod that is commonly found in soil and water (Palleroni, 1984). It has been experimentally shown to induce mortality in the northern leopard frog, *Rana pipiens*, housed under suboptimal conditions (Brodkin et al., 1992). Affected frogs developed crouched posture, produced foam in the mouth, and were less responsive to stimuli. Their skin darkened and appeared more granular, and the limbs became splayed. Splenic mass was higher in the *P. aeruginosa*-inoculated group than in the saline controls.

Acinetobacter. Recurrent mass mortality attributed to *Acinetobacter haemolyticus* (*calcoaceticus*) has been reported in four free-ranging populations of the tiger salamander, *Ambystoma tigrinum*, in the Wasatch Mountains, Utah (Worthylake & Hovingh, 1989). The epizootic occurred in seepage lakes during late summer when extensive lowering of the water levels occurs. This leads to a concentration of nitrogen and results in a bacteria bloom which increased numbers of this

Gram-negative aerobic rod (Juni, 1984). Laboratory-housed salamanders exposed to this bacterium showed significant mortality.

Serratia. Bacteria belonging to the genus *Serratia* are common in the environment and have been recovered from both salt and fresh water, plants, insects, and mammals (Grimont et al., 1984). The organism is believed to affect almost exclusively an already compromised amphibian. *Serratia* spp. have been recovered from both healthy and diseased insects so these should be considered as a potential source of infection for captive amphibians (Hoff, 1984b).

Disease occurred when *Serratia anolium* was experimentally inoculated by intramuscular injection into the northern leopard frog, *Rana pipiens,* and the American toad, *Bufo americanus* (Clausen & Duran-Reynals, 1937). Four days after inoculation, swelling was present at the injection site. One month after inoculation, a postmortem examination indicated the frogs were septicemic.

Gram-positive bacteria. Nonhemolytic, group B *Streptococcus* isolates from amphibians and humans show similar whole-cell protein profiles (Elliott et al., 1990). Although this may indicate a shared common ancestor, frog isolates appear to have phenotypically adapted to amphibians and display both a different CAMP reaction and lack of growth in 4% NaCl. These differences suggest that zoonotic transmission would be unlikely.

A nonhemolytic, group B *Streptococcus* and unidentified stressors were thought to cause a fatal infection in a commercially reared colony of the bullfrog, *Rana catesbeiana* (Amborski et al., 1983). The epizootic resulted in the death of 80% of the estimated 100,000 frog population. Affected animals were characterized by necrotizing splenitis and hepatitis with hepatic and renal hemorrhage.

Staphylococcus epidermis has been implicated in dermatosepticemia of ranid frogs (Gibbs et al., 1966).

13.3.2 *Mycobacterium* spp.

Although the term tuberculosis has often been used when referring to amphibian mycobacterial infections, this is inaccurate and should not be applied to mycobacteria other than tubercle bacilli (Thoen & Schliesser, 1984). Acid-fast bacillary infections of amphibians should be referred to as mycobacterial infections or mycobacterioses. The epidemiology of mycobacterial infection in amphibians is different from the disease in birds and mammals. In amphibians, mycobacteriosis often presents as a disease of the integument, the pathogenesis of which is widely assumed to be secondary to dermal wounds, although ingestion is a proven route of infection in tadpoles (Nonidez & Kahn, 1937). Mycobacteria are ubiquitous in aquatic environments and are likely to be found in most, if not all, aquariums in which amphibians are kept (Brownstein, 1984; Elkan, 1976).

Several species of *Mycobacterium* have been isolated from amphibians. Isolates include *M. chelonei* subsp. *abscessus, M. (giae) fortuitum, M. marinum, M. ranae, M. thamnospheos,* and *M. xenopi,* although one review concluded that *Mycobacterium avium, M. marinum, M. fortuitum,* and *M. xenopi* are the only four species of *Mycobacterium* spp. affecting amphibians that have been isolated and adequately described (Thoen & Schliesser, 1984). This review suggested that all other previously described species are synonymous with these four, or were insufficiently described and the isolates have been lost so that their identities are unknown. The unrecognized or synonymous species are *M. abscessus, M. giae, M. ranae,* and *M. piscium.* Despite this debate, it is apparent that the list of susceptible species of amphibians either in larval or adult life stage is extensive (Table 13.3). Incidence of infections in amphibian populations has been reported as high as 20% (Brownstein, 1984). Several of these species (e.g., *M. chelonei* and *M. fortuitum*) are known to be saprophytic organisms (Mok & Carvalho, 1984). *Mycobacterium xenopi* and *M. marinum* are the most common isolates from the clawed frog, *Xenopus laevis* (Asfari, 1988; Schwabacher, 1959; Thoen & Himes, 1986), but spontaneous infection has not been reported in tadpoles of *X. laevis,* suggesting the incubation period may exceed the larval time period.

Mycobacteriosis often presents as multiple gray nodules of varying sizes in the skin, liver, spleen, respiratory tract, and intestinal tract. The digital tips, digital webs, lips, and the mouth are frequent sites of infection. Miliary lesions on the skin and hindlimbs also may be noted, and widely disseminated lesions may be found internally. The liver and the spleen consistently have granulomata in spontaneous mycobacterioses. The kidneys are often infected when there are lesions on the hindlimbs due to spread by lymphatics. Mucopurulent nasal and oral secretions containing large numbers of acid-fast bacilli have been observed, suggesting that a cephalic infection spreads to the respiratory system. Mycobacteriosis in the clawed frog, *Xenopus* spp., may present as a solitary massive granuloma in nearly any organ or tissue (Elkan, 1976), but this appears to be uncommon in terrestrial adult amphibians. By the time an amphibian is clinically abnormal, generalized disease is usually present. Miliary "tubercles" may be observed in many organs, but in the subclinical or early stages of mycobacteriosis, the intestines and liver are most consistently affected. Weight loss and emaciation are not consistent findings in mycobacteriosis. Wasting may occur in some amphibians despite a good appetite due to the compromise of the intestinal tract and associated organs from mycobacterial granulomas whereas other am-

Table 13.3. Species known to be susceptible to mycobacterioses. (Aronson, 1957; Asfari, 1988; Barros et al., 1988; Brownstein, 1984; Clark and Shepard, 1963; Clothier and Balls, 1973a, b; Elkan, 1960; Griffith, 1928; Joiner and Abrams, 1967; Mok and Carvalho, 1984; Nonidez and Kahn, 1937; Rowlatt and Roe, 1966; Schwabacher, 1959; Shively et al., 1981; Vogel, 1958)

Species	Common Name
Order CAUDATA	
Family Amphiumidae *Amphiuma* spp.	amphiuma
Family Plethodontidae *Desmognathus fuscus fuscus* *Desmognathus ochrophaeus* *Desmognathus monticola* *Desmognathus quadramaculatus* *Gyrinophilus porphyriticus danielsi* *Leurognathus marmoratus* *Plethodon cinereus* *Plethodon glutinosus* *Plethodon jordani* *Pseudotriton ruber ruber*	northern dusky salamander mountain dusky salamander seal salamander blackbelly salamander Blue Ridge spring salamander shovelnose salamander redback salamander northern slimy salamander Jordan's salamander northern red salamander
Family Salamandridae *Cynops pyrrhogaster*	Japanese firebelly newt
Order ANURA	
Family Bufonidae *Bufo bufo* *Bufo cognatous* *Bufo granulosus* *Bufo marinus* *Bufo valliceps* *Bufo woodhousei*	European common toad Great Plains toad common lesser toad giant toad Gulf Coast toad Woodhouse's toad
Family Hylidae *Acris* spp. *Pelodryas (Litoria) caerulea* *Pseudacris ocularis* *Pseudacris triseriata*	cricket frog White's treefrog little grass frog western chorus frog
Family Leptodactylidae *Leptodactylus pentadactylus* *Pleurodema cinerca* *Pleurodema marmoratus*	South American bullfrog Juliaca four-eyed frog marbled four-eyed frog
Family Pipidae *Xenopus borealis* *Xenopus laevis*	Marsabit clawed frog African clawed frog
Family Pseudidae *Pseudis paradoxa*	swimming frog (paradox frog)
Family Ranidae *Rana catesbeiana* *Rana clamitans clamitans* *Rana pipiens* *Rana tigrina*	bullfrog bronze frog northern leopard frog Indian bullfrog

phibians may become anorectic. The fat bodies may undergo serous atrophy and the muscles may be catabolized if the amphibian lives for any length of time once the gastrointestinal tract has been affected.

Culture of *Mycobacterium* spp. is frequently unsuccessful despite their obvious presence in the organs and secretions of the infected amphibian, making a definitive diagnosis difficult. Isolation should be attempted using Lowenstein-Jensen agar, and dual cultures attempted, i.e., one at room temperature and one at 37°C (98°F). Acid-fast staining of the isolate should be attempted, however not all mycobacteria will stain positive. The identification of *Mycobacterium* spp. using PCR technology is under development.

Isolates that grow at 37°C (98°F) are of greater zoonotic concern. Given the zoonotic potential and the fact that there is no known efficacious treatment for any mycobacterioses of amphibians, euthanasia of the affected individual and its cagemates is warranted. The enclosure should be stripped bare and all porous materials discarded. The items to be reused must be thoroughly cleaned with a detergent and sterilized with a tuberculocidal disinfectant or heat. Rinsing must be thorough as any detergent or disinfectant left behind could prove deleterious to future amphibian inhabitants. The enclosure should be evaluated to eliminate predisposing factors (i.e., a rough concrete surface), and the husbandry regimen should also be reviewed to determine any relevant environmental stressors (e.g., excessively cold temperatures, malnutrition, poor water quality, etc.).

The disease can be experimentally transmitted to other amphibians by exposure to suspensions of ground tissue. Rapidly occurring disease may be fatal without any gross pathologic changes (Aronson, 1957). Specimens of the giant toad, *Bufo marinus*, and the common lesser toad, *B. granulosus*, experimentally infected with *Mycobacterium chelonei* had histologically detectable mycobacteria 5 days postinfection, however deaths did not occur until approximately 50 days postinoculation (Mok & Carvalho, 1984). When the inoculum used corn oil as a carrier rather than saline, the severity of infection was increased greatly, attributed to impaired phagocytosis of the mycobacteria suspended in oil. Although irradiation, corticosteriods, and induced hibernation did not significantly alter the pathogenesis of the experimentally induced disease (Joiner & Abrams, 1967), it seems likely that these and other stressors play a role in naturally occurring disease.

Intentional and unintentional intracoelomic injections of mycobacteria have been reported in amphibians (Inoue & Singer, 1963; Mok & Carvalho, 1984). Depending on the dose, species, cultural growth stage of the mycobacteria, and the ambient temperature of the experimental amphibians, death due to generalized mycobacteriosis usually occurs in 60–90 days. Some intracoelomically injected amphibians developed granulomata in nearly all coelomic organs, with the spleen and liver most prominently affected, while in other studies, distinct gross lesions were not evident 60 days postinoculation (see also Section 27.2.3, Alimentary Tract, Infectious Etiologies—*Mycobacterium*).

While there is experimental evidence that zoonotic transmission may occur, evidence to support a widespread public health threat does not exist (Brownstein, 1984). There is no satisfactory treatment regime for infected amphibians. Precautions are warranted for those who choose to work with a suspected or confirmed case of mycobacteriosis. Disposable gloves should be worn whenever handling the amphibian or material contaminated with mycobacteria (i.e., substrate from a contaminated enclosure). Immunosuppressed people should not handle infected amphibians. All open wounds should be covered, preferably with a watertight bandage or gloves, and a germicidal soap should be used to wash hands after working with the amphibian or its enclosure.

13.3.3 *Chlamydia*

Chlamydia psittaci is a Gram-negative, nonmotile, membrane-bound coccoid organism (0.2–1.5 μm) that multiplies within the cells of its host (Moulder, 1984). Infections by *Chlamydia psittaci* have been reported to cause mortality in amphibians. For example, an epizootic caused by *Chlamydia psittaci* led to a mass mortality of approximately 20,000 of 40,000 captive specimens of the African clawed frog, *Xenopus laevis*, which were fed uncooked beef livers (Howerth, 1984; Howerth & Pletcher, 1986; Newcomer et al., 1982; Wilcke et al., 1983). Affected frogs exhibited lethargy, patchy depigmentation and petechiation of cutaneous surfaces, and appeared edematous. Frogs were observed at the surface of the water breathing more frequently. Clinically, this appeared similar to red leg syndrome. Upon necropsy subcutaneous edema, coelomic effusion, and hepatosplenomegaly were noted. Histologic lesions included granulomatous hepatitis, splenic congestion and extensive infiltration of histiocytes, and fibrinopurulent glomerulonephritis and interstitial nephritis. Electron micrographs revealed inclusion-laden livers that were pathognomonic of the genus *Chlamydia*, and isolation studies confirmed the agent to be *C. psittaci*.

Chlamydiosis was diagnosed in wild-caught specimens of Gunther's triangle frog, *Ceratobatrachus guentheri* (Honeyman et al., 1992). Disseminated granulomas and glomerulonephritis, hepatitis, and splenic histiocytosis were noted at necropsy, but these and other findings were complicated by bacterial septicemia attributed to *Bordetella bronchiseptica*. Intracytoplasmic granules compatible with *Chlamydia* spp.

were detected in most granulomas. Concomitant bacterial septicemias may occur often in frogs with chlamydial infection, thus screening postmortem specimens for chlamydial inclusions is recommended prior to assigning a final etiologic diagnosis. Doxycycline (5–10 mg/kg PO SID to BID), oxytetracycline (50–100 mg/kg IM q 48 h, 50 mg/kg PO SID, or 100 mg/L as a 1-h bath SID) or tetracycline (50 mg/kg PO BID) are suggested therapies for chlamydiosis (Wright, 1996). Concomitant therapy aimed at Gram-negative bacteria (e.g., amikacin, enrofloxacin) should be considered. Antibiotic prophylaxis is recommended for cagemates if exposure to chlamydiosis is confirmed.

13.3.4 Rickettsia

Despite several surveys for rickettsia in amphibians, few have been reported to occur (Hoff, 1984a; Yadav & Sethi, 1979). *Aegyptianella ranarum* sp. nov. was recorded from free-ranging specimens of the bullfrog, *Rana catesbeiana*, the green frog, *R. clamitans*, and the mink frog, *R. septentrionalis*, from southern Ontario, Canada (Desser, 1987). This organism occurs within the erythrocyte cytoplasm in membrane-bound vacuoles. No clinical disease was noted in the infected animals. Carriers of this organism were not identified among other amphibian species in this area.

13.4 NONPATHOGENIC ISOLATES WITH ZOONOTIC POTENTIAL

While there are many bacterial species that have been isolated from amphibians that appear nonpathogenic, several bacteria with zoonotic potential have been studied. This should not imply that amphibians are the source of transmission.

13.4.1 *Leptospira*

Isolation or serologic evidence of *Leptospira* spp. has occurred in the giant toad, *Bufo marinus*, the northern leopard frog, *Rana pipiens*, the edible frog, *R. esculenta*, and the rufous frog, *Leptodactylus fuscus* (Babudieri et al., 1973; Everard et al., 1988; Hoff & White, 1984). Kidney isolates from four of 211 free-ranging specimens of the giant toad, *B. marinus*, on Barbados yielded *L. interrogans* serovar bim (*Autumnalis*) (Everard et al., 1988). Serological testing, using the leptospire microscopic agglutination test, from 198 of these toads revealed positive titers of greater than 1:100 in 21% of the animals. The positive serogroups included Australis, Autumnalis, and Panama. Another serologic survey of the long-tailed salamander, *Eurycea longicauda*, the cave salamander, *E. lucifuga*, and the gray treefrog, *Hyla versicolor*, for sera leptospiral agglutins yielded none despite the fact that simultaneously collected reptiles were positive (Andrews et al., 1965).

Disease in amphibians has yet to be attributed to these Gram-negative flexible helicoidal bacteria (Johnson & Faine, 1984). It is not known why *Leptospira* spp. grow in ectothermic hosts, such as amphibians, but parasitize hosts of higher body temperature (Ellinghausen, 1968).

13.4.2 *Listeria*

Listeria monocytogenes has been noted to be long-lived in aquatic ecosystems, and has been isolated from the feces of healthy specimens of the northern leopard frog, *Rana pipiens*, and the bullfrog, *R. catesbeiana* (Botzler et al., 1973). Most of these isolations were made after heavy rains at ponds which were also used frequently by white-tailed deer, *Odocoileus virginiaus*. Experimentally, *L. monocytogenes* has also been shown to transfer between leopard frogs through either direct contact or through contaminated water (Botzler & Cowan, 1985). No lesions were associated with the oral inoculation of this organism. Experimental studies also demonstrated that orally inoculated frogs shed *L. monocytogenes* for 3–6 days, however shedding ceased by day 12 (Botzler et al., 1975).

13.4.3 *Salmonella*

Healthy amphibians have been reported to carry *Salmonella* spp., but there appear to be no reports of it causing clinical disease (Speare, 1990). These Gram-negative straight rods are ubiquitous in the aquatic environment and show no particular host preference (Hoff & Hoff, 1984; Minor, 1984). *Salmonella* spp. have been reported in amphibians from developing countries (Anver & Pond, 1984). The isolation of this bacteria is thought to reflect sewage contamination of their habitats. Amphibians may carry more than one species of *Salmonella* and isolates may exhibit multiple antibiotic resistance (Ang et al., 1973; Trust & Bartlett, 1979). It has been postulated that these animals may transmit the organism to other species which utilize the same water source (Sharma et al., 1974), but this has yet to be documented. Due to the zoonotic potential of many *Salmonella* serotypes, basic hygiene precautions should be taken to prevent transmission. The export trade of frog legs for human consumption is affected by *Salmonella* spp. contamination (Rao & Nandy, 1976).

Free-ranging frogs (unreported species) from India and Istanbul have been found to be healthy carriers of *Salmonella* spp. (Ang et al., 1973; Rao & Nandy, 1976; Saxena et al., 1980; Sharma et al., 1974). Species identified included *S. abony*, *S. anatum*, *S. arizonae*, *S. boecker*, *S. bovis-morbificans*, *S. brijbhumi*, *S. goverdham*, *S. hofit*, *S. hvittingfoss*, *S. kottbus*, *S. london*, *S. mikawaima*, *S. newbrunswick*, *S. newport*, *S. poona*, *S. reading*, *S. richmond*, *S. saint-paul*, *S. stanley*, *S. typhimurium*, *S. worthington*. A lesser treefrog, *Hyla minuta*, was found to carry *S. mendoza* while a South American bullfrog, *Leptodactylus pentadactylus,* from Panama carried *S. rubislaw* (Everard et al., 1979; Kourany et al., 1970). A *Salmonella* spp. was recovered from one hylid frog out of 67 amphibians that were surveyed through fecal culture as part of a routine animal health program at the Vancouver Aquarium (MacNeill & Dorward, 1986).

Aquatic frogs (i.e., clawed frogs, *Xenopus* spp., dwarf clawed frogs, *Hymenochirus* spp., and the Surinam toad, *Pipa pipa*) have been found to carry *Salmonella arizonae, S. bovis-morbificans, S. hadar, S. newport, S. saint-paul, S. typhimurium,* and *S. worthington* (Bartlett et al., 1977; Trust & Bartlett, 1979). Many of these isolates displayed resistance to 18 commonly prescribed antibiotics including erythromycin, kanamycin, nitrofurantoin, novobiocin, streptomycin, tobramycin, and triple sulfa, however all were susceptible to chloramphenicol, colistin, and polymyxin B. Newts (unreported species) have also been found to carry *S. worthington* (Trust et al., 1981).

Intestinal cultures of healthy free-ranging specimens of the giant toad, *Bufo marinus,* from Grenada, Panama, Surinam, and Trinidad, have yielded *Salmonella abaetetuba, S. amherstiana, S. anatum, S. arizonae, S. caracas, S. kaapstad, S. litchfield, S. london, S. mendoza, S. newport, S. oranienburg, S. panama, S. rubislaw, S. san diego, S. thompson,* and *S. typhimurium* (Bool & Kampelmacher, 1958; Everard et al., 1979; Kourany et al., 1970). Toads (unreported species) in India were found to carry *S. bareilly, S. goverdham, S. newport, S. richmond, S. typhimurium,* and *S. weltevreden* (Singh et al., 1979). Antibiotic resistance was found to bacitracin, novobiocin, and oleandomycin while sensitivity occurred to ampicillin, chloramphenicol, carbenicillin, cephaloridine, furazolidone, gentamicin, neomycin, kanamycin, polymyxin B, and streptomycin.

The detection of *Salmonella* spp. in an amphibian is problematic, and the presumption should be made that most, if not all, amphibians carry one or more *Salmonella* sp. at some point. The client should be cautioned about the zoonotic potential of these bacteria and advised on appropriate preventive practices as have been described for reptiles (Johnson-Delaney, 1996) and advocated by the Association for Reptilian and Amphibian Veterinarians (Bradley & Angulo, 1998). It is unlikely that treatment will eliminate *Salmonella* spp. from amphibians, and this should not be attempted. Clinically ill amphibians that are shedding *Salmonella* spp. are likely to have another primary illness and treatment should be aimed at the underlying cause rather than eliminating the *Salmonella* spp.

13.4.4 *Edwardsiella*

Edwardsiella spp. are Gram-negative motile straight rods (Farmer & McWhorter, 1984). Isolates of *Edwardsiella tarda* are commonly obtained from domestic, wild and marine mammals, as well as fish (White, 1984). In addition, the organism can be found in surface waters. Thus it is not surprising that *E. tarda* have been cultured from the intestinal contents of healthy amphibians. Clinical disease has yet to be associated with its recovery from an amphibian. A variety of cases support that this organism exists as an asymptomatic carrier state in amphibians (Sharma et al., 1974; White, 1984).

13.4.5 *Yersinia*

Yersinia enterocolitica has been isolated from free-ranging healthy specimens of the northern leopard frog, *Rana pipiens,* and a *Yersinia*-like sp. has been isolated from two specimens of the green frog, *R. clamitans,* from Michigan (Botzler et al., 1968). *Yersinia* are Gram-negative facultative anaerobes that may be straight rods or coccobacilli. These bacteria may be recovered from a broad range of habitats (Bercovier & Mollaret, 1984).

13.5 GERM-FREE STRAINS OF AMPHIBIANS

Attempts have been made to produce a germ-free strain of the northern leopard frog, *Rana pipiens,* for research, but this has not been achieved in a practical manner (Timmons et al., 1977). Producing a germ-free amphibian is dependent on feeding a germ-free food source, and studies have shown that bacteria isolated from the cloacae of amphibians have originated from the live arthropods offered as food (Vander Waaij et al., 1974). In addition, the amphibian's water source may become contaminated directly from these arthropods. Although the number of bacteria isolated from arthropods may be reduced by keeping these live food sources cold for a week, there is no practical way of eliminating bacteria in living arthropods.

13.6 BACTERIOLOGIC TECHNIQUES FOR THE DIAGNOSTIC LABORATORY

Basic culture techniques and identification characteristics for bacteriology may be found in many references (Carter & Chengappa, 1991; Krieg, 1984; MacFaddin, 1980; Sneath, 1986). It is essential to become familiar with the normal flora of amphibians and their environment. A specific bacterial profile may be developed for a species and its captive environment. While this may seem excessively time and labor consuming, such information may pinpoint sources of bacterial species. If culturing is done prior to a disease outbreak, the normal flora of the amphibian and environment may be compared to the flora associated with disease. Species-specific bacteriologic studies have been conducted or reviewed for the bullfrog, *Rana catesbeiana*, the northern leopard frog, *R. pipiens*, the giant toad, *Bufo marinus*, and the Wyoming toad, *B. hemiophrys baxteri* (Banas et al., 1988; Carr et al., 1976; Glorioso et al., 1974a; Gossling et al., 1982a, b; Speare, 1990; Taylor et al., 1995; Vander Waaij et al., 1974) (Table 13.4).

13.6.1 Specimen Samples

Bacterial cultures collected from live amphibians should include, at a minimum, blood cultures and fluid aspirates or swabs of the ventral skin and the cloaca. Gloves should be worn during sample collection to ensure bacterial cultures reflect the flora of the amphibian and not the hand of the person who restrained it.

Table 13.4. Bacteria generally considered nonpathogenic in amphibians. Although these bacteria may be isolated in diseased amphibians they are usually considered nonpathogenic and part of the normal flora isolated from an amphibian. If any of these species are isolated from blood or coelomic fluid, or are present at high densities, they may be part of the etiology of the illness. This list is based in part on Glorioso et al., 1974a and Taylor et al., 1995. (Compare to Table 10.1.)

- *Achromobacter* sp.
- *Acinetobacter lwoffi*
- *Alcaligenes faecalis*
- *Arizona* sp.
- *Bacillus cereus*
- *Bacillus megaterium*
- *Bacillus sphaericus*
- *Corynebacterium* sp.
- *Eikenella corrodens*
- *Enterobacter cloacae*
- *Enterobacter* sp.
- *Escherichia coli*
- *Gaffkya* sp.
- *Klebsiella ozaenae*
- *Leptospira* sp.
- *Micrococcus* sp.
- *Pasteurella* sp.
- *Pectobacterium* sp.
- *Plesiomonas shigelloides*
- *Proprionibacterium* sp.
- *Pseudomonas alcaligenes*
- *Pseudomonas maltophila*
- *Pseudomonas pickerii*
- *Pseudomonas pseudoalcaligenes*
- *Salmonella* sp.
- *Sarcinia lutea*
- *Shigella* sp.
- *Staphylococcus* sp.
- *Streptococcus* sp.
- *Vibrio* sp.

Sections of tissues or swabs from dead amphibians should include ventral skin, subcutaneous fluid, coelomic fluid, liver, lung, kidney, and intestine. We have found that culture of subcutaneous or coelomic fluid is the most reflective sample of systemic infection and provides the highest recovery of organisms. When collecting samples from postmortem specimens, it is important to alcohol flame necropsy instruments frequently between stages of the prosection. This will assist in preventing cross contamination of tissue samples. Tissues should be placed in separate sterile containers and sealed to prevent desiccation. Blood cultures, if obtainable, may be diagnostic of the etiologic agent involved in a septicemia. Specialized commercially prepared media systems for blood cultures are available (Carter, 1975).

In the event of multiple mortalities within a colony, environmental cultures should be obtained. These should include the surface of the terrestrial substrate, substrate of hiding or hut area, interface of aquatic/terrestrial substrate, exhibit water, water from tap source, water holding tank, food sources, and the caretakers' hands (prior to washing).

Sterile culture swabs containing bacterial transport medium (S/P Brand Culturette Systems, Baxter Diagnostics, Deerfield, IL) may be used to collect samples from these tissues or environments. Recovery of the organisms may be enhanced by moistening the swab first with the transport media and then collecting the sample. Tissues can be collected into sterile containers or plastic bags and sealed to prevent leakage or desiccation. Samples should be kept cold until inoculated onto media if there is a significant interval (i.e., greater than 1 hour) between collection and inoculation.

13.6.2 Culture Media

Most septicemias in amphibians appear to be caused by Gram-negative aerobic or facultative anaerobic organisms. At the Wyoming State Diagnostic Laboratory, the routine bacteriologic protocol for amphibian tissues is to plate the sample onto Columbia agar with 5% sheep blood. The plates are then routinely incubated at 35°C (95°F) in atmospheric air for 96 hours. If an anaerobic agent is suspected, then duplicate plates are placed in the anaerobe chamber.

Incubation temperature trials with samples collected from specimens of the Wyoming toad, *Bufo hemiophrys baxteri*, have supported the use of 35°C (95°F) for best recovery. Cultures incubated at cooler temperatures, such as those recommended for fish isolates, were less successful despite the fact that the Wyoming toad, *B. hemiophrys baxteri*, is a cold climate species. Warmer bacterial incubation temperatures in some species may increase isolation of bacteria because the amphibians bask and their microclimate is actually warmer than the macroclimate (see Chapter 4, Applied Physiology). It may be prudent to conduct incubation trials for a given amphibian species prior to disease outbreaks to determine appropriate incubation temperatures for that species. Each day plates should be examined for bacterial growth and colonies restruck for identification. All plates are held for 96 hours to allow for the culturing of all bacteria in the sample, even slow-growing species. Most veterinary diagnostic laboratories only incubate plates for 24–48 hours and thus extended incubation time should be specially requested for amphibian cultures.

13.6.3 Bacterial Identification

The interpretation of bacteriological reports generated from culturing amphibians may be challenging. The recovery of bacterial isolates is dependant on sample age, transport method, media selection, incubation temperature (Finegold & Baron, 1986), method of identification, and the experience of the microbiologist. To assist with identification by traditional biochemical methods, keys have been developed of known potentially pathogenic isolates (Glorioso et al., 1974b). Recent advances in bacterial identification systems now make this task rapid, affordable, as well as less labor and media intensive. In some instances, labor intensive identification methods are still required.

As with any microbial identification system it is the experience of the microbiologist that assures the quality and accuracy of the results. Experience provides the ability to identify commonly encountered colonies based on characteristics and morphology. It is always advisable to use reference strains from national culture collections for comparative purposes. The purity and use of the appropriate tests and methods with those tests determines accuracy of identification (Holt et al., 1994). Gram stains should be prepared on all isolates and morphology should be noted. Stains, such as Ziehl-Neelsen or Kinyoun, assist in identifying acid-fast bacteria (Carter, 1975; Clothier & Balls, 1973a; Mok & Carvalho, 1984; Shively et al., 1981). If *Chlamydia* spp. or rickettsiae are suspected, then appropriate cell cultures should be initiated (Newcomer et al., 1982).

Biochemical Reactions. Traditional bacterial identification utilizes individual biochemical reactions which characterize the organism. There are numerous references that can assist with identification (Carter & Chengappa, 1991; Krieg, 1984; MacFaddin, 1980; Sneath, 1986) (see also Chapter 10, Microbiological Techniques for the Exotic Practice). Keys have been developed to assist with the laboratory identification of bacterial pathogens of aquatic animals (Glorioso et al., 1974b). However, for small microbiology laboratories, such as those at most zoos and aquariums, identification through these tests may be labor intensive and yield a lengthy isolate identification time.

To assist with bacterial identification there are now commercial systems available that utilize a selected panel of biochemical tests placed in miniwell plates (e.g., Pasco Panels, Difco Laboratories, Detroit, MI). Thus, a miniature plate system combines approximately 20–50 tests onto a small hand-held plate. The range of tests included varies depending on the product and manufacturer, but typically includes tests of fermentation, oxidation, degradation and hydrolysis, and antibiotic sensitivity. The miniwell system, designed for mammalian isolates, uses sensitive indicators to detect metabolic end products (Woods, 1992). The resulting colorimetric changes are easily quantified using specially designed plate readers. In a study performed by the Centers for Disease Control, Gram-positive isolates were compared. This system identified 721/784 (92%) of the cultures correctly, as compared to traditional biochemical tubes. At the Wyoming State Diagnostic Laboratory this rapid system of identification has been accurate for identifying amphibian isolates to the genus level and then usually to the species.

Samples are plated onto blood agar (5% sheep blood) until appropriate growth occurs. Then isolates are placed in brain-heart infusion media and allowed to incubate for 4–6 hours at 37°C (98.6°F) in an enriched air incubator. (Note that this incubation temperature is 2°C (3.6°F) higher than the growing temperature used in the recovery and isolation phase.) A known aliquot of isolate-containing broth is then placed in a sterile solution and mixed. The resultant solution is then poured out on a plate and the inoculator plate is placed in the solution to allow contact with the isolate. The inoculator plate, which now contains the isolate, is dipped into the biochemical test plate to inoculate its wells. The plate is then incubated for 24 hours at 37°C (98.6°F) in atmosphere air. After incubation, the color changes and growth in wells can be recorded into a hand held computer. This compares the results to previously confirmed isolates and usually gives one to three choices with percentages on the most likely identification of the isolate. The computer also indicates test results that do not match up with the most likely choice. This provides the investigator the opportunity to recheck a result or conduct further investigation of the isolate.

The miniwell biochemical system is easy to use with minimal training. The system is rapid, and isolation identification can be obtained in approximately 24 hours. Few materials are needed to run this test, and unused plates can be stored in the freezer for several months. This method eliminates the expense of making and storing many different types of traditional tubes. In addition, it provides the second and third closest matches for comparison. Cost per isolate currently is about $3-5 U.S. dollars. The computer that identifies the isolates is approximately $300-500 U.S. This provides for an affordable system in the laboratory and saves personnel time.

The primary weakness of this system is the limited preselected set of standardized tests on the plate. In addition, reading color changes can be difficult when first becoming familiar with the system. If the plates are jostled, the solutions from adjoining wells can contaminate each other. Plates are stored frozen until use and are ruined if thawed and refrozen. Originally developed for identifying commonly encountered human isolates, it and other similar systems have yet to be evaluated for veterinary isolates (Salmon et al., 1995). It appears more accurate when used to identify isolates to the genus rather than to the species level for veterinary isolates. The computer's library of isolate profiles is not easily updated by the user. However, additional computer chips with increased databases can be purchased from the manufacturer. As with any automated system, experience and familiarity with the cultures provides the microbiologist with a level of expertise in determining whether they believe the colony morphology and characteristics are consistent with the machine's identification.

Carbon Source Utilization Systems. In 1995, the Wyoming State Diagnostic Laboratory began using a carbon source utilization test system (Biolog Panels, Biolog, Inc., Hayward, CA) with great success. After initial isolation of a bacterium, a spectrographically determined suspension is prepared and used to innoculate the miniwell plate, which is then incubated for 4-24 hours. The system is made up of approximately 95 tests in which utilization of a carbon source is detected as an increase in cellular respiration. A resultant color change can either be read manually or with an automated microplate reader. This data is then entered into a software program which compares the pattern to a library of over 800 bacterial species. The system can be customized and updated as needed. The library of this system includes human and veterinary isolates. This system offers rapid identification at a midprice range of $5 U.S. per isolate and a system cost of $15,000 U.S.

Initial trials comparing this method against other bacterial identification systems (miniwell plates or cellular fatty acid methyl ester gas-liquid chromatography) found that the carbon source utilization system is quite accurate. It has provided a rapid identification system that can identify isolates from both amphibians and aquatic/terrestrial environments accurately, usually with only 4 hours of incubation.

Cellular Fatty Acid Gas-Liquid Chromatography. Extremely accurate bacterial identification systems utilize gas-liquid chromatography to analyze cellular fatty acids (Microbial Identification System *MIDI*, Newark, DE). Within the bacterial cells, the fatty acid component is composed of species-specific compositions of methyl esters, dimethyl acetyls, aldehydes and other compounds. After extraction of these components from a bacterial isolate, they can be identified, quantified and compared to the database of bacteria with known compositions (Stoakes, et al., 1994). The gas-liquid chromatograph system utilizes a flame ion detector with an integrator to differentiate these compositions. Computer software is then utilized to rapidly compare the profiles with those known profiles in the database (Ghanem et al., 1991).

The process of extraction is summarized as follows: isolates are streaked into four quadrants on a Trypticase soy broth agar plate. After incubation for 24 hours at 25°C (77°F) in atmospheric air, isolate growth from the third and fourth quadrants are then taken and weighed. A standardized weight for all samples is essential. The cells of the isolate are ruptured, and then processed via saponification, fatty acid methylation, and extraction of methyl esters. Samples are then placed in a small gas-liquid chromatography vial with a crimp cap and can be analyzed immediately or frozen. The chromatograph can process numerous samples on autopilot overnight. The associated computer software is able to match bacterial fatty acid profiles, and provide a first, second, and third most likely choice as well as a percentage of certainty with each match. A known control bacteria is run with each batch of samples for quality assurance.

Cellular fatty acid gas-liquid chromatography appears to be accurate to the genus and species level. An analysis of bacterial fatty acids correctly identified 413/470 (87.8%) isolates of *Staphylococcus* spp. when compared to traditional biochemical methods (Stoakes et al., 1994). Of the 45 misidentified isolates, 36 isolates had the correct identification listed, but not as the first choice. The analysis was unable to identify the remaining twelve isolates. To test reproducibility, 78 isolates were recultured and processed. The identification of 73 isolates remained the same. However, the first and second identification choice was reversed in the remaining five isolates. A study on the identification of 686 isolates of 285 strains of *Clostridium* spp. used fatty acid gas-liquid chromatography (Ghanem et al., 1991). Depending on the strain of *Clostridium,* this system was able to identify the isolates correctly 89–100% of the time. This system has been analyzed for coagulase-negative Staphylococci (Kotilainen et al., 1991). In an analysis of 264 isolates, 92.4% were identified correctly as compared to traditional biochemical methods. Gas-liquid chromatography has been tested for identification of Gram-negative anaerobic bacilli (Stoakes et al., 1991). In an analysis of 225 isolates, it was accurate in identifying to the genus level 93.3% of the time. Further, it was accurate 88.9% of the time to group, and 72.4% to species level.

Strengths of the fatty acid analysis are that the procedure is quick, easy to perform, and highly reproducible. The chemicals involved have a long shelf life. The systems library or database can be constantly updated by the user. In addition, it becomes tailored to the species of isolates that one is investigating. These databases can be shared to expand their capabilities. With minimal training, after initial isolation, samples can be identified in 24–48 hours. The extraction process is labor intensive if only a few samples are being done, however with little experience 100 samples can be processed in 24 hours by one person. The materials and chemicals involved in extractions are relatively inexpensive.

The predominant weakness of fatty acid analysis is the prohibitive cost of the gas-liquid chromatography equipment and software (approximately $60,000–80,000 U.S.). Current commercial prices for isolate extraction and analysis is $50–80 U.S. per isolate, but the actual cost for running a sample is about $5 U.S. However, as the technology becomes more available and libraries of bacterial fatty acid profiles become larger, it is expected that cost per sample will decrease. Currently there are few institutions that are able to afford it, thus fatty acid analysis is predominantly a research tool.

Another weakness with this system is that errors can occur from not harvesting enough cells from the third and fourth quadrants of Trypticase soy broth agar plates. Many of the isolates do not grow proficiently on this media, thus two or more plates must be struck to achieve the desired sample weight. If samples are deficient in cells, then there will not be enough fatty acid components extracted. Errors can also occur if isolates are not pure. Strict adherence to the protocols for extraction are essential. These are precisely timed, and if something happens to delay a step in the extraction protocol, the samples are unusable. (Ghanem et al. 1991; Stoakes et al., 1994).

13.6.4 Bacterial Isolate Preservation

Bacterial isolates can be preserved for years. Once an isolate is pure, it can be placed in 1 ml of sterile brain-heart infusion within a 2 ml sterile cryogenic vial and stored at −70°C (−90°F). Vials that open with the lid fitting over the container, rather then screwing into the container are preferred. This decreases contamination if the lid inadvertently touches something. Room must be left in the vial for the media to expand upon freezing. Vials can be filled aseptically several months ahead of time and stored at room temperature. If there is microbial contamination of the vials, the media turns cloudy and should not be used. This characteristic can also be used to ensure the isolate is alive by leaving the inoculated media out at room temperature for several hours prior to freezing. Thawing can be achieved by placing vials in warm water for a short period of time. Many organisms lose viability during the thawing process and thus it is best to thaw them rapidly and immediately inoculate them onto suitable media (Carter, 1975). Amphibian bacterial cultures have been stored at the Wyoming State Veterinary Laboratory for over 3 years, and thawed and refrozen seven to eight times from the same vial with excellent viability.

13.6.5 Antibiotic Sensitivities

In vitro and in vivo testing needs to be conducted on pathogenic isolates obtained from amphibians to identify an antibiotic agent, dose, and route of administration that are efficacious and safe. Tissue concentrations and excretion rates also need to be determined.

The most common and easiest method of determining bacterial susceptibility to antibiotics is the disc susceptibility test (Carter, 1975; Carter & Chengappa, 1991). This method uses a suitable media placed on a plate which is then uniformly inoculated with a standardized quantity of the organism to be tested. Paper discs which are impregnated with an antimicrobial agent are then placed on the inoculated media. After incubation, the plate is observed for zones of bacterial inhibition around the discs. These areas are measured and the bacteria is determined to be susceptible or resistant to each antibiotic based on the size of the zone of inhibition. However, this process states nothing about the effectiveness of the drug in vivo.

Ideally, isolates are pure and bacterial species are individually plated for antibiotic sensitivity testing. However, in acute epidemics modified sensitivity tests may be done to attempt to obtain more rapid results. This entails taking the sample swab, after identification plating has been performed, and placing it in antibiotic inoculation system directly. Selection of the antibiotic is based on the widest zone of bacterial inhibition as mentioned above. This modified method is potentially useful if identification cultures and sensitivity cultures yield a predominant species, as may occur with a septicemia. If no single species predominates or the septicemia is caused by a slow-growing organism, this method will yield no advantage. In acute epidemics, it may support early decisions in antibiotic choice as plates can often indicate antibiotic sensitivity after only 8–12 hours of incubation.

REFERENCES

Abrams, G.D. 1969. Diseases in an amphibian colony, in Mizell, M. (Ed.): Biology of Amphibian Tumors. Springer-Verlag, New York, pp. 419–428.

Amborski, R.L., T.G. Snider, R.L. Thune, and D.D. Culley. 1983. A nonhemolytic, group B *Streptococcus* infection of cultured bullfrogs, *Rana catesbeiana*, in Brazil. Journal of Wildlife Diseases 19:180–184.

Ambrus, J.L., C.M. Ambrus, and J.W.E. Harrison. 1951. Prevention of *Proteus hydrophilus* infections (red leg disease) in frog colonies. American Journal of Pharmacology 123:129.

Andrews, R.D., J.R. Reilly, D.H. Ferris, and L.E. Hanson. 1965. Leptospiral agglutinins in sera from southern Illinois herpetofauna. Bulletin of the Wildlife Disease Association 1:55–59.

Ang, O., O. Ozek, E.T. Cetin, and K. Toreci. 1973. *Salmonella* serotypes isolated from tortoises and frogs in Istanbul. Journal of Hygiene 71:85–88.

Anver, M.R. and C.L. Pond. 1984. Biology and Diseases of Amphibians, in Fox, J.G., B.J. Cohen, and F. M. Loew (Eds): Laboratory Animal Medicine Academic Press, Inc., Orlando, FL, pp. 427–447.

Aronson, J.D. 1957. Tuberculosis of cold blooded animals: A review. Leprosy Briefs 8:21–32.

Asfari, M. 1988. *Mycobacterium*-induced infectious granuloma in *Xenopus*: Histology and Transmissibility. Cancer Research 48:958–963.

Babudieri, B., E.R. Carlos, and E.T. Carlos. 1973. Pathogenic *Leptospira* isolated from toad kidneys. Tropical and Geographical Medicine 25:297–299.

Banas, J.A., W.J. Loesche, and G.W. Nace. 1988. Classification and distribution of large intestinal bacteria in nonhibernating and hibernating leopard frogs (*Rana pipiens*). Applied and Environmental Microbiology 54:2305–2310.

Barros, G.C.D., C.H. Langenegger, J. Langenegger, and P.V. Peixoto. 1988. Surto de microbacteriose em criacao de ras (*Rana catesbeiana*) caseate per *Mycobacterium marinum*. Pesq. Vet. Braz. 8:75–80.

Bartlett, K. H., T. J. Trust, and H. Lior. 1977. Small pet aquarium frogs as a source of *Salmonella*. Applied Environmental Microbiology 33:1026–1029.

Bercovier, H. and H. H. Mollaret. 1984. Yersinia, in Krieg, N.R. and Holt, J.G. (Eds.): Bergey's Manual of Systemic Bacteriology (Volume 1). Williams and Wilkins Publishing, Baltimore, MD, pp. 489–506.

Blaustein, A.R., P.D. Hoffman, D.G. Hokit, J.M. Kiesecker, S.C. Walls, and J.B. Hayes. 1994. UV repair and resistance to solar UV-B in amphibian eggs: A link to population declines? Proceedings of National Academy of Sciences (USA) 91:1791–1795.

Bool, P.H. and E.H. Kampelmacher. 1958. Some data on the occurrence of *Salmonella* in animals in Surinam. Antonie van Leeuwenhoek 24:76–80.

Botzler, R.G. and A.B. Cowan. 1985. Transfer of *Listeria monocytogenes* between frogs. Journal of Wildlife Diseases 21:173–174.

Botzler, R.G., A.B. Cowan, and T.F. Wetzler. 1975. Rate of *Listeria monocytogenes* shedding from frogs. Journal of Wildlife Diseases 11:277–279.

Botzler, R.G., T.F. Wetzler, and A.B. Cowan. 1968. *Yersinia enterocolitica* and *Yersinia*-like organisms isolated from frogs and snails. Bulletin of the Wildlife Disease Association 4:110–115.

Botzler, R.G., T.F. Wetzler, and A.B. Cowan. 1973. *Listeria* in aquatic animals. Journal of Wildlife Diseases 9:163–170.

Boyer, C.I., K. Blackler, and L.E. Delanney. 1971. *Aeromonas hydrophila* infection in the Mexican axolotl, *Siredon mexicanum*. Laboratory Animal Science 21:372–375.

Bradford, D.F. 1991. Mass mortality and extinction in a high-elevation population of *Rana muscosa*. Journal of Herpetology 25:174–177.

Bradley, T. and F.J. Angulo. 1998. *Salmonella* and reptiles: veterinary guidelines. Bulletin of the Association of Reptilian and Amphibian Veterinarians 8(2):14.

Brodkin, M.A., M.P. Simon, A.M. DeSantis, and K.J. Boyer. 1992. Response of *Rana pipiens* to graded doses of the bacterium *Pseudomonas aeruginosa*. Journal of Herpetology 26:490–495.

Brooks, D.E., E.R. Jacobson, E.D. Wolf, S. Clubb, and J.M. Gaskin. 1983. Panophthalmitis and otitis interna in fire-bellied toads. Journal of the American Veterinary Medical Association 183:1198–1201.

Brownstein, D.G. 1984. Mycobacteriosis, in Hoff, G.L., F.L. Frye, and E.R. Jacobson (Eds.): Diseases of Amphibians and Reptiles. Plenum Press, New York, pp. 1–23.

Bulger, R.J. and J.C. Sherris. 1966. The clinical significance of *Aeromonas hydrophila*. Archives of Internal Medicine 118:562–564.

Cahill, M.M. 1990. A review: Virulence factors in motile *Aeromonas* species. Journal of Applied Bacteriology 69:1–16.

Carey, C. 1993. Hypothesis concerning the causes of the disappearance of boreal toads from the mountains of Colorado. Conservation Biology 7:355–362.

Carr, A.H., R.L. Amborski, D.D. Culley, and G.F. Amborski. 1976. Aerobic bacteria in the intestinal tracts of bullfrogs (*Rana catesbeiana*) maintained at low temperatures. Herpetologica 32:239–244.

Carter, G.R. 1975. Diagnostic Procedures in Veterinary Microbiology. Charles C. Thomas Publisher, Springfield, IL, 362 pp.

Carter, G.R. and M.M. Chengappa. 1991. Essentials of Veterinary Bacteriology and Mycology. Lea & Febiger, Philadelphia, PA, 284 pp.

Cartwright, G.A., D. Chen, P.J. Hanna, N. Gudkovs, and K. Tajima. 1994. Immunodiagnosis of virulent strains of *Aeromonas hydrophila* associated with epizootic ulcerative syndrome (EUS) using a monoclonal antibody. Journal of Fish Disease 17:123–133.

Chopra, A.K., T.N. Vo, and C.W. Houston. 1992. Mechanism of action of a cytotoxic enterotoxin produced by *Aeromonas hydrophila*. Federation of European Microbiological Societies (FEMS) Microbiology Letters 91:15–20.

Clark, H.F. and C.C. Shepard. 1963. Effect of environmental temperatures on infection with *Mycobacterium marinum* (balnei) of mice and a number of poikilothermic species. Journal of Bacteriology 86:1057–1069.

Clausen, H.J. and F. Duran-Reynals. 1937. Studies on the experimental infection of some reptiles, amphibia and fish with *Serratia anolium*. American Journal of Pathology 13:441–451.

Clothier, R.H. and M. Balls. 1973a. Mycobacteria and lymphoreticular tumours in *Xenopus laevis*, the South African clawed toad: Isolation, characterization and pathogenicity for *Xenopus* of *M. marinum* isolated from lymphoreticular tumour cells. Oncology 28:445–457.

Clothier, R.H. and M. Balls. 1973b. Mycobacteria and lymphoreticular tumours in *Xenopus laevis*, the South African clawed toad: Have mycobacteria a role in tumour initiation and development? Oncology 28:458–480.

Colt, J., K. Orwicz, and D. Brooks. 1984. Gas bubble disease in the African clawed frog, *Xenopus laevis*. Journal of Herpetology 18:131–137.

Cooper, J.E., J.R. Needham, and J. Griffin. 1978. A bacterial disease of the Darwin's frog (*Rhinoderma darwini*). Laboratory Animals 12:91–93.

Cunningham, A.A., T.E.S Langton, P.M. Bennett, S.E.N. Drury, R.E. Gough, and J.K. Kirkwood. 1993. Unusual mortality associated with poxvirus-like particles in frogs (*Rana temporaria*). Veterinary Record 133:141–142.

Desser, S.S. 1987. *Aegyptianella ranarum* sp. nov. (Rickettsiales, Anaplasmataceae): Ultrastructure and prevalence in frogs from Ontario. Journal of Wildlife Diseases 23:52–59.

Dusi, J.L. 1949. The natural occurrence of "redleg" *Pseudomonas hydrophila*, in a population of American toads, *Bufo americanus*. Ohio Journal of Science 49:70–71.

Elkan, E. 1960. Some interesting pathological cases in amphibians. Proceedings of the Zoological Society London 134:275–296.

Elkan, E. 1976. Pathology in the Amphibia, Chapter 6, in Lofts, B. (Ed): Physiology of the Amphibia, Volume 3. Academic Press, New York, pp. 273–312.

Ellinghausen, H.C. 1968. Cultural and biochemical characteristics of a Leptospire from a frog kidney. Bulletin of the Wildlife Disease Association 4:41–50.

Elliott, J.A., R.R. Facklam, and C.B. Richter. 1990. Whole-cell protein patterns of nonhemolytic group B, type Ib, Streptococci isolated from humans, mice, cattle, frogs, and fish. Journal of Clinical Microbiology 28:6628–630.

Emerson, H. and C. Norris. 1905. "Red-leg"—An infectious disease of frogs. Journal of Experimental Medicine 7:32–58.

Everard, C.O.R., D. Carrington, H. Korver, and J.D. Everard. 1988. Leptospiras in the marine toad (*Bufo marinus*) on Barbados. Journal of Wildlife Diseases 24:334–338.

Everard, C.O.R., B. Tota, D. Bassett, and C. Ali. 1979. *Salmonella* in wildlife from Trinidad and Grenada, W. I. Journal of Wildlife Diseases 15:213–219.

Farmer, J.J. and A.C. McWhorter. 1984. *Edwardsiella, in* Krieg, N.R. and Holt, J.G. (Eds.): Bergey's Manual of Systemic Bacteriology (Volume 1) Williams and Wilkins Publishing, Baltimore, MD, pp. 486–491.

Finegold, S.M. and E.J. Baron. 1986. Bailey and Scott's Diagnostic Microbiology. The CV. Mosby Co., St. Louis, MO, 914 pp.

Fox, G.A. 1992. Epidemiological and pathobiological evidence of contaminant-induced alterations in sexual development in free-living wildlife, *in* Colborn, T. and C. Clement (Eds.): Chemically-induced Alterations in Sexual and Functional Development: The Wildlife/Human Connection. Advances in Modern Environmental Toxicology, Volume 21. Princeton Scientific Publishing Company, Princeton, NJ, pp. 147–158.

Frye, F.L. 1989. *Aeromonas* and *Citrobacter* epizootics in an institutional amphibian collection [Abstr.] 3rd International Colloquium on Pathology of Reptiles & Amphibians, 13–15 January 1989, Orlando, FL, pp. 31–32.

Ghanem, F.M., A.C. Ridpath, W.E.C. Moore, and L.V.H. Moore. 1991. Identification of *Clostridium botulinum, Clostridium argentinense,* and related organisms by cellular fatty acid analysis. Journal of Clinical Microbiology 29:1114–1124.

Gibbs, E.L. 1963. An effective treatment for red-leg disease in *Rana pipiens*. Laboratory Animal Care 13:781–783.

Gibbs, E.L. 1973. *Rana pipiens*: Health and disease—How little we know. American Zoologist 13:93–96.

Gibbs, E.L., T.J. Giggs, and P.C. Van Dyck. 1966. *Rana pipiens*: Health and disease. Laboratory Animal Care 16:142–160.

Glorioso, J.C., R.L. Amborski, G.F. Amborski, and D.C. Culley. 1974a. Microbiological studies on septicemic bullfrogs (*Rana catesbeiana*). American Journal of Veterinary Research 35:1241–1245.

Glorioso, J.C., R.L. Amborski, J.M. Larkin, G.F. Amborski, and D.C. Culley. 1974b. Laboratory identification of bacterial pathogens of aquatic animals. American Journal of Veterinary Research 35:447–450.

Gossling, J., W.J. Loesche, and G.W. Nace. 1982a. Response of intestinal flora of laboratory-reared leopard frogs (*Rana pipiens*) to cold and fasting. Applied and Environmental Microbiology 44:67–71.

Gossling, J., W.J. Loesche, and G.W. Nace. 1982b. Large intestine bacterial flora of nonhibernating and hibernating leopard frogs (*Rana pipiens*). Applied and Environmental Microbiology 44:59–66.

Griffith, A.S. 1928. Tuberculosis in captive wild animals. Journal of Hygiene 28:198–218.

Grimont, P.A.D., F. Grimont, and M. Popoff 1984. *Serratia, in* Krieg, N.R. and Holt, J.G. (Eds.): Bergey's Manual of Systemic Bacteriology (Volume 1). Williams and Wilkins Publishing, Baltimore, MD, pp. 477–484.

Gross, T.S., L.J. Guillette, H.F. Percival, G.R. Masson, J.M. Matter, and A.R. Woodward. 1994. Contaminant-induced reproductive anomalies in Florida. Comparative Pathology Bulletin 26:1–8.

Gruia-Gray, J. and S.S. Desser, 1992. Cytopathological observations and epizootiology of frog erythrocytic virus in bullfrogs (*Rana catesbeiana*). Journal of Wildlife Diseases 28:34–41.

Hazen, T.C. 1979. Ecology of *Aeromonas hydrophila* in a South Carolina cooling reservoir. Microbial Ecology 5:179–195.

Hazen, T.C., C.B. Fliermans, R.P. Hirsch, and G.W. Esch. 1978. Prevalence and distribution of *Aeromonas hydrophila* in the United States. Applied and Environmental Microbiology 36:731–738.

Hird, D.J., S.L. Diesch, R.G. McKinnell, E. Gorham, F.B. Martin, S.W. Kurtz, and C. Dubrovolny. 1981. *Aeromonas hydrophila* in wild-caught frogs and tadpoles (*Rana pipiens*) in Minnesota. Laboratory Animal Science 31:166–169.

Hoff, G.L. 1984a. Q fever, *in* Hoff, G.L., F.L. Frye, and E.R. Jacobson (Eds.): Diseases of Amphibians and Reptiles. Plenum Press, New York, pp. 101–106.

Hoff, G.L. 1984b. *Serratia, in* Hoff, G.L., F.L. Frye, and E.R. Jacobson (Eds.): Diseases of Amphibians and Reptiles. Plenum Press, New York, pp. 59–67.

Hoff, G.L. and D.M. Hoff. 1984. *Salmonella* and *Arizona, in* Hoff, G.L., F.L. Frye, and E.R. Jacobson (Eds.): Diseases of Amphibians and Reptiles. Plenum Press, New York, pp. 69–82.

Hoff, G.L. and F.H. White. 1984. Leptospirosis, *in* Hoff, G.L., F.L. Frye, and E.R. Jacobson (Eds.): Diseases of Amphibians and Reptiles. Plenum Press, New York, pp. 93–100.

Holmes, B., R.J. Owen, and T.A. McMeekin. 1984. *Flavobacterium, in* Krieg, N.R. and Holt, J.G. (Eds.): Bergey's Manual of Systemic Bacteriology (Volume 1). Williams and Wilkins Publishing, Baltimore, MD, pp. 353–360.

Holt, J.C., N.R. Krieg, P.H.A. Sneath, J.T. Staley, and S.T. Williams. 1994. Bergey's Manual of Determinative Bacteriology, Ninth Edition. Williams and Wilkins Publishing, Baltimore, MD, 787 pp.

Honeyman, V.L., K.G. Mehren, I.K. Barker, and G.J. Crawshaw. 1992. *Bordetella* septicemia and chlamydiosis in eyelash leaf frogs. Proceedings of the Joint Conference of the American Association of Zoo Veterinarians and the American Association of Wildlife Veterinarians, p. 68.

Hoogesteyn, A.L. and M.D. Stetter. 1996. Oral paste, a new bandage for the treatment of skin lesions in amphibians. Bulletin of the Association of Reptilian and Amphibian Veterinarians 6(4):4–5.

Howerth, E.W. 1984. Pathology of naturally occuring chlamydiosis in African clawed frogs, *Xenopus laevis*. Veterinary Pathology 21:28–32.

Howerth, E.W. and J.M. Pletcher. 1986. Diagnostic exercise: death of African clawed frogs. Laboratory Animal Science 36(3):286–287.

Hubbard, G.B. 1981. *Aeromonas hydrophila* infection in *Xenopus laevis*. Laboratory Animal Science 31:297–300.

Hunsaker, D. and F.E. Potter. 1960. "Red leg" in a natural population of amphibians. Herpetologica 16:285–286.

Inoue, S. and H. Singer. 1993. Transmissibility and some histopathology of a spontaneously originated visceral tumor in the newt, *Triturus pyrrhogaster*. Cancer Research 23:1679–1684.

Johnson-Delaney, C.A. 1996. Reptile zoonoses and threats to public health, *in* Mader, D.R. (Ed.): Reptile Medicine and Surgery. W.B. Saunders Co., Philadelphia, PA, pp. 20–33.

Johnson, R.C. and S. Faine. 1984. Leptospiraceae, *in* Krieg, N.R. and Holt, J.G. (Eds.): Bergey's Manual of Systemic Bacteriology (Volume 1). Williams and Wilkins Publishing, Baltimore, MD, pp. 62–67.

Joiner, G.N. and G.D. Abrams. 1967. Experimental tuberculosis in the leopard frog. Journal of the American Veterinary Medical Association 151:942–949.

Joseph, S.W. and A. Carnahan. 1994. The isolation, identification, and systematics of the motile *Aeromonas* species. Annual Review of Fish Diseases 4:315–343.

Juni, E. 1984. *Acinetobacter, in* Krieg, N.R. and Holt, J.G. (Eds.): Bergey's Manual of Systemic Bacteriology (Volume 1). Williams and Wilkins Publishing, Baltimore, MD, pp. 303–307.

Kaplan, H.M. and L. Light. 1955. Evaluation of chemicals used in control and treatment of disease in fish and frogs caused by *Pseudomonas hydrophila*. American Journal of Veterinary Research 59:342–344.

Ketover, B.P., L.S. Young, and D. Armstrong. 1973. Septicemia due to *Aeromonas hydrophila*: Clinical and immunologic aspects. The Journal of Infectious Diseases 127:284–290.

Koivastik, T. 1950. An outbreak of "red-leg" disease in *Xenopus laevis* controlled with penicillin G. American Journal of Clinical Pathology 20:71–74.

Kotilainen, P., P. Huovinen, and E. Eerola. 1991. Application of gas-liquid chromatographic analysis of cellular fatty acids for species identification and typing of coagulase-negative Staphylococci. Journal of Clinical Microbiology 29:315–322.

Kourany, M., C.W. Myers, and C.R. Schneideri. 1970. Panamanian amphibians and reptiles as carriers of *Salmonella*. The American Journal of Tropical Medicine and Hygiene 19:632–638.

Krieg, N.R. 1984. Bergey's Manual of Systemic Bacteriology, Volume 1. Williams and Wilkins Publishing, Baltimore, MD, pp. 1–964.

Kulp, W.L. and D.G. Borden. 1942. Further studies on *Proteus hydrophilus,* the etiological agent in "red leg" disease of frogs. Journal of Bacteriology. 44:673–685.

Li, X. and N.S. Lipman. 1995. Peritoneal gorgoderiasis in a bullfrog (*Rana catesbeiana*). Laboratory Animal Science 45:309–311.

MacFaddin, J.F. 1980. Biochemical Tests for Identification of Medical Bacterial. Williams and Wilkins Publishing, Baltimore, MD, 527 pp.

MacNeill, A.C. and W.J. Dorward. 1986. *Salmonella* prevalence in a captive population of herptiles. Journal of Zoo Animal Medicine 17:110–114.

Martin, D. and H. Hong. 1991. The use of Bactine in the treatment of open wounds and other lesions in captive anurans. Herpetological Review 22:21.

Menard. M.R. 1984. External application of antibiotic to improve survival of adult laboratory frogs (*Rana pipiens*). Laboratory Animal Science 34:94–96.

Mika, J., M. Chadzinska, M. Stosik, and B. Plytycz. 1995. Bacterial survival in spleens of *Bombina variegata*, *B. bombina*, and *Rana esculenta*. Herpetopathologia (Proceedings of the 5th Internation Colloquium on the Pathology of Reptiles and Amphibians) 1995:129–133.

Miles, E.M. 1950. Red-leg in treefrogs caused by *Bacterium alkaligenes*. Journal of General Microbiology 4:434–436.

Minor, L.L. 1984. *Salmonella*, in Krieg, N.R. and J.G. Holt (Eds.): Bergey's Manual of Systemic Bacteriology, Volume 1. Williams and Wilkins Publishing, Baltimore, MD, pp. 427–458.

Mok, W.Y. and C.M. Carvalho. 1984. Occurrence and experimental infection of toads (*Bufo marinus* and *B. granulosus*) with *Mycobacterium chelonei* subsp. *abscessus*. Journal of Medical Microbiology 18:327–333.

Moulder, J.W. 1984. Chlamydiaceae, in Krieg, N.R. and J.G. Holt (Eds.): Bergey's Manual of Systemic Bacteriology, Volume 1. Williams and Wilkins Publishing, Baltimore, MD, pp. 729–739.

Newcomer, C.E., M.R. Anver, J.L. Simmons, B.W. Wilcke, and G.W. Nace. 1982. Spontaneous and experimental infections of *Xenopus laevis* with *Chlamydia psittaci*. Laboratory Animal Science 32(6):680–686.

Nonidez, J.F. and M.C. Kahn. 1937. Experimental tuberculosis infection in the tadpole and the mechanism of its spread. American Review of Tuberculosis 36:191–211.

Nygaard, G.S., M.L. Bissett, and R.M. Wood. 1970. Laboratory identification of Aeromonads from man and other animals. Applied Microbiology 19:618–620.

Nyman, S. 1986. Mass mortality in larval *Rana sylvatica* attributed to the bacterium, *Aeromonas hydrophila*. Journal of Herpetology 20:196–201.

Olson, M.E., S. Gard, M. Brown, R. Hampton, and D.W. Morck. 1992. *Flavobacterium indolgenes* infection in leopard frogs. Journal of the American Veterinary Medical Association 201:1766–1770.

Palleroni, N.J. 1984. Pseudomonadaceae, in Krieg, N.R. and J.G. Holt (Eds.): Bergey's Manual of Systemic Bacteriology (Volume 1). Williams and Wilkins Publishing, Baltimore, MD, pp. 141–218.

Palumbo, S.A. 1993. The occurrence and significance of organisms of the *Aeromonas hydrophila* group in food and water. Medical Microbiology Letters 2:339–346.

Paniagua, C., O. Rivero, J. Anguita, and G. Naharro. 1990. Pathogenecity factors and virulence for rainbow trout (*Salmo gairneri*) of motile *Aeromonas* spp. isolated from a river. Journal of Clinical Microbiology 28:350–355.

Parker, M.W., J.T. Buckley, J.P.M. Postma, A.D. Tucker, K. Leonard, F. Pattus, and D. Tsernoglou. 1994. Structure of the *Aeromonas* toxin proaerolysin in its water-soluble and membrane-channel states. Nature 367:292–299.

Paul, K.S. and D.L. Dillehay. 1991. Diagnostic exercise: High mortality in leopard frogs (*Rana pipiens*). Laboratory Animal Science 41:169–170.

Pazzaglia, G. 1993. Studies of virulence and mechanisms of pathogenesis in *Aeromonas* species. Doctorate of Science Dissertation, Johns Hopkins University, MD, 401 pp.

Penner, J.L. 1984. *Providencia*, in Krieg, N.R. and J.G. Holt (Eds.): Bergey's Manual of Systemic Bacteriology, (Volume 1). Williams and Wilkins Publishing, Baltimore, MD, pp. 495–496.

Popoff, M. 1984. *Aeromonas*, in Krieg, N.R. and J.G. Holt (Eds.): Bergey's Manual of Systemic Bacteriology, (Volume 1). Williams and Wilkins Publishing, Baltimore, MD, pp. 545–548.

Rao, N.M. and S.C. Nandy. 1976. *Salmonella* and other enterobacteriaceae group of organisms associated with meat meal, bone meal and frog legs. Indian Journal of Microbiology 16:120–126.

Reed, G.B. and G.C. Toner. 1942. *Proteus hydrophilus* infections of pike, trout, and frogs. Canadian Journal of Research 20:161–166.

Rigney, M.M., J.W. Zilinsky, and M.A. Rouf. 1978. Pathogenicity of *Aeromonas hydrophila* in red leg disease in frogs. Current Microbiology 1:175–179.

Rouf, M.A. and M.M. Rigney. 1971. Growth temperatures and temperature characteristics of *Aeromonas*. Applied Microbiology 22:501–506.

Rowlatt, U.F. and F.J.C. Roe. 1966. Generalized tuberculosis in a South American frog, *Leptodactylus pentadactylus*. Pathologica Veterinarius 3:451–469.

Russell, F.H. 1898. An epidemic, septicemic disease among frogs due to the *Bacillus hydrophilus fuscus*. Journal of the American Medical Association 30:1442–1449.

Sakazaki, R. 1984. *Citrobacter*, in Krieg, N.R. and J.G. Holt (Eds.): Bergey's Manual of Systemic Bacteriology, (Volume 1). Williams and Wilkins Publishing, Baltimore, MD, pp. 458–461.

Salmon, S.A., J.L. Watts, R.D. Walker, R.J. Yancey, Jr. 1995. Evaluation of a commercial system for the identification of gram-negative, nonfermenting bacteria of veterinary importance. Journal of Veterinary Diagnostic Investigations 7:161–164.

Saxena, S.N., S. Ahuja, M.L. Mago, and H. Singh. 1980. *Salmonella* pattern in India. Indian Journal of Medical Research. 72:159–168.

Schwabacher, H. 1959. A strain of *Mycobacterium* isolated from skin lesions of a cold-blooded animal, *Xenopus laevis*, and its relation to atypical acid-fast bacilli occurring in man. Journal of Hygiene 57:57–67.

Seidler, R.J., D.A. Allen, H. Lockman, R.R. Colwell, S.W. Joseph, and O.P. Daily. 1980. Isolation, enumeration, and characterization of *Aeromonas* from polluted waters encountered in diving operations. Applied and Environmental Microbiology 39:1010–1018.

Sharma, V.K., Y.K. Kaura, and I.P. Singh. 1974. Frogs as carriers of *Salmonella* and *Edwardsiella*. Antonie van Leeuwenhoek 40:171–175.

Shively, J.N., J.G. Songer, S. Prchal, M.S. Keasey, and C.O. Thoen. 1981. *Mycobacterium marinum* infection in Bufonidae. Journal of Wildlife Diseases 17:3–7.

Shotts, E.B. 1984. *Aeromonas*, in Hoff, G.L., F.L. Frye, and E.R. Jacobson (Eds.): Diseases of Amphibians and Reptiles. Plenum Press, New York, pp. 49–57.

Singh, S., V.D. Sharma, and M.S. Sethi. 1979. Toads as reservoirs for salmonellae: Prevalence and antibiogram. International Journal of Zoonoses 6:82–84.

Slotnick, I.J. 1970. *Aeromonas* species isolates. Annals New York Academy of Sciences 174:503–510.

Smith. S.W. 1950. Chloromycetin in the treatment of "Red leg". Science 112:274–275.

Sneath, P.H. 1986. Bergey's Manual of Systemic Bacteriology, (Volume 2). Williams and Wilkins Publishing, Baltimore, MD, pp. 965–1599.

Speare, R. 1990. A review of the diseases of the cane toad, *Bufo marinus*, with comments on biological control. Australian Wildlife Res., 17:387–410.

Speare, R., K. Field, J. Koehler, and K. McDonald. 1994. Disappearing Australian rainforest frogs: Have we found the answer? [Abstr.] FrogLog #9:2.

Stoakes, L., T. Kelly, B. Schieven, D. Harley, M. Ramos, R. Lannigan, D. Groves, and Z. Hussain. 1991. Gas-liquid chromatography of cellular fatty acids for identification of gram-negative anaerobic bacilli. Journal of Clinical Microbiology 29:2636–2638.

Stoakes, L., M.A. John, R. Lannigan, B.C. Schieven, M. Ramos, D. Harley, and Z. Hussain. 1994. Gas-liquid chromatography of cellular fatty acids for identification of Staphylococci. Journal of Clinical Microbiology, 32:1908–1910.

Taylor, F.R., R.C. Simmonds, and D.G. Loeffler. 1993. Isolation of *Flavobacterium meningosepticum* in a colony of leopard frogs (*Rana pipiens*). Laboratory Animal Science 43:105.

Taylor, S.K., E.S. Williams, K.W. Mills, A.M. Boerger-Fields, C.J. Lynn, C.E. Hearne, E.T. Thorne, and S.J. Pistono. 1995. A review of causes of mortality and the diagnostic investigation for pathogens of the Wyoming toad (*Bufo hemiophrys baxteri*). US Fish & Wildlife Service, Cheyenne, WY, 37 pp.

Thoen, C.O. and E.M. Himes. 1986. *Mycobacterium*, chapter 4, in Gyles, C.L. and C.O. Thoen (Eds.): Pathogenesis of Bacterial Infections in Animals. Iowa State University Press, Ames, IA, pp. 26–37.

Thoen, C.O. and T. Schliesser. 1984. Mycobacterial infections in cold-blooded animals, in Kubica, G.F. and L.G. Wayne (Eds.): The Mycobacteria: A Sourcebook. Dekker-Marcel, New York. pp. 1297–1311.

Timmons, E.H., G.M. Olmsted, and H.K. Kaplan. 1977. The germfree leopard frog (*Rana pipiens*): Preliminary report. Laboratory Animal Science 27:518–521.

Trust, T.J. and K.H. Bartlett. 1979. Aquarium pets as a source of antibiotic-resistant salmonellae. Canadian Journal of Microbiology 25:535–541.

Trust, T.J., K.H. Bartlett, and H. Lior. 1981. Importation of salmonellae with aquarium species. Canadian Journal of Microbiology 27:500–504.

Vander Waaij, D., B.J. Cohen, and G.W. Nace. 1974. Colonization patterns of aerobic gram-negative bacteria in the cloaca of *Rana pipiens*. Laboratory Animal Science 24:307–312.

Vogel, H. 1958. Mycobacteria from cold-blooded animals. American Review of Tuberculosis and Pulmonary Disease 77:823–838.

White, F.H. 1984. *Edwardsiella tarda*, in Hoff, G.L., F.L. Frye, and E.R. Jacobson (Eds.): Diseases of Amphibians and Reptiles. Plenum Press, New York, pp. 83–92.

Wilcke, B.W., C.E. Newcomer, M.R. Anver, J.L. Simmons, and G.W. Nace. 1983. Isolation of *Chlamydia psittaci* from naturally infected African clawed frogs, *Xenopus laevis*. Infection and Immunology 41:789–794.

Wolf, K., G.L. Bullock, C.E. Dunbar, and M.C. Quimby. 1968. Tadpole edema virus: A viscerotropic pathogen for anuran amphibians. Journal of Infectious Disease 118:253–262.

Wolf, K., G.L. Bullock, C.E. Dunbar, and M.C. Quimby. 1969. Tadpole edema virus: Pathogenesis and growth studies and additional studies of virus-infected bullfrog tadpoles, *in* Mizell, M. (Ed.): Biology of Amphibian Tumors. Springer-Verlag, New York, pp. 327–336.

Woods, G.L. 1992. Automation in clinical microbiology. American Journal of Clinical Pathology, Supplement 1, 98:S22–S30.

Worthylake, K.M. and P. Hovingh. 1989. Mass mortality of salamanders (*Ambystoma tigrinum*) by bacteria (*Acinetobacter*) in an oligotrophic seepage mountain lake. Great Basin Naturalist 49:364–372.

Wright, K.M. 1996. Chlamydial infections of amphibians. Bulletin of the Association of Reptilian and Amphibian Veterinarians 6(4):8–9.

Yadav, M.P. and M.S. Sethi. 1979. Poikilotherms as reservoirs of Q-fever (*Coxiella burnetii*) in Uttar Pradesh. Journal of Wildlife Diseases 15:15–17.

Zapata, A.G., A. Varas, and M. Torroba. 1992. Seasonal variations in the immune system of lower vertebrates. Immunology Today 13:142–147.

Zasloff, M. 1987. Magainins, a class of antimicrobial peptides from *Xenopus* skin: Isolation, characterization of two active forms, and partial cDNA sequence of a precursor. Proceedings of the National Academy of Science 84:5449–5453.

CHAPTER 14
MYCOSES

Sharon K. Taylor, DVM, PhD

14.1 INTRODUCTION

Although moist soils of the interface between aquatic and terrestrial environments provide favorable conditions for a diversity of potentially pathogenic fungi, the literature contains relatively few reports of amphibian mycoses (e.g., Reichenbach-Klinke & Elkan, 1965). Mycotic infections in mammalian species manifest almost exclusively in those which have undergone severe physical stress, injury, and/or immunosuppression. (Ajello, 1988; Koneman & Roberts, 1985; Rippon, 1982; Roberts, 1986). While there has been little research to evaluate potential predisposing factors, most amphibian mycoses are associated with compromised individuals (Anver & Pond, 1984).

Until recently there have been no mycotic epizootics known to occur in amphibians reported (Marcus, 1981), but current studies have now identified several significant mycotic pathogens in amphibians (Blaustein et al., 1994; Taylor et al., 1995). Epizootics involving horizontal transmission of infections in free-ranging juvenile and adult amphibians are extremely rare. These age classes of animals often live solitary lives and are not as likely to become infected directly from other amphibians as are the larval forms which may be found in large aggregations. The exception to the solitary lifestyle of the postmetamorphic amphibian occurs during the breeding season when congregations may occur around bodies of water such as ponds and ephemeral pools (Anver & Pond, 1984). In captive situations amphibians are often group-housed and horizontal transmission is more likely to occur. Historically, fungi found on egg masses and larva were reported as postmortem growth. However, more recent investigations have demonstrated that some of these same fungi can be primary pathogens to the developing amphibian embryo (Blaustein et al., 1994; Villa, 1979).

Amphibian species have varying immunologic reactions to mycotic infections. Some species have giant cells that appear to engulf fungal elements, apparently a reaction to the presence of the fungus (Elkan & Reichenbach-Klinke, 1974). This cellular response is lacking in other species such as the Wyoming toad, *Bufo hemiophrys baxteri*, which have a 100% fatality associated with untreated mycotic dermatitis (Taylor et al., 1995). There may also be seasonal variations in amphibian immune system structures and susceptibility to infectious organisms (Cooper et al., 1992; Zapata et al., 1992).

Although there has been the opinion that most species of fungi that affect amphibians are not potential human pathogens (Cosgrove, 1977), there is concern that many of the fungi species described within this chapter are capable of being zoonotic (Davis et al., 1994; Rippon, 1982; Schmidt & Hartfiel, 1977). Disposable gloves should always be worn when handling amphibians suspected of mycotic infections to reduce the potential of human exposure. Masks to prevent inhalation of infective elements are suggested as an additional precaution when handling animals with external lesions and during necropsies of infected amphibians.

14.2 LOCALIZED MYCOSES

14.2.1 Mycotic Dermatitis

Mycotic dermatitis should be considered in amphibians displaying signs consistent with red leg syndrome. Organisms known to cause mycotic dermatities are *Basidiobolus ranarum*, *Mucor* spp., *Saprolegnia* spp., *Cladosporium* spp., *Ichthyophonus* sp., a chytridiomycete, and others. Due to its federal status as an endangered species, considerable attention has been given to the Wyoming toad, *Bufo hemiophrys baxteri,* and a large body of knowledge has been established concerning mortality associated with *Basidiobolus* dermatitis. Likewise chromoblastomycosis is heavily represented in the literature because it has been associated with large anurans that are prominent exhibit animals in zoos. Unfortunately there exists broad gaps in the understanding of fungal infections of amphibians, and much of the knowledge is based on pathology rather than treatment of the disease.

Basidiobolus ranarum. *Basidiobolus ranarum* is a widespread saprophytic fungus of the family Entomophthoraceae (Coremans-Pelseneer, 1973; Drechsler 1952, 1964). This organism was first isolated from healthy frog intestines in 1886 and has since been cultured from feces and the intestinal lining of many species of amphibians. *Basidiobolus* spp. isolates have been recovered from feces of a wide variety of healthy amphibians (Drechsler, 1956; Hutchinson & Nickerson, 1970; Nickerson & Hutchinson, 1971; Okafor et al., 1984; Robinow, 1963; Tills, 1974; Zahari et al., 1990) (see Table 14.1). The spores of this fungus have also been identified in cultures from the mouth of the Spanish ribbed newt, *Pleurodeles waltll* (Reichenbach-Klinke & Elkan, 1965).

A fatal cutaneous entomophthoromycosis of amphibians caused by *Basidiobolus ranarum* was first reported in postmetamorphic individuals of the western dwarf clawed frog, *Hymenochirus curtipes*, in a private culture facility (Groff et al., 1991). This epizootic resulted in a morbidity and mortality rate of almost 100% and affected 10,000 animals. Studies conducted during this outbreak indicated that transmission occurred with cohabitation of infected moribund animals but not with exposure to fungal broth culture suspensions. Treatment consisted of baths of benzalkonium chloride (2.0 mg/L for 30 min q 48 h for three treatments, then 5 nontreatment days followed by treatment with the same regimen.) This reqimen reduced mortality to 10%.

Basidiobolus ranarum is the etiologic agent of a fatal mycotic dermatitis in free-ranging and captive specimens of the Wyoming toad, *Bufo hemiophrys baxteri*, captive specimens of the Canadian toad, *B. hemiophrys hemiophrys*, and captive specimens of the northern leopard frog, *Rana pipiens*. These specimens were collected from different geographic locations and housed at separate captive facilities. The condition occurs with a higher incidence in the fall and appears to affect only adults of the population of Wyoming toad, *Bufo hemiophrys baxteri*. First observable signs included sitting in water for a prolonged period, darkening of dorsal skin, and a constant hunching or arching of their backs. Digits became hyperemic (Plate 14.1). Affected toads developed hyperemia and sloughing of the ventral skin (Plate 14.2). These clinical signs commonly progressed until death occurred, usually within 5 days. Hepatomegaly was the only consistent post-mortem finding, with the livers appearing mottled with gray (Plate 14.3). Specimens of the northern leopard frog, *R. pipiens*, displayed hyperemia of ventral abdominal skin but no sloughing.

Periodic acid-Schiff (PAS)-stained impression smears from skin lesions may reveal spherules sugges-

Table 14.1. Amphibians known as asymptomatic carriers of *Basidiobolus ranarum*.

CAUDATA	
Ambystomatidae	
Spotted salamander	*Ambystoma maculatum*
Marbled salamander	*A. opacum*
Smallmouth salamander	*A. texanum*
Plethodontidae	
Dusky salamander	*Desmognathus fuscus*
Seal salamander	*D. monticola*
Northern two-lined salamander	*Eurycea bislineata*
Longtail salamander	*E. longicauda*
Cave salamander	*E. lucifuga*
Many-ribbed salamander	*E. multiplicata*
Redback salamander	*Plethodon cinereus*
Zigzag salamander	*P. dorsalis*
Northern slimy salamander	*P. glutinosus*
Grotto salamander	*Typhlotriton spelaeus*
Proteidae	
Mudpuppy	*Necturus maculosus*
Salamandridae	
Red-spotted newt (efts)	*Notophthalmus viridescens*
Spanish ribbed newt	*Pleurodeles waltll*
ANURA	
Bufonidae	
American toad	*Bufo americanus*
Fowler's toad	*B. woodhousei fowleri*
Giant toad	*B. marinus*
Southern toad	*B. terrestris*
Hylidae	
Northern cricket frog	*Acris crepitans*
Green treefrog	*Hyla cinerea*
Gray treefrog	*H. versicolor*
Microhylidae	
Eastern narrowmouth toad	*Gastrophryne carolinensis*
Pelobatidae	
Eastern spadefoot toad	*Scaphiopus holbrooki*
Ranidae	
Green frog	*Rana clamitans*
Bullfrog	*R. catesbeiana*
Edible frog	*R. esculenta*
Southern leopard frog	*R. utricularia*

tive of *Basidiobolus ranarum* (Plates 14.4, 14.5) while Gomori's methenamine silver (GMS) stained smears were often negative. Histologically, sections of skin from affected specimens of the Wyoming toad, *Bufo hemiophrys baxteri*, were characterized by invasion of numerous fungal spherules and occasional hyphae in the superficial layers of the epidermis without significant inflammatory reaction. The skin of the toes contained fungi which normally did not invade into the underlying dermis. Microscopically, the hepatocytes were swollen but the livers lacked inflammatory reaction, suggesting toxemia or physiologic change caused the hepatocellular swelling. Livers were also noted to contain pigment-bearing macrophages. In fish, this has been reported to be a sign of chronic inflammatory response (Ferguson, 1989). It is likely that these fungal lesions may provide an avenue for secondary bacterial invasion and subsequent toxemia.

Basidiobolus ranarum has been isolated from postmortem mycologic cultures of sections of ventral skin and toes (not scrapings) in approximately 50% of the cases. This organism is easily identified based on its distinctive "beaked" zygospores (Plate 14.6) and *Streptomyces*-like odor (Drechsler, 1958). Postmortem PAS-stained impression smears of the ventral skin can confirm the diagnosis rapidly and allow early treatment of animals. The efficacy of impression smears as a screening tool for detecting subclinically affected animals is under investigation. A negative impression smear should not be used as a rule out for infection.

Although *Basidiobolus ranarum* can be found in apparently healthy amphibians, untreated amphibians showing signs of *Basidiobolus* dermatitis experience 100% mortality. Success has been achieved in initial trials with itraconazole in both subspecies of the Canadian toad, *Bufo hemiophrys* spp. This drug is a synthetic triazole antifungal agent that inhibits the cytochrome P-450 dependent synthesis of ergosterol, which is a vital component of fungal cell membranes. Itraconazole (Sporanox, Janssen Pharmaceutica, Titusville, NJ) was administered as a dose of one bead from an opened 100-mg capsule orally in 0.1 ml of water once a day for 9 d to each toad (average weight 30 g). Within 3 days of treatment the ventral skin showed decreased hyperemia. After 5 days abdominal edema occurred and, when handled, toads urinated large quantities. Dorsal skin darkened progressively and animals also became hunched up and appeared to experience severe pain upon being handled. However, within 48 h of treatment, all skin coloration had returned to normal, the hunching of the back discontinued, and the abdominal edema ceased. The abnormal posture and abdominal edema may be indicators of nephrotoxicity from the drug. No toads were sacrificed to determine possible renal or other pathology and all have survived more than a year following treatment. Specimens of the Wyoming toad, *B. hemiophrys baxteri*, that weighed 25–45 g and given this same dose did not demonstrate the adverse affects seen in the Canadian toad, *B. hemiophrys hemiophrys*. However, since this dose was not very accurate, and there are inactive carriers in the itraconazole beads, the differing reactions and response to treatment may be reflective of widely varying dosages of itraconazole given to different patients. Since itraconazole is more readily dissolved in acidic solutions, a more accurate dosage may be achieved by dissolving a capsule in orange juice and white vinegar and using this solution for oral dosing (personal communication, W. Suedemeyer). Recently, a liquid form of itraconazole has become available. There also may be better bioavailability if taken with a fatty meal. Itraconazole dosages from 2–10 mg/kg PO q 24 h has been used in some amphibians (see Chapter 24, Pharmacotherapeutics).

Basidiobolus ranarum is known to have chitinolytic activity (Gugnani & Okafor, 1980), and the organism has been recovered from feed crickets cultured by this author. Thus the amphibian's predominant food base in captivity, the cricket, may be responsible for the presence of this organism in the gastrointestinal tract of "normal" amphibians.

Human mycoses have been reported from *Basidiobolus* spp. but earlier cases that were attributed to *B. ranarum* were later debated (Eades & Corbel, 1979; Greer & Friedman, 1964, 1966; Hutchinson et al., 1972; Williams, 1969). This etiologic agent has been confirmed to cause clinical disease in humans (Davis et al., 1994).

Mucor spp. Although *Mucor* spp. are usually considered nonpathogenic contaminants (Rippon, 1982), a *Mucor* sp. was identified in four cases of a fatal mycotic dermatitis in captive specimens of the Wyoming toad, *Bufo hemiophrys baxteri*. The affected toads were being hormonally stimulated for breeding when all died within 4 days of each other while toads in nearby tanks were not affected. The condition had a rapid onset and appeared as multiple raised nodules of about 2 mm in circumference on the ventral abdominal skin (Plate 14.7). Mycotic cultures of the nodules from all toads grew pure isolates of a *Mucor* sp. (Plate 14.8). Histological sections of the skin revealed characteristic uniform hyphae (Plate 14.9). Sections of other major organs did not demonstrate systemic mycosis.

Saprolegniasis. Species of watermolds (Oomycetes, Diplomastigomycotine) are common in aquatic environments and are opportunistic pathogens known to infect amphibians with abraded skin. White cottony growths on the skin and gills usually are due to one of several genera of watermolds, including *Saprolegnia, Achyla, Aphanomyces, Leptolegnia,* and others. Watermolds have a complex life cycle that includes multiple propagative stages. During sexual and asexual reproductive stages, oospores, zoospores, gemma, and hyphae may be produced. Some spores are thick-walled to resist environmental extremes (oospores), while others are flagellated and free-swimming (zoospores) and may repeatedly encyst and hatch into zoospores. It is not clear whether both the 5–25 micron diameter oospores and zoospores are infective to aquatic animals (Noga, 1993a). (For additional information on the life cycle of Oomycetes, see Neish & Hughes, 1980; Noga, 1993a). Although infections with watermolds are considered common, isolation and identification of the infecting organisms in amphibians is rarely reported. Cases are reported as consistent with *Saprolegnia* or as *Saprolegnia* spp. (Cooper, 1985; Frye & Gillespie, 1989; Jacobson, 1989), hence the common use of the term saprolegniasis.

Larvae of the spotted salamander, *Ambystoma maculatum,* have a high incidence of saprolegniasis associated with bite wounds from interspecies aggression (Walls & Jaeger, 1987). The mudpuppy, *Necturus maculosus,* is affected commonly (Anver & Pond, 1984), but this may simply reflect the fact that it is a common laboratory species. *Saprolegnia parasitica* and *S. ferax* have been associated with grayish cottony patches overlying injuries in frogs and newts (Reichenbach-Klinke & Elkan, 1965). *Achyla flagellata* and *Dictyuchus monosporus* have been reported from newts (Reichenbach-Klinke & Elkan, 1965).

In aquatic amphibians, the white or grayish-white, cottony, hyphae tangles may be present anywhere on the body (Plate 14.10) including the external gills (Jacobson, 1989). Skin wounds are the site of most watermold infections (Cooper, 1985). The anterior snout, gills, and tail tip (Plate 14.11) are common sites of infection, but infections may occur anywhere on the body and limbs. The underlying skin is discolored, necrotic or ulcerated, and inconsistently reddened. Advanced deep ulcerations which expose underlying musculature or bone (Reichenbach-Klinke & Elkan, 1965) may be hemorrhagic. The delicate cotton mattes collapse when the animal is removed from water. The color of the fungal matte may indicate the length of time the infection has been present. Acute lesions are usually white, while older lesions trap water-borne particles and may darken to a gray, brown, or green color.

Signs of saprolegniasis in salamanders may be multi-systemic and include lethargy, anorexia, vomiting, respiratory distress (gaping), weight loss, and death (Frye & Gillespie, 1989). Tadpoles may have fungal mattes protruding from the mouth and spiracle. Although the hyphae rarely become septicemic, extensive involvement of bone, muscle, spinal cord, and other organs may occur by direct extension from primary epithelial lesions (Bly et al., 1992; Frye & Gillespie, 1989). Tissue edema is variable but it is not clear whether it is a true host inflammatory response, or due to osmosis of water through the devitalized skin. Deep hyphae invasion of underlying soft tissues may be detected but may be due to postmortem growth of the fungi.

Presumptive diagnosis of saprolegniasis is by wet mount examination of skin scrapings (Plate 14.12), but culture is required for definitive diagnosis. Zoospores and hyphae are present in the dermal lesions. Zoospores are thin-walled, roughly spherical, 10–14 microns diameter, and may contain 1–4 internal spores (Frye & Gillespie, 1989; Noga, 1993a). Hyphae are aseptate, occasionally branching, quite variable in stain affinity in PAS and H&E preparations, have parallel walls, and are highly variable in diameter (2–40 microns) (Noga, 1993b). It is not clear whether these variable hyphae diameters represent different growth stages of one species, or mixed watermold infections.

Several treatment regimes have been reported as effective for watermold infections: 1) Malachite green (1:15,000 or 67 mg/L) for no more then 15 seconds once a day for 2–3 days. Immersion for longer then 15 seconds may cause epidermal exfoliation; 2) Copper sulfate (1:2000 or 500 mg/L) immersion for 2 minutes daily for at least 5 days then once a week until healed; 3) Potassium permanganate bath (1:5000 or 200 mg/L) for 5 minutes; and 4) Benzalkonium chloride (1:4,000,000 or 0.0025 mg/L) in water and then change water three times weekly (Fowler, 1986; Marcus, 1981; Raphael, 1993). Other treatments have been efficacious (see Chapter 24, Pharmacotherapeutics, and Table 24.5). It is important to note that supportive care in the form of continuous electrolyte baths and artificial slime is important to prevent a fatal osmotic imbalance resulting from the disrupted integument. Concurrent bacterial infections are common at sites of watermold infection, and parenteral antibiotics may be warranted.

Chytridiomycosis. Dermatitis associated with a chytridiomycete was described from a number of captive anurans (Nichols et al., 1996). It was first noted in captive specimens of the arroyo toad, *Bufo microscaphus californicus,* that displayed nonspecific signs of anorexia and lethargy. The signs progressed to include pupillary miosis and muscle incoordination, and toads died within 2–5 weeks of developing clinical signs. Spherical single-celled intracellular organisms were associated with epidermal hyperplasia/hyperkeratosis and underlying dermal inflammation. In this initial outbreak, treatment consisted of soaks in a trimethoprim-sulfadiazine/saline bath, one part 240 mg/ml injectable TMS (Di-Trim, Syntex Animal Health Inc., West Des Moines, IA) and 250 parts 0.6% saline, for 24 h every other day for 2 weeks. Mortality stopped and was associated with an increased shedding of the skin. The organisms were identified on light microscopy in three distinct stages: a uninucleate vegetative form, a multinucleate endosporulating stage, and a thick-walled multispored cyst. The organisms were stained with both periodic acid-Schiff stain and Gomori's methenamine silver stain but were not acid-fast. Flagella were detected on the spores via transmission electron microscopy. Although originally thought to be a fungal-like protist, this organism was in fact a chytridiomycete, a type of zoosporic fungus related to oomycete watermolds (e.g., *Saprolegnia* spp.). This was an extremely unexpected finding since all other chytridiomycetes described to date are not pathogens of vertebrates! Subsequent cases of fatal chytridiomycotic dermatitis were noted in other anurans including the amargosa toad, *Bufo nelsoni,* Woodhouse's toad, *B. woodhousii woodhousii,* White's treefrog, *Pelodryas caerulea,* and the ornate horned frog, *Ceratophrys ornata.*

Since the original discovery in amphibians, "chytrid" infection has been well studied. The host list has expanded considerably and there have been reports of infection in captive and free-ranging amphibians worldwide (Berger & Speare, 1998; Berger et al., 1998, 1999a, b; Daszak et al., 1999; Nichols et al., 1998; Pessier et al., 1999). The causative agent, *Batrachochytrium dendrobatidis*, was formally described by Longcore et al. (1999). To date, there have been no differences detected in chytrid isolated from a dozen different species of amphibian (Longcore, 2000). Many researchers believe that previous reports of *Basidiobolus* infection may actually be attributed to *Batrachochytrium dendrobatidis,* but this has not been formally refuted.

Batrachochytrium dendrobatidis uses keratin as a substrate. Its growth is restricted to the superficial layers of skin and other structures high in keratin. Typical clinical signs include excessive shedding of the skin, often within 14 days of exposure to the chytrid. Hyperemia of pale skin may be noted. The digits are often affected first. In anuran tadpoles, the keratin beak may be deformed from chytrid infection. In many outbreaks, unexpected deaths were observed before any clinical signs were detected. It is likely that disruption of the skin's osmotic regulation and other biological functions cause the majority of clinical signs. Secondary infection with other pathogens may occur. Chytrid infection should be considered in the rule out list for any ill amphibian.

The organism is readily detected in wet mounts of infected skin and formalin-preserved skin sections (Berger & Speare, 1998; Berger et al., 1999b; Pessier et al., 1999). Toe-clips and skin scrapes may be used to detect chytrid in living amphibians.

Chytridiomycosis has been successfully treated in dendrobatid frogs. Nichols and Lamirande (2000) reported successful treatment of cutaneous chytridiomycosis using a 1% suspension of itraconazole (Sporanox, Janssen Pharmaceutica, Inc., Titusville, NJ). Itraconazole was diluted to a final concentration of 0.01% itraconazole with 0.6% saline. Dyeing poison frogs, *Dendrobates tinctorius,* were exposed to chytrid-infected skin and infection was confirmed by excessive shedding of the skin and observation of chytrid in their skin. Some frogs were bathed in 0.01% itraconazole for 5 minutes SID for 11 days. Frogs that were not treated died 35 days postexposure. Treated frogs were free of infection when euthanized at 68 days postexposure. Frogs treated for only 8 days in a subsequent trial remained healthy 8 months postexposure.

Since chytrid is limited to keratinized (superficial) structures, topical treatment with itraconazole is recommended although other imidazoles (e.g., miconazole, ketaconazole) are likely to be effective. Maintenance of the electrolyte balance is important for stabilization of the patient.

Disinfection of equipment and enclosures may be accomplished with any of the readily available disinfectants. Due to its ready transmission in moist environments, extreme care should be taken to isolate contaminated enclosures and animals from uninfected animals and enclosures.

***Cladosporium* spp.** *Cladosporium* sp. has been reported to cause one case of mycotic dermatitis in a giant toad, *Bufo marinus* (Bube et al., 1992).

14.2.2 Mycotic Myositis

Infections of mycotic origin which are limited to skeletal muscle are rare. Diagnosis is determined histologically in most instances as culture attempts are often unsuccessful.

***Ichthyophonus* spp.** *Ichthyophonus* spp. is a recognized pleomorphic fungi with unsettled taxonomy (Lauckner, 1984; McVicar, 1982; Neish & Hughes, 1980; Rand, 1994). *Ichthyophonus* spp. fungal infections have been mistakenly identified as a microsporidium and thus misnamed *Ichthyosporidium* spp. (Elkan, 1976; Reichenbach-Klinke & Elkan, 1965; Thoen & Schliesser, 1984).

A fungal epizootic limited to the skeletal musculature was noted in free-ranging specimens of the red-spotted newt, *Notophthalmus viridescens,* from West Virginia (Herman, 1984) and Vermont (Green et al., 1995). Affected newts had prominent swellings observable on the body surface, were lethargic, and tended to float just below the water's surface. Lesions occurred dorsolaterally over the caudal half of the body, and ranged from small individual nodules to large multiple nodules which restricted movement. Ulceration was noted on some nodules. The overlying skin is somewhat roughened but normal in color. Newts continued to feed despite infection. Mortality reached close to 100% of the population by the end of summer. Wet mounts of skeletal muscle revealed characteristic light brown torpedo-shaped fungal elements. Histologic evaluation of lesions revealed cysts that appeared similar to the resting stage of *Ichthyophonus hoferi*. Culture attempts were unsuccessful and thus confirmation of histological findings was not possible. Little inflammatory response was observed in the affected tissue. It is likely that the ulcerated lesions were susceptible to secondary mycotic and bacterial infections which were actually responsible for the high incidence of mortality.

Cladosporium spp. A rapidly growing mycotic granuloma caused by a *Cladosporium* sp. occurred in a captive specimen of the barred tiger salamander, *Ambystoma tigrinum mavortium*, but was limited to the lumbar musculature (Migaki & Frye, 1975). The area was excised and submitted for culture but attempts were unsuccessful. Histologically, the granuloma contained round yeastlike budding cells and long septate hyphae which appeared morphologically similar to *Cladosporium* spp.

14.2.3 Mycotic Hepatitis

Candida spp. and *Penicillium* spp. have been isolated from liver granulomas in a black-spined toad, *Bufo melanostictus* (Griner, 1983). *Candida parapsilosis* has been isolated from pustules on the liver surface of a common European toad, *B. bufo,* but the organism did not invade into the liver tissue (Gugnani & Okafor, 1980). One report of hepatitis involved a green treefrog, *Hyla cinerea*, that had no external lesions but a severe diffuse mycosis of the liver from an unidentified etiology (Elkan & Reichenbach-Klinke, 1974). All cases were diagnosed on postmortem evaluation, so no treatment regimes were evaluated.

14.2.4 Mycotic Pneumonia

Reports of fungal pneumonias are surprisingly rare considering the vast opportunity for inhalation of pathogenic spores by amphibians. Postmortem culture of an infected lung yielded an *Aspergillus* spp. in a captive black-spined toad, *Bufo melanostictus* (Griner, 1983). *Geotrichim candidum* and *Candida tropicalis* have been isolated from the lungs of the common lesser toad, *B. granulosus,* and *Candida glabrata* was cultured from the lungs of a giant toad, *B. marinus* (Mok & Moratp de Carvalho, 1985). All cases were diagnosed on postmortem evaluation, so no treatment regimes were evaluated.

14.2.5 Intestinal Mycoses

Mycotic infections of the intestine are usually diagnosed postmortem. *Basidiomycetes* spp. was identified in an intestinal wall granuloma from a captive tiger salamander, *Ambystoma tigrinum* spp. (Griner, 1983). Numerous nematodes were also present in the intestine of this salamander. An unidentified fungus caused an extensive intestinal infection in an American treefrog, *Hyla* spp. (Elkan & Reichenbach-Klinke, 1974).

14.3 SYSTEMIC MYCOSES

14.3.1 Egg Mass and Larval Mycoses

Reports of mycoses affecting egg masses are rare perhaps due to the erroneous assumption that fungi only grow on infertile or dead eggs. Recent studies have shown that fungi such as *Saprolegnia* spp. and *Mycelia sterilia* can be primary pathogens to amphibian eggs.

Saprolegnia spp. *Saprolegnia* spp. are commonly found in fresh water and moist soils and some species are known to be common pathogens in aquarium fish and their eggs (Leibovitz & Pinello, 1980). *Saprolegnia* spp. has been considered postmortem fungi growth affecting only nonviable eggs (Tilley, 1972), however *S. ferax* was the pathogen involved in 95% mortality in an estimated 2.5 million eggs laid by a free-ranging population of the western toads, *Bufo boreas* (Blaustein et al., 1994). Embryos were observed under magnification to be viable and developing normally until the neural plate stage when infection became visible and progressed until mortality ensued. The fungus appeared to progress in a wavelike fashion across egg masses. Transmission was hypothesized to be introduced via fish stocking or from individual amphibians as they migrated or dispersed.

Embryos of the natterjack toad, *Bufo calamita,* have also had developmental failure from *Saprolegnia* spp. infection at low temperatures or at a pH lower than 6 (Banks & Beebee, 1988). Incidence of this infection on eggs of the European common frog, *Rana temporaria,* increased with cold and decreasing calcium concentration (Beattie et al., 1991).

Saprolegnia parasitica and *S. ferax* are the most common isolates from amphibian larval mycosis (Anver & Pond, 1984). Saprolegniasis on free-ranging tadpoles of the Plains spadefoot toad, *Scaphiopus bombifrons,* was reported to cause mass mortality (Bragg & Bragg, 1958). The epizootic occurred in a temporary ditch in southwestern Oklahoma. The tadpoles were observed with white fuzz strands extending from them. Nearby ditches contained unaffected tadpoles.

Tadpoles of the Rio Grande leopard frog, *Rana berlanderi*, died from *Saprolegnia* spp. and it was suspected that tadpoles of the southern toad, *Bufo terrestris*, were also affected (Bragg, 1962). At the same time in the same temporary pond, tadpoles of Strecker's chorus frog, *Pseudacris streckeri streckeri*, were unaffected. Tadpoles of the gray treefrog, *Hyla versicolor*, and the Great Plains narrowmouth toad, *Gastrophryne olivacea*, were observed in the same pond later that season and were followed through metamorphosis, apparently without this disease. This indicated a potential species difference in infection susceptibility.

Treatments for *Saprolegnia* spp. infections in larval stage amphibians historically included baths of a weak solution of potassium permanganate (1:1000 or 1 gm/L), methylene blue (3:10,000 or 0.3 gm/L), or trypaflavin (1:100 or 10 gm/L). Unfortunately the literature does not report the frequency and duration of these regimes (Reichenback-Klinke & Elkan, 1965). See Chapter 24 for currently recommended treatments.

Mycelia spp. A fungi provisionally identified as *Mycelia sterilia* has been found to cause mortality in treefrog egg masses in Central America (Villa, 1979). In experimental trials, treefrog eggs exposed to *Mycelia* spp. demonstrated clinical infections within 5 days.

14.3.2 Chromomycosis

Chromomycosis (chromoblastomycosis) describes a disease caused by pigmented or black fungi (Roberts, 1986), and has been shown to be caused by *Cladosporium carrioni*, *C. cladosporioides*, *C. herbarum*, *Fonsecaea dermatitidis*, *F. pedrosoi*, *Phialophora* spp., *Scolecosbasidium humicola*, and *Wangiella (Hormiscium) dermatitidis* (Anver & Pond, 1984; Bube et al., 1992; Mok & Moratp de Carvalho, 1985). The organisms involved are common worldwide in soils, wood, and decayed vegetation (Gonzalez-Mendoza, 1988). In amphibians the disease may be characterized by ulcerative or granulomatous lesions of the skin (Plate 14.13) or be disseminated systemically (Schmidt, 1984) (Plates 14.14, 14.15). Affected amphibians may show anorexia and weight loss. Culture attempts are often unsuccessful. If growth occurs the fungus frequently will not sporulate, thus eluding identification. Chromomycosis has been reported in bufonid, hylid, leptodactylid, ranid, and rhacophorid anurans (Ackermann & Miller, 1992; Dhaliwal & Griffiths, 1964; Miller et al., 1992; Rush et al., 1974; Schmidt & Hartfiel, 1977; Speare, 1990; Velasquez & Restrepo, 1975) (Table 14.2).

Table 14.2. Species of amphibians reported with chromomycosis.

Bufonidae	
Bufo alvarius	Colorado river toad
Bufo blombergi	Colombian giant toad
Bufo bufo	common European toad
Bufo melanostictus	black-spined toad
Bufo paracnemis	Cururu toad
Leptodactylidae	
Ceratophrys ornata	ornate horned frog
Leptodactylus pentadactylus	South American bullfrog
Hylidae	
Osteopilus septentrionalis	Cuban treefrog
Pelodryas caerulea	White's treefrog
Phyllomedusa trinitatus	Trinidad leaf frog
Pternohyla fodiens	lowland burrowing treefrog
Ranidae	
Pyxicephalus adspersus	Tschudi's African bullfrog
Rana pipiens	northern leopard frog
Rhacophoridae	
Rhacophorus spp.	flying frogs

Captive wild-caught specimens of the northern leopard frog, *Rana pipiens*, have developed chromomycosis (Rush et al., 1974). Clinically affected animals developed cutaneous gray-black nodules and ulcers and distended abdomens. Death occurred 20 days after the first skin lesion was observed. Liver, spleen, and kidneys were enlarged and nodular. These granulomatous lesions contained brown fungal components (Anver, 1980). Wild-caught specimens of the giant toad, *Bufo marinus*, have also been found with internal lesions, but not skin lesions, of chromomycosis (Velasquez & Restrepo, 1975). Other bufonids, including the Colorado River toad, *Bufo alvarius* (Frank & Roester, 1970), the European common toad, *Bufo bufo* (Elkan & Philpot, 1973), and South American toads (the Colombian giant toad, *Bufo blombergi*, the Cururu toad, *B. paracnemis*, and the black-spined toad, *B. melanostictus*) (Correa et al., 1968), have been diagnosed with chromomycosis.

Systemic chromomycosis caused by *Fonsecaea*

pedrosoi can occur and be transmitted between debilitated or stressed amphibians. Experimental transmission has not been demonstrated in animals not stressed. *Fonsecaea pedrosoi* has been reported as the etiologic agent of chromomycosis in free-ranging and captive specimens of the giant toad, *Bufo marinus,* the bullfrog, *Rana catesbeiana,* and a leopard frog, *R. pipiens* (Cicmanec et al., 1973) Upon necropsy, well-circumscribed gray granulomas ranging from 2–30 mm in diameter were found in liver, kidney, heart, skeletal muscle, meninges, or bone marrow tissues. Nodules contained both brown septate fungal cells and hyphae. This disease could be experimentally induced in stressed toads by changing feeding and decreasing temperatures. Spontaneous infection has also been noted to occur.

A *Phialophora*-like fungus, probably *P. gougerotii,* contributed to mortality in a private collection of White's treefrog, *Pelodryas caerulea,* the Cuban treefrog, *Osteopilus septentrionalis,* a Trinidad leaf treefrog, *Phyllomedusa trinitatis,* and a flying frog, *Rhacophorus* spp. (Elkan & Philpot, 1973). Isolates of *Cladosporium herbarum* and *Scolecobasidium humicola* were also cultured. The condition was fatal in all animals which demonstrated clinical signs of poor coloration and ulceration of the digits, hands, feet, rostrum, and ventrum. Anorexia and death ensued in 1–6 months. Histological lesions included local accumulations of histiocytes, in particular, monocytes and fibroblasts in association with fungal hyphae which had invaded the epidermis. The liver and kidney contained tubercles of epithelioid monocytes and fibrocytes. These organs also had areas of central caseous necrosis. Soil samples from the vivaria were negative for fungal growth but this does not preclude presence of the organisms.

Unfortunately, no cases of amphibians surviving chromomycosis have been reported. Amphotericin-B was a successful treatment in the domestic cat (McKeever et al., 1983), and may be attempted in amphibians at a starting dosage of 1 mg/kg ICe q 24 h. Treatment with ketoconazole (10 mg/kg q 24 h) or itraconazole (2–10 mg/kg PO q 24 h) orally every 24 h may be attempted. Higher dosages may prove effective but the risk of toxicity to the patient also increases. Surgical debridement of obvious lesions is a possible ancilliary therapy, however it is unlikely that the infection is limited to these visible external lesions. Ultrasonography, transillumination, or celioscopy may sometimes confirm the internal granulomas. Organisms involved in amphibian chromomycosis have zoonotic potential and thus care should be taken when handling any animal suspected of this disease. In most instances, euthanasia of the infected amphibian should be recommended instead of treatment to reduce the risk of spreading the disease through the collection and to the handlers.

14.3.3 Zygomycoses

Diseases that fall under the term zygomycosis are caused by members of the orders Mucorales and Entomophthorales. These etiologic agents are distributed worldwide and are common in soil and decaying organic matter (Roberts, 1986). Frequently fungi species from these orders are recovered as nonpathogenic contaminants from amphibians. (Taylor et al., 1995) Diseases from these organisms are thought to be acquired by inhalation of the airborne spores or from direct inoculation through the skin or tissue by traumatic incident (Ajello, 1988).

Australian free-ranging specimens of the giant toad, *Bufo marinus,* were systemically infected with *Mucor amphibiorum* (Speare et al., 1994). The overall prevalence of infections was 0.71% of 3518 toads. Granulomas were found in the liver, spleen, mesonephroi, bladder, heart, lung, subcutaneous lymph sacs, skin, gastrointestinal tract, muscle, bone, oral cavity, and cranial cavity (Speare et al., 1997). Histologic examination of the granulomas revealed spherules ranging from 4.9–36.4 μm in diameter observable in internal tissues. Fungal hyphae were not formed. *Mucor amphibiorum* is known to grow well in soil, thus the animals may have become infected when incidentally ingesting soil during feeding.

A systemic *Mucor* spp. infection has also been observed in a White's treefrog, *Pelodryas caerulea* (Frank, 1975). White nodules were found on the surface of the liver and spleen.

Culture of these nodules yielded an undermined species of *Mucor*. The organism was experimentally inoculated into common toads (presumably the common European toad, *Bufo bufo*) which resulted in transmission of the disease.

Rhizopus spp. were isolated from six specimens of the Colorado River toad, *Bufo alverius* (Fowler, 1986). The toads demonstrated skin ulcerations, and necropsy of two toads revealed fungal mycelium in lungs, liver, spleen, kidneys, and myocardial tissue.

Regression of the skin lesions was observed after treatment with sulfadiazine (132 mg/kg), once a day for 6 weeks. However, the animals died within 2 weeks of fulminating mycosis after treatment was prematurely terminated.

14.3.4 Candidiasis

Candida spp. are usually associated with endogenous infections of warm-blooded animals and cause the most frequently encountered opportunistic fungal infection in humans (Roberts, 1986). It is unknown if *Candida* spp. are normal endogenous flora of amphibians, but some species do exist in water, soil, plants, and fish, making exogenous infections possible (Ahearn, 1988).

Candidiasis has occurred in a giant toad, *Bufo*

marinus (Hill, 1954). The unspeciated organism was isolated from cultures of the kidney, lung, liver, and spleen. *Candida guilliermondii* has caused disease in the giant toad, *Bufo marinus,* the common lesser toad, *B. granulosus,* and the basin treefrog, *Hyla lanciformis* (Mok & Moratp de Carvalho, 1985).

Crusts resembling dead skin may develop on some amphibians (Plate 14.16). *Candida* sp. may be cultured from the underside of these crusts. The significance of this finding is unknown, but topical application of an antifungal agent to the lesion is recommended.

14.4 SPECIMEN SAMPLES

Impression smears of the skin of amphibians are recommended if mycotic dermatitis is suspected (Plate 14.17). The skin should be slightly moistened with water, and a microscope slide is pressed gently against the skin surface. The slide is then air dried and stained with Periodic acid-Schiff stain. Microscopic evaluation can be conducted for evidence of fungi and identifying morphologic characteristics. Currently, impression smears are an effective rapid tool for postmortem confirmation of clinical cases of this disease, but their use in subclinical mycotic dermatitises is unproven.

Skin scrapings can be taken for mycotic culture samples from live amphibians. Culture of suspected mycoses from postmortem cases usually involves a section of skin, liver, intestine, and lung. Sections of both ventral abdominal skin and the distal digits improve isolate recovery from cases of mycotic dermatitis in amphibians. Other specimens such as blood, urine, bone marrow, cerebrospinal fluid, coelomic fluid, and synovial fluid can also be cultured. Samples should be collected with alcohol flamed instruments to prevent cross contamination of tissues and placed in sterile transport containers.

Increased recovery of mycotic isolates may also occur when sections of tissue or digits are placed on the media directly, rather than using scrapings. Samples should not be homogenized as this will destroy the viable hyphae elements in zygomycetes infections (Roberts et al., 1985). Cotton can be placed in the top of the tube before the lid is placed on to catch any spores from becoming airborne when tube is uncapped in the future. Culture tube lids are then loosely screwed on to allow for oxygen for growth.

14.5 MEDIA AND INCUBATION

There are many commercially available media for fungal isolation as well as references with media recipes (Rippon, 1982). Most fungal isolates from amphibians will grow on Sabouraud dextrose agar. Slants which are prepared and capped tightly to prevent dehydration will last for more then 6 months. While Sabouraud dextrose agar may not provide all the essential nutrients that a specific species of fungi may need, excellent results have been noted.

Room temperature is usually adequate for incubation of mycotic cultures. Racks of culture-inoculated tubes should be placed away from drafts or outside walls to prevent fluctuations in temperatures. Caps of culture tubes must be loosely screwed on to allow for oxygen for growth.

14.6 IDENTIFICATION OF FUNGI

Identification of mycotic cultures is a relatively quick and easy procedure. Cultures should be checked at 5 days and then biweekly (Rippon, 1982). Cultures should be allowed to incubate at least 4 weeks before being reported as negative (Roberts et al., 1985). If growth occurs, the gross morphology of the colony growth should be described as it occurs on both the up and down side against the media slant. Subculturing can be performed to purify mycotic species. Frequently this is not necessary if cultures are watched and identified as growth occurs.

Slide preparation requires a laminar flow hood or microbiological glove box in which the culture tube should be uncapped and a small amount of the culture media and mycelium strands removed. Two microbiology probes work effectively for this procedure. The specimen is then placed on a microscope slide and gently teased apart. A drop of stain such as lactophenol cotton blue is placed on the slide and a coverslip is placed on top. Examination can then be conducted to observe microscopic conidia morphology, size, arrangement, and mycelial appendages (Rippon, 1982). Numerous references with drawings and photos to assist in identification of fungi are available (McGinnis et al., 1982; Moss & McQuown, 1953; Rippon, 1982; Roberts, 1986; Roberts et al., 1985).

An atlas exists to assist with identification of fungi in histologic sections (Chandler et al., 1980), but confirmation of the identity of the fungus requires recovery and isolation of the organism in culture. Culture slides can be preserved for future reference by gently sealing the edges around the coverslip with clear nail polish. Slides must be stored in a horizontal position to prevent the fungi and stain from pooling on one end as the stain remains in a liquid state even when sealed.

14.7 CULTURE PRESERVATION

Short-term preservation of cultures can be achieved by subculturing onto another Sabouraud slant every 6 weeks. To provide for long-term preservation of cultures, sterile heavy mineral oil can be added to the to the culture tube to cover the mycotic growth and agar (Cooper, 1985). The tube is then tightly capped and a sheet of paraffin is wrapped around the cap-tube interface. Cultures can then be stored at room temperature for a year without subculturing. Lyophilization and freezing techniques can also provide longer term culture storage (Carter, 1975).

REFERENCES

Ackermann, J. and E. Miller. 1992. Chromomycosis in an African bullfrog, *Pyxicephalus adspersus*. Bulletin of the Association of Reptilian and Amphibian Veterinarians 2(2):8–9.

Ahearn, D.G. 1988. Candidiasis, *in* Balows, A., W.J. Hausler, and E.H. Lennette (Eds.): Laboratory Diagnosis of Infectious Diseases—Principles and Practice. Springer-Verlag, New York, pp. 584–589.

Ajello, L. 1988. Zygomycosis, *in* Balows, A., W.J. Hausler, and E.H. Lennette (Eds.): Laboratory Diagnosis of Infectious Diseases—Principles and Practice. Springer-Verlag, New York, pp. 715–722.

Anver, M.R. 1980. Diagnostic exercise. Laboratory Animal Science 30: 165–166.

Anver, M.R. and C.L. Pond. 1984. Biology and diseases of amphibians, *in* Fox, J.G., B. J. Cohen, and F. M. Loew (Eds.): Laboratory Animal Medicine. Academic Press Inc., Orlando, FL, pp. 427–447.

Banks, B. and T.J.C. Beebee. 1988. Reproductive success of natterjack toads (*Bufo calamita*) in two contrasting habitats. Journal of Animal Ecology 57:475–492.

Beattie, R.C., R.J. Aston, and A.G.P. Milner. 1991. A field study of fertilization and embryonic development in the common frog (*Rana temporaria*) with particular reference to acidity and temperature. Journal of Applied Ecology 28:346–357.

Berger L., and R. Speare 1998. Chytridiomycosis: a new disease of wild and captive amphibians. ANZCCART Newsletter (11(4):1–3.

Berger, L., R. Speare, and A. Hyatt. 1999a. Chytrid fungi and amphibian declines: Overview, implications and future directions, *in* A. Campbell (Ed.): Declines and Disappearances of Australian Frogs. Environment Australia: Canberra. 1999:21–31.

Berger, L., R. Speare, and A. Kent. 1999b. Diagnosis of chytridiomycosis of amphibians by histological examination. Zoos Print Journal 15:184–190.

Berger, L., R. Speare, P. Daszak, D.E. Green, A.A. Cunningham, C.L. Goggin, R. Slocombe, M.A. Ragan, A.D. Hyatt, K.R. McDonald, H.B. Hines, K.R. Lips, G. Marantelli, and H. Parkes. 1998. Chytridiomycosis causes amphibian mortality associated with population declines in the rain forests of Australia and Central America. Proceedings of the National Academy of Science, USA 95:9031–9036.

Blaustein, A.R., D.G. Hokit, R.K. O'Hara, and R.A. Holt. 1994. Pathogenic fungus contributes to amphibian losses in the Pacific Northwest. Biological Conservation 67:251–254.

Bly, J.E., L.A. Lawson, D.J. Dale, A.J. Szalai, R.M. Durborow, and L.W. Clem. 1992. Winter saprolegniasis in channel catfish. Diseases of Aquatic Organisms 13:155–164.

Bragg, A.N. 1962. *Saprolegnia* on tadpoles again in Oklahoma. The Southwestern Naturalist 7:79–80.

Bragg, A.N. and W.N. Bragg. 1958. Parasitism of spadefoot tadpoles by *Saprolegnia*. Herpetologica 14:34.

Bube, A., E. Burkhardt, and R. Weib. 1992. Spontaneous chromomycosis in the Marine toad (*Bufo marinus*). J. Comp. Path. 106:73–77.

Carter, G.R. 1975. Diagnostic Procedures in Veterinary Microbiology. Charles C. Thomas Publisher, Springfield, IL, 362 pp.

Chandler, F.W., W. Kaplan, and L. Ajello. 1980. A Colour Atlas and Textbook of the Histopathology of Mycotic Diseases. Wolfe Medical Publications Ltd., London, UK, 333 pp.

Cicmanec, J.L., D.H. Ringler, and E.S. Beneke. 1973. Spontaneous occurrence and experimental transmission of the fungus, *Fonsecaea pedrosol*, in the marine toad, *Bufo marinus*. Laboratory Animal Sciences 23:43–47.

Cooper, B.H. 1985. Taxonomy, classification, and nomenclature of fungi, *in* Lennett, E.H., A. Balows, W.J. Hausler, and H.J. Shadomy (Eds.): Manual of Clinical Microbiology. American Society for Microbiologists, Washington, DC, pp. 495–499.

Cooper, E.L., R.K. Wright, A.E. Klempau, and C.T. Smith. 1992. Hibernation alters the frog's immune system. Cryobiology 29:616–631.

Coremans-Pelseneer, J. 1973. Isolation of *Basidiobolus meristosporus* from natural sources. Mycopathologia et Mycologia applicata 49:173–176.

Correa, R., I. Correa, G. Garces, D. Mender, L.F. Morales, and A. Restrepp. 1968. Lesiones microticas (cromomicosis?) observades en sapos (*Bufo sp.*). Antioquia Med. 18:175–184.

Cosgrove, G.E. 1977. Amphibian diseases, *in* Current Veterinary Therapy VI Small Animal Practice. W.B. Saunders Co., Philadelphia, PA, pp. 769–772.

Daszak P., L. Berger, A.A. Cunningham, A.D. Hyatt, D.E. Green, and R. Speare. 1999. Emerging infectious diseases and amphibian population declines. Emerging Infectious Diseases 5:735–748.

Davis, S.R., D.H. Ellis, P. Goldwater, S. Dimitriou, and R. Byard. 1994. First human culture-proven Australian case of entomophthoromycosis caused by *Basidiobolus ranarum*. Journal of Medical and Veterinary Mycology 31:225–230.

Dhaliwal, S.S. and D.A. Griffiths. 1964. Fungal Disease of Malayan toads (*Bufo melanostictus*). Sabouraudia 3:279–287.

Drechsler, C. 1952. Widespread distribution of *Delacroixia coronata* and other saprophytic entomophthoraceae in plant detritus. Science 115:575–576.

Drechsler, C. 1956. Supplementary developmental stages of *Basidiobolus ranarum* and *Basidiobolus haptosporus*. Mycologia 48:655–676.

Drechsler, C. 1958. Formation of sporangia from conidia and hypha segments in an Indonesian *Basidiobolus*. American Journal of Botany 45:632–638.

Drechsler, C. 1964. An odorous *Basidiobolus* often producing conidia plurally and forming some diclinous sexual apparatus. American Journal of Botany 51:770–777.

Eades, S.M. and M.J. Corbel. 1979. Experimental cerebral lesions produced by inoculation with *Basidiobolus* strains. Mycopathologia 67:187–192.

Elkan, E. 1976. Pathology in the Amphibia, Chapter 6, *in* Lofts, B. (Ed): Physiology of the Amphibia, Volume 3. Academic Press, New York, NY, pp. 273–312.

Elkan, E. and C.M. Philpot. 1973. Mycotic infections in frogs due to a *Phialophora*-like fungus. Sabouraudia 11:99–105.

Elkan, E. and H. Reichenbach-Klinke. 1974. Color Atlas of the Diseases of Fishes, Amphibians and Reptiles. TFH Publications, Inc., Neptune City, NJ, 256 pp.

Ferguson, H.W. 1989. Systemic Pathology of Fish. Iowa State University Press, Ames, IA, 263 pp.

Fowler, M.E. 1986. Amphibians, *in* Fowler, M.E.: Zoo & Wild Animal Medicine, 2nd Edition. W.B. Saunders Co., Philadelphia, PA, pp. 99–184.

Frank, W. 1975. Mycotic infections in amphibians and reptiles, *in* Page, L.E. (Ed.): Wildlife Diseases. Plenum Press, New York, pp. 73–87.

Frank, W. and U. Roester. 1970. Amphibien als Trager von *Hormiscium (Hormodendrum) dermatidis*, KANO, 1937, Einen Erreger der Chromoblastomykose (Chromomykose) des Menschen. Z. Tropenmed. Parasitol. 21:93–108.

Frye, F.L. and D.S. Gillespie. 1989. Saprolegniasis in a zoo collection of aquatic amphibians. Proceedings of the 3rd International Colloquium on the Pathology of Reptiles and Amphibians, p. 43.

Gonzalez-Mendoza, A. 1988. Chromoblastomycosis, *in* Balows, A., W.J. Hausler, and E.H. Lennette (Eds.): Laboratory Diagnosis of Infectious Diseases—Principles and Practice. Springer-Verlag, New York, NY, pp. 590–599.

Green, D.E., J. Andrews, and J. Abell. 1995. Preliminary investigations on mycotic myositis in red-spotted newts, *Notophthalmus viridescens*, from Vermont. Herpetopathologia 1995 (Proceedings of the 5th International Colloquium on the Pathology of Reptiles and Amphibians), pp. 201–214.

Greer, D.L. and L. Friedman. 1964. Effect of temperature on growth as a differentiating characteristic between human and nonhuman isolates of *Basidiobolus* species. J. Bacteriol. 88:812–813.

Greer, D.L. and L. Friedman. 1966. Studies on the genus *Basidiobolus* with reclassification of the species pathogenic for man. Sabouraudia 4:231–241.

Griner, L.A. 1983. Amphibia, *in* Pathology of Zoo Animals. Zoological Society of San Diego, San Diego, California, pp. 1–17.

Groff, J.M., A. Mughannam, T.S. McDowell, A. Wong, M.J. Dykstra, F.L. Frye, and R.P. Hedrick. 1991. An epizootic of cutaneous zygomycosis in cultured dwarf African clawed frogs (*Hymenochirus curtipes*) due to *Basidiobolus ranarum*. Journal of Medical and Veterinary Mycology 29:215–223.

Gugnani, H.C. and J.I. Okafor. 1980. Mycotic flora of the intestine and other internal organs of certain reptiles and amphibians with special reference to characterization of *Basidiobolus* isolates. Mykosen 23:260–268.

Herman, R.L. 1984. *Ichthyophonus*-like infection in newts (*Notophthalmus viridescens* Rafinesque). Journal of Wildlife Diseases 20:55–56.

Hill, W.C.O. 1954. Report of the Society's Prosector for the Year. Proceedings of the Zoological Society of London 124:304–311.

Hutchinson, J.A., and M.A. Nickerson. 1970. Comments on the distribution of *Basidiobolus ranarum*. Mycologia 60:585–587.

Hutchinson, J.A., D.S. King, and M.A. Nickerson. 1972. Studies on the temperature requirements, odor production and zygospore wall undulation of the genus *Basidiobolus*. Mycologia 64:467–474.

Jacobson, E. 1989. Mycotic diseases of amphibians and reptiles. Proceedings of the 3rd International Colloquium on the Pathology of Reptiles and Amphibians, pp. 41–42.

Koneman, E.W. and G.D. Roberts. 1985. Practical Laboratory Mycology—Third Edition. Williams & Williams, Baltimore, MD, 211 pp.

Lauckner, G. 1984. Agents: Fungi, *in* Kinne, O. (Ed.): Diseases of Marine Animals, Part 1, Volume IV. Biologische Anstalt Helgoland, Hamburg, Germany, pp. 89–113.

Leibovitz, L. and C. Pinello. 1980. Mycotic infections. Journal of the American Veterinary Medical Association 177:1110–1111.

Longcore, J.E. 2000. ABSTRACT—*Batrachochytrium dendrobatidis*, the "frog chytrid." Getting the Jump! on Amphibian Diseases Conference.

Longcore, J.E., A.P. Pessier, and D.K. Nichols. 1999. *Batrachochytrium dendrobatidis* gen. et sp. nov., a chytrid pathogenic to amphibians. Mycologia 91:219–227.

Marcus, L.C. 1981. Veterinary Biology and Medicine of Captive Amphibians and Reptiles. Lea & Febiger, Philadelphia, PA, p. 239.

McGinnis, M.R., R.F. D'Amato, and G.A. Land. 1982. Pictorial Handbook of Medically Important Fungi and Aerobic Actinomycetes. Praeger, New York, 160 pp.

McKeever, P., D.D. Caywood, and V. Perman. 1983. Chromomycosis in a cat: successful medical therapy. Journal of the American Animal Hospital Association 19:533–536.

McVicar, A.H. 1982. *Ichthyophonus* infection of fish, *in* Roberts, R.J. (Ed.): Microbial Diseases of Fish. Academic Press, London, pp. 243–269.

Migaki, G. and F.L. Frye. 1975. Mycotic granuloma in a tiger salamander. Journal of Wildlife Diseases 11:525–528.

Miller, E.A., R.J. Montali, E.C. Ramsay, and B.A. Rideout. 1992. Disseminated chromoblastomycosis in a colony of ornate-horned frogs (*Ceratophrys ornata*). Journal of Zoo and Wildlife Medicine 23:433–438.

Mok, W.Y. and C. Moratp de Carvalho. 1985. Association of anurans with pathogenic fungi. Mycopathologia 92: 37–43.

Moss, E.S. and A.L. McQuown. 1953. Atlas of Medical Mycology. Williams and Wilkins Publishing, Baltimore, MD, 245 pp.

Neish, G.A. and G.C. Hughes. 1980. Fungal Diseases of Fishes, Book 6, *in* Sniesko, S.F. and H.R. Axelrod (Eds.): Diseases of Fishes. TFH Publications, Inc., Neptune City, NJ. 159 pp.

Nichols, D.K. and E.W. Lamirande. 2000. POSTER—Treatment of cutaneous chytridiomycosis in blue-and-yellow poison dart frogs (*Dendrobates tinctorius*). Getting the Jump! on Amphibian Diseases Conference.

Nichols, D.K., A.P. Pessier, and J.E. Longcore. 1998. Cutaneous chytridiomycosis: an emerging disease? Proceedings of the American Association of Zoo Veterinarians, pp. 269–271.

Nichols, D.K., A.J. Smith, and C.H. Gardiner. 1996. Dermatitis of anurans caused by fungal-like protists. Proceedings of the American Association of Zoo Veterinarians, pp. 220–222.

Nickerson, M.A. and J.A. Hutchinson. 1971. The distribution of the fungus *Basidiobolus ranarum* Eidam in fish, amphibians and reptiles. The American Midland Naturalist 86:500–502.

Noga, E.J. 1993a. Watermold infections of freshwater fish: Recent advances. Annual Review of Fish Diseases 3:291–304

Noga, E.J. 1993b. Fungal and algal diseases of temperate freshwater and estuarine fishes, *in* Stoskpof, M.K. (Ed.): Fish Medicine, W.B. Saunders Co., Philadelphia, PA, pp. 278–283.

Okafor, J.I., D. Testrake, H.R. Mushinsky, and B.G. Yangco. 1984. A *Basidiobolus* sp. and its association with reptiles and amphibians in southern Florida. Sabouraudia 22:47–51.

Pessier, A.P., Nichols, D.K., Longcore, J.E., and Fuller, M.S. 1999. Cutaneous chytridiomycosis in poison dart frogs (*Dendrobates* spp.) and White's treefrogs (*Litoria caerulea*). Journal of Veterinary Diagnostic Investigation 11:194–199.

Rand, T.G. 1994. An unusual form of *Ichthyophonus hoferi* (Ichthyophonales: Ichthyophonaceae) from yellowtail flounder *Limanda ferruginea* from the Nova Scotia shelf. Diseases of Aquatic Organisms 18:21–28.

Raphael, B.L. 1993. Amphibians, *in* The Veterinary Clinics of North America—Small Animal Practice—Exotic Pet Medicine I. W. B. Saunders Co., Philadelphia, PA, pp. 1271–1286.

Reichenbach-Klinke, H. and E. Elkan. 1965. Amphibia, *in* The Principal Diseases of Lower Vertebrates. Academic Press, New York, pp. 209–384.

Rippon, J.W. 1982. Medical Mycology: The Pathogenic Fungi and the Pathogenic Actinomycetes. W. B. Saunders Co., Philadelphia, PA, 842 pp.

Roberts, G.D. 1986. Laboratory methods in basic mycology, *in* Finegold, S.M. and E.J. Baron (Eds.): Bailey and Scott's Diagnostic Microbiology. The C.V. Mosby Company, St. Louis, MO, pp. 678–774.

Roberts, G.D., N.L. Goodman, G.A. Land, H.W. Larsh, and M.R. McGinnis. 1985. Detection and recovery of fungi in clinical specimens, *in* Lennett, E.H., A. Balows, W.J. Hausler, and H.J. Shadomy (Eds.): Manual of Clinical Microbiology. American Society for Microbiologists, Washington, DC. pp. 500–513.

Robinow, C.F. 1963. Observations on cell growth, mitosis, and division in the fungus *Basidiobolus ranarum*. The Journal of Cell Biology 17:123–152.

Rush, H.G., M.R. Anver, and E.S. Beneke. 1974. Systemic chromomycosis in *Rana pipiens*. Laboratory Animal Science 24:646–655.

Schmidt, R.E. 1984. Amphibian chromomycosis, *in* Hoff, G.L., F.R. Frye, and E.R. Jacobson (Eds.): Diseases of Amphibians and Reptiles. Plenum Press, New York, pp. 169–181.

Schmidt, R.E. and D.A. Hartfiel. 1977. Chromomycosis in amphibians. Journal of Zoo Animal Medicine 8:26–28.

Speare, R. 1990. A review of the diseases of the Cane Toad, *Bufo marinus*, with comments on biological control. Australian Wildlife Res. 17: 387–410.

Speare, R., L. Berger, P. O'Shea, P.W. Ladds, and A.D. Thomas. 1997. Pathology of mucormycosis of cane toads of Australia. Journal of Wildlife Diseases 33(1):105–111.

Speare, R., A.D. Thomas, P. O'Shea, and W.A. Shipton. 1994. *Mucor amphibiorum* in the toad, *Bufo marinus*, in Australia. Journal of Wildlife Diseases 30:399–407.

Taylor, S.K., E.S. Williams, K.W. Mills, A.M. Boerger-Fields, C.J. Lynn, C.E. Hearne, E.T. Thorne, and S.J. Pistono. 1995. A review of causes of mortality and the diagnostic investigation for pathogens of the Wyoming toad (*Bufo hemiophrys baxteri*). US Fish & Wildlife Service, Cheyenne, WY, 37 pp.

Thoen, C.O. and T. Schliesser. 1984. Mycobacterial infection in cold-blooded animals, *in* Kubica, G.P. and L.G. Wayne (Eds.): The Mycobacteria: A Sourcebook. Dekker-Marcel, New York, pp. 1297–1311.

Tilley, S.G. 1972. Aspects of parental care and embryonic development in *Desmognathus ochrophaeus*. Copeia 1972(3):532–540.

Tills, D.W. 1974. The distribution of the fungus, *Basidiobolus ranarum* Eidam, in fish, amphibians and reptiles of the southern Appalachian region. Transactions of the Kansas Academy of Science 80:75–77.

Velasquez, L.F. and A. Restrepo. 1975. Chromomycosis in the toad (*Bufo marinus*) and a comparison of the etiologic agent with fungi causing human chromomycosis. Sabouraudia 13:1–9.

Villa, J. 1979. Two fungi lethal to frog eggs in Central America. Copeia 1979(4):650–655.

Walls, S.C. and R.G. Jaeger. 1987. Aggression and exploitation as mechanisms of competition in larval salamanders. Can. J. Zool. 65:2938–2944.

Williams, A.O. 1969. Pathology of phycomycosis due to *Entomophthora* and *Basidiobolus* species. Arch. Path. 87:13–20.

Zahari, P., R.G. Hirst, W.A. Shipton, and R.S.F. Campbell. 1990. The origin and pathogenicity of *Basidiobolus* species in northern Australia. Journal of Medical and Veterinary Mycology 28:461–468.

Zapata, A.G., A. Varas, and M. Torroba. 1992. Seasonal variations in the immune system of lower vertebrates. Immunology Today 13:142–147.

CHAPTER 15

PROTOZOA AND METAZOA INFECTING AMPHIBIANS

Sarah L. Poynton, PhD and Brent R. Whitaker, MS, DVM

15.1 INTRODUCTION

Protozoa and metazoa frequently utilize amphibians as hosts, yet clinical diseases are relatively rare (Crawshaw, 1992b). There is a wide variety of interrelationships, ranging from commensal—which is harmless and may even be beneficial, to parasitic—where the protozoa or metazoa is nutritionally dependent upon its host, and where the infection may have pathogenic consequences for the host. Since many protozoa, metazoa, and amphibians have coevolved, it is usual to find infections in clinically healthy amphibians, and treatment is not always advisable or necessary.

Aquatic and terrestrial amphibians, as eggs, tadpoles and adults, are hosts to a wide variety of protozoa and metazoa (Figure 15.1 and Table 15.1). The fauna infecting larval amphibians and aquatic species has many similarities to that infecting fish. Some protozoa and metazoa have direct (or monoxenous) life cycles, requiring only the amphibian host. Others have indirect (or heteroxenous) life cycles requiring at least two kinds of hosts, in which case the amphibian can serve as the intermediate host carrying immature stages, or it can serve as the final host with sexually mature stages. Wild amphibians typically carry a diversity of protozoan and metazoan species, some of which have direct life cycles, and some have indirect life cycles. Typically when wild hosts are brought into captivity, their protozoan and metazoan fauna change. Species having indirect life cycles tend to die out, due to the absence of vectors or other hosts necessary for completion of the life cycles. In contrast, direct life cycle species may increase in prevalence, intensity and density; this is because exposure is amplified in captivity, due to confined conditions and the potential for constant reinfection. Captive-born amphibians tend to have fauna dominated by protozoa and metazoa having direct life cycles.

Most of our knowledge of the protozoa and metazoa that infect amphibians comes from parasite-host checklists and clinical pathology reports. Within this literature, there is a very uneven distribution of knowledge for the different amphibian groups, with the greatest amount of information for the Anura pertaining to the families Bufonidae, Hylidae, Leptodactylidae, and Ranidae; for the Caudata, most information is available for the families Plethodontidae and Salamandridae (Baker, 1987). Overviews of protozoan and metazoan infections in amphibians include the following: Brannian, 1984; Brooks, 1984; Crawshaw 1992a, b; Duellman & Trueb, 1986, 1994; Elkan & Reichenbach-Klinke, 1974; Flynn, 1973; Frank, 1984; Griner, 1983; Marcus, 1981; Reichenbach-Klinke & Elkan, 1965; Wallach & Boever, 1983; Wright, 1996. Checklists of parasites of amphibians have been published by Baker, 1987; Canning & Lom, 1986; Flynn, 1973; Frank, 1984; Reichenbach-Klinke & Elkan, 1965; and Walton, 1964, 1966, 1967.

Amphibian medicine is not yet as sophisticated as that for other vertebrate groups including fish (Crawshaw 1992b; Wright, 1996). There are relatively few studies of the interrelationships between the amphibian host, the protozoan or metazoan, and the environment. Similarly, there are few rigorous experimental studies of pathogenesis despite the availability of some protozoans in pure cultures, which could be used for experimental infections. There are relatively few comprehensive surveys and detailed studies of therapeutic regimes, and this is especially true for the small and exotic host species (Poynton & Whitaker, 1994).

Recently, Munson (1990) has made recommendations for advances in captive animal medicine, and these can certainly be applied to amphibians. The guidelines include the study of noncaptive cohorts, comparative studies of disease prevalence at different locations, and study of endangered species. The latter is becoming increasingly important as a number of amphibian species are listed by CITES (Convention on International Trade in Endangered Species).

The overview that follows begins with a discussion of management and treatment strategies. This is followed by a discussion of the intricate interrelationships

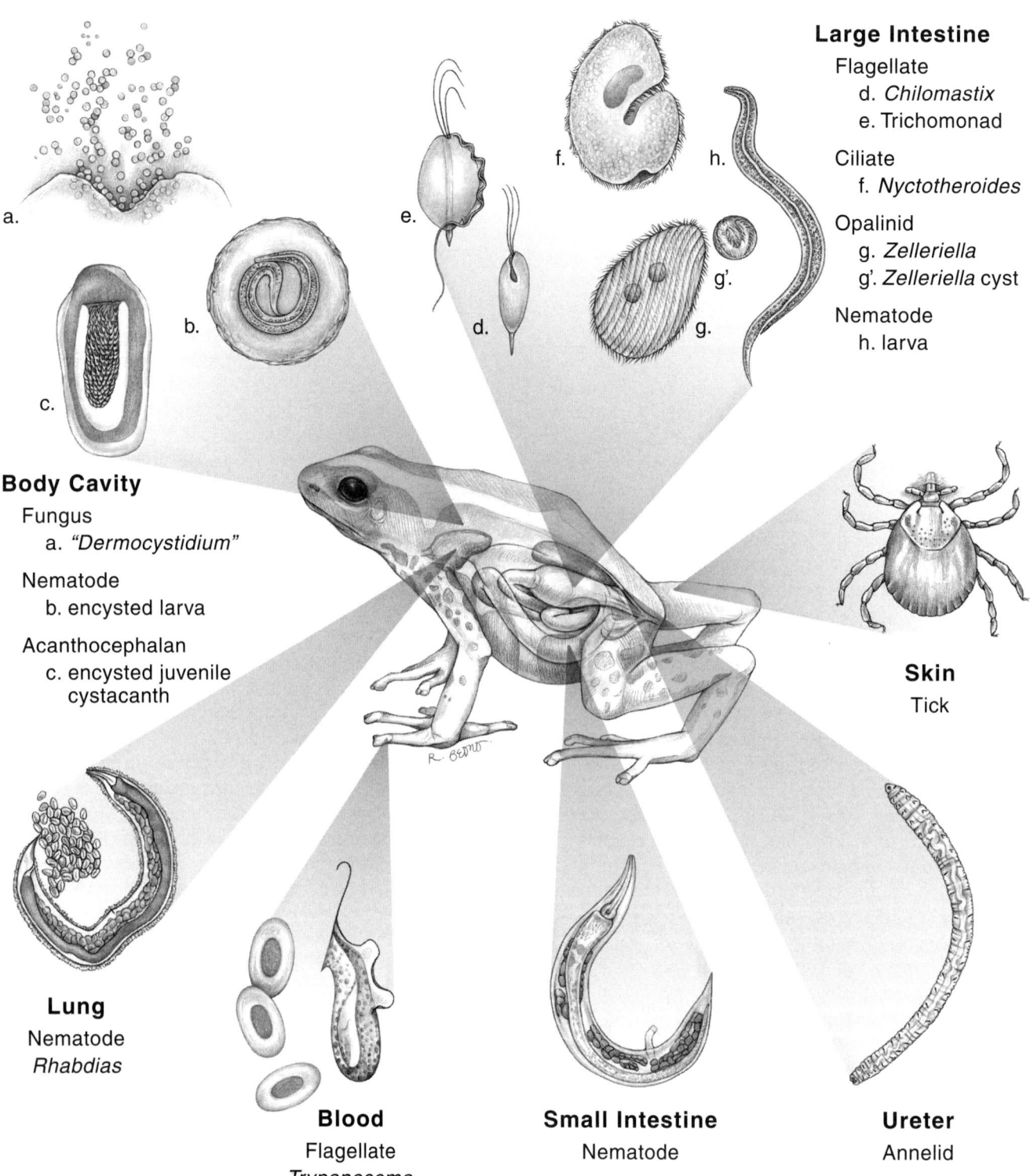

Figure 15.1. A diversity of protozoa and metazoa that infect adult poison frogs (Dendrobatidae). For further details see Poynton and Whitaker (1994). (Rachel Bedno-Robinson, Johns Hopkins University Department of Art as Applied to Medicine)

Table 15.1. Common distribution of protozoa and metazoa in the organ systems of amphibians.

	Skin	Gills	Lungs	Gastro-intestinal	Viscera	Gonads	Urinary bladder	Gall bladder	Blood	Muscle	Coelom
Protozoa											
Ciliates	+	+		+			+				
Opalinids				+ + +							
Flagellates	+	+		+ + +	+ + +				+		
Amoebae				+ +	+ +						
Apicomplexa								+	+		
Microsporidia						+				+	
Metazoa											
Myxosporidia	+ +	+ +		+ + +	+	+	+ +	+		+	+
Monogeans	+ +		+	+ + +	+ +		+ +				+ + +
Digeneans	+ +		+								
Cestodes	+			+	+ +					+ +	+ +
Nematodes									+ (microfilaria)		
Acanthocephala	+	+									+
Leeches	+	+									
Crustaceans											
Fungi											
Dermocystidium	+	+									

Although organisms from the *Dermocystidium* group are fungi, they are considered here for convenience.

between the protozoa, metazoa, and their amphibian hosts, with presentation of some of the most commonly encountered protozoan and metazoan groups, with descriptions of their appearance, life cycles, relationships with their hosts, and management strategies. For several groups of organisms such as the hemogregarines, myxosporeans, and the *Dermocystidium* group (the latter a fungus but considered here for convenience), we are able to present new information on identification, life cycles, and treatments which can be used for guidance in preparing management plans. For pathogenic organisms, clinical signs and treatments are explained. Also included are simple keys and recommendations for techniques and literature that should enable nonspecialists to undertake identification of many of the protozoa and metazoa that will be found, thus providing a sound basis for management and treatment decisions. It is hoped that this will be both of immediate benefit and will help in furthering the science and medicine of amphibian care.

15.2 CONSIDERATIONS FOR MANAGEMENT AND TREATMENT

Our experience with a variety of captive amphibians has shown that protozoan and metazoan infections are commonly encountered, and the use of therapeutics to eliminate true parasites is best accomplished during the quarantine period, thus protecting colony animals from infection. In most cases, the finding of protozoans in the feces of otherwise healthy animals does not require treatment. However, some circumstances, such as recent transportation, changes in environment associated with captivity, and onset of illness, can upset the delicate balance that exists between the protozoa and their amphibian host, and clinical intervention may then be necessary to safeguard the hosts. The presence of metazoa may be more difficult to assess due to internal migration, and subsequent formation of encysted stages. As a result of this, one approach is to treat newly acquired amphibians with a combination of anthelmintics. Rapid destruction of metazoa in the animal's tissues can, in rare cases, cause more harm than good, as inflammatory or even anaphylactic conditions may transpire.

A sound understanding of their life cycles and interrelationships with the host are crucial to effective management and treatment of protozoa and metazoa infection. For example, the likelihood of successfully eliminating metazoa with direct life cycles by using anthelmintics is greatly increased by moving amphibians into a clean vivarium after each treatment. Repetition of this labor intensive process two or three times interrupts the parasite's life cycle, and minimizes reinfection of the host with free-living larvae. Alternatively, amphibians kept in the same vivarium may require more frequent treatments over an extended period of time. The routine use of anthelmintics may be necessary to control metazoan infection in some populations. The prompt removal of excess organic material including sloughed skin, as well as dead or dying animals, is an important management strategy, as this reduces sources of reinfection.

When using medications for the first time in an unfamiliar species, it makes good sense to be conservative. If treating a group, select one or more representative animals to receive therapy. Once comfortable that your course of action is sound, the remainder of the group can be treated. Development of effective treatment regimes should also be guided by the knowledge that different species of parasites, sometimes even within the same family, vary in their susceptibility to treatment (Cone, 1995). It is also important to bear in mind that metazoan parasites have an uneven (over dispersed) distribution among their hosts, with most hosts being lightly infected, and a few hosts being heavily infected. Awareness of this is important when evaluating the need for, and efficacy of, treatments.

Many of the therapies used to treat amphibians have been modified from those used successfully in fish and reptiles. In many cases, doses presented in the literature have been derived for adult amphibians. The clinician should be aware that young larval amphibians may be particularly sensitive to these chemicals, resulting in failure to grow or death if used at the levels recommended for adult amphibians. Recommended doses for many of the chemicals mentioned in the following sections are found in Chapter 24, Pharmacotherapeutics.

15.3 CILIATES

15.3.1 Ciliates in the Gastrointestinal Tract

The gastrointestinal tract of amphibians is commonly infected with commensal ciliates such as *Balantidium, Cepedietta, Nyctotheroides* (listed as *Nyctotherus* in some older literature), *Tetrahymena* and *Sicuophora,* which swim among the contents of the lumen. These ciliates have direct life cycles and reproduce by transverse binary fission.

Nyctotheroides is one of the most frequently encountered ciliates, and can easily be recognized by its flattened body, kidney bean-shaped macronucleus, numerous longitudinal rows of cilia, tufts of compound buccal cilia, and a long curved infundibulum (the inner portion of the buccal cavity) (Plates 15.1A, 15.1B). The genus *Cepedietta* (listed as *Haptophyra* in some older literature), can be recognized by its special method of reproduction in which there is binary fission without separation of the young, thus giving rise to temporary lines or strings of individuals.

Diagnosis. Gastrointestinal ciliates are readily detected in a wet mount prepared from fresh feces. Care must be taken not to confuse them with opalinids. In ciliates, a macronucleus and infundibulum can often be seen (see Plate 15.1A) but these structures are absent from opalinids (see Figure 15.4A).

Treatment. Amphibians rarely require treatment for ciliate infections. In cases where ciliates are thought to be harming the host, metronidazole may be administered orally at a dose of 10–20 mg/kg once a day for 5 d. Paromomycin at a dose of 50–75 mg/kg PO may also reduce levels of ciliates in the gastrointestinal tract.

15.3.2 External Ciliates, and Those in the Urinary Bladder

In the aquatic environment, the skin and gills of the axolotl, *Ambystoma mexicanum,* and anuran tadpoles may be infected with trichodinid ciliates (Wright, 1996) (Figures 15.2A, 15.2B), and heavy infections can be problematic. Since these ciliates feed upon suspended organic material, and have direct life cycles, poor water quality and crowded conditions allow them to thrive, and they may then damage their hosts. Harm occurs when the density of infection is high and the action of the sharp rim of the adhesive discs of numerous ciliates damages the hosts' tissues, causing sloughing of cells upon which the ciliates can also feed. Clinical signs of ectoparasitic trichodinid infection are skin lesions, excess mucus coating the skin, and reddened gills.

Some trichodinids, such as *Trichodina urinicola,* can also exploit the urinary bladder of frogs, toads, and newts, as a site for infection. Such infections are rarely identified and are not believed to be pathogenic.

In addition to trichodinids, other ciliates such as *Carchesium* and *Vorticella* (which are normally free-

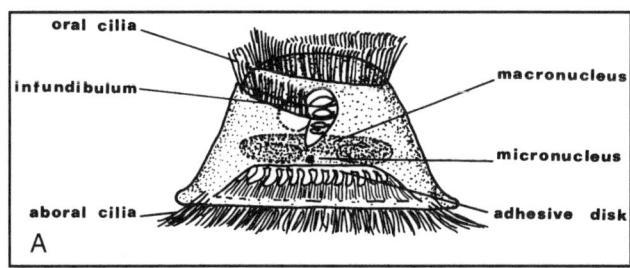

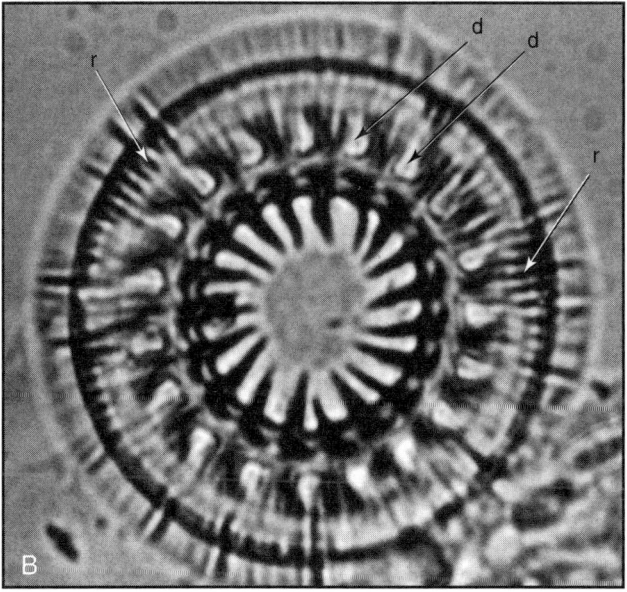

Figure 15.2. A trichodinid ciliate. **A.** Side view showing the spiral of oral cilia, the girdle of cilia at the aboral surface which is in contact with the host, the distinctive adhesive disc, and the macronucleus and micronucleus. **B.** The adhesive disc, with interconnecting denticles (d) and radial pins (r). The coordination of these elements contracts the disc, allowing the ciliate to attach to the host. Diameter of adhesive disc of trichodinids (i.e., distal margin of radial pins to distal margin of radial pins) ranges from 15 to 135 μm. (Sarah L. Poynton, Johns Hopkins University School of Medicine, taken from Stoskopf 1993)

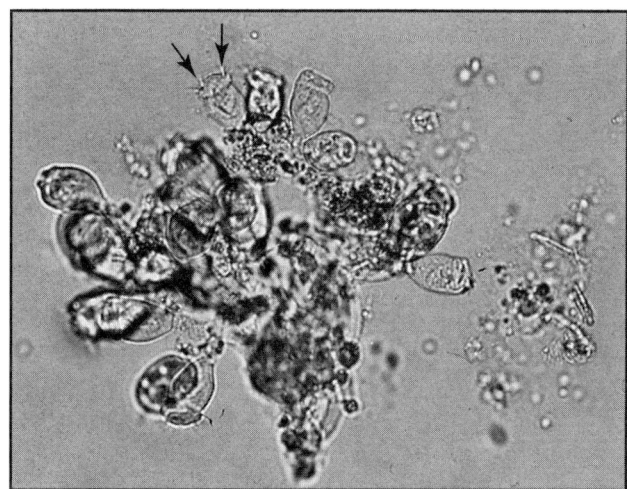

Figure 15.3. A colony of sessile peritrich ciliates from the skin of an aquatic caecilian, *Typhlonectes* sp. Note that in actively feeding individuals, the spiral of oral cilia is cleary visible (arrows). Length of individual sessile peritrichs ranges from 35 to 110 μm. (Kevin Wright, Philadelphia Zoological Garden)

living) and a variety of sessile peritrichs (Figure 15.3) can also colonize the surface of aquatic amphibians, especially those that are young or debilitated. Similar colonization is also seen in fish (Lom & Dykova, 1992).

Diagnosis. External infections by ciliates are easily diagnosed by finding the organisms on a skin scrape of epidermal lesions or a squash preparation of gill tissue. Trichodinids are readily recognized in wet mounts by their whirling motion and distinctive morphology, particularly the adhesive disc and spiral of oral cilia (Plate 15.2; see Figures 15.2A, 15.2B).

Trichodinid urinary infections may be identified by

direct examination of urine using the light microscope. Some anurans will void urine when handled while others may be stimulated to provide a sample (See also Chapter 8, Clinical Techniques).

Treatment. Numerous treatments have been reported to be effective in controlling external trichodinids. In all cases, maintaining excellent water quality will greatly increase the likelihood of success. Before beginning any of the following therapeutic regimes, at least 50% of the vivarium's water should be replaced.

One of the most benign therapies that can be used is to disrupt the parasite's water balance. This can often be accomplished, without placing undue stress on the amphibian's homeostasis, using either distilled water or salt baths. One treatment is to place the amphibian in a distilled water bath for 2–3 h. A salt bath using sea salt or sodium chloride may also be effective at 10–25 g/L as a bath for 5–30 min (at the higher doses, the bath should not exceed 10 min duration) (Wright, 1996). Alternatively, the salt treatment can be administered at 4–6 g/L for a 24 h bath (Raphael, 1993). Other treatments that should be considered include a bath in malachite green, 0.15 mg/L for 1 h daily to effect (Raphael, 1993); or potassium permanganate (7 mg/L bath for up to 5 min every 24 h to effect) (Raphael, 1993). Though potentially more toxic, copper sulfate, 500 mg/L 2 min dip daily to effect (Raphael, 1993), or formalin baths, 10% formalin diluted 1.5 ml in 1 liter water as a 10 min bath every 48 h (Crawshaw, 1992a), may also be effective. Copper sulfate should only be used in hard water to reduce the likelihood of toxicity, while additional aeration is necessary when using formalin treatments. Formalin should not be used for animals with ulcerative lesions. Sodium chlorite ($NaOCl_2$ 20 mg/L for a 6–8 h bath daily to effect) (Dempster et al., 1988) may also be effective against external protozoans, and has proven safe in some anuran tadpoles (personal communication, M. Greenwell). Steinberg's solution or modified Holtfreter's solution (100%) as a bath for 3–5 d may also be used (Maruska, 1994). Since malachite green and formalin are considered potential carcinogens, they should be handled with extra care. Young tadpoles exposed to malachite green may cease to grow during the treatment period.

15.4 OPALINIDS

Opalinids are commensals that are commonly found living in the large intestine of amphibians (principally anurans), and they derive their name from their beautiful opalescent appearance. Although opalinids superficially resemble ciliates, they are considered distinct because: a) they have nuclei of the same size and type (in contrast, ciliates have a large macronucleus and a small micronucleus); and b) they do not have a cell mouth. The five opalinid genera *Cepedea, Opalina, Protoopalina, Protozelleriella,* and *Zelleriella,* are distinguished by the number of nuclei (two or many) and the shape of the cell in transverse section (circular or flattened).

The life cycle of the opalinids is direct, and it is elaborately coordinated with that of their hosts. In the lu-

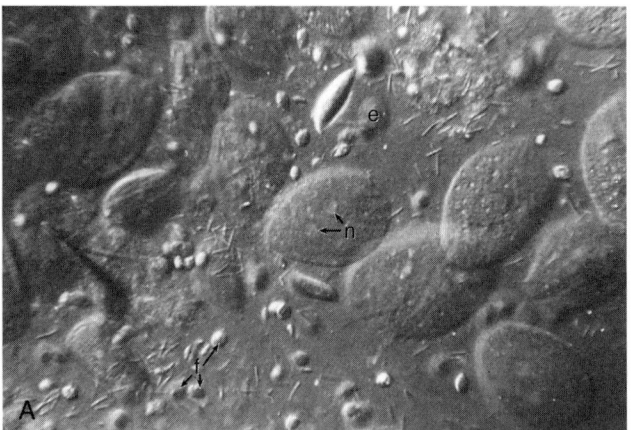

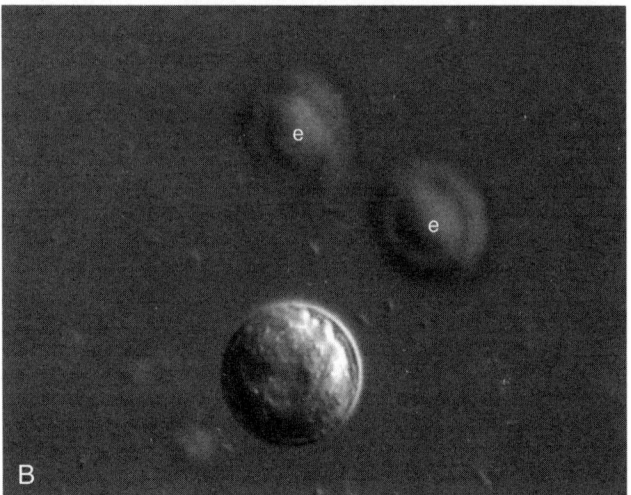

Figure 15.4. The opalinid *Zelleriella* sp. from the lumen of the large intestine of a dendrobatid frog. **A.** The live trophonts (the swimming stage). The rows of flagella covering the body can be clearly seen. The genus *Zelleriella* is flattened and has two equally sized nuclei (n), features that can easily be seen when observing the living cells. *Zelleriella* sp. swims with a tumbling motion, flipping over, so that sometimes it is broad and flat, other times the narrow flattened profile is seen. The relative size of the different inhabitants of the lumen of the large intestine can be appreciated by comparing the size of the opalinids to the flagellates (f), and an erythrocyte (e). **B.** A *Zelleriella* cyst, containing a single infectious individual covered with rows of flagella. Note size in relation to erythrocytes (e). *Zelleriella* trophonts may reach 150 μm in length, cysts are 20 mm in diameter. Viewed with Normarski illumination which gives a three-dimensional appearance. (Sarah L. Poynton, Johns Hopkins University School of Medicine, taken from Poynton and Whitaker 1994)

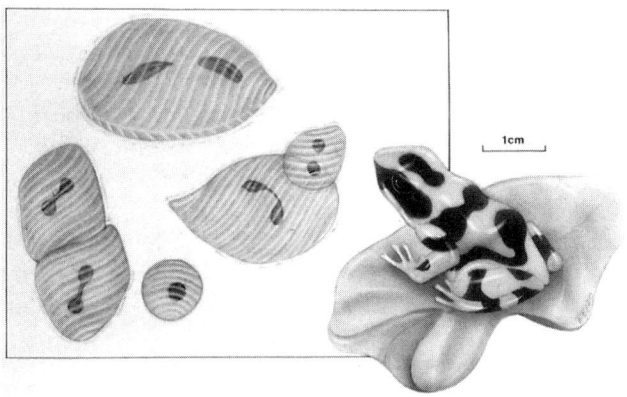

Figure 15.5. Developing and mature stages of the opalinid, *Zelleriella* sp., in the green and black poison frog, *Dendrobates auratus*. In the lumen of the intestine are found the large swimming trophonts, many of which divide and grow to produce new trophonts. However, some trophonts divide without growth, thus giving rise to very small individuals that encyst. Such infective cysts are passed with the feces and await ingestion by newly hatched tadpoles. (Brent Bauer, Johns Hopkins University Department of Art as Applied to Medicine)

men of the adult amphibian's large intestine is found the adult swimming stage of the opalinid called the trophont (Figures 15.4A, 15.5). At any time some of the trophonts will be dividing. However, during the breeding season of the host, some opalinids undergo division without growth (now called tomonts), ultimately becoming very small and encysting (Figures 15.4B; 15.5). These infective cysts are passed with the feces and remain viable for some weeks, during which time they may be eaten by newly hatched tadpoles. In the tadpoles there is a sexual phase, with production of gamonts and then zygocysts, which pass into the water with the tadpole feces. If ingested by a tadpole approaching metamorphosis, an ingested zygocyst will develop to an adult trophont, thus completing the life cycle.

The opalinid trophonts do not have a cell mouth, but instead absorb nutrient-containing fluid by pinocytosis. In the relatively inactive posterior intestine of the host, opalinids and other protozoans feed upon materials which would otherwise pass in the feces, and thus are not believed to compete with the host for nutrition.

Diagnosis. Opalinids can be detected in fresh fecal samples. The active swimming of the large trophonts and smaller tomonts aids in their identification. Spherical cysts can be distinguished from helminth eggs because they contain a small opalinid (with its distinctive rows of flagella clearly visible), which can sometimes be seen moving inside the cyst. It may also be possible to see the two or more characteristic nuclei by focusing through the cyst. In rare cases, hatching of the cyst may be observed in a wet mount, confirming the diagnosis.

Opalinids may be confused with ciliates, however opalinids lack the macronucleus and infundibulum often seen in ciliates (see Plate 15.1A and Figure 15.4A for comparison).

Treatment. Treatment of opalinid infection is not necessary.

15.5 FLAGELLATES

15.5.1 Ectoparasitic Flagellates

Dinoflagellates belonging to the family Oodinidae can infect the skin and gills of amphibians, especially larvae. Their presence causes lesions, osmoregulatory dysfunction, respiratory distress, and debilitation. This irritation can lead to excess mucous production, giving the animals a grayish hue. Severe infections can be fatal, especially in captive animals. A common genus referred to in the literature is *Oodinium*, however, this is now considered incorrect with regard to infection in amphibians, because *Oodinium* is ectoparasitic on marine invertebrates. A related genus, *Piscinoodinium,* is known from larval amphibians (Woo, 1994).

The life cycle of dinoflagellates is direct. The parasitic stage attached to the surface of the host, called the trophont, is a dark or opaque spherical or pyriform structure which lacks flagella (Plate 15.3). It is nourished by absorption of host cytoplasm via its attachment structure. After feeding and growing, the mature trophont detaches, enlarges, and forms a cyst within which numerous flagellated dinospores are formed. When the cyst ruptures, the dinospore swarmers swim with the aid of their two flagella until they locate a suitable host. They then transform into trophonts, thus completing the life cycle. The direct life cycle, with extensive multiplication in the cyst, means that dinoflagellates can be a major problem in captive animals.

The clinical appearance of dinoflagellate infection is in part dependent upon the exact species of parasite present, and may include a velvet or dustlike surface on the body or grayish lesions. The distinctive chromatophores and chlorophyll, which may be present in the trophonts, determine the color of the infected area.

In addition to dinoflagellates, the external surfaces of aquatic amphibians can also be infected with the kinetoplastid flagellate *Ichthyobodo* (synonym = *Costia*). These organisms have a direct life cycle with an attached feeding stage and a free-swimming stage. As with dinoflagellates, the infection results in destruction of epithelial or epidermal cells, hemodilution, and osmoregulatory and circulatory failure (Lom & Dykova, 1992).

Diagnosis. Diagnosis of a dinoflagellate infection is made by collecting skin scrapings of the affected areas and finding the trophonts (see Plate 15.3). Gill clips can also be performed in larger animals or postmortem specimens. Dinospore swarmers and *Ichthyobodo* may be found on both skin and gills.

Treatment. Treatment should be initiated immediately following a large water change designed to reduce the number of infective dinospores and minimize the likelihood of reinfection. A better alternative, however, is to treat affected animals and then move them into a completely new tank. Distilled water or salt baths (using sea salt, Steinberg's solution, or modified Holtfreter's solution) may be effective at reducing or eliminating external flagellates (see "Treatment" in Section 15.3.2, External Ciliates, and Those in the Urinary Bladder). Freshwater animals with serious damage to the gills and skin may be osmotically compromised and benefit from the addition of salts rather than distilled water. Malachite green or sodium chlorite ($NaOCl_2$) baths should also be considered. Though potentially more toxic, copper sulfate or formalin baths may also be effective. Metronidazole baths may be efficacious. Any of these therapeutic regimes must be performed on a regular basis (daily to every other day) in order to eliminate the susceptible dinospore hatchlings (swarmers). A final consideration is the use of oral chloroquine. Although fish have been successfully treated using chloroquine orally at 50 mg/kg once weekly (Lewis et al., 1988), there is no data on its use in amphibians. Clients should be informed that despite treatment, heavily infected animals may perish.

15.5.2 Flagellates in the Blood

The blood of amphibians can be infected by the diplomonads *Brugerolleia* and possibly also *Hexamita* (Desser et al., 1993), and more commonly by the kinetoplastid flagellate *Trypanosoma*. Diplomonad flagellates have been reported from the blood of several species of *Bufo* and *Rana*. Initially such flagellates were all believed to be the same as those from the gastrointestinal tract due to its opportunistic invasion (see Section 15.5.3, Intestinal Flagellates). However, recent ultrastructural studies have clearly shown that a distinct genus, *Brugerolleia,* lives in the blood of the green frog, *Rana clamitans* (Desser et al., 1993). All of the diplomonads can be readily recognized in fresh preparations by their energetic swimming, spherical to ovoid body, six anterior flagella, and two trailing posterior flagella (Figure 15.6). The pathogenecity of diplomonads in the blood of amphibians has not been determined.

Trypanosomes are readily recognized in blood smears by their energetic swimming, the distinctive undulating membrane, and a flagellum that extends freely at the anterior end (Figure 15.7). The pathogenicity associated with infection is variable, most infections being benign while only a few are considered problematic.

Trypanosomes have an indirect life cycle, requiring a vertebrate host and a hematophagous (blood-sucking) vector, which may be a leech or an insect. Thus, once a wild-caught animal is maintained in captivity, infections will usually decrease due to the absence of vectors necessary for completion of the life cycles.

Across all classes of animals, a heavy infection of trypanosomes can cause animals to become anemic, anorectic, and debilitated. It is likely that in some cases, even subclinical infections hamper performance and reproductive success (Wright, 1996). In amphibians, the following species of trypanosomes are reported as pathogenic: *Trypanosoma inopinatum* causes destruction of the spleen and may be fatal in Old World amphibians; *T. pipientis* causes enlargement of the spleen in the leopard frog, *Rana pipiens*; *T. ranarum* infection may result in anorexia, degeneration of erythrocytes, and death of the host; and, *T. diemyctyli* is pathogenic in newts (Marcus, 1981).

Diagnosis. Flagellates often are detected first by their active swimming in a wet mount of whole blood, but identification requires smears stained with Wright-Giemsa stain or protargol. Diplomonads can be distinguished from trypanosomes by the presence of six anterior flagella and two trailing posterior flagella (see Figure 15.7); diplomonads lack an undulating membrane.

Trypanosomes are commonly found when examining blood smears. An undulating membrane is characteristic of these protozoans. Impression smears of the liver, kidney, and spleen, in conjunction with blood smears, aid in the diagnosis. Splenomegaly and splenic necrosis are often found at postmortem of clinically ill amphibians.

Treatment. Treatments using antimalarial compounds, such as quinine sulfate or quinine bisulfate, 30 mg/L bath for up to one hour, or oral chloroquine, 50 mg/kg PO once weekly, should be considered only in clinically ill amphibians showing evidence of anemia (pale mucous membranes, low hematocrit and red blood cell count) and the presence of trypanosomes.

15.5.3 Intestinal Flagellates

A wide variety of flagellates, including proteromonads, retortamonads, diplomonads, oxymonads, and trichomonads, inhabit the anaerobic environment of the amphibian digestive tract. Usually they are found swimming in the intestinal contents in the posterior regions (such as the large intestine and cloacal ampulla), the exceptions being some diplomonads which may be present in the gall bladder, and *Giardia* sp. which attach to the epithelial cells of the small intestine of anuran tadpoles. Most of these flagellates are commensals and should be regarded as a normal component of the

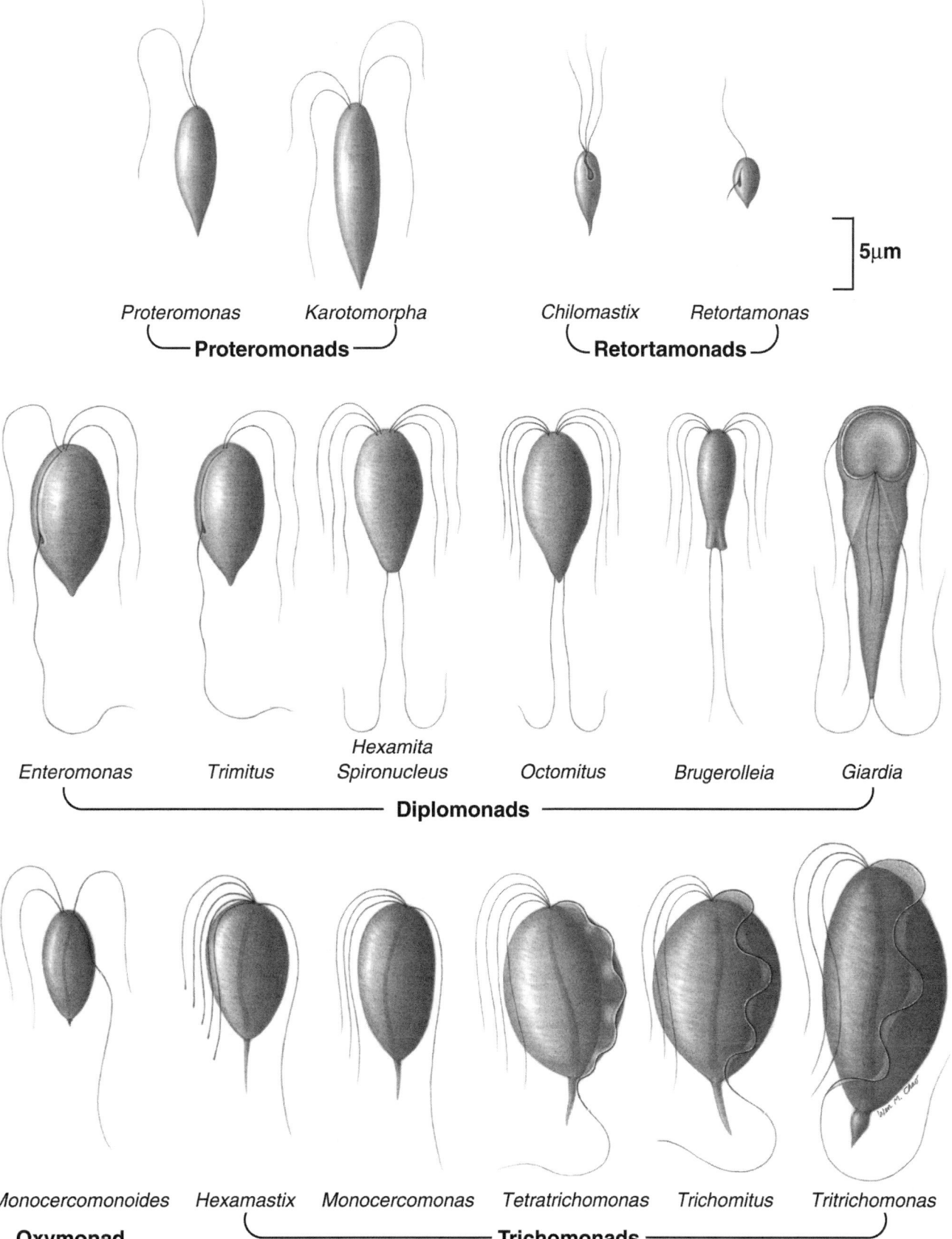

Figure 15.6. A variety of flagellates from the lumen of the large intestine, showing the distinctive features of the five families commonly encountered. Additional information is given in Table 15.2. Note that the diplomonad *Brugerolleia*, normally living in the blood, may be found as a contaminant following dissection of the intestine. All flagellates are shown at same magnification. (Wen-Min Chao, Johns Hopkins University Department of Art as Applied to Medicine)

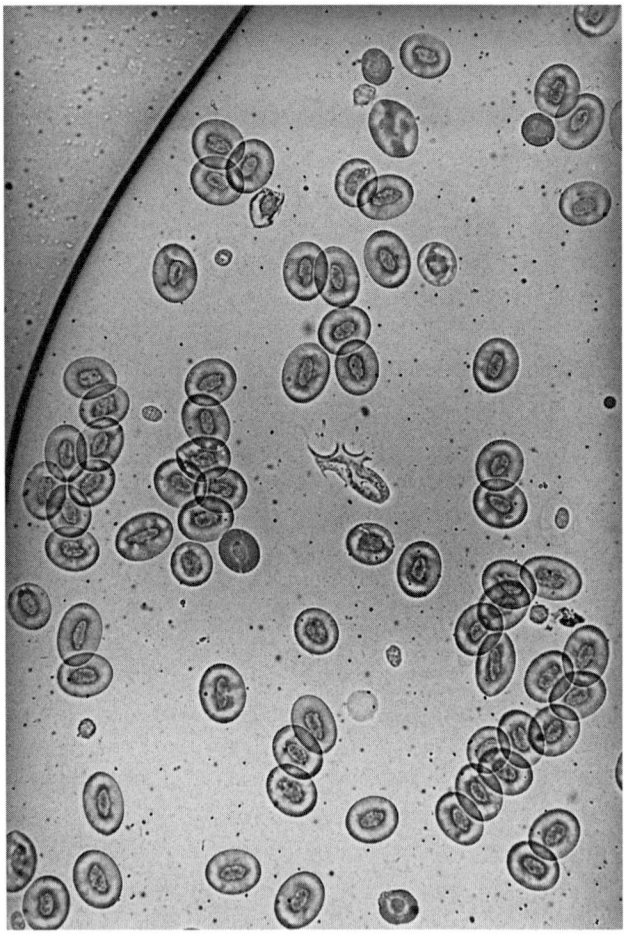

Figure 15.7. A hemoflagellate, *Trypanosoma* sp., from the blood of a poison frog *Dendrobates* sp. The characteristic diagnostic features of this genus, namely the membrane that undulates and the single anterior flagellum, are evident. Length of *Trypanosoma* species ranges from 20–80 mm. (Sarah L. Poynton, Johns Hopkins University School of Medicine, taken from Poynton and Whitaker 1994)

terson, 1960). These factors can influence the nutritional status of the flagellates. Some groups, such as the retortamonads and some of the diplomonads, are bactivorous, feeding by phagocytosis. Other flagellate groups, such as the proteromonads and some trichomonads, feed on dissolved matter by pinocytosis.

Intestinal flagellates normally have a commensal relationship with their amphibian hosts, however, under stressful circumstances such as recent shipping, inadequate nutrition, and improper environmental conditions, the homeostasis that exists in healthy amphibians can be disrupted. Abundant intestinal protozoa, although not the primary cause of illness, are often associated with amphibians that are failing to thrive or are ill. The increased presence of intestinal protozoa is therefore an indication of stress and potential susceptibility to other pathogens. Frogs housed at the National Aquarium in Baltimore showed a decreasing prevalence of intestinal protozoa between arrival, holding in quarantine, and departure from the aquarium (Poynton & Whitaker, 1994).

Diagnosis. Intestinal protozoa are commonly identified in feces and may also be found in samples collected by stomach or cloacal wash. Samples must be fresh in order to fully appreciate the flora present, as many protozoans become encysted or die in unfavorable environments. In some cases, after moistening with warm 0.9% saline and incubating at room temperature for 1–2 h, dried feces may provide limited information by allowing encysted protozoa to emerge. A modified Wright-Giemsa stain, which also preserves flagellates for future viewing, can be utilized as an aid in identification (see Section 15.19, Identification of Protozoa and Metazoa). Although major groups such as trichomonads and

fauna of the amphibian host. However, many gastrointestinal and blood protozoans that are considered nonpathogenic for terrestrial amphibians may cause disease in salamanders (Crawshaw, 1992b). Evidence from other hosts, including fish, shows that some species of diplomonads and trichomonads can be pathogenic (Frank, 1984; Woo & Poynton, 1995), thus it is reasonable to expect that some species infecting amphibians may be pathogenic.

The life cycle of the intestinal flagellates is direct, involving only the amphibian host, which becomes infected by ingestion of contaminated food and water. Inside the amphibian's gut or gall bladder, the swimming trophozoite stages of the flagellates multiply by longitudinal binary fission, and in many genera a resting cyst stage is present. The establishment and equilibrium of the flagellate communities is believed to be influenced by a variety of factors including the host's diet and the bacterial flora in the digestive tract (Pe-

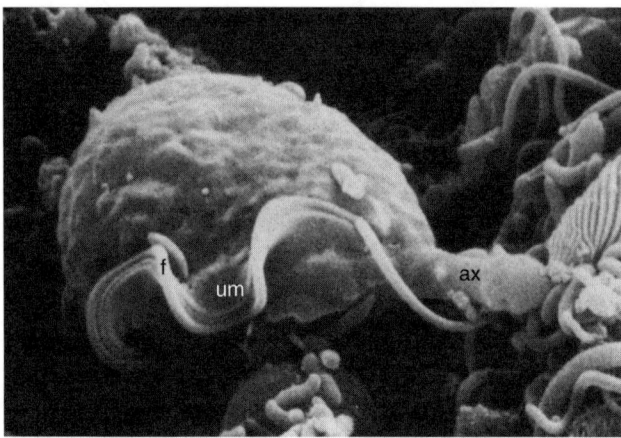

Figure 15.8. A trichomonad, probably *Tritrichomonas*, from the large intestine of a poison frog, *Dendrobates* sp. Note the undulating membrane (um) bordered by a flagellum (f), and the prominent broad protruding axostyle (ax) in this scanning electron micrograph. Length of trichomonads ranges from 10–35 μm. (Phillip Rutledge, University of Maryland at Baltimore County, taken from Poynton and Whitaker 1994)

Table 15.2. Identification of protozoa: preparation methods for smears and imprints, and keys and host-parasite checklists.

	Giemsa Lom & Dykova, 1992	Protargol Lom & Dykova, 1992	Silver Nitrate Lom & Dykova, 1992	Gram	2.5% Potassium Dichromate Barnard & Upton, 1994	Keys and host-parasite checklists
Ciliates	+	+				Lee et al., In press.
trichodinids		+	+			Lom & Dykova, 1992
Opalinids		+				Lee et al., In press.
Flagellates		+				Lee et al., In press.
hemoflagellates	+	+				Diamond, 1965
Apicomplexa in blood*	+					Lee et al., 1985; Levine, 1988a, b
Apicomplexa in tissues					+	Levine, 1988a, b
Microsporidia				+		Canning & Lom, 1986

Note: For additional information on stain or preparation and description of protocol, the reader is referred to Barnard & Upton, 1994; Lee & Soldo, 1992; Pritchard & Kruse, 1982.
*For the hemogregarines, identification to genus depends on characteristics of development in the invertebrate vector (Desser et al., 1995).

diplomonads can be easily differentiated using the light microscope (see Figure 15.6; Table 15.2), further identification to genus and species usually requires special stains and use of electron microscopy (Figure 15.8).

It is common to find mixed infections of different genera from the following groups: proteromonads (*Karotomorpha, Proteromonas*); retortamonads (*Chilomastix, Retortamonas*); diplomonads (*Enteromonas, Trimitus, Hexamita, Spironucleus, Octomitus, Giardia*); oxymonads (*Monocercomonoides*); and, trichomonads (*Hexamastix, Monocercomonas, Tetratrichomonas, Trichomitus,* and *Tritrichomonas*) (see Table 15.2 and Figure 15.6).

Treatment. Amphibians that show evidence of clinical disease concurrent with greater than usual flagellate infections may benefit from daily treatment with metronidazole. Adult amphibians are best treated orally (10 mg/kg daily for 5–10 d), while larval forms are given a 6–8 h bath with powdered metronidazole dissolved in tank water (250 mg/37.8 L or 250 mg/10 gal) once weekly for up to three treatments. The purpose of this therapy is to allow the amphibian to regain its natural flagellate "homeostasis" and not to eliminate the organisms.

15.6 AMOEBAE

A variety of amoebae have been reported from the intestinal tract, liver, and kidney of amphibians. Only a few species of amoebae are reported to be pathogenic, including *Entamoeba ranarum* from the digestive tract and liver of both tadpoles and adults, and *E. ilowaiskii*. Some species of *Naegleria* and *Acanthamoeba* can cause ocular lesions and/or direct penetration of the cribiform plate with central nervous system extension. Other amoebae reported from amphibians include the genera *Copramoeba, Hartmanella, Mastigamoeba,* and *Vahlkampfia*. It should be borne in mind that identification of amoebae is difficult, thus a cautious and critical approach should be taken with regard to investigation and to interpreting the literature.

The amoebae can be recognized by their characteristic formation of pseudopodia (which are protrusions of the cytoplasm) in the trophozoite stage. Formation of resistant cysts is seen in some species, and the genera *Naegleria, Acanthamoeba* and *Vahlkampfia* produce flagella when in contact with water. Their life cycle is direct, and infection is usually via ingestion.

Many factors probably predispose amphibians to amoebiasis, including stress, inappropriate food, lack of ingesta, and other concurrent infections (Wright, 1996). While pathogenic organisms typically cause damage to the mucosa of the stomach and colon, hepatic and renal lesions may also be seen. In some cases, this may be consistent with hematological spread, however, in one group of the giant toad, *Bufo marinus,* diagnosed with renal amoebiasis, no evidence of intestinal infection was found (Valentine & Stoskopf, 1984). Ulcerative lesions of the gastrointestinal tract are likely to lead to secondary bacterial septicemia if left untreated.

Amphibians with intestinal amoebiasis are often anorexic and show obvious weight loss. As the infection progresses, feces become increasingly fluid and mixed with blood, leading to rapid dehydration of the animal. In cases of renal or hepatic ameobiasis, dehydration, anasarca, and ascites may be present.

Diagnosis. Finding amoebae in fecal or cloacal wash samples should be considered a preliminary diagnosis only, as it is difficult to differentiate pathogenic from nonpathogenic organisms. If concomitant leukocytes and erythrocytes are found in the fecal sample or cloacal wash, a presumptive diagnosis of amoebic infection can be assessed. A definitive diagnosis requires a thorough postmortem examination. Confirmation of suspected renal or hepatic amoebiasis is made upon finding the organisms histologically.

Treatment. The successful treatment of amoebiasis requires a multifaceted approach. First, fluid therapy in the form of a shallow water or dilute electrolyte bath should be given to terrestrial species to re-establish hydration. Aquatic amphibians may be suffering from over-hydration if renal function is compromised, and electrolyte baths (e.g., amphibian lactated Ringer's solution, modified Holtfreter's solution) may be necessary. Second, metronidazole is administered orally at a dose of 100 mg/kg every 14 d well beyond evidence of clinical infection. Larval amphibians may be placed in concentrated metronidazole baths (500 mg/L) every 5 d for 15–30 min. Less concentrated baths of 250 mg/37.8 L (250 mg/10 gal) for up to 8 h may be used for sensitive species. Since a large quantity of metronidazole is excreted unchanged in the urine, this drug is a good choice for renal amoebiasis. Third, the animals should be placed in a clean environment free of infective cysts within 24 hours of each treatment. While time consuming and costly, this approach helps to minimize reinfection. Finally, treatment of any other infections should be instituted simultaneously.

15.7 APICOMPLEXA

Apicomplexa infections in amphibians may be recognized in a variety of different sites and forms. In the blood, the genera *Hemogregarina, Hepatozoon, Lankesterella, Schellackia, Babesiosoma,* and *Dactylosoma,* are found. In the erythrocytes, the hemogregarines and lankesterellids can be recognized as banana-shaped inclusions (Desser, 1993) while dactylostomatids appear as oval to round, small inclusions. In the tissues, genera such as *Eimeria* and *Isospora* occur. The morphology of the different apicomplexa parasites is very diverse, and the main unifying feature of the phylum is the possession (at some stage of development) of an apical complex of organelles which may be used for locomotion and penetration of the host cell. However, this feature can only be seen with the transmission electron microscope.

The life cycles of apicomplexa are variable, and may involve vectors or intermediate hosts. Asexual and sexual phases may be involved. The three different phases of multiple fission are: merogony, the production of meronts; gametogony, the production of gametes; and sporogony, the production of spores.

All members of the Apicomplexa are parasitic, some of them important disease agents, while others are apparently nonpathogenic. Pathogenicity is determined by a number of factors including the extent of multiplication that can occur in the host, and the nature and abundance of the host cells in which the parasites develop.

15.7.1 Apicomplexa in the Blood

The blood of amphibians can be infected by apicomplexa belonging to several different groups. The hemogregarines, *Hemogregarina* and *Hepatozoon,* the lankesterellids, *Lankesterella* and *Schellackia,* and dactylosomatids, such as *Babesiosoma* and *Dactylosoma,* have indirect life cycles with vertebrate hosts and invertebrate vectors. In most amphibian infections, details of the apicomplexan life cycles are incompletely known. For hemogregarines, the amphibian is the host for merogony which takes place in the internal organs, and for gametogony, the development from merozoites to gamonts taking place in the erythrocytes. The leech or arthropod host is utilized for sporogony. In a recent study, it was shown that *Hepatozoon catesbianae* infects the bullfrog, *Rana catesbeiana,* when a frog ingests an infected mosquito, *Culex territans,* containing sporocysts; mosquitoes are infected by feeding on frogs infected with gamonts (Desser et al., 1995). For lankesterellids, the amphibian is the host for the entire replicative portion of the life cycle: merogony, gametogony and sporogony (Desser, 1993). Merogony takes place in the small intestine, the connective tissues and the endothelium of blood vessels. Sporozoites are present in the blood cells. The infection is transferred by hematophagous invertebrates such as leeches, mites, and mosquitoes. Amphibians become infected by inoculation of sporozoites when fed upon by leeches, or ingestion of mites or mosquitos. For dactylosomatids the vectors for infection are rhynchobdellid leeches (Barta, 1991).

The pathogenic status of these protozoa is uncertain; some authors report anemia and death (Reichenbach-Klinke & Elkan, 1965; Wallach & Boever, 1983) while others report that they do not cause significant illness (Desser, 1993; Marcus, 1981). As general guidance, the presence of apicomplexan parasites without clinical signs is not an indication for treatment.

Diagnosis. Diagnosis of apicomplexa in the blood is made from Wright-Giemsa stained blood smears. Organisms are found in the cytoplasm of infected red blood cells. Identification to genus and species is difficult because of the confused taxonomy, especially in hemogregarines from amphibians (Desser, 1993). For hemogregarines, identification to genus is dependent on the nature of sporogony in the invertebrate vector (Desser et al., 1995).

Treatment. Treatment is not recommended for blood-borne hemogregarine infections unless associated with life-threatening anemia.

15.7.2 Apicomplexa in the Tissues

In addition to the tissue phases of the apicomplexans described above, typical coccidian parasites belonging to the family Eimeriidae (including *Eimeria* and *Isospora*) are also found in the tissues. *Eimeria* spp. are the most commonly found coccidians in amphibians having been described in frogs, toads, and salamanders. Two species of *Isospora* have been described in the North American salamander (Upton et al., 1993) and only a small number have been identified in frogs and toads (McAllister & Upton, 1996). These parasites are intracellular, with epithelial cells being the preferred site of infection. Most commonly the intestine is infected, but disease may also be found in other locations such as the gall bladder and kidneys.

Within the host, the merogony and gametogony stages of the life cycle take place. In most anuran coccidia, sporulation of oocysts also takes place within the host, frequently with disintegration of the delicate oocysts in the gut, and subsequent release of sporocysts (Paperna & Lainson, 1995b; Upton & McAllister, 1988). In other species, oocysts may be shed with feces, and sporulation takes place outside of the host. In *Eimeria,* the oocyst contains four sporocysts, each with two sporozoites. In *Isospora,* the oocyst contains only two sporocysts, each of which has four sporozoites. Ingestion of sporulated oocysts results in infection.

In general, coccidian infections are relatively benign in adult hosts, and coccidia may be seen in the feces of apparently healthy animals. Pathology associated with infection is most commonly seen in young or compromised animals, and may include weight loss and diarrhea. Renal coccidia are associated with nephritis.

Diagnosis. Coccidial infections can be difficult to diagnose because oocysts are not readily found during examination of the feces, due to their rupture in the gut and/or the abundance of lumen protozoa. Fecal smears stained with Wright-Giemsa contain leukocytes and erythrocytes, which are indicative of mucosal damage associated with possible coccidial (or amoebic) infection. To aid in indentification to genus level, coccidial oocysts may be sporulated by placing the feces into a solution of 1.0–2.5% potassium dichromate or tapwater containing a small amount of an antibiotic solution (100 IU/ml penicillin G, 100 µg/ml streptomycin-fungizone). The samples are then incubated at room temperature (McAllister & Upton, 1996) and checked for sporulation once or twice a day for up to a week by pipetting a small amount of the sample onto a microslide for light microscopy.

Eimeria, with four sporocysts, can be differentiated from *Isospora,* with only two sporocysts.

Infections may be detected by examination of squash preparations of gut tissue, Giemsa-stained smears and histological sections of the intestine (Paperna & Lainson, 1995b).

Treatment. Treatment with coccidiostats such as amprolium have been unrewarding. However, many anurans treated with trimethoprim sulfamethoxazole (TMS), 15 mg/kg of the combined pharmaceuticals PO daily for 7–14 d, have improved clinically yet continued infection was found on subsequent necropsy. It is therefore likely that the benefits of TMS are due to its action as an antibiotic effective against acute alimentary tract bacterial infection, in addition to the anticoccidial activity of the sulfonamide component. Hydration and electrolyte status may be compromised with severe infection. Terrestrial amphibians may require concomitant baths in shallow water or dilute electrolyte solutions, while aquatic amphibians may benefit from concomitant baths in amphibian's lactated Ringer's solution or modified Holtfreter's solution.

15.8 MICROSPORIDIA

Microsporidia are very small spore-forming protozoa (Plate 15.4) that are obligate intracellular parasites. Although microsporidia do not commonly infect amphibians, spores may be concentrated in areas appearing as pale or white streaks in the striated muscle, connective tissue, oocytes, and Bidder's organ, which is a rudimentary ovary in male toads *Bufo* sp. In many cases the spores are present in greatly enlarged host cells called xenomas, which have a cystlike appearance. The xenoma is a greatly hypertrophied host cell, which absorbs nutrients through its modified surface, and enlarges to accommodate the multiplying parasites within. Such xenomas may become so large that they can be seen grossly. Because of their intracellular nature, extensive reproduction, and direct life cycles, microsporidia can be serious pathogens in captive amphibians.

Microsporidia are believed to have a direct life cycle, with transmission via ingestion of spores which hatch in the gut. Development may occur within the intestine or the parasites may be transported to an alternative site (Canning & Lom, 1986). Upon hatching, the spore everts a polar tube which penetrates the host cell, and passes an infectious sporoplasm into it. There then follows proliferation and the production of spores, which fill the host cell. There are many different patterns of development within the host cell, and identification of microsporidia depends in part upon these patterns. The genera *Pleistophora, Alloglugea,* and *Microsporidium* have been reported from amphibians. *Pleistophora* is a well characterized genus, while *Microsporidium* is a collective name used when there is insufficient information to confirm the exact genus to which a certain microsporidian belongs.

A striking microsporidian infection of the common toad, *Bufo bufo,* in England was described by Canning et al. (1964). Wild-caught toads maintained in the laboratory for 2 years became emaciated, and many animals died. Their striated muscles, except the heart, bore white streaks, examination of which revealed that they were packed full of the developing microsporidian, *Pleistophora myotropica.* Although the amphibians were able to regenerate muscle, this process was not able to keep pace with the lysis of the myofibrils and atrophy of the muscles caused by the parasite.

A new microsporidian, *Alloglugea bufonis,* has recently been reported from tadpoles and newly metamorphosed specimens of the giant toad, *Bufo marinus* (Paperna & Lainson, 1995a). Xenomas were present either singly in the lamina propria of the intestine, or aggregated into cystic bodies up to 0.2 mm in diameter which emerged above the intestine's surface. Even though spores from the mature xenomas were accumulated in reticuloendothelial cells of the liver, spleen, and kidneys of tadpoles, metamorphosis was not impeded. It was suggested that tadpoles become infected by eating spores released from dead companions, or by cannibalism, and furthermore that the spores cannot survive dessication (Paperna & Lainson, 1995a).

Recently Graczyk et al. (1996) have described a novel pathogenic microsporidian infection in a captive South American giant tree frog, *Phyllomedusa bicolor.* The host had progressive ulcerative erythematous dermatitis with a mass of microsporidian spores, 12 × 9 μm in size, evident in tissue imprints from the lesion.

Diagnosis. Transillumination may reveal pale or white streaks in muscle and organs. Diagnosis may be made by the finding of microsporidian spores in impression smears or squashed tissue from lesions, and in impression smears of the cloaca. Spores may also be found in the feces. The spores are 5–20 μm in length and are typically pyriform or pear-shaped, having a distinct posterior vacuole (Plate 15.4). Before hatching, the spores are refractile and green when viewed with transmitted light, and bright under phase contrast. They stain reddish purple with Gram's stain; this positive reaction is in contrast to all other protozoan spores or cysts (see Table 15.2, and Section 15.19, Identification of Protozoa and Metazoa from Amphibians). Transmission electron microscopy is needed to confirm genus identification of microsporidians.

Treatment. Once a diagnosis of microsporidiosis has been reached, a decision must be made between depopulation of seriously affected individuals or attempted therapy. At present there is no generally accepted treatment for microsporidiosis, and thus the quarantine of new animals is very important in management of these infections. However, Graczyk et al. (1996) reported injectable chloramphenicol sodium succinate (Lymphomed™, Division of Fujisawa USA, Deerfield, IL) and topical oxytetracycline hydrochloride with polymyxin B sulfate (Terramycin®, Pfizer, New York, NY) inhibited spore production.

15.9 *DERMOCYSTIDIUM,* THE PROTOZOAN-LIKE FUNGI

The small size and sporelike appearance of the lower fungi, *Dermocystidium,* often resulted in their classification as spore-forming protozoan parasites. Although the development and life cycles of *Dermocystidium* from amphibians are poorly understood, similar infections in fish can include development of hyphae, plasmodia, sporoblasts, and spores containing uniflagellated zoospores (Lom & Dykova, 1992). These developmental stages, along with the cell structure and metabolism, are more akin to that of the fungi than the protozoa.

The spores of *Dermocystidium* are present in cysts less than 1 mm in diameter (Plate 15.5), which may be found on the skin and gills. Heavy infections can be debilitating, as is the case in *Dermocystidium pusula* infection in alpine newts, *Triturus* spp. Cutaneous nodules (or cysts) which contain the spores are distributed over the body and gills. Affected animals may have elevated respiratory rates because the cysts interfere with the normal functioning of the gills.

Diagnosis. Diagnosis is made by examining skin scrapings of affected areas allowing recognition of the spherical spores, which have a large central vacuole or refractile body. Gills should be examined in moribund or dead specimens. The spores are contained within small white nodules or cysts, less than 1 mm in diameter (see Plate 15.5). Differentiation of the different organisms within this group is difficult, and many are assigned to the genus *Dermocystidium.* Related or perhaps synonymous genera are *Dermosporidium* and *Dermomycoides* (see also Section 27.2.2, Integumentary System—Infectious Etiologies—Protozoan-like Fungi—*Dermocystidium, Dermosporidium,* and *Dermomycoides*).

Treatment. A reliable treatment regime has not been developed for *Dermocystidium.* An elevation in temperature to 25°C (77°F) has been reported effective in the axolotl, *Ambystoma mexicanum* (Crawshaw, 1992a). Other treatments to consider include ketoconazole given at 10–20 mg/kg PO once a day for 14–28 d and itraconazole given at 2 mg/kg PO or higher once a day for 14–28 d or a benzalkonium bath.

15.10 MYXOSPOREA

Myxosporea (such as the genera *Chloromyxum, Leptotheca, Myxidium,* and *Myxobolus*) are not commonly encountered in amphibians (McAllister & Trauth, 1995), and most infections in the natural hosts are not pathogenic (which implies a long history of association between the host and the myxosporea). Nonetheless, they are particularly interesting organisms. Myxosporea are obligate parasites characterized by their distinctive multicellular infectious spores which contain polar capsules with coiled ejectable filaments and one or two mobile infectious sporoplasms. Their small size and habitats meant that for many years myxosporea were classified as protozoans. This was incorrect as they are multicellular with differentiated cells. Recent molecular biology studies have confirmed that myxosporea are metazoans (Smothers et al., 1994), possibly closely related to bilateral animals.

Although our knowledge of the life cycles of myxosporea affecting amphibians is rudimentary, the life cycles of some myxosporidians affecting fish have been intensively studied and may indicate some likely patterns in amphibians. Some species of *Myxobolus* have indirect life cycles, with typical myxosporean stages in the fish being acquired through contact with actinosporean stages from an invertebrate host such as an aquatic oligochaete worm (Smothers et al., 1994). Thus both myxosporeans and achinosporeans are considered members of the phylum Myxozoa.

The myxosporea, including a *Chloromyxum* sp. newly reported from amphibians (Upton et al., 1995), may be present in hollow organs such as the gall bladder and urinary tract, in which case they are referred to as coelozoic. They may also infect solid tissues, such as the muscles, kidneys, testes and ovary, in which case they are referred to as histozoic. Histozoic organisms may be surrounded by a capsule, thus forming a cyst-like structure. Coelozoic myxosporea are generally less pathogenic than histozoic species.

Diagnosis. Diagnosis of myxosporea infection is made by biopsy of affected tissues or necropsy examination. At postmortem, squash preparations should be examined from all organs, urine, and bile. Diagnosis is simplified if the spores are found, since their characteristic polar capsules are typically pyriform (pear-shaped) or spherical, and refractile. Commonly there are two polar capsules per spore. In addition, proliferative trophozoite stages may also be seen in the amphibian host.

Treatment. Good husbandry plays an important role in preventing myxosporean disease. Treatment of infections is complicated by the extremely resistant nature of the spore. Although we are not aware of any successful treatments for myxosporea infections in amphibians, a variety of approaches have been used with some success in fish (Lom & Dykova, 1995; Moser & Kent, 1994). Effective strategies have included the use of disinfectants (e.g., calcium hydroxide or chlorine) to kill spores at the bottom of ponds and tanks and to sanitize mud, ultraviolet radiation against spores in the water supply, and administration of chemotherapeutics such as furazolidone, proguanil, fumagillin, and toltrazuril to infected fish. A recent report (El-Matbouli & Hoffman, 1991) described reduction of infection rate and prevention of clinical outbreaks of whirling diease in fish (caused by *Myxobolus cerebralis*) by feeding medicated pellets containing 0.1% fumagillin DCH.

15.11 MONOGENEA

Monogenea can infect the skin and gills of larval frogs and salamanders, and are also present in the urinary bladder, stomach, and intestine of adult amphibians. These flatworms are characterized by adhesive organs at their anterior and posterior ends. The posterior organ, or haptor, is frequently equipped with hamuli (also called hooks or anchors), hooklets, suckers or clamps, by which it firmly attaches to the host. Monogenea having a haptor with hamuli (Order Monopisthocotylea) are found internally and externally as parasites on tadpoles (Figure 15.9; Plate 15.6). Monogenea having a haptor with suckers or clamps (Order Polyopisthocotylea) infect the urinary

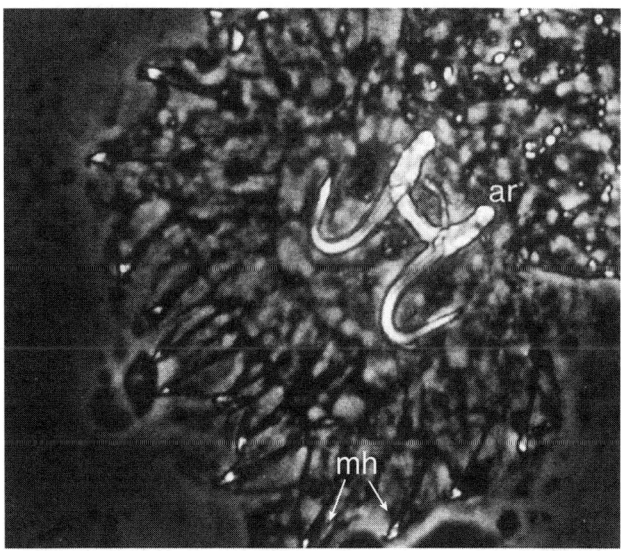

Figure 15.9. The monogenean *Gyrodactylus* sp. showing the posterior haptor armed with a large central pair of hamuli (ar), and 16 marginal hooklets (mh). This organ is used to attach to the outside of the host. Length of *Gyrodactylus* species ranges from 300–800 μm. (Sarah L. Poynton, Johns Hopkins University School of Medicine)

bladder of anurans and less commonly of salamanders. They are also found externally on the skin and gills of salamanders.

The life cycle of monogeneans is direct, requiring only one host. A variation of this simple cycle is seen in the polystomes, which have one generation of larvae infecting the gills of tadpoles and a generation of adults in the urinary bladder of the adult host. Most monogeneans produce eggs from each of which hatches a free-swimming larvae, the oncomiracidium, which usually has cilia and eye-spots, to assist in location of another host. In contrast, in the gyrodactylid group, reproduction is by viviparous polyembryony, production of live young with multiple embryos (Plate 15.6). It has been suggested that some monogenea, such as *Gyrodactylus*, are primarily fish parasites that use tadpoles as paratenic hosts.

The monogeneans are extremely variable in the amount of damage that they induce in their hosts. Some monogeneans cause significant tissue damage because of their robust attachment by hamuli which can provide portals for secondary infections, or because they feed by grazing on host tissues (monopisthocotyleans). Others do not produce significant damage because of their delicate attachment by suckers and their subtle drawing of blood from vessels (polyopisthocotyleans) (Cone, 1995). Hosts with heavy external infection can show signs of irritation, such as increased mucous production on the skin, and increased respiratory rate.

Diagnosis. Diagnosis of ectoparasitic monogeneans may be made by performing a skin scraping. Several areas of the skin should be sampled and if available, more than one animal should be sampled. Transillumination may reveal monogeans in the urinary bladder or intestine. Freshly dead amphibians should be kept in a portion of tank water until necropsy when skin scrapings and wet mounts of gill tissue (if present) can be examined.

Treatment. The finding of an occasional monogenean on an amphibian living in a well balanced ecosystem should not be a cause for alarm or treatment. However, heavy infections, especially of *Gyrodactylus* (which is viviparous, has a high reproductive rate, and harsh attachment mechanisms), do require appropriate management and care. Viviparous monogeneans (easily recognized by the presence of a juvenile within the body of the adult) are relatively easy to treat because both adults and newly emerging larvae are susceptible to the chemicals used. It is more difficult to treat monogeneans that produce eggs because the eggs are usually resistant to therapeutics, and treatment must be directed to the adults and the larvae that emerge from the eggs. In this case, it is advisable to treat the amphibian in a bath and move it to a new, clean environment where reinfection can not occur. This should be repeated once a week for at least three treatments, thus eliminating the parasites as they hatch.

Praziquantel baths, up to 10 mg/L for a 3-h period, may be effective at killing both young and adult *Gyrodactylus*, thus disrupting their life cycle. Placing crushed praziquantel tablets in a nylon stocking and gently massaging the medication into the water works well, although it will appear that not all of the material has dissolved. The use of a formalin bath, 1.5 ml 10% formalin/liter water for up to 10 min, once a week for three treatments, may also be effective. Organophosphates used for treatment of this disease in fish are unsafe for amphibians, and thus should be avoided.

15.12 DIGENEAN TREMATODES

Digenean trematodes are the most commonly encountered platyhelminths in amphibians. Unlike monogeneans which have direct life cycles, digenean trematodes have indirect life cycles, and amphibians can serve as hosts for both larval and adult worms. Larval worms may be found encysted in the subcutaneous tissues and skin, often surrounded by melanophores around the encysted or encapsulated worm. Common sites of infection include the heart, liver, and intestinal wall. Most adult digeneans are found in the lumen of their host's digestive tract. Other locations include the cloaca, urinary bladder (infected by *Gorgodera* and *Gorgoderina*), eyes, central nervous system, body cavity, eustachian tubes (infected by the Hemiuridae), and lungs (infected by the Haematoloechidae, such as *Hematoloechus*). In general, amphibians have a high tolerance of helminth parasites, and pathology associated with infections is uncommon (Brooks, 1984; Prudhoe & Bray, 1982). It has been suggested that the trematodes present in the large intestine might be regarded as commensal, rather than parasitic, since the worm population benefits by the availability of habitat and nutrients and the amphibian host is not harmed, and may even benefit by the ingestion of potentially harmful microorganisms by the worms (Prudhoe & Bray, 1982). Heavy infections by *Gorgodera* and *Gorgoderina* can cause renal damage leading to uremia and death.

Digenean trematodes adopt a variety of indirect life cycle strategies, and the amphibian may become infected via ingestion of infected hosts such as insect larvae, tadpoles, and snails. Infection may also be via penetration of the skin by cercariae (swimming larvae). In the simplest two-host life cycle, an aquatic invertebrate, such as a mollusk, serves as the intermediate host, and the amphibian is the final host. In more complex life cycles, there may be three or four hosts required (Schell, 1985; Wallach & Boever, 1983). Tadpole and adult amphibians may serve as hosts for different life stages of the same digeneans. For example, *Gorgodera* and *Gorgoderina* both utilize clams as a first intermediate host. Tadpoles are the second intermediate host, with *Gorgodera* worms encysting in the intestinal wall, and *Gorgoderina* worms encysting in the heart and liver. Adult amphibians are the final hosts, with adult worms found in the urinary bladder and kidneys.

Development of a digenean trematode requiring three different hosts generally proceeds as follows. The embryonated egg is ingested by a mollusk or hatches to release a miracidium which penetrates the molluscan host. In this host, a series of multiplying larval stages occurs, culminating in the production of cercariae. Dragonfly nymphs or diving beetles, the second intermediate host, are penetrated by the mobile cercaria, which then develop into metacercaria. This larva secretes material for a cyst membrane around which the host may produce a capsule of connective tissue preventing the larva from further migration through the insect's tissues. The amphibian, which is the final host, becomes infected by consuming the second intermediate host in which the metacercaria have fully developed.

A variation of this general development pattern is the production by some digenean trematodes of an extra larval stage, the mesocercaria, immediately after the cercaria. Mesocercaria are known from the genera *Alaria, Procyotrema,* and *Strigea*, with infection occurring in the muscle and connective tissue of tadpoles of toads, *Bufo* spp., and true frogs, *Rana* spp., and of larvae of the tiger salamander, *Ambystoma tigrinum* (Schell, 1985).

Although uncommon, pathogenic infections of digenean trematodes are known and are usually associated with high density infection, such as when there is a large number of parasites in relation to the volume of host tissue. Larvae may cause damage by migration through the host tissues. For example, larvae of *Diplostomum scheuringi* are found in the brain of newts (Etges, 1961), and larvae of *Clinostomum attenuatum* infect the eye of toads (Etges, 1991). Adult worms may cause damage when they are present in a particularly vulnerable organ or when they are present in high numbers. For example, *Haematoloechus* spp., which are ubiquitous in frogs, affect the lungs causing compression of the occupied alveolar tissue, chronic inflammation, edema, and increased mucous production. Dead parasites occupy alveolar nodules and fibrous cysts (Shields, 1987).

Diagnosis. Diagnosis of digenean trematodes is most often made at postmortem, although ova may be detected by direct fecal examination or in tracheal washes. Transillumination antemortem may reveal the presence of verminous granulomas or adult trematodes. Small whitish cysts may be seen grossly in a variety of tissues at necropsy. A squash preparation of all major organs will reveal migrating larvae if present, leading to a rapid diagnosis.

Treatment. The treatment of digenean trematodes can be very difficult, potentially dangerous to the host, and in many cases it is unsuccessful. The rapid killing of parasites throughout the amphibian's tissues can lead to degeneration of dead organisms causing inflammatory and potentially life-threatening reactions. If therapeutics are deemed necessary, prophylactic treatment of the host with corticosteroids beginning at least three days before administration of the anthelmintic is advisable. Praziquantel, given at 8–14 mg/kg PO, IM, or ICe every 14 d for three treatments, may be effective against adults, but immature and encysted forms are resistant. Repeated treatments may be necessary to eliminate recently matured or excysted adults.

15.13 CESTODES

Cestode infections in amphibians are not very common, nonetheless amphibians can serve as both intermediate and final hosts. Larvae, such as *Diphyllobothrium*, may be found in the muscle, skin, connective tissue, viscera, and body cavity (Plate 15.7). Adult cestodes are found in the intestine. *Bothricephalus* spp. in newts and salamanders, and *Cephalochlamys* spp. in clawed frogs, *Xenopus* spp., are a few examples. Three orders of cestodes are represented in the amphibians: Pseudophyllidea, Proteocephalidea, and Cyclophyllidea. Among the Cyclophyllidea is a family specific to the amphibians and reptiles, the Nematotaeniidae. The amount of damage caused by cestode infection in amphibians is generally low, although in newly caught wild animals, the stress of acclimation may allow the worms to become potentially life threatening.

Two different life cycle strategies are employed. For the pseudophyllids and proteocephalids, the embryo hatches in water to become a ciliated larvae, the coracidium, which is subsequently ingested by a crustacean. In this first intermediate host, the parasite develops into the first stage larva called the procercoid. Development to both the second stage larva, called the plerocercoid, and to the adult can take place in intermediate or definitive amphibian hosts (Bray et al., 1994). For cyclophyllids, their life cycle involves hatching of the embryo when the egg containing it is swallowed by a suitable intermediate host. The resulting larva may be a cysticercoid, the host of which may be an invertebrate or vertebrate, or a cysticercus, the host of which is a vertebrate.

Tadpoles heavily infected with larval cestodes cease to grow, and migration of larvae such as *Diphyl-*

lobothrium through the intestinal wall of the amphibian is likely to cause damage. Heavy infections of adult worms in the intestine may result in intestinal obstruction and death, such as that caused by *Nematotaenia* in frogs, toads, and salamanders.

Diagnosis. Adult worms or worm segments (proglottids) may be found trailing from the cloaca of heavily infected animals, and eggs or portions of adult worms may be found during routine fecal analysis. Transillumination may reveal verminous granulomas or adults in the intestine. Encysted tapeworms are often incidental findings at necropsy.

Treatment. Praziquantel given orally (see digenean trematodes above), is the treatment of choice for adult cestodes. Larval forms are more difficult to control as they are often encysted, and are therefore well protected from chemotherapeutics.

15.14 NEMATODES

Nematodes comprise the largest and most diverse of the helminth groups. Their infections in amphibians are well known, with *Rhabdias bufonis* from the amphibian lung being the subject of some of the earliest studies on development and transmission of parasitic nematodes in the middle of the last century (Anderson, 1992). Both larval and adult nematodes commonly infect amphibians (Plates 15.8A, B, 15.9A, B). Larvae are found in many organs including the skin, gastrointestinal tract, skeletal muscle, and mesentery. The larvae may be free or encysted. Adults are most commonly encountered in the lungs and the gastrointestinal tract.

The life cycles of nematodes involves an egg, four larval stages (punctuated development), and adults. Development from one stage to the next is accompanied by molting. Usually there are separate male and female sexes as adults, but in some genera, such *Rhabdias*, the adults are hermaphrodites. Some of the nematodes infecting amphibians have direct life cycles, requiring only the amphibian host. Examples of such worms are members of the Order Rhabditida (*Rhabdias, Strongyloides*) (Plates 15.8A, B), the Superfamily Cosmocercoidea (*Aplectana, Cosmocerca, Cosmocercoides*), and the Superfamily Heterakoidea. The remainder have indirect life cycles, where the amphibian can serve as an intermediate host facilitating development of the nematode larvae, or as a paratenic host, transporting the larvae without further development (Eberhard & Brandt, 1995). Amphibians may also serve as the final host in which the nematodes reach maturity.

The vertebrate host can become infected with nematode parasites via penetration of the skin (*Rhabdias, Cosmocerca, Cosmocercoides*), or orally after ingestion of eggs containing infective larvae, food contaminated with infective larvae, or intermediate or paratenic hosts containing infective larvae.

The commonly encountered genus *Rhabdias* can become problematic in captive amphibians, where heavy loads cause pulmonary damage and predispose amphibians to secondary infections. Captive conditions exacerbate the infections through amplification of the direct life cycle. The confined conditions allow a build up of infective larvae, leading to repeated reinfection of the vulnerable hosts. The superinfected hosts become increasingly debilitated and will shed more infective larvae, further potentiating the problem.

The direct life cycle of *Rhabdias* has both parasitic and free-living phases. The hermaphroditic adults live in the amphibian lung where they deposit eggs which contain the first stage (L1) larvae. These are coughed up and subsequently swallowed and passed out in the feces. After hatching, the larvae can develop into infective larvae or into a free-living generation of adult worms which eventually produce infective third stage larvae. The entire process can occur within two days. Larval migration to the body cavity occurs over several days after penetration of the host's skin, where they develop to the fourth stage and then the subadult. The subadult must invade the lungs in order to mature and produce eggs. Although wild tadpoles of frogs and toads are not known to be infected with *Rhabdias*, experimental infections have been successful, indicating an ecological rather than physiological basis for the absence of this nematode from tadpoles (Anderson, 1992).

A capillarid nematode, *Pseudocapillaroides xenopi* (syn = *Capillaria xenopodis*), lives in the epidermis of the South African clawed frog, *Xenopus laevis* (Stephens et al., 1987). Its presence, especially the burrowing activities of the adults, is damaging and results in pitting and increased sloughing of the skin. As the erosive dermatitis progresses, fluid overload (electrolyte loss), chronic debilitation, anorexia, and secondary bacterial infections result, and ultimately the host may be killed. The direct life cycle allowing completion within the epidermis of the frog contributes to the severity of this infection.

Fatal nematode infection of the skin has also been reported by Colwell and Watkins (1993) in an Indonesian White's treefrog, *Pelodryas caerulea*. Inflamed swellings on the limbs contained guinea worms belonging to the genus *Dracunculus*. The ovoviviparous females, obtained via ingestion of infected copepods, had migrated from the abdomen to the subcutaneous tissues of the limbs when the eggs were mature. Subsequent birth of the young resulted in an allergic reaction inducing skin blistering, allowing the release of immature worms into water. Colwell and Watkins (1993) speculate that the infection may have been fatal due to the stress of importation and captivity, and also suggest that this species of frog may not have been a natural host for this species of *Dracunculus*. Subcutaneous nematode infections are extremely common in imported specimens of the Indonesian White's treefrog, *Pelodryas caerulea*, and Indonesian giant treefrog, *Litoria infrafrenata* (personal communication, K. Wright, 1997).

An unidentified nematode was recovered in skin scrapings of the Cayenne caecilian, *Typhlonectes compressicauda*, at the Philadelphia Zoo (personal communication K. Wright, 1997).

Filarial nematodes such as *Foleyella* infect amphibians, with adults present in the tissues, body cavity, vessels, and lymph spaces, and microfilaria (verminous embryos) present in the blood (Figure 15.10). The nematodes have an indirect life cycle, with mosquitoes serving as the intermediate host. Once ingested by an insect, the microfilaria molt twice within eighteen days before they become infective via insect

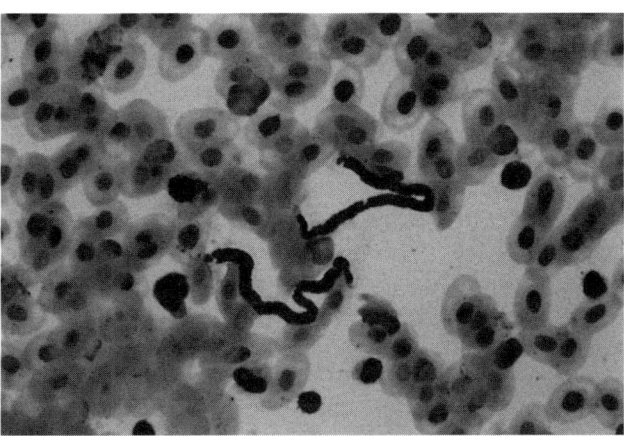

Figure 15.10. Microfilaria (verminous embryos of filarial nematodes) in the blood of a giant toad, *Bufo marinus*. Microfilaria range from 100 to 200 μm in length. (Sharon K. Taylor, Florida Game and Freshwater Fish Commission)

bite to other amphibians. Heavy infections of adult filariae in a debilitated amphibian are thought to be pathogenic (Crawshaw, 1992a; Wright, 1996). Microfilaria may cause lethargy and even death, while adult worms can cause dermal tumors (Flynn, 1973).

On occasion, amphibians may be infected by nematodes that normally infect insects (Poinar & Thomas, 1988). Larval nematodes such as *Neoaplectana* and *Heterorhabditis* can penetrate the gastrointestinal tract of tadpoles and enter the body cavity. During the migration, bacteria from the intestine may pass into the body cavity resulting in fatal septicemia.

Diagnosis. Nematode eggs and larvae are readily found in amphibian feces by both direct and flotation examination. Differentiating nematode infections through fecal analysis is highly challenging, with the morphology of eggs and larvae being of utmost importance (Plates 15.8B, 15.9B). It may be difficult to distinguish between genera other than to distinguish between embryonated ova (e.g., thin-shelled eggs containing L1 larvae which may have been produced by *Rhabdias* in the lung or by *Aplectana* in the intestine) and nonembryonated eggs (e.g., thin-shelled eggs of the intestinal nematode *Cosmocercoides*) (Anderson, 1992). The presence of larvae in the feces will depend upon which gravid nematodes are present in the host, the temperature, humidity, and the time between passing of the feces and its examination. Examination of fresh fecal samples is highly recommended in order to facilitate diagnosis, since in old samples some eggs will develop and larvae will hatch. Active strongyloid larvae in the feces are most likely to be *Rhabdias* spp. (Crawshaw, 1992b); however, other larvae that may be found include *Aplectana*, *Cosmocerca*, and *Cosmocercoides* (Anderson, 1992). *Aplectana* produce eggs that larvate *in utero*, they usually do not hatch until 3–4 hours after being laid. In contrast, *Cosmocercoides* eggs are not larvated in utero, but they develop rapidly to produce L1 larvae in feces (Anderson, 1992).

Ova, larvae, and adult nematodes may be recovered from tracheal washes of infected frogs. Adult *Rhabdias* may sometimes be visualized through transillumination of the frog.

Adult capillarid nematodes and their eggs are easily recognized in skin scrapings. The eggs are typically thick-shelled with two polar pluglike structures, thus giving them a lemonlike appearance. Filarial nematodes are diagnosed by finding microfilaria in samples of blood or coelomic fluid.

Treatment. Amphibians with respiratory difficulty, ulcerative skin lesions, weight loss, diarrhea, intestinal prolapse, anemia, or nonspecific failure to thrive concurrent with evidence of nematode infection are likely to require treatment. Anthelmintics are often incorporated into the quarantine program. In most cases this approach is safe, however, there is a risk of anaphylaxis and inflammation as nematodes die throughout the host's tissues.

Fenbendazole at a dose of 100 mg/kg body weight PO every 10 d for two or three treatments is reportedly safe. Resistant nematodes may be more susceptible to ivermectin. Doses for this drug begin at 200 μg/kg body weight PO or topically, repeated in two weeks. In many species this dose can be increased to 400 μg/kg. Extra care must be taken when preparing this drug for administration to small amphibians as dilutional errors are easily made and can be fatal. Levamisole hydrochloride given at 8–10 mg/kg body weight ICe or topically may also be effective. Levamisole has been effective when used as a bath at concentrations of 100 mg/L or higher. All of these drugs must be repeated every 14 days for a minimum of two to three treatments to be effective. Multiple attempts to eliminate some nematode infections can lead to frustration for the caregiver, as well as for the practitioner. The rotation of anthelmintics is recommended when resistance is detected, and in some cases, a combination of therapeutics may be required. Because the life cycle of most nematodes affecting amphibians is direct, greater success can be achieved by moving treated animals to a new and unaffected vivarium within 24 hours of receiving medication. Aquatic amphibians infected with epidermal capillariasis may be treated with thiabendazole at 0.1 gm/L of aquarium water (Cosgrove & Jared, 1977), although levamisole baths have been effective in treating epidermal nematodiasis in other species. Frequent water changes and removal of all sloughed skin is an important part of the management plan (Cosgrove & Jared, 1977). For those nematodes with indirect life cycles, the intermediate host must be eliminated. Serial stool samples or, in the case of capillariasis, skin scrapings, should be used to monitor the effectiveness of the treatment regime. In addition to anthelmintics, antibiotic therapy should be considered in cases where secondary bacterial infection is suspected.

15.15 ACANTHOCEPHALA

This group of worms is characterized by, and derives its name from, the thorny head—which in fact is an eversible proboscis—that is covered with thornlike hooks. Amphibians can carry adult acanthocephalans in their intestine and may also be infected with the encysted juvenile worms (cystacanths).

Acanthocephalans have indirect life cycles requiring at least one intermediate host. The eggs are very distinctive, being typically spindle-shaped (resembling diatoms) and containing a hooked larvae called the acanthor. This stage must be eaten by an intermediate host, often a crustacean or insect, where it develops to an acanthella. Further development produces an encysted infective juvenile called the cystacanth, which is the second infective stage (Figure 15.11). The final hosts are vertebrates. There appear to be a number of variations on this simple life cycle scheme, including the incorporation of transport hosts in which the cystacanths may re-encyst. Furthermore, the cystacanths may again encyst in the same host in which the adult worms are found.

Amphibians may serve as transport or possibly second intermediate hosts for acanthocephalans. Encysted cystacanths in the genus *Porrochis*, from Australian amphibians, may be found in the body cavity and have birds as the final host (Duellman & Trueb, 1986). Amphibians also serve as definitive hosts, carrying adult acanthocephalans such as *Acanthocephalus ranae*.

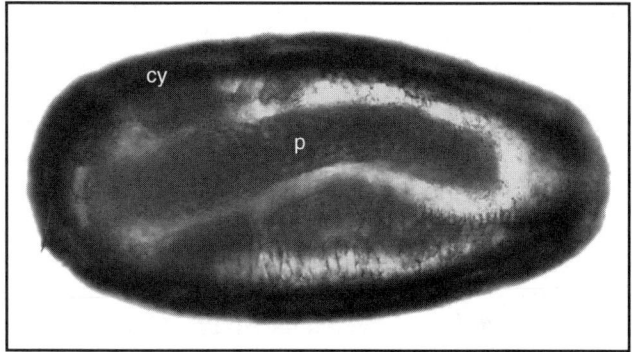

Figure 15.11. A cystacanth of an acanthocephalan (spiny-headed worm) from the body cavity of a dendrobatid frog. The juvenile worm is in an oval cyst (cy), with its distinctive spiny proboscis (p) inverted. Length of cyst is 1 mm. (Sarah L. Poynton, Johns Hopkins University School of Medicine)

The damage caused by adult acanthocephalans is mainly due to their armed proboscis, which they attach firmly to the intestinal epithelium, causing intestinal perforation, coelomitis, sepsis, and weight loss.

Diagnosis. Acanthocephalan infection may be diagnosed by the presence of the distinct spindle-shaped eggs in the feces. Alternatively the adults and encysted juvenile cystacanths may sometimes be seen by transillumination or at necropsy.

Treatment. We are unaware of an effective treatment for acanthocephalan infections in amphibians, however the antidiarrheic drug loperamide, 50 mg/kg PO mixed with food for 3 consecutive days, has been used successfully in fish (Taraschewski et al., 1990). Animals showing clinical signs of secondary bacterial infection should be treated with appropriate antibiotics.

15.16 LEECHES

Aquatic and terrestrial amphibians may be fed upon by leeches, which are annelid worms belonging to the class Hirudinea. These blood feeding organisms are typically ectoparasitic (e.g., Waite, 1925). Less commonly, leeches are endoparasitic, gaining entry via the cloaca to the lymph sacs and body cavity where they may feed upon the blood in the liver and heart (Mann & Tyler, 1963; Richardson, 1974; Tyler et al., 1966). Leeches may leave the host after feeding.

Leeches have direct life cycles with hermaphroditic adults. After mating, which may occur on or off the host, cocoons are deposited, each of which typically contains a single egg. From each egg will hatch a young leech.

The pathogenic consequences of leech infection

arise from their attachment and feeding activities, their transmission of hemoflagellates and blood-inhabiting apicomplexans, and their transmission of viruses and bacteria (Burreson, 1995).

Diagnosis. Leeches can easily be recognized by their distinctive looping movements and the possession of anterior and posterior suckers for locomotion and movement. Ectoparasitic leeches are easily seen attached to the skin of the amphibian, however, they often leave the host after feeding and may not be detected. Endoparasitic leeches are diagnosed via transillumination or at necropsy.

Treatment. External leeches are removed manually from the hosts using forceps or hemostats. The amphibian should be examined daily for leeches which, if found, must be removed in order to disrupt the parasite's life cycle. Moving the amphibian to a clean habitat after leeches have been removed minimizes the likelihood of reinfection by young emerging from cocoons.

15.17 ARTHROPODS: CRUSTACEANS, ARACHNIDS, AND INSECTS

15.17.1 Branchiurans

Branchiuran crustaceans may be found temporarily attached to the epidermis of aquatic amphibians such as tadpoles and salamanders. They are frequently encountered on fish, which gives rise to their common name of "lice" or "fish lice." The most distinctive feature of these creatures is the bilobed dorsal shield, which is carapacelike and covers the dorsal surface of the body. The ventral surface of a branchiuran is not shielded to facilitate grasping the host. (Figure 15.12). Distinctive features on the ventral surface, which is in contact with the aquatic host, are two pairs of antennae, two pairs of maxillae (the first of which, in the common genus, *Argulis,* are modified into suckers), and four pairs of legs (see Figure 15.12).

The life cycle of branchiuran crustaceans is direct. Eggs are deposited on objects such as stones and wood. The hatched larvae are mobile, and both males and females are parasitic on amphibians and fish.

Damage to the skin of the host occurs due to the attachment and feeding activities of the crustaceans. Many branchiuran species feed on the blood of the host, which they obtain by piercing the skin with their proboscis and penetrating to a blood vessel. Other branchiurans feed on sloughed epithelial cells and mucous. The parasite's activities can result in a loss of epithelial integrity with subsequent loss of osmotic homeostasis, secondary bacterial or fungal infections, and anorexia.

Diagnosis. Branchiurans are large and readily identified on the surface of their host, however, they can easily leave the host when it is handled.

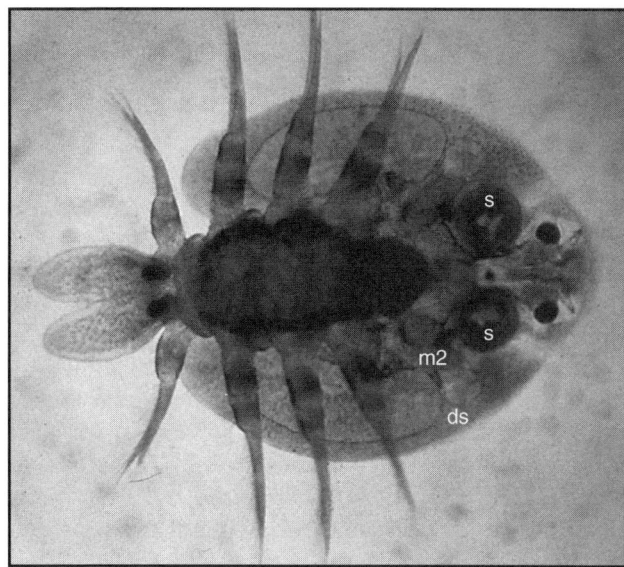

Figure 15.12. The branchiuran crustacean, *Argulus,* which may be found on the surface of tadpoles and salamanders. Ventral surface showing the first maxillae, which are modified into circular suckers (s), the second maxillae (m2), modified for attachment, and four pairs of legs. The abdomen is bilobed. The distinctive dorsal shield (ds), which covers the surface of the body away from the host, can also be seen. Length of *Argulus* species is 5–12 mm. (Heino Möller, Institut für Meereskunde, Kiel, Germany)

Treatment. The crustaceans should be removed manually and the amphibians moved to a clean habitat. This procedure should be repeated as needed. Exposure to a salt bath (10–25 g salt/liter water) for 5–10 min may cause the crustaceans to leave their host, although examination of the amphibian host should follow so that any remaining specimens can be manually removed. Exposure to an ivermectin bath (10 mg/L) for 30–60 min may also be effective. Treatments should be repeated weekly until no further crustaceans are detected. Systemic antibiotic therapy may be necessary if septicemia is suspected.

15.17.2 Pentastomids

Pentastomids have an oral region with a mouth and four retractile hooks, hence the name pentastome ("five mouths"). They also posses an elongate body, with annulations or rings (they are not true segments). The tonguelike shape of some species has given rise to the common name of "tongue-worms." Although the wormlike body of pentastomes might suggest that these organisms are helminths, other evidence, such as embryogenesis, structure of the integument, and gametogenesis, places these bizarre organisms closer to the crustaceans. Adult pentastomes feed on blood and mucosal cells and usually live in the respiratory passages, mouth and esophagus of their hosts, which are typically predatory reptiles, birds, and mammals. Damage to the epithelial lining of these tissues may lead to anemia and hypoproteinemia, and possibly secondary infection.

Strict hygienic practices should be used when handling infected amphibians due to the potential for zoonotic infection.

Life cycles of pentastomids may be direct or indirect. Development includes eggs, larvae, nymphs, and adults. The larvae have two or three pairs of stumpy legs and can migrate through the intestine of the intermediate host to encyst in the viscera where they then develop into wormlike nymphs.

Diagnosis. Transillumination may reveal adult pentastomes in the lungs, while endoscopy may reveal esophageal or gastric-dwelling pentastomes. Adults of small pentastome species may be found via tracheal or gastric wash samples. Characteristic ova containing larvae with legs may be found on fecal examination, or from tracheal or gastric wash samples.

Treatment. Levamisole hydrochloride has been recommended for treatment of adult pentastomes infecting snakes (5 mg/kg SQ or ICe) (Frye, 1981). Levamisole is safe at higher dosages (8–10 mg/kg ICe) used for treating nematode parasites in amphibians, but no specific indications are known for its efficacy against amphibian pentastomes. Jackson (1972) has recommended thiabendazole, 110 mg/kg PO, for pentastomes in snakes. Multiple treatments are suggested when attempting to eliminate pentastomes. Ivermectin may have some efficacy, and may be tried as an alternative treatment. It has stopped the shedding of pentastome ova in some gecko species when used at a dosage of 1 mg/kg PO (Wright, 1997). There are no successful treatments of nymphal pentastomes reported.

15.17.3 Mites

The larvae (chiggers) of trombiculid mites, such as *Hannemania,* are common ectoparasites. A chigger attaches to the host's skin and then feeds by constructing a tube (stylostome) which is inserted into the host's tissues. Saliva from the parasite dissolves surrounding tissues whereupon capillary action draws blood and other fluid through the stylostome. Components of the chigger's saliva provoke an inflammatory reaction in the host. Frequently these parasites are bright orange or red, and may be readily recognized. These infections are usually present only on newly acquired animals, since the free-living nymphs and adults do not readily survive indoors. However, *Hannemania* sp. were detected in specimens of the green salamander, *Aenedes aeneus,* that had been kept on paper towels for over four months (personal communication, K. Wright, 1998). Ereynetid mites can be found in the nasal passages.

Diagnosis. Infection should be evident upon close examination of the skin. A skin scrape or biopsy may also reveal larval mites. In some infections, such as *Hannemania,* orange-red vesicles approximately 1–2 mm in diameter are indicative of infection. Mite eggs are frequently found in stool analysis of terrestrial amphibians. Most often these represent nonpathogenic, free-ranging organisms that were ingested with food and substrate.

Treatment. Mite-infected animals should be kept isolated from uninfected animals, and separate equipment should be used to prevent the spread of the infection. Since some trombiculid mites, such as *Eutrombicula* and *Neotrombicula,* can infect both amphibians and reptiles, vigilance is necessary, especially in mixed species vivariums. Ivermectin at 0.2–0.4 mg/kg body weight given orally or topically may be effective at eliminating cutaneous infections. Dosages up to 2 mg/kg topically may be safe in some species of amphibians. Other options include bathing the amphibian in dilute ivermectin (10 mg ivermectin/1 liter water for 30–60 min). Weekly ivermectin treatments may need to be continued for 12 weeks or more to eliminate mites. Hypertonic electrolyte solutions, such as Holtfreter's or Steinberg's solutions may also be effective when used as a bath (see Chapter 24, Pharmacotherapeutics, for formulas of these solutions). Heat treatment of the soil should prevent introduction of mites into an established vivarium (see Chapter 5, Amphibian Husbandry and Housing).

15.17.4 Ticks

Ticks (family Ixodidiae) are blood-sucking ectoparasites rarely found on amphibians. Most species are host-specific and cannot be transmitted to mammals such as dogs, cats and humans, therefore recently acquired amphibians should not be blamed for ticks that suddenly appear on pets or family members. Some species of tick, such as the iguana tick, *Amblyomma dissimile,* can infect amphibians and reptiles.

Diagnosis. Ticks are easily identified upon gross observation of the amphibian. All limbs should be extended to ensure that no parasites go undetected.

Treatment. Using a sturdy pair of forceps or hemostats to grasp the tick's cephalothorax, the entire parasite is removed by gently pulling. Alternatively, ivermectin at 0.–0.4 mg/kg body weight given orally, subcutaneously, intramuscularly, or topically may kill ticks. Dosages up to 2 mg/kg topically may be safe in some species of amphibians.

15.17.5 Insects

Flies, or Diptera, are the only order of insect that are known to parasitize amphibians. Fly larvae (maggots) can parasitize eggs, larvae, and adult amphibians. Larvae may infest any wound (Plates 15.10A, B). *Notochaeta bufonivora,* a sarcophagid fly, parasitized the Veragoa Stubfoot toad, *Atelopus varius* (Pounds & Crump, 1987). In some cases, such as the toad fly,

Bufolucillia spp., which infests the nasal passages of frogs, larvae can feed so voraciously that the host is killed (Janzen, 1994; Zumpt, 1965). Eggs of the frog fly, *Batrachomyia mertensi*, are laid on the substrate and larvae are ingested by the White's treefrog, *Pelodryas caerulea*, or any of several other genera of frogs. Ingested larvae migrate, often ending up in a subcutaneous lymph sac, and the last larval instars feed on the blood of the host, (Ferrar, 1987; Zumpt, 1965). Infections of White's treefrog, *Pelodryas caerulea*, often are noted at the tympanic membrane (Vogelnest, 1994).

Diagnosis. Larval flies are often collected and identified from scrapings or biopsies of active lesions.

Treatment. Successful treatment of myiasis requires the manual removal of maggots (Janzen, 1994). Hydrogen peroxide can be instilled into the wound to assist in flushing out the larvae. Levamisole, 8–10 mg/kg topically, applied directly to the wound may kill some larvae (Wright, 1996) as may ivermectin, 0.2–0.4 mg/kg topically, applied directly to the wound. Ivermectin baths (10 mg/L for 30–60 min) may also kill larvae. Short exposure (less than 60 min) to organophosphates such as diclorvos (Atgard®) may kill fly larvae, but may be toxic to the amphibian (Wright, 1996). Maggot removal often induces allergic reactions in mammals, but this is unreported in amphibians. The wound should be flushed with an antibiotic solution, and systemic antibiotic therapy is recommended. Mortality rate of infected hosts may be 10% or higher (Ferrar, 1987; Zumpt, 1965).

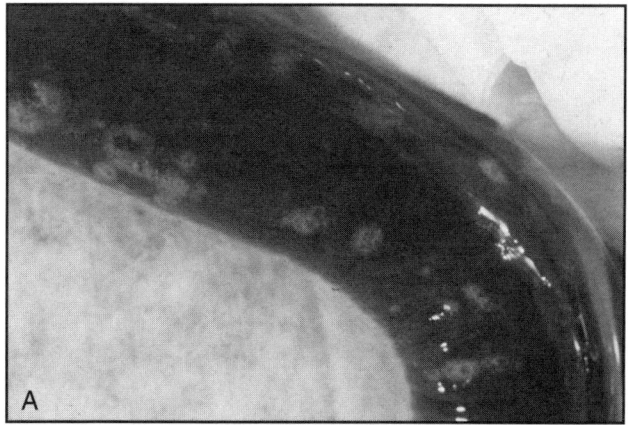

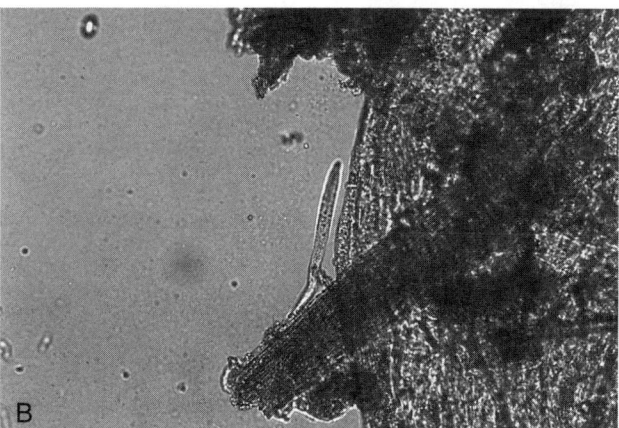

Figure 15.13. Nematode-associated dermatitis. **A.** White elevated lesions on the skin of a Rio Cauca caecilian, *Typhlonectes natans*. **B.** Nematode larvae were identified in skin scrapings of these lesions. (Kevin Wright, Philadelphia Zoological Garden)

15.18 MOLLUSCA

The larvae of the tiger salamander, *Ambystoma tigrinum*, have been experimentally infected with the glochidia larvae of the freshwater mussel, *Lampsilis cardium* (Watters, 1997). The glochidia attached to the gills and tail fins of the salamander larvae, but the pathology associated with gloccidial cysts was not described.

15.19 IDENTIFICATION OF PROTOZOA AND METAZOA FROM AMPHIBIANS

Protozoans and metazoans are easily found in skin scrapings (Figures 15.13A, 15.13B), tracheal washings, blood, lymph, urine, feces (Figures 15.14A, 15.14B, 15.15), and tissues collected surgically (Figures 15.16A, 15.16B) or at necropsy (Figures 15.17A, 15.17B). (See Chapter 8, Clinical Techniques; Chapter 11, Amphibian Hematology; and Chapter 25, Necropsy.) In the case of small amphibians, it may be necessary to sacrifice several animals in order to yield sufficient material for examination. Using the light microscope, most organisms can be seen and identified to order or family, which in many cases is sufficient to determine a course of action. If a more precise identification is desired, there are a number of useful special stains and procedures which are inexpensive and simple to perform. We recommend that these be included in the standard routine of the veterinary diagnostic laboratory. Such simple procedures include Giemsa, silver nitrate, potassium dichromate and Gram stain for protozoa (Table 15.3), and staining and clearing of whole mounts for helminths (Table 15.4). Other preparations are more complex, including protargol silver protein stain and electron microscopy. In a routine laboratory, initial fixation for these procedures may be performed prior to further processing and determination by a specialist.

Wherever possible, it is advisable to examine fresh material, either from a live or freshly dead host (meaning one that has been dead for minutes rather than

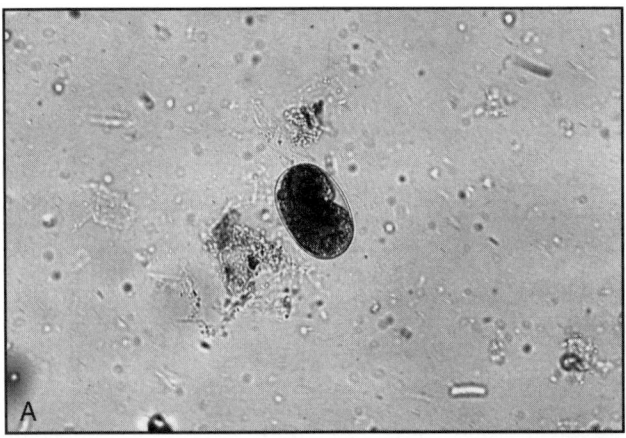

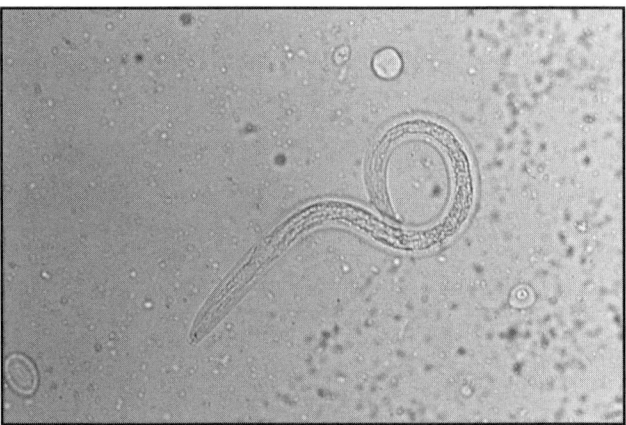

Figure 15.15. Nematodes and larvae may be found in close association with ova or alone as seen in this fecal sample from a polkadot treefrog, *Hyla punctata*. Identification of the ova or larvae is most easily achieved in conjunction with identification of the mature nematode. (George Grall, National Aquarium in Baltimore)

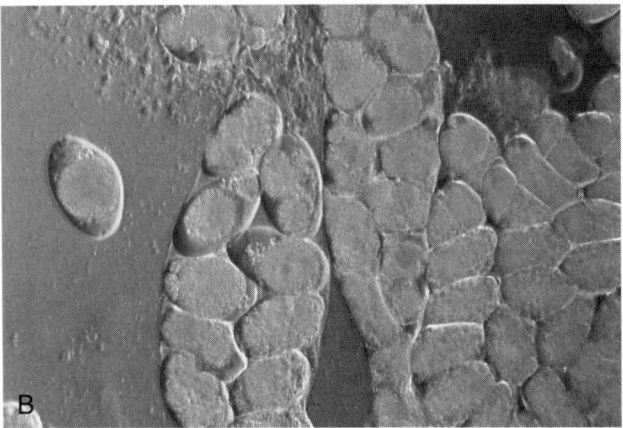

Figure 15.14. **A.** Nematode ova recovered from the feces of a Gunther's triangle frog, *Ceratobatrachus guentheri*. (Sandy McCampbell, Philadelphia Zoological Garden) **B.** Nematode ova recovered from the feces of polkadot treefrog, *Hyla punctata*. More detailed identification requires recovery of whole adult worms. (George Grall, National Aquarium in Baltimore)

hours). Old samples will show confusing postmortem changes, which may include death or encystment of delicate protozoa such as the ciliates, opalinids, and flagellates, and hatching of nematode larvae (Poynton & Whitaker, 1994). Storing samples in a refrigerator may also be detrimental, especially for samples from tropical hosts, where the temperature changes may kill the protozoa.

Observation of the living protozoa or metazoa, which may need to be freed from a cyst, is very valuable. The morphological features and characteristic motility are noted, and should be documented by drawings, photographs, video recordings, and measurements. The rate of movement of active protozoa can be reduced by the addition of a viscous medium such as Methocel® (Fischer Scientific, Pittsburgh, PA) or Detain® (Ward's Natural Science Establishment, Inc., Rochester, NY) to the preparation. Measurements of coccidian and microsporidian spores should always be done using fresh material. Unsporulated coccidian oocysts can be prompted to sporulate by incubation for 1-2 days in an aqueous solution of potassium dichromate (1.0–2.5% is effective) at room temperature. Alternatively, the feces can be placed in tap water containing a small amount of antibiotic (100 IU/ml penicillin G, 100 μg/ml streptomycin/fungizone solution) (McAllister & Upton, 1996).

Further identification methods vary according to the type of organism and the amount of information required (see Table 15.2). In many cases, it is important to immobilize, preserve, and stain the organism in order to visualize its distinguishing features. For ciliates, opalinids, and flagellates, two stains are recommended, a simple modified Giemsa and a more complicated protargol silver protein stain. The former technique is performed by taking the dried smear (e.g., blood, feces) and fixing it for 1 min in methanol. Once dry, the smear is then fixed in 10% neutral buffered formalin for 2 min and dried before staining with Wright-Giemsa. The protargol silver protein stain, although time consuming and costly, is recommended because it stains the cilia, flagella, and nuclear membranes, which are the most important diagnostic features. For the trichodinid ciliates, a silver nitrate stain is essential in order to visualize the structures of the proteinaceous adhesive disc. The small size of many protozoa and the paucity of their features visible with the light microscope necessitates use of scanning and electron microscopy for their identification. Thus it is helpful to have electron microscopy fixatives routinely available, such as 2% paraformaldehyde and 3% glutaraldehyde in phosphate buffered saline at pH 7.35. In some unusual cases, such as the hemogregarines, identification to genus is not possible solely on the basis of the appearance of the parasite in

PROTOZOA AND METAZOA INFECTING AMPHIBIANS —— 217

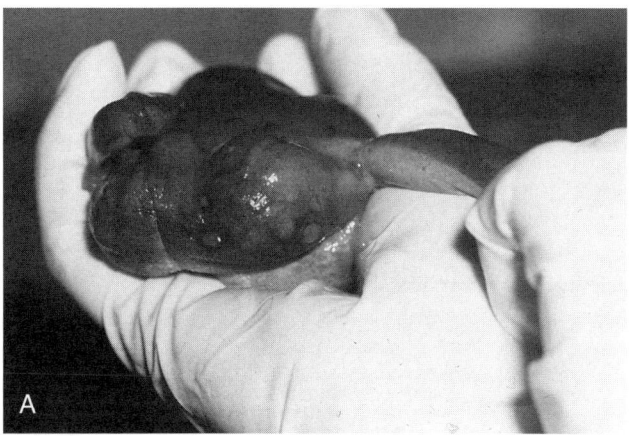

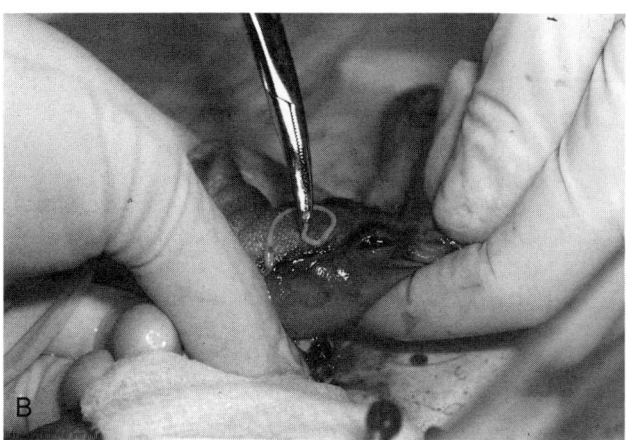

Figure 15.16. **A.** Verminous cysts distending from the skin and thigh musculature of a White's treefrog, *Pelodryas caerulea*. **B.** Surgical removal of a worm. Worm must be submitted intact for identification. (Kevin Wright, Philadelphia Zoological Garden)

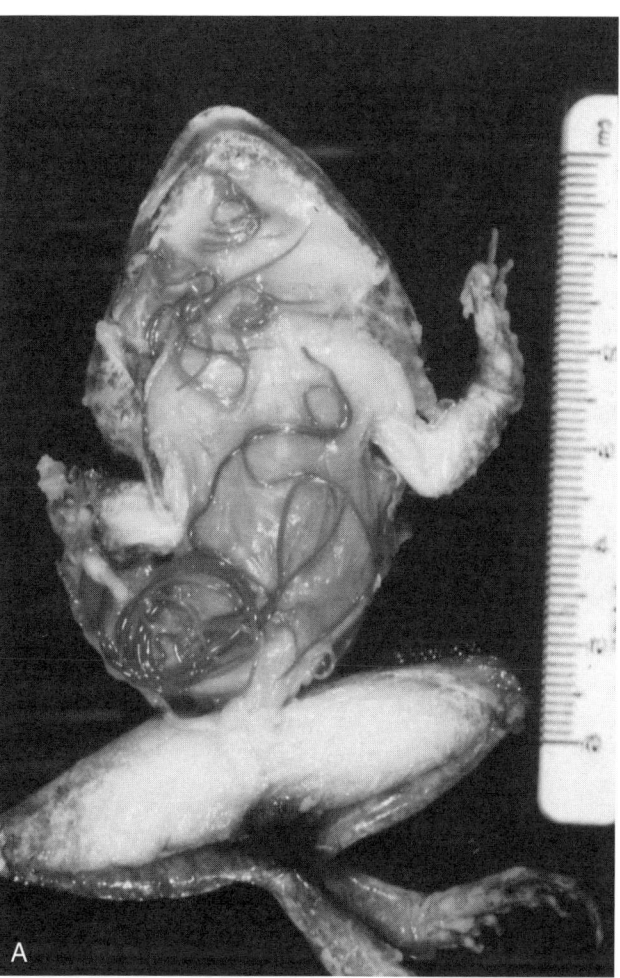

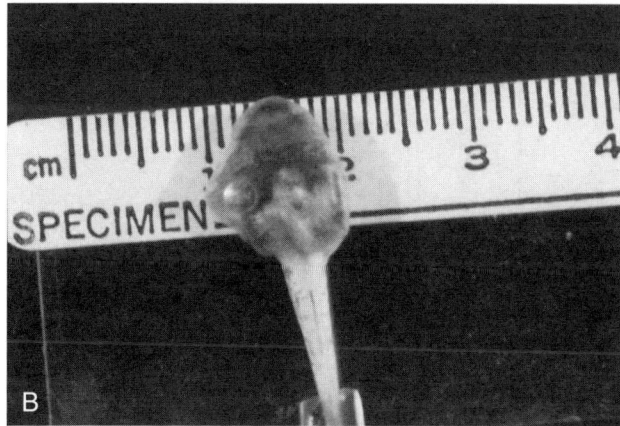

Figure 15.17. **A.** These nematodes were not eliminated despite numerous treatments of this Gunther's triangle frog, *Ceratobatrachus guentheri*, with anthelmintics. Whole worms recovered at necropsy and placed in 10% buffered formalin for over 4 hours were still mobile. **B.** The gas bubble noted in the coelom of this New Granada cross-banded treefrog tadpole, *Smilisca phaeota*, was caused by nematodes. (Virginia Pierce, Philadelphia Zoological Garden)

Table 15.3. Features used to distinguish the different flagellate groups living in the digestive tract of amphibians. These features can be seen using light microscopy with bright field illumination, 100x objective lens, and a viscous medium to slow movement of flagellates. Identification is based on Frank (1984) and Lee et al. (1985).

Order and genera	Flagella	Axostyle	Undulating membrane	Posterior end pointed	Length in μm	Comments
Proteromonadida proteromonads *Karotomorpha* *Proteromonas*	1 or 2 pairs	–	–	+	10–30	
Retortamonadida retortamonads *Chilomastix* *Retortamonas*	2 or 4	–	–	+	5–20	posterior end may be a spike
Diplomonadida diplomonads *Enteromonas* (E) *Trimitus* (E) *Hexamita* (H) *Spironucleus* (H) *Octomitus* (H) *Giardia* (H)	Enteromonadidae have 3 or 4 Hexamitidae have 8	– –	– –	– ±	5–20 5–20	hexamitids bilaterally symmetric *Octomitus* has a columna seen as a posterior spike *Giardia* has a sucking disk bacteria frequently attach to surface
				+	5–15	
Oxymonadida oxymonads *Monocercomonoides*	4 in 2 pairs	+	–	+		
Trichomonadida trichomonads *Hexamastix* (M) *Monocercomonas* (M) *Tetratrichomonas* (T) *Trichomitus* (T) *Tritrichomonas* (T)	4–6	+ +	– in M + in T	+ +		

Key: E—Enteromonadidae; H—Hexamitidae; M—Monocercomonadidae; T—Trichomonadidae

Table 15.4. Identification of metazoa from amphibians: preparation methods, keys, and host-parasite check lists.

Organism	Stain or preparation			Literature**
	Hematoxylin or Carmine	Clearing	External features*	
Myxosporea				Lom & Arthur, 1989; Lom & Dykova, 1995; Lom & Noble, 1989.
Monogenea	+			Prudhoe & Bray, 1982; Schell, 1985.
Digenean trematodes	+			Johnson, 1970; Prudhoe & Bray, 1982; Schell, 1985.
Cestoda	+			Khalil et al., 1994; Prudhoe & Bray, 1982.
Nematoda		+		Anderson, 1992; Anderson et al. 1974–1983; Baker, 1987.
Acanthocephala		+		McAlpine, 1996
Leeches	+			
Arthropods: crustaceans			+	
arachnids			+	
insects			+	

*Most identifying features are external so no special preparations are needed to show internal features.
**In addition, the reader is referred to Pritchard & Kruse, 1982.

the amphibian. Instead, identification depends on the characteristics of development in the vector (Desser et al., 1995). The most frequently used preparation methods for identification of protozoa are given in Table 15.3. A simple identification scheme for intestinal flagellates is presented in Figure 15.6.

For platyhelminths (monogenea, digenean trematodes, and cestodes) whole mounts are prepared and stained with hematoxylin or carmine in order to see the internal features of the organism. For nematodes, whole worm and sometimes *en face* (head uppermost) preparations of the anterior end are made. Usually, such preparations are cleared rather than stained. Many metazoa, especially the nematodes and acanthocephalans, must be relaxed by refrigeration in saline solution prior to fixation, staining, and storage (Pritchard & Kruse, 1982). Relaxation allows curled nematodes to straighten, and the retracted proboscises of acanthocephalans to evert, allowing important taxonomic characteristics to be visualized. For metazoan parasites, it is particularly important to observe multiple organisms of both sexes in order to make accurate identifications. The most frequently used preparation methods for metazoa are given in Table 15.4.

Protozoa and metazoa can also be identified in tissue sections. However, the limited amount of morphological information (a 5-μm section of the organism) precludes identification to genus and species in some cases. For identification of organisms in tissue sections, the following literature is recommended: for protozoans, Gardiner et al., 1988; for metazoans, Chitwood & Lichtenfels, 1972; Gardiner & Poynton, 1999.

In order to provide the best veterinary care for amphibians, an accurate diagnosis of their protozoan and metazoan infections is critical. It is therefore a wise investment of time to equip a laboratory with the fixatives, stains, and literature that will allow the organisms to be identified, either in-house or by outside specialists.

ACKNOWLEDGMENTS

We would like to thank Dr. Wayne Coats of the Smithsonian Environmental Research Center for use of photomicroscopy facilities. The work was supported in part by the National Science Foundation (grant no. HRD-9104020) awarded to Sarah L. Poynton.

REFERENCES

Anderson, R.C. 1992. Nematode Parasites of Vertebrates: Their Development and Transmission. CAB International, Wallingford, UK, 578 pp.
Anderson, R.C., A.G. Chabaud, and S. Wilmott 1974–1983. CIH Keys to

the Nematode Parasites of Vertebrates. Nos. 1–10. CAB International, Wallingford, UK, 470 pp.

Baker, M.R. 1987. Synopsis of the Nematoda Parasitic in Amphibians and Reptiles. Memorial University of Newfoundland, Occasional Papers in Biology No.11, 325pp.

Barnard, S.M. and S.J. Upton. 1994. A Veterinary Guide to the Parasites of Reptiles. Krieger Publishing Co., Malabar, FL, 154 pp.

Barta, J.R. 1991. The Dactylosomatidae. Advances in Parasitology 30:1–32.

Brannian, R.E. 1984. Lungworms, in Hoff, G.L., F.L. Frye, and E.R. Jacobson (Eds.): Diseases of Amphibians and Reptiles. Plenum Press, New York, pp. 213–218.

Bray, R.A., A. Jones, and K.I. Andersen. 1994. Order Pseudophyllidea Carus, 1863, in Khalil, L.F., A. Jones, and R.A. Bray (Eds): Keys to the Cestode Parasites of Vertebrates. CAB International, Wallingford, UK, pp. 205–247.

Brooks, D.R. 1984. Platyhelminths, in Hoff, G.L., F.L. Frye, and E.R. Jacobson (Eds.): Diseases of Amphibians and Reptiles. Plenum Press, New York, pp. 247–258.

Burreson, E.M. 1995. Phylum Annelida: Hirudinea as vectors and disease agents, in Woo, P.T.K. (Ed.): Fish Diseases and Disorders. Volume 1. Protozoan and Metazoan Infections. CAB International, Wallingford, UK, pp. 599–629.

Canning, E.U., E. Elkan, and P.I. Trigg. 1964. *Plistophora myotropica* spec. nov. causing high mortality in the common toad *Bufo bufo* L., with notes on the maintenance of *Bufo* and *Xenopus* in the laboratory. Journal of Protozoology 11:157–166.

Canning, E.U. and J. Lom. 1986. The Microsporidia of Vertebrates. Academic Press, Orlando, FL, 289 pp.

Chitwood, M. and J.R Lichtenfels. 1972. Identification of parasitic metazoa in tissue section. Experimental Parasitology 32:407–515.

Colwell, G.J. and K.A. Watkins. 1993. An incidence of fatal subcutaneous parasite load in an imported Indonesian White's tree frog (*Litoria caerulea*). Bulletin of the Chicago Herpetological Society 28:164.

Cone, D.K. 1995. Monogenea (Phylum Platyhelminthes), in Woo, P.T.K. (Ed.): Fish Diseases and Disorders. Volume 1. Protozoa and Metazoa Infections. CAB International, Wallingford, UK, pp. 289–327.

Cosgrove, G.E. and D.W. Jared. 1977. Treatment of skin-invading capillarid nematode in a colony of South African clawed frogs (*Xenopus laevis*). Laboratory Animal Science 27:526–527.

Crawshaw, G.J. 1992a. Amphibian medicine, in Kirk, R.W. and J.D. Bonagura (Eds.): Current Veterinary Therapy. XI. Small Animal Practice. W.B. Saunders Co., Philadelphia, PA, pp. 1219–1230.

Crawshaw, G.J. 1992b. Medicine and diseases of amphibians, in Schaffer, D.O. (Ed.): The care and use of amphibians, reptiles and fish in research. Scientists Center for Animal Welfare, Bethesda, MD, pp. 41–48.

Dempster, R.P., T. Morales, and F.X. Glennon. 1988. Use of sodium chlorite to combat anchor worm infestation of fish. Progressive Fish Culturist 50:51–55.

Desser, S.S. 1993. The Haemogregarinidae and Lankesterellidae, in Kreier, J.P. (Ed.): Parasitic Protozoa. Second Edition, Volume 4. Academic Press, San Diego, CA, pp. 247–272.

Desser, S.S., H. Hong, and D.S. Martin. 1995. The life history, ultrastructure and experimental transmission of *Hepatozoon catesbianae* n. comb., an apicomplexan parasite of the bullfrog, *Rana catesbeiana* and the mosquito, *Culex territans* in Algonquin Park, Ontario. Journal of Parasitology 81:212–222.

Desser, S.S., H. Hong, M.E. Siddall, and J.R. Barta. 1993. An ultrastructural study of *Brugerolleia algonquinensis* gen. nov., sp. nov. (Diplomonadina; Diplomonadida) a flagellate parasite in the blood of frogs from Ontario, Canada. European Journal of Protistology 29:72–80.

Diamond, L.S. 1965. A study on the morphology, biology and taxonomy of the trypanosomes of Anura. Wildlife Diseases 44:85 pp. (Microfiche).

Duellman, W.E. and L. Trueb. 1986. Biology of Amphibians. McGraw-Hill Book Co., New York, 670 pp.

Duellman, W.E. and L. Trueb. 1994. Biology of the Amphibians. Johns Hopkins University Press, Baltimore, MD, 690 pp.

Eberhard, M.L. and F.H. Brandt. 1995. The role of tadpoles and frogs as paratenic hosts in the life cycle of *Dracunculus insignis* (Nematoda: Dracunculoidea). Journal of Parasitology 81:792–793.

Elkan, E. and H.H. Reichenbach-Klinke. 1974. Color Atlas of the Diseases of Fishes, Amphibians and Reptiles. TFH Publications, Inc., Neptune City, NJ, 256 pp.

El-Matbouli, M. and R.W. Hoffman. 1991. Prevention of experimentally induced whirling disease in rainbow trout *Oncorhynchus mytuss* by fumagillin. Diseases of Aquatic Organisms 2:109–113.

Etges, F.J. 1961. Contributions to the life history of the brain fluke of newts and fish, *Diplostomum scheuringi* Hughes, 1929 (Trematoda, Diplostomatidae). Journal of Parasitology 47:453–458.

Etges, F.J. 1991. *Clinostomum attenuatum* (Digenea) from the eye of *Bufo marinus*. Journal of Parasitology 77:634–635.

Ferrar, P. 1987. A Guide to the Breeding Habits and Immature Stages of Diptera Cyclorrhapha. Entomonograph 8. E.J. Brill, Leiden, The Netherlands, 907 pp.

Flynn, R.J. 1973. Parasites of Laboratory Animals. Iowa State University Press, Ames, IA, pp. 507–645.

Frank, W. 1984. Non-hemoparasitic protozoans, in Hoff, G.L., Frye, F.L., and E.R. Jacobson (Eds.): Diseases of Amphibians and Reptiles. Plenum Press, New York, pp. 259–384.

Frye, F.L. 1981. Biomedical and surgical aspects of captive reptile husbandry. Veterinary Medicine Publishing Company, Edwardsville, KS, pp. 218–219.

Gardiner, C.H. and S.L. Poynton. 1999. An Atlas of Metazoan Parasites in Animal Tissues. Armed Forces Institute of Pathology. American Registry of Pathology. Washington, DC, 63 pp.

Gardiner, C.H., R. Fayer, and J.P. Dubey. 1988. An Atlas of Protozoan Parasites in Animal Tissues. U.S. Department of Agriculture, Washington, DC, 83 pp.

Graczyk, T.K., M.R. Cranfield, E.J. Bicknese, and A.P. Wisnieski. 1996. Progressive ulcerative dermatitis in a captive, wild-caught, South American giant tree frog (*Phyllomedusa bicolor*) with microsporidial septicemia. Journal of Zoo and Wildlife Medicine 27(4):522–527.

Griner, L.A. 1983. Pathology of Zoo Animals. Zoological Society of San Diego, San Diego, CA, 608 pp.

Jackson, O.F. 1972. Helminth infestation in snakes. Veterinary Record 90:51.

Janzen, P. 1994. Healing success by *Bufo bufo* with *Lucilia* infestation (Diptera: Calliphoridae). Salamandra 30:265–267.

Johnson, A.D. 1970. *Alaria mustelae*: description of mesocercaria and key to related species. Transactions of the American Microscopical Society 89:250–253.

Khalil, L.F., A. Jones, and R.A. Bray. 1994. Keys to the Cestode Parasites of Vertebrates. CAB International, Wallingford, UK, 751 pp.

Lee, J.J. and A.T. Soldo. 1992. Protocols in Protozoology. Society of Protozoologists, Lawrence, KS.

Lee, J.J., S.H. Hutner, and E.C. Bovee. 1985. An Illustrated Guide to the Protozoa. Society of Protozoologists, Lawrence, KS, 629 pp.

Lee, J.J., G.F. Leedale, and P. Bradbury. In press. An Illustrated Guide to the Protozoa (2nd edition). Society of Protozoologists. Lawrence, KS.

Levine, N.D. 1988a. The Protozoan Phylum Apicomplexa. Volume 1. CRC Press, Boca Raton, FL, 203 pp.

Levine, N.D. 1988b. The Protozoan Phylum Apicomplexa. Volume 2. CRC Press, Boca Raton, FL, 154 pp.

Lewis, D.H., W. Wang, A. Ayers, and C.R. Arnold. 1988. Preliminary studies on the use of chloroquin as a systemic chemotherapeutic agent for amyloodinosis in the red drum (*Sciaenops ocellatus*). Contributions in Marine Science 30:183–189.

Lom, J. and J.R. Arthur. 1989. A guideline for the preparation of species description in Myxosporea. Journal of Fish Diseases 12:151–156.

Lom, J. and I. Dykova. 1992. Protozoan Parasites of Fishes. Elsevier Press, Amsterdam, The Netherlands, 315 pp.

Lom, J. and I. Dykova. 1995. Myxosporea (Phylum Myxozoa), in Woo, P.T.K. (Ed.): Fish Diseases and Disorders, Volume 1 Protozoan and Metazoan Infections. CAB International, Wallingford, UK, pp. 97–148.

Lom, J. and E.R. Noble. 1989. Revised classification of the Myxosporea Butschli, 1881. Folia Parasitologica 31:193–205.

Mann, K.H. and M.J. Tyler. 1963. Leeches as endoparasites of frogs. Nature 190:1224–1225.

Marcus, L.C. 1981. Veterinary Biology and Medicine of Captive Amphibians and Reptiles. Lea & Febiger, Philadelphia, PA, 239 pp.

Maruska, E.J. 1994. Procedure for setting up and maintaining a salamander colony, in Murphy, J.B., K. Adler, and J.T. Collins (Eds.): Captive Management and Conservation of Amphibians and Reptiles. Society for the Study of Amphibians and Reptiles, Ithaca, NY, Contributions to Herpetology 11:229–242.

McAllister, C.T. and S.E. Trauth. 1995. New host records for *Myxidium serotinum* (Protozoa: Myxosporea) from North American Amphibians. Journal of Parasitology 81:485–488.

McAllister, C.T. and S.J. Upton. 1996. Identification of coccidian genera in amphibians and reptiles. Vivarium 7(5):44–48.

McAlpine, D.F. 1996. Acanthocephala parasitic in North American amphibians: a review with new records. Alytes 14(3):115–121.

Moser, M. and M.L. Kent. 1994. Myxosporea, *in* Kreier, J.P. (Ed): Parasitic Protozoa Second Edition, Volume 8. Academic Press, San Diego, CA, pp. 265–318.

Munson, L.L. 1990. Future directions for zoological pathology. Journal of Zoo and Wildlife Medicine 21:385–390.

Paperna, I. and R. Lainson. 1995a. *Alloglugea bufonis* nov. gen., nov. sp. (Microsporidia: Glugeidae), a microsporidian of *Bufo marinus* tadpoles and metamorphosing toads (Amphibia: Anura) from Amazon Brazil. Diseases of Aquatic Organisms 23:7–16.

Paperna, I. and R. Lainson. 1995b. Life history and ultrastructure of *Eimeria bufonis* n. sp. (Apicomplexa: Eimeriidae) of the giant toad, *Bufo marinus* (Amphibia: Anura) from Amazonian Brazil. Parasite 2:141–148.

Peterson, W.J. 1960. Population changes in the cecal protozoa of rats and some factors influencing them. Experimental Parasitology 10:293–312.

Poinar, G.O. and G.M. Thomas. 1988. Infection of frog tadpoles (Amphibia) by insect parasitic nematodes (Rhabditia). Experientia 44:528–531.

Pounds, J.A. and M.L. Crump. 1987. Harlequin frogs along a tropical montane stream: aggregation and the risk of predation by frog-eating flies. Biotropica 19:306–309.

Poynton, S.L. and B.R. Whitaker. 1994. Protozoa in poison dart frogs (Dendrobatidae): clinical assessment and identification. Journal of Zoo and Wildlife Medicine 25(1):29–39.

Pritchard, M.H. and G.O.W. Kruse. 1982. The Collection and Preservation of Animal Parasites. University of Nebraska Press, Lincoln, NE, 141 pp.

Prudhoe, S. and R.A. Bray. 1982. Platyhelminth Parasites of the Amphibia. British Museum (Natural History) and Oxford University Press, London and Oxford, UK, 217 pp.

Raphael, B.L. 1993. Amphibians. Veterinary Clinics of North America, Small Animal Practice (Exotic Pet Medicine 1) 23(6):1271–1286.

Reichenbach-Klinke, H. and E. Elkan. 1965. The Principal Diseases of Lower Vertebrates. Book II. Diseases of Amphibians. TFH Publications, Inc., Neptune City, NJ, 381 pp.

Richardson, L.R. 1974. A contribution to the general zoology of the land leeches (Hirudinea: Haemadypsoidea *superfam. nov.*) Acta. Zoologica Academy of Science, Hungary 21:119–152.

Schell, S.C. 1985. Trematodes of North America. University Press of Idaho, Moscow, ID, 263 pp.

Shields, J.D. 1987. Pathology and mortality of the lungfluke *Haematoloechus longiplexus* (Trematoda) in *Rana catesbeiana*. Journal of Parasitology 73:1005–1013.

Smothers, J.F., C.D. von Dohlen, L.H. Smith, and R.D. Spall. 1994. Molecular evidence that the Myxozoan protists are metazoans. Science 265:1719–1721.

Stephens, L.C., D.M. Cromeens, V.W. Robbins, P.C. Stromberg, and J.H. Jardine. 1987. Epidermal capillariasis in South African clawed frogs (*Xenopus laevis*). Laboratory Animal Science 37:341–344.

Stoskopf, M.K. 1993. Fish Medicine. W. B. Saunders Co., Philadelphia, PA, 882 pp.

Taraschewski, H., H. Mehlhorn, and W. Raether. 1990. Loperamide, an efficaceous drug against fish-pathogenic acanthocephalans. Parasitology Research 76:619–623.

Tyler, M.J., F. Parker, and R.N.H. Bulmer. 1966. Observations on endoparasitic leeches infesting frogs in New Guinea. Record of the South Australia Museum 15(2):356–359.

Upton, S.J. and C.T. McAllister. 1988. The Coccidia (Apicomplexa: Eimeriidae) of Anura, with descriptions of four new species. Canadian Journal of Zoology 66:1822–1830.

Upton, S.J., C.T. McAllister, and S.E. Trauth. 1993. The coccidia (Apicomplexa: Eimeriidae) of Caudata (Amphibia) with descriptions of two new species from North America. Can. J. Zool. 71:2410–2418.

Upton, S.J., C.T. McAllister, and S.E. Trauth. 1995. A new species of *Chloromyxum* (Myxozoa: Chloromyxidae) from the gall bladder of *Eurycea* spp. (Caudata: Plethodontidae) in North America. Journal of Wildlife Diseases 31:394–396.

Valentine, B.A. and M.K. Stoskopf. 1984. Amebiasis in a neotropical toad. Journal of the American Veterinary Medical Association 185:1418–1419.

Vogelnest, L. 1994. Myiasis in a green tree frog, *Littoria caerulea*. Bulletin of the Association of Reptile and Amphibian Veterinarians 4(1):4.

Waite, E.R. 1925. Fieldnotes on some Australian reptiles and a batrachian. Records of the South Australia Museum 3(1):17–32.

Wallach, J.D. and W.J. Boever. 1983. Diseases of Exotic Animals. W.B. Saunders Co., Philadelphia, PA, 1159 pp.

Walton, A.C. 1964. The parasites of amphibia. Journal of Wildlife Diseases #39 and #40 (Micro cards).

Walton, A.C. 1966. Supplemental catalogue of the parasites of amphibia. Journal of Wildlife Diseases #48 (Micro card, 58 pp.).

Walton, A.C. 1967. Supplemental catalogue of the parasites of amphibia. Journal of Wildlife Disease # 49 (Micro card, 10 pp.).

Watters, G.T. 1997. Glochidial metamorphosis of the freshwater mussel *Lampsilis cardium* (Bivalvia: Unionidae) on larval tiger salamanders, *Ambystoma tigrinum* ssp. (Amphibia: Ambystomatidae). Canadian Journal of Zoology 75:505–508.

Woo, P.T.K. 1994. Flagellate parasites of fish, *in* Kreier, J.P. (Ed.): Parasitic Protozoa, Second Edition Vol 8. Academic Press, San Diego, CA, pp. 1–80.

Woo, P.T.K. and S.L. Poynton. 1995. Diplomonadida, Kinetoplastida and Amoebida (Phylum Sarcomastigophora), *in* Fish Diseases and Disorders. Volume 1. Protozoan and Metazoan Infections. CAB International, Wallingford, UK, pp. 27–96.

Wright, K.M. 1996. Amphibian husbandry and medicine, *in* Mader, D.R. (Ed.): Reptile Medicine and Surgery. W.B. Saunders Co., Philadelphia, PA, pp. 436–459.

Wright, K.M. 1997. Treatment of pentastomids in Standing's day geckoes *Phelsuma standingii*. Bulletin of the Association of Amphibian and Reptilian Veterinarians 7(1):5.

Zumpt, F. 1965. Myiasis in Man and Animals in the Old World; A Textbook for Physicians, Veterinarians, and Zoologists. Butterworths, London, UK, 267 pp.

CHAPTER 16
CLINICAL TOXICOLOGY

Stephen G. Diana, MS, DVM, Val B. Beasley, DVM, PhD, Diplomate ABVT, and Kevin M. Wright, DVM

16.1 INTRODUCTION

Amphibians may be exposed to toxic compounds via contamination of food, water, air, soil, sediment, enclosures, handling equipment, the skin or gloves of handlers, and other sources. Acute toxicosis is not a common cause of death or clinical disease in well-managed amphibian populations whether captive or free-ranging. Nevertheless, an amphibian population may be devastated due to lethal exposure to a toxic agent. Also, chronic subclinical toxicoses may play a substantial role in the development of infectious, neoplastic, developmental, reproductive, nutritional, and other disorders.

Several aspects of amphibian physiology and husbandry make these animals particularly sensitive to chemical exposure. Amphibian skin is a highly permeable organ. While skin of mammals, reptiles, and birds is generally an effective barrier to all but highly lipid-soluble compounds, amphibian integument admits a wide variety of substances. Oxygen, carbon dioxide, water, urea, glucose, sodium, chloride, calcium, potassium, hydrogen, ammonium, and hydroxide ion among others, have all been reported to cross amphibian integument via either active or passive transport (Boutilier et al., 1992). Additional uptake is possible through the gills of larval and neotenic amphibians. Unless proved otherwise, it must be assumed that any chemical in the aquatic or terrestrial portion of the amphibian environment is a candidate for absorption.

Amphibian eggs are contaminated easily by toxicants. The permeability of the outer layers of the egg allows relatively easy penetration by waterborne toxicants. Moreover, the reliance of embryos and young larvae on egg yolk for their nutritive needs results in substantial exposure to contaminants stored prior to oviposition. This is particularly relevant for highly lipid-soluble, metabolically recalcitrant compounds. These chemicals can slowly accumulate to high concentrations in lipid stores of adult animals, and subsequently be loaded into yolk during the vitellogenic phase of egg development. The resulting embryos may be exposed to higher concentrations of the toxicant, and at a more vulnerable stage in development, than were the parents. Lipophilic compounds also may accumulate slowly in the tail of larval anurans. These compounds may be rapidly mobilized during tail resorption at metamorphic climax, resulting in high plasma concentrations of the toxicant.

Most of the drug metabolizing enzyme systems described in amphibians are less active than in mammals. This is especially true in the larval amphibians (Doherty & Khan, 1980; Marty et al., 1992). When a xenobiotic is toxic in its original form, this slow rate of metabolism may cause amphibians to be more sensitive to exposure than mammals, due to the prolonged half-life of the compound in the amphibian. However, the toxicity of some compounds (e.g., the organophosphorus insecticide malathion) is increased by metabolic change, a process known as bioactivation. In this situation, the slow rate of toxicant metabolism may allow for more complete excretion of the parent compound before substantial metabolic toxification. Since amphibians are ectothermic, their rate of drug and toxicant metabolism varies with ambient temperature. Manipulation of ambient temperature may prove to be a useful ancillary treatment for amphibian toxicoses, in attempt either to hasten metabolic degradation or retard bioactivation.

In many captive situations, numerous individual habitats share a common water supply as well as a common water treatment or filtration system. The use of a shared treatment facility, water supply, or food source can potentially result in widespread toxicosis from a single incident of contamination.

16.2 PRINCIPLES OF DIAGNOSIS

Definitive diagnosis of a toxicologic disease is dependent upon a history of exposure to a compound at a potentially toxic dose, an appropriate time of onset and duration of effects, the development of clinical signs and lesions compatible with the toxic potential of the agent, and ruling out of other plausible explanations for the observed abnormalities. In most cases, components of the definitive diagnosis are unfulfilled, and a plan of action must be formulated based on a tentative diagnosis. Despite the many limitations associated with diagnostic toxicology of amphibian species, it remains important to avoid premature or inaccurate diagnoses of toxicologic disease. Infectious and nutritional diseases are likely more common, and both may cause incidence patterns similar to those of toxicologic diseases. Therefore, a thorough differential diagnosis list should be considered before toxicosis is assumed.

In live amphibians, a general approach to toxicologic diagnosis should involve the collection, when possible, of urine, feces, serum, and blood with EDTA as anticoagulant. Urine, feces, and serum should be frozen, and blood refrigerated until analysis.

For dead amphibians, specimens that should be collected routinely for histological examination include brain, tail when present, gills if present, lungs if present, skin, heart, liver, kidney, all parts of the reproductive tract, all segments of the digestive tract, eyes, skeletal muscle, bone and bone marrow, and any other organs in which lesions are observed or suspected. Blocks of tissue approximately 3 mm in thickness should be fixed in neutral buffered formalin and subsequently processed for histologic examination. In addition, specimens of brain, liver, kidney, digestive tract contents, urine, and skin should be collected for chemical analysis. These specimens should be maintained continuously in a frozen state until they are analyzed. Specimens of all types of food items, water, soil, sediment, and other potential sources of contaminants, as well as excreta, also should be collected and frozen. Great care must be taken to avoid cross contamination (e.g., from amphibian to amphibian, from digestive tract or skin to internal organs, or from toxicant source to any other specimen).

Research concerning amphibian toxicology has focused largely on the acute and usually lethal effects of toxicants on larval amphibians of only a relatively few species. The existing data has been compiled in a detailed review and may be used to evaluate the significance of chemical concentrations identified by chemical analyses of samples (Harfenist et al., 1989).

16.3 PRINCIPLES OF TREATMENT

Treatment of acute toxicoses in amphibians include stabilization of vital signs, removal of the toxicant, administration of an antidote or antagonist when available, facilitation of the metabolic detoxification and/or removal of absorbed toxicant from the amphibian, and supportive therapy.

When toxicant exposure is suspected or confirmed, a high priority must be prevention of further exposure to, and absorption of, the toxicant by the amphibians. If the toxicant source cannot be identified, the amphibians should be transferred to new quarters, and *given food and water from different sources than those previously used*. Once exposure ceases, affected amphibians should be held under optimal conditions to allow recovery.

Antidotes or antagonists of toxicants are available and commonly used in veterinary practice. These compounds, however, have not yet been evaluated thoroughly, if at all, for use in amphibians. Sodium thiosulfate soaks have been used as a 1% solution without adverse effects for cases of halogen toxicosis, to convert Cl^0 or I^0 to Cl^- or I^-, respectively (Stoskopf et al., 1985), but their efficacy has not been established.

Increasing or decreasing the body temperature of the amphibian may affect the course of the toxicosis. If an antidote is known but not immediately available, cooling the amphibian may slow the progression of toxicosis or at least reduce the metabolism enough so that the amphibian survives until treatment is available. Once the antidote is available, it can be administered and the amphibian brought back to its preferred body temperature. If no antidote is available, elevating the body temperature may increase the metabolism and elimination of the toxicant. However, changing the body temperature is not routinely recommended due to its profound effects on physiologic and immunologic function.

16.4 ORGANOPHOSPHORUS AND CARBAMATE INSECTICIDES

Organophosphorus (OP) and carbamate insecticides are the active ingredients of many home and garden products. These compounds are used widely and often in an indiscriminate manner. Toxicosis in amphibians is commonly seen following use of these compounds in the home, or after placing recently collected materials such as plants or moss in the vivarium. Consumption of contaminated insects (i.e., wild-caught insects) also may result in toxicosis.

Reported effects of organophosphorus toxicosis in amphibians include reduced mobility or paralysis of larvae, increased hematocrit and mean red blood cell volume, increased or decreased reticulocyte and erythroblast count, decreased cholinesterase activity, delayed metamorphosis, developmental abnormalities, increased activity, hemorrhages, edema and color change, as well as death (Honorubia et al., 1993; Lyons et al., 1976; Mohanty-Hejmadi & Dutta, 1981; Pawar et al., 1983; Rzehak et al., 1977).

Organophosphorus and carbamate insecticides inhibit hydrolysis of acetylcholine by phosphorylating or carbamylating the enzyme acetylcholinesterase (AChE). The resulting accumulation of acetylcholine induces continuous stimulation of nervous, muscular, and glandular acetylcholine receptors. Nicotinic receptors may experience a depolarizing blockade. Abnormal body posture, failure to right itself, tetany, seizures, and other neurologic signs may occur in the adult amphibian exposed to either class of AChE-inhibiting compound (Figures 16.1, 16.2).

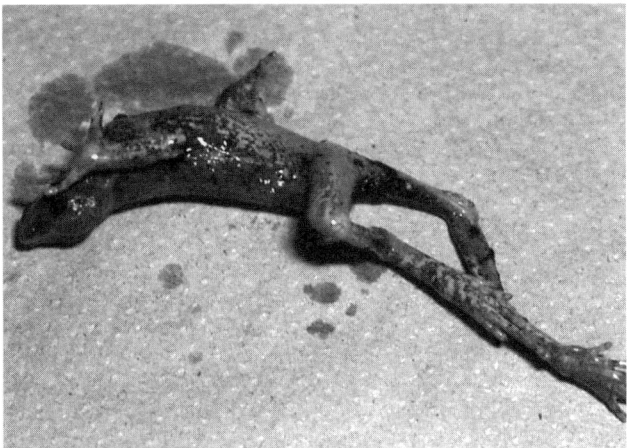

Figure 16.1. An Asian spadefoot toad, *Megophrys montana*, that is unable to right itself. This is suggestive of either organophosphate or carbamate intoxication, as well as other neurological disorders. (Kevin M. Wright, Philadelphia Zoological Gardens)

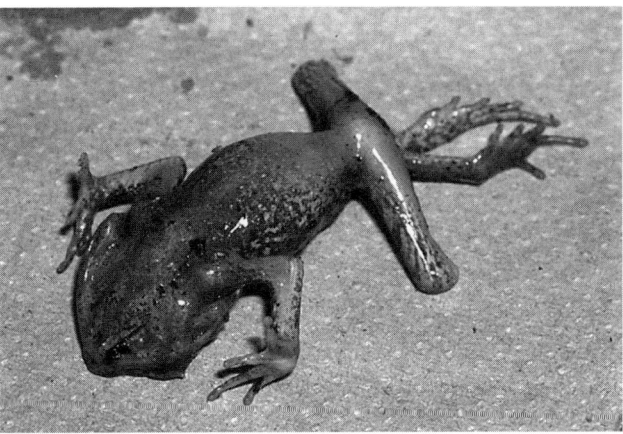

Figure 16.2. Opisthotonos in the Asian spadefoot toad, *Megophrys montana*, from Figure 16.1. (Kevin M. Wright, Philadelphia Zoological Garden)

The relative potencies and rank orders of the various organophosphorus insecticides differ substantially when tested in different vertebrate classes. This appears to be due to differences among affinities of the inhibitors for, and the subsequent rates of phosphorylation of, AChE. The concentrations of methyl paraoxon, paraoxon, gutoxon, and ethyl gutoxon required to induce 50% inhibition of AChE activity in vitro were approximately 10- to 100-fold greater for ranids than for monkeys, rats or chickens. The relative sensitivity of each species' AChE to each OP insecticide was apparently related to both the affinity of the compound for the enzyme and the rate of its phosphorylation (Wang & Murphy, 1982). Similarly, the dose of trichlorfon, ekatin and fenitrothion required to kill 50% of treated amphibians (LD_{50}) was approximately 10-fold greater than that for mammals (Gromysz-Kalkowska & Szubartowska, 1993). Differences in metabolic pathways involved in toxification of OP insecticides with $-P=S$ groups (must be converted to $-P=O$ before they are effective cholinesterase inhibitors), as well as in detoxification pathways that result in conversion to more readily excreted compounds, are also likely to play a role in the comparative sensitivity of amphibian species to organophosphorus insecticides.

An additional possible cause for amphibian resistance to AChE inhibitors is the capacity of many amphibians for cutaneous respiration. A common cause of death in OP-exposed mammals is suffocation secondary to respiratory paralysis, bronchoconstriction, and/or increased bronchial secretions. Although lethality occurs due to other mechanisms as well, amphibians may be more tolerant of OP and carbamate insecticide exposure due to their reduced reliance on pulmonary respiration.

Although there is evidence that organophosphorus compounds and carbamates induce measurable reductions in AChE activity in amphibians, this indicator has not been adequately validated for use in amphibian species. Furthermore, although organophosphorus toxicoses sometimes induce prolonged reductions in whole blood AChE activity in mammals, the decrease caused by carbamate toxicosis is more transient, potentially resulting in false negative diagnoses. Therefore, any attempt to use AChE activity to strengthen the certainty of diagnosis of OP or carbamate toxicosis in amphibians must be considered in view of the limitations of both the assay and the current knowledge regarding amphibian toxicology. Given the fact that neither the range of AChE activities found in normal amphibians nor the magnitude of AChE suppression that is clinically relevant have been described, specimens from apparently normal, non-exposed amphibians of the same species should be submitted with those from the potentially poisoned amphibians. AChE activity determination is typically performed on whole blood (with EDTA as an anticoagulant) and brain, and this determination should be performed as promptly as possible. Blood drawn for AChE determination should be refrigerated until assay, while brain tissue should be frozen.

Another component in the diagnosis of organophosphorus and carbamate toxicoses is the detection of the toxicant in environmental specimens, excreta, and in amphibian tissues at postmortem. Hydrolysis of carbamates may result in false negatives, especially if specimens are not collected and frozen shortly after death.

The utility of atropine (i.e., 0.1 mg/kg IM, SQ, or ICe as a starting dose) for OP or carbamate toxicoses, or pralidoxime chloride (i.e., protopam chloride) for OP toxicosis in amphibians, has not been examined, to the authors' knowledge. Since they can each induce toxicosis in their own right, use of these drugs should be avoided except with life-threatening toxicoses, and then they should be administered carefully and titrated to effect.

16.5 PYRETHRIN AND PYRETHROID INSECTICIDES

Pyrethrins are natural insecticidal products of exotic chrysanthemums (*Pyrethrum* spp.), and pyrethroids are man-made compounds of similar structure. Pyrethrins are a common ingredient of many commercially available pest control products, including flea control products for cats and dogs. In mammals, these compounds act largely by decreasing and prolonging axonal transmembrane sodium conductance and decreasing potassium conductance in peripheral nerves, resulting in repetitive firing of motor nerves. Pyrethroids bearing α-cyano groups also interfere with binding of the inhibitory neurotransmitter GABA, and sometimes glutamic acid, to their receptors.

Hyperactivity, swimming in spirals, tremors, or spasms in response to prodding, lateral or dorsal recumbency, lateral deformity of the tail, and death have been reported in larvae (stages 26–30) of the common toad, *Bufo arenarum*, exposed to deltamethrin via the water (Salibian, 1992). The aqueous concentration inducing 50% mortality (LC_{50}) in this study ranged from 4–17 ppb, depending on metamorphic stage and length of exposure. Unfortunately, the deltamethrin concentration at which these effects were first observed (i.e., the threshold toxic concentration) was not reported.

Decreased activity has been noted in the northern leopard frog, *Rana pipiens*, the southern leopard frog, *R. sphenocephala,* and the plains leopard frog, *R. blairi,* exposed to esfenvalerate in water at 1.3 ppb for 24 h, and spasmodic twitching and twisting at a concentration of 3.6 ppb or higher for 36 h. In this study, larvae that survived the milder effects of acute exposure generally recovered after 1 week in uncontaminated water, however, those that had displayed spasmodic behavior ultimately died (Materna et al., 1995).

Permethrin and fenvalerate induced an abnormal twisting response to prodding, rather than typical escape behavior, in larvae of the green frog, *Rana clamitans,* and the leopard frog, *R. pipiens,* which were held for 22 h in water containing as little as 10 ppb of either compound. Larvae exposed to permethrin at 100–2000 ppb for 96 h were significantly more likely to develop scoliosis than controls. Addition of the synergist and inhibitor of P450 metabolism, piperonyl butoxide, apparently did not increase the potency of either pyrethroid compound. Hatching success of embryos of the wood frog, *R. sylvatica,* the northern leopard frog, *R. pipiens,* the green frog, *R. clamitans,* and the American toad, *Bufo americanus,* was not affected by exposure of embryos to permethrin at up to 100 ppb for 22 h (Berrill et al., 1993).

16.6 ROTENONE

Rotenone is an insecticidal and piscicidal compound extracted from plants of the genus *Derris* or *Lonchocarpus* that acts by blocking NADH-initiated mitochondrial oxidative phosphorylation. The inability of tissues to utilize oxygen as a terminal electron acceptor results in signs of hypoxia, even in the presence of adequate blood oxygen concentrations. Poisoned animals typically rise to the surface of the water to gasp for air. Larval amphibians are more sensitive to rotenone toxicosis than are adults, apparently due to their reliance upon gill and cutaneous respiration (Fontenot et al., 1994). Aqueous LC_{50} values (96-h exposures) for various adult amphibians range from 3.2–5.8 ppm, while for larvae of the Florida leopard frog, *Rana utricularia sphenocephala,* the value was 0.5 ppm (Chandler & Marking, 1982; Farringer, 1972). It seems likely that neotenic salamanders may retain a high sensitivity to rotenone into adulthood.

Detection of rotenone in tissues is difficult and not commonly performed by most diagnostic laboratories. However, qualitative or semiquantitative detection of rotenone in tissue or water is possible and may be helpful when confirmation of exposure is required. Fortunately, rotenone degrades as a consequence of exposure to summer sunlight after a period of a few days.

16.7 HERBICIDES

Recent studies by our research group (Beasely & Diana) seem to suggest that concentrations of herbicides toxic to aquatic plants may secondarily harm wild populations of amphibians via deprivation of cover and reduced oxygen production. A reduction in algal food may seriously compromise large numbers of tadpoles, placing the future of that population at risk.

16.8 HALOGENS

Halogens are most likely to contaminate amphibian quarters via cleaning or disinfectant solutions, or as constituents of municipally supplied water. Twelve specimens of the harlequin poison frog, *Dendrobates histrionicus*, died when held for 3 h in plastic containers that had been soaked overnight in povidone iodine solution and subsequently rinsed with water (Stoskopf et al., 1985). Iodine-containing disinfectants readily stain many plastics. If used to disinfect items used for the amphibian enclosure, iodine can leach from the stain and contaminate the captive environment. Frogs that did not die acutely were noted to be lethargic and anorectic. Also, they assumed positions that minimized contact of their ventral skin with the substrate. A 1% sodium thiosulfate bath was prepared for treatment for the toxicosis, but all of the frogs died before it was administered. Only nonspecific liver changes were noted on postmortem examination. It was noted that frogs had been routinely held in the same type of containers, disinfected in the same manner. However, previous holding times lasted a maximum of only 30 min (Stoskopf et al., 1985). When new containers were disinfected and rinsed in a similar manner as the offending containers, iodine concentrations of the standing water ranged from 0.179–0.358 ppm. The total available iodine extracted from the containers ranged from 89–179 μg per container.

The toxicity of iodine to amphibians appears to be related to the form of iodine (iodide salts or iodine), the amount of iodine absorbed or ingested, and species-specific tolerances. "Iodine nibbles for caged birds" have been used by one herpetoculturist to reduce the incidence of spindly leg syndrome in offspring of the dyeing poison frog, *Dendrobates tinctorius* (Halfpenny, 1992). "Iodine nibbles" presumably contains potassium iodide, a common oral iodine supplement used in domestic animals. Iodine requirements of amphibians are unknown. In other species, there is a significant difference between nutritive and toxic doses. For example, a concentration of iodine as low as 0.14 mg/kg feed (0.14 ppm) prevents iodine deficiency in immature swine, whereas 800 mg/kg feed (800 ppm) causes iodine toxicity in immature swine with resultant anemia, anorexia, poor growth, and ocular lesions (Anonymous, 1979). No specific concentration of iodide (or iodine) can be determined for the "iodine nibbles," but the potassium iodide level ingested or absorbed by the tadpoles was presumably extremely low.

Potassium iodide is very different from povidone-iodine, which was implicated in the death of specimens of the harlequin poison frog, *Dendrobates histrionicus* (Stoskopf et al., 1985). Povidone-iodine is a complex of the suspending and dispersing agent povidone (a synthetic polymer formerly named polyvinylpyrrolidone) and iodine. Povidone-iodine has a concentration between 9 and 12% available iodine, and this solution appeared to form a reversible bond with the plastic of the holding containers. There do appear to be species-specific differences in iodine tolerance as povidone-iodine has been used as a surgical scrub without adverse effects in the mudpuppy, *Necturus maculosus* (Jacobson, 1975), and the green treefrog, *Hyla cinerea* (Brown, 1995).

It is generally accepted that chlorine is toxic to amphibians, especially gilled amphibians, and it is recommended that tap water be used for their culture only after dechlorination. Chlorine concentrations of 0.1–0.3 ppm are commonly found in municipal drinking water, and values may approach or exceed 1 ppm in cold winter months. Hyperplasia of the gill epithelium is the most common postmortem finding in affected fish. Chronic exposure to chlorine at concentrations as low as 0.002 ppm, while typically sublethal in fish, can induce branchial epithelial hyperplasia (Stoskopf, 1993a, b). While it appears that many amphibians can tolerate exposure to levels of chlorine found in tap water for 24 hours or more, it is prudent to avoid this on a regular basis. One of the main reasons for exposure to lethal levels of chlorine is incompletely rinsed cages or furnishings following disinfection with household bleach (Figure 16.3).

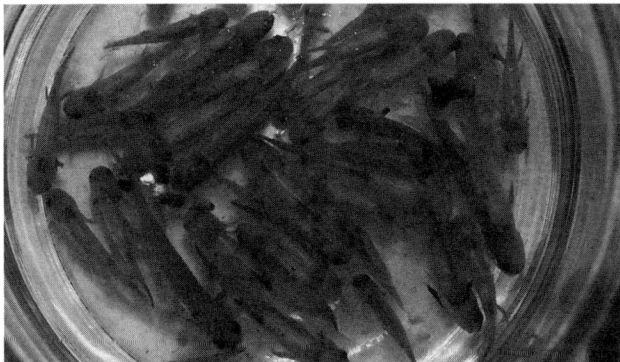

Figure 16.3. Larvae of the spotted salamander, *Ambystoma maculatum*, that suffered mass mortality following exposure to a disinfectant solution composed of household bleach. (Kevin Wright, Philadelphia Zoological Garden)

16.9 METALS

The most likely sources of metal contamination of amphibian quarters are tainted water and overzealous use of copper-containing therapeutics. Metal screening and other metal fixtures are to be avoided in the amphibian enclosure to eliminate the risk of metal ions leaching into the system (Figure 16.4). Plumbing

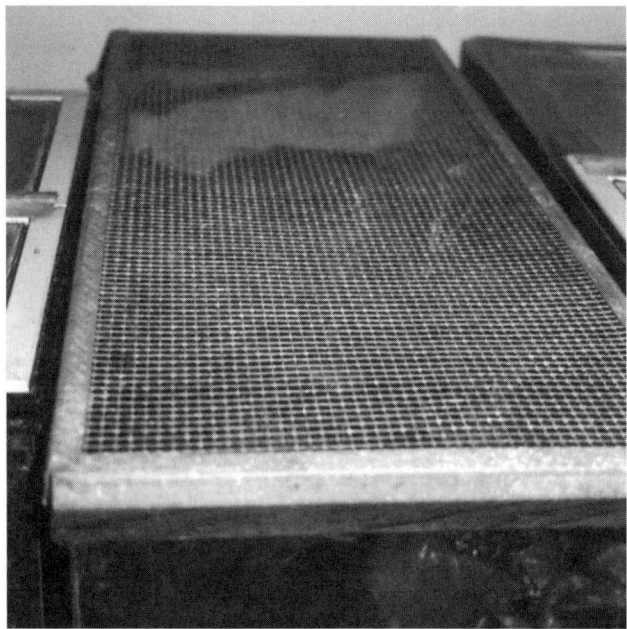

Figure 16.4. Metal screen tops are sold to convert aquariums into enclosures suitable for amphibians and reptiles. This is not recommended for amphibians as the screen may be a source of metal contamination of the captive environment. (Brent Whitaker, National Aquarium in Baltimore)

fixtures composed of copper or zinc may leach enough metal into the water, particularly in recirculating systems, to cause toxicoses in fish (Klontz, 1993). Activated carbon is not a reliable adsorbent to remove all metal ions from water. Lead, cadmium, silver, selenium, and chromium also have poisoned cultured fish (Klontz, 1993; Post, 1987). Lesions associated with chronic metal toxicosis in fish are most often associated with renal and hepatic failure (Klontz, 1993). Aqueous metal concentrations believed to be safe for salmonid culture have been published (Post, 1987), however, similar parameters have not been determined for amphibians. Acidification of aqueous environments readily increases the solubility, and thus the bioavailability of heavy metals.

Published reports of metal toxicoses in amphibians are limited to either laboratory studies, typically involving high-concentration, short-duration exposures, or environmental exposures. As a general rule, sensitivity to lethal metal toxicosis varies widely with stage of larval development. Also, developmental abnormalities are induced by lower concentrations than are required to cause mortality. For example, cadmium, at an aqueous concentration of 0.25 ppm, was 100% lethal in embryos of the common toad, *Bufo arenarum*, when exposed as neurulae, while 4 ppm and 1 ppm were required to cause death in blastulae and larvae with complete opercula, respectively (Herkovitz & Perez Coll, 1993). By contrast, mortality was minimal, but developmental abnormalities consistently occurred in larvae of the African clawed frog, *Xenopus laevis*, as a result of exposure to cadmium at 0.001 ppm (Miller & Landesman, 1978).

Diagnosis of metal toxicosis is strengthened by demonstration of high metal concentration in water and tissues. Samples recommended for submission to the toxicology laboratory include frozen liver, kidney, muscle, and potential source materials (e.g., water, soil, and food), as well as a wide range of formalin-fixed tissues (brain, liver, kidney, heart, digestive tract, bone marrow, etc.).

16.10 SALT

Amphibians are adapted to life in, or in association with, fresh water, with the exception of a limited number of species which tolerate brackish water. Few species survive in a salinity that exceeds their own body fluids (200–300 mOsm) (Shoemaker et al., 1992). Immersion of the northern leopard frog, *Rana pipiens*, in sea water is lethal (Bentley & Schmidt-Nielsen, 1971). Among the better known species that tolerate relatively high salinity are the crab-eating frog, *Rana cancrivora*, the European green toad, *Bufo viridis*, the African clawed frog, *Xenopus laevis*, the California slender salamander, *Batrachoseps attenuatus*, and the garden slender salamander, *Batrachoseps major* (Gordon, 1962; Gordon et al., 1961; Jones & Hillman, 1978; Schlisio et al., 1973). The slender salamanders, *B. attenuatus* and *B. major*, have been acclimated to salt concentrations as high as 600 mOsm (Jones & Hillman, 1978), while the crab-eating frog, *R. cancrivora*, can live in environments of 930 mOsm (Gordon & Tucker, 1965). Larvae of the African clawed frog, *X. laevis*, are able to tolerate salinities only up to approximately 330 mOsm (Seiter et al., 1978). In general, larvae of salt-tolerant species are less able to withstand high salinity than their adult counterparts (Balinsky, 1981). Salt toxicosis is rare in captive amphibians, but may occur if marine aquaria are kept nearby. Amphibians suffering from salt toxicosis should be immediately placed in fresh water. Parenteral hypotonic fluids may be beneficial.

16.11 DISSOLVED GAS SUPERSATURATION

Dissolved gases may cause toxicoses (termed "gas bubble disease") in fish when aqueous gas concentration rises above the saturation level of the water (Weitkamp & Katz, 1980). In a captive management situation, dissolved gas supersaturation is likely to result from defects or malfunctions in the water handling and delivery systems. Air leaks on the suction side of the water supply system can allow entrance of air, which is subsequently forced into solution when the air/water mixture is pressurized. Partial obstruction of the water intake system can increase the vacuum on the intake side of the system, encouraging air entrance into an otherwise airtight system. It is also possible for water drawn from a deep well to be supersaturated with gas when raised to the level of the containment facility.

An outbreak of gas bubble disease was reported in a colony of the African clawed frog, *Xenopus laevis*, held in water drawn from a deep well and naturally supersaturated to 151 mm Hg above local barometric pressure, largely due to nitrogen and argon partial pressures (Colt et al., 1984a). Affected frogs had gas bubbles, progressing to hyperemia in the interdigital webbing and legs, petechial and ecchymotic hemorrhages progressing to erosions in the skin of the legs and abdomen, and partial loss of the mucous coat. The animals were noted to float, and to be secondarily infected with a bacteria identified as *Aeromonas hydrophila*. When gas partial pressures were reduced by packed column aeration of incoming water, affected animals recovered within 1–2 days. Subcutaneous emphysema and air embolism also were reported in animals killed after a 5-day experimental exposure to water with a similar degree of supersaturation (Colt et al., 1984a).

Larvae of the bullfrog, *Rana catesbeiana*, exposed to deep well water, naturally supersaturated to 160 to 180 mm Hg above local barometric pressure, floated within 24 h of exposure but had no gas bubbles evident on external body surfaces. Larvae transferred to equilibrated water after a 4-day exposure to supersaturated water recovered within 24–48 h, with no significant mortality. A 10-fold increase in *Aeromonas hydrophila* isolated from the kidneys was noted in larvae exposed for 6–7 days (Colt et al., 1984b).

16.12 POLYVINYL CHLORIDE GLUES

Polyvinyl chloride (PVC) plumbing is relatively common in animal housing facilities (Figure 16.5) and occasionally found in domestic and commercial dwellings. Joining of pipes and fittings is accomplished using a primer-glue system containing methyl-ethyl-ketone, tetrahydrofuran, and cyclohexanone. Thorough curing and flushing of the plumbed system is necessary to avoid contamination of water with these compounds.

Toxicosis associated with these volatile compounds has been reported in dendrobatid frogs exposed via a newly constructed PVC misting system (Whitaker, 1993). Affected frogs climbed the enclosure walls, abraded their rostra while attempting to escape, and lost weight (Figure 16.6). Tetrahydrofuran, methyl-ethyl-ketone, and cyclohexanone were detected in the wa-

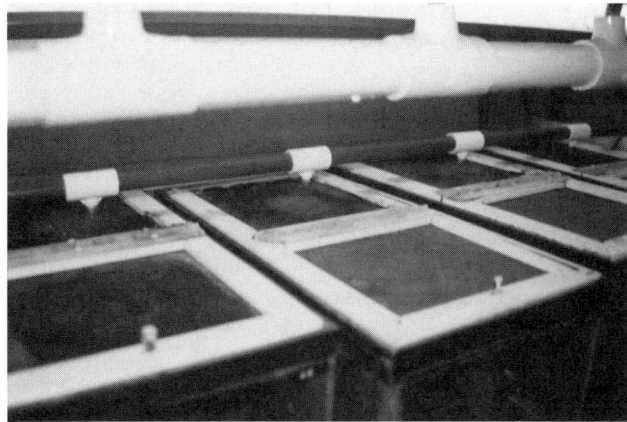

Figure 16.5. The PVC pipe used to plumb this misting system required the use of glues that contained volatile organics toxic to amphibians. (Brent Whitaker, National Aquarium in Baltimore)

ter mist emitted from these pipes at concentrations of 25 ppm, 2 ppm, and 16 ppm, respectively.

Some recommendations for using PVC glues in water delivery systems include minimizing the number of glued joints, allowing 14 days for air curing with or without forced air, flushing the system with hot water for 7 days, reflushing the system if malodor is detected, using carbon filtration, chemical analysis of

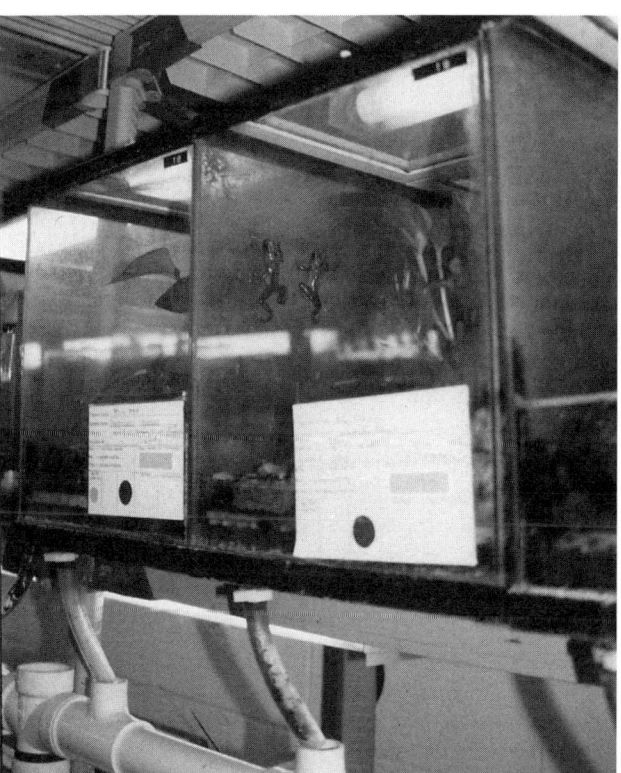

Figure 16.6. Toxins from polyvinyl chloride glues caused these dendrobatid frogs to climb the walls of their vivarium trying to escape contact with these irritating compounds. (Brent Whitaker, National Aquarium in Baltimore)

water during early use of the system, and using sentinel animals to test for adverse reactions (Whitaker, 1993).

16.13 NICOTINE

There are no published reports of nicotine toxicosis in amphibians, however tobacco smoking in the vicinity of aquaria or intakes to air pumping systems has caused nicotine toxicosis in fish. Acutely affected fish typically display rigidity and tremors of pectoral fins prior to death (Stoskopf, 1993b). Signs of nicotine toxicosis in other vertebrates include vomiting, diarrhea, respiratory depression, and death. Although no specific treatment is known for amphibians, affected amphibians should be removed from the contaminated environment and given supportive care in the form of supplemental oxygen and copious baths in clean water. Additional treatments may include small intracoelomic doses of a baributurate to provide relief of convulsions if they develop. Gentle gavage with activated charcoal may speed recovery.

16.14 AMMONIA, NITRITE AND NITRATE

Ammonia toxicosis is often associated with problems of the biological filter used in a vivarium. A newly established tank may have an insufficient number of bacteria to handle the nitrogen load excreted by the amphibian inhabitants resulting in toxic levels of ammonia in the water. The use of antibiotics and copper-containing therapeutics can disrupt the equilibrium of the biological filter resulting in elevated levels of ammonia and nitrite in the water. Unfiltered spartan enclosures do nothing to reduce the level of ammonia or urea excreted by an amphibian, and it is not uncommon for a large amphibian (e.g., Tschudi's African bullfrog, *Pyxicephalus adspersus*) to display signs of ammonia toxicosis within a few days after a large meal if its water is not changed (Figure 16.7). Un-ionized ammonia (NH_3) is more toxic than the ionized form of ammonia (NH_4^+), and the equilibrium between the two forms is dependent on the pH of the water (see Chapter 12, Water Quality) with a pH above 7.0 promoting the un-ionized (more toxic) form. A healthy established enclosure should have undetectable levels of ammonia so, if any ammonia is detected it should be considered a contributing factor to an amphibian's illness. Levels above 0.02 ppm of NH_3 are definitely of concern, and levels exceeding 0.1 ppm require immediate corrective action.

Clinical signs of ammonia toxicosis include excess mucous production and escape behavior as the amphibian attempts to get away from the irritant. Ter-

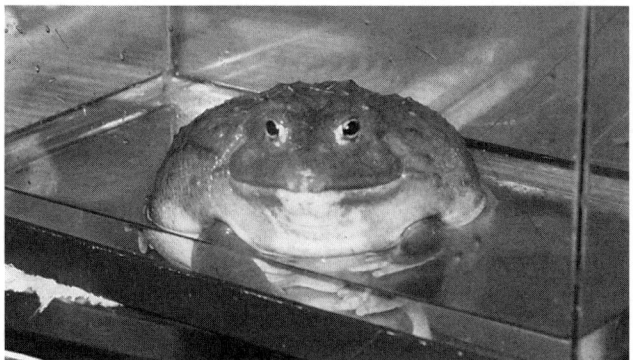

Figure 16.7. Large amphibians such as this Tschudi's African bullfrog, *Pyxicephalus adspersus,* can produce large amounts of ammonia in their urine. This can quickly lead to ammonia intoxication in an unfiltered spartan enclosure. (Kevin Wright, Philadelphia Zoological Garden)

restrial amphibians will adopt a body posture that minimizes contact with the ammonia-contaminated water, while aquatic amphibians may gulp and attempt to leave the water. Treatment consists of immediate removal of the amphibian from the contaminated water, and flushing with copious amounts of clean water. If it is impractical to do a full water change in the contaminated system, ammonia-trapping resins and clays can be used in a canister filter to reduce the ammonia concentrations to an acceptable level (i.e., below 0.02 ppm).

Nitrite toxicosis may occur concomitantly with ammonia toxicosis or as a separate entity. Nitrite is the second product in the cycle of biological nitrification, and should not exceed 0.1 ppm in a vivarium with an established biological filter. Although the LC_{50} (96 h) of the small-mouthed salamander, *Ambystoma texanum*, is 1.06 ppm nitrite (Huey & Beitinger, 1980), brief exposure to lower levels of nitrite also may evoke serious metabolic derangements. Nitrite causes the formation of methemoglobin which impedes normal oxygen delivery to tissues. Chocolate brown blood in combination with elevated nitrite levels in the enclosure's water support a diagnosis of nitrite toxicosis. Therapy should include immediate placement of the amphibian in an aerated bath of methylene blue (2 mg/L for larvae, 4 mg/L for adults) and provision of supplemental oxygen. This should continue until the amphibian appears to be breathing normally. If a pulse oximeter is available, it can be used to monitor the oxygen saturation of the amphibian. If an amphibian is respiring normally and the oxygen saturation plateaus at a level above 70% (a normal level for the bullfrog, *Rana catesbeiana*, (Pinder et al., 1992)), the treatment may be considered effective.

Nitrate is the least toxic of the nitrogen compounds involved in the nitrogen cycle of a healthy biological filter, however elevated levels (>100 ppm) are toxic to many fish and cause ionic imbalances similar to those evoked by exposure to hypertonic salt solution. Amphibians exposed to elevated nitrate levels should be placed in freshwater baths for 24 hours or more, and water changes should be performed on the original enclosures.

16.15 FROG EMBRYO TERATOGENESIS ASSAY USING *XENOPUS* (FETAX)

Experimental teratogenesis assessments have been studied as a method of predicting toxic effects of substances on amphibians. One standardized approach to evaluating the teratogenic potential of substances is the Frog Embryo Teratogenesis Assay of *Xenopus* (FETAX) (American Society for Testing and Materials Standard, 1991). This assay has evaluated hundreds of substances since its inception. The prolific nature of the African clawed frog, *Xenopus laevis*, ensures a ready supply of laboratory-produced embryos for statistically significant toxicologic studies. Various induced abnormalities have been catalogued (Bantle et al., undated), and this atlas serves as a reference to assist in interpretation of results.

16.16 SUMMARY

When evaluating a case toxicologically, it is important to take adequate samples and to choose the appropriate analytic technique. Water, substrate, and food samples should be carefully collected, stored, transported, and analyzed. Tissues of both affected and unaffected amphibians should be submitted, taking care to avoid cross-contamination. Both formalin-preserved and frozen samples should be held until a diagnosis is obtained. Affected amphibians should be transferred immediately to a completely new system with different water and food sources than used previously.

The paucity of published case reports of amphibian toxicoses necessarily limits the scope of this clinically-directed text. Much of the information presented has been extracted from reports of laboratory studies, often involving acute, high-dose exposures, or has been extrapolated from fish toxicology reports. The importance of publishing well-documented case reports in amphibian toxicology, and the evolving field of amphibian health management in general, cannot be overstated.

REFERENCES

American Society for Testing and Materials. 1991. Standard guide for conducting the frog embryo teratogenesis assay-*Xenopus* (FETAX), Designation E-1439-91, *in* Annual Book of ASTM Standards, Philadelphia, PA.

Anonymous. 1979. Swine nutrition, *in* The Merck Veterinary Manual, 5th Edition. Merck and Co., Rahway, NJ, pp. 1310–1324.

Balinsky, J.B. 1981. Adaptation of nitrogen metabolism to hyperosmotic environment in Amphibia. Journal of Experimental Zoology 215:335–350.

Bantle, J.A., J.N. Dumont, R.A. Finch, and G. Linder. Undated. Atlas of Abnormalities: A guide for the Performance of FETAX. [Available from J.A. Bantle, Department of Zoology, 430 LSW, Oklahoma State University, Stillwater, OK 74078.]

Bentley, P.J. and K. Schmidt-Nielsen. 1971. Acute effects of sea water on frogs (*Rana pipiens*). Comparative Biochemistry and Physiology 40A:547–548.

Berrill, M., S. Bertram, A. Wilson, S. Louis, D. Brigham, and C. Stromberg. 1993. Lethal and sublethal impacts of pyrethroid insecticides on amphibian embryos and tadpoles. Environmental Toxicology and Chemistry 12:525–539.

Boutilier, R.G., D.F. Stiffler, and D.P. Toews. 1992. Exchange of respiratory gases, ions, and water in amphibious and aquatic amphibians, *in* Feder, M.E. and W.W. Burggren (Eds.): Environmental Physiology of the Amphibians. University of Chicago Press, Chicago, pp. 81–124.

Brown, C.S. 1995. Rear leg amputation and subsequent adaptive behavior during reintroduction of a green treefrog, *Hyla cinerea*. Bulletin of the Association of Reptilian and Amphibian Veterinarians 5(2):6–7.

Chandler, L.H. and L.L. Marking. 1982. Toxicity of rotenone to selected aquatic invertebrates and frog larvae. Progressive Fish Culture 44:78–80.

Colt, J., K. Orwicz, and D. Brooks. 1984a. Gas bubble disease in the African clawed frog, *Xenopus laevis*. Journal of Herpetology 18:131–137.

Colt, J., K. Orwicz, and D. Brooks. 1984b. Effects of gas-supersaturated water on *Rana catesbeiana* tadpoles. Aquaculture 38:127–136.

Doherty, M.J. and M.A.Q. Khan. 1980. Hepatic microsomal mixed-function oxidase in the frog, *Xenopus laevis*. Compendium of Biochemistry and Physiology 68C:221–228.

Farringer, J.E. 1972. The determination of acute toxicity of rotenone and bayer 73 to selected aquatic organisms. M.S. Thesis, University of Wisconsin-La Crosse.

Fontenot, L.W., G.P. Noblet, and S.G. Platt. 1994. Rotenone hazards to amphibians and reptiles. Herpetological Review 25:150–156.

Gordon, M.S. 1962. Osmotic regulation in the green toad (*Bufo viridis*). Journal of Experimental Biology 39:261–270.

Gordon, M.S. and V.A. Tucker. 1965. Osmotic regulation in the tadpoles of the crab-eating frog (*Rana cancrivora*). Journal of Experimental Biology 42:437–445.

Gordon, M.S., K. Schmidt-Nielsen, and H.M. Kelly. 1961. Osmotic regulation in the crab-eating frog (*Rana cancrivora*). Journal of Experimental Biology 38:659–678.

Gromysz-Kalkowska, K. and E. Szubartowska. 1993. Toxicity of tetrachlorwinfos to *Rana temporaria* L. Comparative Biochemistry and Physiology 105C:285–290.

Halfpenny, S. 1992. Spindly-leg syndrome. British Dendrobatid Group Newsletter #13 as reprinted in American Dendrobatid Society Newsletter 12:1–2.

Harfenist, A., T. Power, K.L. Clark, and D.B. Peakall. 1989. A Review and Evaluation of the Amphibian Toxicological Literature. Technical Report No. 61, Canadian Wildlife Service, Environment Canada, Ottowa.

Herkovitz, J. and C.S. Perez Coll. 1993. Stage-dependent susceptibility of *Bufo arenarum* embryos to cadmium. Bulletin of Environmental Contamination and Toxicology 50:608–611.

Honorubia, M.P., M. Hernandez, and R. Alvarez. 1993. The carbamate insecticide ZZ-Aphox induced structural changes of gills, liver, gall-bladder, heart, and notochord of *Rana perezi* tadpoles. Archives of Environmental Contamination and Toxicology 25:184–191.

Huey, D.W. and T.L. Beitinger. 1980. Toxicity of nitrite to larvae of the salamander *Ambystoma texanum*. Bulletin of Environmental Contamination and Toxicology 25:909–912.

Jacobson, E. 1975. The effects of ACTH, glucagon, and norepinephrine on plasma glucose levels in the mud puppy, *Necturus maculosus*. PhD dissertation, University of Missouri.

Jones, R.M. and S.S. Hillman. 1978. Salinity adaptation in the salamander *Batrachoseps*. Journal of Experimental Biology 76:1–10.

Klontz, G.W. 1993. Environmental requirements and environmental diseases of salmonids, *in* Stoskopf, M.K. (Ed.): Fish Medicine. W.B. Saunders Co., Philadelphia, PA, pp. 333–343.

Lyons, D.B., C.H. Buckner, B.B. McLeod, and K.M.S. Sundaram. 1976. The effects of Fenitrothion, Matacil and Orthene on frog larvae. Chemical Control Research Institute, Environment Canada, Report CC-X-129.

Marty, J., J.L. Riviere, M.J. Guinaudy, P. Kremers, and P. Lesca. 1992. Induction and characterization of cytochromes P450IA and -IIB in the newt, *Pleurodeles waltl*. Ecotoxicology and Environmental Safety. 24:144–154.

Materna, E.J., C.F. Rabeni, and T.W. LaPoint. 1995. Effects of the synthetic pyrethroid insecticide, esfenvalerate, on larval leopard frogs (*Rana* spp.). Environmental Toxicology and Chemistry 14:613–622.

Miller, J.C. and R. Landesman. 1978. Reduction of heavy metal toxicity to *Xenopus* embryos by magnesium ions. Bulletin of Environmental Contamination and Toxicology 20:93–95.

Mohanty-Hejmadi, P. and S.K. Dutta. 1981. Effects of some pesticides on the development of the Indian bull frog *Rana tigrina*. Environmental Pollution Ser. A 24:145–161.

Pawar, K.R., H.V. Ghate, and M. Katdare. 1983. Effect of malathion on embryonic development of the frog *Microhyla ornata* (Dumeril and Bibron). Bulletin of Environmental Contamination and Toxicology 31:170–176.

Pinder, A.W., K.R. Storey, and G.R. Ultsch. 1992. Estivation and hibernation, *in* Feder, M.E. and W.W. Burggren (Eds.): Environmental Physiology of the Amphibians. University of Chicago Press, Chicago, pp. 250–274.

Post, G. 1987. Textbook of Fish Health. TFH Publications, Inc., Neptune City, NJ, 288 pp.

Rzehak, K., A. Maryanska-Nadachowska, and M. Jordan. 1977. The effect of Karbatox 75, a carbaryl insecticide, upon the development of tadpoles of *Rana temporaria* and *Xenopus laevis*. Folia Biologica 25:391–399.

Salibian, A. 1992. Effects of deltamethrin on the South American toad, *Bufo arenarum*, tadpoles. Bulletin of Environmental Contamination and Toxicology 48:616–621.

Schlisio, V.W., K. Jurss, and L. Spannhof. 1973. Osmo- und ionenregulation von *Xenopus laevis* Daud. Nach adaptation in verschiedenen osmotisch wirksamin losungen: 1. Taleranz und wasserhaushalt. Zoologische Jahrbucher, Abteilung fur allgemeine Zoologie und Physiologie der Tiere 77:275–290.

Seiter, P., H. Schultheiss, and W. Hanke. 1978. Osmotic stress and excretion of ammonia and urea in *Xenopus laevis*. Comparative Biochemistry and Physiology 61A:571–576.

Shoemaker, V.H., S.S. Hillman, S.D. Hillyard, D.C. Jackson, L.L. McClanahan, P.C. Withers, and M.L. Wygoda. 1992. Exchange of water, ions, and respiratory gases in terrestrial amphibians, *in* Feder, M.E. and W.W. Burggren (Eds.): Environmental Physiology of the Amphibians. University of Chicago Press, Chicago, pp. 125–150.

Stoskopf, M.K. 1993a. Environmental requirements and diseases of carp, koi and goldfish, *in* Stoskopf, M.K. (Ed.): Fish Medicine. W.B. Saunders Co., Philadelphia, PA, pp. 454–460.

Stoskopf, M.K. 1993b. Environmental requirements of freshwater tropical fishes, *in* Stoskopf, M.K. (Ed.): Fish Medicine. W.B. Saunders Co., Philadelphia, PA, pp. 545–553.

Stoskopf, M.K., A. Wisneski, and L. Pieper. 1985. Iodine toxicity in poison arrow frogs. Proceedings of the American Association of Zoo Veterinarians, pp. 86–88.

Wang, C. and S.D. Murphy. 1982. Kinetic analysis of species difference in acetylcholinesterase sensitivity to organophosphate insecticides. Toxicology and Applied Pharmacology 66:409–419.

Weitkamp, D.E. and M. Katz. 1980. A review of dissolved gas supersaturation literature. Transactions of the American Fisheries Society 109:659–702.

Whitaker, B.R. 1993. The use of polyvinyl chloride glues and their potential toxicity to amphibians. Proceeding of the American Association of Zoo Veterinarians, pp. 16–18.

CHAPTER 17
TRAUMA

Kevin M. Wright, DVM

17.1 ABRASIONS

The rostral abrasion is one of the more common traumatic lesions noted in captive amphibians. Abrasions are commonly noted on the rostrum of animals following shipment (Plate 17.1), but may also be noted in fractious anurans that jump and hit the glass when startled (Figure 17.1), and in amphibians that explore their enclosure and contact screen or other rough surfaces (Plates 17.2, 17.3). Evaluation of the situation and correction of the underlying cause is essential. Buffer panels of opaque plastic, bubble wrap, or foam should be hung on the inside walls of the enclosure until nervous anurans have adapted to the enclosure and are no longer prone to explosive jumps. Paper with a bold pattern may be hung on the outside of the glass of an enclosure until the amphibians learn to recognize glass as a barrier. Rough surfaces should be removed if possible, or coated with silicon rubber or other smooth nontoxic coating agent to minimize the abrasive quality of the object. Care should be taken to allow proper curing of the coating agent to avoid risk of chemical irritation or intoxication!

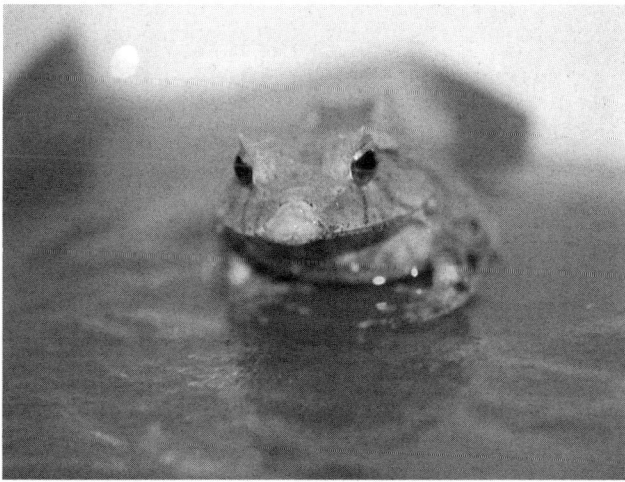

Figure 17.1. Chronic rostral abrasion in Gunther's triangle frog, *Ceratobatrchus guentheri*. The skittish nature of some species causes them to repeatedly hit the glass wall of their enclosure. (Kevin Wright, Philadelphia Zoological Garden)

Acute clean abrasions require minimal treatment, and some abrasions will granulate and re-epithelialize without any effort by the clinician. Evaluation of the abrasion should include documenting the size of the lesion using vernier calipers so that its appearance may be objectively evaluated on re-examination. If the abrasion increases in size over a 24–48 hour period, it should be debrided by gently rolling a dry cotton tip applicator across the surface of the wound. Do not rub or swab the lesion as this may damage and remove the new cell growth! Saline solutions (e.g., adding 20 to 25 g of sea salt to 1 liter of fresh water to yield a solution with a specific gravity of 1.020–1.025 or hyperosmotic ophthalmic solutions) may be applied topically 1–3 times a day. The salt solution should be rinsed off using fresh water after 10–15 min. Do not apply this solution to the amphibian while it is in its normal enclosure or salt intoxication may occur. If salt solutions appear irritating, this treatment should be discontinued and antibiotic ophthalmic solutions, ophthalmic ointments, or antibiotic cremes may be used instead. Gentamicin-based ophthalmic preparations are a recommended initial therapy, starting at a dosage of 1–2 drops applied twice daily to the lesion. Silver sulfadiazine cream (e.g., Sylvadene® cream, Marion Merrell Dow, Kansas City, MO) or human oral care gels (e.g., Orabase® gel) are alternative treatment options. Resolution of uncomplicated rostral abrasions occurs within 5–14 days, although return of normal epithelium may take considerably longer.

Chronic abrasions require more aggressive therapy. Cytologic and microbiologic evaluation should be undertaken using the debrided material on the cotton tip applicator. A rolled swab from normal-appearing skin may be submitted for microbiological evaluation to better assess the bacterial flora cultured from the lesion (see also Sections 13.2.2, Superficial Wounds, Ulcers, and Abscesses, and 13.6, Bacteriologic Techniques for the Diagnostic Laboratory). Skin scrapes of the lesion's periphery are recommended to evaluate possible presence of pathologic organisms in the subcutaneous layers. Daily rolling debridement using a cotton tip applicator is recommended. Topical antibiotics should be applied TID to QID, and antifungals such as miconazole solution or ketoconozole cream may be applied BID to TID. A silver sulfadiazine cream is an excellent first choice for chronic abrasions due to its broad spectrum of activity against Gram-negative bacteria and fungi. Systemic antibiotic and antifungals may be warranted, as may topical anthelmintics such as ivermectin or levamisole in case larval nematodes are contributing to the lesion or inhibiting its healing. Re-evaluation of the enclosure for contributing factors is recommended.

Foot abrasions are another common injury. Treatment includes antibiotic baths creams and parenteral therapy where appropriate. Plastic bubble wrap, such as is used to protect delicate equipment during shipment, has proven especially helpful in resolving these lesions. Multiple pieces of bubble wrap should be cut to fit the enclosure housing the amphibian so that each piece can be disinfected and dried between uses. The bubble wrap is best secured when it is is long enough to drape over the top edges of the enclosure, hang down the sides, and cover the floor. The ends hanging outside the enclosure can be secured with tape, or the lid of the enclosure itself. The bubble wrap seems to help relieve pressure on these abrasions, and the size of the amphibian determines the size (diameter) of the bubbles to be used.

A syndrome was noted in captive specimens of the redback salamander, *Plethodon cinereus,* termed atrophic mandibular stomatitis (see Section 27.2.2, Atrophic Mandibular Stomatitis). These salamanders were maintained in plastic dishes with paper towels as a substrate. It is assumed that the skin over the mandible was eroded by the salamanders attempting to burrow into the enclosure's floor. In some instances, mandiblular fractures occurred at or near the symphysis. A similar condition occurred in specimens of the crocodile newt, *Tylototriton shanjing* (Plates 17.4, 17.5, 17.6), at the Philadelphia Zoo. These animals were part of a confiscated shipment, and arrived with varying degrees of rostral and mandibular abrasions. Several were managed long-term with tube-feeding and antibiotics. Many of the crocodile newts that arrived at the Zoo with mandibular fractures succumbed, but all those that had solely epidermal damage recovered when treated with either Sylvadene® cream or Orabase® gel and maintained in a warm 25°C (80°F) environment. Other management techniques included a change in substrate to accommodate the species' burrowing behavior. Some newts received antibiotic baths and parenteral treatment. Assist feeding was necessary since the anatomy of the oropharynx is compromised (e.g., mandibular fracture) making suction feeding impossible. Pharyngostomy tubes in the form of intravenous catheters can be used for easier feeding. The prognosis for this condition in an amphibian is grave, but some do recover completely.

17.2 LACERATIONS

Lacerations generally result from inappropriate handling of an amphibian, cagemate bites, injuries from live rodent prey, or inappropriate cage furnishings (Plate 17.7). Incautious skin scrapes can result in lacerations, as may venipuncture attempts. Bites may result in severe damge to the digits, limbs, tail or torso. Debridement of the wound is recommended, and a culture of the deep tissues may be submitted for microbial culture. A flush of the wound with an antibiotic solution (e.g., gentamicin) is recommended. Hemostasis is generally achieved with direct pressure using a cotton tip applicator. Corn starch can be used as a coagulant, but rarely needs to be used. Parenteral supplemental fluids may be given in the face of severe hemorrhage. The need for corticosteroids to treat shock in amphibians is undocumented, but a dose of 1 mg/kg prednisolone IM may be given without obvious ill effect. Closure of the wound can be accomplished using tissue glue. Small lacerations may be left to heal by second intention. The amphibian needs to be assessed for sepsis, and prophylactic antibiotics should be initiated for severe or problematic wounds.

17.3 TRAUMATIC AMPUTATIONS

Traumatic amputations are not uncommon in captive amphibians. Cagemate aggression can result in the amputation of digits, limbs, and tails. Often times the limbs get caught as the lid to an enclosure is being shut (Figure 17.2). In one bizarre case a gray treefrog, *Hyla versicolor-chrysoscelis,* held at the Philadelphia Zoo actually ate its own front foot. In many cases, hemostasis is achieved physiologically before the

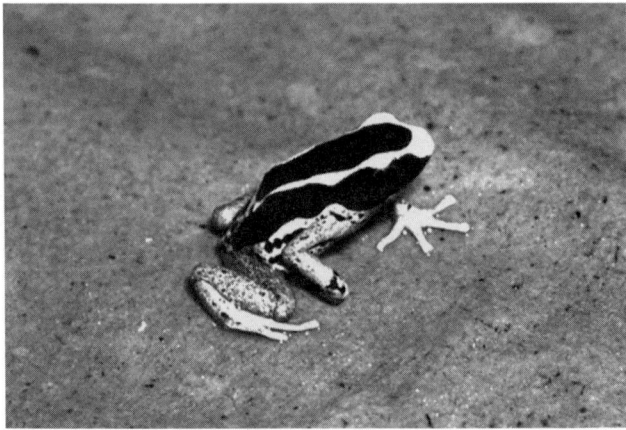

Figure 17.2. Traumatic amputation of the forelimb in a young dyeing poison frog, *Dendrobates tinctorius.* (Kevin Wright, Philadelphia Zoological Garden)

amphibian is evaluated. However, direct pressure to the bleeding site is recommended as first aid. Hemostatic clips can be applied to the digit or limb to achieve hemostasis. Corn starch may be used as a coagulant for small wounds. In most instances the clinician can do little other than to debride the wound and administer antibiotics if needed. In some cases the wound may heal by primary intent if the wound edges are opposed by tissue glue or fine sutures (see Section 21.5.1, Amputation). If the amphibian appears in shock, corticosteroids may be administered as may intracoelomic fluids.

17.4 SKELETAL FRACTURES

Any amphibian with a diagnosis of a bone fracture should be evaluated for metabolic bone disease, and appropriate supplementation of calcium and vitamin D begun immediately (see Section 7.1, Metabolic Bone Disease). A postural abnormality may be the first indication that a fracture has occurred (Figures 17.3, 17.4). Fresh closed fractures generally heal well if stabilized whereas old closed fractures and open fractures may require amputation. Fracture repair of the long bones of the European common frog, *Rana temporaria*, has been studied (Pritchard & Ruzicka, 1950). Although this study did not document the length of time required for mineralization of the callus and return to normal bone architecture, union of the fracture ends was apparent at 70 days postfracture, primarily as a result of the formation of a cartilaginous callus.

A fresh closed fracture of the long bones is often suspected upon palpation and the diagnosis is confirmed by radiographs. Limbs may be stabilized using a variety

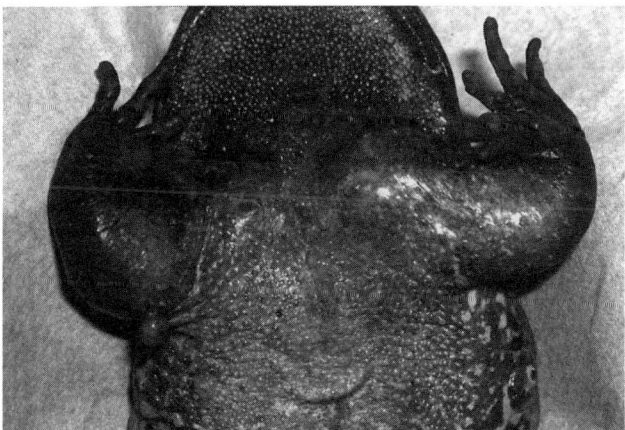

Figure 17.3. Postural abnormalities may be indicative of a fracture such as this coracoid fracture (right) in a South American bullfrog, *Leptodactylus pentadactylus*. This frog had metabolic bone disease. Note the papilloma on its elbow (left). (Kevin Wright, Philadelphia Zoological Garden)

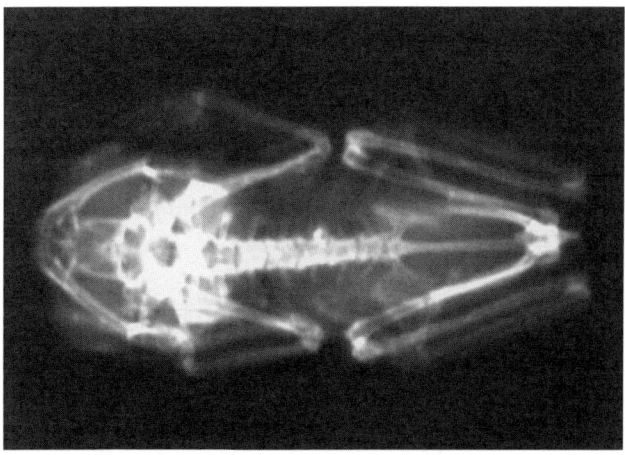

Figure 17.4. Fracture of the ilium in a hylid frog. Ambulation is often impaired with this type of fracture. (National Aquarium in Baltimore)

of methods. The close apposition of the bony cortices is not necessary for callus formation and resolution of the fracture, but provision of a stable external support or internal support is recommended in amphibians of sufficient body size. The application of a splint or Robert-Jones bandage is best made while the patient is under general anesthesia. A water soluble gel (e.g. KY Gel™) should coat the limb prior to application of the coaptation device. Soft cotton gauze rolls may be used as an initial base, and elastic bandages (e.g., Vetrap™, St. Paul, MN) can be used for the external wrap. Some bandages will shrink or expand when moistened, so the material should be wetted prior to application. Weekly assessment of the coaptation device is recommended, and changing of the device done as needed. Callus formation can be assessed by a radiograph of the patient with the coaptation device in place.

The use of intramedullary pins and other fixation devices have not been documented in amphibians.

Fractures of the vertebral column carry a grave prognosis. Corticosteroid therapy is recommended to mitigate further spinal cord injury associated with inflammation and swelling. Suggested corticosteroid therapy includes prednisolone acetate at 2 mg/kg IM or IV q 6 h for 24 h after presentation. Dexamethasone may prove an acceptable substitute. Corticosteroid therapy should be tapered in diminishing doses after the first 24 h of therapy. Supportive care that includes confinement to minimize movement of the vertebral column and assist feeding if necessary is recommended. If the amphibian is unable to defecate on its own 28 days after injury, euthanasia is recommended. Spinal cords may regenerate in some salamanders, but its occurrence in other orders is unknown.

Fractures of the mandible (Plate 17.5) or hyoid bone carry a grave prognosis as this may alter the kinetics of the mouth in a way the precludes capture and ingestion of prey. Tube feeding is necessary as supportive care. Tube feeding is necessary as supportive care. The author attempted to use a polypropylene 22 gauge intravenous catheter as a pharyngostomy tube in a crocodile newt, *Tylototriton shanjing*, but was unable to secure the tube and the salamander could pull it out.

17.5 HYPERTHERMIA

The succession of signs of hyperthermia can occur quite rapidly and quickly lead to death or permanent neurological dysfunction. An amphibian exposed to inappropriately high temperatures typically acts somewhat agitated and shows unusual levels of exploratory activity and possible changes in skin coloration. This is followed by excitation with uncoordinated movements (i.e., random hopping as opposed to purposeful hopping), lethargy, seizures, failure to right itself, and death. Excess mucous production is noted in aquatic amphibians during the excitation phase. Corrective action should include immediate exposure to the lower range of that species' preferred body temperature, usually by removing the amphibian from its overly hot enclosure and placing it in a bath of cool water, artificial pond water, amphibian Ringer's solution, or 10% modified Holtfreter's solution. In general, aquatic amphibians should be provided with an electrolyte-containing solution and terrestrial amphibians should be given access to water or dilute electrolyte solutions. Artificial slime (e.g., Shieldex®, Aquatronics, Malibu, CA) may be added to the bath to soothe the injured epidermis. Topical or systemic corticosteroids may be administered for severely stressed amphibians in conjunction with parenteral fluids for extremely hypovolemic patients. Prophylactic antibiotic baths and parenteral antibiotics are recommended for 5 days following a hyperthermic episode.

Localized burns or scalds are rare unless the caretaker fails to monitor the enclosure's heating devices such as submersible aquarium heaters or heat tape. Erythema or discoloration of the epidermis is seen with minor thermal injuries, whereas blistering and skin sloughing are noted with more severe thermal injuries. Typically burns and scalds disrupt the osmotic imbalance of the amphibian through damage to the skin and exposure of the lymphatics, as well as providing an ideal route for bacterial colonization and subsequent septicemia. Minor thermal injuries can be treated with cool baths of water, artificial pond water, amphibian Ringer's solution, or 10% modified Holtfreter's solution, and artificial slime may be added. Topical antibiotics are warranted for minor injuries, and parenteral antibiotics should be used if infection is suspected. Major thermal injuries generally are fatal, although supportive care as outlined above should be instituted. Large doses of corticosteroids and intracoelomic injection of colloidal suspensions may offset the osmotic imbalance, but despite this therapy this injury carries a grave prognosis.

17.6 HYPOTHERMIA

Hypothermia is less readily defined as a clinical entity than hyperthermia, although cases of frostbite and "freezer burn" are sometimes seen. Most hypothermic injuries are the result of inappropriate hibernation techniques. Many cold-adapted amphibian species produce antifreeze particles in their blood, and will freeze and thaw without consequence (e.g., wood frog, *Rana sylvatica*). However, this ability may not hold true for every population within a species, and frostbite or death can result from exposure to freezing or near freezing temperatures. "Freezer burn" results from a combination of cold and desiccation. Hibernated amphibians should be kept damp at all times to prevent this condition. Treatment of freezer burn is supportive, and may include amputation of affected digits to remove a potential nidus of infection. Baths in artificial slime are recommended.

It is likely that exposure to inappropriately cool temperatures can result in immunosuppression of the amphibian. There is some evidence that complement activity in the northern leopard frog, *Rana pipiens,* is influenced by temperature (Green & Cohen, 1977), thus a hypothermic amphibian may be more susceptible to infectious diseases and should be closely monitored for signs for several weeks after apparent recovery from the hypothermia. Fecal samples should be obtained and examined to detect any parasite outbreaks resulting from the immunosuppression, and careful monitoring of appetite and behavior is recommended.

17.7 DEHYDRATION AND DESICCATION

The majority of amphibians readily lose water when exposed to an arid environment. Dehydration and subsequent desiccation can occur quite rapidly if the captive environment is too dry or the water source is inappropriately presented. Some burrowing salamanders will not enter a water bowl when the substrate (e.g., soil) is drying out, instead burrowing deeper into the substrate. Thus an amphibian can dehydrate and desiccate despite the presence of a bowl of water in its enclosure. The decreased humidity in the home associated with radiant or central heating and air conditioning may promote evaporation in a vivarium at a much faster rate than anticipated. Pet sitters may not recognize the need to monitor the humidity of an amphibian's enclosure with the unpleasant surprise of a dehydrated or desiccated amphibian awaiting the client upon return to their home. Temperatures above the preferred body temperature require increased water turnover in the amphibian to cope with the metabolic stress, thus promoting dehydration in the amphibian.

The dehydrated amphibian is tacky to the touch (Plates 17.8, 17.9). The protective layer of slime becomes more viscous as the amphibian conserves bodily water for maintaining normovolemia. The slime may become opaque or even grayish in cast. Extremities become desiccated before the trunk of the amphibian. The skin takes on a darker hue and becomes wrinkled and shriveled as the protective slime dries. Desiccated amphibians may feel leathery to the touch (Plate 17.10).

If given access to mud, some amphibians (e.g., lesser siren, *Siren intermedia,* horned frogs, *Ceratophrys* spp.) respond to desiccation by forming protective water-conserving cocoons and estivating until favorable water conditions resume. The majority of amphibians in the pet trade do not form cocoons and cannot escape the onslaught of dry conditions in this manner.

The dehydrated and desiccated amphibian should be placed in a shallow bath of cool (i.e., temperatures at or slightly below the preferred body temperature of the species), well-oxygenated, aged, or filtered water. Shock may be concurrently treated with corticosteroids and intracoelomic administration of hypotonic fluids. Obtain a quick weight on the amphibian patient and immediately place it in the water bath. The next step of treatment is to administer 1–2 mg/kg dexamethasone IM and a fluid volume equal to 2–5% of the amphibian's body weight. This author uses two parts lactate-free electrolyte solution (e.g., Plasmalyte-A, Baxter Pharmaceuticals) or saline to one part 5% dextrose as the initial fluid therapy, and if needed follows with a subsequent solution of nine parts LRS (or sterilized amphibian Ringer's solution) or saline to one part sterile water. Artificial slime (e.g., Shieldex®) may be added to the bath after 12 h to soothe the injured epidermis. Prophylactic antibiotic baths are recommended as aftercare. If the amphibian survives the first 24 h, additional supportive care should include topical antibiotic gels or ointments to the damaged skin and parenteral antibiotics.

17.8 DROWNING

Drowning is a risk to many species of amphibians. Species that are entirely aquatic (e.g., axolotl, *Ambystoma mexicanum*) may switch to pulmonary respiration when faced with low dissolved oxygen, and if the amphibian cannot readily access the surface it may drown. Drowning may also occur during mating attempts if the water source is too deep or too crowded with other cagemates. In some species (e.g., tomato frog, *Dyscophis guinetti*), drowning may occur in a shallow pool if an amplexed couple flips upside down and are unable to right themselves.

Immediately attempt to clear the airways of the drowned amphibian. Cup the amphibian in your hands with the head facing distally. Sling your hands forcefully back and forth several times. If done correctly this promotes the expulsion of fluids from the lungs and trachea. Gentle massage of the abdomen may milk additional fluid out of the lungs and trachea. Following these efforts to clear the airways, the drowned amphibian should immediately be treated by forced ventilation with oxygen if its glottis is large enough for intubation. Polypropylene intravenous catheters can be used as endotracheal tubes for small amphibians. If intubation is impossible, maintain the amphibian in a shallow bath of water with oxygen bubbling into it, making sure to keep the nares and mouth above water. Doxapram hydrochloride may be placed in the trachea, dripped on the skin, or given parenterally. If there is no cardiac impulse, gentle cardiac massage should be instituted at a rate of 10–20 beats per min. Epinephrine can be administered intratracheally, topically, or parenterally. Decreasing the body temperature by immersing the amphibian in a cold water bath may decrease the metabolic demands of the tissue until circulation and ventilation is restored. If the amphibian is resuscitated successfully, parenteral antibiotics are recommended to decrease risk of respiratory tract infections. Use of corticosteroids and parenteral hypertonic solutions (e.g., 0.1 ml hypertonic/10 g body weight as a guideline) may help mobilize any remaining pulmonary fluid.

17.9 ELECTRICAL SHOCK

Ground fault interrupted electrical circuits and Underwriter Labs approved electrical devices should be used around amphibian enclosures to protect the amphibian and the caretaker against risk of electrical shock. Resuscitation of the electrocuted amphibian should include intubation where practical, ventilation (either pulmonic or cutenously by bathing in cool well oxygenated water), and cardiac massage. Artificial slime (Shieldex®), topical antibiotics, and parenteral antibiotics are recommended for accompanying burns.

17.10 RADIATION

Radiation injuries are uncommon in the pet amphibian. Diffuse corneal opacity has been suspected to be linked to the use of ultraviolet-emitting bulbs as a light sources for an amphibian's vivarium (e.g., black lamps, sunlamps). Discontinue use of these or similar bulbs if this is suspected as a contributing factor to corneal or skin discoloration. Ophthalmic corticosteroids and antibiotics are recommended for a minimum of 7–10 days.

Sunburn may occur if an amphibian is exposed to direct sunlight and possibly to certain types of ultraviolet-emitting bulbs. Erythema, excess mucus production, discoloration, sloughing, blistering, and ulceration are signs of sunburn. Treatment as appropriate for hyperthermia is indicated, but the artificial slime (e.g. Shieldex®) and topical antibiotics should be administered until the skin returns to normal coloration. Every effort should be made to prevent dehydration from fluid loss through the damaged skin.

Amphibians can be radiographed with standard radiograph and mammography units without risk of radiation injury.

Clinical signs associated with radiation poisoning are initially limited to skin lesions and depigmentation in the roughskin newt, *Taricha granulosa*, when exposed to 2.5 Gy, but half of the exposed group died within 200 days of exposure (Willis & Lappenbusch, 1976). Progressive anemia was reported in those newts exposed to a single dose higher than 6.5 Gy, and at levels of 80 Gy or above, half of the exposed group died within 100 days of exposure. Red-spotted newts, *Notophthalmus viridescens*, exhibited suppression of forelimb regeneration when exposed to 20 Gy (Sicard & Lombard, 1990). Half of the frogs (*Rana* spp.) died within 150 days of exposure to 7.8 Gy (Hinton & Scott, 1990). Treatment of radiation poisoning in amphibians was not documented in these reports. Amphibians have received scant attention with regard to radiation pollution of the environment (Eisler, 1994).

REFERENCES

Eisler, R. 1994. Radiation hazards to fish, wildlife, and invertebrates: a synoptic review. Biological Report 26, December 1994; Contaminant Hazard Reviews Report 29. U.S. Department of the Interior, National Biological Service, Washington, DC, 124 pp.

Green, N. and N. Cohen. 1977. Effect of temperature on serum complement levels in the leopard frog, *Rana pipiens*. Developmental and Comparative Immunology 1:59–64.

Hinton, T.G. and D.E. Scott. 1990. Radioecological techniques for herpetology, with an emphasis in freshwater turtles, *in* Gibbons, J.W. (Ed.): Life history and ecology of the slider turtle. Smithsonian Institution Press, Washington, DC, pp. 267–287.

Pritchard, J.J. and A.J. Ruzicka. 1950. Comparison of fracture repair in the frog, lizard, and rat. Journal of Anatomy 84:236–261.

Sicard, R.E. and M.F. Lombard. 1990. Putative immunological influence upon amphibian forelimb regeneration II. Effects of X-irradiation on regeneration and autograft rejection. Biological Bulletin 178:21–24.

Willis, D.L. and W.L. Lappenbusch. 1976. The radiosensitivity of the rough-skinned newt (*Taricha granulosa*), *in* Cushing, C.E. (Ed.): Radioecology and energy resources. Proceedings of the fourth national symposium on radioecology, 12–14 May 1975, Oregon State University, Corvallis. The Ecological Society of America, Special Publication 1, pp. 363–375.

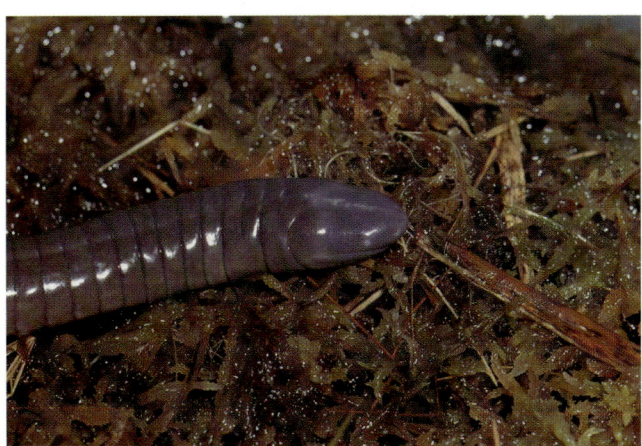

Plate 2.1. The Mexican caecilian, *Dermophis mexicanus*, is one of the most common terrestrial caecilians in captivity at this time. (Kevin Wright, Philadelphia Zoological Garden)

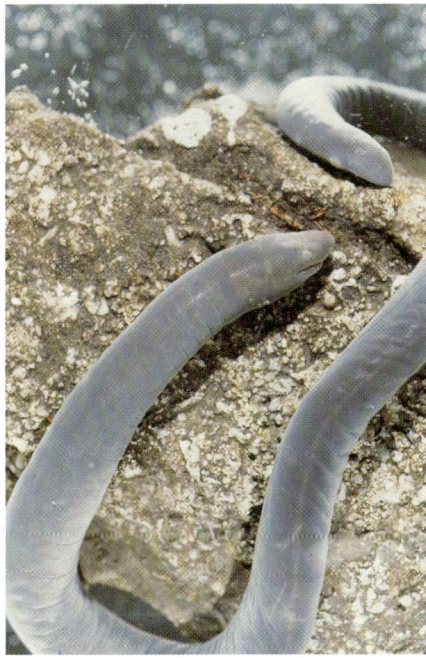

Plate 2.2. Aquatic caecilians, such as the Rio Cauca caecilian, *Typhlonectes natans*, are often sold in pet stores as "rubber eels." (Kevin Wright, Philadelphia Zoological Garden)

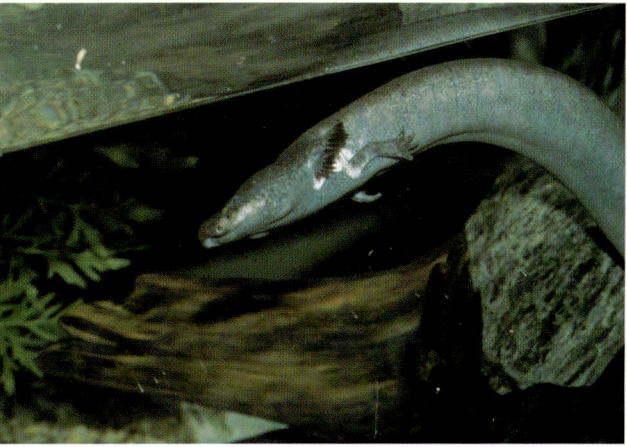

Plate 2.3. The lesser siren, *Siren intermedia*. A forelimb and the external gills are visible. (Kevin Wright, Philadelphia Zoological Garden)

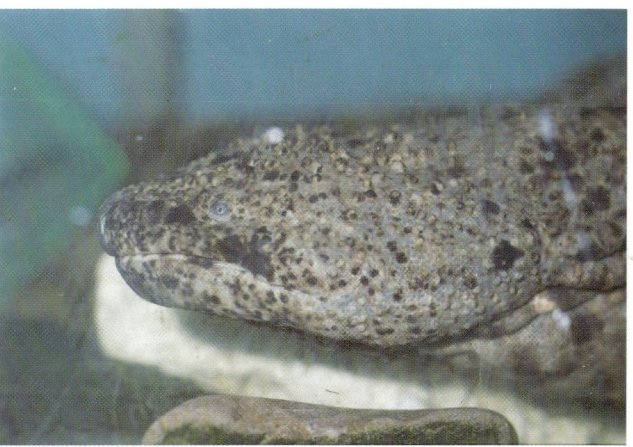

Plate 2.4. Head of a Japanese giant salamander, *Andrias japonicus*, which may reach a weight in excess of 45 kg (100 lbs.). (Steve Walker, Philadelphia Zoological Garden)

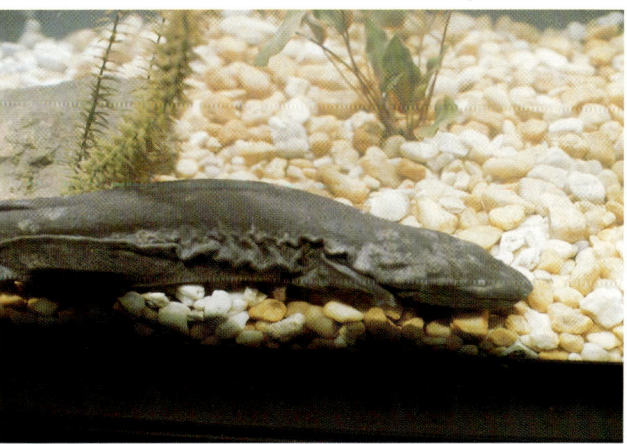

Plate 2.5. The skin folds on the side of this hellbender, *Cryptobranchus alleganiensis*, serve as respiratory surfaces. (Philadelphia Zoological Garden)

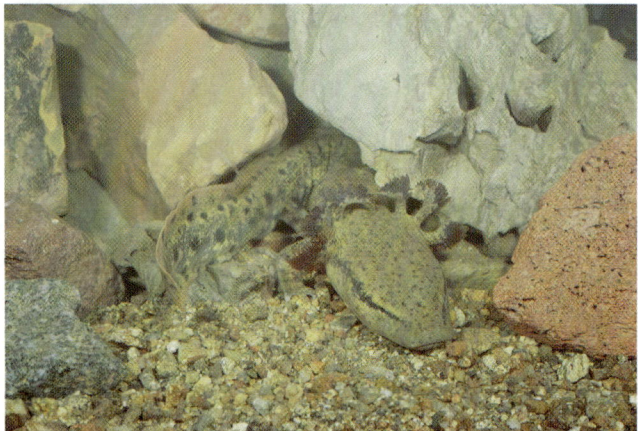

Plate 2.6. The Alabama waterdog, *Necturus alabamensis*, is a close relative of the mudpuppy, *Necturus maculosus*. (R. Andrew Odum, Toledo Zoological Society)

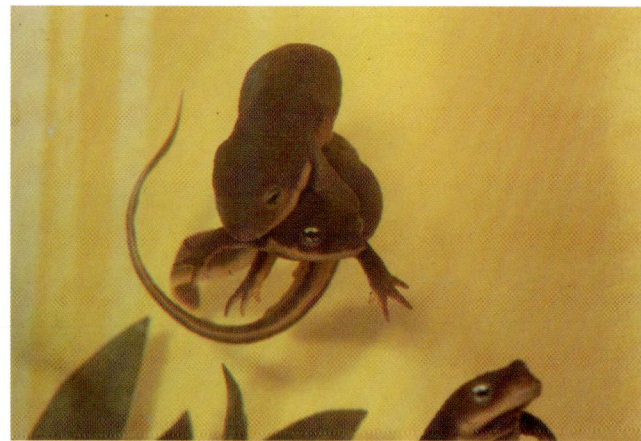

Plate 2.9. Roughskin newts, *Taricha* spp., are commonly available, but few are set up for captive breeding. This is a courting pair. (Robert Dougan)

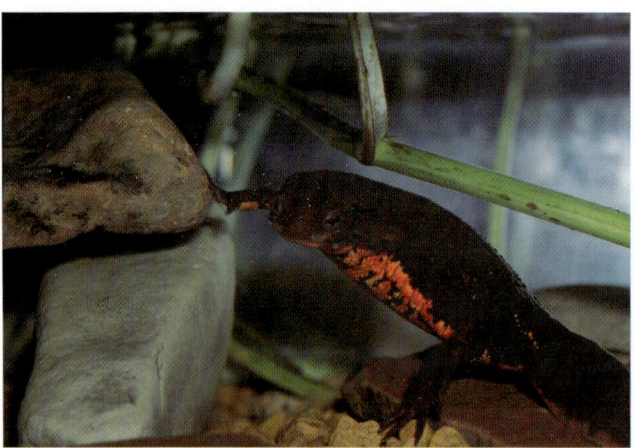

Plate 2.7. The Japanese firebelly newt, *Cynops pyrrhogaster*, is commonly sold in pet stores. (Kevin Wright, Philadelphia Zoological Garden)

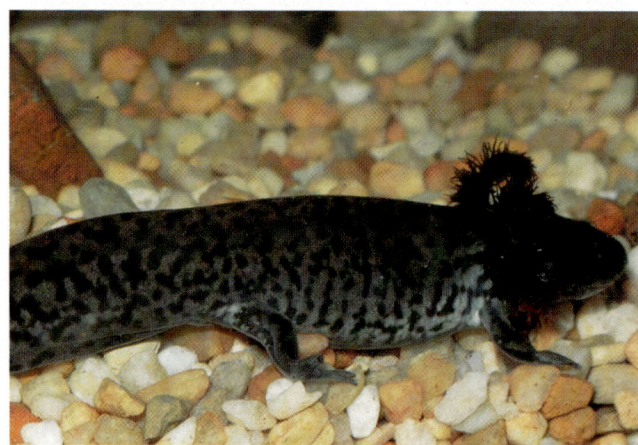

Plate 2.10. Anderson's axolotl, *Ambystoma andersoni*, has a more punctate pattern but is otherwise similar in appearance to the common axolotl, *A. mexicanum*. (Robert Dougan)

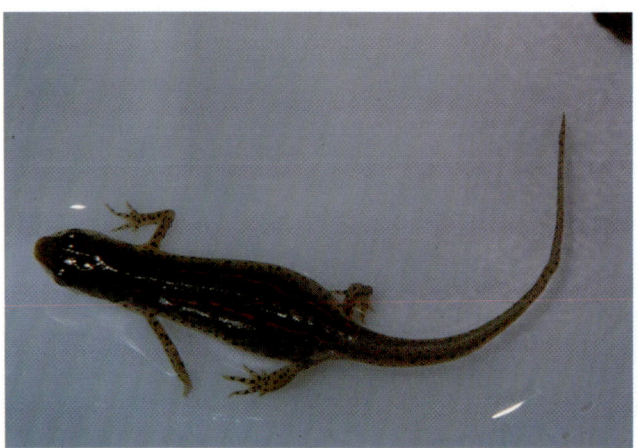

Plate 2.8. The red-spotted newt, *Notophthalmus viridescens viridescens*, is commonly available. (Robert Dougan)

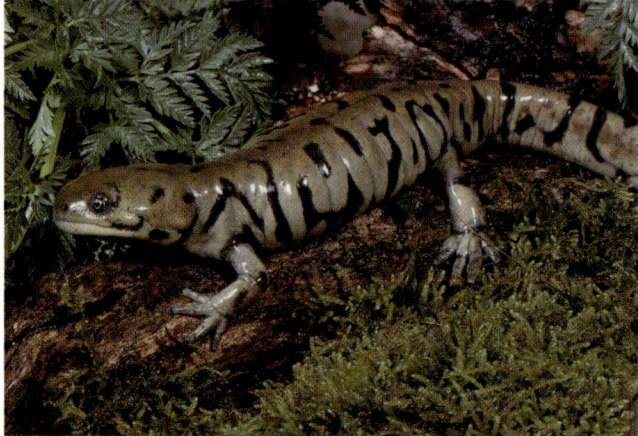

Plate 2.11. The Eastern tiger salamander, *Ambystoma tigrinum tigrinum*, is one of the more common salamanders in the pet trade. (R. Andrew Odum, Toledo Zoological Society)

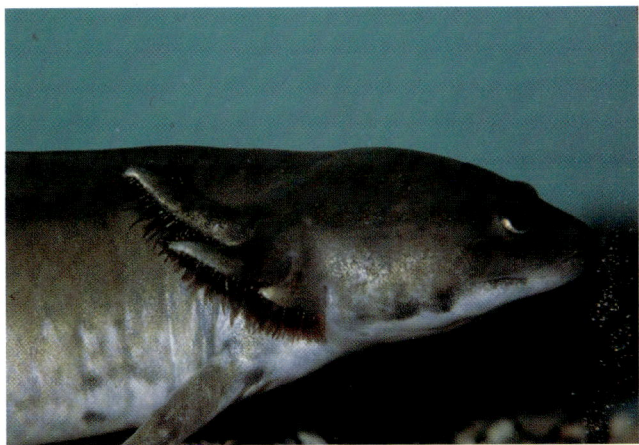

Plate 2.12. Larva of the tiger salamander, *Ambystoma tigrinum*, are often sold under the name "waterdog." These should not be confused with true waterdogs, family Proteidae. (Robert Dougan)

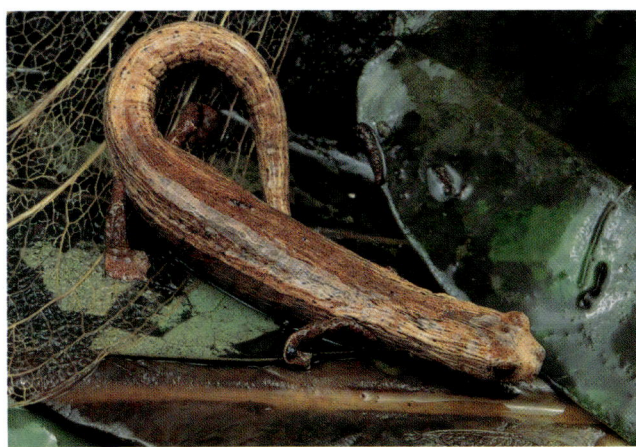

Plate 2.15. A tropical lungless salamander, *Bolitoglossa* sp. Identification of many species is problematic without locality data due to the lack of a comprehensive key for this genus. (George Grall, National Aquarium in Baltimore)

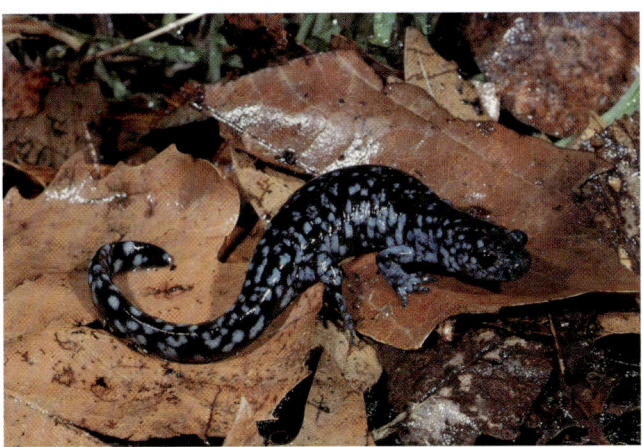

Plate 2.13. The blue-spotted salamander, *Ambystoma laterale*, is occasionally found in pet stores. It is sometimes erroneously labeled as a "spotted salamander" (i.e., *Ambystoma maculatum*). (R. Andrew Odum, Toledo Zoological Society)

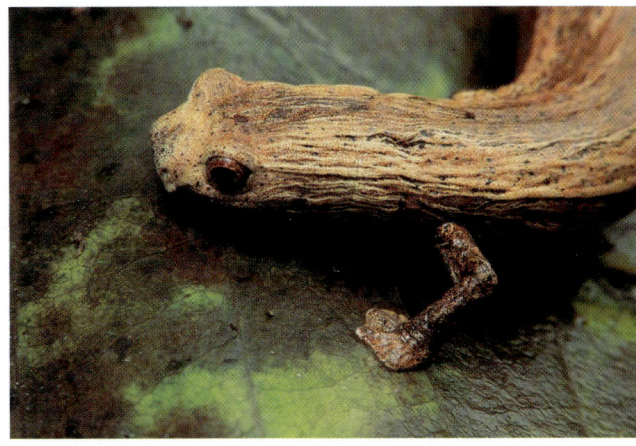

Plate 2.16. The feet of tropical lungless salamanders, *Bolitoglossa* spp., are shaped like suction cups, an adaptation for climbing. (George Grall, National Aquarium in Baltimore)

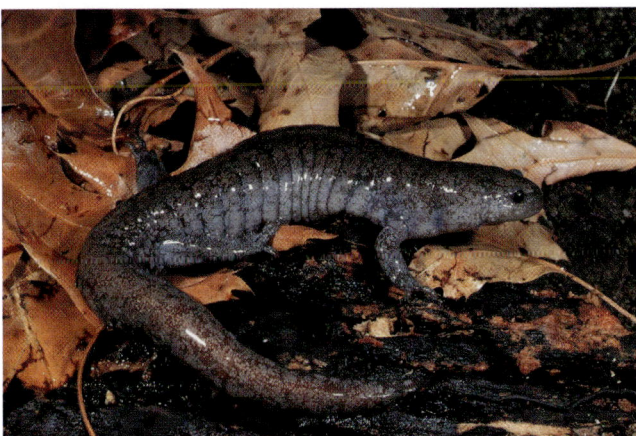

Plate 2.14. The small-mouthed salamander, *Ambystoma texanum*, is rarely seen in captivity. (R. Andrew Odum, Toledo Zoological Society)

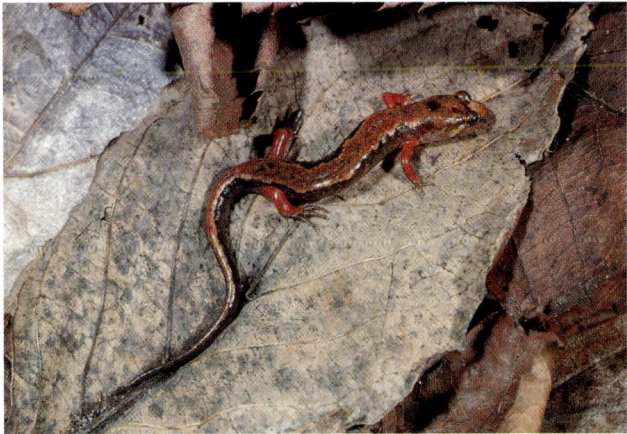

Plate 2.17. The imitator salamander, *Desmognathus imitator*, is an attractive North American plethodontid. (R. Andrew Odum, Toledo Zoological Society)

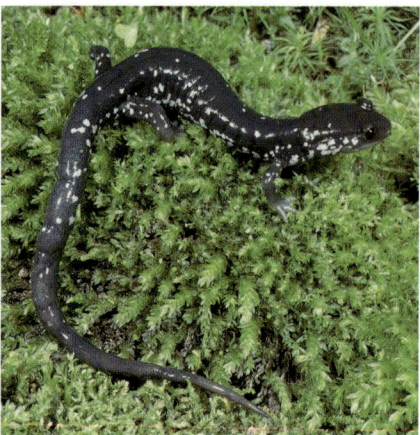

Plate 2.18. Slimy salamanders (*Plethodon glutinosus* complex) are difficult to speciate without locality data. These species produce mucilaginous skin secretions as an antipredator mechanism. (R. Andrew Odum, Toledo Zoological Society)

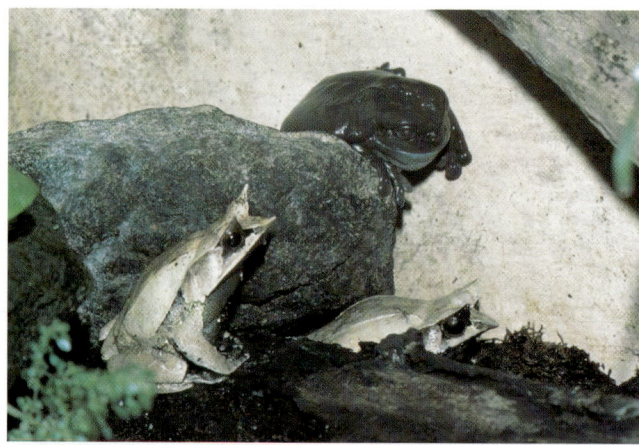

Plate 2.21. Females of the Asian spadefoot toad, *Megophrys montana*, are much larger than males. A White's treefrog, *Pelodryas caerulea*, shares the cage, but mixing species from such disparate locales is not advised due to possibility of disease transmission. (Robert Dougan)

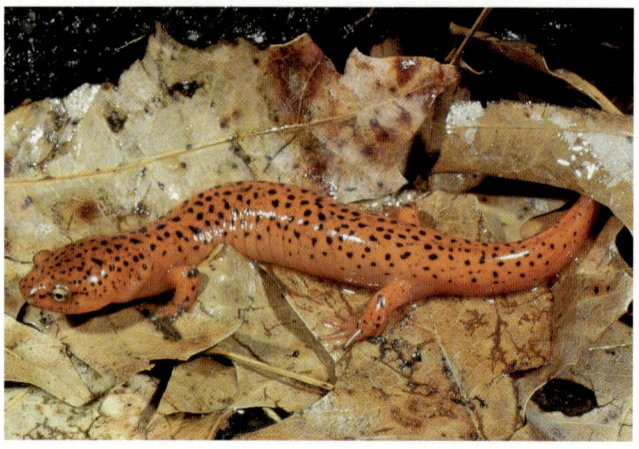

Plate 2.19. The red salamander, *Pseudotriton ruber*, is a semiaquatic lungless salamander. (R. Andrew Odum, Toledo Zoological Society)

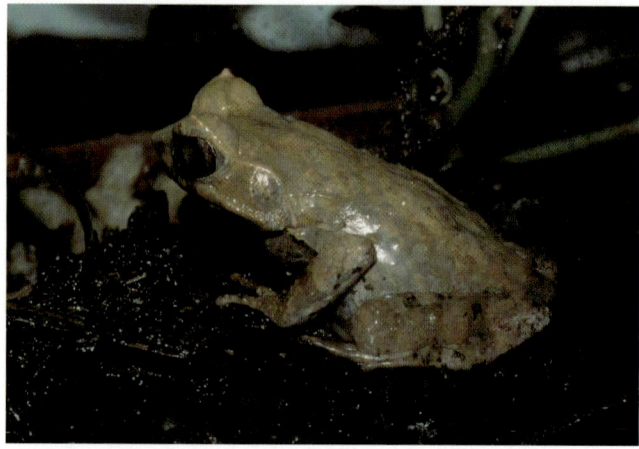

Plate 2.22. A male Asian spadefoot toad, *Megophrys montana*. (Robert Dougan)

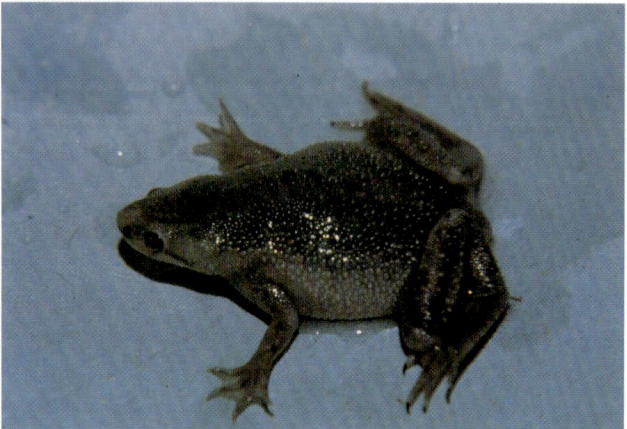

Plate 2.20. Dwarf clawed frogs, *Hymenochirus* spp., are commonly sold in tropical fish stores. This species rarely leaves water voluntarily. (Robert Dougan)

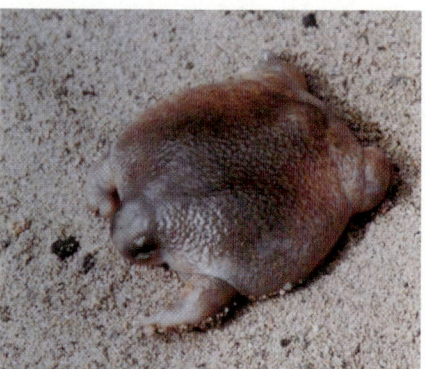

Plate 2.23. The turtle frog, *Myobatrachus gouldi*, is a poorly known myobatrachid frog from Australia. (Philadelphia Zoological Garden)

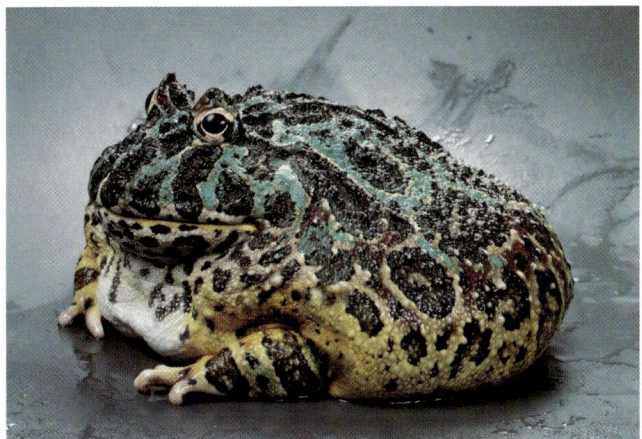

Plate 2.24. The captive-bred babies of the ornate horned frog, *Ceratophrys ornata*, are often sold under the name "Pac-man frog." (George Grall, National Aquarium in Baltimore)

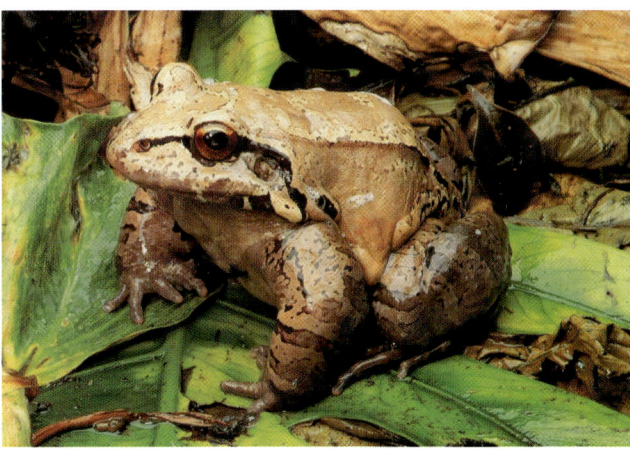

Plate 2.27. The South American bullfrog, *Leptodactylus pentadactylus*. (George Grall, National Aquarium in Baltimore)

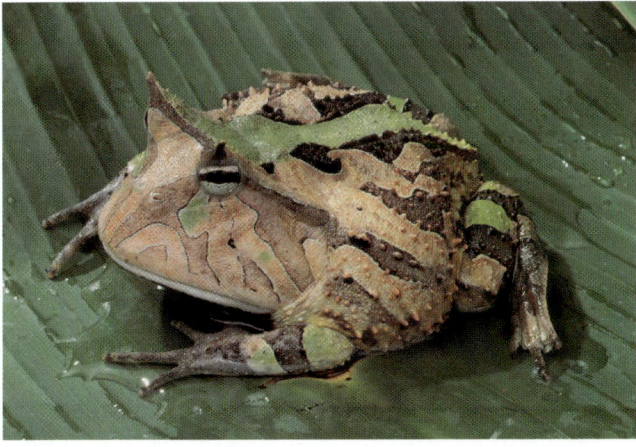

Plate 2.25. Wild-caught specimens of the Surinam horned frog, *Ceratophrys cornuta*, are difficult to establish in captivity and not recommended for the average herpetoculturist. (George Grall, National Aquarium in Baltimore)

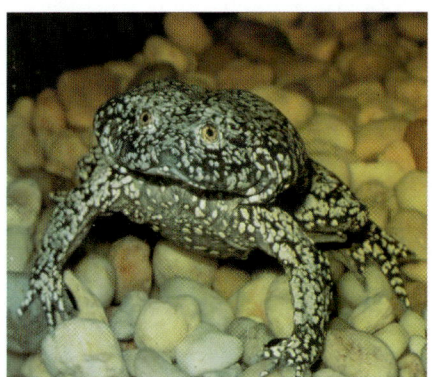

Plate 2.28. The Lake Titicaca water frog, *Telmatobius culeus*, is a frog highly adapted for an aquatic existence. (Robert Dougan)

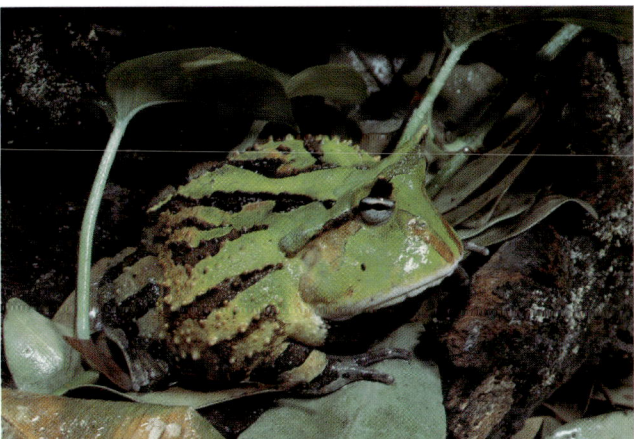

Plate 2.26. Specimens of the Surinam horned frog, *Ceratophrys cornuta*, may be quite variable in coloration. (R. Andrew Odum, Toledo Zoological Society)

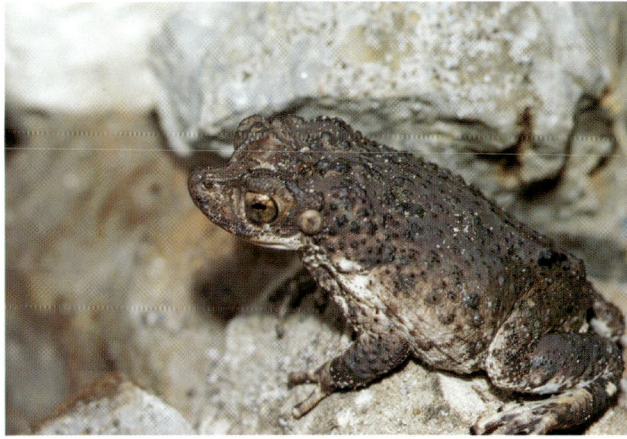

Plate 2.29. The lowland Caribbean toad, *Peltophryne lemur*, also known as the Puerto Rican crested toad, has been successfully reintroduced to the wild as a result of cooperative efforts among zoos. (Kevin Wright, Philadelphia Zoological Garden)

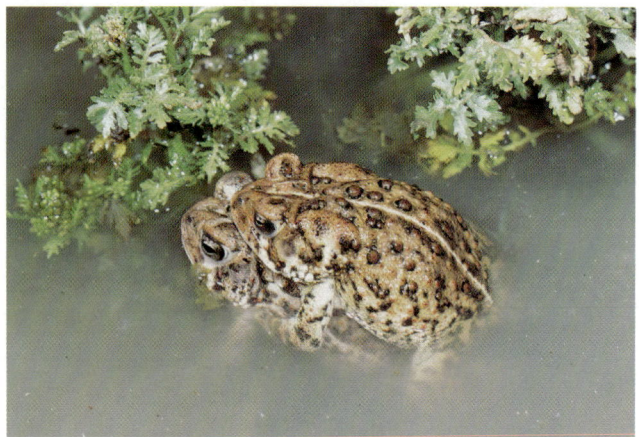

Plate 2.30. An amplexing pair of Houston toads, *Bufo houstonensis*, a highly endangered species. (R. Andrew Odum, Toledo Zoological Society)

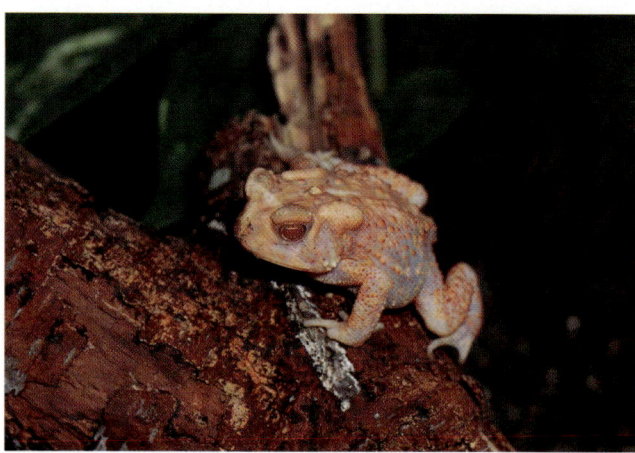

Plate 2.33. An albino specimen of the American toad, *Bufo americanus*. (Kevin Wright, courtesy of the Detroit Zoological Garden)

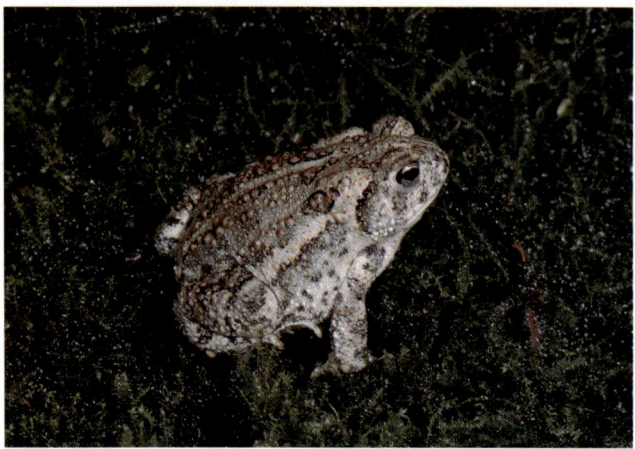

Plate 2.31. The Wyoming toad, *Bufo hemiophrys baxteri*, is the subject of a recovery plan that involves captive breeding and release of specimens. (R. Andrew Odum, Toledo Zoological Society)

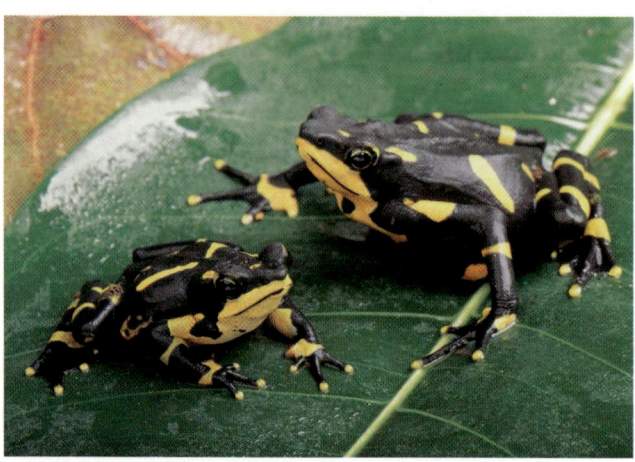

Plate 2.34. The Veragua stubfoot toad, *Atelopus varius*, is also known as the harlequin frog. This species exhibits sexual dimorphism, with females being much larger than males. (George Grall, National Aquarium in Baltimore)

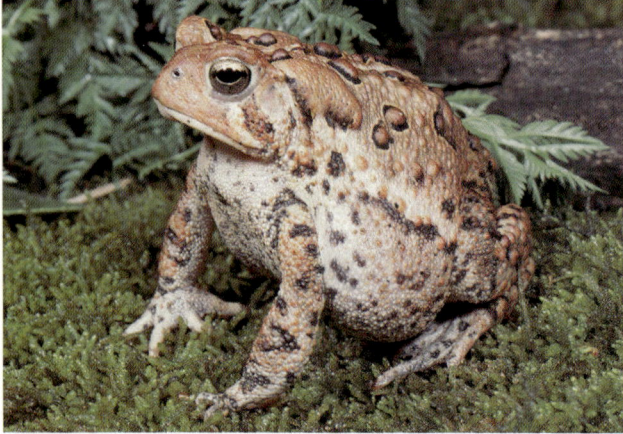

Plate 2.32. The American toad, *Bufo americanus*, is still quite common throughout most of its range. (R. Andrew Odum, Toledo Zoological Society)

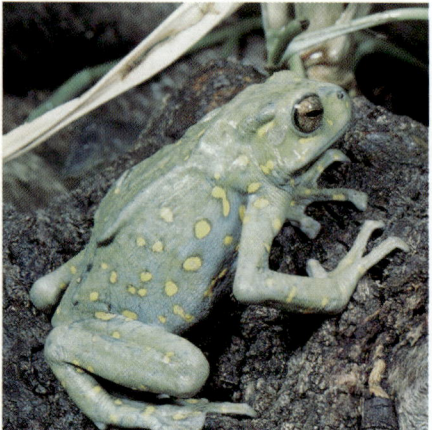

Plate 2.35. Boulenger's Asian tree toad, *Pedostibes hosii*, is difficult to acclimate to captivity and not recommended for the average herpetoculturist. (R. Andrew Odum, Toledo Zoological Society)

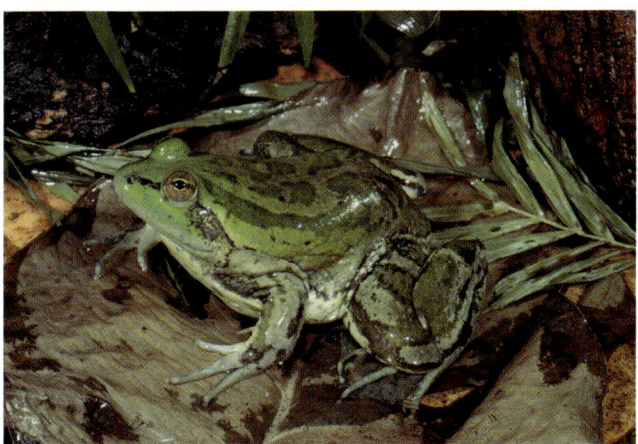

Plate 2.36. The swimming frog, *Pseudis paradoxa*, is also known as the paradox frog since its tadpoles grow to a larger size than the adult frog. (R. Andrew Odum, Toledo Zoological Society)

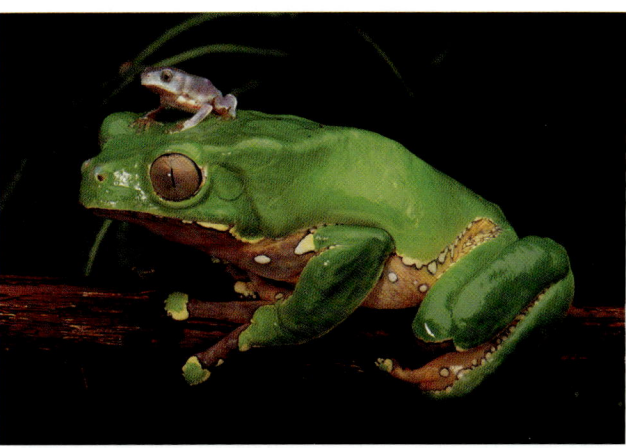

Plate 2.38. An adult giant monkey frog, *Phyllomedusa bicolor*, and its captive-born offspring. (George Grall, National Aquarium in Baltimore)

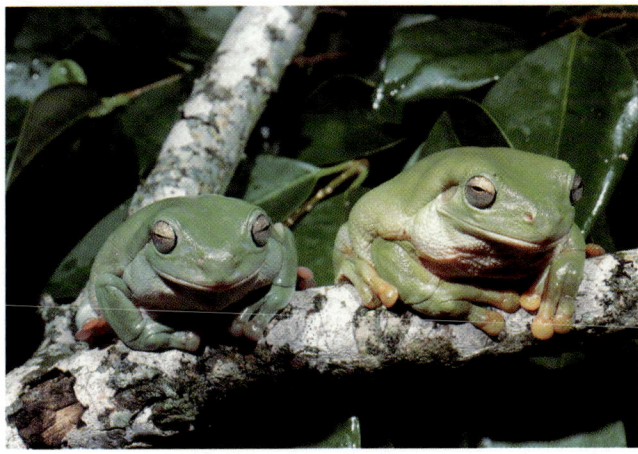

Plate 2.37. A. White's treefrog, *Pelodryas (Litoria) caerulea*, is an extremely popular pet. (R. Andrew Odum, Toledo Zoological Society)

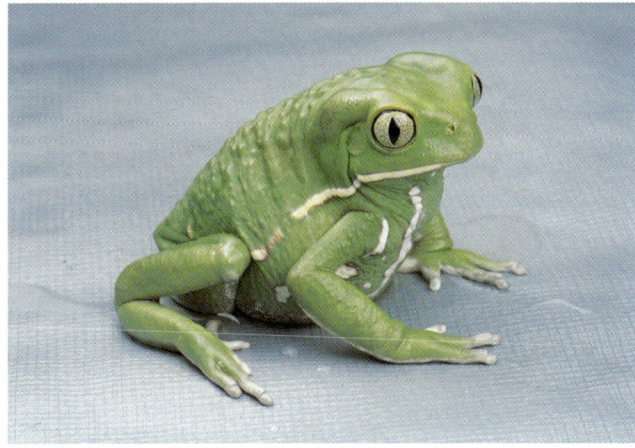

Plate 2.39. The painted-belly monkey frog, *Phyllomedusa sauvagii*, produces uric acid as its main nitrogenous waste. (George Grall, National Aquarium in Baltimore)

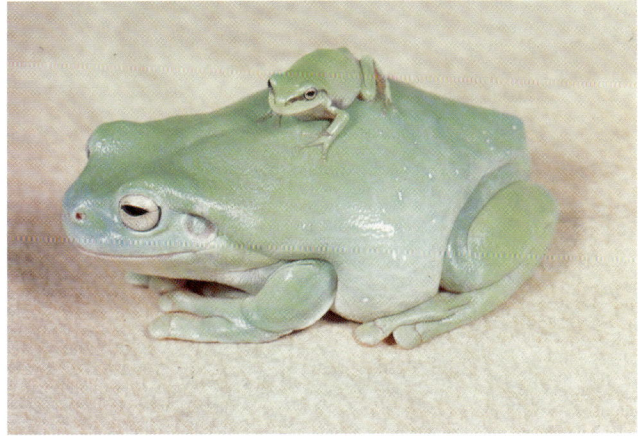

Plate 2.37. B. Captive-bred specimens of White's treefrog, *Pelodryas caerulea*, are readily available in the pet trade. The young lose their eye stripes as they mature. (R. Andrew Odum, Toledo Zoological Society)

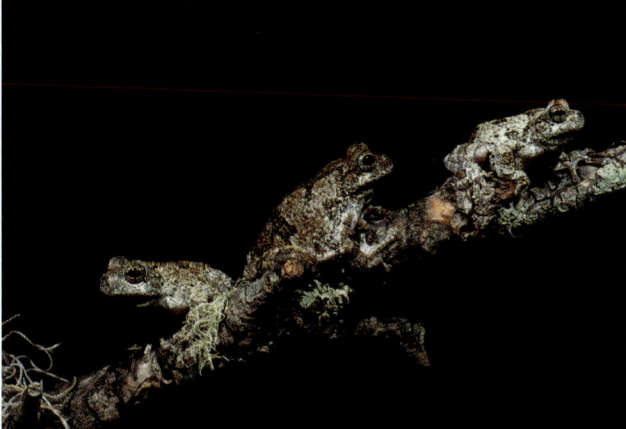

Plate 2.40. The gray treefrog, *Hyla versicolor*, is a commonly available North American hylid. (R. Andrew Odum, Toledo Zoological Society)

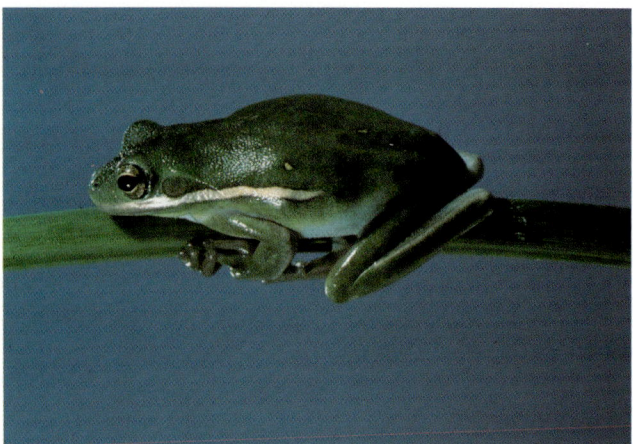

Plate 2.41. The green treefrog, *Hyla cinerea*, is an attractive frog from the southeastern United States. (Robert Dougan)

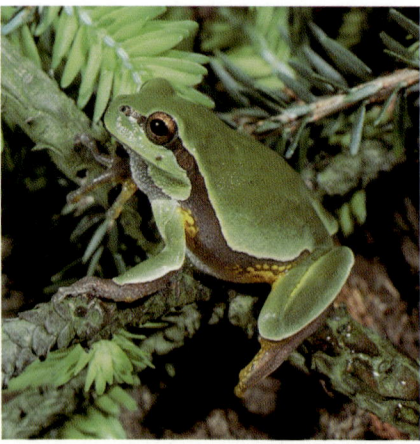

Plate 2.42. The Pine Barrens treefrog, *Hyla andersoni*, is an endangered North American hylid, and special permits are required to possess this species. (R. Andrew Odum, Toledo Zoological Society)

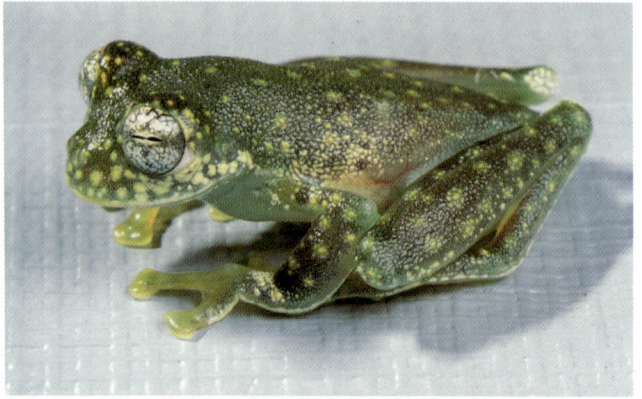

Plate 2.43. The white-spotted glass frog, *Centrolenella (Cochranella) albomaculata*, from Costa Rica. (George Grall, National Aquarium in Baltimore)

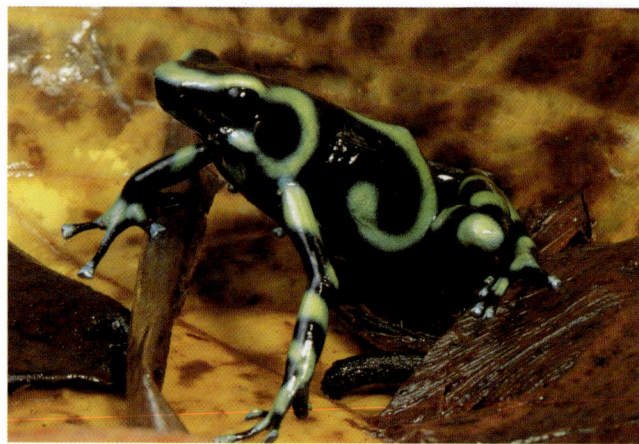

Plate 2.44. The green and black poison frog, *Dendrobates auratus*, is one the most common captive-bred dendrobatids. Free-ranging populations have been established in the state of Hawaii. (George Grall, National Aquarium in Baltimore)

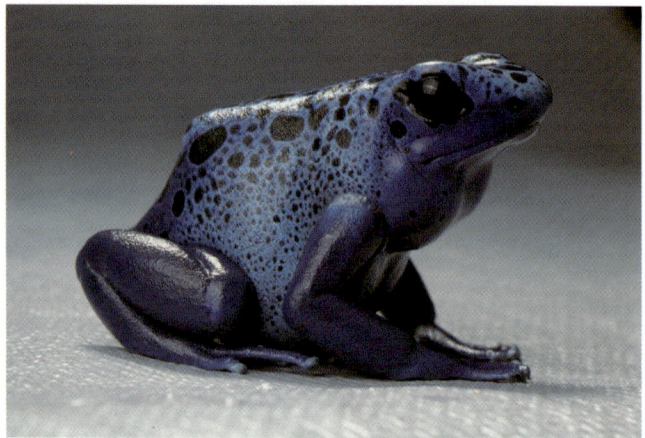

Plate 2.45. The blue poison frog, *Dendrobates azureus*, is now protected and should not be collected from the wild for the pet trade. This specimen is obese. (George Grall, National Aquarium in Baltimore)

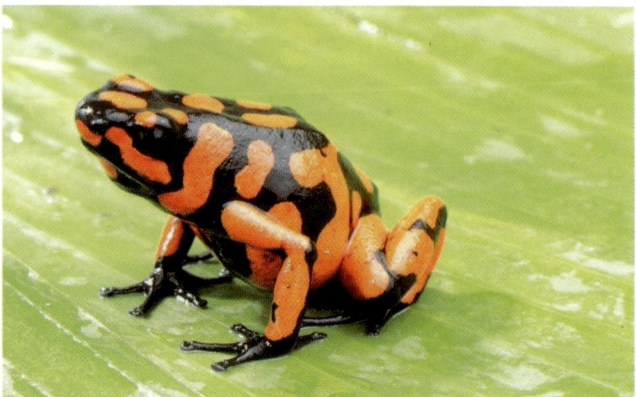

Plate 2.46. The colors of captive-bred specimens of the harlequin poison frog, *Dendrobates histrionicus*, are not as colorful as this wild-caught specimen. (George Grall, National Aquarium in Baltimore)

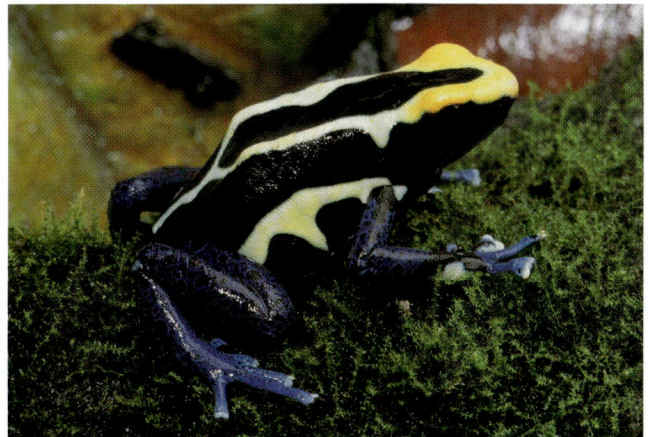

Plate 2.47. Captive-bred offspring of several color morphs of the dyeing poison frog, *Dendrobates tinctorius*, are regularly available. (George Grall, National Aquarium in Baltimore)

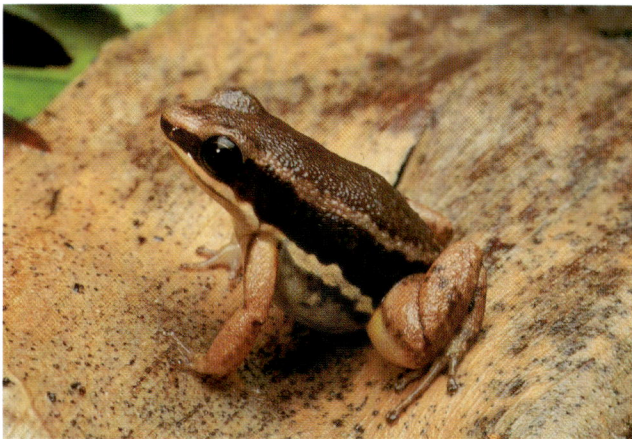

Plate 2.50. Not all dendrobatid frogs are colorful. The Talmanaca rocket frog, *Colestethus talmanacae*, is a typical representative of this genus. (George Grall, National Aquarium in Baltimore)

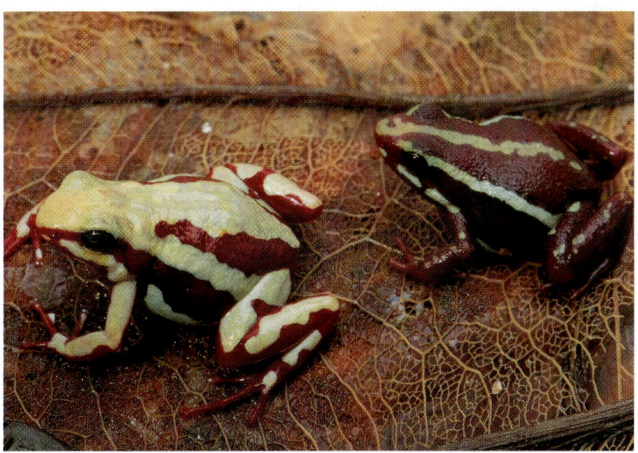

Plate 2.48. The color pattern of the wild-caught phantasmal poison frog, *Epipedobates tricolor*, includes much more green than the captive-bred specimen on the right. (George Grall, National Aquarium in Baltimore)

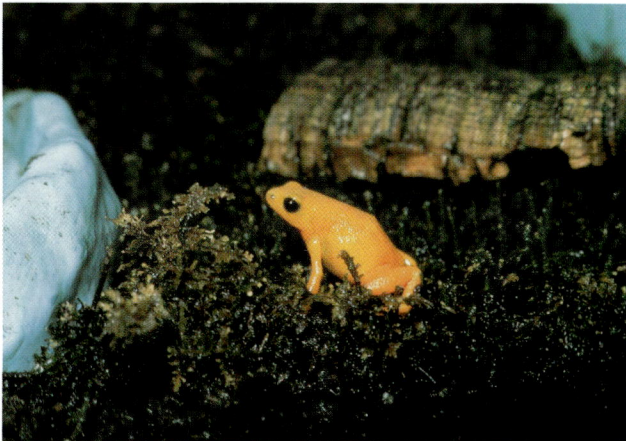

Plate 2.51. The golden mantella, *Mantella aurantiaca*, is readily available in the pet trade due to heavy exploitation of this species, a practice which appears to be unsustainable. (Robert Dougan)

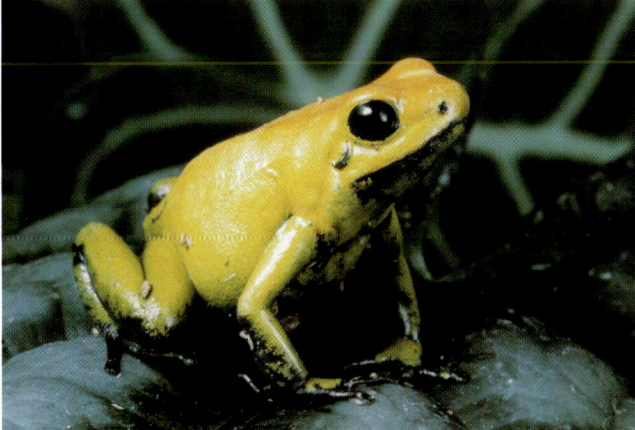

Plate 2.49. The black-legged poison frog, *Phyllobates bicolor*. (George Grall, National Aquarium in Baltimore)

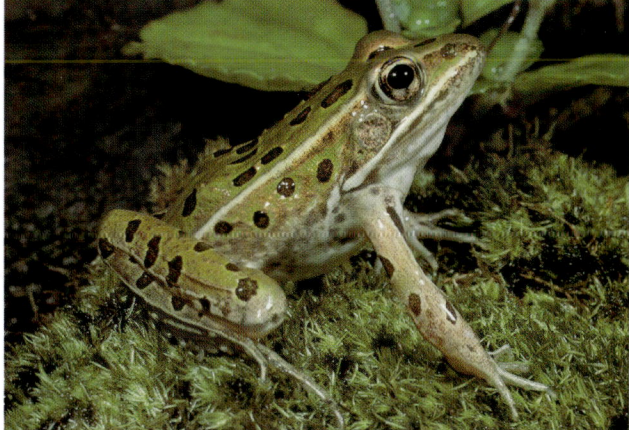

Plate 2.52. The northern leopard frog, *Rana pipiens*, is extensively used in biomedical research. (R. Andrew Odum, Toledo Zoological Society)

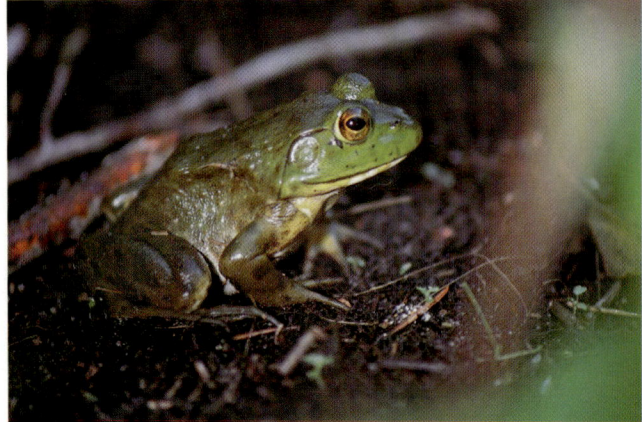

Plate 2.53. The bullfrog, *Rana catesbeiana*, is a popular research frog. (Florence Robin, Philadelphia Zoological Garden)

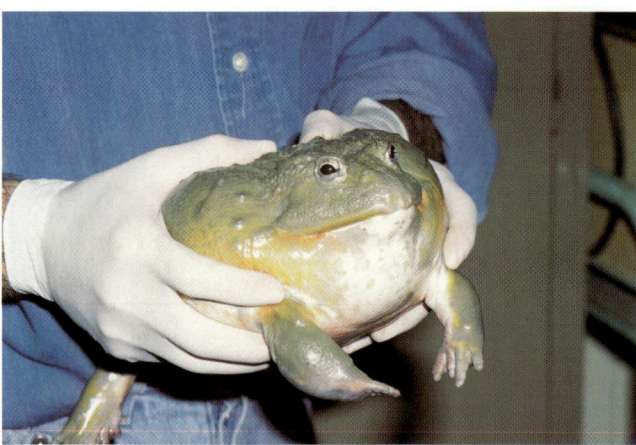

Plate 2.56. Tschudi's African bullfrog, *Pyxicephalus adspersus*. (Kevin Wright, Philadelphia Zoological Garden)

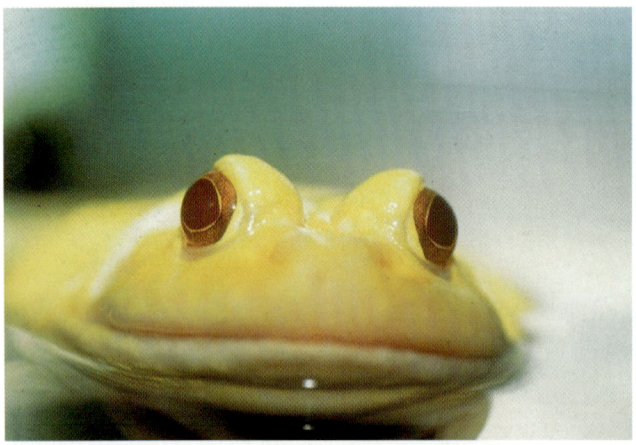

Plate 2.54. Albino specimens of the bullfrog, *Rana catesbeiana*, are readily available in the pet trade. (Philadelphia Zoological Garden)

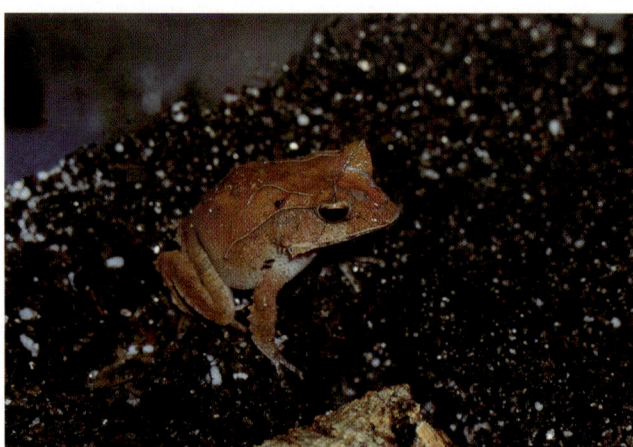

Plate 2.57. Gunther's triangle frog, *Ceratobatrachus guentheri*, does not have a tadpole stage. Froglets hatch directly from eggs which are buried underground. (Kevin Wright, Philadelphia Zoological Garden)

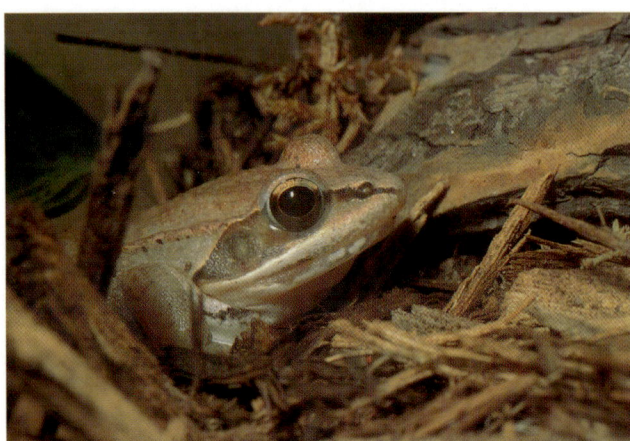

Plate 2.55. The wood frog, *Rana sylvatica*, is the subject of physiological research due to its ability to endure freezing temperatures. (Tom Dewey, Philadelphia Zoological Garden)

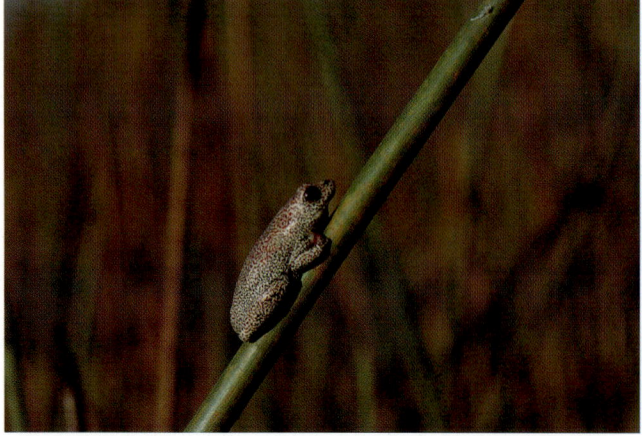

Plate 2.58. A marbled reed frog, *Hyperolius marmoratus*. (Robert Dougan)

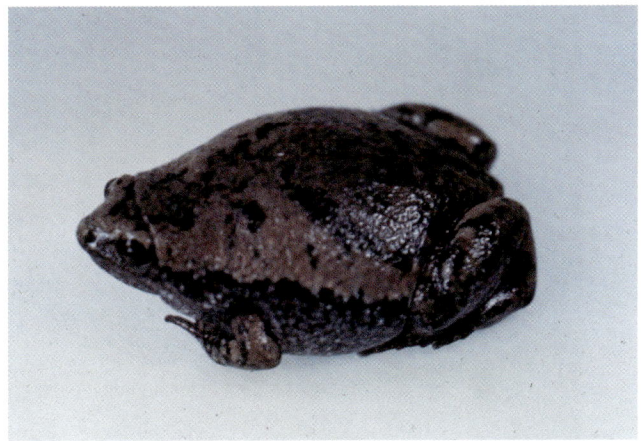

Plate 2.59. The eastern narrowmouth toad, *Gastrophryne caroliniensis*, is a North American microhylid that feeds on ants. (Philadelphia Zoological Garden)

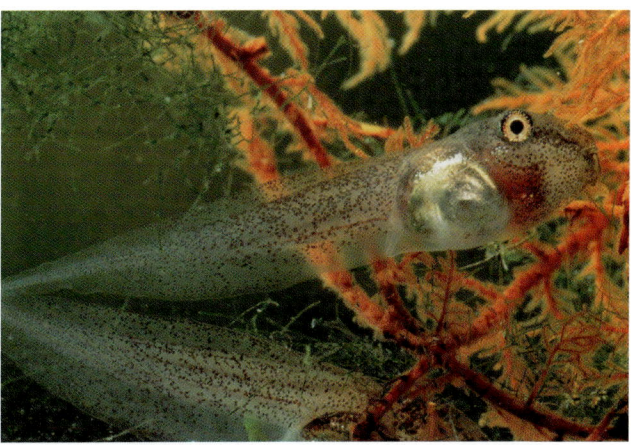

Plate 3.2. Tadpole of a red-eyed treefrog, *Agalychnis callidryas*. (George Grall, National Aquarium in Baltimore)

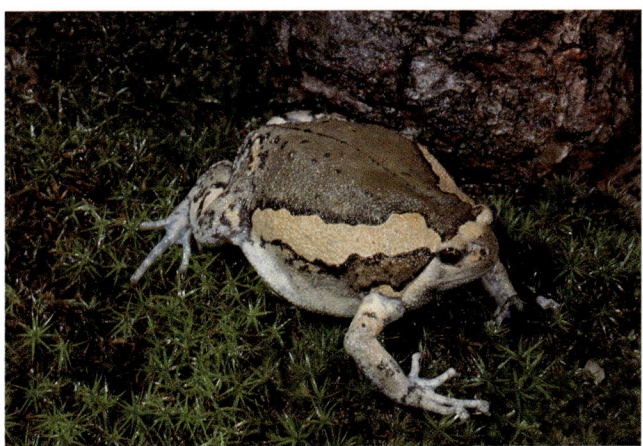

Plate 2.60. The Malaysian narrowmouth toad, *Kaloula pulchra*, is an inexpensive and hardy species. (R. Andrew Odum, Toledo Zoological Society)

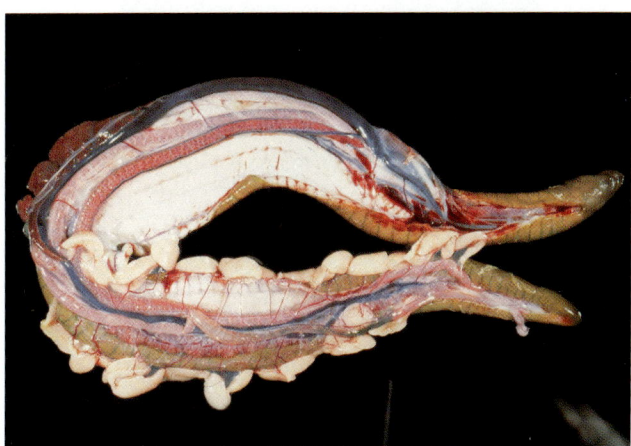

Plate 3.3. Visceral anatomy of a female Rio Cauca caecilian, *Typhlonectes natans*. (Kevin Wright, Philadelphia Zoological Garden)

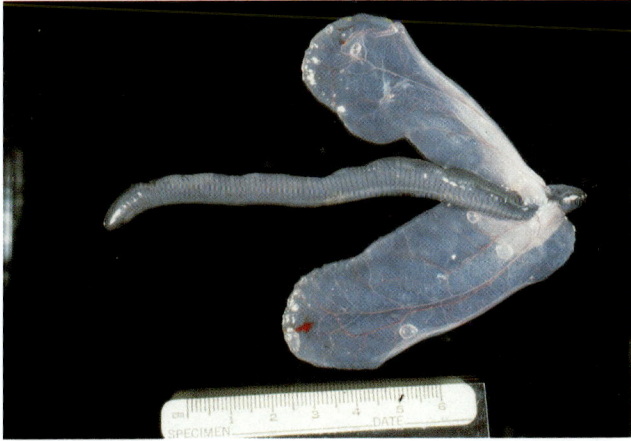

Plate 3.1. Gills of a neonatal Rio Cauca caecilian, *Typhlonectes natans*. (Virginia Pierce, Philadelphia Zoological Garden)

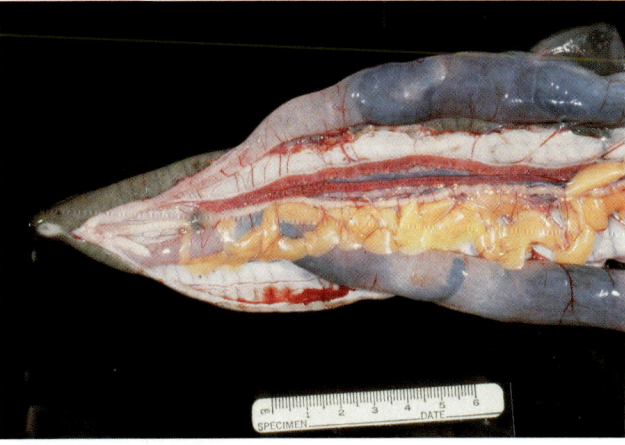

Plate 3.4. Cloacal anatomy of a gravid female Rio Cauca caecilian, *Typhlonectes natans*. (Kevin Wright, Philadelphia Zoological Garden)

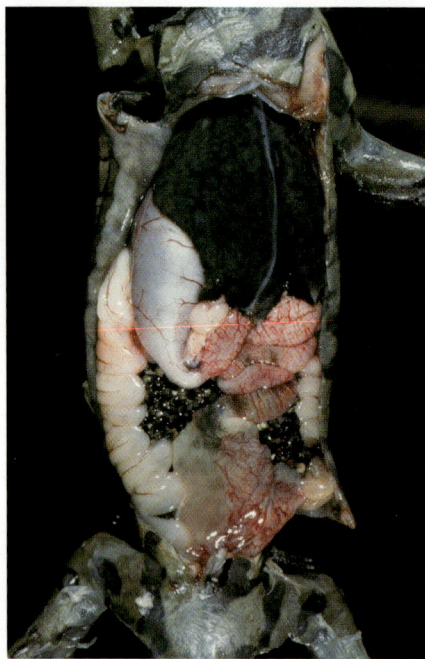

Plate 3.5. Visceral anatomy of a female tiger salamander, *Ambystoma tigrinum*. (Kevin Wright, Philadelphia Zoological Garden)

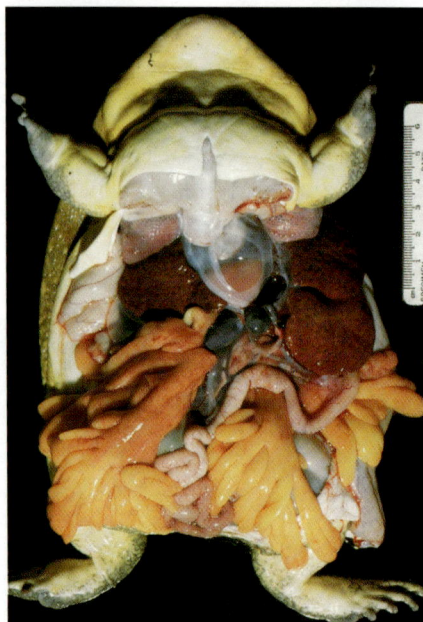

Plate 3.6. Visceral anatomy of a Tschudi's African bullfrog, *Pyxicephalus adspersus*. (Virginia Pierce, Philadelphia Zoological Garden)

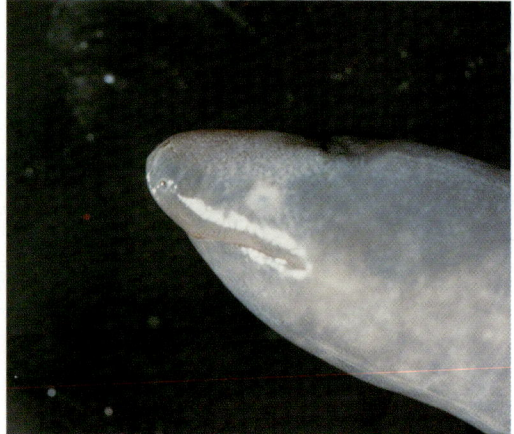

Plate 3.7. The eye is covered with skin in this Rio Cauca caecilian, *Typhlonectes natans*. The tentacle is retracted in the tentacular groove rostral to the eye. (Kevin Wright, Philadelphia Zoological Garden)

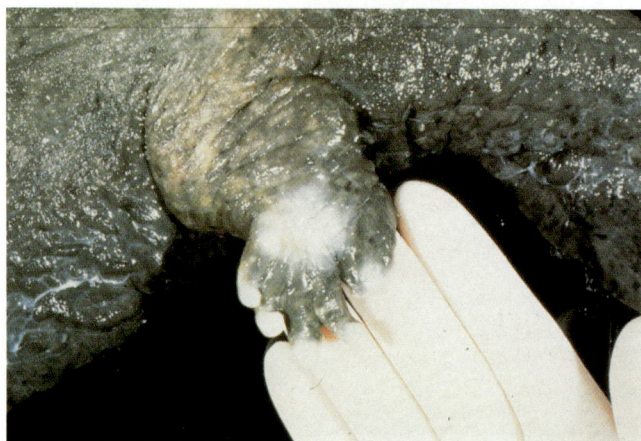

Plate 3.8. The white area on the plantar surface of the foot of this hellbender, *Cryptobranchus alleganiensis*, is normal. (Kevin Wright, Philadelphia Zoological Garden)

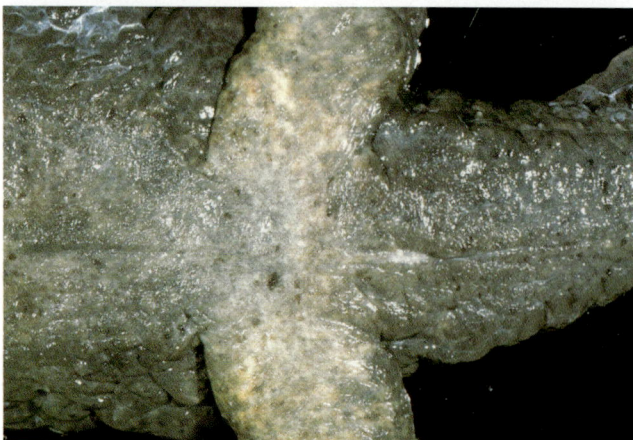

Plate 3.9. Cloacal lips of a female hellbender, *Cryptobranchus alleganiensis*. (Kevin Wright, Philadelphia Zoological Garden)

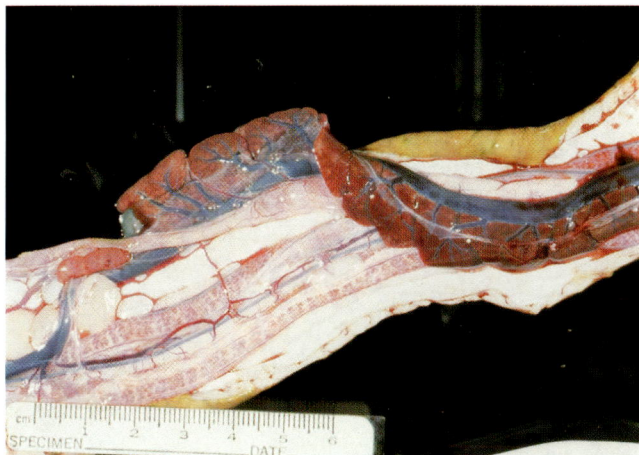

Plate 3.10. Segmented kidneys of a Rio Cauca caecilian, *Typhlonectes natans*. (Virginia Pierce, Philadelphia Zoological Garden)

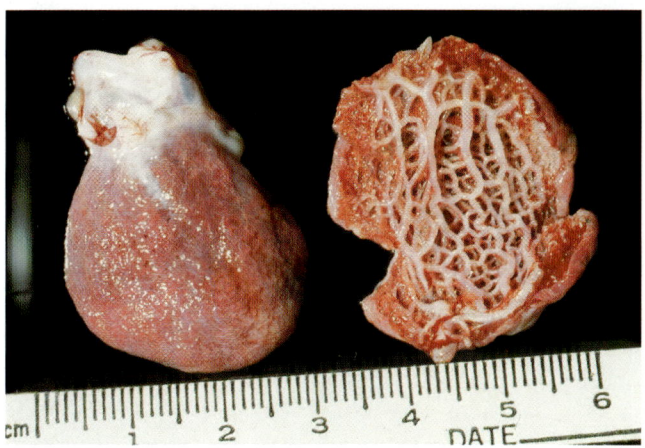

Plate 3.11. Ventricular trabeculae of a Tschudi's African bullfrog, *Pyxicephalus adspersus*. (Virginia Pierce, Philadelphia Zoological Garden)

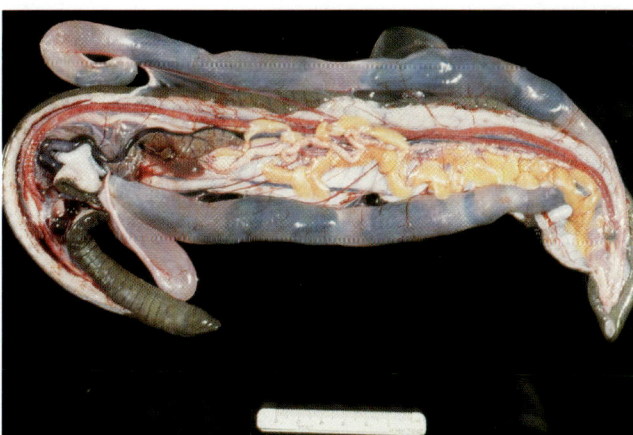

Plate 3.12. Dilated oviducts of a gravid Rio Cauca caecilian, *Typhlonectes natans*. (Virginia Pierce, Philadelphia Zoological Garden)

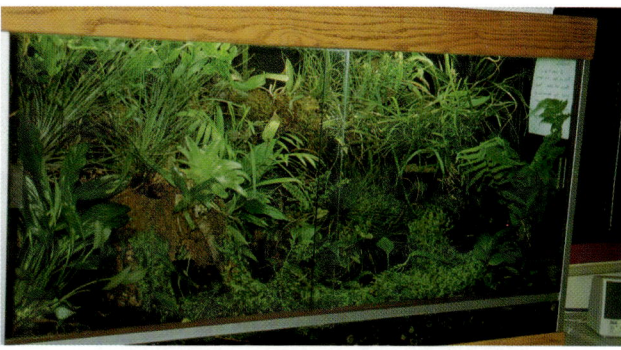

Plate 5.1. Lush, naturalistic terrariums can be created using little soil; ground plants are kept in hidden pots, and liberal use is made of epiphytic and hydroponic plants. (Brent Whitaker, National Aquarium in Baltimore)

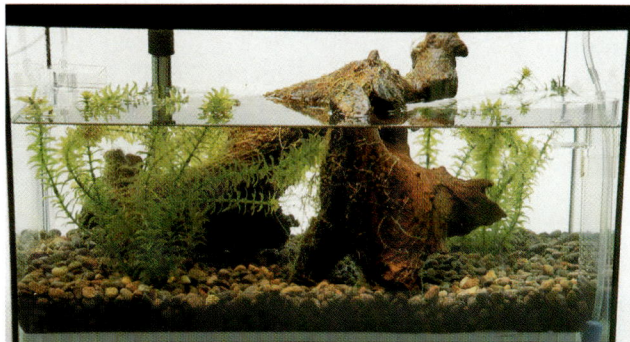

Plate 5.2. Gnarled grape wood and emergent aquatic plants provide underwater retreats as well as above-water resting sites in this basic amphibian pond enclosure. (George Grall, National Aquarium in Baltimore)

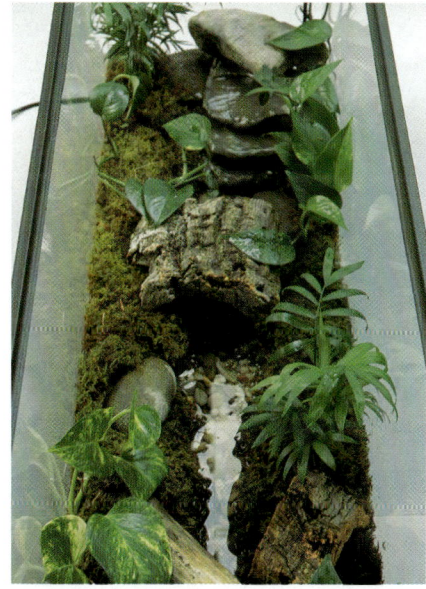

Plate 5.3. A pump-fed waterfall feeds the waterway running through this mossy stream-side enclosure. Plants and cork caves provide retreats for small amphibians on both land and in the water. (George Grall, National Aquarium in Baltimore)

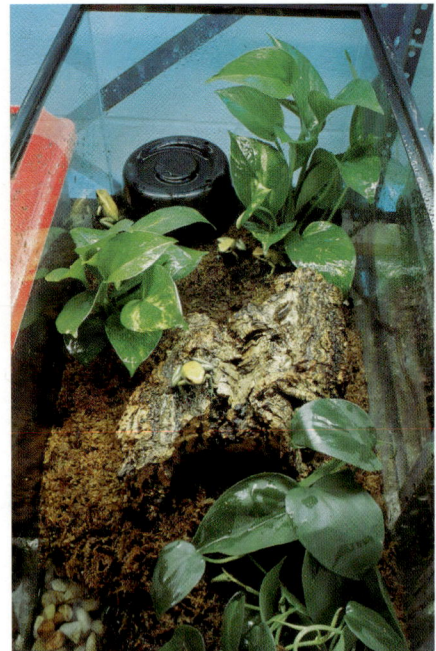

Plate 5.4. This basic forest floor enclosure, enriched with a sheet moss substrate, several *Pothos* plants, and cork and plastic retreats is appropriate for many terrestrial amphibians, such as these dendrobatid frogs, *Phyllobates bicolor*. (George Grall, National Aquarium in Baltimore)

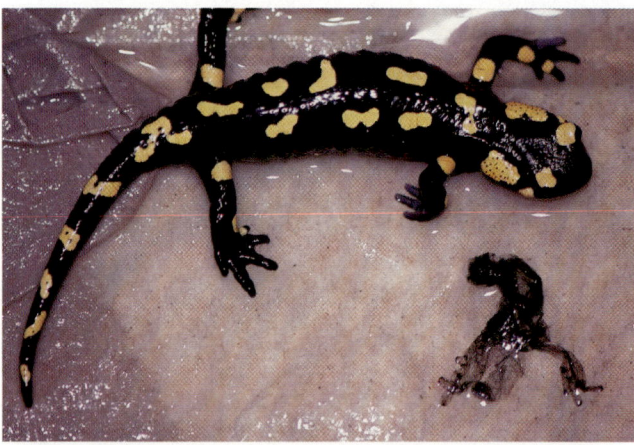

Plate 6.1. Fire salamander, *Salamandra salamandra*, and its freshly shed skin. Many species of amphibian consume their shed skin. Failure to consume the skin may be a sign of illness in these species. (Kevin Wright, Philadelphia Zoological Garden)

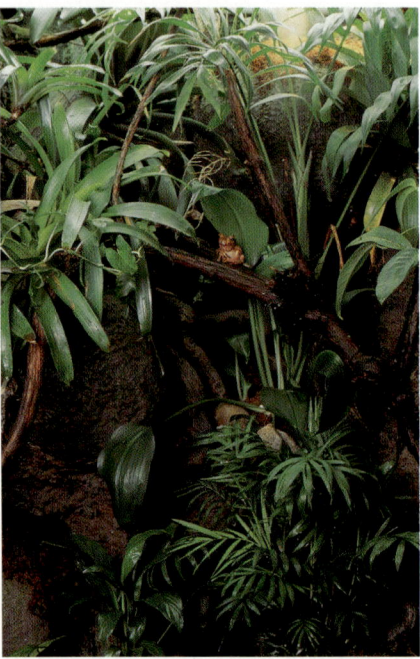

Plate 5.5. Cut grapevine, bromeliads anchored to branches and rockwork, and plants potted in elevated soil beds provide excellent habitat for tree-dwelling frogs in this complex arboreal enclosure. (George Grall, National Aquarium in Baltimore)

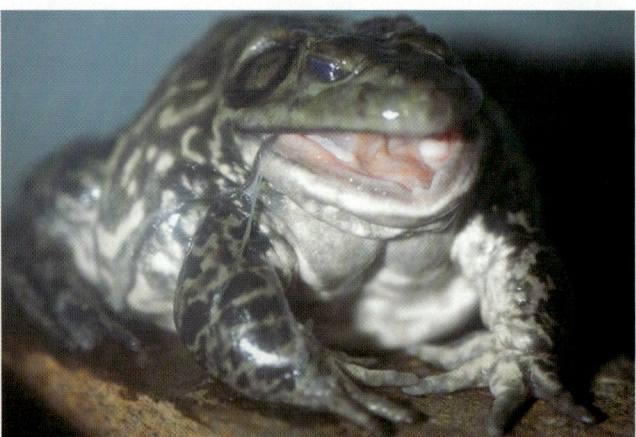

Plate 6.2. Healthy amphibians such as this bullfrog, *Rana catesbeiana*, readily consume shed skin. Sometimes this is misinterpreted as gagging or an abnormal behavior. (Philadelphia Zoological Garden)

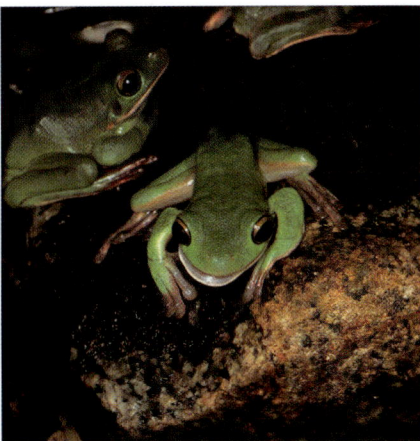

Plate 7.1. Australian giant treefrog, *Litoria infrafrenata*, with mandibular and forelimb deformities from metabolic bone disease. (Philadelphia Zoological Garden)

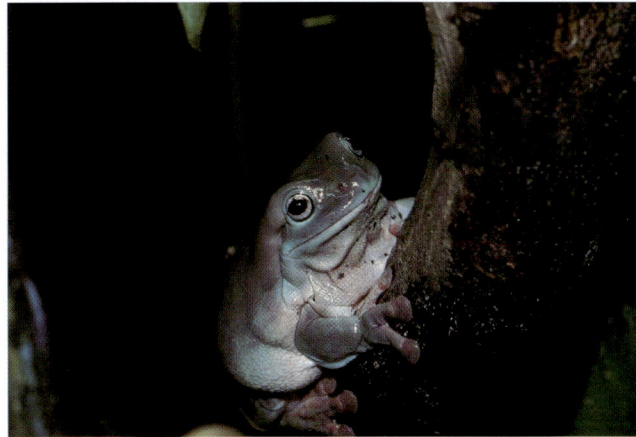

Plate 7.4. An obese White's treefrog, *Pelodryas caerulea*. The supraocular skin folds are becoming quite prominent and the abdomen appears distended as a result of large intra-abdominal fat pads. (Kevin Wright, Philadelphia Zoological Garden)

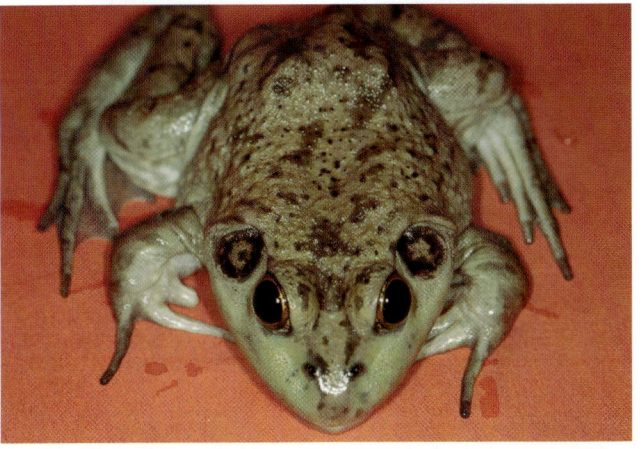

Plate 7.2. Bullfrog, *Rana catesbeiana*, with metabolic bone disease. It cannot elevate its head due to pathologic fractures of the long bones, as well as the spine and pelvis. Note that the sacrum is not aligned with the spine. A slight mandibular deformity is present. (Kevin Wright, Philadelphia Zoological Garden)

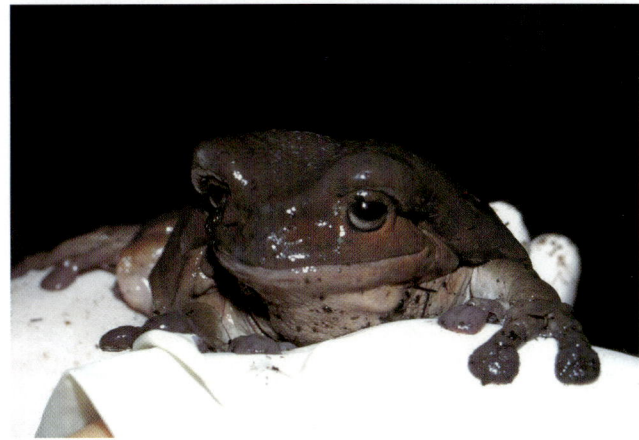

Plate 7.5. A severely obese White's treefrog, *Pelodryas caerulea*. The supraocular skin folds are starting to obscure its vision. (Kevin Wright, Philadelphia Zoological Garden)

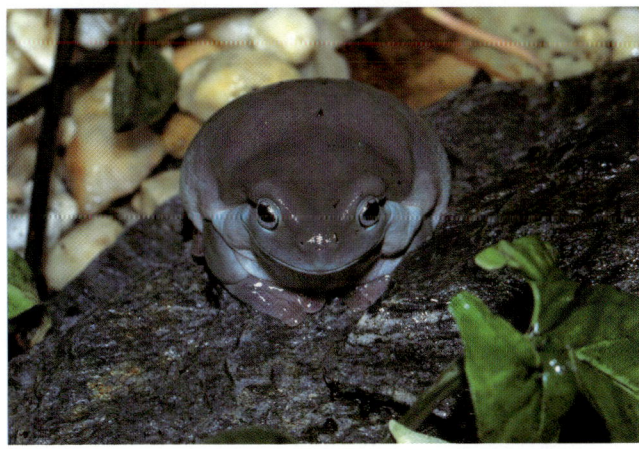

Plate 7.3. A slightly overweight White's treefrog, *Pelodryas caerulea*. (Kevin Wright, Philadelphia Zoological Garden)

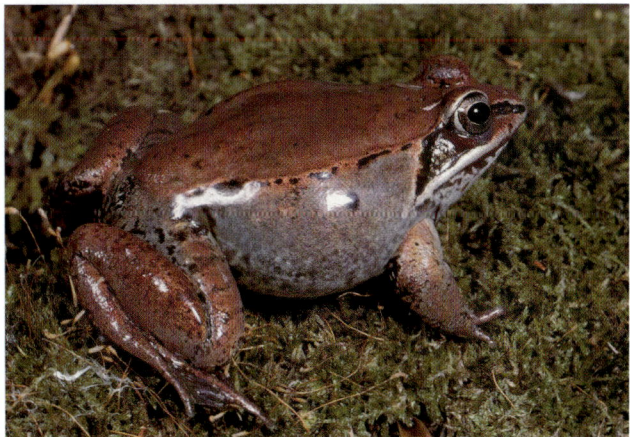

Plate 7.6. Obese wood frog, *Rana sylvatica*, with distended abdomen. (R. Andrew Odum, Toledo Zoological Society)

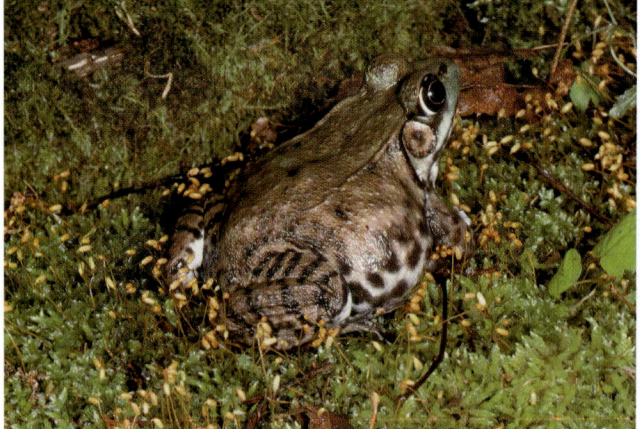

Plate 7.7. Obese green frog, *Rana clamitans melanota*, with distended abdomen. Note that legs appear small compared to body girth. (R. Andrew Odum, Toledo Zoological Society)

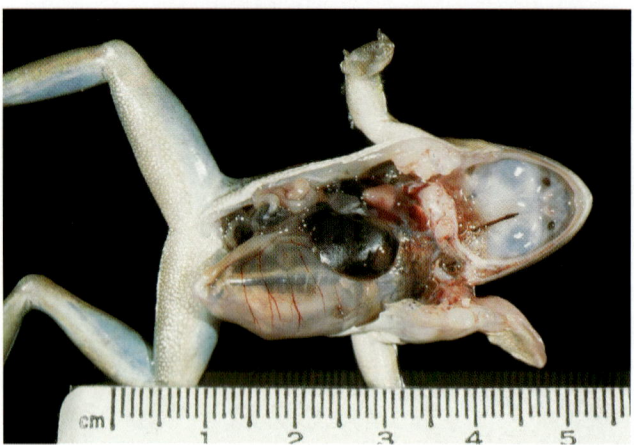

Plate 7.8. A green and golden bell frog, *Litoria aurea*, that died from gastric overload caused by ingestion of adult crickets. The ovipositor of one cricket was visible in the oropharynx next to the optic bulge. (Virginia Pierce, Philadelphia Zoological Garden)

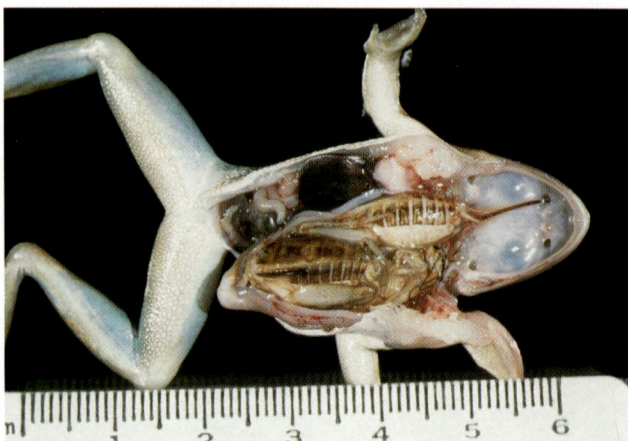

Plate 7.9. The green and golden bell frog, *Litoria aurea*, from Plate 7.8. The stomach has been incised to reveal its contents. Minimal digestion of the ingested crickets has occurred. (Virginia Pierce, Philadelphia Zoological Garden)

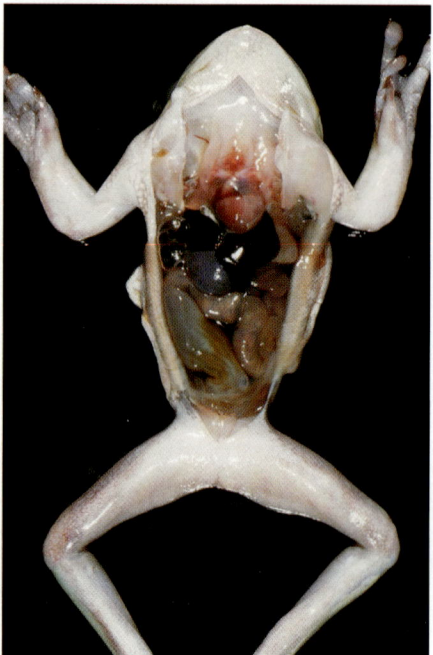

Plate 7.10. Cachectic Australian giant treefrog, *Litoria infrafrenata*. No abdominal fat bodies are detected. (Viriginia Pierce, Philadelphia Zoological Garden)

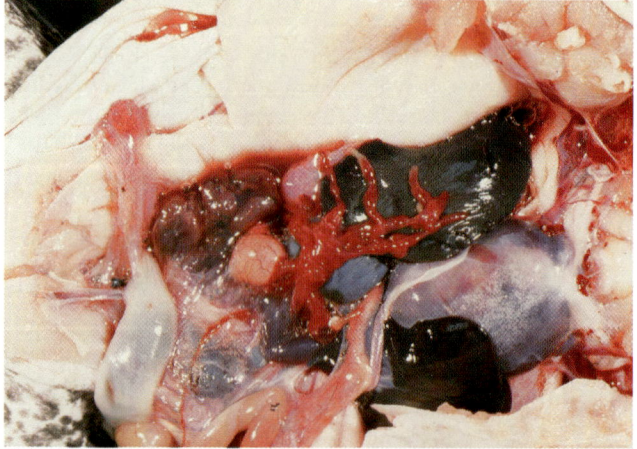

Plate 7.11. Cachectic bullfrog, *Rana catesbeiana*, with atrophy of the fat bodies. The normally large, yellow, fingerlike fat bodies become small and bright red as the fat is used. (Virginia Pierce, Philadelphia Zoological Garden)

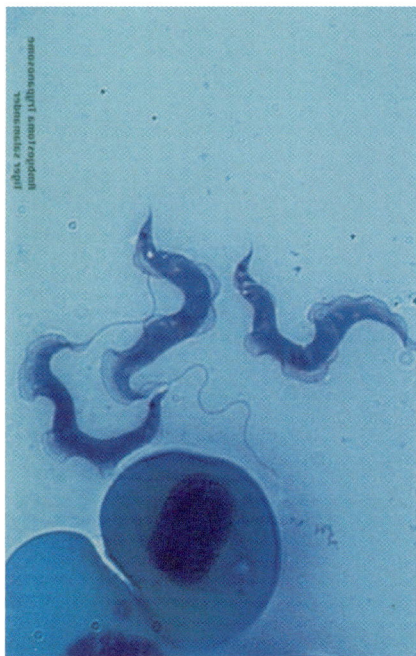

Plate 11.1. Trypanosomes are extracellular parasites often detected in the blood of amphibians. This trypanosome is from the blood of a tiger salamander, *Ambystoma tigrinum*. Modified May-Grunwald Wright-Giemsa stain. (Jenni Jenkins, National Aquarium in Baltimore)

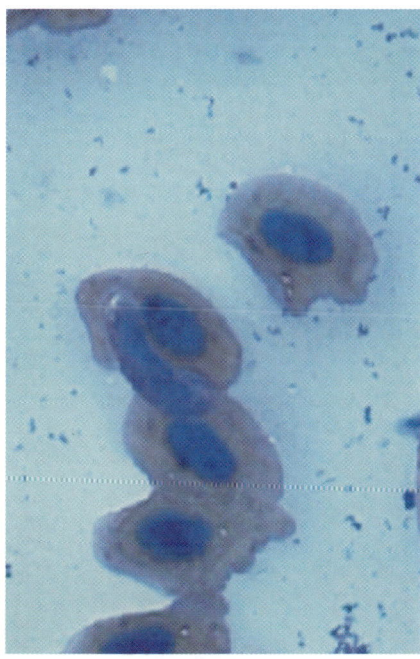

Plate 11.2. Hemogregarines are intracellular parasites frequently encountered in the blood of amphibians. Modified Wright-Giemsa stain. (Jenni Jenkins, National Aquarium in Baltimore)

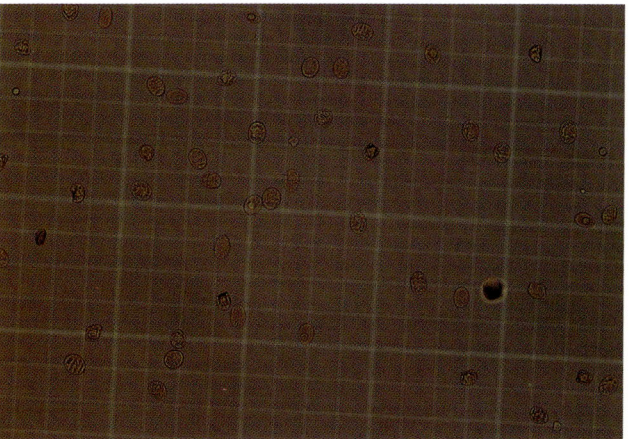

Plate 11.3. Hemocytometer charged with the blood of the Anderson's axolotl, *Ambystoma andersoni*. (Sandy McCampbell, Philadelphia Zoological Garden)

Plate 11.4. Eosinopette charged with the blood of the Anderson's axolotl, *Ambystoma andersoni*. (Sandy McCampbell, Philadelphia Zoological Garden)

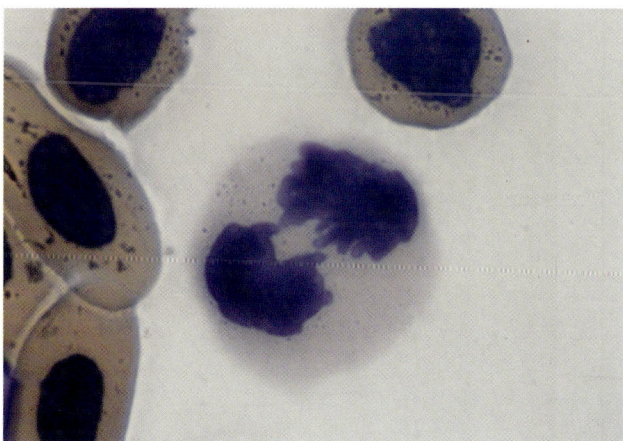

Plate 11.5. Mitotic erythrocytes are occasionally seen as in this Japanese giant salamander, *Andrias japonicus*. Wright-Giemsa stain. (Sandy McCampbell, Philadelphia Zoological Garden)

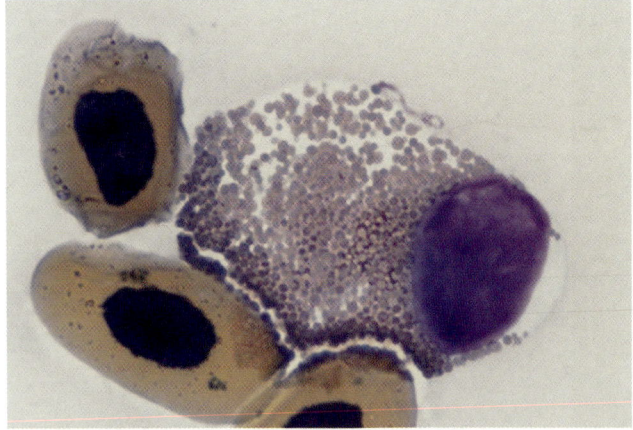

Plate 11.6. Heterophil, Japanese giant salamander, *Andrias japonicus*. Wright-Giemsa stain. (Sandy McCampbell, Philadelphia Zoological Garden)

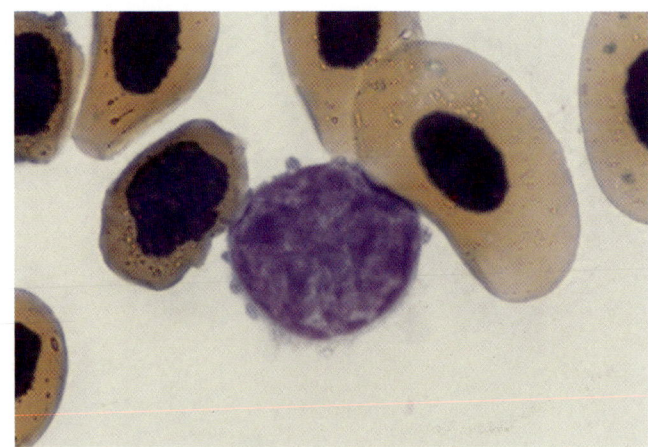

Plate 11.9. Lymphocyte, Japanese giant salamander, *Andrias japonicus*. Wright-Giemsa stain. (Sandy McCampbell, Philadelphia Zoological Garden)

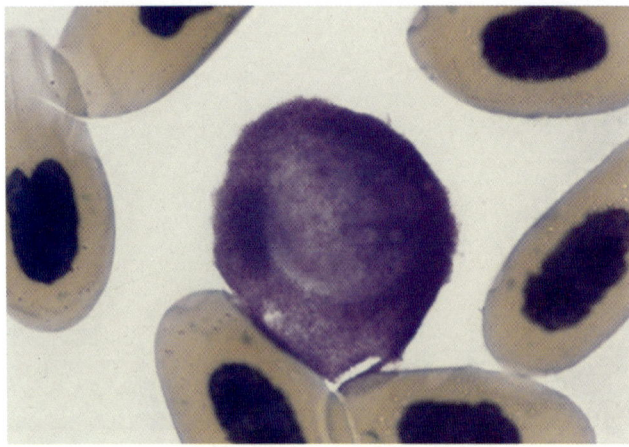

Plate 11.7. Basophil, Japanese giant salamander, *Andrias japonicus*. Wright-Giemsa stain. (Sandy McCampbell, Philadelphia Zoological Garden)

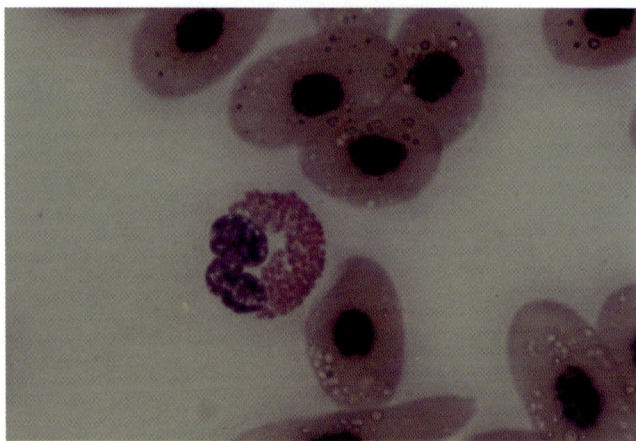

Plate 11.10. Heterophil, bullfrog, *Rana catesbeiana*. Wright-Giemsa stain. (Sandy McCampbell, Philadelphia Zoological Garden)

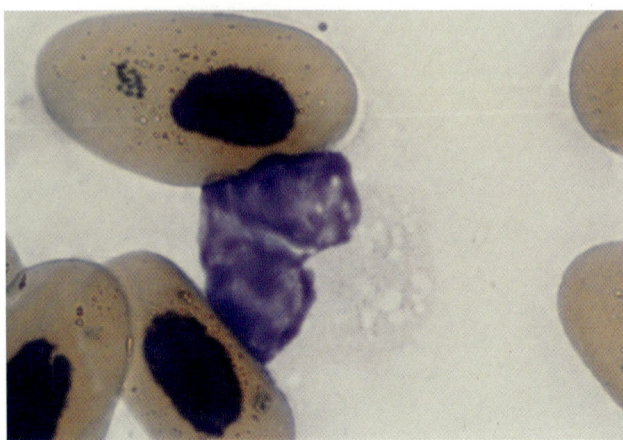

Plate 11.8. Azurophil, Japanese giant salamander, *Andrias japonicus*. Wright-Giemsa stain. (Sandy McCampbell, Philadelphia Zoological Garden)

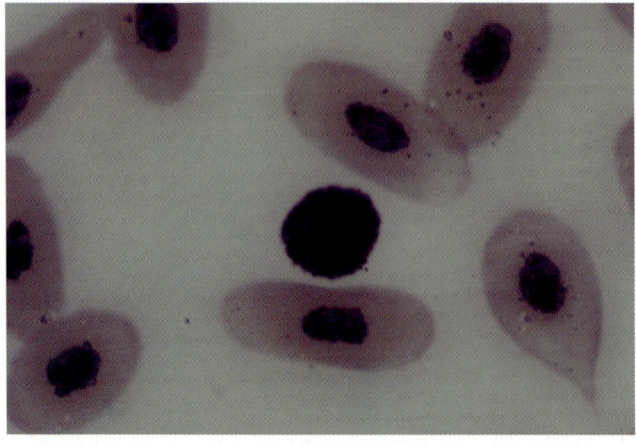

Plate 11.11. Basophil, bullfrog, *Rana catesbeiana*. Wright-Giemsa stain. (Sandy McCampbell, Philadelphia Zoological Garden).

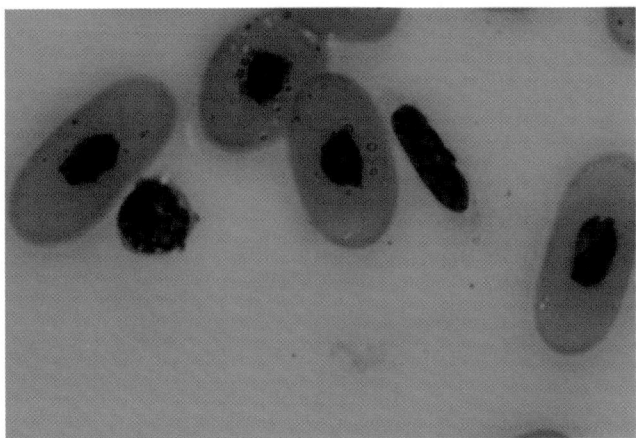

Plate 11.12. Lymphocyte and thrombocyte, bullfrog, *Rana catesbeiana*. Wright-Giemsa stain. (Sandy McCampbell, Philadelphia Zoological Garden)

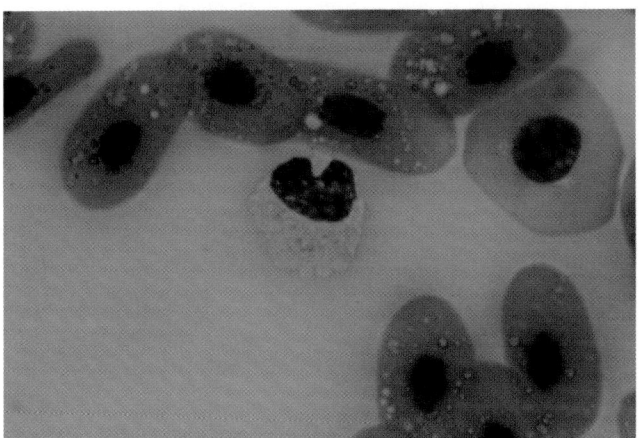

Plate 11.13. Neutrophil, bullfrog, *Rana catesbeiana*. Wright-Giemsa stain. (Sandy McCampbell, Philadelphia Zoological Garden)

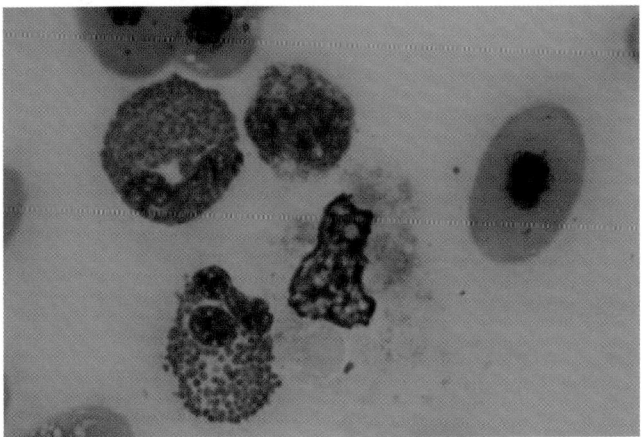

Plate 11.14. Heterophil, azurophil, and monocyte, bullfrog, *Rana catesbeiana*. Wright-Giemsa stain. (Sandy McCampbell, Philadelphia Zoological Garden)

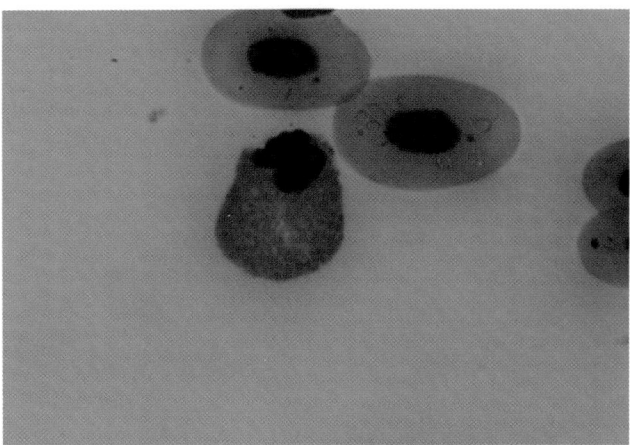

Plate 11.15. Heterophil, ornate horned frog, *Ceratophrys ornata*. Wright-Giemsa stain. (Sandy McCampbell, Philadelphia Zoological Garden)

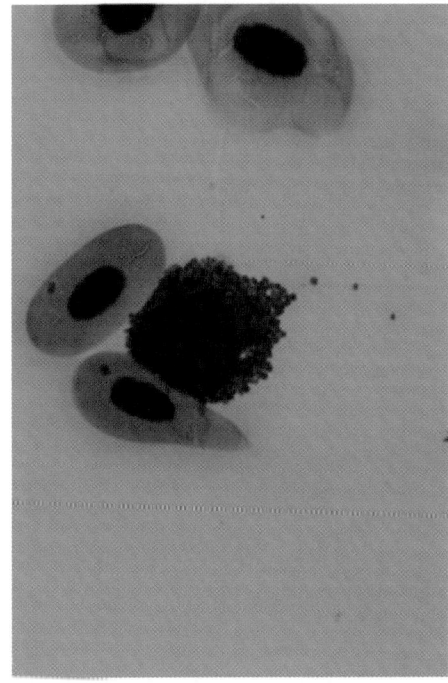

Plate 11.16. Basophil, ornate horned frog, *Ceratophrys ornata*. Wright-Giemsa stain. (Sandy McCampbell, Philadelphia Zoological Garden)

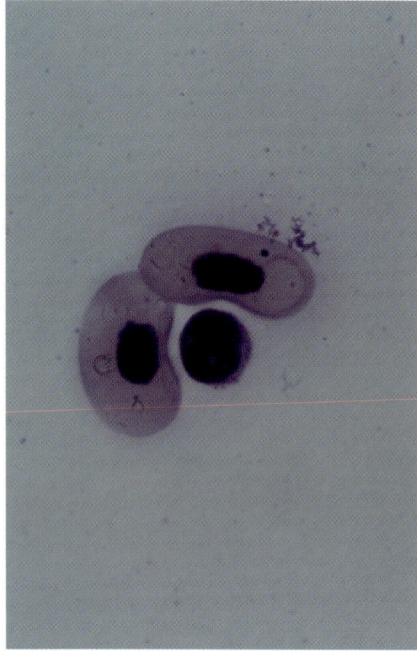

Plate 11.17. Lymphocyte, ornate horned frog, *Ceratophrys ornata*. Wright-Giemsa stain. (Sandy McCampbell, Philadelphia Zoological Garden)

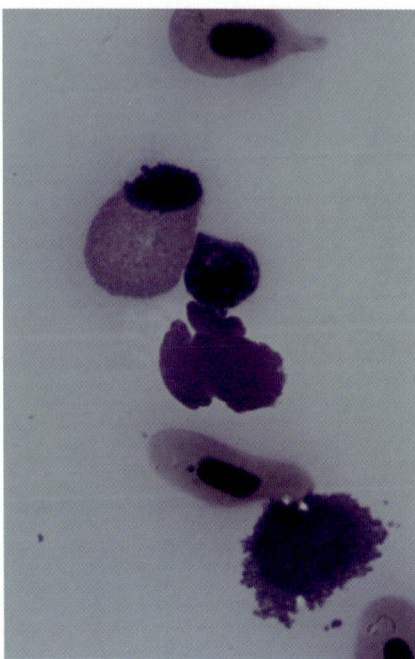

Plate 11.18. Basophil, lymphocyte, heterophil, ornate horned frog, *Ceratophrys ornata*. Wright-Giemsa stain. (Sandy McCampbell, Philadelphia Zoological Garden)

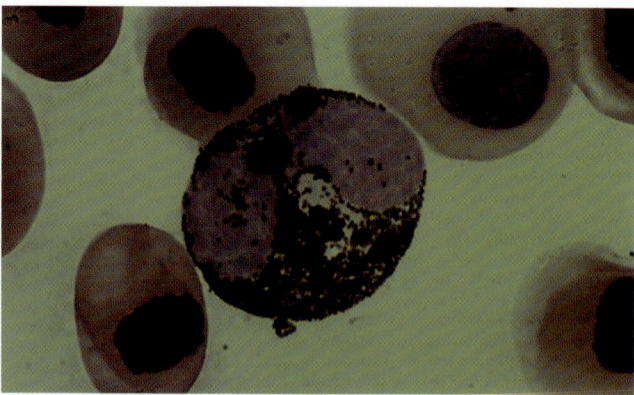

Plate 11.19. Phagocytic monocyte, Anderson's axolotl, *Ambystoma andersoni*. Wright-Giemsa stain. (Sandy McCampbell, Philadelphia Zoological Garden)

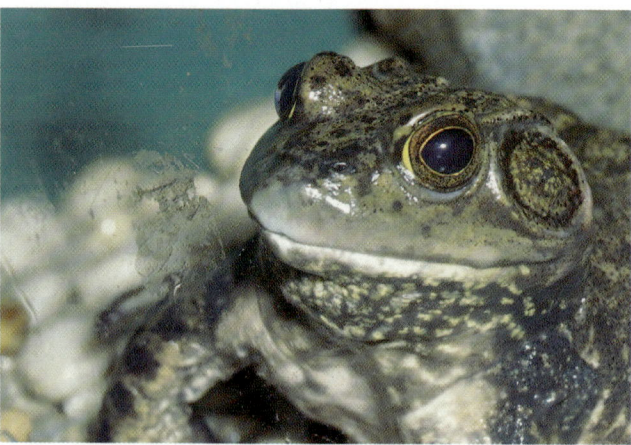

Plate 12.1. A. Increased mucous production in a North American bullfrog, *Rana catesbeiana*, exposed to high levels of ammonia in its water. Mucous is also seen smeared on the glass as the animal attempted to escape its noxious environment. (Kevin Wright, Philadelphia Zoological Garden)

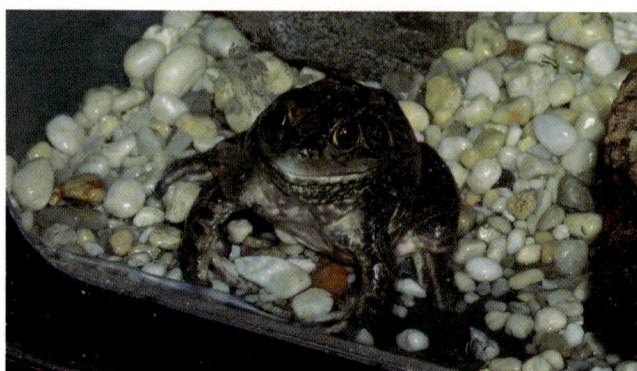

Plate 12.1. B. Ammonia toxicity in a North American bullfrog, *Rana catesbeiana*, resulting from inadequate biological and chemical filtration. Dull skin pigmentation, increased mucous production, adopting a body posture that minimizes contact with the water, and repeated attempts to escape from the enclosure are common signs of exposure to ammonia. (Kevin Wright, Philadelphia Zoological Garden)

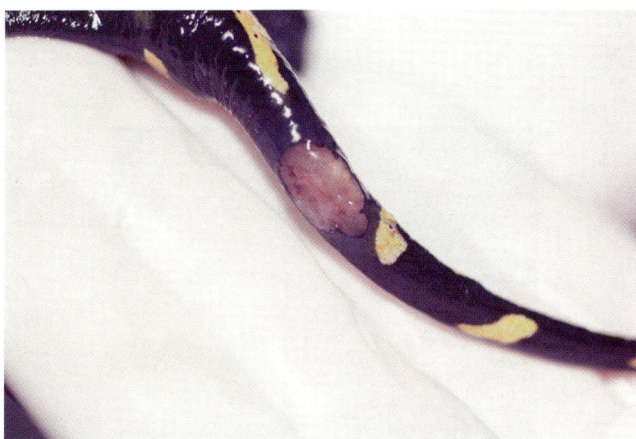

Plate 13.1. Cutaneous ulcer in a European fire salamander, *Salamandra salamandra*. This responded well to topical gentamicin. (Kevin Wright, Philadelphia Zoological Garden)

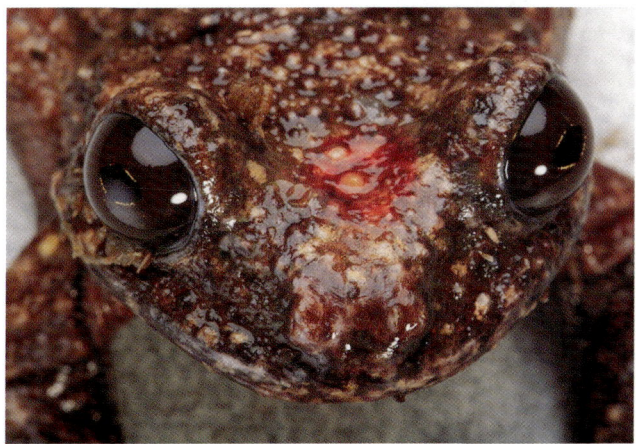

Plate 13.2. Rostral ulcer on a Tungara frog, *Physalaemus pustulosus*. (George Grall, National Aquarium in Baltimore)

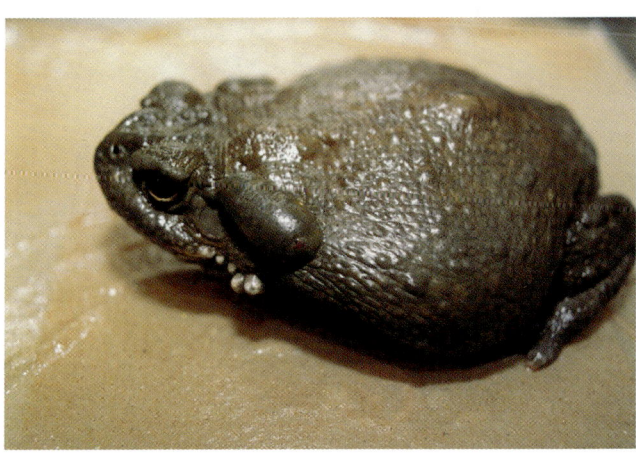

Plate 13.3. Punctate ulcer on caudal aspect of parotid gland of a Colorado River toad, *Bufo alvarius*. (Kevin Wright, Philadelphia Zoological Garden)

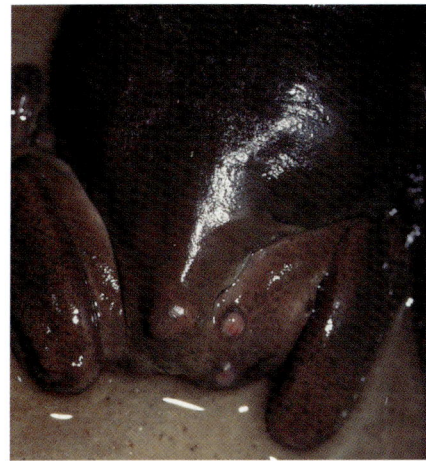

Plate 13.4. A *Staphylococcus* spp. was isolated from these circumscribed lesions on the hindlimb of a White's treefrog, *Pelodryas caerulea*. These lesions occurred above verminous cysts. (Kevin Wright, Philadelphia Zoological Garden)

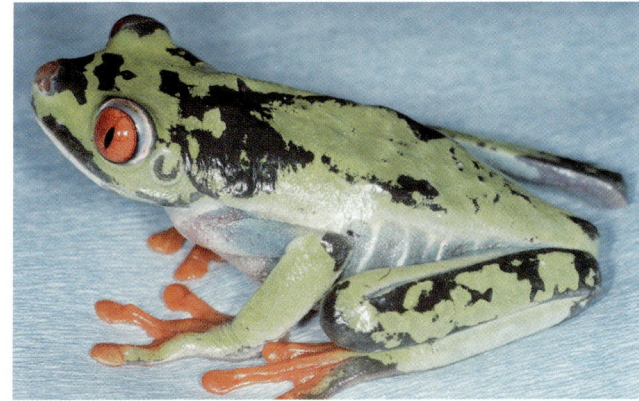

Plate 13.5. A red-eyed treefrog, *Agalychnis callidryas*, with a skin discoloration suggestive of a bacterial dermatitis. This disorder responded to antibiotic treatment. This frog also has a rostral abrasion. (Steve Barten)

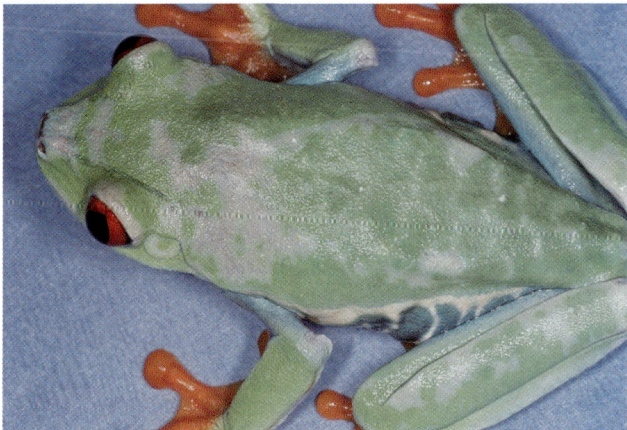

Plate 13.6. Post-treatment resolution of lesions in the red-eyed treefrog, *Agalychnis callidryas*, depicted in Plate 13.5. (Steve Barten)

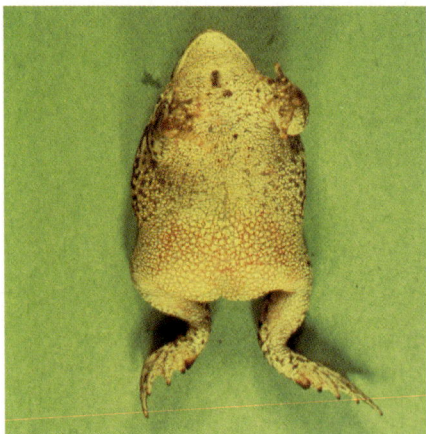

Plate 13.7. Wyoming toad, *Bufo hemiophrys baxteri*, with red leg syndrome. (Sharon K. Taylor, Wyoming State Veterinary Lab)

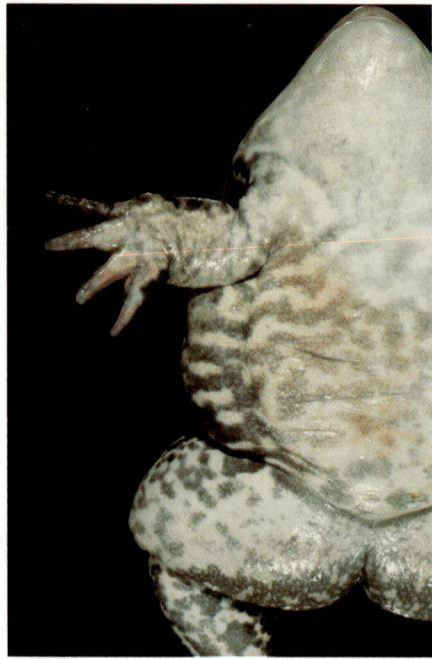

Plate 13.10. A bullfrog, *Rana catesbeiana*, that died of red leg syndrome (bacterial dermatosepticemia). Note the erythema of the ventrum, forearm, and digits. This frog also has profound subcutaneous edema and hydrocoelom. (Kevin Wright, Philadelphia Zoological Garden)

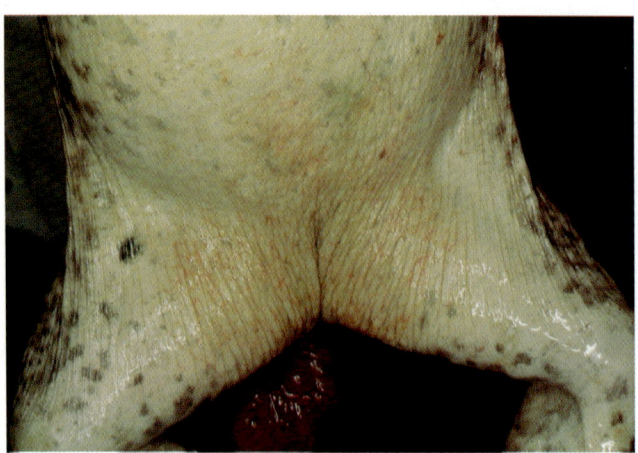

Plate 13.8. Ventral erythema associated with rectal prolapse of a giant toad, *Bufo marinus*. The chronicity of the prolapse allowed systemic infection. (Kevin Wright, Philadelphia Zoological Garden)

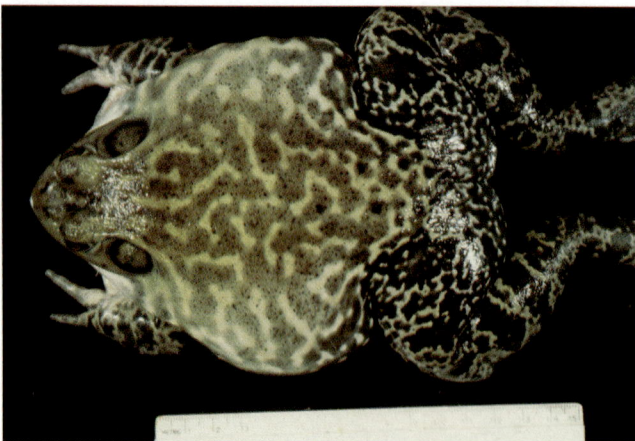

Plate 13.11. Dorsal view of the bullfrog, *Rana catesbeiana*, from Plate 13.10 with hydrocoelom and subcutaneous edema from red leg syndrome. (Kevin Wright, Philadelphia Zoological Garden)

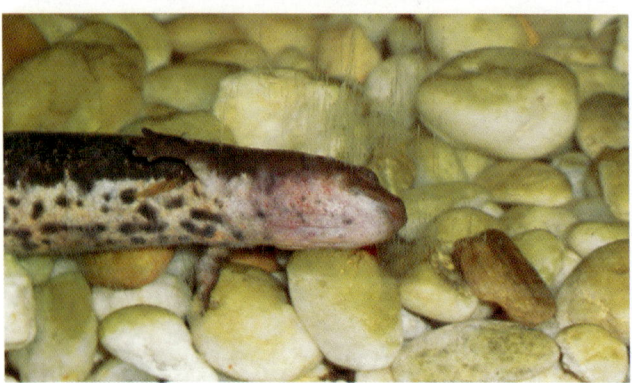

Plate 13.9. A septicemic Tsitou newt, *Pachytriton brevipes*. Note the hyperemia of the throat, legs, and abdomen. (Kevin Wright, Philadelphia Zoological Garden)

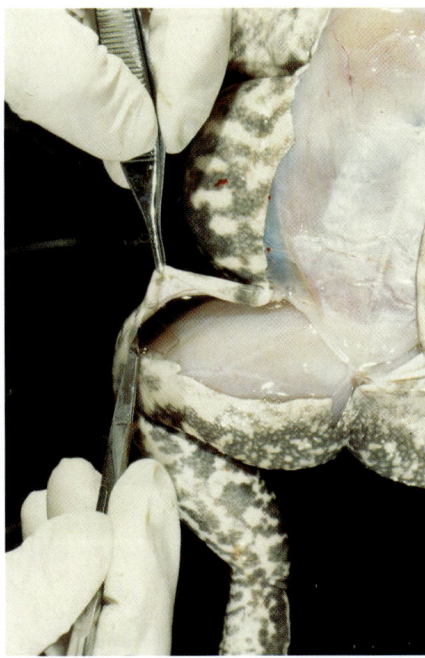

Plate 13.12. Subcutaneous edema over the hindlimb of the septic bullfrog, *Rana catesbeiana* from Plate 13.10. (Kevin Wright, Philadelphia Zoological Garden)

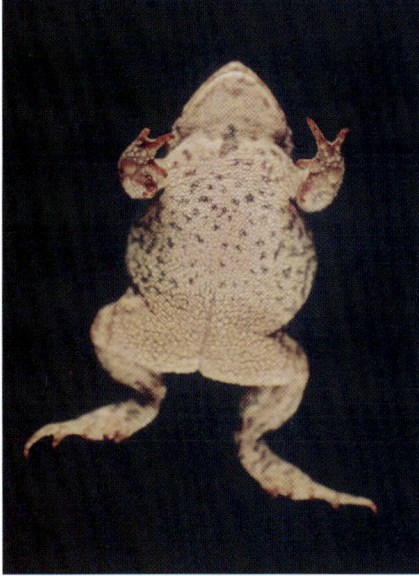

Plate 14.1. Wyoming toad, *Bufo hemiophrys baxteri*, with erythema and sloughing of the skin on the digits. The etiological agent involved was *Basidiobolus ranarum*. Many researchers now believe this organism is actually *Batrachochytrium dendrobatidis*. (Sharon K. Taylor)

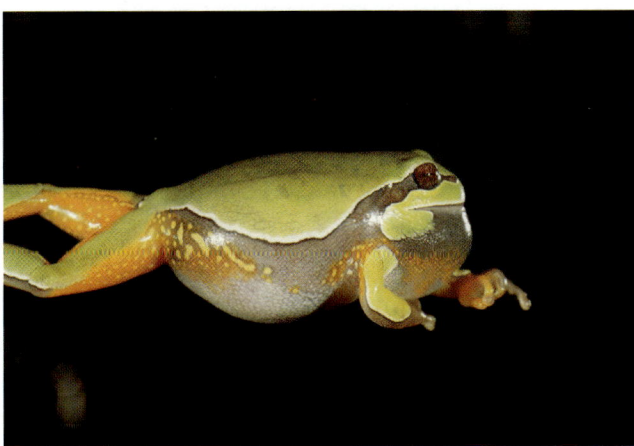

Plate 13.13. Edema syndrome in a Pine Barrens treefrog, *Hyla andersoni*. Subcutaneous edema and hydrocoelom are not pathognomic for an infectious etiology. (Kevin Wright, Philadelphia Zoological Garden).

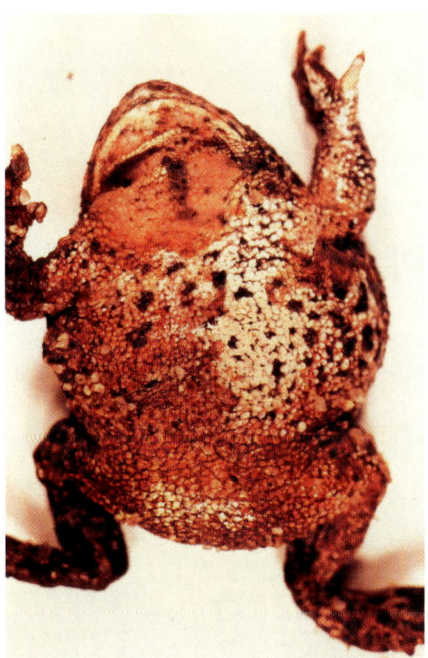

Plate 14.2. Fatal mycotic dermatitis caused by *Basidiobolus ranarum* in a Wyoming toad, *Bufo hemiophrys baxteri*. Severe generalized erythema and sloughing of the skin is present, especially on the throat. Normal skin can be seen on the left side of the sternum. (Sharon K. Taylor)

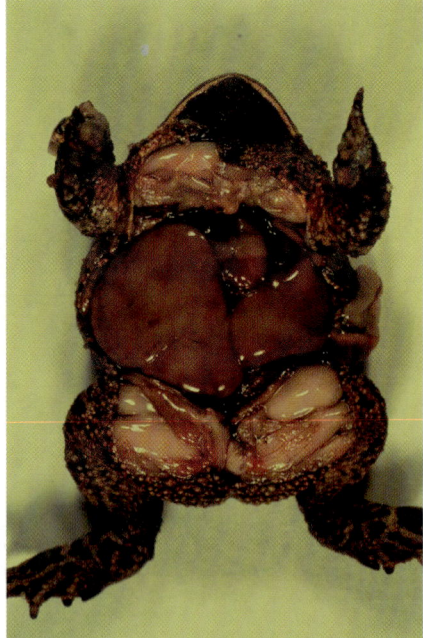

Plate 14.3. Hepatomegaly in a Wyoming toad, *Bufo hemiophrys baxteri*, that died from a mycotic dermatitis caused by *Basidiobolus ranarum*. Hepatomegaly was the only consistent gross finding in these cases. (Sharon K. Taylor)

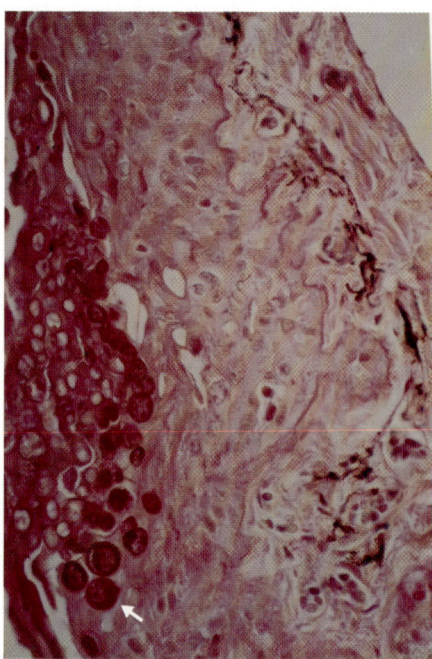

Plate 14.5. Periodic acid-Schiff-stained section of the ventral skin of a Wyoming toad, *Bufo hemiophrys baxteri*, with mycotic dermatitis. The spherules in the outermost layers of the skin are indicative of *Basidiobolus ranarum*, which was confirmed by recovery of the organism in culture. (Sharon K. Taylor)

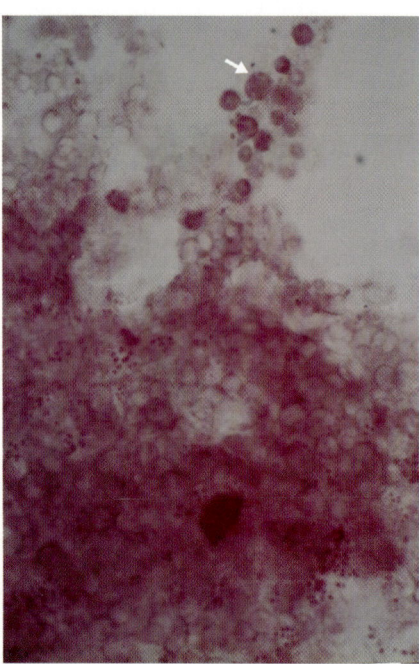

Plate 14.4. Periodic acid-Schiff-stained impression smear of the skin lesion of a Wyoming toad, *Bufo hemiophrys baxteri*. The spherules are indicative of *Basidiobolus ranarum*, which was confirmed by recovery of the organism in culture. (Sharon K. Taylor)

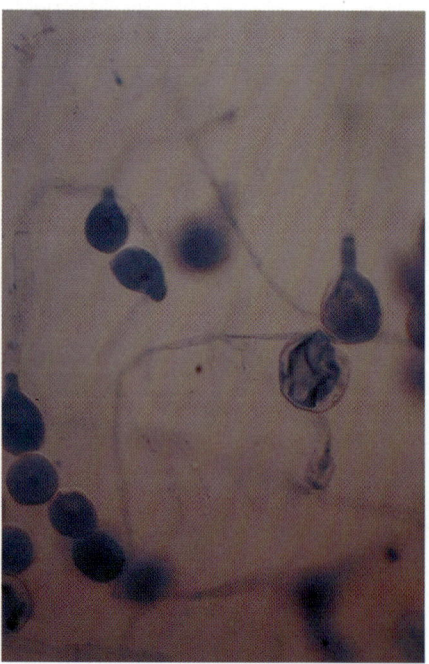

Plate 14.6. Lacto-phenol blue wet mount of *Basidiobolus ranarum* cultured from the ventral skin of a Wyoming toad, *Bufo hemiophrys baxteri*. Note the beaked zygospores. (Sharon K. Taylor)

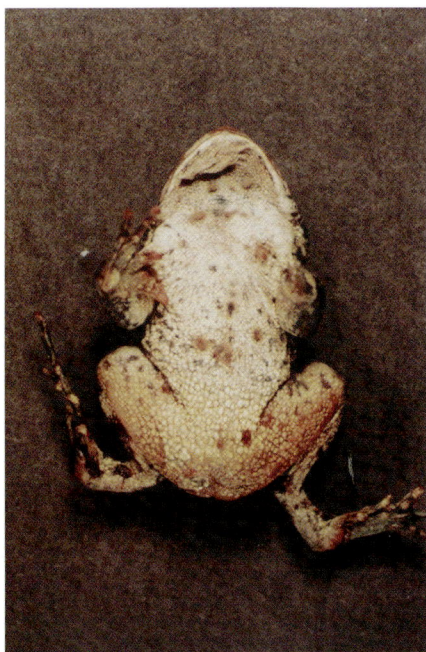

Plate 14.7. Lethal nodular mycotic dermatitis in a Wyoming toad, *Bufo hemiophrys baxteri*, caused by a *Mucor* sp. The digits were erythemic. (Sharon K. Taylor)

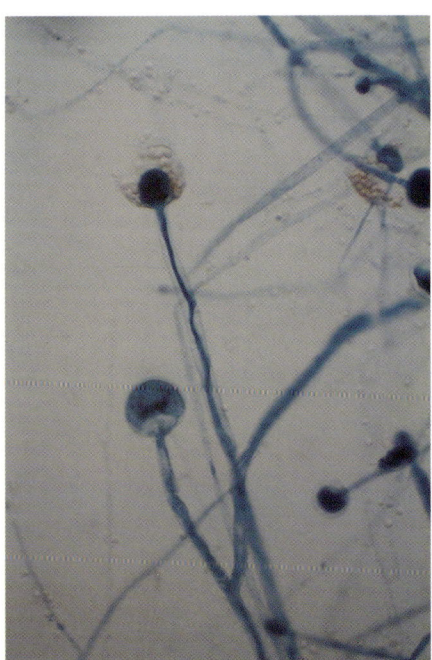

Plate 14.8. Lacto-phenol blue wet mount of the *Mucor* sp. recovered from a skin nodule of a Wyoming toad, *Bufo hemiophrys baxteri*. Note the uniform diameter fungal hyphae, hyphae branching, and mucor columella. (Sharon K. Taylor)

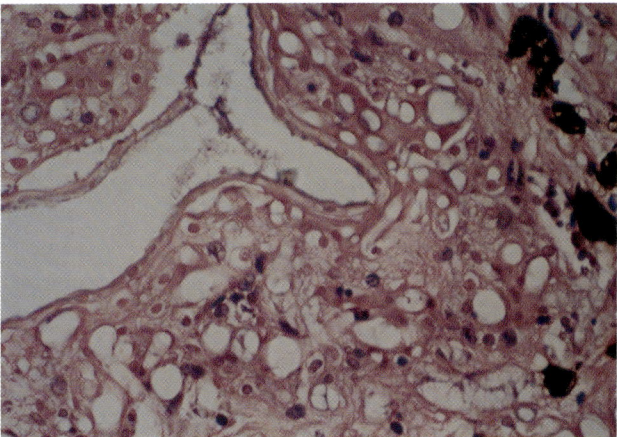

Plate 14.9. Hematoxylin and eosin-stained skin section of nodular mycotic dermatitis in a Wyoming toad, *Bufo hemiophrys baxteri*. The organism involved was a *Mucor* sp., which was confirmed by culture. (Sharon K. Taylor)

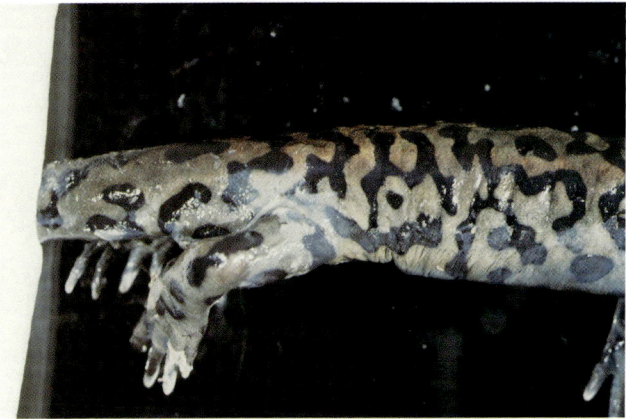

Plate 14.10. Saprolegniasis in a tiger salamander, *Ambystoma tigrinum*. (Kevin Wright, Philadelphia Zoological Garden)

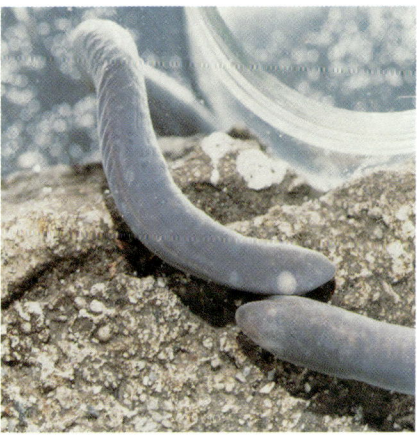

Plate 14.11. Saprolegniasis in an aquatic caecilian, *Typhlonectes* sp. (Kevin Wright, Philadelphia Zoological Garden)

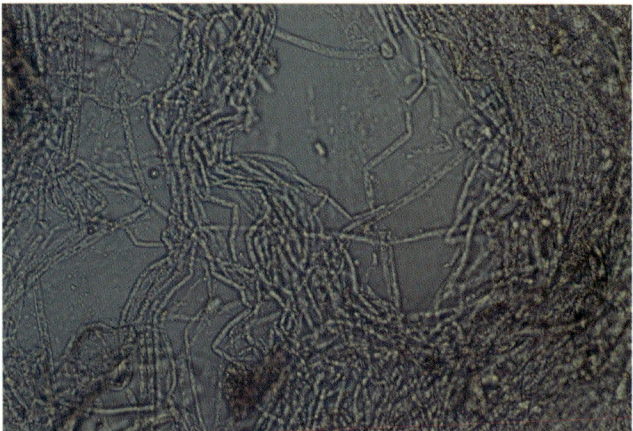

Plate 14.12. Fungal hyphae and zoospores in the wet mount of a skin scraping of an aquatic caecilian, *Typhlonectes* sp. The presumptive diagnosis is saprolegniasis. This disease is more common in cold water (<70°F). (Kevin Wright, Philadelphia Zoological Garden)

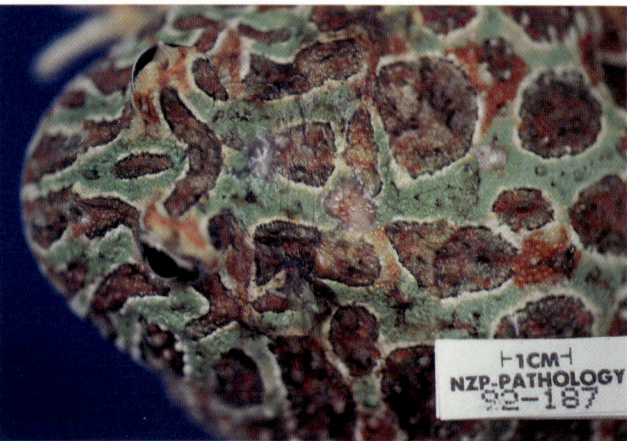

Plate 14.13. Tan to grayish cutaneous nodules caused by chromoblastomycosis in an ornate horned frog, *Ceratophrys ornata*. (Lisa Tell, courtesy of the U.S. Govt.)

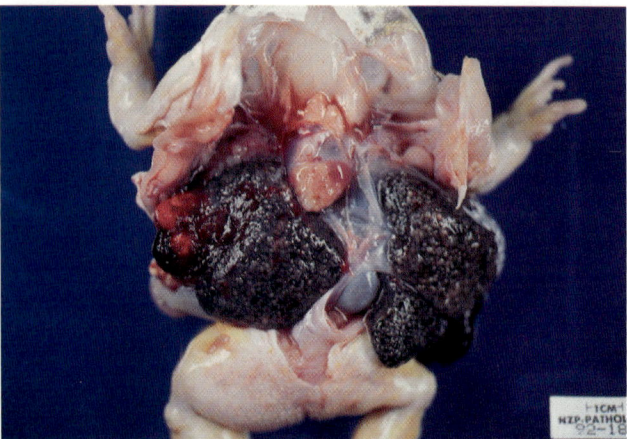

Plate 14.14. Visceral dissemination of chromoblastomycosis in an ornate horned frog, *Ceratophrys ornata*. (Lisa Tell, courtesy of the U.S. Govt.)

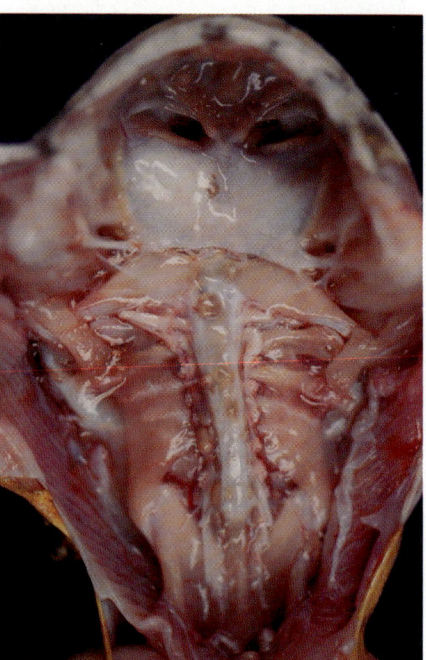

Plate 14.15. Nodules caused by chromoblastomycosis are visible on the ventral aspect of the vertebral column in this ornate horned frog, *Ceratoprhys ornata*. (Lisa Tell, courtesy of the U.S. Govt.)

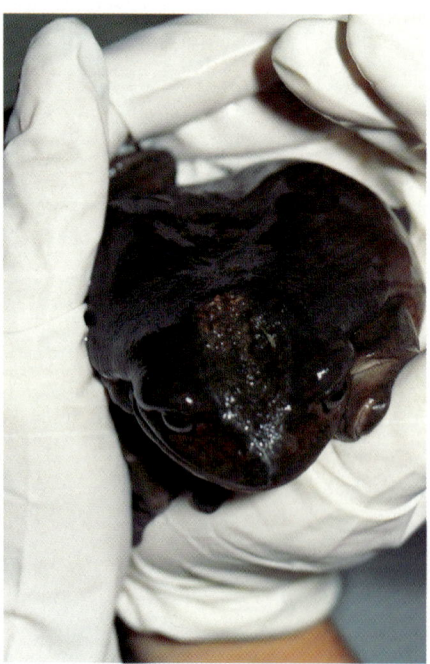

Plate 14.16. Crust on the head of a White's treefrog, *Pelodryas caerulea*. *Candida* sp. can often be recovered from the underside of the crust. (Kevin Wright, Philadelphia Zoological Garden)

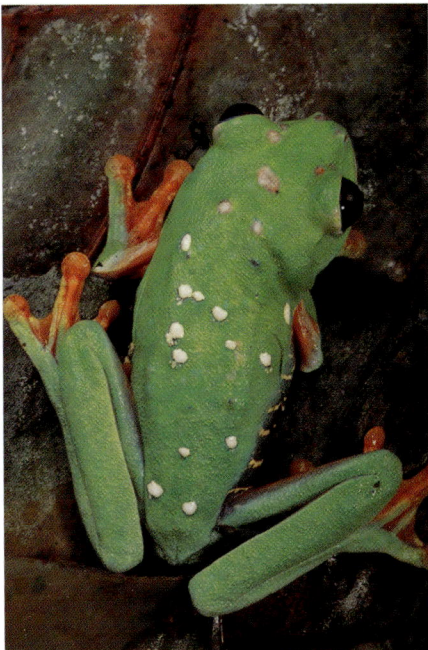

Plate 14.17. Ulcerated nodules on the head of a red-eyed treefrog, *Agalychnis callidryas*, that are consistent with localized bacterial infection, mycobacteriosis, nodular fungal dermatitis, and other etiologies. Impression smears, cultures, and biopsies may be needed to diagnose the underlying etiology. The white elevated nodules on the rest of the body are normal structures and should not be confused with lesions. (George Grall, National Aquarium in Baltimore)

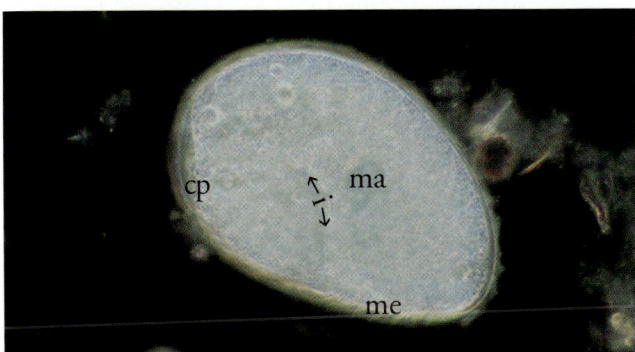

Plate 15.1. A. The ciliate *Nyctotheroides* sp. from the lumen of the large intestine of a dendrobatid frog. Live organism viewed by dark-field illumination. Note the kidney bean-shaped macronucleus (ma), the tufts of compound buccal cilia called membranelles (me), the beating of which transport food into the cell, and the long curved infundibulum (the inner portion of the buccal cavity) (i). The cell anus or cytoproct (cp) is visible at the posterior end, and can be seen actively emptying in live specimens. Note that the same features could be seen in bright-field illumination, where the ciliate would appear dark against a light background. (Sarah L. Poynton, Johns Hopkins University School of Medicine, taken from Poynton and Whitaker, 1994)

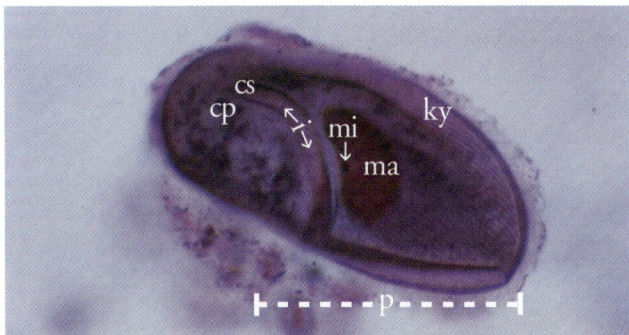

Plate 15.1 B. Organism stained by protargol impregnation (silver protein). Note how elegantly this stain shows the longitudinal rows of cilia, also called the kineties (ky), the kidney bean-shaped macronucleus (ma) and the much smaller micronucleus (mi); and the full extent of the buccal apparatus, which comprises the external peristome (p), and the internal infundibulum (i), leading to the cytostome (cs) and cytopharynx (cp). Length of *Nyctotheroides* species is 150–200 μm. (Sarah L. Poynton, Johns Hopkins University School of Medicine, taken from Poynton and Whitaker, 1994)

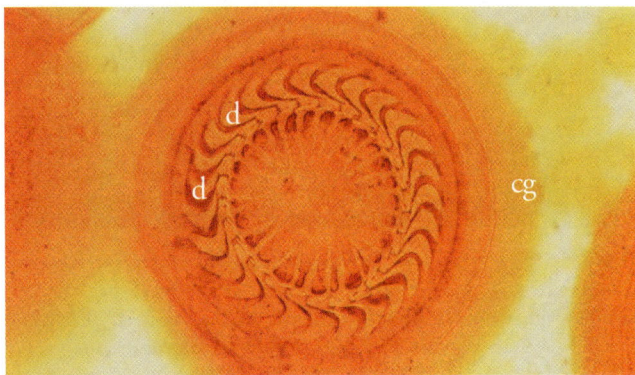

Plate 15.2. A trichodinid ciliate showing the distinctive adhesive disc by which the organism attaches to the amphibian host. The disc is made of proteinaceous elements, the most distinctive of which are the large interconnecting denticles (d). A girdle of cilia (cg) can be seen at the margin of the body. Diameter of adhesive disc is 15–135 μm (see Figure 15.2). Smear preparation was stained with silver nitrate. (Sarah L. Poynton, Johns Hopkins University School of Medicine)

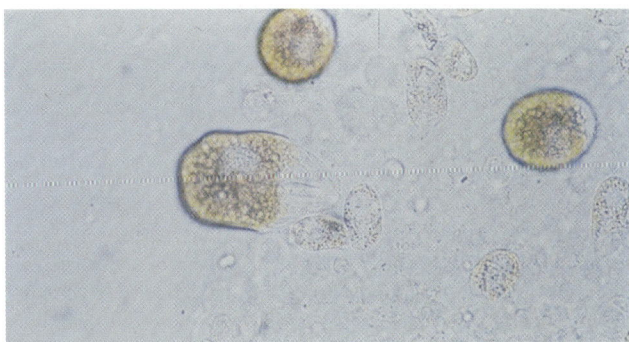

Plate 15.3. Trophont stages of a dinoflagellate, which were attached to the host's skin cells and fed upon their cytoplasm. Trophonts may reach 670 μm in length. (Scott Citino)

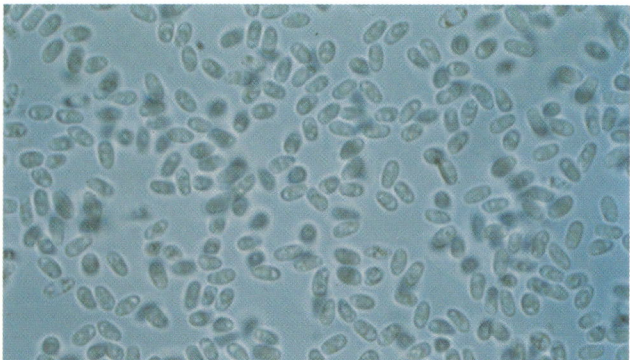

Plate 15.4. Microsporidian spores. Note the typical pyriform (pear-shaped) outline, and refractile vacuole. Length of microsporidian spores ranges 2–20 µm. (Heino Möller, Institut für Meereskunde, Kiel, Germany)

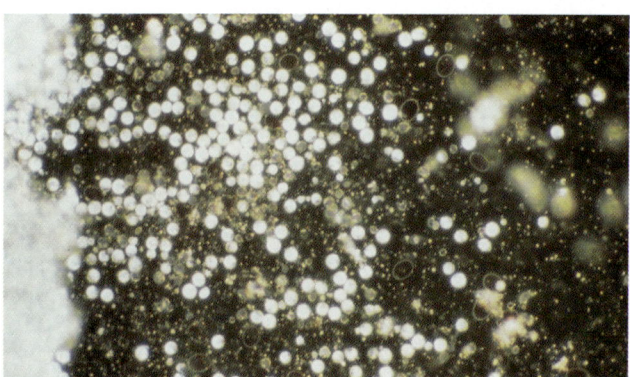

Plate 15.5. Spores of a *Dermocystidium*-like organism from a dendrobatid frog. Numerous spherical stages were packed inside a small white nodule. *Dermocystidium* and its relatives are believed to be akin to fungi. Diameter of spores ranges 12–14 µm. (Sarah L. Poynton, Johns Hopkins University School of Medicine)

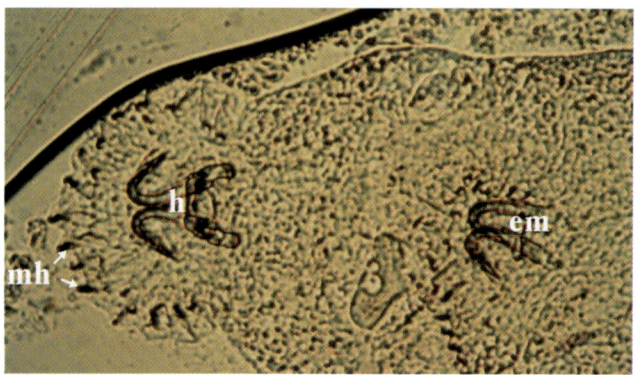

Plate 15.6. The monogenean *Gyrodactylus* sp., which can be found as an ectoparasite on tadpoles. This worm attaches to its host via a posterior haptor armed with hamuli (h) and marginal hooklets (mh), features characteristic of the monopisthocotylean group. The gyrodactylid family is further distinguished by giving birth to live young. Note the hamuli and marginal hooklets of the embryo (em) that can be seen within this parent worm. Length of *Gyrodactylus* species is 300–800 µm. (Sarah L. Poynton, John Hopkins University School of Medicine)

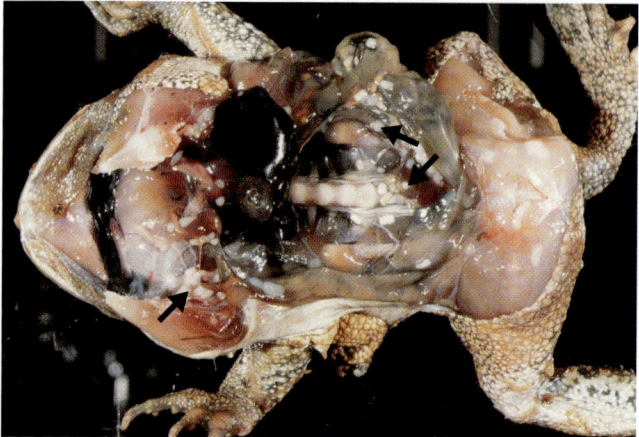

Plate 15.7. The body cavity of an American toad, *Bufo americanus*, infected with cestodes. In this instance, the toad serves as an intermediate host and carries numerous encysted cestode larvae (arrows). (Kevin Wright, Philadelphia Zoological Garden)

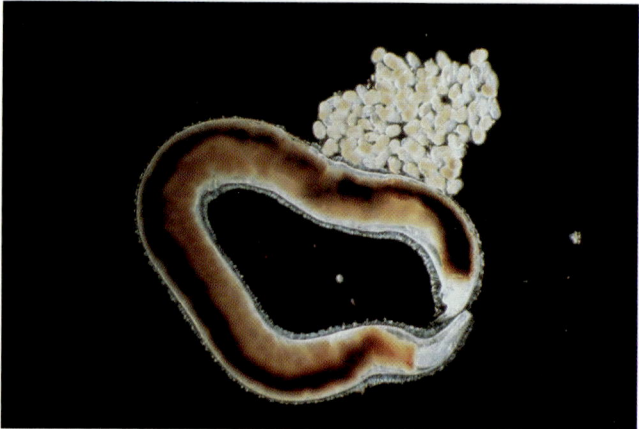

Plate 15.8. A. The nematode *Rhabdias* from the lungs of a dendrobatid frog. A hermaphrodite adult which has just released eggs. (Sarah L. Poynton, Johns Hopkins University School of Medicine)

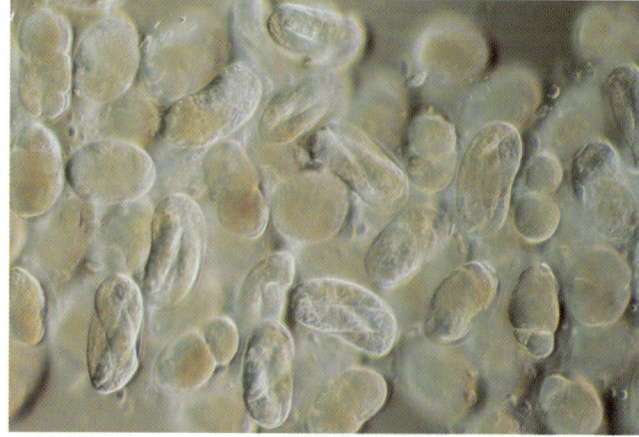

Plate 15.8. B. The thin-shelled eggs which contain a first stage (L1) larvae. The adult may reach 13 mm in length, eggs are 110–120 µm long. (Sarah L. Poynton, Johns Hopkins University School of Medicine)

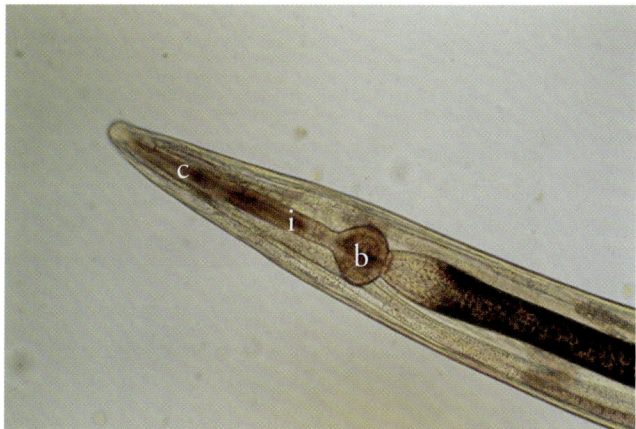

Plate 15.9. A. An adult nematode from the lumen of the gastrointestinal tract of a dendrobatid frog. Anterior end, showing the distinctive esophagus, which has a cylindrical corpus (c), an elongated isthmus (i), and a spherical bulb (b). (Sarah L. Poynton, Johns Hopkins University School of Medicine)

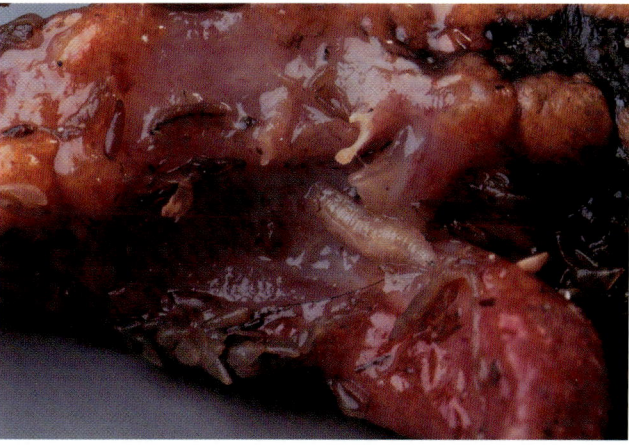

Plate 15.10. B. Fly larvae are aggressively debriding the wound on the pelvis of the crocodile newt depicted in Plate 15.10A. In some instances the larvae begin to consume healthy tissue, too. (George Grall, National Aquarium in Baltimore)

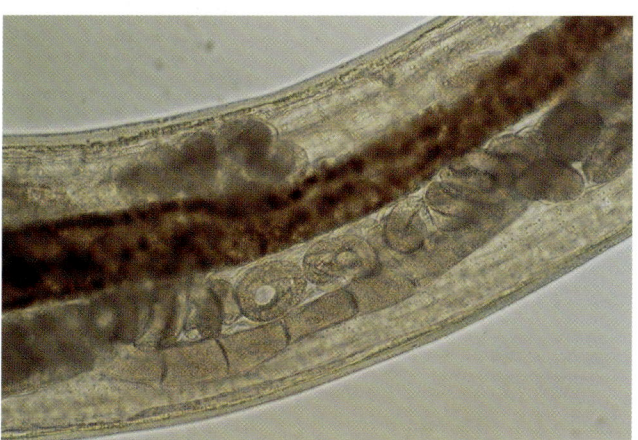

Plate 15.9. B. Mid-region of a female nematode showing the eggs which are thin-shelled and contain a first stage (L1) larvae. The eggs are 80–100 μm long. (Sarah L. Poynton, Johns Hopkins University School of Medicine)

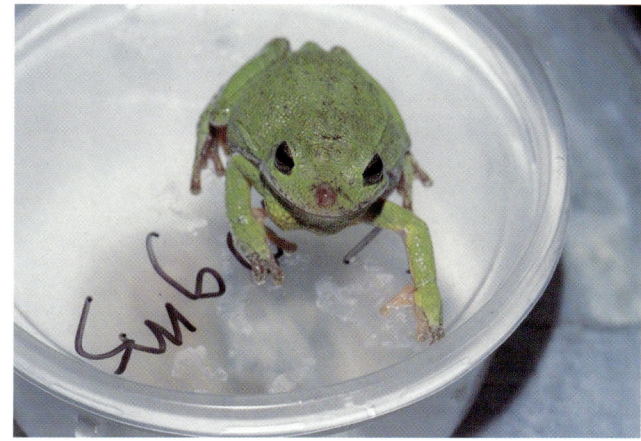

Plate 17.1. Acute rostral abrasion on a barking treefrog, *Hyla gratiosa*, that was shipped in a deli cup. (Kevin Wright, Philadelphia Zoological Garden)

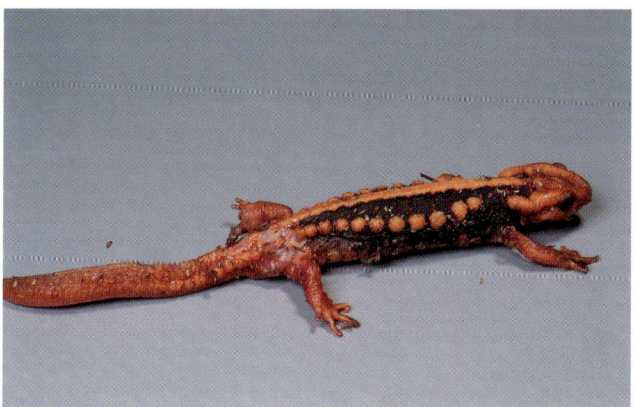

Plate 15.10. A. Myasis of a pelvic wound on a crocodile newt, *Tylototriton shanjing*. (George Grall, National Aquarium in Baltimore)

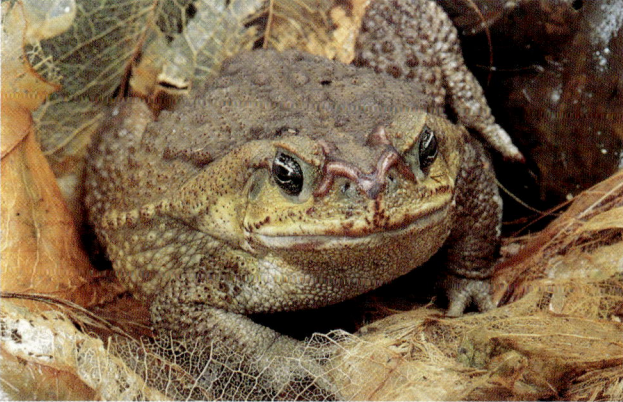

Plate 17.2. Rostral abrasion on a giant toad, *Bufo marinus*. Enclosures that are too small may result in this injury as the anuran hops around. (George Grall, National Aquarium in Baltimore)

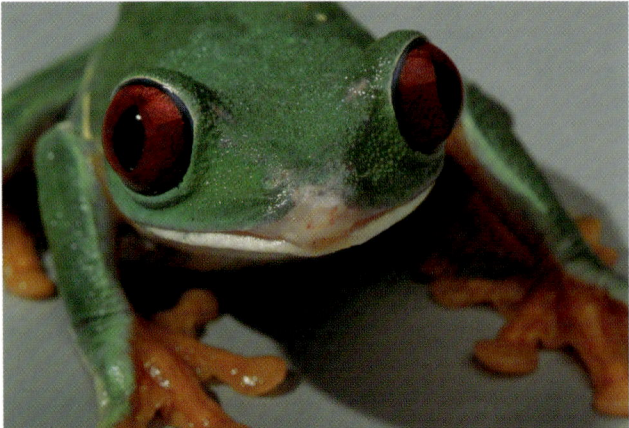

Plate 17.3. Healing rostral abrasion in a red-eyed treefrog, *Agalychnis callidryas*. (George Grall, National Aquarium in Baltimore)

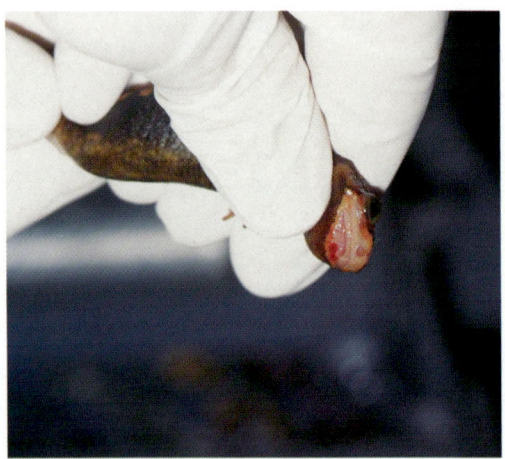

Plate 17.4. Mild atrophic mandibular stomatitis in a crocodile newt, *Tylototriton shanjing*. (Kevin Wright, Philadephia Zoological Garden)

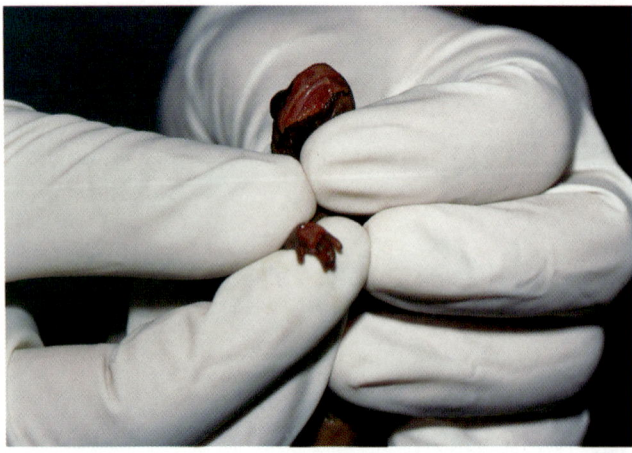

Plate 17.5. Mild atrophic mandibular stomatitis in a crocodile newt, *Tylototriton shanjing*. The mandible has been fractured. (Kevin Wright, Philadelphia Zoological Garden)

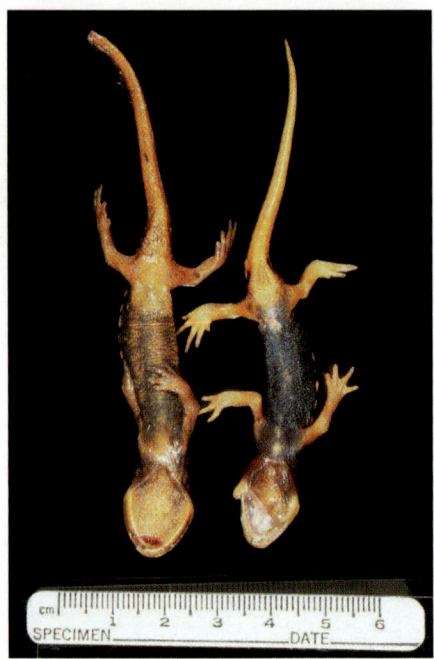

Plate 17.6. Damage to the mandible can be severe enough to starve the amphibian, such as occurred with these two crocodile newts, *Tylototriton shanjing*. (Kevin Wright, Philadelphia Zoological Garden)

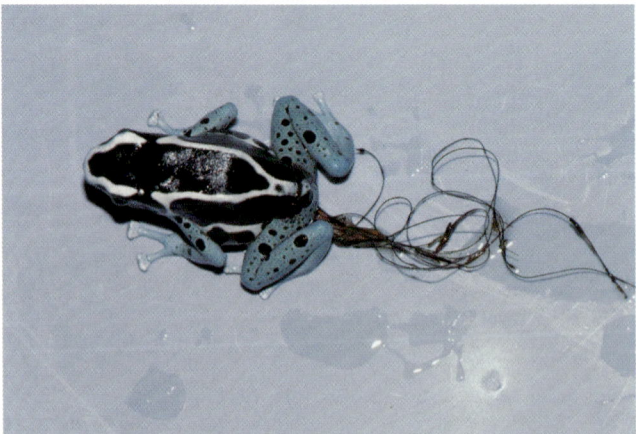

Plate 17.7. Dyeing poison frog, *Dendrobates tinctorius*, with full-thickness skin laceration due to entanglement in fibers of Spanish moss. Inappropriate cage furnishings are a common source of injury for amphibians. (Kevin Wright, Philadelphia Zoological Garden)

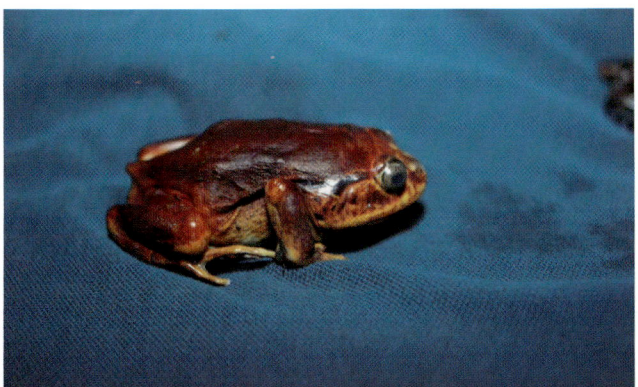

Plate 17.8. Sambava tomato frog, *Dyscophus guineti*, in a state of advanced dehydration. Although tacky to the touch, the coloration is near normal. (Kevin Wright, Philadelphia Zoological Garden)

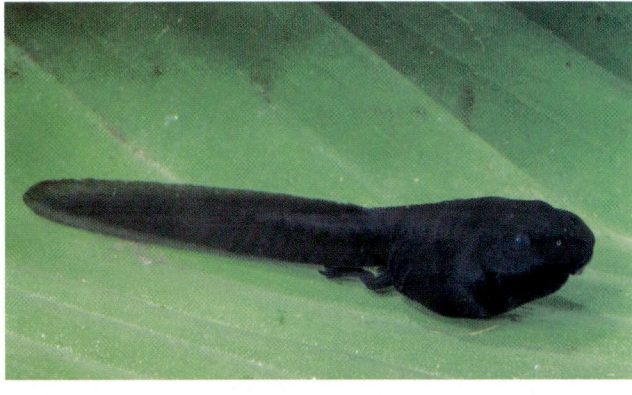

Plate 18.1. Normal hindlimb development in a tadpole of the blue poison frog, *Dendrobates azureus*. (George Grall, National Aquarium in Baltimore)

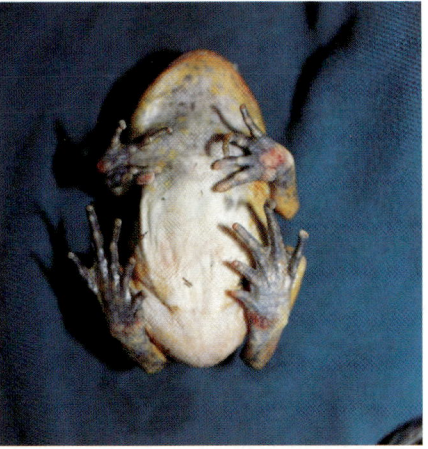

Plate 17.9. Sambava tomato frog, *Dyscophus guineti*, from Plate 17.8. A cardiac impulse could be detected ventrally, but the frog died within minutes of detection. The ventral skin typically stays moist even in a state of advanced dehydration. (Kevin Wright, Philadelphia Zoological Garden)

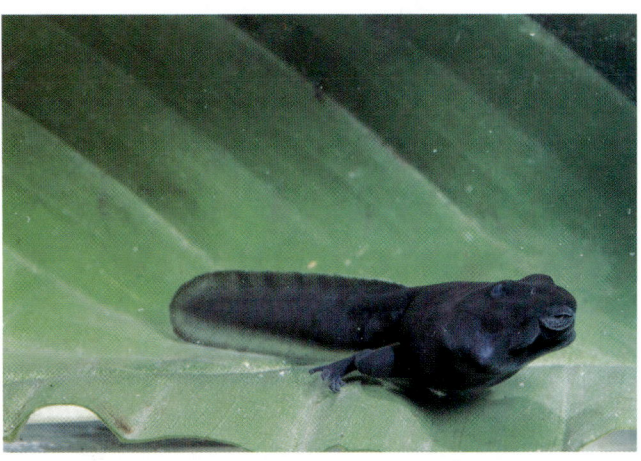

Plate 18.2. Forelimb bud development in a tadpole of the blue poison frog, *Dendrobates azureus*. (George Grall, National Aquarium in Baltimore)

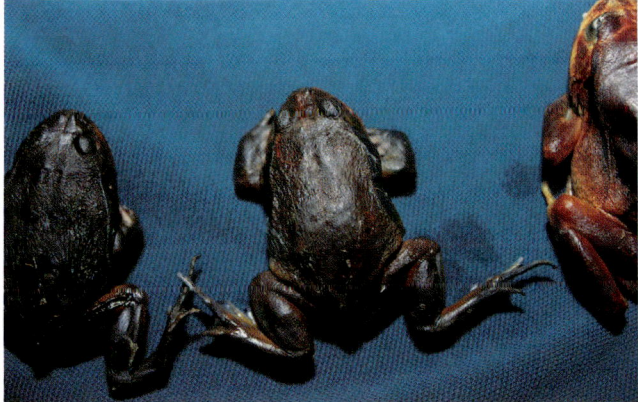

Plate 17.10. Advanced dehydration and desiccation in the Samabava tomato frog, *Dyscophus guineti*. The skin darkens and becomes leathery to the touch with the onset of desiccation. (Kevin Wright, Philadelphia Zoological Garden)

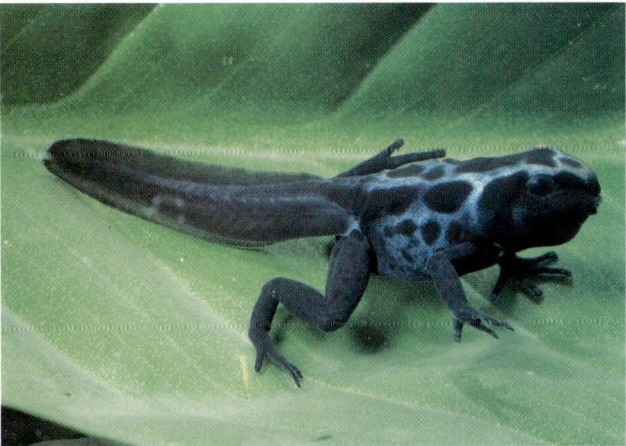

Plate 18.3. Normal forelimbs and hindlimbs in a late stage tadpole of the blue poison frog, *Dendrobates azureus*. (George Grall, National Aquarium in Baltimore)

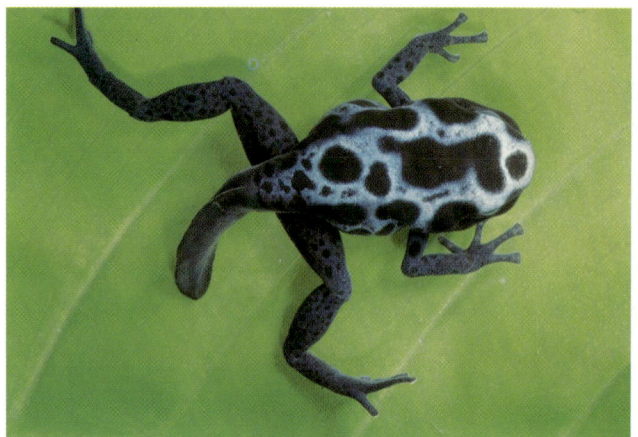

Plate 18.4. Premetamorphic tadpole of the blue poison frog, *Dendrobates azureus*, with normal limb development. (George Grall, National Aquarium in Baltimore)

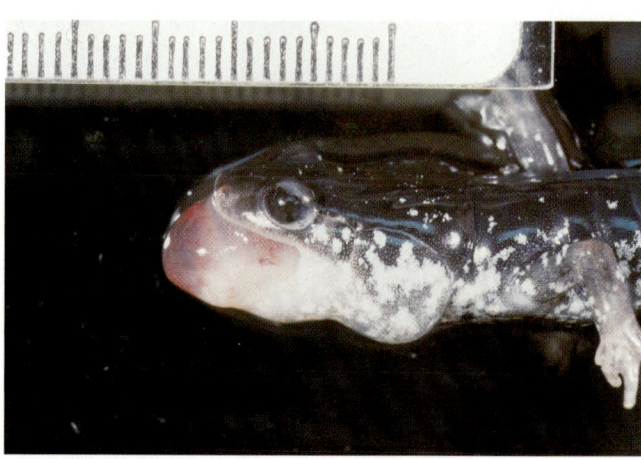

Plate 18.7. Gastric prolapse in a northern slimy salamander, *Plethodon cylindraceous*. (Kevin Wright, Philadelphia Zoological Garden)

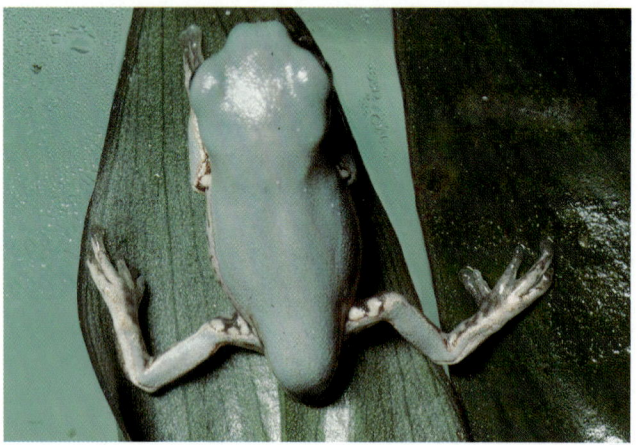

Plate 18.5. Spindly leg in a newly metamorphed orange-legged leaf frog, *Phyllomedusa hypochondrialis*. (Tracy Barker, Vida Preciosa)

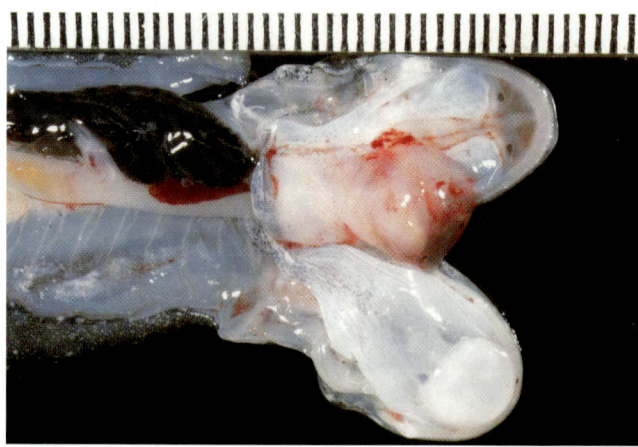

Plate 18.8. Gastric prolapse in a northern slimy salamander, *Plethodon cylindraceous*. The mandible has been reflected to allow visualization of the upper gastrointestinal tract. (Kevin Wright, Philadelphia Zoological Garden)

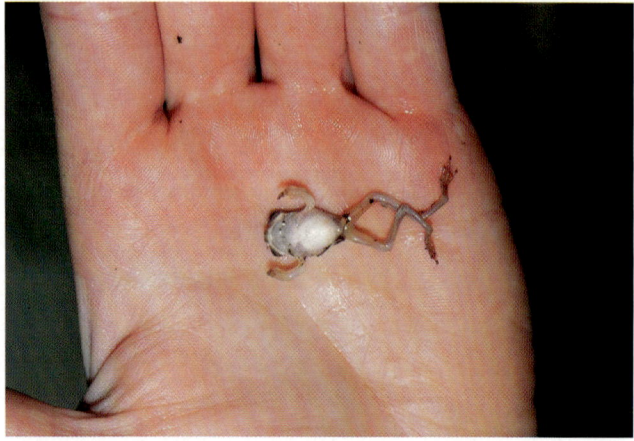

Plate 18.6. Spindly leg in a newly metamorphed New Granada cross-banded frog, *Smilisca phaeota*. (Kevin Wright, Philadelphia Zoological Garden)

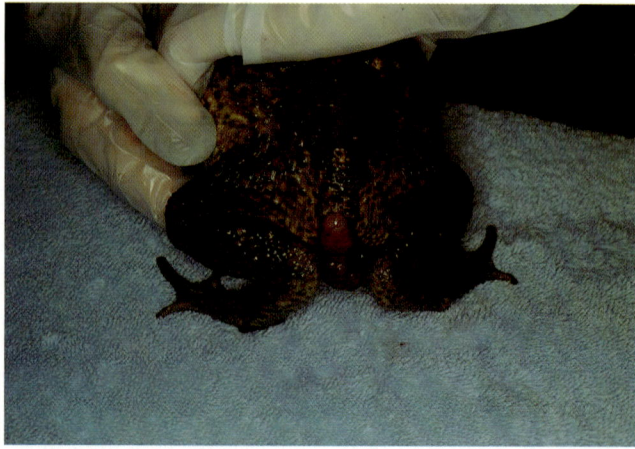

Plate 18.9. Rectal prolapse in a giant toad, *Bufo marinus*. (Kevin Wright, Philadelphia Zoological Garden)

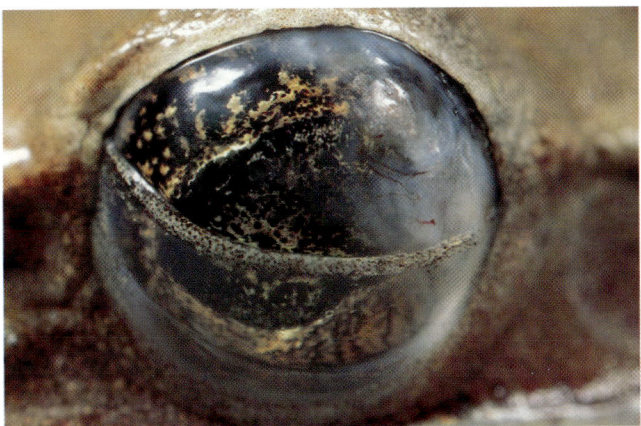

Plate 19.1. The thin transluscent eyelid of the masked treefrog, *Hyla lanciformis*, partially covers the cornea. Stromal corneal opacity of unknown etiology and neovascularization are present adjacent to the medial canthus. (George Grall, National Aquarium in Baltimore)

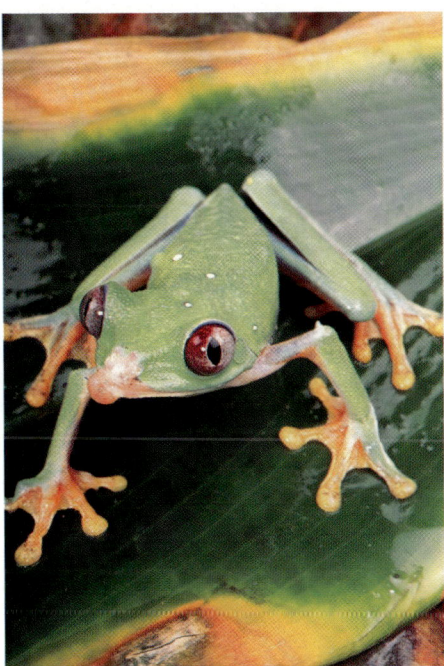

Plate 19.2. Bilateral loss of iridial pigment associated with terminal illness in the red-eyed treefrog, *Agalychnis callidryas*. (George Grall, National Aquarium in Baltimore)

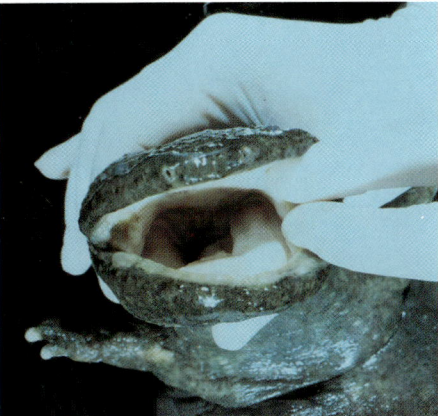

Plate 19.3. Examination of the oral cavity and thin membrane separating the back of the globe from the oropharynx. (Kevin Wright, Philadelphia Zoological Garden)

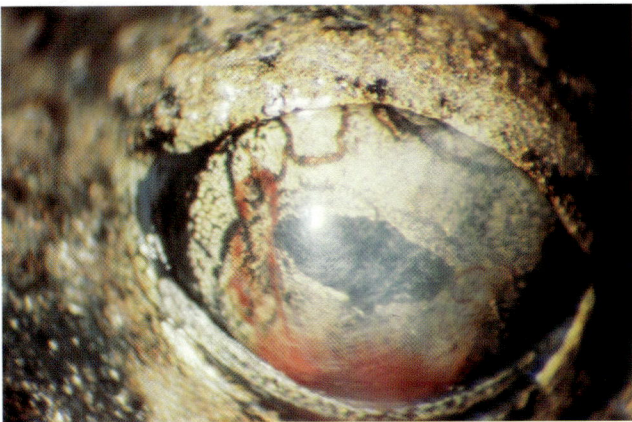

Plate 19.4. Rupture of an iridial blood vessel during handling for photodocumentation of superficial keratitis in a tungara frog, *Physalaemus pustulosus*. (Wilmer Photography, Johns Hopkins University)

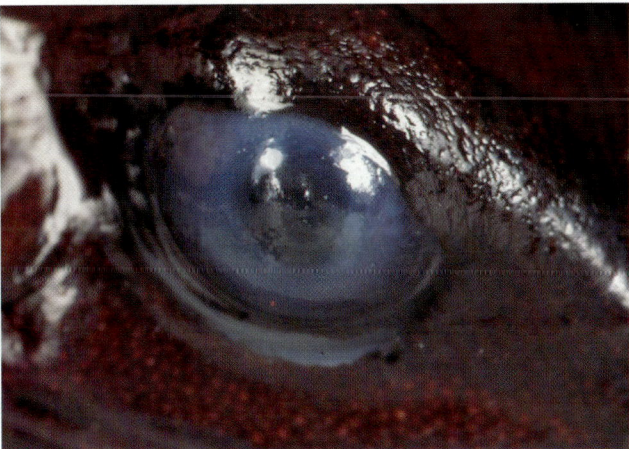

Plate 19.5. Fungal uveitis in a red-and-black poison frog, *Dendrobates histrionicus*. (George Grall, National Aquarium in Baltimore)

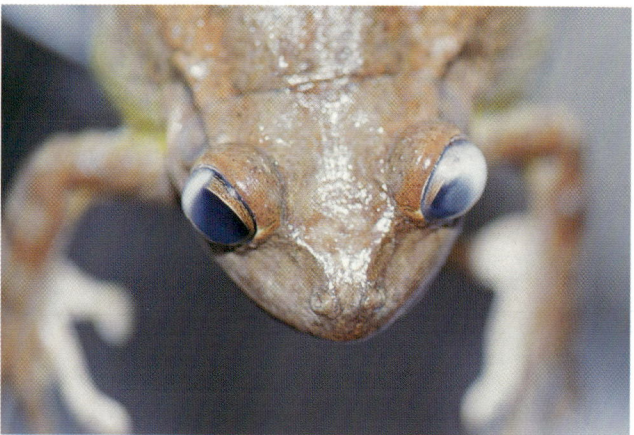

Plate 19.6. Early lesions resulting from corneal lipidosis in a Cuban treefrog, *Osteopilus septentrionalis*. (Kevin Wright, Philadelphia Zoological Garden)

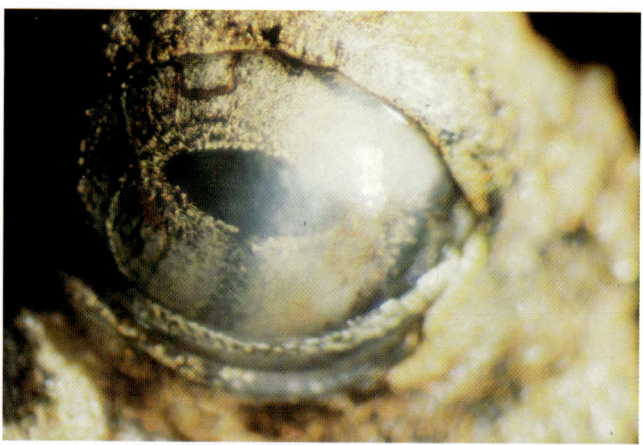

Plate 19.9. Neovascularization of the cornea is seen as superficial circular keratitis progresses in this tungara frog, *Physalaemus pustulosus*. (National Aquarium in Baltimore)

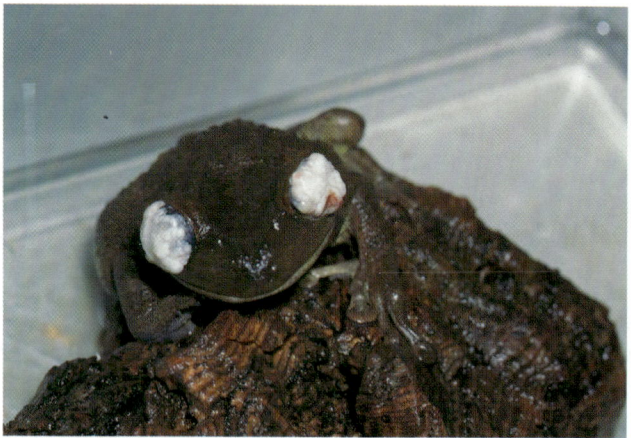

Plate 19.7. Corneal lipidosis 19 months later in the same Cuban treefrog, *Osteopilus septentrionalis*, from Plate 19.6. (Kevin Wright, Philadelphia Zoological Garden)

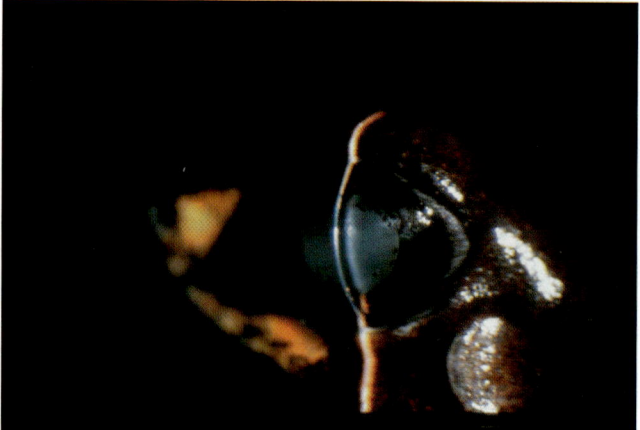

Plate 19.10. Cataract in the eye of a red-and-black poison frog, *Dendrobates histrionicus*, is examined using a slit lamp. (National Aquarium in Baltimore)

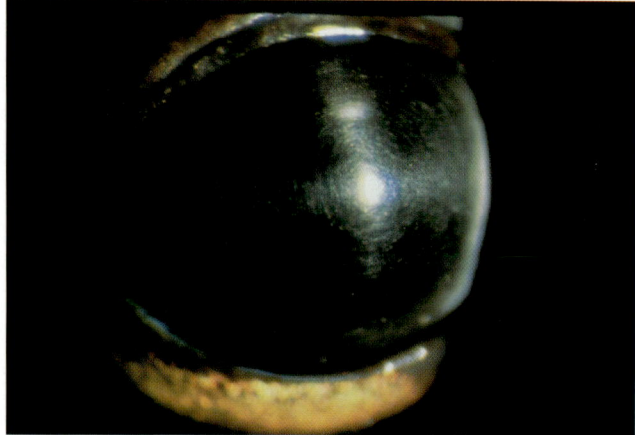

Plate 19.8. The "ground glass" appearance of superficial keratitis of unknown etiology. (National Aquarium in Baltimore)

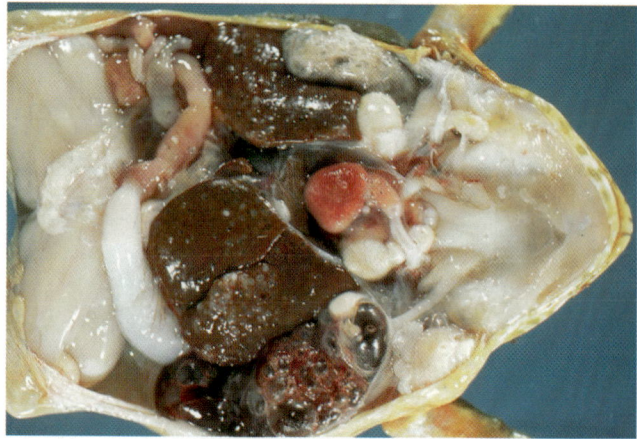

Plate 20.1. Postmortem picture revealing several pericardial granulomas surrounding the heart. Histopathology revealed intralesional acid-fast organisms within the granulomatous tissue. (Tracey McNamara)

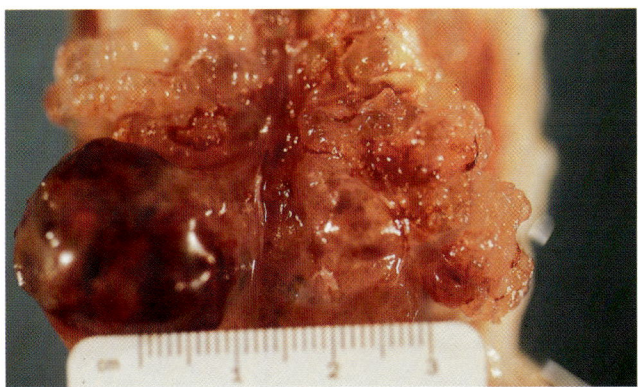

Plate 20.2. Postmortem picture revealing severe bilateral polycystic kidneys. No grossly normal renal tissue could be identified. The large hematoma on the right kidney is a blood-filled cyst induced during ultrasound-guided cyst aspiration. (Mike Lynn)

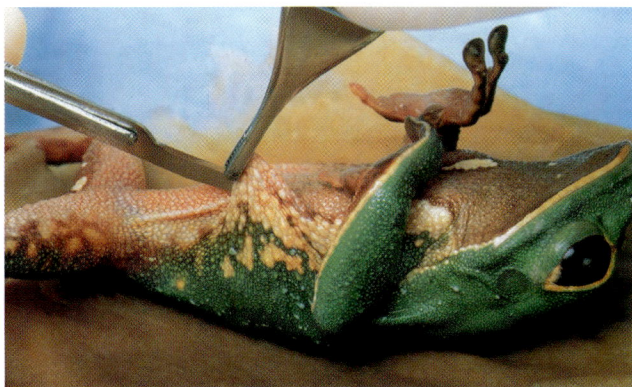

Plate 21.2. Initial skin incision on the leaf frog undergoing a celiotomy.

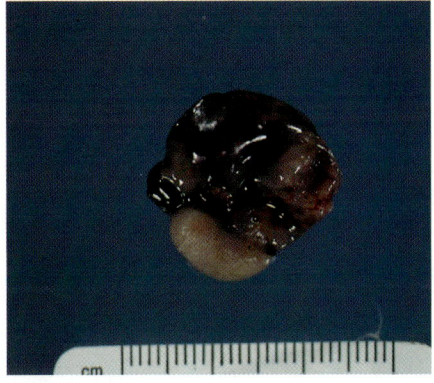

Plate 20.3. Postmortem picture of the heart. The small white structure is the ventricle. The large red structures are the enlarged atrias. Histopathology revealed ventricular myocardial fibrosis and severe dilated atrial cardiomyopathy. Within the atrial lumen was a large well-organized thrombus firmly attached to the endocardial wall. (Jim Walberg)

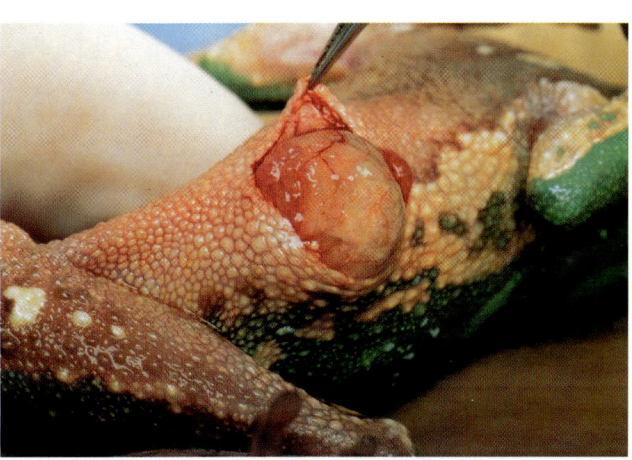

Plate 21.3. Urate stone within the bladder.

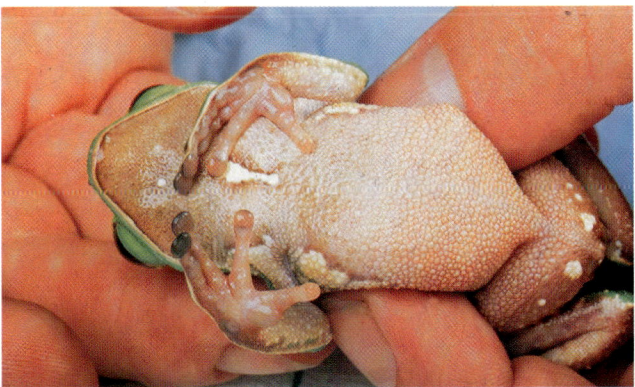

Plate 21.1. Leaf frog, *Phyllomedusa* sp., with a palpable bladder stone. Plates 21.2–21.12 illustrate excising the stone from this frog's bladder. (Plates 21.1–21.12, George Grall, National Aquarium in Baltimore)

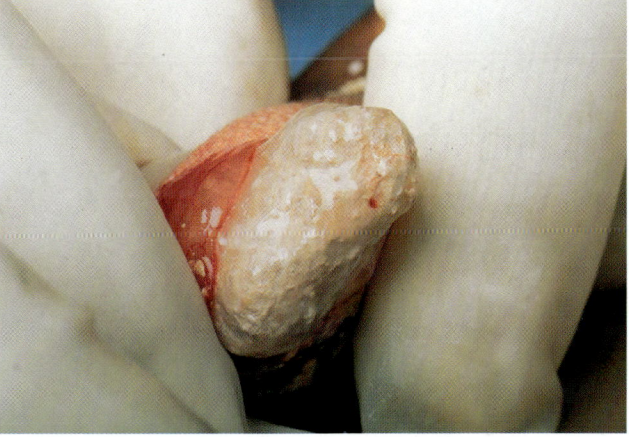

Plate 21.4. Urate stone being removed from the bladder.

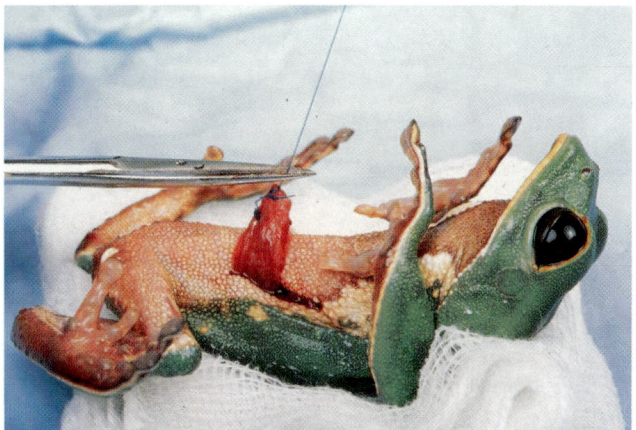

Plate 21.5. Closing the bladder.

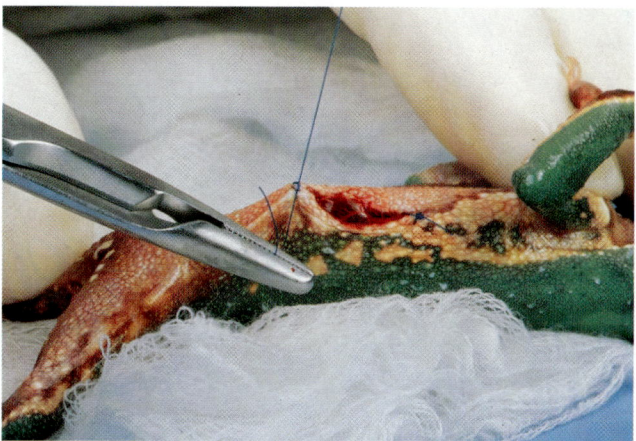

Plate 21.8. Knotting the first suture for skin closure. Care should be taken to avoid inverting the edge of the skin.

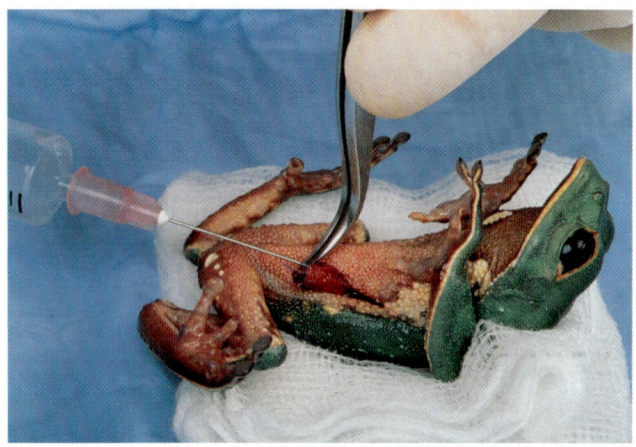

Plate 21.6. Testing the seal on the closed incision by injecting the bladder with sterile saline.

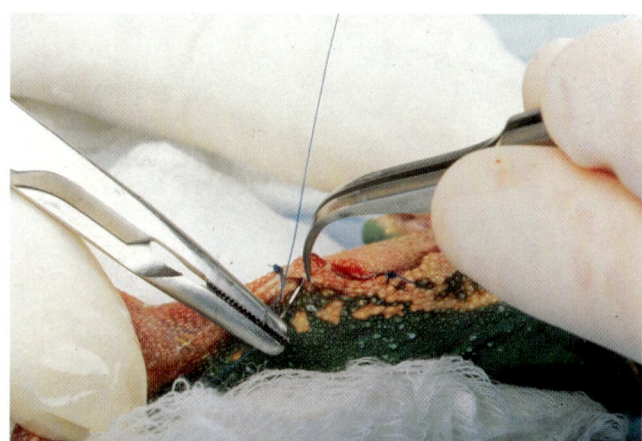

Plate 21.9. Continuing the interrupted suture pattern.

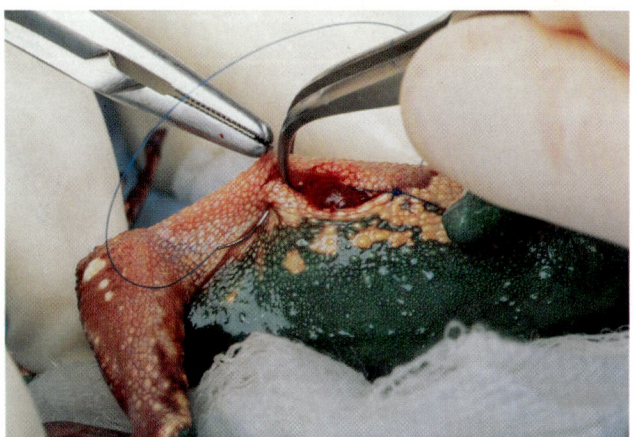

Plate 21.7. Initial placement of a simple interrupted suture for skin closure.

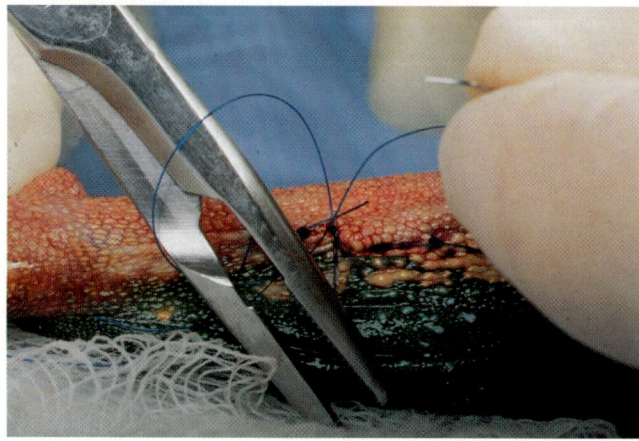

Plate 21.10. Tying the simple interrupted suture.

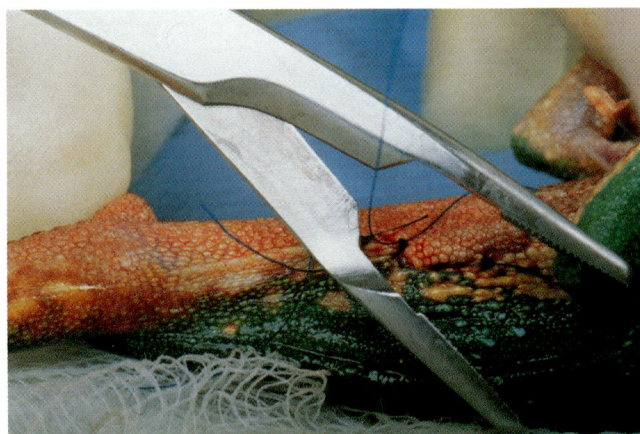

Plate 21.11. Clipping the ends of the suture.

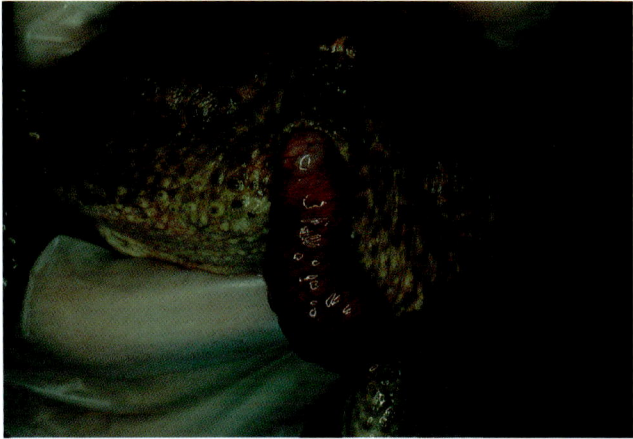

Plate 21.14. Intestinal prolapse in a giant toad, *Bufo marinus*. The deep red color of the tissue suggests that this tissue has been exposed for several hours. A pursestring suture of the cloacal opening is recommended following reduction of the prolapse. (Kevin Wright, Philadelphia Zoological Garden)

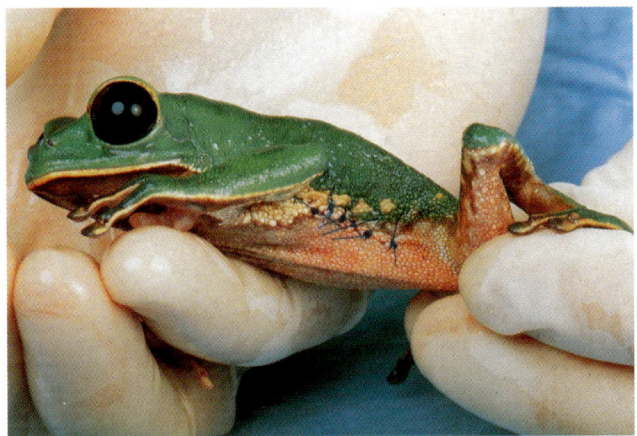

Plate 21.12. Sutured skin incision. Tissue glue can be placed over the incision line for added waterproofing and strength.

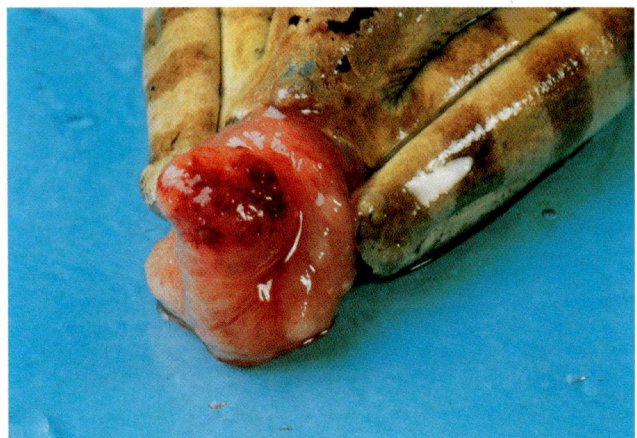

Plate 21.15. Intestinal prolapse in a New Granada cross-banded treefrog, *Smilisca phaeota*, with severe nematodiasis and intestinal adenocarcinoma. (George Grall, National Aquarium in Baltimore)

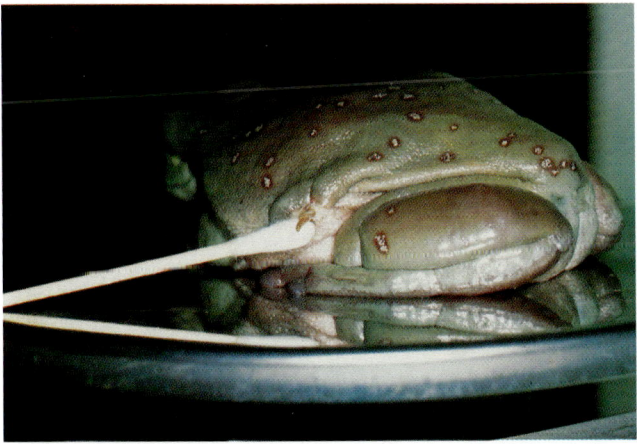

Plate 21.13. Plant awn protruding through the stomach wall of a White's treefrog, *Pelodryas caerulea*. (Kevin Wright, Philadelphia Zoological Garden)

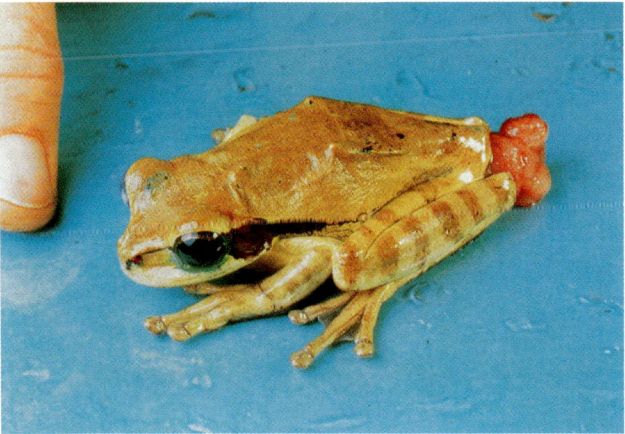

Plate 21.16. Many similarly afflicted anurans with intestinal prolapse appear bright and alert, such as this New Granada cross-banded treefrog. (George Grall, National Aquarium in Baltimore)

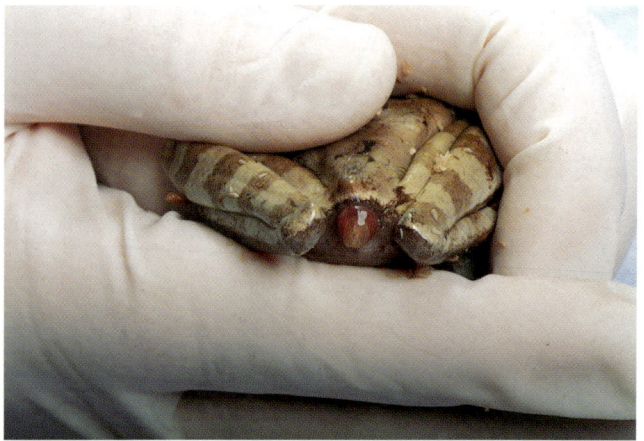

Plate 21.17. Mild cloacal prolapse in a New Granada cross-banded treefrog, *Smilisca phaeota*, with nematodiasis. A pursestring suture is optional following reduction of a minor prolapse. (Plates 21.17–21.23, George Grall, National Aquarium in Baltimore)

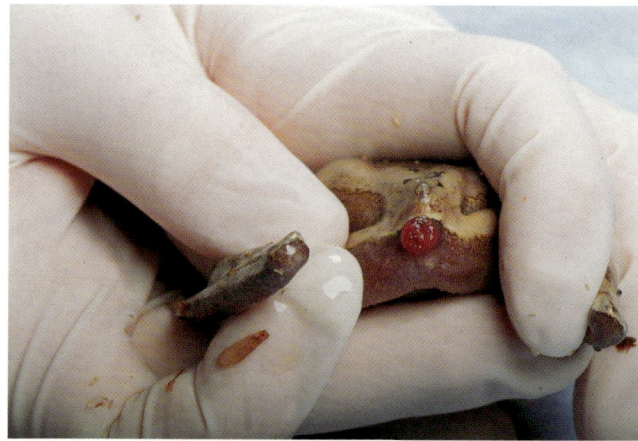

Plate 21.20. The prolapse is firmer and less edematous following treatment with hyperosmotic saline.

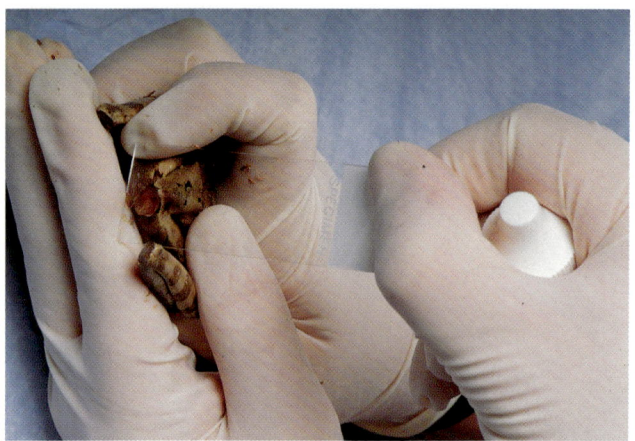

Plate 21.18. A touch prep of the prolapsed tissue may reveal helminths and their ova.

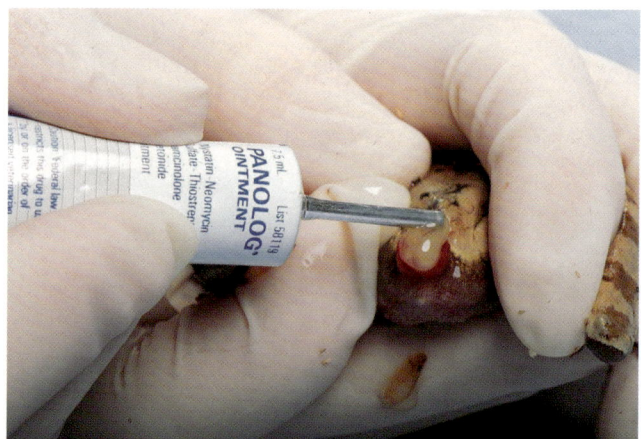

Plate 21.21. The tissue should be lubricated prior to replacement within the amphibian's body.

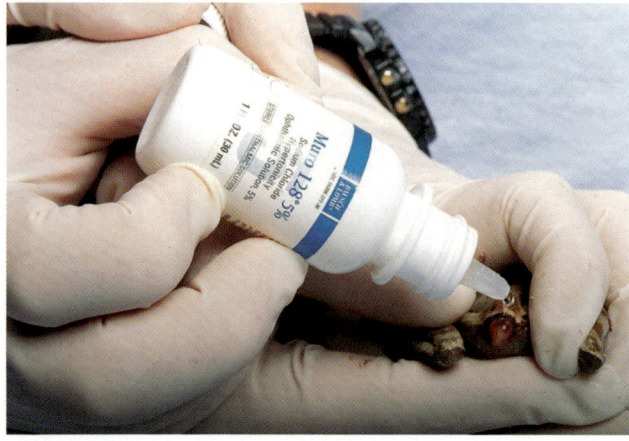

Plate 21.19. Hyperosmotic saline ophthalmic solution can be used to reduce swelling of the prolapsed tissue.

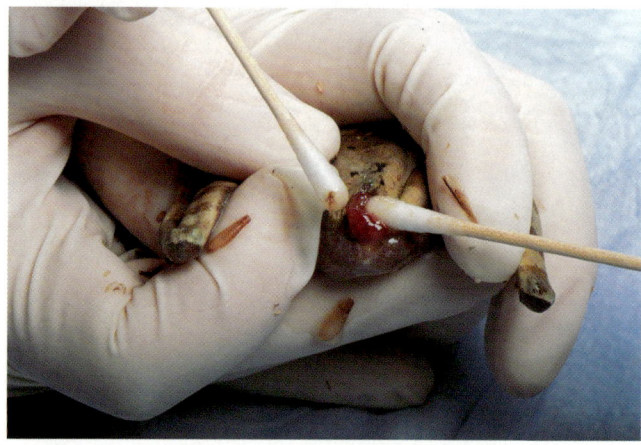

Plate 21.22. Replacing the prolapsed tissue.

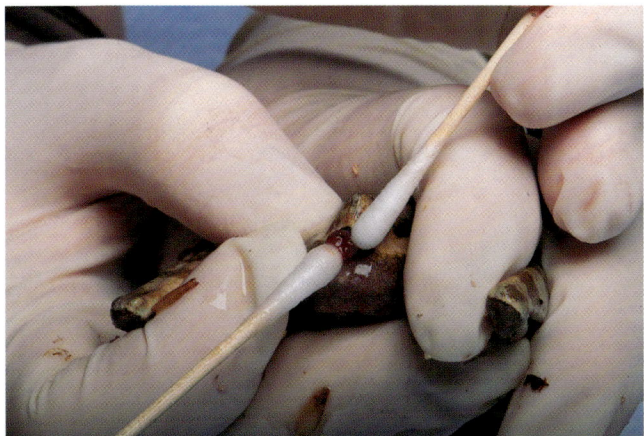

Plate 21.23. Final positioning of the tissue.

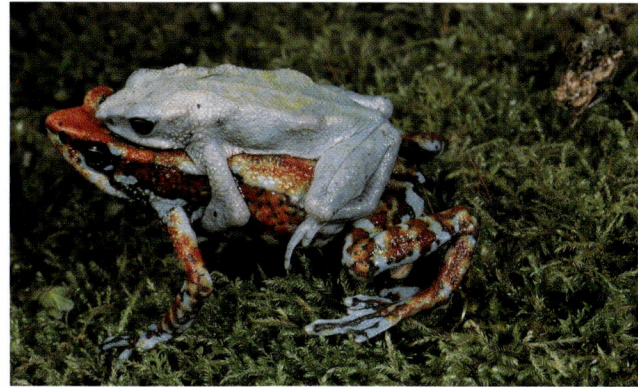

Plate 22.3. Some anurans, like this amplexed pair of the Lewis' stubfoot toad, *Atelopus chiriquiensis*, are sexually dimorphic in coloration and size. The male is the smaller of the frogs. (George Grall, National Aquarium in Baltimore)

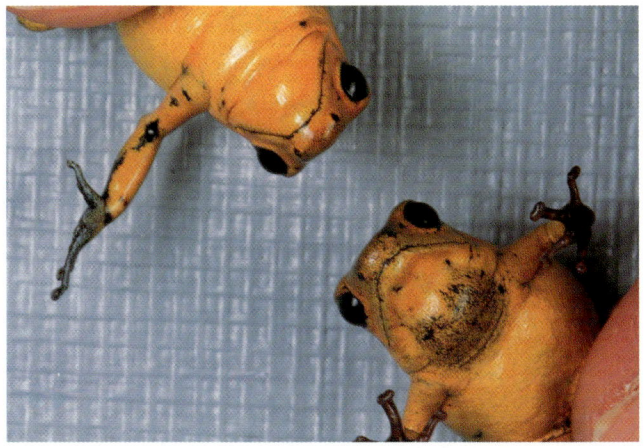

Plate 22.1. The permanently pigmented throat of the male and the unpigmented throat of the female are seen in some populations of the strawberry poison frog, *Dendrobates pumilio*. (George Grall, National Aquarium in Baltimore)

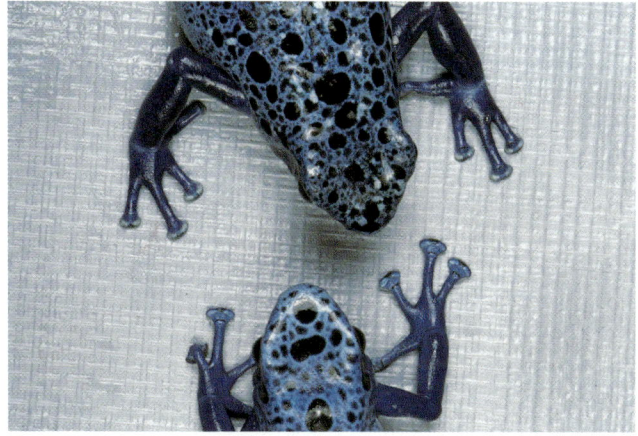

Plate 22.4. A. Some male dendrobatid frogs, such as this *Dendrobates azureus*, possess enlarged digital toe pads. (George Grall, National Aquarium in Baltimore)

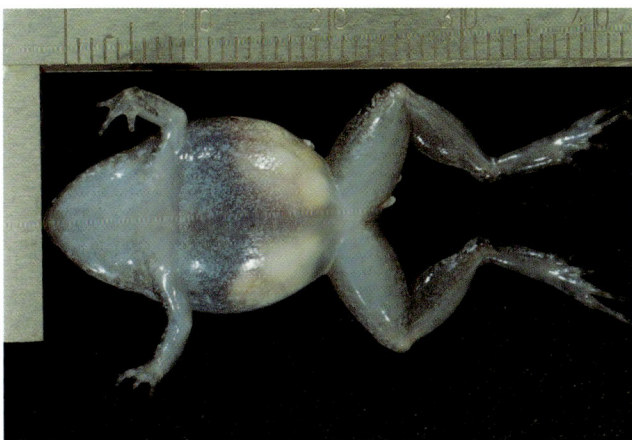

Plate 22.2. Eggs within the coelomic cavity are visible through the abdominal skin and muscles of some frogs and salamanders. (Virginia Pierce, Philadelphia Zoological Garden)

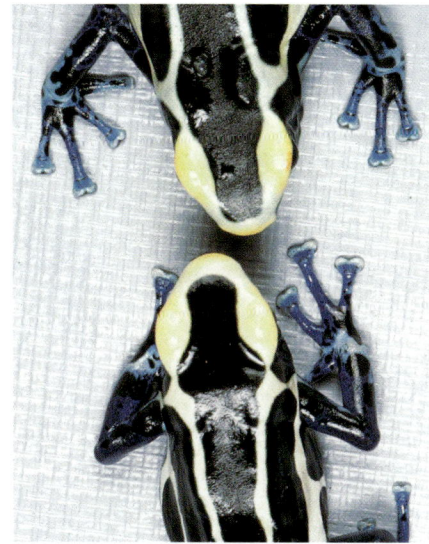

Plate 22.4. B. *Dendrobates tinctorius* with enlarged toe pads. Males are at the bottom of each plate. (George Grall, National Aquarium in Baltimore)

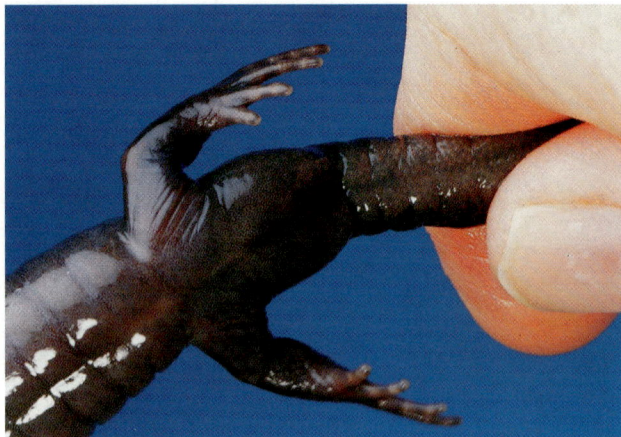

Plate 22.5. Cloacal glands of male salamanders, such as this spotted salamander, *Ambystoma maculatum*, are necessary for the production of spermatophores. (George Grall, National Aquarium in Baltimore)

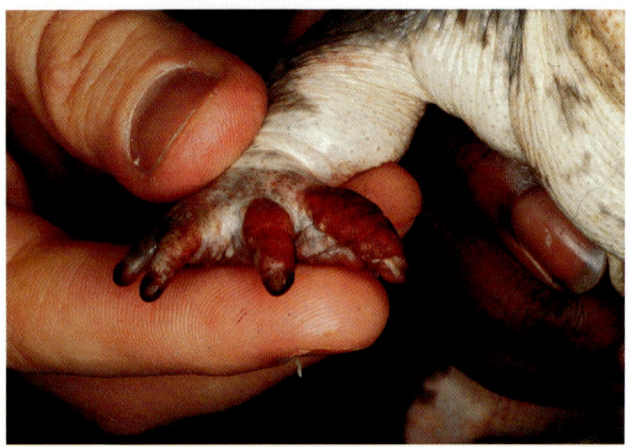

Plate 22.6. Nuptial pads of a male Colorado river toad, *Bufo alvarius*. (Kevin Wright, Philadelphia Zoological Garden)

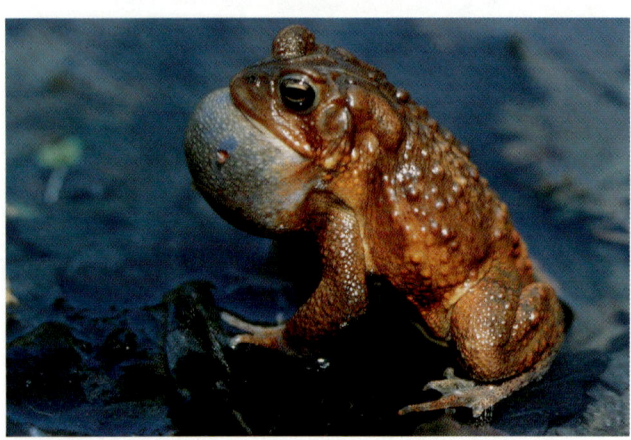

Plate 22.7. Inflated vocal sac of a male American toad, *Bufo americanus*. (Robert Dougan)

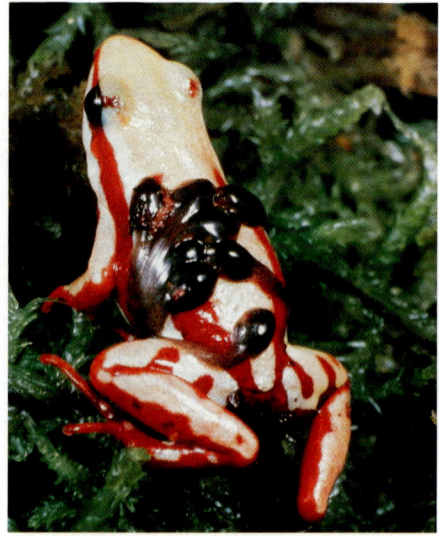

Plate 22.8. The male phantasmal poison frog, *Epipedobates tricolor*, provides parental care as it carries its young on its back through the forest. (National Aquarium in Baltimore)

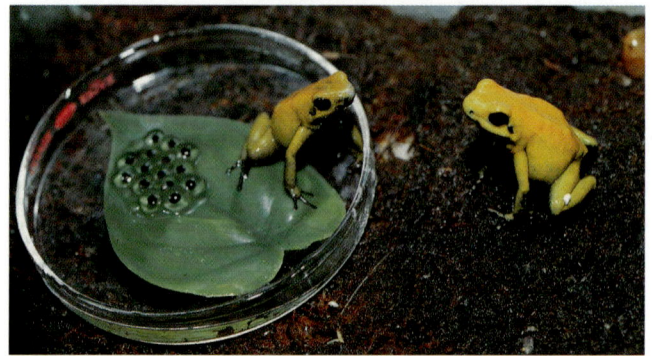

Plate 22.9. In captivity, broad plastic leaves function as oviposition sites for leaf spawners such as the black-legged poison frog, *Phyllobates bicolor*. The plastic hut normally covering the dish has been removed. (National Aquarium in Baltimore)

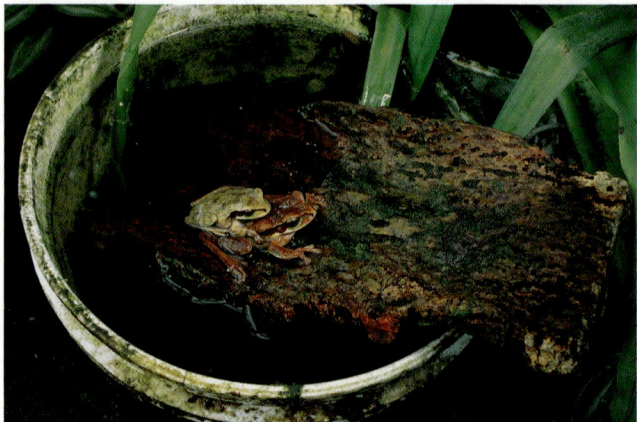

Plate 22.10. New Granada cross-banded treefrog, *Smilisca phaeota*, in amplexus prior to oviposition into water. (George Grall, National Aquarium in Baltimore)

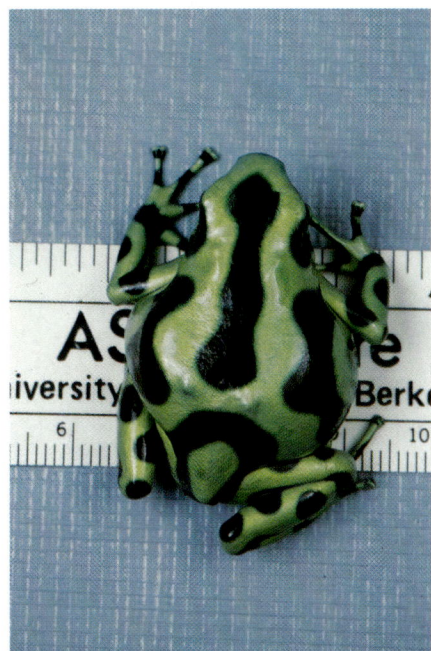

Plate 22.11. The rapid accumulation of fluid in this green and black poison frog, *Dendrobates auratus*, was associated with the gradual cessation of egg laying. The etiology of this condition is unknown. (George Grall, National Aquarium in Baltimore)

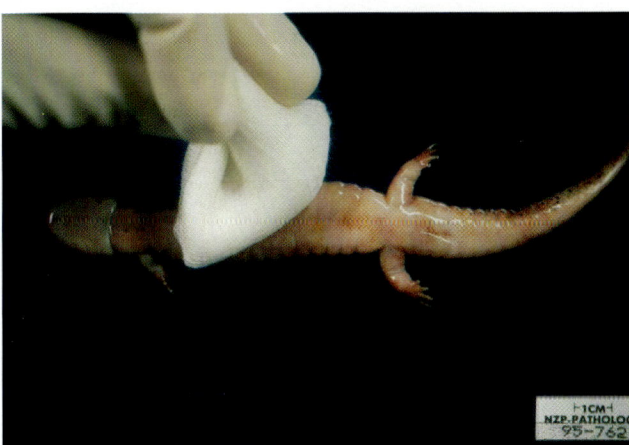

Plate 25.1. Disinfection of the skin of a red salamander, *Pseudotriton ruber*, prior to incision for gross necropsy. Carcass is placed in dorsal recumbency and the ventral surface is disinfected using a gauze swab soaked in 70% ethanol or iodine solution. (Donald K. Nichols, National Zoological Park)

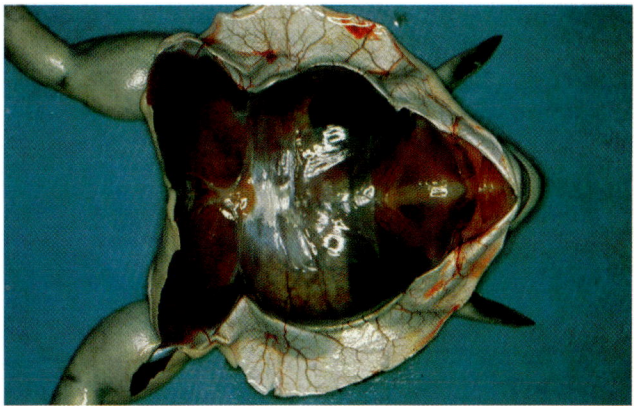

Plate 25.2. Carcass of an African clawed frog, *Xenopus laevis*, in dorsal recumbency. Initial incisions of the ventral skin have been made and the skin has been reflected laterally to expose the underlying musculature. Note: Necropsy instruments should be sterilized or exchanged for a new set of instruments before opening the coelomic cavity. (Donald K. Nichols, National Zoological Park)

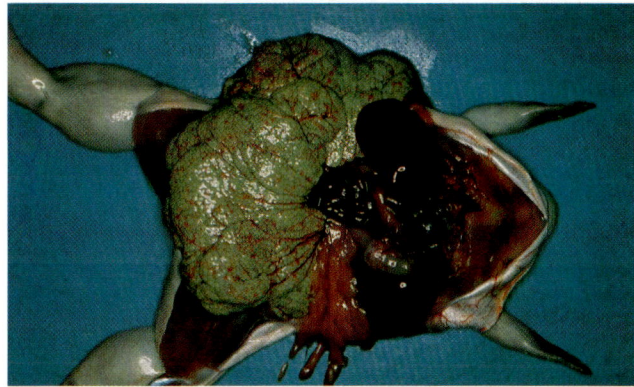

Plate 25.3. Following ventral midline incision of the musculature and sternum, the musculature has been reflected laterally to expose the viscera in this African clawed frog, *Xenopus laevis*. (Donald K. Nichols, National Zoological Park)

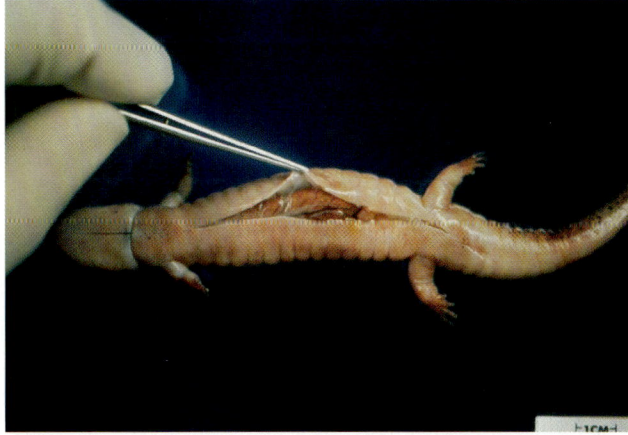

Plate 25.4. Carcass of a red salamander, *Pseudotriton ruber*, in dorsal recumbency. A ventral midline incision extends from the mandibular symphysis to the cloacal opening; the skin and underlying musculature are being reflected laterally. (Donald K. Nichols, National Zoological Park)

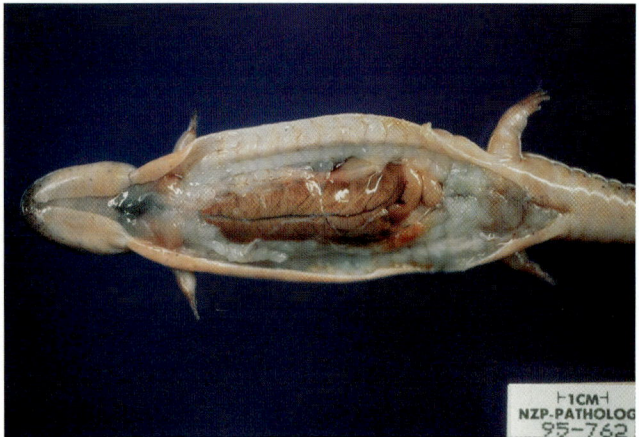

Plate 25.5. Lateral reflection of the ventral skin and musculature reveals the viscera of this red salamander, *Pseudotriton ruber*. (Donald K. Nichols, National Zoological Park)

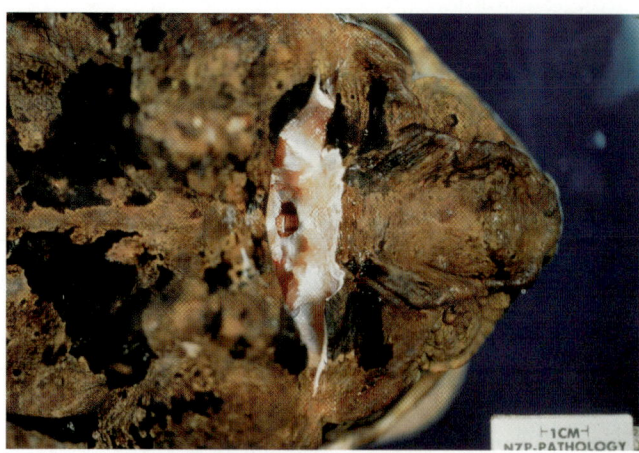

Plate 25.8. A. Brain removal from the carcass of a giant toad, *Bufo marinus*, using a dorsal approach. An incision has been made at the atlanto-occipital joint, exposing the foramen magnum. (Donald K. Nichols, National Zoological Park)

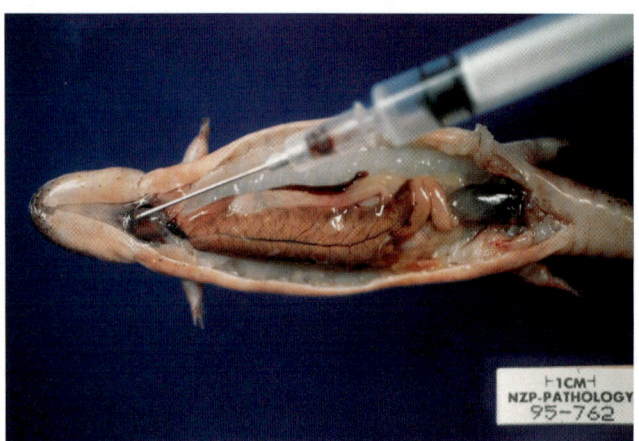

Plate 25.6. Heart blood collection from the carcass of a red salamander, *Pseudotriton ruber*. (Donald K. Nichols, National Zoological Park)

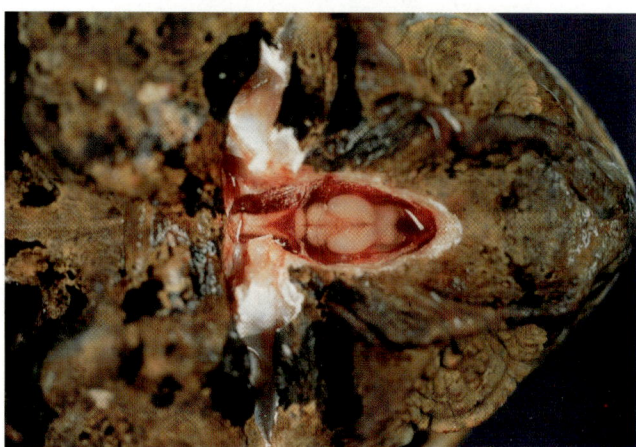

Plate 25.8. B. The brain has been exposed by carefully removing the overlying skull and soft tissues using scissors and forceps. (Donald K. Nichols, National Zoological Park)

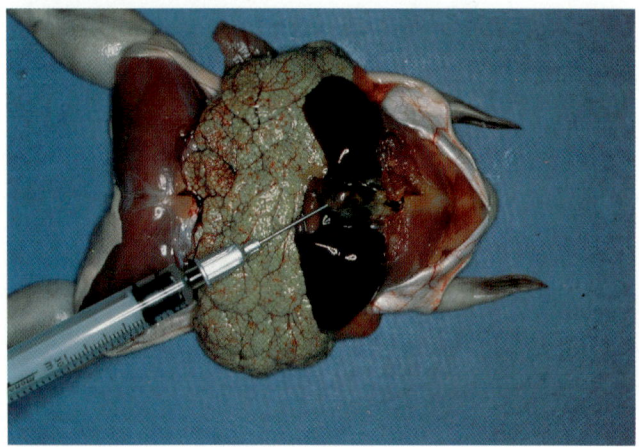

Plate 25.7. Heart blood collection from the carcass of an African clawed frog, *Xenopus laevis*. (Donald K. Nichols, National Zoological Park)

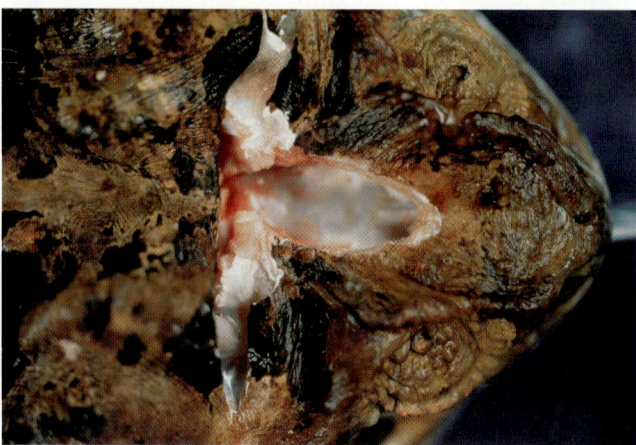

Plate 25.8. C. The brain has been removed, exposing the ventral calvarium. (Donald K. Nichols, National Zoological Park)

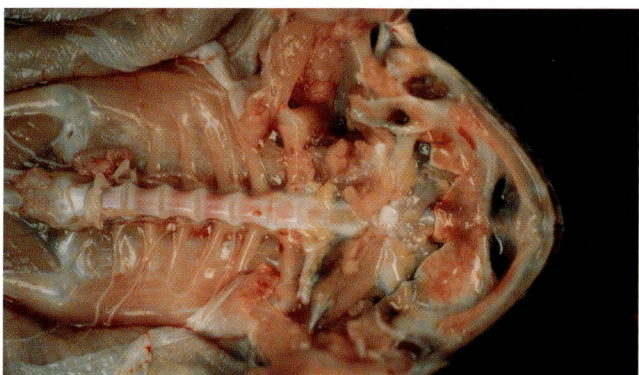

Plate 25.9. A. Brain removal from the carcass of a giant toad, *Bufo marinus*, using a ventral approach. The toad is in dorsal recumbency and the tongue, pharynx, and coelomic viscera have been removed, exposing the vertebral column. (Donald K. Nichols, National Zoological Park)

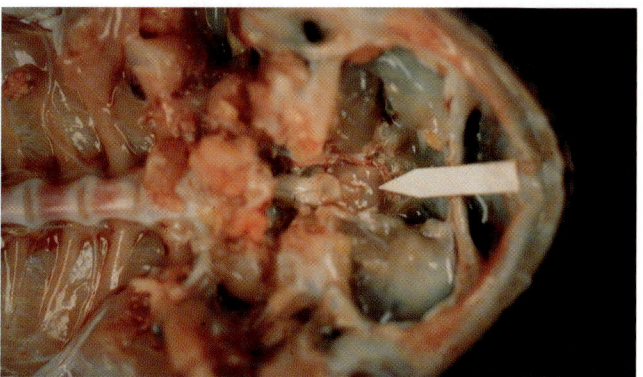

Plate 25.9. B. Scissors and forceps have been used to remove the ventral calvarium, exposing the brain (arrow). (Donald K. Nichols, National Zoological Park)

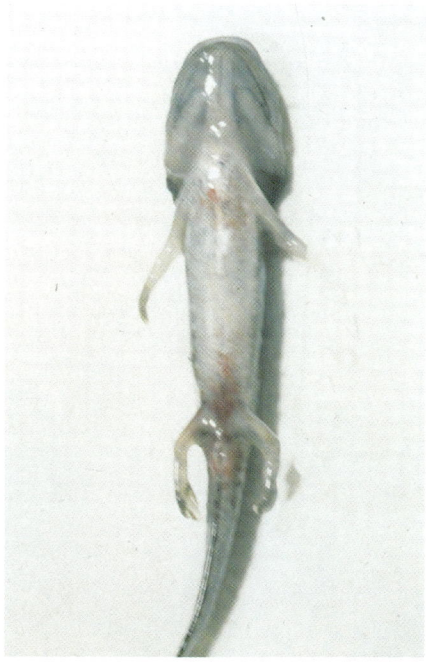

Plate 27.2. Acute red leglike syndrome in a captive larval Arizona tiger salamander, *Ambystoma tigrinum nebulosum*. Note the miliary red petechia in the ventral skin of the pectoral, inguinal, and vent regions. (D.E. Green)

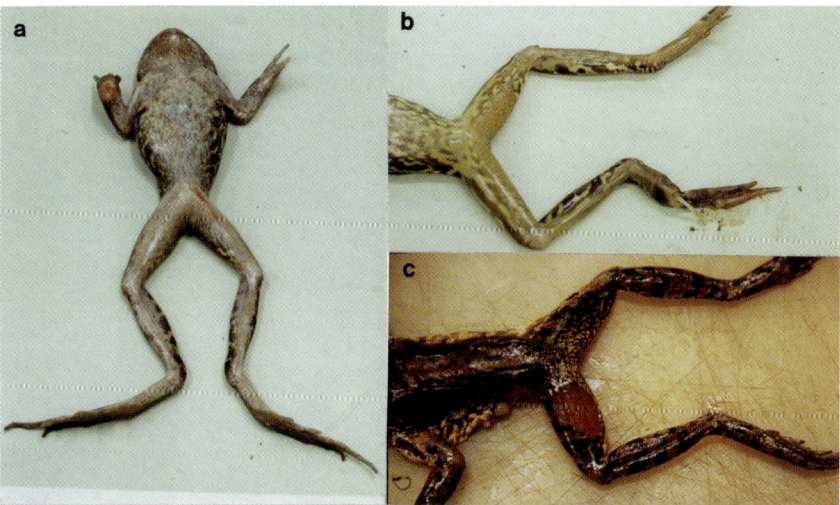

Plate 27.1. Ulcerative skin syndrome in three wild specimens of the European common frog, *Rana temporaria*. Multiple ranaviruses were isolated from these frogs. **a.** Ventrum of frog with a linear ulcer of the upper left femoral region and extensive ulceration of the right carpus and digits. **b.** Necrosis of soft tissues of the right hindlimb with exposed bones. **c.** Dorsum of frog with a large ulcer of the left femoral region. (A.A. Cunningham, The Zoological Society of London, taken from Cunningham et al., 1996b, with permission)

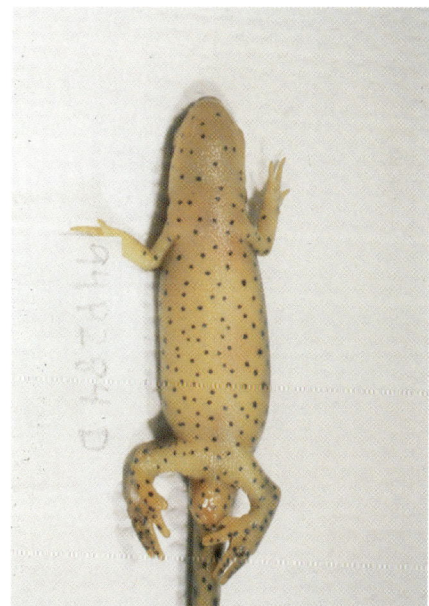

Plate 27.3. Acute red leglike syndrome in a red-spotted newt, *Notophthalmus viridescens viridescens*. This newt shows prominent swelling of the gular region and body. Pure cultures of *Citrobacter freundii* were obtained from the lymphatic sacs, coelom, and internal organs. (D.E. Green)

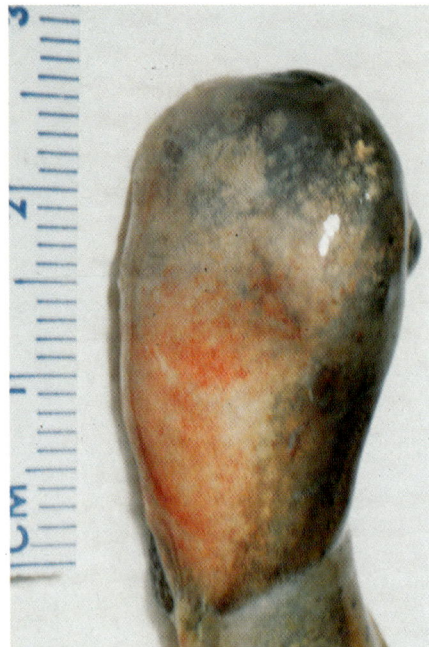

Plate 27.4. Acute red leglike syndrome in a tadpole of the green frog, *Rana clamitans*. The ventral body shows disseminated erythema of the skin and moderate swelling. *Aeromonas hydrophila* was isolated from the coelom. (D.E. Green)

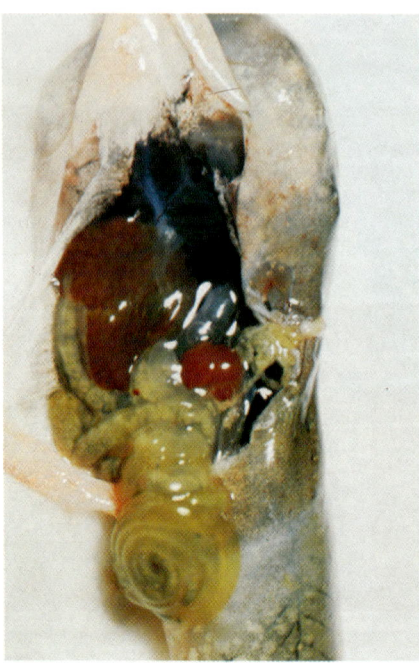

Plate 27.5. Same tadpole as in Plate 27.4. Note the enlarged and bright red spleen (splenomegaly), and minute petechia in the serosa of the intestine. (D.E. Green)

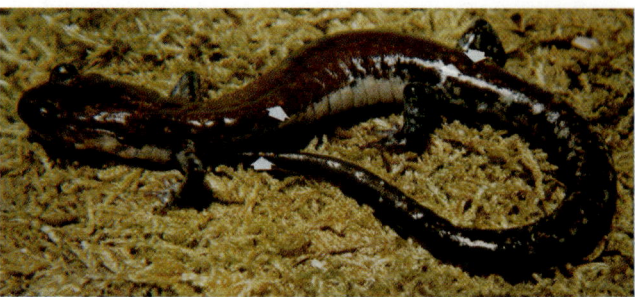

Plate 27.6. Nymphal chigger infection (*Hannemania dunni*) in a wild Rich Mountain salamander, *Plethodon ouachitae*. Note the bright red slightly raised nodules in the skin of the back and tail (arrows). (Scott Highton)

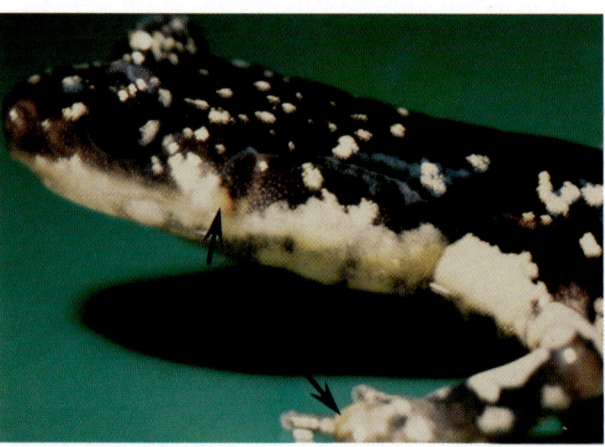

Plate 27.7. Nymphal chigger infection (*Hannemania dunni*) in a wild Fourche Mountain salamander, *Plethodon fourchensis*. Note the raised red nodules caused by the nymphs burrowing in webs between the toes and on the cheek (arrows). (D.E. Green)

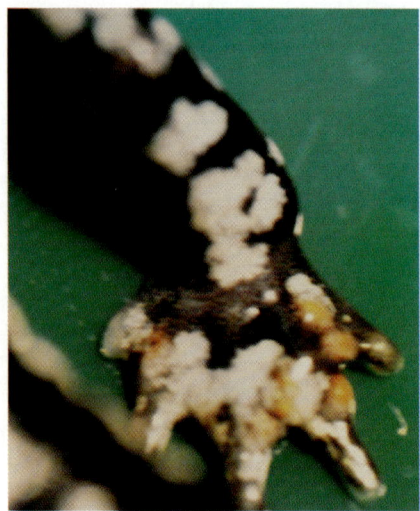

Plate 27.8. Same animal as Plate 27.7. Numerous raised red nodules in the toe webs are caused by *Hannemania dunni*. These lesions were present for over 3 months. (D.E. Green)

CHAPTER 18

IDIOPATHIC SYNDROMES

Kevin M. Wright, DVM

Despite aggressive diagnostic efforts, the underlying etiology of an amphibian's illness may remain unknown. The necropsy may yield essentially normal results, or results that are in conflict with the findings from amphibians with similar-appearing clinical signs. There are several idiopathic syndromes that have received considerable attention, and while some may yield to classification within standard pathologic etiologies (i.e., nutritional, infectious, etc.), undoubtedly other idiopathic syndromes will be encountered and reported as interest in amphibian medicine expands.

18.1 SPINDLY LEG

Many captive anuran larvae fail to metamorphose properly or die shortly after metamorphosis is complete. In some instances there are obvious anatomic deformities that would seem to decrease survival. Some of these deformities have been so prevalent in captive anuran breeding programs that they are often called spindly leg or spindly leg syndrome, although the phrase skeletal and muscular underdevelopment (SMUD) is preferred by some (Hakvoort & Gouda, 1995). Spindly leg syndrome is described solely from captive anurans while postmetamorphic death syndrome (described below) has only been applied to wild anurans, although there are similarities between the two syndromes. It is likely that multiple etiologies are involved in both syndromes, and these may be overlapping terms. The relative abundance of frog propagation in captivity, especially dendrobatids, when compared to the successful propagation of all salamanders and caecilians combined has inextricably linked spindly leg syndrome with anurans, although it was recently noted in the metamorph of a crocodile newt, *Tylototriton shanjing*, at the Philadelphia Zoo. Furthermore, although caecilians lack limbs, there may be failures in their anatomic development during the transitional stage from larva to adult. The complexity involved in the proper sequencing of metamorphosis is not elucidated well, and failures at any point for any reason may result in metamorph defects (For a review of normal and abnormal metamorphosis, see Etkin & Gilbert, 1968; Weber, 1965a; Weber, 1965b). Known interrupters of metamorphosis include antibiotics (presumably interfering with cyanocobalamine production by gastrointestinal flora although a direct action is known for actinomycin D), goitrogenic substances, and various toxins. The etiology for a birth defect such as phocomelus (flipper foot) in humans is multifactorial, and, using humans as a model for amphibian disease, it seems highly likely that spindly leg syndrome is a panoply of diseases with a common gross pathology.

The classic development of spindly leg syndrome in a dendrobatid begins with an apparently healthy tadpole sprouting hindlegs (For normal development see Plates 18.1, 18.2, 18.3, 18.4). The hindlegs may be normal, but generally by the time the foreleg buds appear the hindlegs exhibit valgus or varus deformity or both (Plates 18.5, 18.6). One or both of the forelegs may fail to erupt, and the developing foreleg will be extremely thin and delicate, hence the term "spindly leg." If it survives the metamorphosis, the froglet usually dies within a few days. The stomach is usually empty at necropsy, although whether this is the result of an inability to pursue prey, to ingest prey, or both, is unclear. Histopathologic reports of spindly leg victims are poorly documented, as is the incidence of spindly leg in wild populations of anurans.

There are several factors that have been implicated in the malformation of limbs in froglets: nutrition (tadpole, parents), genetics (inbreeding, line senescence, interspecific hybridization, interracial hybridization), environment (toxins, crowding, low dissolved oxygen, illumination), and trauma. Little attention has been focused on the milieu of the egg and its link to spindly leg, for seemingly all the attention has been focused on the posthatching husbandry.

The link between diet and the development of spindly leg is fairly clear, yet the exact nutrients involved are undefined. It seems likely that a deficiency of one or more of the B vitamins can cause spindly leg in the African clawed frog, *Xenopus laevis* (Pollack & Liebig, 1989), dendrobatids, and some hylids. Supplementation of the water with B complex is recommended for egg and larvae unless there is evidence to suggest otherwise (see Chapter 7, Nutritional Disorders).

Tadpoles fed one diet can develop normally, yet clutchmates will develop spindly leg if fed a different diet or if the parents are on a different diet (e.g., Davies, 1993; Peaker, 1993; Powell, 1993). Given the reliance on manufactured fish foods, this can be frustrating as the nutritional composition of most brands, if available, is considered proprietary information and inaccessible. Furthermore, these fish foods are similar to dog foods in that the nutritional analysis listed on the package is not a guarantee of the actual ingredients but is rather a guarantee of minimum levels of broad classes of nutrients, therefore the exact levels of fat, crude protein, vitamins, and minerals can vary significantly between batches. The ratio of nutrients available and the timing of its uptake by the fetus drastically influence the fetal development. This batch variability may be the result of failures between cohorts as might the degradation of nutrients within the food with time. Batch variability may be an underlying factor for some of the anecdotes concerning the influence of genetics and parental reproductive senescence on the development of spindly leg in cohorts produced over the course of a parent frog's lifetime. Thus the recipe used by one herpetoculturist, although a good starting point, is no guarantee of success for another herpetoculturist, and the clinician is advised to avoid errant promises to the client about a particular diet being the spindly leg panacea.

One herpetoculturist reported the complete elimination of spindly leg in the offspring of a group of the dyeing poison frog, *Dendrobates tinctorius,* upon the addition of "iodine nibbles for caged birds" to the water of the tadpoles and dusted onto the diet of the parent frogs (Halfpenny, 1992) (see Section 16.8, Halogens, for discussion of iodine toxicosis). This report and others (e.g., Davies, 1993; Peaker, 1993) supports the hypothesis that the nutrition of the parent frogs is also linked to the development of spindly leg. The female frog invests considerable energy (i.e., nutrient stores such as fat and vitamins) in the development of the egg and associated yolk and gel capsule. A diet lacking in a critical nutrient will result in an egg that may not support proper embryonic growth. The nutrition of the male is often overlooked given the relative contributions of the egg cytoplasm to the sperm cytoplasm, but undoubtedly the sperm resultant from malnutrition can be lacking in enzymes and other critical factors necessary for embryonic development. Thus a varied diet with vitamin and mineral supplementation is recommended for the prospective parents. Any illness should be fully resolved and all weight gained back prior to attempting breeding.

The genetic link of spindly leg is also supported in that the offspring from one parental group consistently developed spindly leg when raised contemporaneously with the offspring of another parental group (Powell, 1993). This raises the possibility of interspecific hybridization, a likely possibility given the taxonomic uncertainty of many amphibian species (e.g., generic status of dendrobatid frogs is in question) and the lack of locality data for many captive specimens. The diploid/triploid status of the North American gray treefrog complex (*Hyla versicolor* × *H. chrysocoelius*) is illustrative of the difficulties that may exist in other taxons. These two species are visually identical but have different chromosomal numbers as well as different vocalizations. Thus the females of this species can only be distinguished on a cytopathological level. The North American slimy salamander complex (*Plethodon glutinosus*) is another documented problematical group, virtually indistinguishable on a gross phenotypic level. It is likely that several other species complexes exist, and the result of interspecific hybridization may be spindly leg syndrome or other developmental abnormalities. Other possibilities include line senescence and inbreeding. Some female dendrobatid frogs have produced normal offspring over the course of 5 years or more and simply started producing fewer eggs or gelatinous capsules without ova as they aged, yet spindly leg of the offspring was not noted. This is not to discount this possibility, only to suggest that it is probably a rarer etiology for this syndrome than many others discussed. Inbreeding over ten generations or more has not increased the incidence of spindly leg in groups of the dyeing poison frog, *Dendrobates tinctorius,* so inbreeding as an etiology for spindly leg in lower generations (e.g., F1 offspring) seems unlikely.

Exposure to toxins, low oxygen, suboptimal temperatures, and teratogens may promote the development of spindly leg. One study of the spotted salamander, *Ambystoma maculatum,* demonstrated a clear link between elevated temperatures and a smaller size of newly hatched larvae, as well as death of embryoes at inappropriately low temperatures (Ross, 1993). Water quality and environmental parameters should always be assessed when spindly leg is detected.

Prototheca algae have been implicated as an agent retarding tadpole growth, but the exact correlation is subject to debate (Beebee, 1995; Petranka, 1995).

It is likely that viral infections and other infectious diseases can interfere with the normal development of larvae. Histopathology and culture efforts for a broad spectrum of disease agents are needed to elucidate these as underlying causes.

The effect of spacial restrictions on the development of tadpoles is documented. Crowded conditions will result in slower tadpole growth, delayed metamorphosis, and smaller animals at metamorphosis (Wilbur, 1977). It should be noted that cannibalism is not an infrequent result of crowding, especially in carnivorous larvae such as salamander larvae. The wild populations of some species routinely have cannibalistic morphs among clutches. Thus attention should be given to the needs of each species, and when in doubt raise the offspring in isolation with as much room as is practical.

Illumination has been investigated as an influence on growth of fish and amphibians since the 1880s. This is a problematic issue as the optimal spectral needs of all species held in captivity are unknown. There are reports of techniques that work, but the link to the lighting has not been unequivocally proven (e.g., Rugh, 1935). In some instances, it is the lighting that promotes algal growth which the tadpoles feed upon and thus is not a true spectral effect.

Traumatic injuries to the tail of tadpoles of the firebelly toad, *Bombina orientalis,* have been demonstrated to have serious consequences for the subsequent development throughout metamorphosis (Parichy & Kaplan, 1992). Although this study does not demonstrate a clear link to spindly leg syndrome, the time till metamorphosis was prolonged and the size of the froglets after metamorphosis were smaller than in the larvae that did not have any injuries. Unlimited access to high quality food mediated the effects somewhat, as did a high maternal investment (i.e., large yolk amount). A study on larvae of the bullfrog, *Rana catesbeiana,* demonstrated similar consequences as a result of tail injury. Undoubtedly the investment needed for a larval amphibian to recover from even minor injuries (i.e., those injuries undetected by the herpetoculturist or veterinarian) will have potentially deleterious effects on metamorphosis, and this diversion of energy, protein, and other nutrients may alter the normal development of the larvae. An interesting study would be to compare the incidence of spindly leg in anurans raised under "rougher" conditions (e.g., the dump-and-fill water changing system used for some dendrobatids) to those raised in undisturbed conditions (e.g., left tended by parents or raised in a chamber with filtered water).

18.2 POSTMETAMORPHIC DEATH SYNDROME

There have been die-offs of ranid and bufonid metamorphs in certain free-ranging populations. The western toad, *Bufo boreas,* the Yosemite toad, *B. canorus,* and the Wyoming toad, *B. hemiophrys baxteri,* appear to have lower mortality rates than noted for the Tarahumara leopard frog, *Rana tarahumarae,* and the Chirichua leopard frog, *R. chiricahuensis.* The metamorphs are without reported anatomic abnormalities, suggestive of an infectious disease. No organisms have as yet been reported in these die-offs, and the phrase postmetamorphic death syndrome (PDS) has been applied to these circumstances (Scott, 1993). Key features of this syndrome are the fact that the majority of the metamorphs die within a brief span of time, although it may not affect all areas inhabited by a given taxon's popualtion. Cold weather is linked to outbreaks of PDS, and breeding adults as well as tadpoles and metamorphs are affected. Closely related species may be spared the disease. Complete viral, bacterial, fungal, parasitological, and toxicological studies are needed, but given the species-specificity of PDS it seems likely that a pathogen rather than a toxin is involved. Chytridiomycosis is currently considered a likely etiology. The link between this syndrome and that of spindly leg syndrome is tentative, but it is likely that both syndromes have multifactorial and possible overlapping etiologies.

18.3 GOUT

Articular and periarticular gout has been reported in an African bullfrog, *Tomopterna (Pyxicephalus) delalandii* (Frye, 1989; Frye & Williams, 1995). The reported clinical sign was a swollen pollux that was discolored and painful upon palpation. A wet mount of material expressed from the swelling revealed urate crystals. The digit was amputated and submitted for histopathology. A chronic inflammatory response was seen surrounding urate crystals. The frog remained healthy a minimum of 2.5 years following the amputation. The etiology for this incident of gout remains unknown. The diet reported was typical for this species in captive collections and included crickets, goldfish, and mice. It is tempting to speculate that there may be a defect in the protein metabolism of this particular anuran that interfered with the transport and clearance of certain proteins contained within these domestic prey items that are not present in the natural diet of this species, but given the solitary nature of the lesion and the survival of the patient after surgery this seems unlikely, or at best an incomplete explanation.

Renal gout and bladder stones are sporadically encountered in uricotelic anurans following prolonged periods of dehydration, exposure to xeric to mesic conditions, and possibly from ingesting prey that have fed upon oxalate-containing plants (see Chapter 7, Nutritional Disorders). Urinary bladder calculi designated calcium hydroxylapatite were noted in the green and golden bell frog, *Litoria aurea* (Richardson & Truscoe, 1963). The author is aware of several cases of renal gout or bladder stones in specimens of the painted-belly monkey frog, *Phyllomedusa sauvagii*, held in zoos and private collections, as well as other phyllomedusine frogs. Exploratory celiotomy has been performed to remove the bladder stone. Survival postoperatively is over 3 months, although in one case the frog succumbed to a second stone that developed (personal communication, W. Brant, 1995). Specimens of the painted-belly monkey frog, *Phyllomedusa sauvagii*, kept under more humid conditions have yet to develop this condition (personal communication, A. Snider, 1996). Supportive care for the gout patient should include unlimited access to water. The use of allopurinol in amphibians appears undocumented.

Aminoglycosides have not been a documented source of renal gout in amphibians at this time, but caution should be used when administering aminoglycosides to uricotelic species of amphibians. Prolonged followup of cases after aminoglycoside therapy is warranted by the clinician, given the extended length of time required prior to onset of clinical signs in reptiles, and the client should be asked to provide the body for necropsy in the event of death so that the histopathology of the kidneys and joints may be documented.

18.4 MOLCHPEST

Molchpest is the term that was used to describe disease in European newts (Salamandridae) (Reichenbach-Klinke & Elkan, 1965). The initial sign reported was incomplete shedding or failure to consume shed skin. This is typically followed by development of lethargy, anorexia, and equilibrium problems. Shortly thereafter skin lesions develop. Hyperemia is noted, followed by small white nodules and edema. The disease is invariably fatal. Until further work is published, molchpest is not considered a valid disease by this author, for the signs described are typical for the progression of a variety of infectious diseases in salamanders.

18.5 EDEMA SYNDROME

Edema syndrome refers to the development of hydrops and generalized subcutaneous fluid in amphibians, and this syndrome is often the result of a bacterial infection or other infectious process that affects the skin's ability to maintain water homeostasis (see *Edema Syndrome* in Section 13.3.1, Bacterial Dermatosepticemia). However, there are other possible etiologies for this syndrome including but not limited to ovarian neoplasia, hepatic failure, renal failure, malnutrition (hypoproteinemia), and osmotic imbalance such as exposure to water with low dissolved solutes (e.g., distilled water). Hypocalcemia may diminish the frequency and force of the lymph heart contractions and cause subcutaneous edema. The etiology behind some cases remains unknown. Specimens of the strawberry poison frog, *Dendrobates pumilio*, have developed edema syndrome which spontaneously resolved (Figures 18.1, 18.2), and this has been noted in several other anurans.

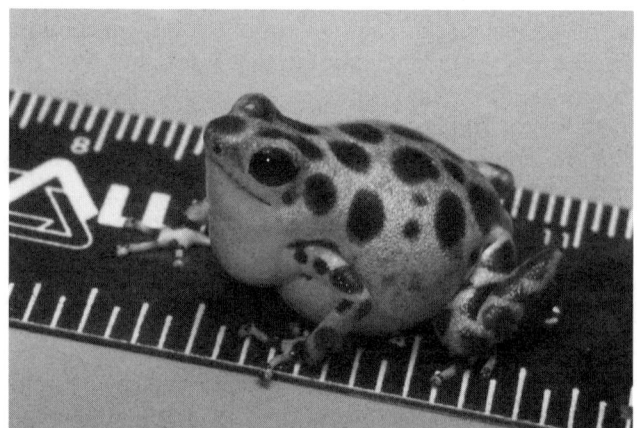

Figure 18.1. Spontaneously resolving edema syndrome of unknown etiology in a strawberry poison frog, *Dendrobates pumilio*. (George Grall, National Aquarium in Baltimore)

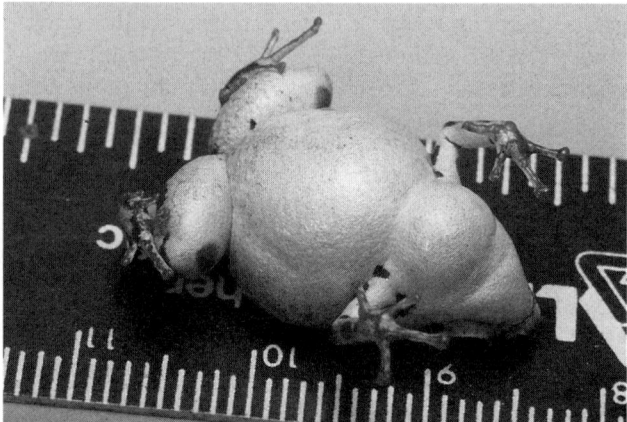

Figure 18.2. Ventral view of spontaneously resolving edema syndrome of unknown etiology in a strawberry poison frog, *Dendrobates pumilio*. (George Grall, National Aquarium in Baltimore)

Horn frogs, *Ceratophrys* spp., are often noted to have subcutaneous edema with or without hydrocoelom. This may serve as a fluid reserve for this and other frogs, but often it is linked to a problem such as metabolic bone disease and concomitant hypocalcemia (presumably due to alteration of the lymph heart function), acute bacterial infection, renal failure, hepatic failure (low plasma protein), or exposure to water with low dissolved solutes (often suggested by low levels of plasma sodium and/or potassium and protein). Supportive care should include bathing the frog in electrolyte solutions such as amphibian Ringer's solution along with treatment of the underlying etiology if known (see Section 24.9, Maintaining the Electrolyte Balance of the Ill Amphibian).

Localized edema has been noted in a number of anurans (Figures 18.3, 18.4). This often is indicative of paralyzation of the lymph heart that drains a given area, as may happen with curare and other toxins. The lymph heart may be damaged by rough handling, purposeful injection, and trauma. Obstruction of the lymph heart outflow is another possible cause of localized edema. Oxalate crystals, uric acid crystals (gout), protozoal cysts, filarid nematodes, abscesses, tumors, and scar tissue may decrease the size of the lymphatic channel. Aspiration of the lymph fluid for analysis may prove useful. The fluid can be examined by light microscopy for the presence of crystals, bacteria, fungi, protozoa, metazoa, or inflammatory or neoplastic cells. The chemistries of the lymph can be compared to the plasma of the amphibian. If the lymph shows an elevated uric acid level with respect to the plasma, or if both fluids have a high uric acid level, this suggests gout as a possible underlying etiology. Elevated CPK levels may suggest an acute traumatic injury. Providing that the etiology of the obstruction is not representative of a dangerous underlying condition (i.e., oxalate toxicosis), most amphibians survive quite well with these localized fluid accumulations which may even spontaneously regress.

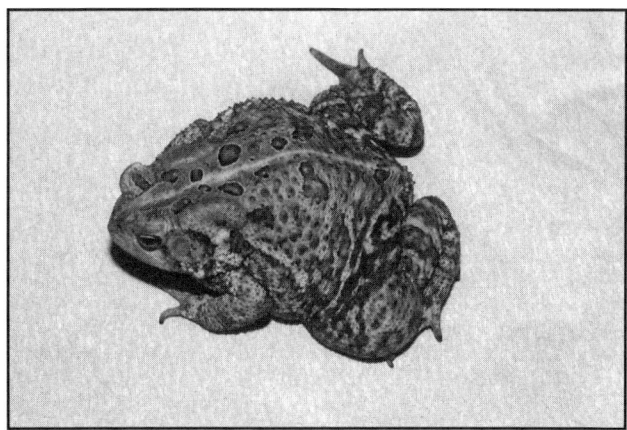

Figure 18.4. American toad, *Bufo americanus*, with localized edema of its hindlimb. (Steve Barten)

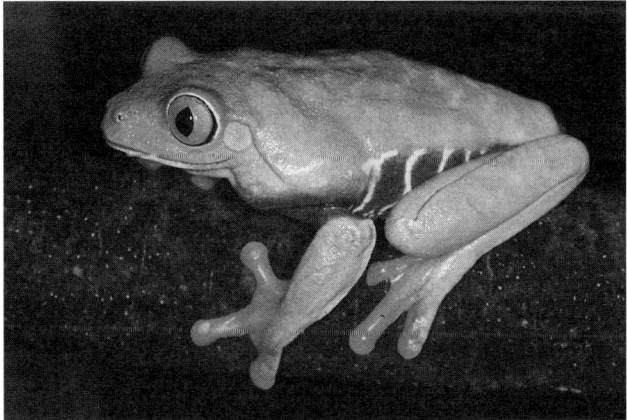

Figure 18.3. Red-eyed treefrog, *Agalychnis callidryas*, with localized edema. (Steve Barten)

Hydrocoelom has been reported in tadpoles infected with various strains of ranaviruses (e.g., tadpole edema virus) and in larvae with surgically extirpated pronephroi (Fox, 1963). Hydrocoelom is regularly encountered in tadpoles if sufficient numbers are examined, but rarely is the pathogenesis demonstrated. Induced ovulation in frogs may result in eggs that are insufficiently invested with capsules and therefore the developing tadpoles are much more prone to imbibe water and develop hydrocoelom (Reichenbach-Klinke & Elkan, 1965).

18.6 RECTAL, CLOACAL, AND GASTRIC PROLAPSE

The underlying cause for prolapse of rectal, gastric or cloacal tissue is often unknown (Plates 18.7, 18.8, 18.9). Hypocalcemia, gastrointestinal impaction or obstruction, parasitism, and toxins are among the more common etiologies. These conditions are considered a surgical emergency (see Section 21.5.6, Cloacal and Rectal Prolapse).

REFERENCES

Beebee, T.J.C. 1995. Tadpole growth: Is there an interference effect in nature? Herpetological Journal 5:204–205.

Davies, B. 1993. More on spindly-leg. British Dendrobatid Group Newsletter 15 as reprinted in American Dendrobatid Group Newsletter 12: 3–4.

Etkin, W. and L.I. Gilbert. 1968. Metamorphosis, a Problem in Developmental Biology. Appleton-Century-Crofts, New York, 459 pp.

Fox, H. 1963. The amphibian pronephros. Quarterly Review of Biology 38.1–25.

Frye, F.L. 1989. Periarticular gout in a pixie frog, *Pyxicephalus delandii*. Abstracts of the Third International Colloquium on the Pathology of Reptiles and Amphibians, p. 108.

Frye, F.L. and D.L. Williams. 1995. Self-Assessment Color Review of Reptiles and Amphibians. Iowa State University Press, Ames, IA, pp. 27–28.

Hakvoort, H. and E. Gouda. 1995. Skeletal and muscular underdevelopment (SMUD) in Dendrobatidae. Herpetopathologica (Proceedings of the Fifth International Colloquium on Pathology of Reptiles and Amphibians), pp. 271–275.

Halfpenny, S. 1992. Spindly-leg syndrome. British Dendrobatid Group Newsletter #13 as reprinted in American Dendrobatid Society Newsletter 12:1–2.

Parichy, D.M. and R.H. Kaplan. 1992. Developmental consequences of tail injury on larvae of the oriental fire-bellied toad, *Bombina orientalis*. Copeia 1992(1):129–137.

Peaker, M. 1993. More on spindly leg disease. American Dendrobatid Group Newsletter 12:2–3.

Petranka, J.W. 1995. Interference competition in tadpoles: Are multiple agents involved? Herpetological Journal 5:206–207.

Pollack, E.D. and V. Liebig. 1989. An induced developmental disorder of limbs and motor neurons in *Xenopus*. American Zoologist 29:163A.

Powell, C.L. 1993. Conformation of adult frogs causing spindly-leg in tadpoles. American Dendrobatid Group Newsletter 12:4–5.

Reichenbach-Klinke, H. and E. Elkan. 1965. Syndromes from various causes, *in* Diseases of Amphibians. TFH Publications, Inc., Neptune City, NJ, pp. 358–367.

Richardson, L.R. and R. Truscoe. 1963. Vesical calculus in the frog *Hyla aurea*. Trans. Roy. Soc. N.Z. Zool. 3(1):1–3 as cited in Reichenbach-Klinke, H. and E. Elkan. 1965. Diseases of Amphibians, TFH Publications, Inc., Neptune City, NJ, pp. 366.

Ross, S.R. 1993. Effect of temperature on body size, developmental stage, and timing of hatching in *Ambystoma maculatum*. Journal of Herpetology 27(3):329–333.

Rugh, R. 1935. The spectral effect on the growth rate of tadpoles. Physiological Zoology 8:186–195.

Scott, N.J. 1993. Postmetamorphic death syndrome. FROGLOG 7:1–2.

Weber, R. 1965a. The Biochemistry of Animal Development, Vol.1 Descriptive Biochemistry of Animal Development. Academic Press, New York, 648 pp.

Weber, R. 1965b. The Biochemistry of Animal Development, Vol. 2 Biochemical Control Mechanisms and Adaptations in Development. Academic Press, New York, 481 pp.

Wilbur, H.M. 1977. Density-dependent aspects of growth and metamorphosis in *Bufo americanus*. Ecology 58:196–200.

CHAPTER 19
THE AMPHIBIAN EYE

Brent R. Whitaker, MS, DVM

19.1 INTRODUCTION

The amphibian eye has long been the subject of many anatomical and functional studies. With the exception of corneal lipidosis, relatively little has been written on the diseases that affect the amphibian eye. In most cases of corneal and lenticular disease, the etiology of such lesions remains unknown. Ocular lesions may be the result of either primary or secondary disease. An understanding of ocular anatomy, techniques used to examine the eye, commonly observed lesions, and appropriate therapeutic usage is therefore helpful in formulating the overall clinical approach to ocular disease in amphibians.

19.2 ANATOMY

Amphibians by definition live at least part of their life closely associated with water. While some are truly aquatic, others spend the majority of their life on land. Adaptations enabling the transition between water and land have therefore evolved. Most aquatic and all larval amphibians lack eyelids. Obligatory neotenic salamanders never develop functional lids, while subterranean species acquire lids that degenerate. Many adult salamanders, however, have well developed, movable lids. Most anurans that become land dwelling at metamorphosis develop short lids and a translucent false nictitating membrane that protects the eye. The upper lid is a thick fold of integument while the lower lid is thin, often translucent, and folded upon itself (Plate 19.1). The latter, referred to as the nictitating membrane, is connected to both ends of the upper lid so that when the globe is retracted it is pulled tightly over the cornea. As the eye returns, the membrane is folded with the help of a special muscle that arises from the levator bulbi (Noble, 1954). In other animals such as the red-eyed treefrog, *Agalychnis callidryas*, the membrane forms a net which camouflages its colorful eye while allowing vision through it (Figure 19.1). While a Harderian gland and superior eyelid margin gland are found in most species of amphibians, the nasolacrimal duct is absent.

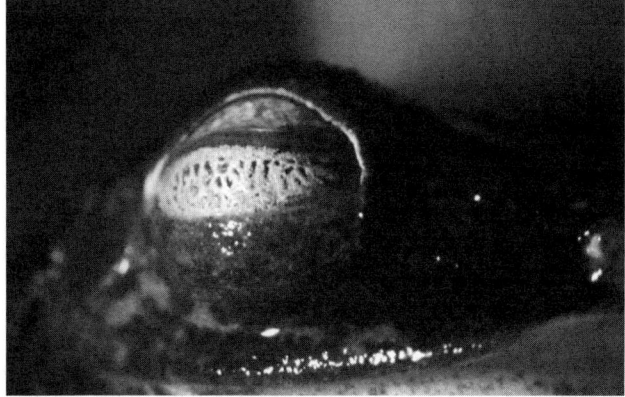

Figure 19.1. The eyelid of the red-eyed treefrog, *Agalychnis callidryas*, provides protection and camouflage of its brightly colored eye while allowing vision. (Wilmer Photography, Johns Hopkins University)

A powerful retractor bulbi muscle provides added protection as it pulls the globe back into the orbit. Anurans posses a large, membranous orbit which has a very poorly developed lacrimal bone. Because the circumorbital bones, and interorbital septum have been modified or have disappeared completely (Prince, 1956), the globe is separated from the buccal cavity by only a thin membrane. The eye is therefore actively pulled into the pharynx by the retractor bulbi muscle when swallowing food or providing protection for the globe. Another muscle, the levator bulbi, returns the eye to its prior position. No other movement of the eye occurs as the remaining extraocular muscles are vestigial.

The amphibian globe is spherical (Figure 19.2). Unlike the cornea of fish, which has the same refractive index as water, the cornea of the terrestrial amphibian acts as a dioptic focusing structure. The amphibian cornea is analogous to that of other vertebrates with a multicellular epithelium, stroma, descemets membrane, and single cell layer endothelium. Two Asian giant salamanders, *Andrias davidianus* and *A. japonicus*, show unusual stromal vascularization, the significance of which is unknown. While the sclera of the salamander is fibrous, that of the adult anuran

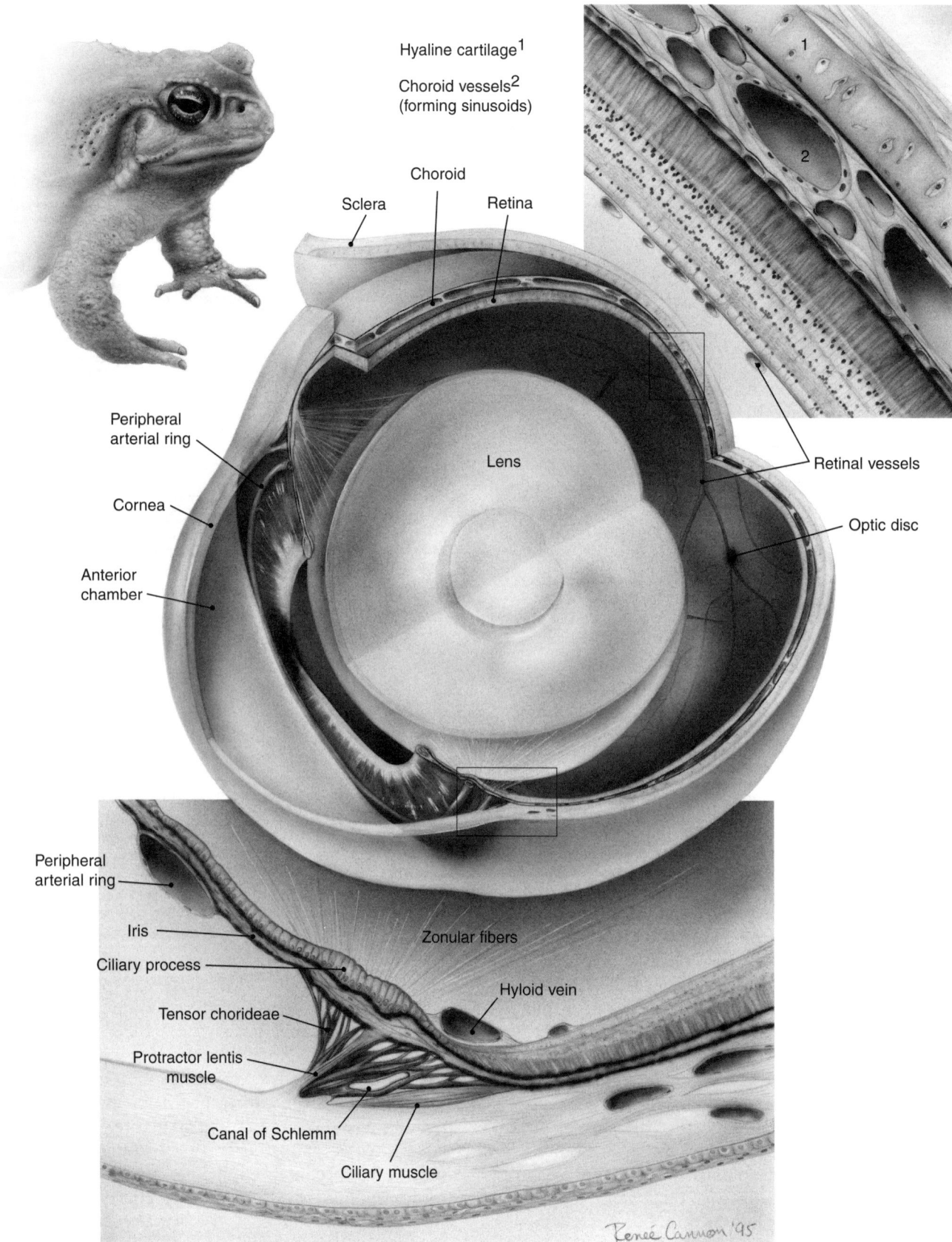

Figure 19.2. Ocular anatomy of the giant toad, *Bufo marinus*. (Reneé Cannon, Johns Hopkins University Department of Art as Applied to Medicine)

includes a posterior cup of hyaline cartilage extending from the posterior pole to the equator, and in some cases an anterior ring of scleral bone. These modifications provide the eye with needed protection from food items passing through the buccal cavity.

The iris is often iridescent as a result of the many colors produced by melanophores, carotenoid pigments, and guanine crystals. Pupils are found in a variety of shapes. Like fish, the iris of many amphibians has a vertical inferior stripe thought to be a remnant of the fetal cleft (Mann, 1931) (Figure 19.3). Vasculature of the iris is easily viewed as it protrudes through the anterior mesothelium and appears to sit on the surface (Walls, 1942). Myoepithelial cells in some may constrict autonomically when stimulated by light, while the pupillary light reflexes under conscious control are sluggish and not a good measure of light response.

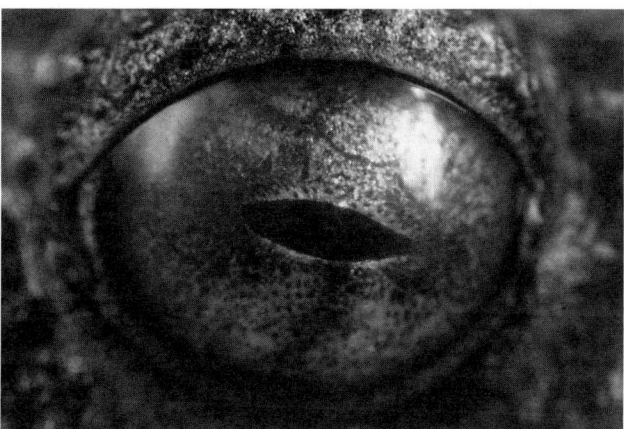

Figure 19.3. Nonspecific superficial keratitis in the tungara frog, *Physalaemus pustulatus*. The inferior vertical stripe is easily seen in this species. (George Grall, National Aquarium in Baltimore)

The amphibian lens lies directly behind the iris where it is held in place by radiating fibers which extend from the edge of the lens to the ciliary body. Except for some larval amphibians, the lens is not completely spherical due to a flattened anterior surface which is more pronounced in anurans than urodeles (Noble, 1954). Flattening of the lens at metamorphosis increases the distance to the overlying cornea thus making the animal farsighted, an advantage lost in water due to turbidity. Accommodation is achieved by contraction of the protractor lentis muscle, which originates from the corneal periphery and inserts into the ciliary body. Anurans have both a dorsal and ventral protractor lentis while salamanders have only a ventral muscle. Unlike reptiles and birds which alter the shape of their lens to focus, amphibians contract the protractor lentis muscle moving the entire lens forward thus allowing for distant vision. Drainage of the aqueous humor occurs through the iridocorneal angle. Dorsal and ventral ciliary venous sinuses are present (Williams & Whitaker, 1994).

The vitreous humor is a clear, gelatinous, connective tissue that fills the space between the posterior lens and the retina. In anurans, the avascular retina is nourished by choroidal capillary plexuses and the membrana vasculosa retinae which lies between the retina and the vitreous, and may be viewed using an opthalmoscope. Salamanders do not possess a membrana vasculosa retinae, but many have a pecten (Michaelson, 1954).

The amphibian retina is similar to that of other animals in general structure and includes the internal limiting membrane at the vitreoretinal junction, the ganglion cell layer, the inner plexiform layer, the inner nuclear layer, the outer plexiform layer, the outer nuclear layer, the photoreceptors, and the outer pigmented epithelium. Anurans have at least four different photoreceptors: the single cone, the double cone, the red rod and the green rod. Green rods are unique to amphibians although caecilians, and some subterranean and obligate neotenic salamanders lack them (Duellman & Trueb, 1994; Prince, 1956). In bufonids, hylids and possibly other nocturnal frogs, oil droplets may be found within the cones (Walls, 1942). Sudden exposure to bright light causes the iris to constrict, albeit slowly, and the retinal pigment epithelial cells to send out processes that further protect the rods and cones. Concurrent elongation of the cones, contraction of the rods for optimum exposure to light, and regression of the pigment cells are present in the dark-adapted eye (Noble, 1954).

19.3 CLINICAL EVALUATION

A thorough examination of the amphibian eye is an important component of health assessment. Bilateral ocular changes are often indicative of systemic disease while unilateral changes may implicate a local condition. The sudden, partial loss of red iridal pigment in both eyes of the red-eyed treefrog, *Agalychnis callidryas,* for example has been associated with terminal disease although the mechanisms causing this observation are unknown (Plate 19.2). Before handling, the clinician should attempt to observe the amphibian's conformation, behavior, and mobility in its own environment. Visual impairment may be determined by watching the animal as it attempts to feed. The body, eyes, and head should be symmetrical and in proper proportion. Because the oral cavity is separated from the globe by a thin membrane, it is especially important to check this area for signs of trauma, foreign bodies or inflammation (Plate 19.3). Handling can be very stressful to the animal and can result in the rupture of iridal vessels (Plate 19.4). The exam should be concluded immediately and the animal returned to its habitat.

A focal light source, such as a penlight, ophthalmoscope or slit lamp, as well as magnification are necessary for proper examination. Pupillary light reflexes are sluggish at best and are generally not useful in the assessment of neuro-ophthalmic function. A slit lamp provides illumination, excellent magnification, and accurate location and depth of lesions commonly observed in the cornea, anterior chamber, iris, and lens (Figure 19.4).

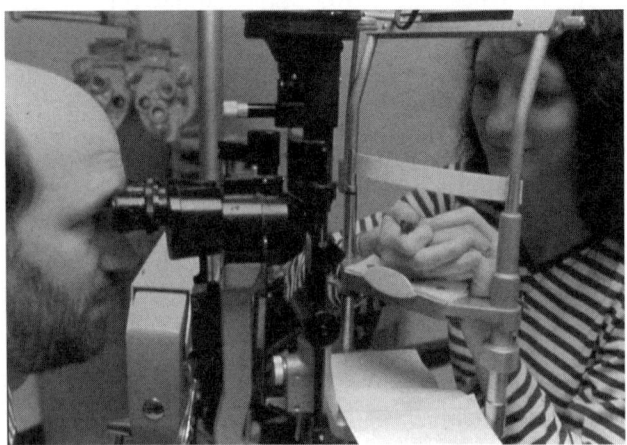

Figure 19.4. A slit lamp provides illumination, excellent magnification, and accurate location and depth of lesions observed in the cornea, anterior chamber, iris, and lens in the smallest of amphibian patients such as this dendrobatid frog. (Wilmer Photography, Johns Hopkins University)

The pupillary sphincter muscles are striated and therefore nonresponsive to parasympatholytic drugs such as atropine. Mydriasis may be attained using a combination of the muscle relaxant D-tubocurarine and benzalkonium chloride as a carrier topically, but the dilutions used and contact time needed for mydriasis have not been established. The commonly available dilutions of D-tubocurarine have not been effective in selected anuran species. Rarely, an intracameral injection of D-tubocurarine, succinyl choline or vecuronium may be used, and is best achieved in amphibians anesthetized with tricaine methanesulfonate. Due to the potential toxicity and empirical dosing of these drugs, pupillary dilatation is not commonly performed unless there is a specific indication to do so.

Corneal disease may be defined using special stains such as fluorescein to demarcate loss of epithelium and ulceration. This water-soluble dye is not absorbed by the healthy cornea due to the high lipid content of the epithelium. Once this protective layer has been compromised, however, the stain readily adheres to the underlying water-soluble stroma imparting a fluorescent green color to the eye. Care should be taken to completely wash all excess stain off the animal using sterile saline. While large defects are easily seen, smaller ones are better evaluated in a dimly lit room using a cobalt blue light and magnification. This allows the clinician to differentiate fluorescein dye that has adhered to a roughened cornea or mucus from true erosions. Rose Bengal stain highlights devitalized epithelial cells of the cornea and conjunctiva. Conditions that alter the normal metabolism of these cells, such as keratoconjunctivitis sicca, cause retention of this stain.

Impression smears may further define corneal disease. This is accomplished by lightly touching several dry, methanol-cleaned glass slides to the lesion. Both Gram and Wright-Giemsa stains may show bacteria, fungi, and/or parasites as well as cells associated with specific disease processes. A light corneal scraping in the anesthetized amphibian using the back of a scalpel blade or a Kimura spatula may also produce material for cytological examination. Samples of intraocular fluid may be obtained under anesthesia using a 25–30 gauge needle directed into either the anterior or posterior chamber. A small drop of cyanoacrylate glue may be used to seal the site of entry. Bacterial and fungal organisms are commonly identified through cytology and culture.

19.4 OCULAR DISEASE

Ocular disease is common in amphibians. Etiologies most commonly include metabolic, nutritional, infectious, traumatic, and environmental factors. With the exception of cave-dwelling animals, most terrestrial amphibians depend upon vision to capture prey. The development of cataracts, corneal opacities, or other conditions that impair their sight most often result in starvation and eventual death. For these reasons, amphibians that present with ocular disease are often thin as they are unable to efficiently capture their prey.

19.4.1 Panophthalmitis and Uveitis

Panophthalmitis or uveitis is often associated with systemic disease (Plate 19.5). Red leg syndrome, which is caused by ubiquitous Gram-negative organisms such as *Aeromonas hydrophila,* frequently causes infection of the eyes as well as other tissues. Conjunctivitis has been seen in septicemic frogs. Ocular lesions may include corneal edema, scleritis, hyphema, hypopyon, iridocyclitis, cataract, chorioretinitis, and anterior chamber fibrin deposits (Millichamp, 1991; Williams & Whitaker, 1994). Periocular blood-filled blisters have also been noted in tadpoles (Glorioso et al., 1974). Intraocular inflammation is most likely a result of septic emboli disseminating to uveal vessels, bacterial toxins, and the host's immunological response (Brooks et al., 1983). Panophthalmitis is often associated with poor husbandry practices (Millichamp, 1991). Gram-positive organisms, such as B *Streptococcus* and fungi have been associated with uveitis in both fish and amphibia (Brooks et al., 1983).

19.4.2 Corneal Lipidosis

Corneal lipidosis or lipid keratopathy has been described in several species of hylid treefrog including the Cuban treefrog, *Osteopilus septentrionalis,* the veined treefrog, *Phrynohyas venulosa,* the Mexican leaf frog, *Pachymedusa dacnicolor,* White's treefrog, *Pelodryas caerulea,* and one leptodactylid frog, the Sabinal frog, *Leptodactylus melanonotus* (Dziezyc & Millichamp, 1989). This disease has also been observed in bufonids (personal communication, G. Crawshaw, 1996), the South American bullfrog, *Leptodactylus pentadactylus,* the New Granada cross-banded treefrog, *Smilisca phaeota,* and suspected in a tiger salamander, *Ambystoma tigrinum* (personal communication, K. Wright, 1996). Lesions associated with this degenerative disorder may vary in severity from focal, opaque corneal opacities within the superficial stroma to dense, raised, white plaques that invade both deep and superficial stroma. Early stages of this disease may be recognized as fine crystalline deposits that sparkle when examined with high magnification. Neovascularization and superficial pigmentation may develop as well as bullous keratopathy. Although the corneal stroma becomes thickened and irregular as the disease progresses (Plates 19.6, 19.7), the epithelium typically remains intact. Histopathologically, cholesterol clefts, granulocytes, melanocytes, and macrophages containing fat further characterize this disease as stromal degeneration and necrosis occur (Dziezyc & Millichamp, 1989). The formation of granulomas at the limbus, mineralization adjacent to Bowman's membrane, and endothelial cell vacuolation have also been observed (Williams & Whitaker, 1994). While often bilateral, these lesions are not necessarily symmetrical. Concurrently, cataracts have also been noted in some frogs (Zwart & van der Linde-Sipmand, 1989).

The etiology of corneal lipidosis remains unclear. The majority of frogs severely affected are mature females with developing eggs that have been in captivity three or more years. In some cases, a generalized xanthomatosis has been associated with the corneal lesions which is indicative of a metabolic disturbance (Millichamp, 1990). Xanthomas, which are white to yellow foci containing cholesterol, cholesterol esters, or other lipids, have been found in many soft tissues including the skin, brain, nerves, ovaries, gastric submucosa, liver, kidney, and lungs (Carpenter et al., 1986; Russell et al., 1990). Moderate to extreme hypercholesterolemia has also been associated with the formation of xanthomas. The severity of these lesions appears to be directly related to the degree and duration of elevated serum cholesterol (Russell et al., 1990). Serum biochemistries of some Cuban treefrogs, *Osteopilus septentrionalis,* show hypercholesterolemia of 600–800 mg/dl (Russell et al., 1990), and a South American bullfrog, *Leptodactylus pentadactylus,* consistently had hypercholesterolemia in excess of 1000 mg/dl (personal communication, K. Wright, 1996). Values for triglycerides, high density lipoproteins and low-density lipoproteins were 47–94 mg/dl, 22–80 mg/dl, and 62–702 mg/dl, respectively (Carpenter et al., 1986; Russell et al., 1990). Dietary composition may contribute, at least in part, to hypercholesterolemia. Lesions have developed in frogs given newborn mice containing high levels of maternally derived milk lipids. Alternatively, other frogs have developed similar lesions fed only mineral-supplemented crickets (Williams & Whitaker, 1994). The accumulation of cholesterol crystals within the cornea may also occur as a result of prior injury or inflammation. During the healing process newly formed blood vessels deposit cholesterol. Inherited dystrophies, toxicosis, or injury resulting in pathological changes to corneal cell metabolism may lead to the improper utilization of these lipids (personal communication, 1996, K. Corcoran). Examination of these animals may show evidence of corneal scarring and ghost vessels.

19.4.3 Keratitis

Corneal lipidosis must be differentiated from other corneal conditions which have been observed in a large number of captive frogs including hylids, dendrobatids, and leptodactylids. Frequently observed opacities range from subtle, diffuse clouding of the cornea to focal, vascularizing keratitis. The cause of these lesions is unknown and is most likely multifactorial. Environmental and nutritional factors, chronic disease affecting normal metabolic function, and immune mediated processes should be considered. Exposure to long periods of ultraviolet light used to prevent metabolic bone disease has been suspected in some cases of keratitis. Typically, a superficial keratopathy is noted grossly in one or both eyes. The "ground glass" appearance of the superiocentral opacities is best appreciated using a slit lamp (Plate 19.8). As this superficial circular keratitis progresses, the corneal surface may either remain smooth or become irregular. Mild neovascularization may develop as the disease progresses (Plate 19.9). Eventually, more of the cornea becomes involved and the animal's ability to capture prey is diminished to the point that death results from starvation or secondary systemic infection. Histopathology of corneal lesions show an accumulation of histiocytes and lymphocytes. To date, no effective treatment has been found.

Ulcerative keratitis has been noted on rare occasion in amphibians. Diagnosis of early or minor lesions may require the use of fluorescein. In some cases, trauma is suspected, unless bacterial and fungal organisms are found. Often however, the etiology is unknown. Despite treatment, ulceration in some cases may progress rapidly resulting in a descemetocele. This syndrome of corneal melting is similar to that seen in other species with collagenolytic ulcers. Once diagnosed, treatment should begin immediately after collecting diagnostic samples. Topical antibiotic and antifungal agents should be administered three to four times daily if possible. In refractory cases, the addition of a cyanoacrylate patch may provide protection while allowing healing to occur.

Vascularizing keratitis (pannus) has been detected in a captive ornate horned frog, *Ceratophrys ornata*, and other species (Williams & Whitaker, 1994). The vascularization can progress to impair vision. Etiology remains unknown, but infections and exposure to ultraviolet lighting are possible contributing factors.

19.4.4 Cataracts

Cataracts are occasionally observed and easily diagnosed (Plate 19.10). They may be described according to position as capsular, subcapsular, cortical, or nuclear, and by stage as either immature, intumescent, mature, or hypermature. The cause of their formation is not always clear, but appears to be associated with other disease processes that have infectious, toxic, parasitic, or nutritional etiologies. In some cases, cataract development may be associated with age (Figure 19.5). Environmental factors may also play a role as exposure to excessive sunlight and cold-induced precipitation of lens proteins have been documented to cause cataracts in fish and rats (Millichamp, 1991; Wilcock & Dukes, 1989). Dendrobatid frogs treated with 5% dextrose during systemic illness have developed cataracts which subsequently resolved once sugar supplements ceased. Removal of the lens has been accomplished in a dendrobatid frog and remains an option if necessary.

19.4.5 Parasites

Parasitic infection of the amphibian eye has been described (Etges, 1961, 1991; Flynn, 1973). The trematodes *Diplostomum scheuringi*, *D. flexicaudum*, and *Clinostomum attenuatum* have been found in the eye of adult anurans, sirens, newts, and tadpoles. Wild populations of the red-spotted newt, *Notophthalmus viridescens*, commonly harbor the fluke *Diplostomum scheuringi* with up to 100% of the animals infected. Cercaria that enter through the skin typically migrate to the brain. Upon penetration of the cornea, cercaria of this fluke are found unencysted in the vitreous, perhaps in an effort to reach the brain via the optic nerve. The lens remains unaffected by this metazoan (Flynn, 1973). Occasionally, migrating nematode larva may be found in the eye as they are in other tissues throughout the host.

19.4.6 Neoplasia

Neoplasia of ocular tissues is uncommon. Amphibians, in general, appear less susceptible to malignant neoplasia which in part may be due to their great ability to reconstruct normal tissues (Balls, 1962; Balls et al., 1989). Ocular neoplasia, however, should always be considered when presented with ocular or periocular lesions.

19.4.7 Glaucoma

Glaucoma in amphibians has rarely been reported. In one European common toad, *Bufo bufo*, it was necessary to suture the false nictitating membrane across the cornea as the animal could no longer fully retract its globe into the orbit (Williams & Whitaker, 1994). Similarly, there has been little recognition of retinal disease. In part, this is likely due to the lack of proper equipment, training, and routine ophthalmic examinations required to make a definitive diagnosis.

19.5 THERAPEUTIC CONSIDERATIONS

Once ocular disease has been recognized, a therapeutic strategy should be developed and implemented as quickly as possible. This plan may range from simple supportive care to aggressive medical therapy. Factors that should be considered are the disease process, the nutritional state of the animal, the species of amphibian and its reaction to frequent handling. Oral and/or injectable antibiotics should begin immediately when systemic disease or uveitis of bacterial

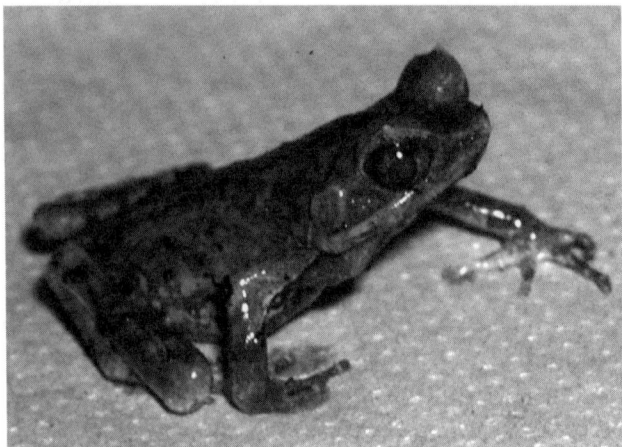

Figure 19.5. Cataracts may develop in elderly amphibians such as this Asian spadefoot toad, *Megophrys montana*. (Kevin Wright, Philadelphia Zoological Garden)

origin is suspected. Culture and sensitivity testing is highly recommended to confirm that the best drug has been selected. Although conjunctivitis and corneal ulceration may result from systemic disease, topical therapy is usually employed as well. Because amphibians have a semipermeable skin, medications applied topically may ultimately be absorbed systemically. This is especially important to remember when medicating the eye of very small patients on a frequent basis. Ophthalmic preparations including tobramycin, cefazolin, gentamicin, tetracycline, chloramphenicol, and triple antibiotic (neomycin, polymixin B and bacitracin) have all been used successfully. Microliter syringes or pipettes may help to meter small amounts of medication directly to the eye. An alternative is to dilute potentially toxic medications such as gentamicin drops, which when diluted to 2 mg/ml reduces the likelihood of an overdose (Williams & Whitaker, 1994).

N-butyl cyanoacrylate (Nexaband® ophthalmic, Veterinary Products Laboratories, Phoenix, AZ) has been used in conjunction with medications to successfully treat corneal ulcers in fish (Whitaker, 1993) and frogs (Bicknese & Cranfield, 1995). The "patch" that is created serves as a watertight barrier, thus protecting the damaged cornea from further infection and irritation during the healing process. Mid to deep corneal ulcers may require chemical restraint allowing for proper debridement of tissue and placement of the cyanoacrylate. The surface of the cornea is prepared by copious lavage with an antibiotic that has good stromal penetration, such as chloramphenicol. After one minute the surface is dried by rolling a sterile cotton tip swab to remove necrotic debris. A thin layer of n-butyl cyanoacrylate is then applied to the defect using a 30 gauge needle and tuberculin syringe. Excessive glue will likely peel off prematurely. In larger animals, the false nictitating membrane may be sutured to the upper lid providing protection to the cornea while healing occurs.

19.6. CONCLUSION

Despite detailed studies of the amphibian eye, relatively little is known about the diseases that affect it. Herpetologists who note changes in the appearance of an eye or the animal's visual ability can help further our knowledge by immediately engaging an experienced practitioner or veterinary ophthalmologist to perform a complete ophthalmic examination. Additionally, veterinarians should include a thorough ocular examination as part of every routine health assessment. With practice and appropriate equipment, these examinations can provide valuable information that is essential in the diagnosis of disease and monitoring of patients undergoing therapy. Further research and clinical trials are needed to understand the reason some individuals develop ocular disease while others remain asymptomatic. As our knowledge grows, it may become clear that we can prevent many diseases of the amphibian eye.

ACKNOWLEDGMENTS

Dr. Walter Stark, Professor of Ophthalmology and Director of Corneal Service at Johns Hopkins University's Wilmer Eye Institute, has contributed greatly to our understanding of the amphibian eye and its diseases. The enthusiasm and interest he and his residents have shown for our small patients has made it possible for us to study the amphibian eye and gain a better understanding of the diseases that affect it.

REFERENCES

Balls, M. 1962. Spontaneous neoplasms in amphibia: A review and descriptions of six new cases. Cancer Research 22:1142–1161.

Balls, M., R.H. Clothier, L.N. Ruben, and J.C. Harshbarger. 1989. The incidence and significance of malignant neoplasia in amphibians. Proc. 3rd Int. Colloq. Path. Rept. Amphib. p. 70.

Bicknese, E.J. and M.J. Cranfield. 1995. Cyanoacrylate treatment for corneal ulcers in Kokoe-Pa Poison dart frogs (*Dendrobates histrionicus*). Proceedings of the Association of Reptilian and Amphibian Veterinarians: 67.

Brooks, D.E., E.R. Jacobson, E.D. Wolf, S. Clubb, and J.M. Gaskin. 1983. Panophthalmitis and otitus interna in fire-bellied toads. JAVMA 183:1198–1201.

Carpenter, J.L., A. Bachtrach, Jr., D.M. Albert, S.J. Vainisi, and M.A. Goldstein. 1986. Xanthomatous keratitis, disseminated xanthomatosis, and atherosclerosis in Cuban treefrogs. Vet. Pathol. 23:337–339.

Duellman, W.E. and L. Trueb. 1994. Biology of Amphibians. The Johns Hopkins University Press, Baltimore, MD, 670 pp.

Dziezyc, J. and N.J. Millichamp. 1989. Lipid keratopathy of frogs. Proc. 3rd Intl. Colloq. Pathol. Reptiles Amphib. 3:95–96.

Etges, F.J. 1961. Contributions to the life history of the brain fluke of newts and fish, *Diplostomum scheuringi* Huges, 1929 (Trematoda: Diplostomatidae). J. of Parasit. 47:453–458.

Etges, F.J. 1991. *Clinostomum attenuatum* (Digenea) from the eye of *Bufo marinus*. J. of Parasit. 77:634–635.

Flynn, R.J. 1973. Parasites of Laboratory Animals. Iowa State University Press, Ames, IA, pp. 507–645.

Glorioso, J.C., R.L. Amborski, G.F. Amborski, and D.D. Culley. 1974. Microbiological studies on septicemic bullfrogs (*Rana catesbeiana*). Am. J. Vet. Res. 35:1241–1245.

Mann, I. 1931. Iris pattern in the vertebrates. Trans. Ophthalmol. Soc. UK 21:355–408.

Michaelson, I.C. 1954. Retinal Circulation in Man and Animals. Charles C. Thomas, Springfield, IL, pp. 12–15.

Millichamp, N.J. 1990. Ocular disease in captive amphibians and reptiles. Proceedings of the American Association of Zoo Veterinarians, pp. 297–301.

Millichamp, N.J. 1991. Exotic animal ophthalmology, in Gelatt, K.N. (Ed.): Veterinary Ophthalmology second edition. Lea & Febiger, Philadelphia, PA, pp. 685–686.

Noble, G.K. 1954. The Biology of the Amphibia. Dover Publications, Inc., New York.

Prince, J.H. 1956. Comparative Anatomy of the Eye. Charles C. Thomas, Springfield, IL, pp. 11–12.

Russell, W.C., D.L. Edwards, E.L. Stair, and D.C. Hubner. 1990. Corneal lipidosis, disseminated xanthomatosis, and hypercholesterolemia in Cuban treefrogs (*Osteopilus septentrionalis*). J. Zoo Wild. Med. 21(1):99–104.

Walls, G.L. 1942. The Vertebrate Eye and its Adaptive Radiation. Cranbrook Institute of Science Bulletin No. 19.

Whitaker, B.R. 1993. The diagnosis and treatment of corneal ulcers in fish. Proc. Amer. Assoc. Zoo Vet. pp. 92–95.

Wilcock, B.P. and T.W. Dukes. 1989. The Eye, *in* Ferguson, H. W. (Ed.): Systemic Pathology of Fish. Iowa State University Press, Ames, IA, pp. 168–194.

Williams, D.L. and B.R. Whitaker. 1994. The amphibian eye—A clinical review. J. Zoo Wild. Med. 25(1):18–28.

Zwart, P. and J.S. van der Linde-Sipmand. 1989. Lipid keratopathy in a European treefrog. Proc. 3rd Intl. Colloq. Pathol. Reptiles Amphib. Orlando, FL 3:91–94.

CHAPTER 20

DIAGNOSTIC IMAGING OF AMPHIBIANS

Mark D. Stetter, DVM, Diplomate ACZM

20.1 INTRODUCTION

Radiography and ultrasonography are two readily available diagnostic tools that are exceedingly useful for diagnosing and monitoring amphibian diseases. Diagnostic imaging has become one of the most commonly utilized and helpful tools in human and veterinary medicine. Radiography was historically the standard for anatomical imaging in veterinary medicine, and radiographs of amphibians yield excellent images of skeletal anatomy, lungs (if present) and, to a lesser extent, the gastrointestinal system. Radiographic detail is poor when imaging visceral organs of amphibians as there are neither contrasting fat dense tissue nor air separating the different organs. Unlike mammalian or avian radiography, it is rare that coelomic anatomic structures can be individually identified.

Ultrasonography is an excellent adjunct to radiography and can provide outstanding images of visceral anatomy. Ultrasonography provides real time images enabling the operator to thoroughly assess the coelomic cavity, soft tissues, and their relationship to one another. Movement such as blood flow and contractility of the heart can be visualized and provide valuable information. Ultrasound may also be used to safely guide needles to their desired target for aspiration or biopsy while avoiding large vessels or other important structures. The hand-held transducer contains piezoelectric crystals which both emit and receive the sound waves. These ultrasound pulses pass through water and soft tissues but are blocked by air or bone. Amphibians provide excellent ultrasound images since they can be placed in water which removes the usual air interface between patient and probe. The primary limitations of ultrasonic imaging are the capabilities of the equipment and the experience of the operator. Once these are overcome, high quality images of normal and abnormal anatomy can be easily obtained by the clinician.

CT scans and MR images have been performed on amphibians and provide excellent anatomical detail of organ location and structure. This chapter includes radiographs, CT scans, ultrasound images, and six case studies.

20.2 RADIOGRAPHY

Most radiographs can be obtained without chemical restraint. The easiest and least stressful restraint technique is to place the patient in a moistened sealable plastic bag. The plastic bag should be large enough to hold the animal comfortably without allowing the animal to turn around. This method will allow the animal to be positioned without excessive handling. Amphibians can be kept in the restraint bag until the radiographs have been processed. For prolonged procedures, small holes can be placed in the bag or the animal should be returned to its environment.

Chemical restraint using either tricaine methanesulfonate or isoflurane will allow better positioning and visualization of the limbs which are otherwise often pulled tightly underneath the nonsedated anuran. Sedation will also facilitate positioning if the x-ray tube is stationary and cannot be rotated for horizontal beam lateral and craniocaudal views.

A minimum of two views taken at 90° angles to each other, such as a dorsoventral view (DV) and

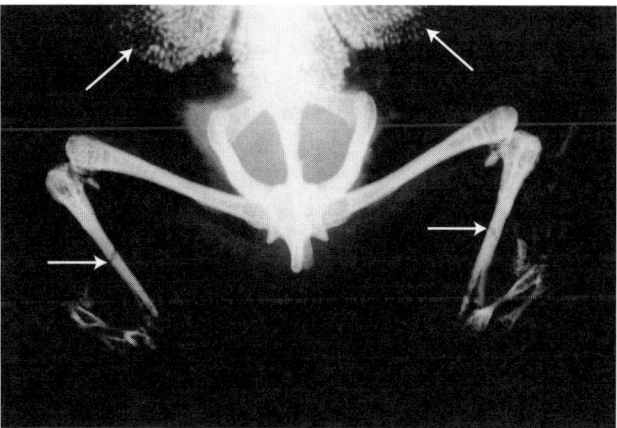

Figure 20.1. Normal radiographic appearance. Dorsoventral view. Horned frog, *Ceratophrys* sp. Note the prominent nutrient foramen (arrows) which are commonly visualized in the tibiofibula bone. This normal anatomical structure should not be confused with a fracture. *Ceratophrys* frogs have large bony plates which project laterally from the thoracic vertebrae (arrows). (Mark Stetter)

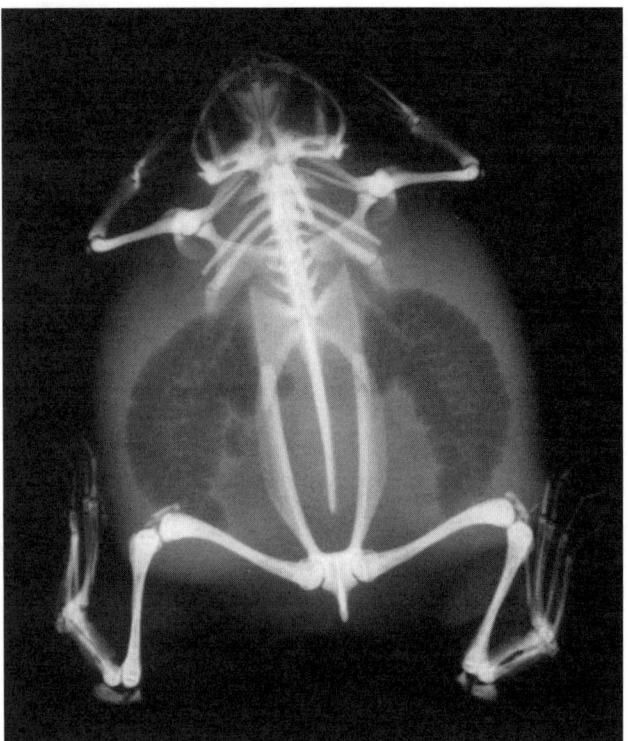

Figure 20.2. Normal radiographic appearance. Dorsoventral view. Surinam toad, *Pipa pipa*. Note the radiographic detail of the air-filled lungs compared to the complete lack of contrast in visualizing other visceral organs. (Mark Stetter)

horizontal beam lateral, are required to form a multidimensional image and help the clinician decipher possible artifacts. The easiest and most useful diagnostic view is the dorsoventral (DV), with the patient resting in a normal sternal position (Figures 20.1, 20.2). Laterally recumbent views are useful in amphibians, as are horizontal beam lateral, craniocaudal, obliques, and ventrodorsal (VD) views. In a nonsedated amphibian, these views can be acquired by placing the animal on a foam block and moving the x-ray tube (Figure 20.3). Amphibians can also be gently placed between moistened foam blocks to aid in restraint and positioning.

20.2.1 Radiographic Techniques

Standard Radiograph Units. (Figures 20.4–20.7) Direct exposure of film produces the best images, but intensifying screens are needed in clinical practice due to the limitations of radiograph machines and to reduce the risk of patient motion during an exposure.

A single emulsion film in combination with a compatible high detail rare earth screen is most practical for imaging amphibians. Calcium tungstate screens may provide better quality images, but they are slower than rare earth screens.

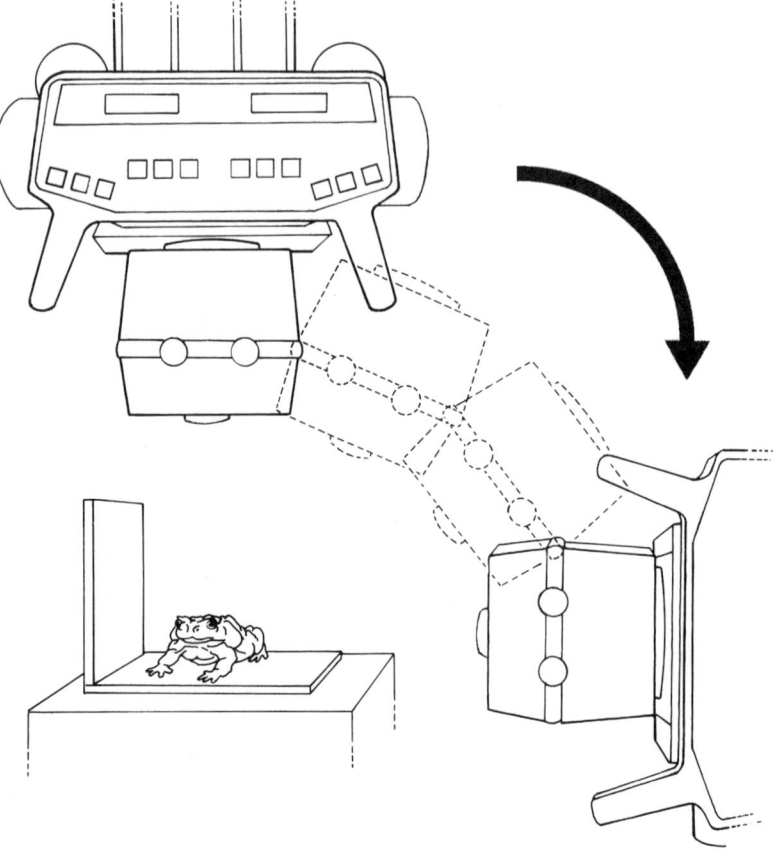

Figure 20.3. Illustration depicting radiographic positioning in an amphibian. Two views (ventrodorsal and lateral) can be acquired without manual restraint of the patient. The animal can be placed within a moistened sealable plastic bag to prevent movement. (Emiko-Rose Koike, Johns Hopkins University Department of Art as Applied to Medicine)

DIAGNOSTIC IMAGING OF AMPHIBIANS — 255

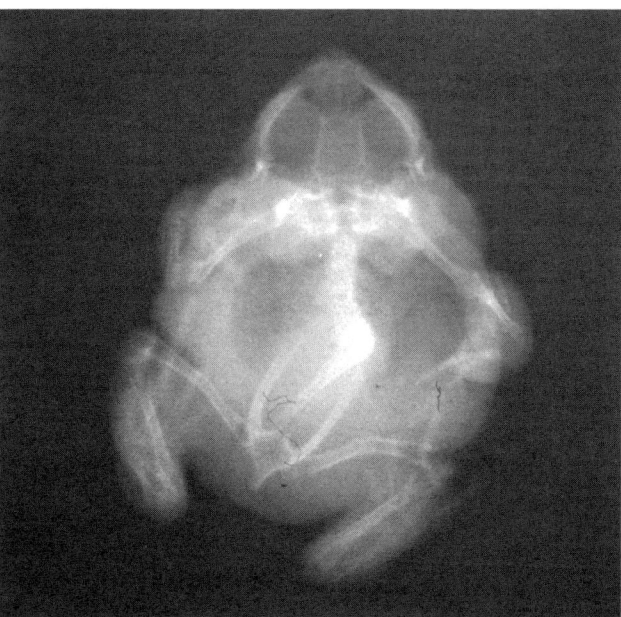

Figure 20.4. Metabolic bone disease. Dorsoventral view. Horned frog, *Ceratophrys* sp. Note the generalized osteopenia, bowing of the femurs, severe scoliosis, and spinal fracture. (Mark Stetter)

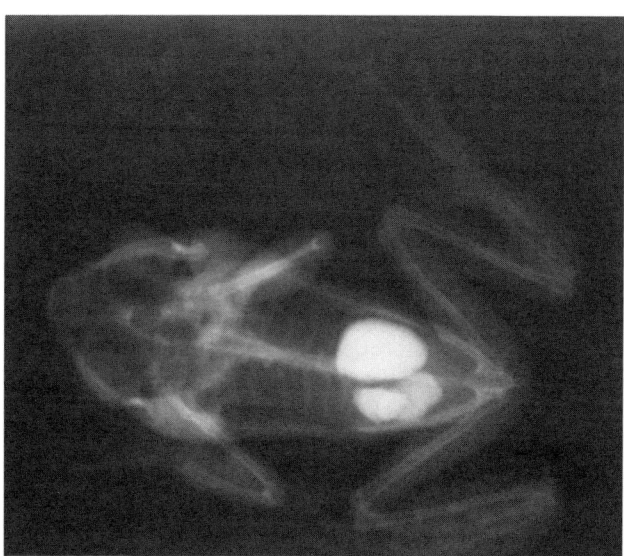

Figure 20.6. Gastrointestinal foreign bodies. Dorsoventral view. Cope's brown treefrog, *Hyla miliaria*. Note the prominent radiodense objects (rocks) in the upper gastrointestinal tract. Various substrates from the environment are commonly ingested and are not always associated with clinical disease. (Mark Stetter)

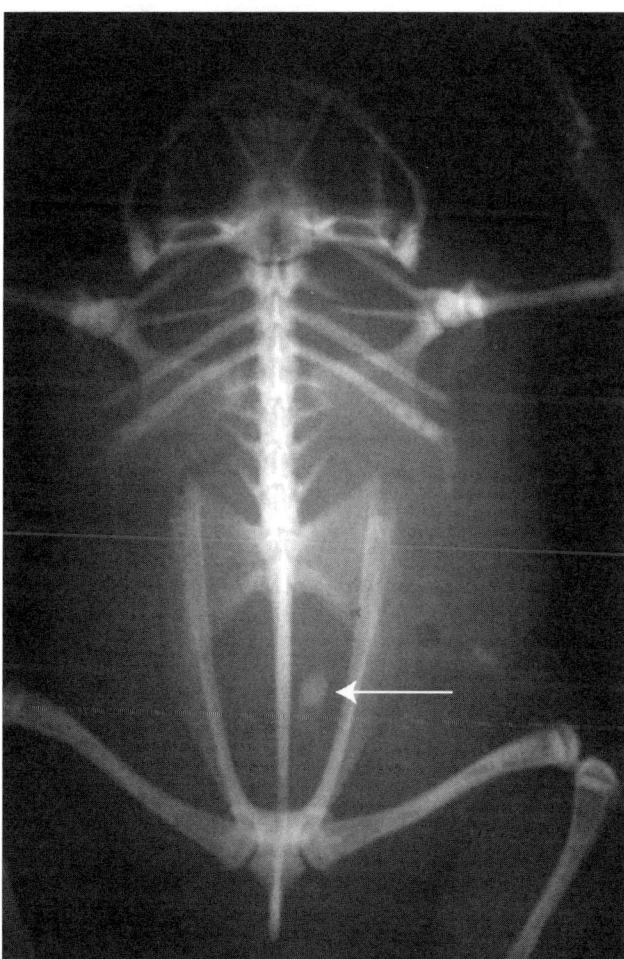

Figure 20.5. Cystic calculus. Dorsoventral view. Surinam toad, *Pipa pipa*. Note the round radiodense object in the right caudal coelom (arrow). This could easily be confused with material within the colon. A lower gastrointestinal series or ultrasonography can be used to better delineate the object's location. (Mark Stetter)

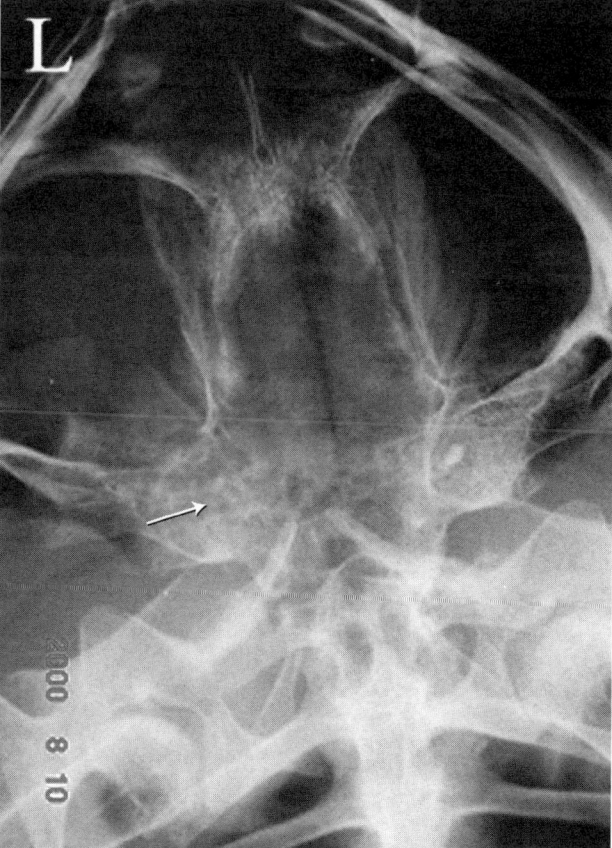

Figure 20.7. Otitis media. Dorsoventral view. Smooth-sided toad, *Bufo guttatus*. Notice the osteolyses of the left otolith (arrow). This animal demonstrated a left head tilt upon clinical examination. (Barbara Mangold)

Radiographic quality is improved by using the shortest possible exposure times, the largest practical focal film distance, keeping the patient as close to the film cassette as possible, and using the smallest focal spot available. Magnification radiography can be performed with any radiograph machine that has a focal spot of 0.3 mm or less by placing the patient a given distance away from the film. Specific imaging techniques for normal and magnification radiography will vary with the machine, type of film, intensifying screen, and the patient's size. The clinician is encouraged to take the time to develop a technique table for various sized amphibians.

Mammography Radiograph Units. Mammography x-ray machines have great application for veterinary diagnostics (Figure 20.8). Older units can frequently be acquired from human hospitals. While specialized mammography film and cassettes are available, routine film and cassettes can also be used. The images produced are of very high quality and refined detail. As with standard radiographic units, magnification can be achieved while maintaining image quality with these units by positioning the patient several inches above film. Routine automatic processing machines can be used, but may need to be adjusted to a higher temperature if using mammography film. If available, mammography x-ray machines are preferred over standard radiography units due to the greater detail and quality of the images. Interpretation of mammographic images takes practice as the image quality is of long latitude (lots of shades of gray).

Dental Radiographic Film. Use of dental radiographic film for amphibian radiography has a number of advantages. Dental film is a nonscreen film that is high speed compared to other nonscreen films. It comes in a variety of sizes which makes it particularly useful for whole body radiographs of small amphibians or for focal areas of interest in larger species (Figure 20.9A, B). Dental film can be used with standard radiographic units or with more specialized dental units.

A focal-film distance of 20 cm is commonly utilized with dental units. Specific technique settings will depend upon the film, machine, and patient. A focal-film distance of 20 cm and a mAs of 5.0 in conjunction with a kVp of 60 is an appropriate starting point for obtaining a good image of an amphibian using a dental unit. There is no need to changed the focal-film distance from 40 cm if the dental film is used in conjunction with a standard radiographic unit.

Dental film can be developed either by manual processing (dip tanks or tabletop dental processor) or with an automatic processor. Processing times and temperature are different from standard film thus individual product information should be consulted.

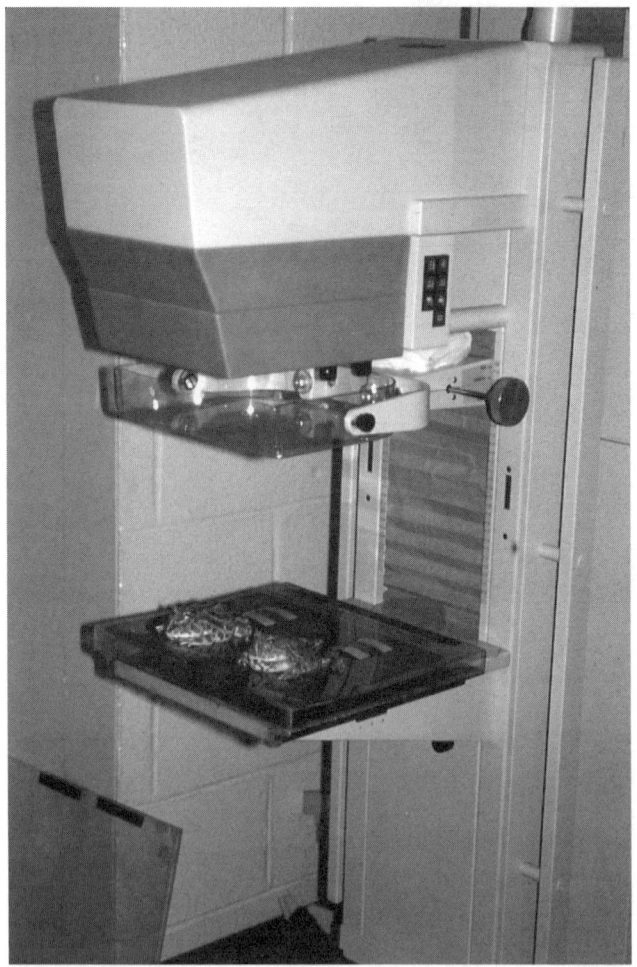

Figure 20.8. Mammography radiographic unit. Radiographs of normal and abnormal individuals can be taken simultaneously to help interpret true lesions from normal anatomy. (Mark Stetter)

Radiographic Contrast Studies. Contrast radiography is often a helpful technique when attempting to identify organ position or pathologic lesions. A gastrointestinal (GI) series is the most frequently performed contrast study and is useful for identifying the location of the stomach and intestines as well as identifying foreign bodies (Figure 20.10). Gastrointestinal obstruction in amphibians may result from a variety of causes including, but not limited to, foreign bodies, gastric, intestinal or coelomic masses, intussusception, and torsions. Displacement of the stomach and intestines due to organomegaly or a coelomic mass may be identified and characterized with a GI series. The author usually uses barium sulfate for gastrointestinal contrast material. Organic iodinated compounds have also been used and provide excellent imaging, however their potential systemic toxic effects in amphibians have not been evaluated. In other animals, the nonionic, water-soluble, iodinated compounds are considered to be safer than ionic, water-soluble, iodinated

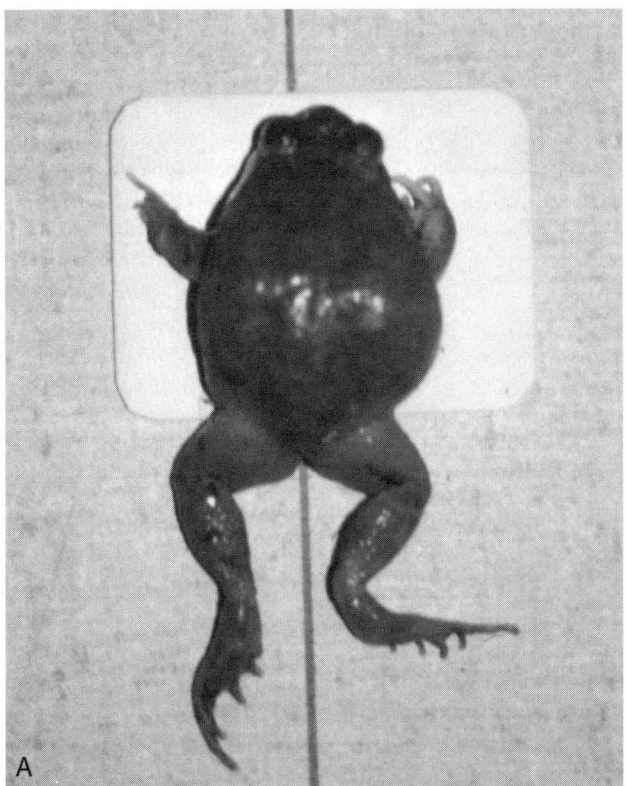

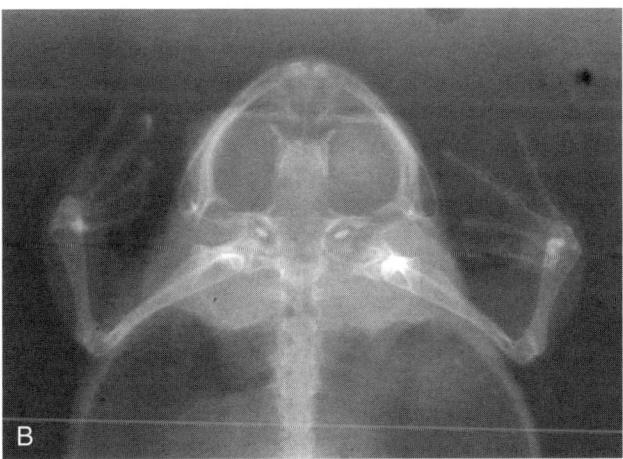

Figure 20.9. Use of dental radiographic film for radiography in amphibians. **A.** A tomato frog, *Dyscophus antongili*, is placed directly on a piece of dental radiographic film to acquire a dorsoventral view of the cranial half of the frog. **B.** Dorsoventral radiograph of the tomato frog using dental film. Note the anatomical detail provided by dental film. (Mark Stetter)

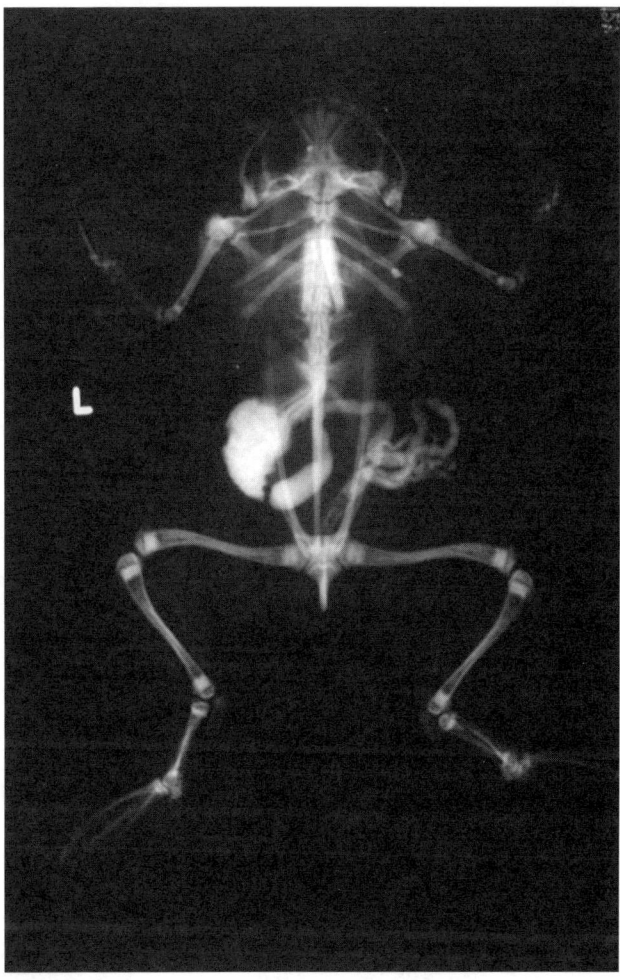

Figure 20.10. Gastrointestinal contrast study. Dorsoventral view. Surinam toad, *Pipa pipa*. Note the normal position of the stomach on the left (L) side with passage of contrast media into the intestine. Normal transit times for amphibians have not been established and are highly dependent upon the animal's physiological state. (Mark Stetter)

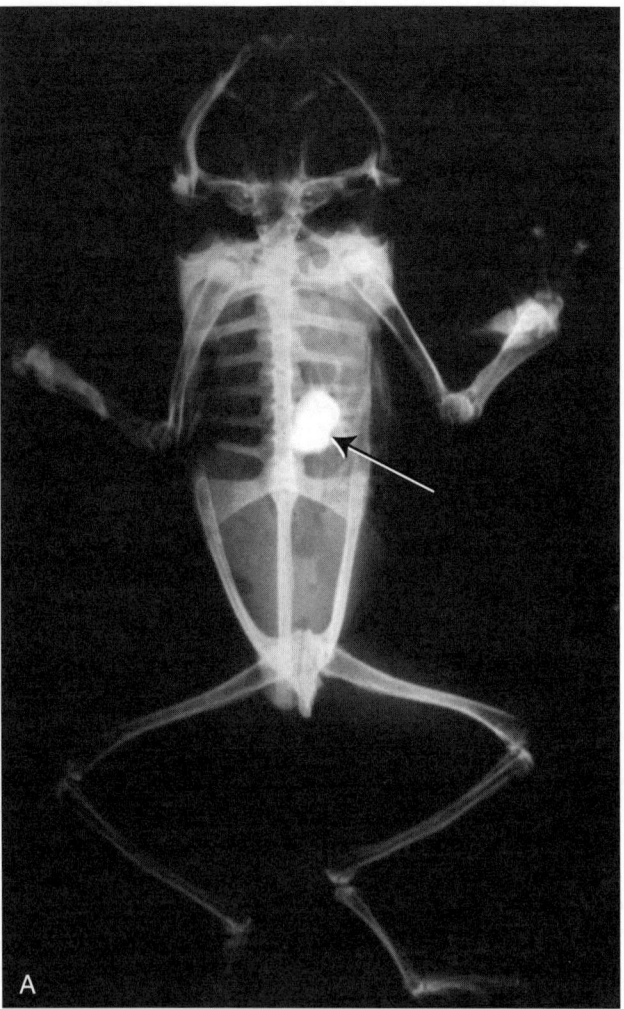

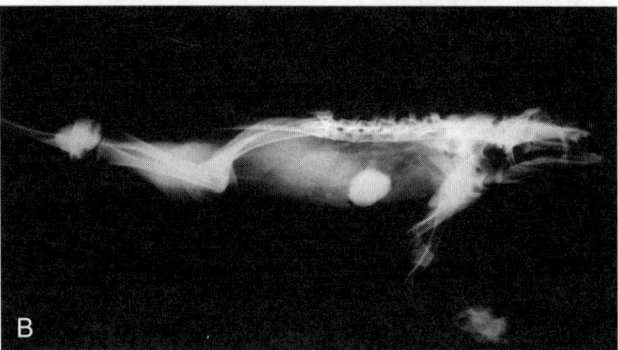

Figure 20.11. Contrast radiography showing postmortem cholecystogram in a spotted toad, *Bufo guttatus*. **A.** Dorsoventral view. Iodinated contrast media was infused into the gall bladder. The gall bladder (arrow) commonly lies just to the right of midline adjacent to the stomach, liver, and heart. **B.** Lateral view. (Mark Stetter)

compounds. Other specialized contrast studies include barium enemas, pneumocoelograms, cholecystograms (Figure 20.11A, B), and double contrast coelograms (Figure 20.12). While the author has performed these

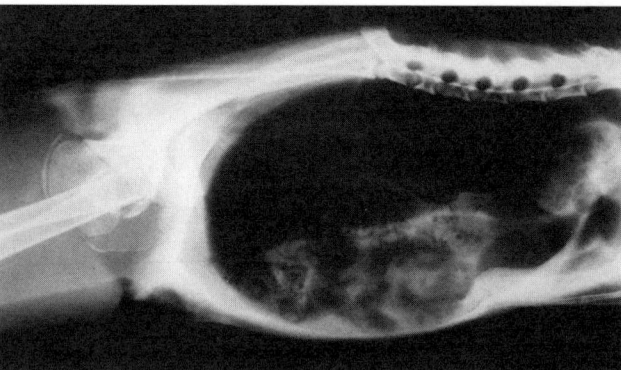

Figure 20.12. Double contrast coelography. Right lateral view. Bullfrog, *Rana catesbeiana*. A butterfly catheter is used to inject and then aspirate iodinated contrast material followed by the injection of a small amount of air into the coelomic cavity. Note the numerous coiled radiolucent structures in the caudal ventral coelom. These are encysted nematodes within the mesentery. (Mark Stetter)

studies only on a limited basis, the diagnostic images have been excellent and identified lesions (e.g., coelomic nematodiasis) which would have gone unrecognized utilizing routine radiographic techniques.

20.3 AMPHIBIAN ULTRASONOGRAPHY

Most ultrasonographic exams can be accomplished without direct manual or chemical restraint of the amphibian (Figure 20.13A, B, C). The amphibian can be placed in a rigid plastic container holding enough water to cover ½–¾ of the patient (see Figure 20.13A, B). Care should be taken to use water free of toxic substances (e.g., chlorine, copper, etc.) and to ensure that any disinfectants have been copiously rinsed from all of the equipment before use. The restraint container should be thoroughly cleaned between animals. This is particularly important with amphibians because of the potential spread of infectious diseases and exposure to toxins which can be released from the amphibian dermis. Toxicities have occurred when using an inadequately cleaned container between two different anuran species.

Imaging is accomplished by either placing the ultrasound probe in direct contact with the bottom of the plastic container (see Figure 20.13A) or on the side of the container for a dorsal view. Coupling gel should be used between the probe and the plastic container. For a sagittal or transverse view, the probe can be placed directly in the water adjacent to the patient (see Figure 20.13B), although care should be taken not to submerge the entire probe if connections are not waterproof. When placing the probe directly in the water, coupling gel need not be used. The presence

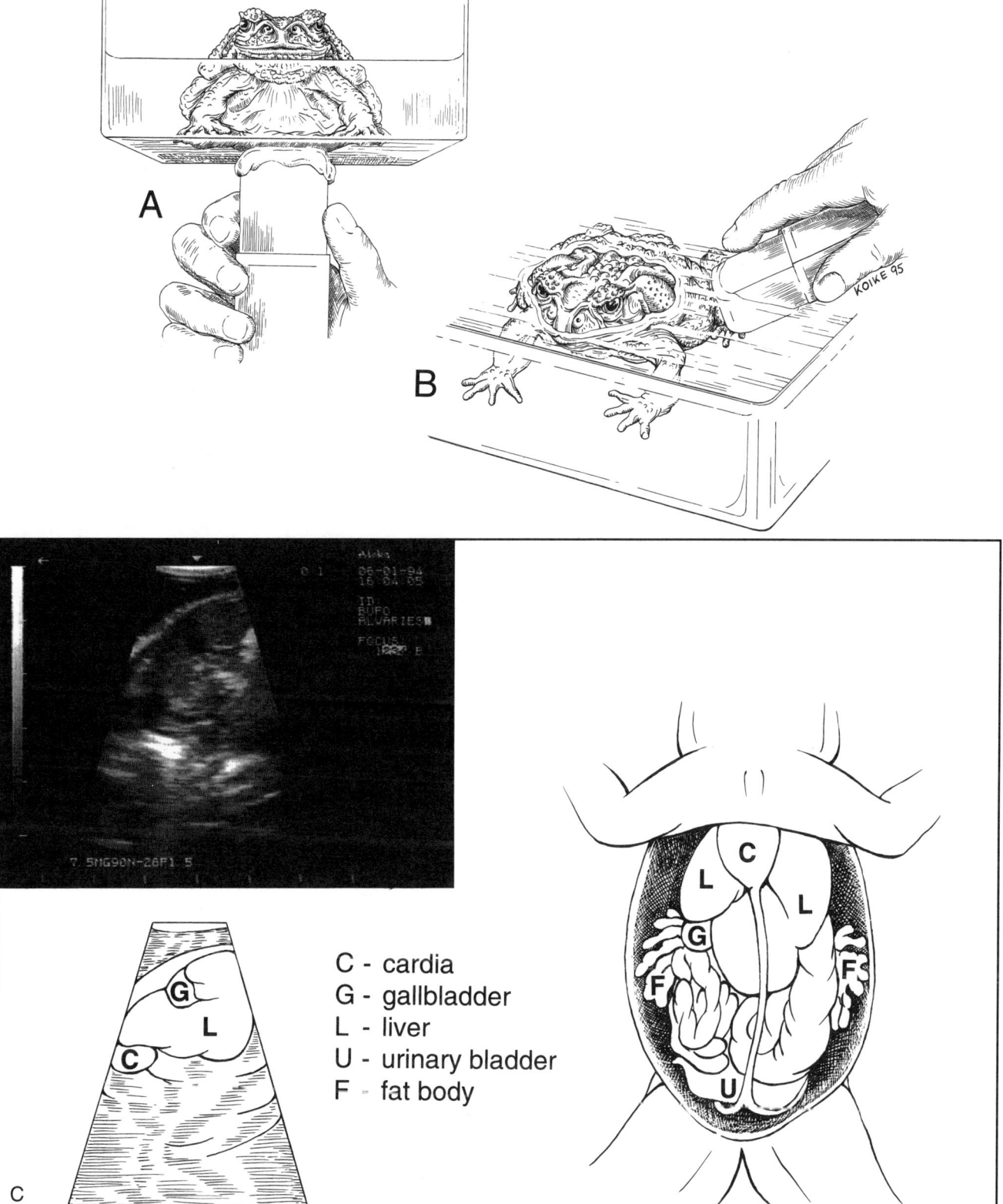

Figure 20.13. Ultrasonography in amphibians may be readily accomplished with minimal restraint. **A.** An amphibian is placed within a plastic container that is filled with water. The ultrasound probe is placed against the container with coupling gel. **B.** A dorsolateral approach using the water bath as an acoustic window. **C.** Visceral and cardiac anatomy of a typical ranid frog. The cardiac anatomy corresponds in orientation to the ultrasonogram of the heart. (Emiko-Rose Koike, Johns Hopkins University Department of Art as Applied to Medicine)

of the water between the probe and patient acts as a coupling medium enhancing the ultrasound image. Most thin plastic food containers will provide unobstructed imaging with minimal artifacts.

Amphibians usually remain quiet when placed in an aquatic environment. Increased activity in the water bath may be due to an inappropriate water temperature or presence of an irritant. Smaller containers with lids and foam blocks can also be used to reduce movement in very active animals. Strictly arboreal species (e.g. hylid frogs) will usually remain quiet if given a small branch or similar object to perch upon while in the water.

20.3.1 Equipment

B-mode real time ultrasound machines are frequently used for amphibian imaging. These machines are becoming increasingly affordable and thus more commonly used in veterinary medicine. Additional options which have not been routinely utilized by the author include doppler, color flow doppler, and M-mode imaging.

The small size of most amphibian patients usually requires that a 7.5 megahertz (MHz) probe be used. Large animals can be visualized albeit with less resolution using a 5.0 MHz probe. Higher frequency 10.0 MHz probes have become available and offer the most detailed imaging of amphibians. Both linear array or convex probes can be used with amphibian patients.

Ultrasound images should be recorded on video tape. This is an important part of the individual animal's medical record and provides future documentation of the normal anatomy of different species and pathologic ultrasonographic findings. Video taping also allows the clinician and consultants to review the images at a later date and correlate clinicopathologic findings with the ultrasound images. A printed image can be made either during the examination or later, when the video is being reviewed. This hard copy should be kept with the patient's medical record.

20.3.2 Patient Examination

The heart is the most reliable anatomical landmark to begin the ultrasound exam. The heart is located on the ventral midline at the level of the forelimbs (see Figure 20.13C). Amphibian species have two thin-walled atria and a single thick-walled ventricle (Figure 20.14A, B). The pericardial sac can often be visualized and normally contains a small amount of fluid. In various disease states, increased amounts of pericardial fluid can be detected (see case 20.5.4). Pericardial effusion can be recognized as an anechoic (black) region immediately surrounding the epicardium.

Amphibians lack a diaphragm thus all visceral organs are located within the coelomic cavity. Once the

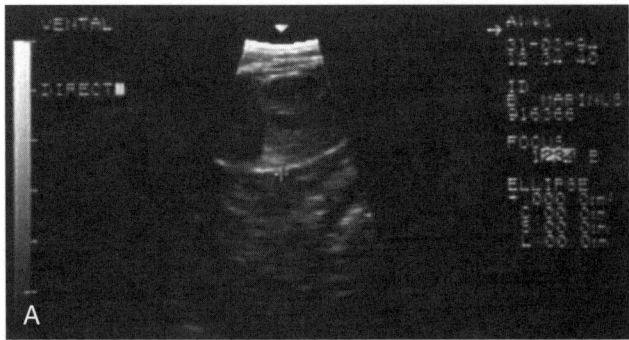

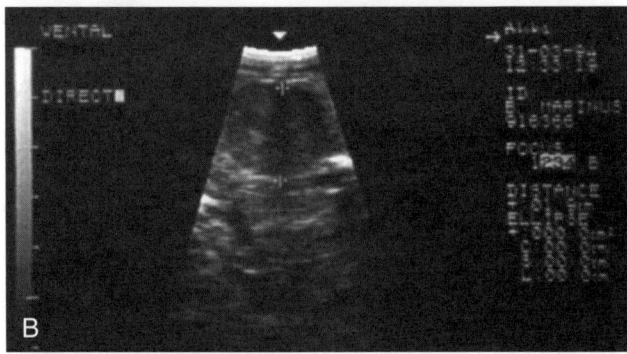

Figure 20.14. Normal ultrasound appearance of the heart of a giant toad, *Bufo marinus*. Ventral probe placement. **A.** Long axis view with the thin-walled, fluid-filled, hypoechoic atria on the left and the thick-walled ventricle on the right. **B.** Short axis view of ventricle from left to right. Note the thin black shadow through the center of the heart which is an artifact caused by blockage of the ultrasound waves as they reflect off the sternum which lies between the ultrasound probe and the heart. (Mark Stetter)

heart has been located and evaluated, the liver can be found adjacent to and on either side of the ventricular apex. In anurans, the liver is usually bilobed while in salamanders the liver is a often a simple elongate structure (Figure 20.15). A characteristic hypoechoic ring (Figure 20.16A, B) readily defines the gastrointestinal tract.

The extrahepatic gall bladder is visualized as a well delineated spherical anechoic mass adjacent to the heart and liver (Figure 20.17). A full gall bladder may approximate the size of the heart in some individuals.

Anurans and salamanders in good body condition have fat bodies within their coelomic cavity. These structures can be quite large, especially in well fed animals just before hibernation. The anuran fat bodies are composed of fingerlike projections which emerge from a common stalk at the base of each gonad. The salamander fat bodies are longitudinal structures located between the kidney and gonad and are not routinely visualized on ultrasound. In anurans, the fat tissue is hyperechoic (white) in relation to other visceral organs (liver), while in other species fat may be hypoechoic depending on its location.

DIAGNOSTIC IMAGING OF AMPHIBIANS —— 261

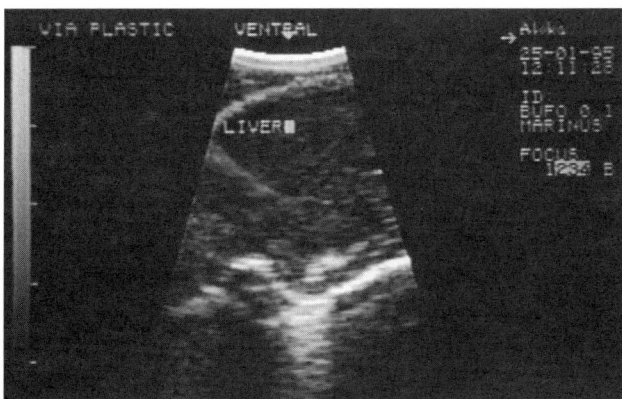

Figure 20.15. Normal ultrasound appearance of the liver of a giant toad, *Bufo marinus*. Ventral probe placement. The liver is located just caudal to the heart and commonly extends from the left to right lateral body walls. Amphibian hepatic ultrasound appearance is similar to mammals with various sized hepatic vessels coursing through an otherwise uniform hepatic architecture. (Mark Stetter)

The urinary bladder can be easily recognized if it is filled with urine. It is visualized as a thin-walled, smooth-surfaced, spherical, anechoic structure in the caudal abdomen. Some salamander species have a cylinderlike or bilobate bladder. Anurans commonly empty their urinary bladder when manually restrained.

Changes associated with reproduction can be dramatic and are influenced by the species, age, sex, and reproductive status of the animal. Gravid females often produce large numbers of ova which can occupy more than half of the coelomic cavity. Grossly, these animals may be noted to have marked coelomic distension. Upon physical and radiographic examination, it may be difficult to differentiate a gravid animal from an animal with ascites (Figure 20.18). It is not uncommon for gravid amphibians to demonstrate nonspecific clinical signs associated with illness (anorexia, lethargy, etc.). Ultrasonography is a very useful means of differentiating gravid animals from those which have ascites (Figure 20.19). Gravid females will have a uniform echogenic area in the caudal ventral abdomen, which extends cranially to the liver. In large animals, the numerous ova create a mixed alternating anechoic/hyperechoic pattern. The small anechoic areas represent the fluid portion of the egg while the more hyperechoic areas are thought to represent the yolk. In small animals, a uniform diffuse mottled density is visualized occupying the entire caudal coelomic cavity. The reproductive tract in a nongravid female usually cannot be visualized. If the animal is of adequate size, the testes can be visualized as oval structures attached to the dorsum at the base of the fat bodies, next to the urinary bladder.

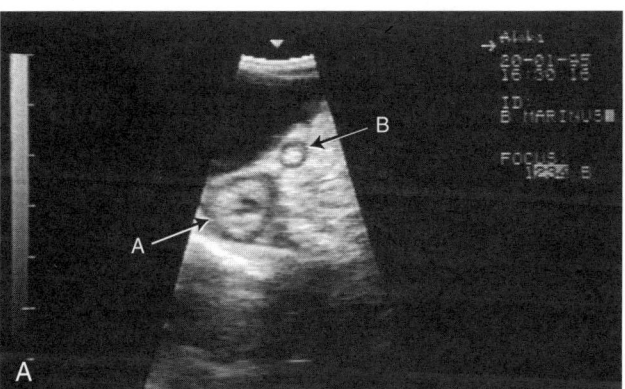

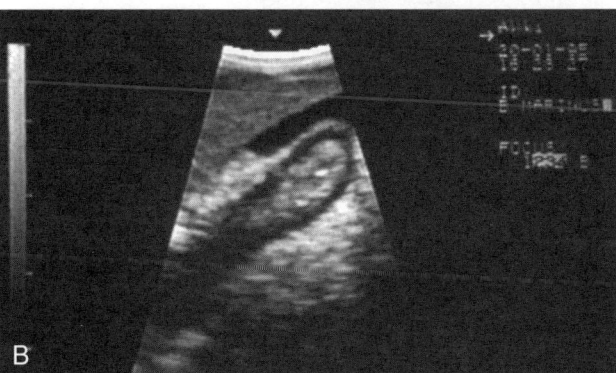

Figure 20.16. Ultrasonographic appearance of the gastrointestinal tract and hydrocoelom in a giant toad, *Bufo marinus*. **A.** Ventral probe placement with a cross-sectional view of the stomach (A arrow) and intestines (B arrow). Note the characteristic hypoechoic ring that is commonly seen when imaging the GI tract. **B.** Longitudinal view of stomach. The tip of the left liver lobe can be seen to the left of the stomach. Note that a moderate amount of coelomic fluid can be seen as anechoic (black) areas adjacent to the GI tract. (Mark Stetter)

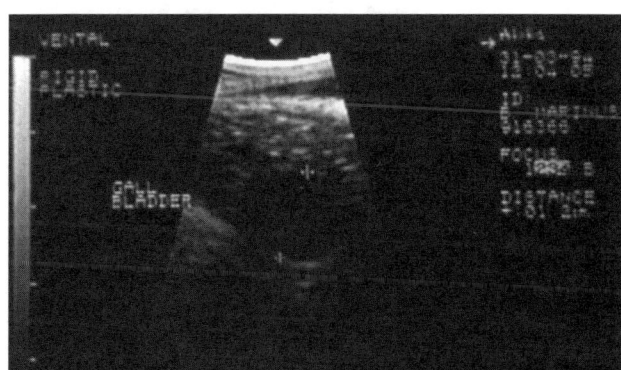

Figure 20.17. Normal ultrasound of the gall bladder and liver of a giant toad, *Bufo marinus*. Ventral probe placement. The gall bladder is outside of, but adjacent to the liver. It can be seen as a round anechoic (black) structure varying in size. Calculi and sludge may be seen as hyperechoic particulate matter floating in the bile. Note that size measurements of normal anatomical structures should be made for documentation and future use in establishing normal parameters. (Mark Stetter)

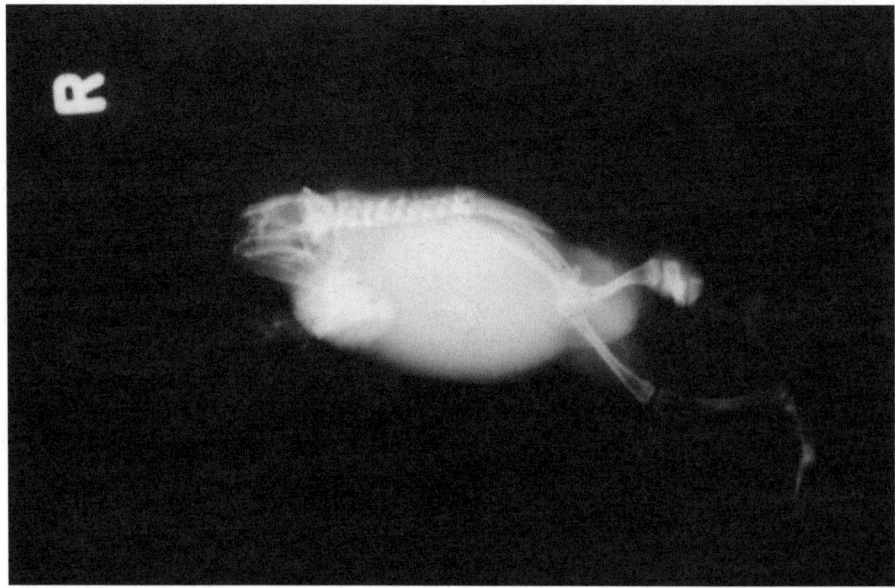

Figure 20.18. Left lateral view of a gravid Fowler's toad, *Bufo woodhousei fowleri*. Note the marked abdominal distention and lack of visceral detail. Ascites and organomegaly have a similar appearance radiographically. Ultrasound can be used to better visualize coelomic viscera. (Mark Stetter)

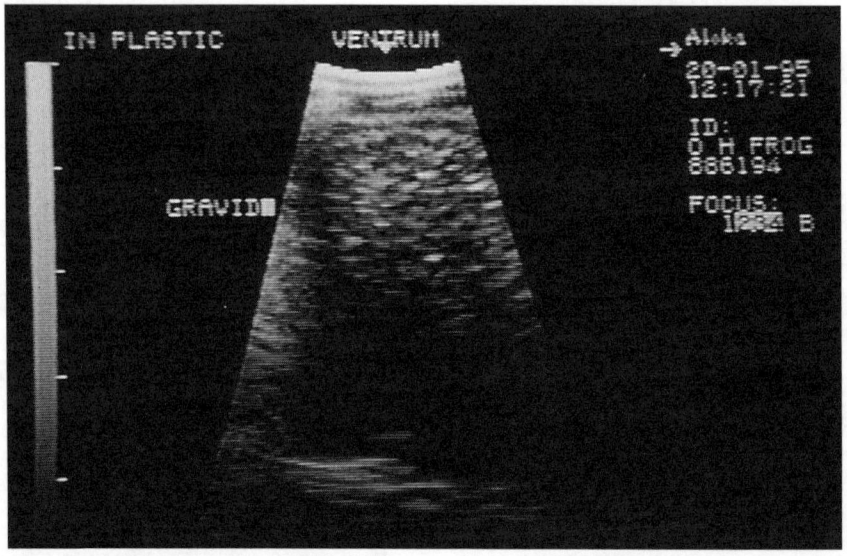

Figure 20.19. Normal ultrasound appearance of a gravid horned frog, *Ceratophrys* sp. Ventral probe placement. Ova can be seen on ultrasound as a uniform structure from the edge of the liver to the caudal limits of the coelom. The ova are slightly hyperechoic in comparison to the liver. Ova commonly will have a granular appearance with an intermingling of pinpoint hypoechoic and hyperechoic areas. (Mark Stetter)

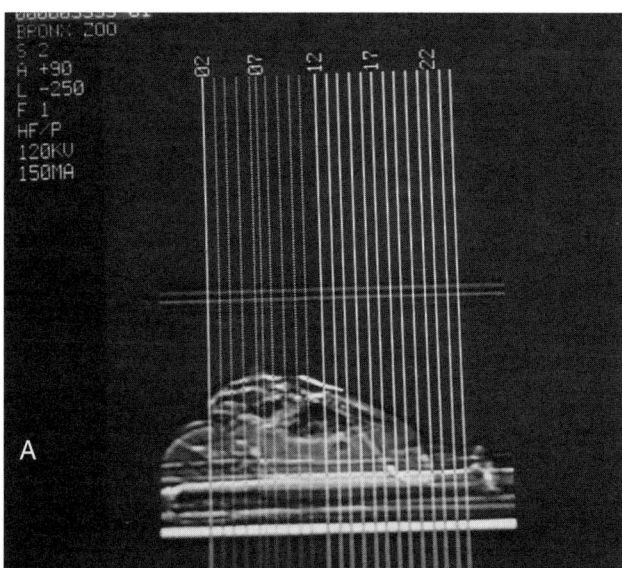
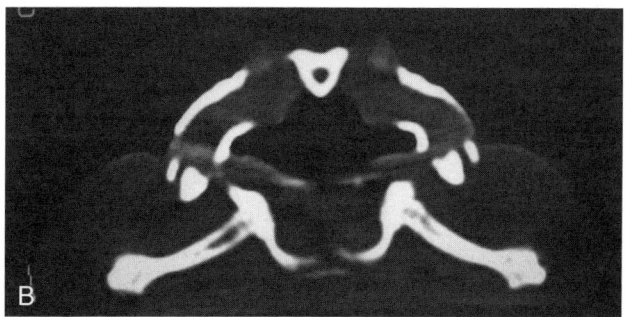
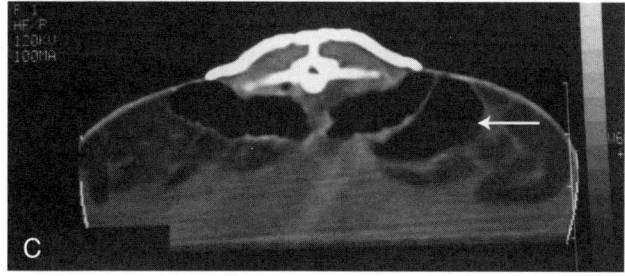

Figure 20.20. Normal CT Scan. Horned frog, *Ceratophrys* sp. Initial survey image. A. Left lateral view. White lines indicate the location of the 1 cm horizontal slices. The frog's head is supported by roll gauze and located to the left of the picture. B. Dorsal image at the mid cranium. The eyes, skull, oral cavity, and humeral bones can be easily seen. C. Transverse slice at the midbody. The vertebrae, lungs, stomach (arrow), and fat bodies can be distinguished. Other visceral organs cannot be individually identified. (Mark Stetter)

Coelomic effusion is a common, nonspecific indication of illness in amphibians. The presence of coelomic fluid provides an acoustic window which greatly enhances visualization of visceral organ details. Ascites can be recognized as an anechoic area with no discrete borders (unlike the gall or urinary bladders). Small amounts of coelomic fluid are commonly noted in clinically normal individuals. Large amounts of fluid can completely fill the coelomic cavity leaving the liver, gastrointestinal tract, and fat bodies floating in the fluid.

20.4 AMPHIBIAN CT SCAN AND MR IMAGING

Computerized axial tomography (CT scans) and magnetic resonance imaging (MRI) provide cross-sectional anatomical images that allow visualization of internal anatomy. The primary disadvantages of these two modalities are their cost, accessibility, and the patient must remain immobile during imaging thus sedation is commonly required. The images created by CT and MRI are thin anatomical slices of specific designated areas (Figures 20.20–20.22). Radiology and CT are best suited for imaging bone, while ultrasound and MRI are best suited for evaluation of soft tissue. Radiology and ultrasonography are better suited for routine scanning procedures while CT and MRI can be used to provide additional information concerning the fluid composition of a lesion and its precise anatomic location.

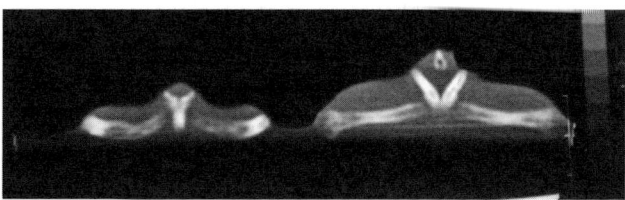

Figure 20.21. CT Scan. Horned frog, *Ceratophrys* sp. Transverse slices of normal (right) and abnormal (left) frogs at the area of the hind limbs. The animal on the left has metabolic bone disease with bowed femurs which appear to have thin radiolucent cortices. (Jay Stefanacci)

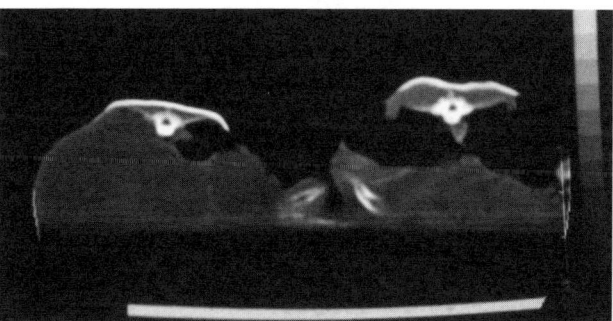

Figure 20.22. CT Scan. Horned frog, *Ceratophrys* sp. Transverse slices of normal (right) and abnormal (left) frogs. Note the large structure occupying most of the coelomic cavity and displacing the lungs and other viscera dorsally and to the right. Histopathology revealed the cystic structure to be ovarian in origin. (Jay Stefanacci)

20.5 CASE STUDIES

The following six case studies help to illustrate the value of radiography and ultrasonography in the evaluation of amphibian patients. For a self-assessment review, examine the plates and figures mentioned (without reviewing the captions) before reading the case summation (see Plates 3.1–3.3, and Figures 3.1A, B and 3.2A, B for illustrations of normal soft tissue and skeletal anatomy).

20.5.1 Tiger Salamander, *Ambystoma tigrinum*, Abdominal Distension

Initial survey of this tiger salamander, *Ambystoma tigrinum* (Figure 20.23A–F), utilized a standard dorsoventral view and lateral views. In the dorsoventral radiograph there is a noticeable cranial displacement of the right lung lobe suggesting a space-occupying lesion in the right caudal coelom. A gastrointestinal contrast series was used to further delimit the lesion. The contrast study revealed dorsocranial displacement of the stomach with a marked left displacement and partial obstruction of the intestinal tract. Ultrasonography revealed a uniformly echogenic mass in the coelomic cavity and minimal coelomic fluid. An exploratory celiotomy was performed which allowed removal of the mass. The mass was determined to be a neoplastic tumor of gonadal origin. Although this was a large solid gonadal tumor with concomitant scant coelomic fluid, it is not uncommon for gonadal tumors to result in large amounts of coelomic fluid. Small gonadal tumors can be accompanied by severe hydrocoelom, rendering detection of the tumor problematic without surgical exploration.

20.5.2 Colorado River Toad, *Bufo alvarius*, Ulcerative Dermatitis

Diagnostic evaluation of this Colorado River toad, *Bufo alvarius* (Figure 20.24A, B), included ultrasonography as ulcerative dermatitis can be a sign of systemic granulomatous disease. Two well delineated hyperechoic structures were noted in the ventricular myocardium. A 4.8 cm fluid-filled renal mass was also noted. The cardiac lesions were partially calcified granulomas containing fungal organisms. The renal lesion was an abscess. Generalized granulomatous disease carries a poor prognosis and in this case the final diagnosis for this toad was generalized chromomycosis.

20.5.3 New Guinea Giant Treefrog, *Litoria infrafrenata*, Anorexia

Once common husbandry errors have been eliminated as a cause for anorexia, parasitic disease, septicemia, malnutrition, and gastrointestinal foreign bodies should be considered as probable causes. Survey radiographs of this New Guinea giant treefrog, *Litoria infrafrenata* (Figure 20.25A–C), revealed radiopaque material occupying most of the caudal coelomic cavity indicative of a foreign body gastric impaction. Surgical intervention is recommended for many foreign bodies, although a CT scan may help determine if endoscopic retrieval via the mouth is possible. Surgical exploration confirmed a severe gastric impaction in this frog. The foreign body consisted of sand used as a substrate in the frog's exhibit.

20.5.4 Tschudi's African Bullfrog, *Pyxicephalus adspersus*, Routine Examination

A thorough quarantine examination should include survey radiographs (and ultrasonography) as many amphibians with granulomatous disease may not display overt signs of poor health until late in the course of the infection. A routine radiography survey of this Tschudi's African bullfrog, *Pyxicephalus adpsersus* (Figure 20.26A–C, Plate 20.1), revealed numerous round radiodense masses (arrows) in the cranial coelom. Ultrasonography revealed mild pericardial effusion and a pericardial mass. Given the grave nature of granulomatous diseases in amphibians, this frog was euthanized. Necropsy confirmed the presence of multiple pericardial granulomas (Plate 20.1). A diagnosis of mycobacteriosis was confirmed when histopathology revealed intralesional acid-fast organisms within the granulomatous tissue.

20.5.5 Bullfrog, *Rana catesbeiana*, Hydrocoelom and Edema

Fluid accumulation in the subcutaneous space of anurans is often accompanied by abdominal distension from coelomic fluid or a mass. This bullfrog, *Rana catesbeiana* (Figure 20.27A–E, Plate 20.2), was examined ultrasonographically to determine the underlying cause of hydrocoelom and edema. Multiple fluid-filled structures were noted in the area of the kidneys suggestive of cysts (parasitic, neoplastic, or congenital) or abscesses. An ultrasound-guided needle biopsy was attempted but was nondiagnostic. The lack of identifiable normal kidney tissue supported a grave prognosis. Necropsy revealed polycystic kidneys and one iatrogenic hematoma attributed to the biopsy attempt (Plate 20.2).

20.5.6 Surinam Toad, *Pipa pipa*, Abdominal Distension

A Surinam toad, *Pipa pipa* (Figure 20.28A–E, Plate 20.3), was presented for abdominal distension suggestive of hydrocoelom. Survey radiographs using a mammography machine revealed normal appearing lungs and a generalized lack of visceral organ detail.

DIAGNOSTIC IMAGING OF AMPHIBIANS —— 265

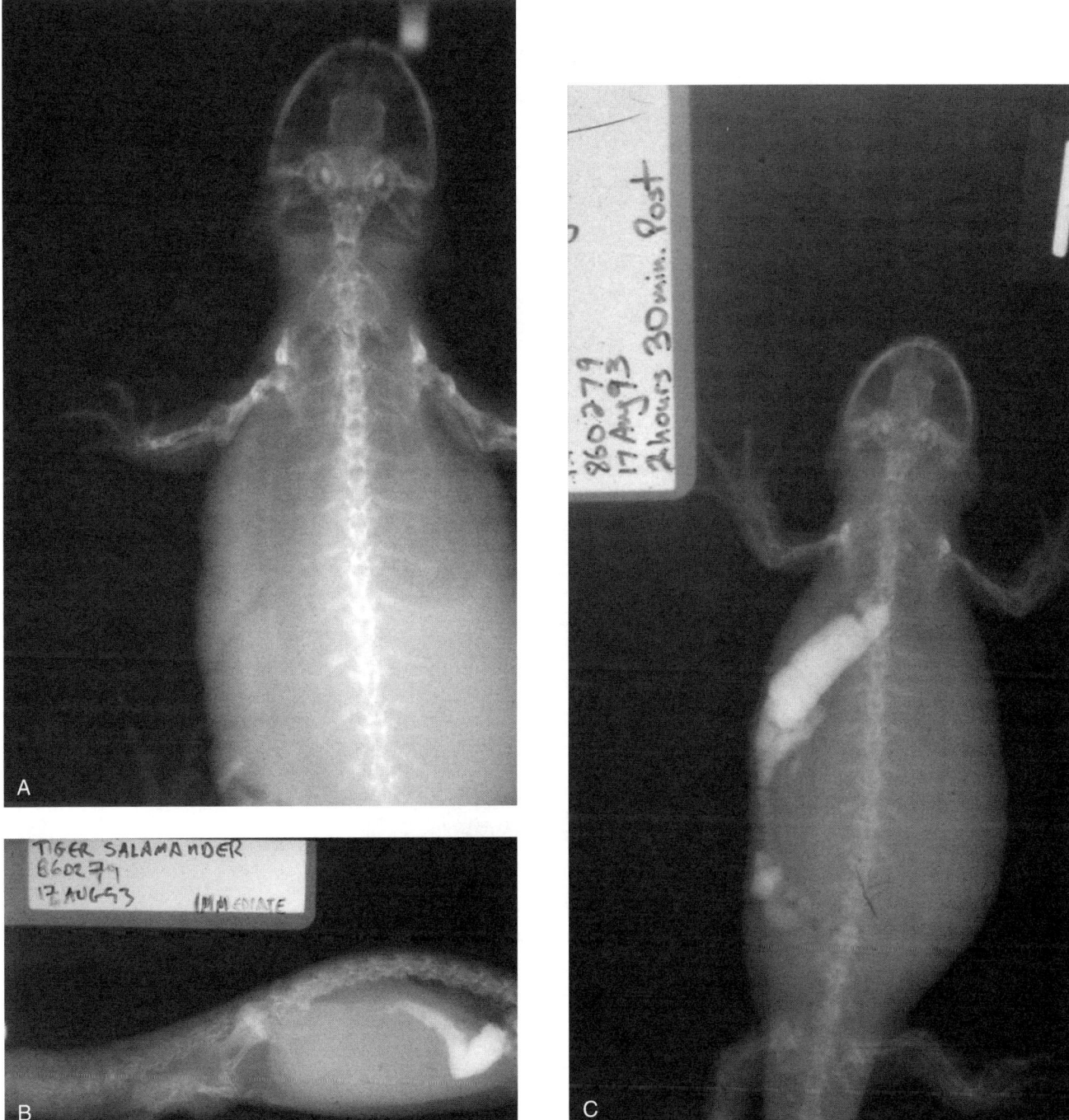

Figure 20.23. Tiger salamander, *Ambystoma tigrinum*. History of abdominal distension. **A.** Dorsoventral radiograph. Note the mass effect in right caudal coelom with cranial displacement of the right lung lobe. **B.** Gastrointestinal contrast series with barium sulfate. Lateral view demonstrates a mass effect with dorsocranial displacement of the stomach. **C.** Gastrointestinal contrast series with barium sulfate. Dorsoventral view demonstrates a marked left displacement and partial obstruction of the intestinal tract.

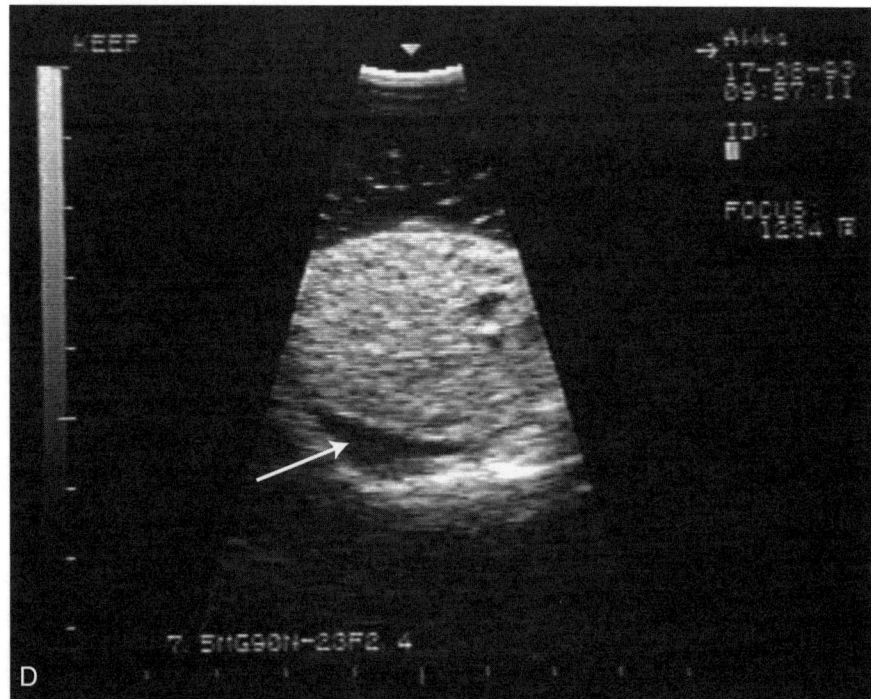

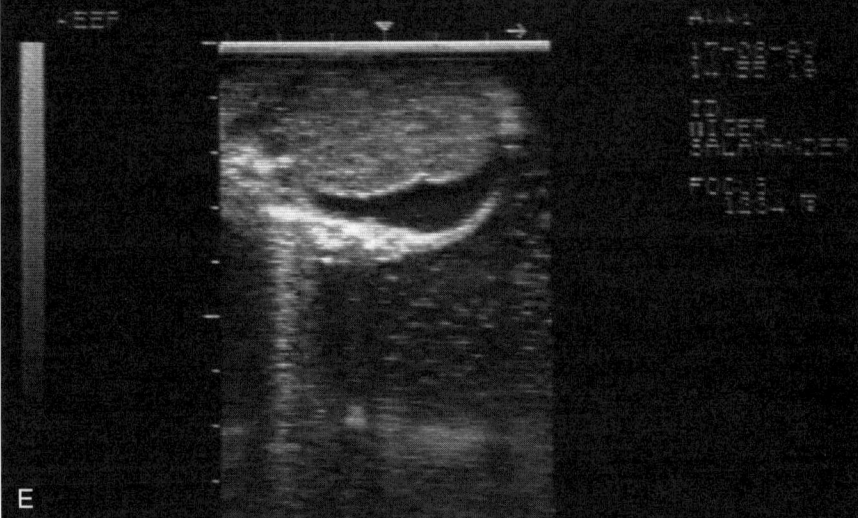

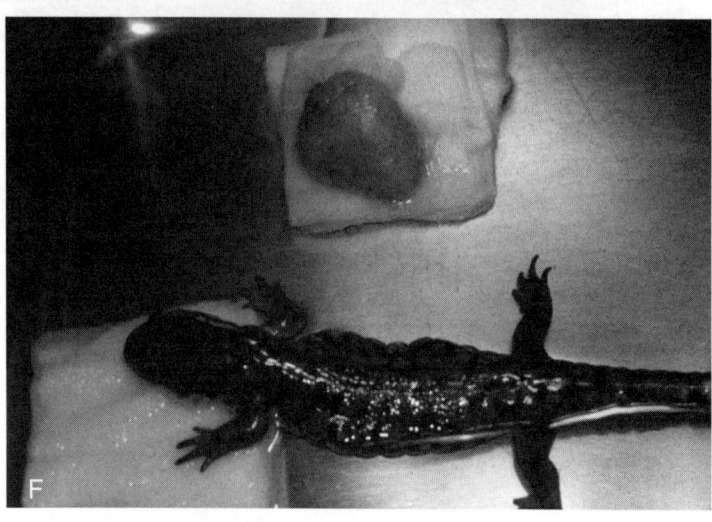

Figure 20.23 (*Continued*). D. Ultrasound image of a large coelomic mass. Dorsal plane midbody view with 7.5 MHz sector probe. The patient was imaged while in a water bath. The anechoic (black) area between the probe and the animal is the water bath. Note the fairly uniform echogenicity of the mass which occupies most of the coelomic cavity. A small amount of coelomic fluid can be seen between the mass and the dorsolateral body wall (arrow). E. Longitudinal ultrasound view of the midcoelom with a 5.0 MHz linear array probe. The animal's head is to the left and the animal's ventral surface is at the top of the image. Note the mass occupying most of the coelomic cavity with some coelomic fluid dorsally. F. The tiger salamander immediately after surgical removal of the mass. Histopathology revealed a neoplastic tumor of gonadal origin. (Mark Stetter)

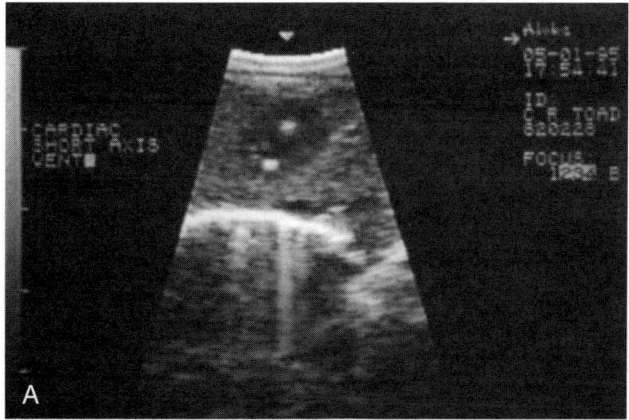
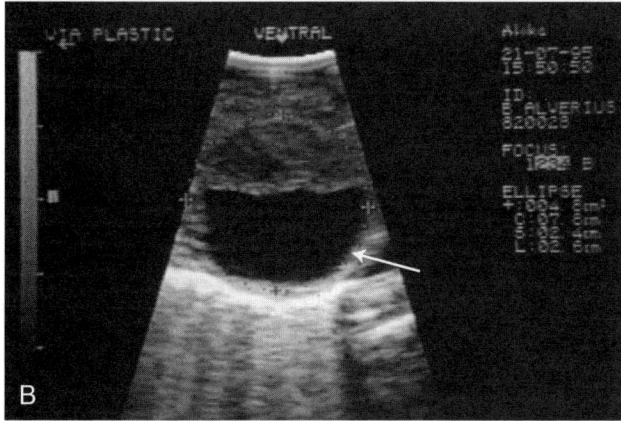

Figure 20.24. Colorado River toad, *Bufo alvarius*. History of ulcerative dermatitis. **A.** Short axis ultrasound image of the ventricle. Note the two well delineated hyperechoic (white) structures within the myocardium. Histological evaluation revealed partially calcified granulomas with intralesional fungal organisms (chromomycosis). **B.** Ultrasound view of a 4.8-cm renal mass. Note the round shape and thick wall (arrow). Within the mass, heavier particulate material has settled ventrally while clear anechoic fluid is dorsal. Histopathology revealed a renal abscess associated with a generalized chromomycosis infection. (Mark Stetter)

septicemia, fluid imbalances associated with renal disease, skin disease, or water quality issues, and neoplasia. Ultrasonography revealed severe hydrocoelom, however the short axis ultrasound view through the atria revealed a dilated atria containing a soft-tissue dense mass. The atria is markedly dilated and filled with a tissue mass displaying varying degrees of echogenicity. Cardiac disease is rarely reported in amphibians, perhaps due to the limited use of ultrasonography at present. Necropsy revealed ventricular myocardial fibrosis and severe dilated atrial cardiomyopathy (Plate 20.3). A large well organized thrombus was firmly attached to the endocardial wall.

ACKNOWLEDGMENTS

The author is indebted to Emiko Koike for her medical illustrations. I would also like to thank Dolores Sanginito for her tremendous help with manuscript preparation. The amphibians cited in this chapter are part of the Department of Herpetology at the Wildlife Conservation Park and the Central Park Conservation Center. A special thanks to the veterinary clinicians and pathologist at the Wildlife Health Center for their help with manuscript review and documentation of pathologic lesions.

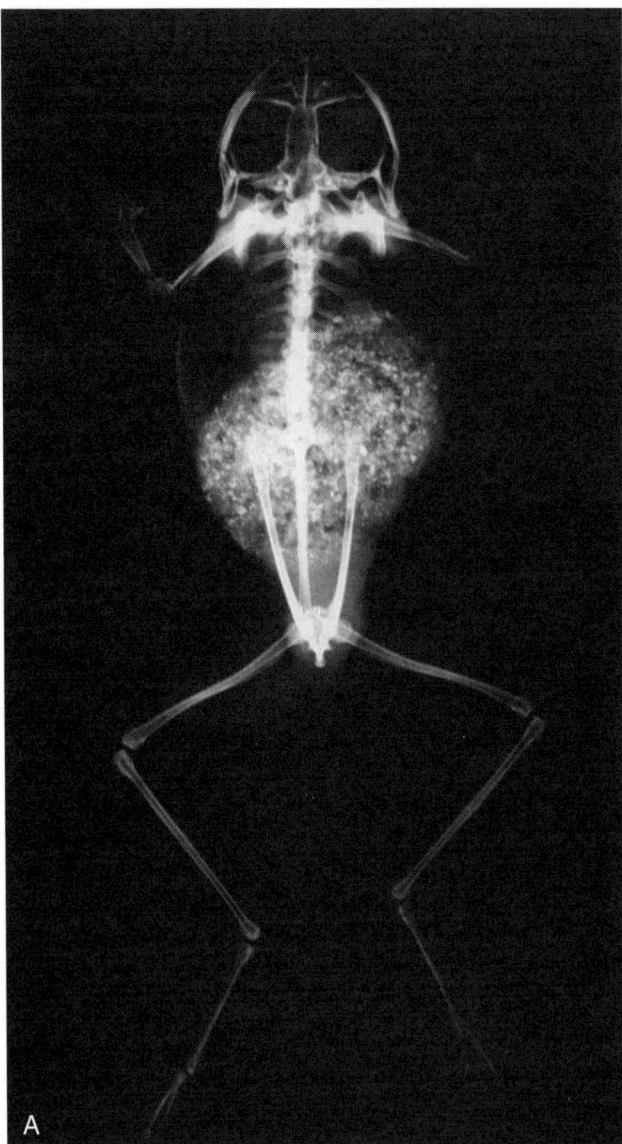
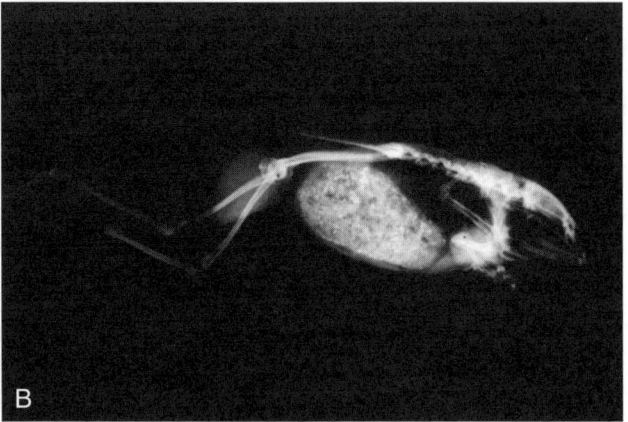
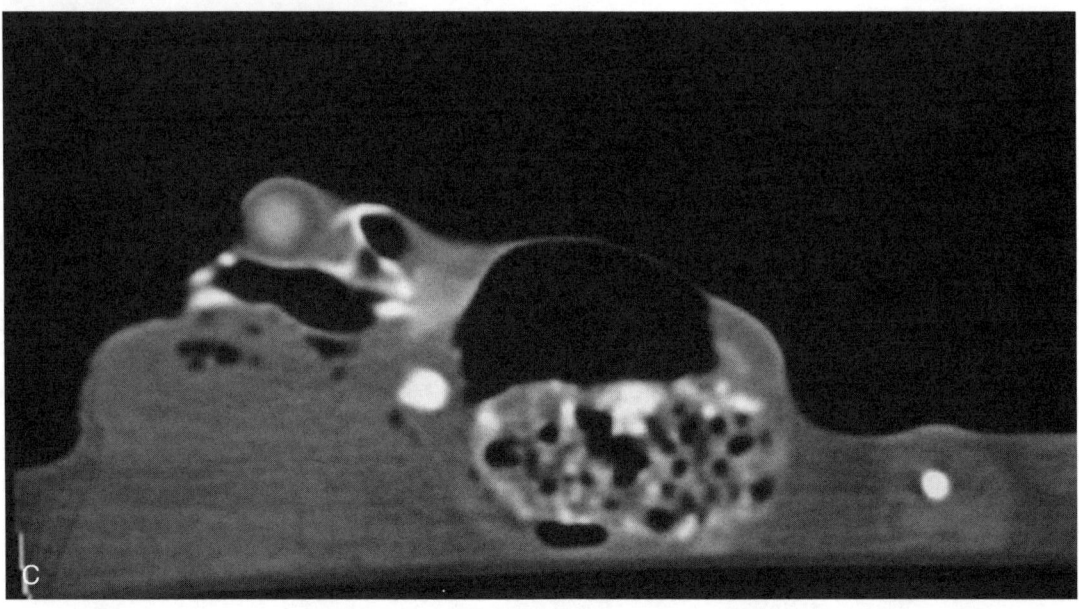

Figure 20.25. New Guinea giant treefrog, *Litoria infrafrenata*. History of anorexia. A. Ventrodorsal radiograph. Note the radiopaque material filling most of the caudal coelomic cavity suggestive of foreign body gastric impaction. B. Lateral radiograph. Radiopaque material occupies most of the caudal coelomic cavity. Surgical exploratory revealed severe gastric impaction with sand substrate from the exhibit. C. Left sagittal CT image with the head to the left. The head has been elevated and rests on gauze. The orbit, oral cavity, lung, stomach, and long bones can be identified. Note the impacted stomach filled with sand and gravel. (Mark Stetter and Jay Stefanacci)

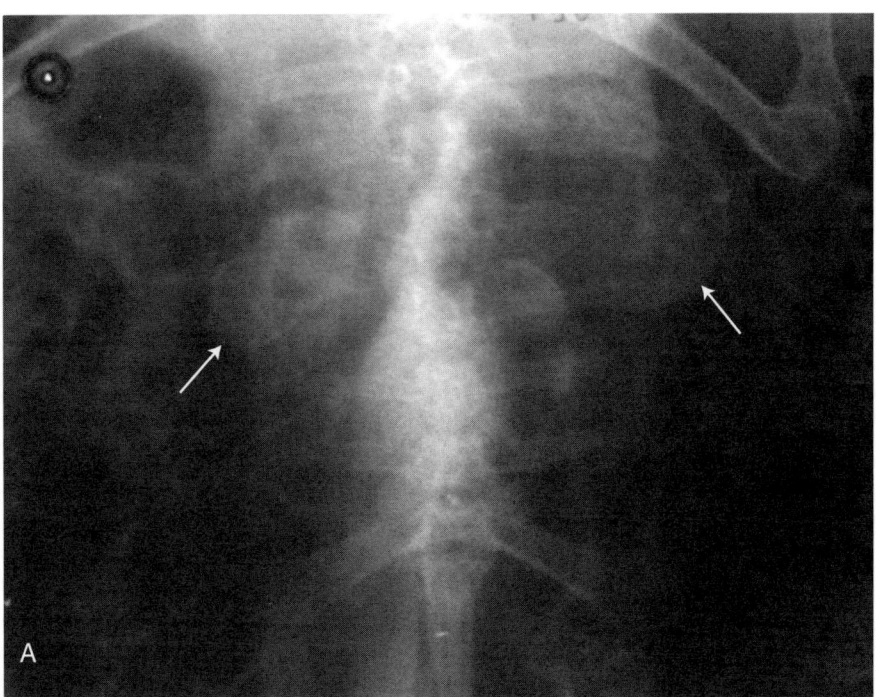
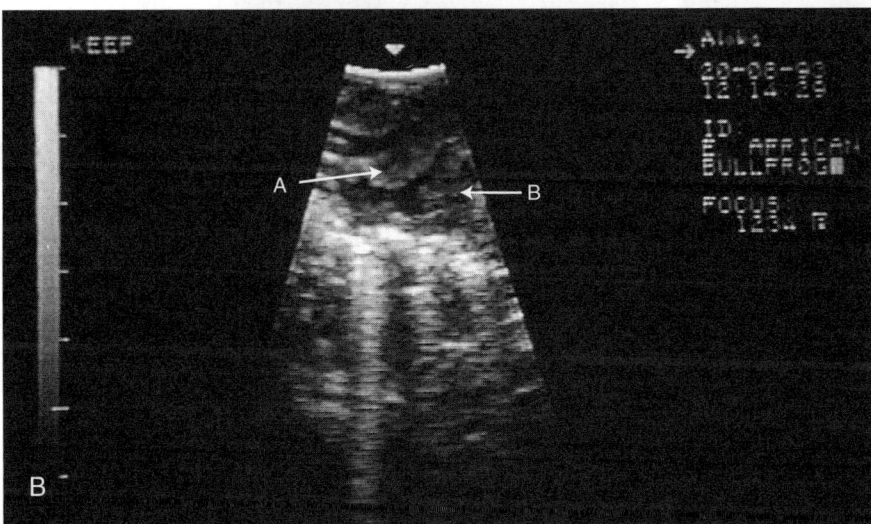
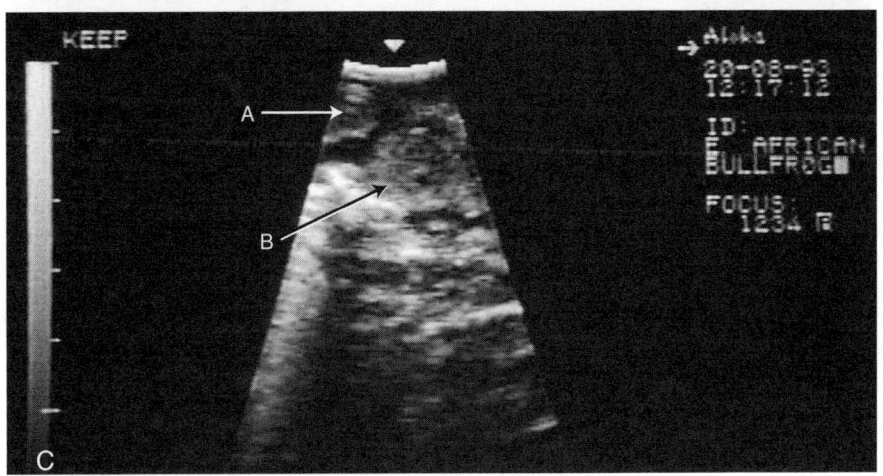

Figure 20.26. Tschudi's African bullfrog, *Pyxicephalus adspersus*. Routine quarantine examination. **A.** Dorsoventral view using dental radiograph film. Note the numerous round radiodense masses (arrows) in the cranial cavity. **B.** Long axis ultrasound image of the ventricle (A arrow) and surrounding tissue. Note the mild pericardial effusion (black area surrounding the heart) and round mass attached to the pericardial sac (B arrow). **C.** This image was captured 1.5 cm caudal to the cardiac image in Figure 20.26B. The apex of the ventricle (A arrow) can be seen in the upper left corner and the pericardial mass can be seen just caudal to the heart (B arrow). (Mark Stetter)

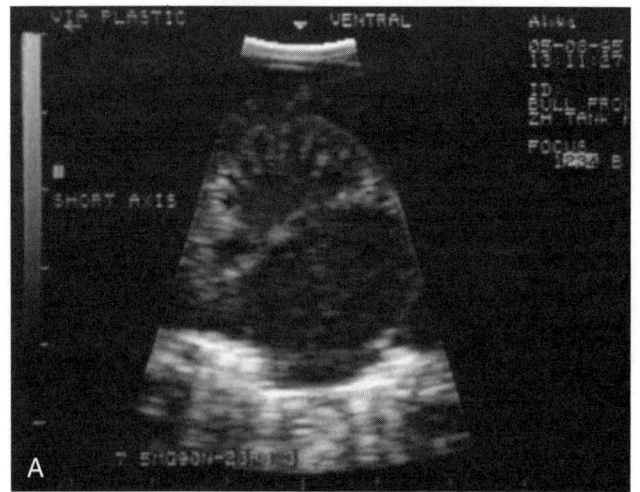
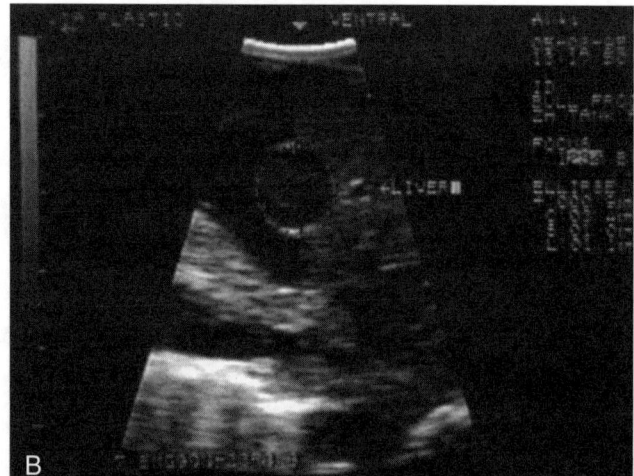
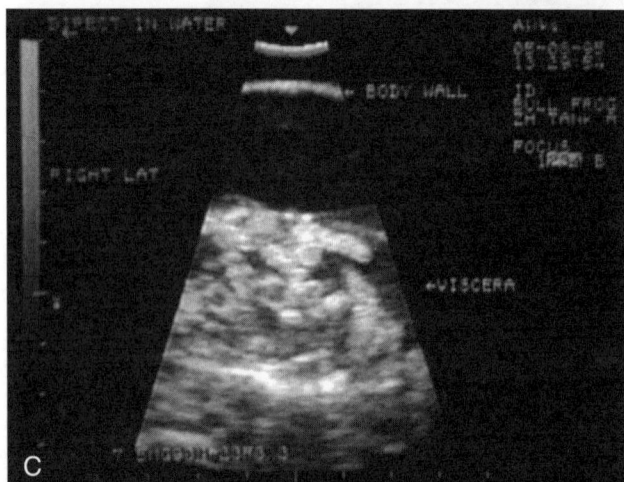
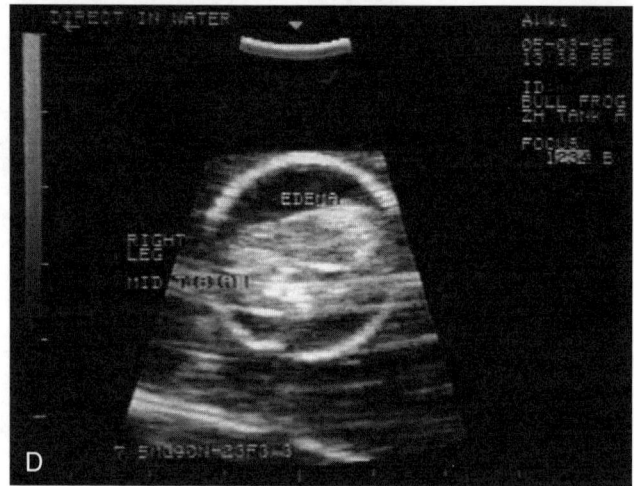
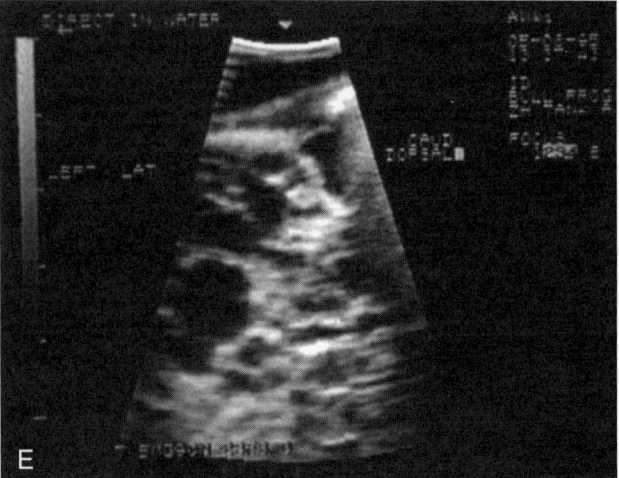

Figure 20.27. Bullfrog, *Rana catesbeiana*. History of hydrocoelom and edema. **A.** Short axis ultrasound view of the heart. Note the anechoic (black) pericardial fluid surrounding the heart. The thick-walled ventricle and thin-walled atria can be easily visualized. **B.** Ultrasound of midcoelomic area. The gall bladder (circled) and liver (arrow) can be seen floating in the copious amount of coelomic fluid (black). **C.** Ultrasound of the right dorsolateral coelom. Note the marked accumulation of anechoic fluid between the body wall and coelomic cavity. Fat bodies and intestinal loops can be seen floating within the coelomic fluid. **D.** Cross-section ultrasound view of the right leg at the midtibial region. Note the accumulation of fluid between the skin and underlying musculature. **E.** Ultrasound image through the caudal left lateral wall. Multiple fluid-filled cysts of various sizes are noted in the area of the kidneys. (Mark Stetter)

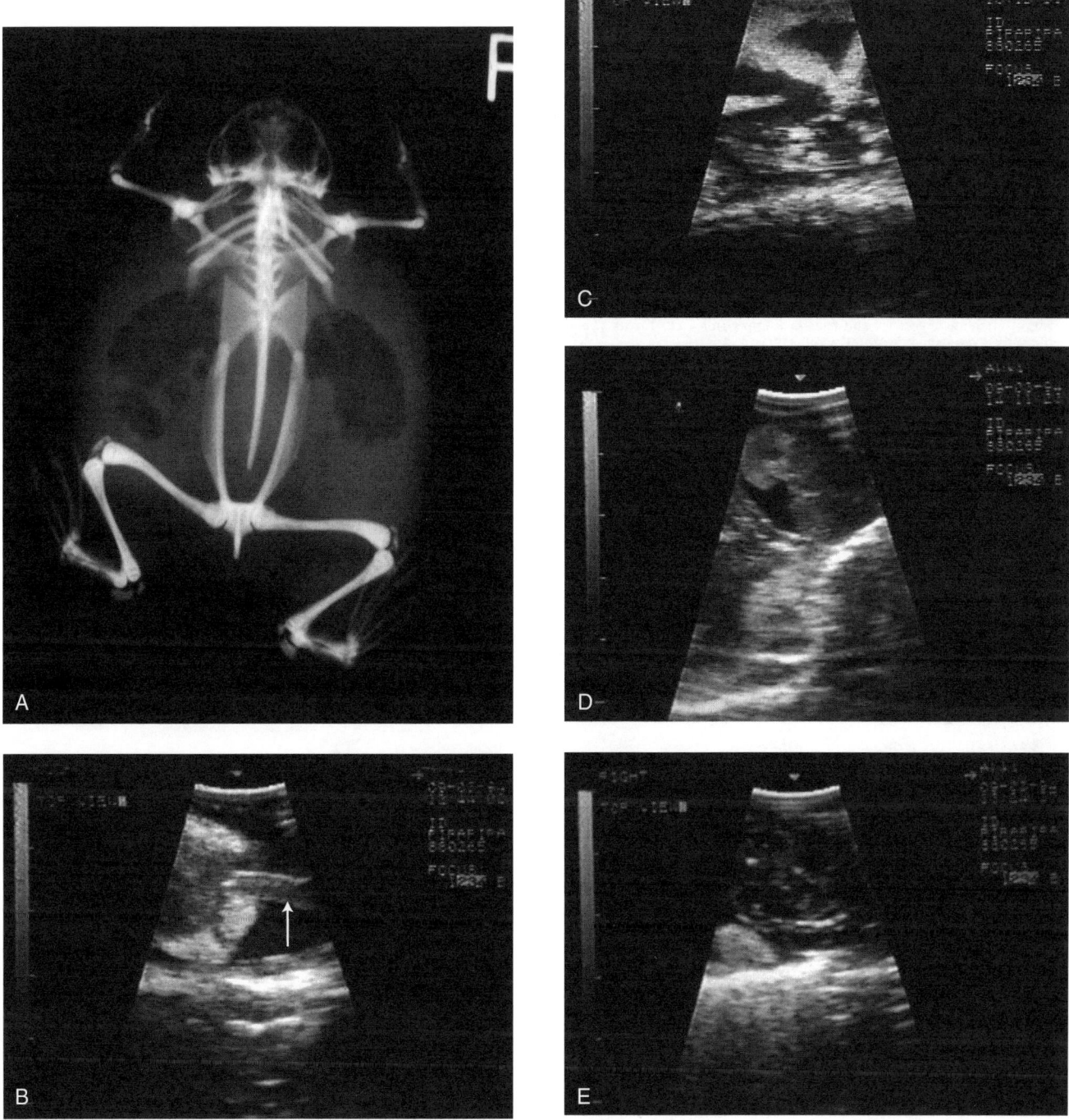

Figure 20.28. Surinam toad, *Pipa pipa*. History of abdominal distension and lethargy. **A.** Whole body dorsoventral radiograph using mammography machine. Note the abnormal appearing lungs and the generalized lack of visceral organ contrast. **B.** Ultrasound image of mid-coelom. A liver lobe can be seen floating within the coelomic fluid. The large hepatic portal vessel can be seen entering the liver (arrow). **C.** Ultrasound of caudal coelom. Intestines and fat bodies can be seen floating in the anechoic coelomic fluid. **D.** Long axis ultrasound view of the heart. The ventricle can be seen as a small ball on the left. The ventricle is surrounded by anechoic pericardial fluid and attached on the right to a markedly enlarged atria. **E.** Short axis ultrasound view through the atria. The atria is markedly dilated and filled with a complex tissue mass. This mass fills most of the lumen and has various degrees of echogenicity. (Mark Stetter)

REFERENCES

Blackband, S.J. and M.K. Stoskopf. 1990. In vivo nuclear magnetic resonance imaging and spectroscopy of aquatic organisms. Magnetic Resonance Imaging. Vol. 8, pp. 191–198.

Crawshaw, G.J. 1993. Amphibian medicine, in Fowler, M.E. (Ed.): Zoo and Wild Animal Medicine. 3rd ed. W.B. Saunders Co., Philadelphia, PA, pp. 131–139.

Duellman, W.E. and L. Trueb. 1986. Biology of Amphibians. McGraw-Hill Company, New York, pp. 287–414.

Kuchling, G. 1989. Assessment of ovarian follicles and oviductal eggs by ultrasound scanning in live freshwater turtles, *Chelodina oblonga*. Herpetologica 45:89–94.

O'Grady, J.P., C.H. Yeager, W. Thomas, G. Esra, and L. Findleton. 1978. Practical applications of real time ultrasound scanning to problems of zoo veterinary medicine. J. Zoo Anim. Med. 9:52–56.

Robeck, T.R., D.C. Rostal, P.M. Burchfield, D.W. Owens, and D.C. Kraemer. 1990. Ultrasound imaging of reproductive organs and eggs in Galapagos tortoises (*Geochelone elephantopus* sp.). Zoo Biology 9:349–359.

Rostal, D.C., T.R. Robeck, D.W. Owens, and D.C. Kraemer. 1990. Ultrasound imaging of ovaries and eggs in Kemp's ridley sea turtles (*Lepidochelys kempi*). J. Zoo Wildl. Med. 21(1):27–35.

Rübel, G.A., E. Isenbügel, and P. Wolverkamp. 1993. Atlas of Diagnostic Radiology of Exotic Pets. W.B. Saunders Co., Philadelphia, PA, 224 pp.

Rübel, A., W. Kuoni, and F.L. Frye. 1992. Radiology and imaging, in Frye, F.L. (Ed.): Biomedical and Surgical Aspects of Captive Reptile Husbandry. Krieger Publishing Co., Malabar, FL, pp. 185–208.

Rübel, A., W. Kuoni, and N. Augustiny. 1994. Emerging Techniques: CT Scan and MRI in Reptile Medicine. Seminars in Avian and Exotic Pet Medicine 3(3):156–160.

Sainsbury, A.W. and C. Gili. 1991. Ultrasonographic anatomy and scanning technique of the coelomic organs of the bosc monitor (*Varanus exanthematicus*). J. Zoo Wildl. Med. 22(4):421–433.

Schildger, B.J., M. Casares, M. Kramer, H. Spörle, M. Gerwing, A. Rübel, H. Tentiu, and T. Göbel. 1994. Technique of ultrasonography in lizards, snakes, and chelonians. Seminars in Avian and Exotic Pet Medicine 3(3):147–155.

Stetter, M.D. 1993. Use of dental x-ray film for non-dental radiography in zoological medicine. 1993. Proceedings American Association of Zoo Veterinarians, p. 123.

Stetter, M.D. and R.A. Cook. 1994. Normal and pathological ultrasonographic anatomy of amphibians. 1994 Proceedings American Association of Zoo Veterinarians, p. 76.

Stoskopf, M.K. 1989. Clinical imaging in zoological medicine: A review. J. Zoo Wildl. Med. 20(4):396–412.

Underhill, R.A. 1969. Laboratory Anatomy of the Frog. Wm. C. Brown Publishers, Dubuque, IA, 56 pp.

CHAPTER 21

SURGICAL TECHNIQUES

Kevin M. Wright, DVM

21.1. INTRODUCTION

Clinicians may experience unwarranted trepidation when faced with their first amphibian surgical case. Amphibians are generally good candidates for surgery. As an example, amphibians are generally more resistant to blood loss than birds or mammals. Furthermore, postoperative infections are rare, attributable, in part, to the antimicrobial properties of amphibian skin secretions. Amphibians must be kept moist during surgery, but this is easily accomplished in clinical practice for all but the largest aquatic specimens. The instruments used in amphibian surgeries are routinely used in other orders of animals including domestic species.

21.2 PRESURGICAL PREPARATION OF THE AMPHIBIAN PATIENT

Before the presurgical preparation of the amphibian patient, the clinician must take into account some of the unique aspects of amphibians such as their fluid needs and their susceptibility to water-soluble toxins such as iodine.

The amphibian should be well hydrated and have as normal an electrolyte balance as possible prior to surgery. Soaking the amphibian in a shallow water bath for 60 minutes or so prior to surgery will help ensure adequate hydration. An accurate weight should be obtained prior to surgery and immediately postoperatively so that hydration and nutritional status can be readily monitored.

Prophylactic antimicrobial therapy is recommended prior to any major surgery such as a celiotomy or limb amputation. The requisite moist environment necessary for the amphibian patient does not lend itself to maintaining a sterile surgical field. Although it appears that amphibians are remarkably resistant to postoperative infection, there has been no quantitative assessment of postoperative infections in amphibians versus other orders of animals. Although amphibian skin secretions may have antimicrobial effects, the cell-mediated immune response may be subdued following surgery allowing pathogens to flourish in the coelom or bloodstream. Antibiotics effective against anaerobes and with a Gram-negative spectrum of activity should be used.

To avoid emesis associated complications, the stomach should be empty of ingesta for elective surgeries (see also Section 9.2.1, Patient Preparation). Gastric emptying occurs within 4 hours for many small amphibians (<20 g). Larger insectivorous amphibians should be fasted a minimum of 48 h preoperatively, while vertebrate-eating amphibians should be fasted a minimum of 7 days. Fasting times should be prolonged if the amphibian is below its preferred body temperature. However, emergency surgeries should not be delayed as the risk of emesis is minimal.

Once an amphibian has been anesthetized with tricaine methanesulfonate, it should be removed from the anesthetic solution to avoid excessively prolonged anesthesia. Removal from isoflurane baths or removal of isoflurane gel is likewise recommended. The amphibian's hydration should be maintained via well-oxygenated clean water, and additional anesthetic used only if the amphibian shows signs of recovery intraoperatively (see Chapter 9, Restraint Techniques and Euthanasia).

Following induction of anesthesia, artificial slime, such as Shieldex® (Aquatronics, Malibu, CA) or Poly-Aqua (Kordon Division of Novalek Corp., Hayward, CA), may be used to coat the amphibian prior to surgical preparation. Water-soluble eye protectant may be needed if the surgery is to be prolonged. Sterile water-soluble gels (e.g., KY Jelly) should not be used to coat the skin as they might inhibit cutaneous respiration.

A surgical board made of plastic is recommended to contain the moist environment. A piece of plastic with a raised lip border will suffice. Meat-thawing trays sold in kitchen sundries stores work well. Oxygen may be bubbled though the water within the tray to assist respiration. The water should be changed periodically to remove any anesthetic excreted by the amphibian into solution.

A more complex surgical board can be custom-made by routing channels into a section of ⅜" thick plexiglass and gluing plexiglass edges to the board. The board can be rigged with a drain on one end to allow a constant flow of fresh water to contact the patient without flooding the surgical field.

The actual surgical bed needs to fix the position of the amphibian patient. A thin layer of sterilized foam rubber or filter floss can be used to support the body. A hollow that fits the amphibian's body should be made to secure the patient in place.

Surgical scrubs, that is those products that contain soaps or detergents, should not be used. Iodine-containing products are not recommended due to possible toxic reactions associated with their use, however the use of tamed-iodine compounds has been documented in the literature without any apparent untoward effect (Brown, 1995; Jacobson, 1975). Isopropyl alcohol is not recommended due to its toxicity in amphibians. The recommended surgical disinfectant is 0.75% chlorhexidine (e.g., diluted from 2% Nolvasan®, Fort Dodge Labs) which has a broader spectrum of antimicrobial activity and an increased residual activity than the iodine compounds. Flaccid paralysis and death occurred in aquatic turtles soaked in a bath of 0.024% chlorhexidine for 45 minutes (Lloyd, 1996), and may have similar adverse effects in some amphibians. Benzalkonium chloride (2 mg/L) may be used to prepare the surgical site. The site should be wiped clean of debris and excess skin secretions before the surgical site disinfectant is applied. The disinfectant should be left in contact with the skin for a minimum of 10 min prior to surgery. This can be accomplished by soaking a clean sterile gauze with the disinfectant solution and placing the soaked gauze onto the surgical site for the duration of the needed contact time. Replacement of the gauze with freshly soaked gauze should occur at least once during the surgical site preparation. A rinse of sterile saline is recommended immediately prior to draping the amphibian.

The amphibian patient is difficult to drape due to the nature of the anesthetic most commonly used (e.g., a solution of tricaine methanesulfonate), its usually small body size, and its moist body surface. A sterile, clear plastic drape (e.g., Barrier Incise Drape®, Surgikos) can be placed across the entire tray. In most instances all that is recommended is to place a sterile field around the surgical board so that instruments and supplies can be left on the operating table with minimal additional contamination. Amphibian surgeries are considered to be clean-contaminated surgeries. Draping of the patient and full gowning of the surgeon may help reduce the contamination of the surgical field, but are deemed of little practical benefit in most instances.

In addition to standard surgical instruments, ophthalmic and microsurgical instruments should be available. Eyelid retractors can be used as coelomic retractors in many amphibian patients. Iris forceps, iris scissors, and micro-mosquito hemostats may be used to manipulate tissue, but finer control such as afforded by retinal forceps and spring-handled scissors is often needed. Castroviejo needleholders are recommended for manipulating the fine suture material needed in many small amphibian patients. Magnification of the surgical field may be provided by operating microscopes or binocular magnification loupes.

Hemostasis may be provided by standard techniques. Hemostatic clips (e.g., Hemoclip®, Weck; Ligaclip®, Pittman Moore) are useful in amphibians, and are more easily manipulated in the small patient than surgical ligatures. Cotton tip applicators, microtip applicators, and small surgical spears (e.g., Weck-Cell Surgical Spears, Weck) can be used to absorb fluid as well as to apply direct pressure to stem any hemorrhage. Absorbable gelatin sponges (Gelfoam, Upjohn, Kalamazoo, MI) can be packed into a space to quell hemorrhage. Electrocautery (electrosurgery) can be used to coagulate hemorrhage sites as well as being used for many other surgical procedures.

Many different types of suture materials have been used in amphibians including but not limited to polyglactin-910 (Vicryl®, Ethicon, Johnson & Johnson, Somerville, NJ) (Wright, 1994) polyglycolic acid (Dexon®, Davis & Geck) (Emerson, 1983) and nylon 3–0 polydioxanone (PDS II®) (Brown, 1995). The breakdown of absorbable sutures has been documented, and these materials are not recommended for skin closure (Brown, 1995; Wright, 1994). Absorbable sutures can be used for closure of hollow organs and muscle layers. Nonabsorbable monofilament suture materials (e.g., nylon) and tissue adhesives should be on hand for skin closure. Suture material 3–0 and 4–0 is recommended, although thicker and thinner material may be needed depending on the patient's body size and surgical needs.

Emergency drugs to deal with life-threatening metabolic disorders should be on hand during any surgical procedure. Dexamethasone, doxapram, prednisolone, epinephrine, glucose, and electrolyte solutions should be on hand in premeasured amounts tailored to the surgical patient's body size.

21.3 SURGICAL PROCEDURES

21.3.1. Incision

The amphibian integument is much tougher to penetrate than one would infer from its few cell layers. A number 15 scalpel blade is most appropriate for initial skin incisions (Plates 21.1–21.4), but the number 11 blade is useful for stab incisions such as are needed for celioscopic procedures. It is best to make one bold stroke leaving a clean long incision rather than several tentative strokes that yield a ragged incision. Avoid transecting macroscopic glands, lymph hearts, and blood vessels with the incision.

21.3.2 Skin Closure

Everting-type suture patterns such as the simple interrupted pattern (Plates 21.5–21.11) or the horizontal mattress pattern is recommended for skin closure. Although other types of suture materials have been used, nonabsorbable monofilament suture material is recommended as many absorbable products dissolve in a moist environment (Brown, 1995; Wright, 1994). An interrupted pattern is recommended over continuous patterns due to the high incidence of dehiscence in the amphibian patient, and the fact that an interrupted pattern may not dehisce as completely as a continuous pattern.

Stent sutures may be needed to relieve pressure on the skin incision. Small cylinders of cured silicon rubber can be manufactured ahead of time to meet the needs of the amphibian patient, or small silastic tubing can be used.

Cyanoacrylate tissue adhesives (e.g., n-butyl-2-cyanoacrylate, isobutyl-2-cyanoacrylate) are being used with increasing frequency in amphibians because the polymerization product is water-resistant (Olson & Bruce, 1987). These glues can serve as hemostatic agents not only for skin closure but also for bleeding from the spleen, liver, kidney, and other organs. Tissue glues may be placed over a suture line for added protection from dehiscence and to serve as a waterproof coating (Plate 21.12).

Only those products marketed for surgical use should be used on amphibians. In some instances short chain industrial adhesives ("superglues") have been used but these products are not recommended as they are documented as the cause of inflammation and tissue death in rodents (Woodward et al., 1965).

21.4 MINOR SURGERIES

Many minor surgeries can be performed using local anesthesia via direct application of 2% lidocaine to the surgical site. The lack of deep pain can be tested via pinprick of the anesthetized area.

21.4.1 Identification Techniques

Toe-clipping. Toe-clipping has been one of the more popular methods of identifying anurans for field studies ever since its formal description 50 years ago (Bogert, 1947). One extensive study of the European common toad, *Bufo bufo,* utilized toe-clipping to mark its study specimens. Based on this study, the first three digits of the hand of male anurans should not be clipped as they are essential for grasping the female during amplexus, nor should the fourth digit of the foot for either sex as this digit is important for removing shed skin (Heusser, 1958).

This technique is not without criticism. Toe-clipping has had an impact on the survival of amphibians in field studies. Site inflammation, site necrosis, and generalized infection was documented in toe-clipped specimens of the natterjack toad, *Bufo calamita,* and up to one month lapsed between the date of toe-clipping and onset of inflammation (Golay & Durrer, 1994). Mortality rates were significantly increased for toe-clipped specimens of the Fowler's toad, *Bufo woodhousei fowleri* (Clarke, 1972). Weight loss occurred in specimens of the northern leopard frog, *Rana pipiens,* that were toe-clipped (Honegger, 1979) One author argues that the reasons for the differential mortality and anorexia noted in these two studies are not conclusively linked with the toe-clipping, and suggests a standardized protocol be developed to minimize the impact of surgical technique on interpreting mortality in a population of toe-clipped amphibians (Reaser, 1995). This argument is supported by another study which followed 61 specimens of the European common toad, *Bufo bufo,* that were toe-clipped with no evidence of inflammation reported over a 10-month observation period (Van Gelder & Strijbosch, 1996). Healing of the toe-clip sites was temperature-dependent, ranging from "a few days" during summer months to 2 weeks in the autumn, and physical fitness, as measured by food intake and mass, showed no significant difference between toe-clipped and intact toads in this study.

Toe-clipping in field studies usually has been done without analgesia and with little attention given to aseptic technique, but this is not recommended in veterinary practice. The amphibian patient either should be anesthetized or provided a suitable level of analgesia via an opioid. Surgical disinfection of the limb which is to be toe-clipped should be performed using chlorhexidine or benzalkonium chloride. Sterile stainless steel clips (e.g., Hemoclips®) can be used to constrict the phalanx to be severed and the digit distal to the ligation can be amputated (Figure 21.1). The amputation should occur at the

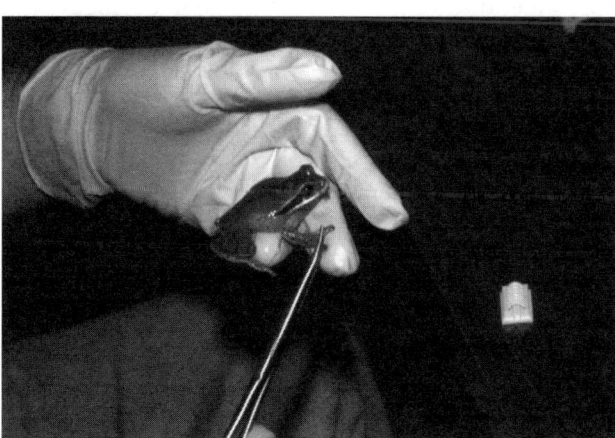

Figure 21.1. Use of a vascular clamp to toe-clip a New Granada cross-banded treefrog, *Smilisca phaeota.* (Ron Conti, Philadelphia Zoological Garden)

interphalangeal joint if possible rather than involving the phalangeal bone. The clip will fall off as the wound heals, a process that may take 7–30 days. Small anurans can be toe-clipped without use of these clips, and direct pressure can be used to stop the bleeding. Absorbable monofilament suture (e.g., PDS®, Ethicon, Johnson & Johnson, Somerville, NJ) may be used to ligate in place of the clips. Tissue glue or Nue-Skin™ may be used to seal the wound and prevent bleeding when the anuran recovers and begins to hop around. Stainless steel clips should not be used on amphibians destined for immediate release as the clip may become entangled and trap the amphibian.

Some anurans, most notably dendrobatids (e.g., dyeing poison frog, *Dendrobates tinctorius*), use their toes to signal each other. Other species, such as the horned frogs, *Ceratophrys* spp., may use their toes for pedal luring to entice prey. Toe-clipping is not recommended for any species with these or similar behaviors.

Some amphibians have remarkable regenerative abilities and the toe-clip may be difficult to distinguish within the span of 12 months. The author has encountered problems distinguishing individuals of the White's treefrog, *Pelodryas caerulea*, by their toe-clips, as well as specimens of the Australian dwarf treefrog, *Litoria fallax*, the oak toad, *Bufo quercicus*, and the golden mantella, *Mantella aurantiaca*. In general the toepad is somewhat deformed and discolored when compared to uninjured toes, and the distal phalanx is shortened, but these changes can be difficult to read with confidence in very small specimens. Newts and salamanders are even more renowned for their regenerative abilities.

Toe-clipping is a relatively inexpensive method of identification, and for this reason will continue to be a popular method of identification in field studies. It can be recommended as a short-term method of identification and in those circumstances where it can be repeated on a regular basis. As there are other methods of identification available that do not disfigure the animal, toe-clipping should be considered one of the least desirable methods.

Implantation of Passive Integrated Transponder Tags (PIT Tags). Passive integrated transponder (PIT) tags have been used in amphibians as a means of permanent identification (Corn, 1992; Fasola et al., 1993; Sinsch, 1992a, b; Vogelnest, 1994). The PIT tags were successfully implanted intracoelomically in newly metamorphosed specimens (body mass >2 g) of the alpine newt, *Triturus alpestris*, and the northern crested newt, *Triturus carnifex*, and specimens of the natterjack toad, *Bufo calamita* with a snout-vent length greater than 30 mm. The use of PIT tags has also been documented in the Australian giant treefrog, *Litoria infrafrenata*, and White's treefrog, *Pelodryas caerulea* (Vogelnest, 1994). This author has used or knows of the use of PIT tags in a variety of amphibian species including the spotted toad, *Bufo guttata*, the lowland Caribbean toad, *Peltophryne lemur*, Tschudi's African bullfrog, *Pyxicephalus adspersus*, the ornate horned frog, *Ceratophrys ornata*, the Surinam toad, *Pipa pipa*, the tiger salamander, *Ambystoma tigrinum*, the axolotl, *Ambystoma mexicanum*, and others. Since caecilians and salamanders lack the subcutaneous space found in anurans, the PIT tag should be placed intracoelomically in members of those two orders, Gymnophiona and Caudata. Intracoelomic placement can be done directly using the trochar needle provided with most PIT tags, or a 3-mm paramedian incision can be made and the PIT tag implanted through the incision. The second method is less likely to inflict damage on internal organs for the trochar is not blindly inserted into the coelom and the exact placement of the PIT tag can be visualized. In anurans the placement of the PIT tag can be either intracoelomic or subcutaneous. Intracoelomic placement is cosmetic, but concern has been raised about possible complications arising from abdominal adhesions. Subcutaneous placement of the PIT tag underneath the parotid (paratoid) gland of bufonids is a cosmetic site, while placement on the proximal ventral thigh is another possible site for other anurans destined for display purposes. The site of PIT tag injection should be closed with tissue glue to prevent ejection of the PIT tag prior to full wound healing. Other difficulties have been noted concerning PIT tag use in reptiles including migration of the PIT tag, breakage of the PIT tag, and loss of the PIT tag's signal (Germano & Williams, 1993).

Microtags. Microtags consisting of binary coded wire have been used to identify amphibians (Sinsch, 1992b). Microtags may be used in the same manner as PIT tags.

Loop and beads. Stainless steel wire may be passed through the muscles of the thigh to circumnavigate the femur. Glass beads of different colors may be threaded onto the wire to serve as visual markers differentiating individual amphibians. A similar technique has also been used on the tail of salamanders that do not autotomize their tails. This has been used to tag the jaw also. One caution is that the wire loop may become entangled on cage furniture in complex enclosures (Joly & Miaud, 1989), thus this is a technique most applicable to research purposes and is not recommended for pet amphibians or those to be used in zoological displays. Improper attachment of the loop may cause necrosis of the encircled bone and muscle. The offending loop should be removed.

21.4.2 Biopsy

Techniques for obtaining biopsies of amphibians vary little from that used in other animals (Cooper, 1994).

Few reports document the specifics of amphibian biopsy techniques (Emerson, 1983). Excisional skin biopsies can be obtained by tenting the skin with forceps and snipping the area to be sampled with iris scissors. This can be used to treat skin cysts and other localized skin lesions. Skin suture or tissue glue can be used to close the defect. Healing of the wound by second intention generally occurs within 21 days. Excisional biopsies are also useful for debulking large masses, and in some instances may be therapeutic. For example, the author treated an Australian giant treefrog, *Litoria infrafrenata,* for a mandibular fibrosarcoma by debulking the mass periodically over the course of several months. Hemorrhage may occur from the biopsy site and is best treated by direct pressure.

Punch biopsy needles (e.g., Anchor® soft tissue biopsy device, Anchor Products Co., Addison, IL) can be used for percutaneous biopsy of the liver in reptiles (Frye, 1997), and may also be used in amphibians. There is a danger that other organs may be sampled even if the needle biopsy is guided by celioscopy or ultrasound, thus celiotomy may be appropriate for better visualization of the desired organ. Biopsy forceps are often the most appropriate sampling device for parenchymatous organ biopsies (Cooper, 1994).

21.4.3 Cryosurgery (Debulking)

Cryosurgery is most useful for cutaneous masses that will create an excessively large skin defect when removed (Figure 21.2). A triple freeze-thaw cycle (30 seconds of liquid nitrogen application, 30 second rest) is recommended to insure cellular death, but this technique may prove less effective in freeze-adapted species such as the wood frog, *Rana sylvatica,* or spring peeper, *Pseudacris crucifer.* In one instance a Tschudi's African bullfrog, *Pyxicephalus adspersus,* died within an hour of cryosurgical debulking of a chromomycotic lesion (Ackerman & Miller, 1992). It is doubtful that the cryosurgery caused the death, but it is possible that topical application of liquid nitrogen could affect respiration.

21.5 MAJOR SURGERIES

21.5.1 Amputation

There are documented reports of anurans that survive quite well after full limbs have been amputated (Brown, 1995; Frye & Williams, 1995). In the case of hind limbs, it is recommended that the entire femur be removed by disarticulating its attachment to the pelvis. The entire femur should be removed rather than leave a bone-containing stump which might become abraded from movement. Anurans should be contained in a small spartan enclosure until the incision has healed to prevent activity that may cause dehiscence of the surgical site. A green treefrog *Hyla cinerea,* adapted quite well to its three-legged condition, fed on its own within 4 weeks postoperatively, and was returned to exhibit 7 weeks postoperatively (Brown, 1995). Since the hindfoot is used to remove skin during ecdysis, retained skin may become a problem in some three-legged anurans. The lack of a hindlimb may render some anurans unsuitable for reproduction as there is no grip for the male during inguinal amplexus. Additionally the hindlimbs are often used to manipulate the expelled ova by the male or the female, and the hind limbs are essential to create an appropriate nest for the ova in some anurans (e.g., foam nesting members of the Rhacophoridae).

An aged grey treefrog, *Hyla versicolor × chrysocelus,* at the Philadelphia Zoo was found with its left forelimb in its mouth. When the mouth was opened, it was apparent that the frog had ingested and digested its own left hand and part of the forearm. The frog managed well without the hand, and skin gradually regrew over the stump. In many species the forelimb is used for postural support of the body, locomotion, manipulating prey items, and grasping, thus a stump is best left in place. The humerus should be removed completely only if abrasions or other adverse consequences are noted. Complete lack of a forelimb renders most male anurans unfit for reproduction as they cannot amplex with the female. Assist feeding may be necessary for anurans lacking a forelimb as they may be unable to grasp and shove prey items into their mouth, a behavior well noted in hylids and bufonids.

Many newts and salamanders can regenerate lost limbs, so amputation is generally without long-term consequence as the limbs regrows. This ability has made certain species the subject of intense biomedical research to determine the exact nature of the nerve re-

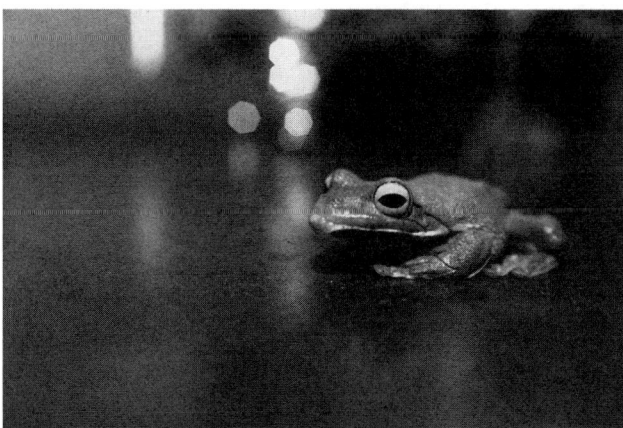

Figure 21.2. Fibrosarcoma on the mandible of a Australian giant treefrog, *Litoria infrafrenata.* This is an excellent candidate for debulking surgery. (David Wood)

generation in the new limb (e.g., Borgens et al., 1977; 1984), but these investigations are beyond the scope of this text. Most of the species of newts and salamanders commonly held in captivity possess the ability to regenerate normal appearing limbs. A Japanese giant salamander, *Andrias japonicus,* at the Philadelphia Zoo had its forelimb bitten off as a result of cagemate aggression. The limb grew back over the course of several years, but despite the normal outward appearance the skeletal structures remained cartilaginous. In this entirely aquatic species this cartilaginous replacement did not affect locomotion or mobility.

Tail amputations can occur through autotomy (e.g., Arntzen, 1994). In nonautotomic species tail amputation is sometimes necessary. Amputation should occur at the intervertebral joint, and if possible enough skin should be retained for flap closure and healing by primary intention. Dehiscence was a problem noted on an amphiuma, but healing by second intention proved successful although it took 70 days for complete reepithelialization (Wright, 1994). In a healthy aquatic system with an active biological filter, the wound may heal despite the appearance of fuzzy or slimy growths (Wright, 1994). If the wounds appears to be enlarging, not healing, or a change in the amphibian's demeanor is noted, then the wound should be reevaluated and debrided. Antibiotic therapy is warranted at this point.

Amputation has major implications for the development and survival of young growing amphibians or reproductively active amphibians. Injuries to the tail of the tadpoles of the firebelly toad, *Bombina orientalis,* reduced survivorship, extended the larval period, and decreased the size of the metamorph (Parichy & Kaplan, 1992). The energy needed to regrow the tail takes away from the energy needed to increase size during the tadpole stage and ultimately affects the size of the metamorph. Likewise injuries to reproductively active amphibians are repaired at the expense of energy put into reproduction, so amphibians that have sustained even mild injuries may not be suitable for propagation efforts for several months. If sufficient food is available, the consequences of injury are mitigated (Parichy & Kaplan, 1992).

Antibiotic therapy is warranted for at least 14 days postoperatively although this may not always be practical nor necessary, and, in some cases of severe infection prior to amputation, it may need to be prolonged for 6 weeks or more.

Assist feeding may be needed postoperatively for one or more meals (Brown, 1995) although other individuals may recover and feed on their own (Wright, 1994). Monitored reintroduction of the altered amphibian is recommended to insure that normal behaviors are expressed such as feeding, thermoregulation, water-seeking, and cagemate interactions.

In the case of amphibians brought in for rehabilitation and release, there has been the suggestion that amputee amphibians with toxic skin secretions may be released and survive as predators will not attack them (Frye & Williams, 1995). Studies supporting this statement are lacking. Furthermore, the ability of a three-legged amphibian to find or build proper shelter and to capture prey may be significantly less efficient than normal members of this species. Beyond the concern for the individual amphibian's well-being, one should consider the negative impact of a nonreproducing individual as it competes for resources from the wild population. This practice can not be condoned until studies supporting the viability of the release of amputee amphibians and validating their contribution to the wild population have been published.

21.5.2 Other Orthopedic Procedures

Although there are no published reports documenting their use in amphibians, intramedullary pins of a suitable size may be used to repair simple fractures of the long bones, along with the judicious use of bone cement, but osteomyelitis is a possible complication due to the difficulties inherent in obtaining a sterile surgical field in amphibians. Antibiotic therapy is warranted for a minimum of 21 days postoperatively, or anytime a fracture or exposure of the bone occurs. Antibiotic therapy may need to be extended for 6 weeks or longer for open fractures. Compound comminuted fractures are best treated with amputation, especially in newts and salamanders given their regenerative abilities. External fixtures are problematic in amphibians due to the posture of their limbs.

Mandibular fractures may result from attempts to open the mouth, and may be treated by applying bone cement in a layer across the reset edges of the bone rather than directly onto the ends. In species that do not rely on "gulping" for respiration, tissue glue may be used to seal the mouth shut for a few days. These fractures carry a grave prognosis as it can be difficult to provide nutritional support until the jaw is healed. Placement of a pharyngostomy tube may be attempted, but the small size of most amphibians precludes the use of all but narrow bore silastic tubing or intravenous catheters, which may be too narrow to permit passage of tube feeding formulas.

21.5.3 Laparoscopy and Endoscopy

Laparoscopy (celioscopy) has been used to determine the gender of the hellbender, *Cryptobranchus alleganiensis,* and the Chinese giant salamander, *Andrias davidianus* (Kramer et al., 1983). Presurgical fasting was 7 days in length. The anesthetized salamanders were placed in dorsal recumbency. The coelom was insufflated with CO_2 through a 2.0-mm incision made through the skin on the lateral side midway between the fore and hind limb. A second incision was made on the contralateral side approximately 3.0 cm anterior to the first incision, and a 5.0-mm endoscope was advanced through this incision. In some cases the abdominal organs had to be manipulated with the insufflating needle to permit viewing of the testicles. The testicles of the hellbender, *Cryptobranchus alleganiensis*, were yellow whereas the testicles of the Chinese giant salamander, *Andrias davidianus*, were tan. The oviduct appeared as a translucent convoluted structure, and the eggs ranged in appearance from small white immature ova to large yellow mature ova. All stages of ova maturation were noted within a salamander. Following identification of the gonads, the remaining CO_2 was vented through the incisions, skins sutures were placed, and the salamanders allowed to recover. The procedure took approximately 10 minutes. Laparoscopy has also been used to determine the gender of ranids such as the goliath frog, *Conraua goliath* (Figure 21.3). Insufflation can be hard to maintain in some amphibians due to the inelasticity of the skin and body wall. Repeated insufflation of gas may be needed to keep the field of view clear.

Laparoscopy has been a useful method of confirming the presence of visceral granulomatous diseases as well as various tumors in amphibians. Biopsies of parenchymatous organs may be obtained by laparoscopy. A paramedian approach allows access to the heart, the liver, the ova in the case of ovulating females, the bladder, and the stomach and intestines. Tilting the surgical table may allow views of the lungs and deeper structures, but often a lateral incision is needed for observation of the gonads, adrenal glands, and kidneys. Tissue glue may be used in place of skin sutures for most laparoscopic incisions.

Complications resulting from a properly performed laparoscopic procedure are rare. Infectious coelomitis may result from introduction of pathogens through the instruments, while sterile coelomitis may result from trauma to the organs by the instruments. Hemorrhage may occur from instrumental trauma, and seeding of neoplasia may be effected by biopsying or other manipulation of the neoplastic mass. If sufficient CO_2 is left behind in an aquatic amphibian, the amphibian may be unable to submerge or swim properly until the gas has been absorbed and dissipated. Antibiotic therapy is warranted for any laparoscopic procedure as it is possible that pathogens are introduced into the coelom via the trochar or the fiber optics of the laparascope.

Endoscopy has been used to retrieve foreign bodies from the upper gastrointestinal tract of a number of amphibians (see Section 7.7, Gastric Overload and Impaction).

21.5.4 Celiotomy

Exploratory celiotomy can be used if laparoscopic equipment is unavailable, if the laparoscopic view is unhelpful, or if further surgery is warranted to diagnose or treat a given condition. Exploratory celiotomy is recommended to evaluate inexplicable anasarca, abnormal coelomic masses and neoplasia, suspected visceral granulomatous disease, gastrointestinal foreign bodies, and many other conditions. Antibiotic therapy is warranted with any celiotomy.

This author is unaware of exploratory celiotomies of ill caecilians, and the very nature of their elongated body plan and musculoskeletal system would make this procedure problematic. It would be best to make several small paramedian incisions rather than one large incision to surgically explore a caecilian. Caesarian sections have been performed on caecilians to remove embryos for histologic study (personal communication, M. Wake, 1996), but the survival of the mothers was not of concern in these studies.

The surgical approach to the anuran or salamander coelom is best accomplished through a paramedian

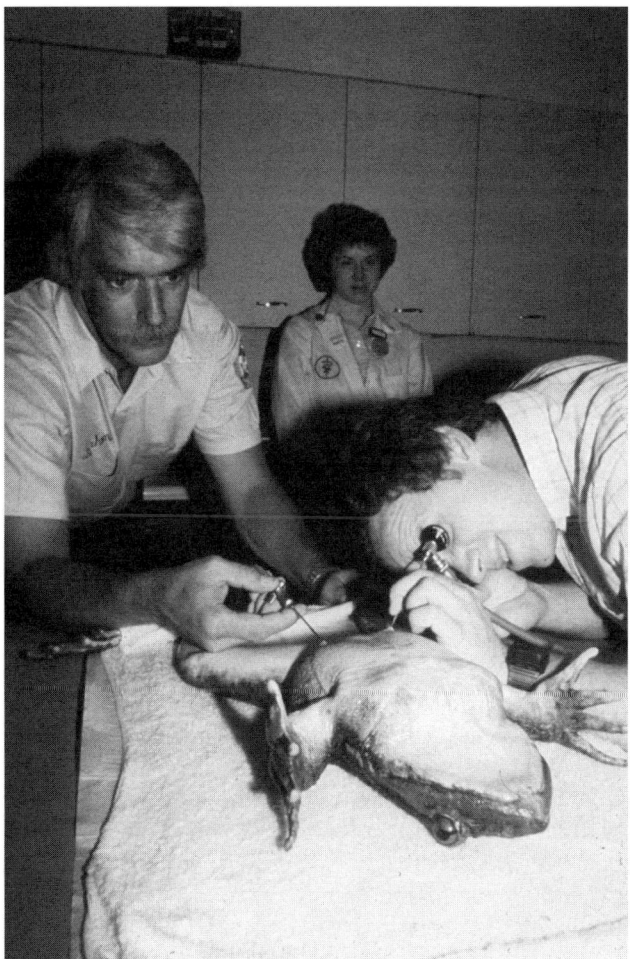

Figure 21.3. Laparoscopy for gender determination in a goliath frog, *Conraua goliath*. (Don Gillespie)

approach or midventral approach while the amphibian is in dorsal recumbency. Care must be taken to avoid damaging the midline abdominal vein during the transection of the muscle layer. Rather than focusing on the suspected underlying etiology of the amphibian's illness, a thorough survey of the organs should commence upon exposure of the coelom so that no lesions or abnormalities are missed. In some instances a lateral approach may be used with the amphibian in lateral recumbency, but damage to the muscle layer is greater than with a paramedian approach.

Closure of the celiotomy should occur in two layers when possible. Muscle layers should be closed if possible. Absorbable gelatin sponges may be placed on the coelomic surface of the muscle and suture placed through this sponge and muscle layer to reduce the likelihood of muscle tearing, a technique that was described for the surgical repair of a ventral abdominal hernia in a tomato frog, *Dyscophus antongili* (Meier, 1982). In this frog, polyglycolic acid absorbable sutures (Dexon®, Davis & Geck Co.) for skin closure were removed 14 days postoperatively without dehiscence occurring. An ovarian herniation in an African clawed frog, *Xenopus laevis,* caused it to be euthanized without surgical intervention (Foley et al., 1995).

A gastrotomy may be performed to remove ingested objects that could not be removed by gavage or endoscopic retrieval. Gastric overload is a surgical emergency, and pre-operative corticosteroids are recommended. Stay sutures should be used to secure the stomach prior to the gastrotomy, and care should be taken to avoid damaging any of the larger gastric vessels. The coelom may be packed with sterile gauze to minimize contamination by spilled gastric contents. Standard closure techniques are recommended using absorbable synthetic monofilament suture material. Postoperative fluids are recommended. If the patient's condition permits, the amphibian should not be fed for a minimum of 7 days postoperatively, and only small meals should be offered for 4–6 weeks thereafter. Maintenance on a liquid diet may be prudent.

On occasion a foreign object such as a plant awn may penetrate through the stomach and body wall (Plate 21.13). These can often be pulled through the skin and the wound debrided and left to heal by second intention. A gastrotomy may be needed to remove the object(s).

This author discovered an intestinal intussusception in a tiger salamander, *Ambystoma tigrinum,* during necropsy. This salamander had shown signs of cachexia and anorexia, and had been maintained on tube-feeding formula. An intestinal obstruction was suspected among other etiologies due to the emaciated appearance of the animal despite an enlarged abdomen (Figures 21.4, 21.5). A small firm cylindrical mass was palpable in the caudal abdomen. The salamander died during an exploratory celiotomy, but an earlier diagnosis via radiograph contrast study or ultrasonography would have merited bowel resection as treatment. Intestinal resection of amphibians has been performed in the course of biomedical research, but the long-term survivorship of these animals is difficult to ascertain.

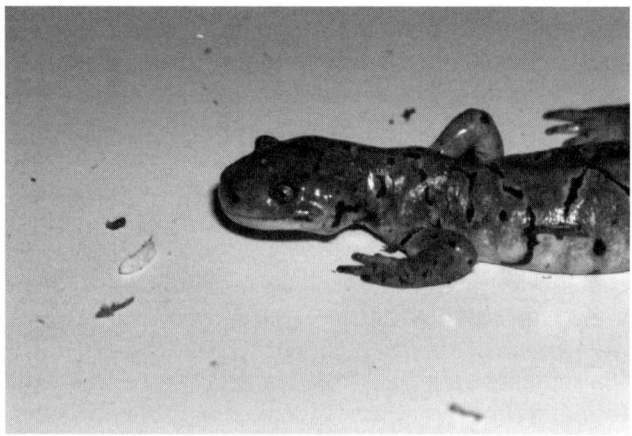

Figure 21.4. A tiger salamander, *Ambystoma tigrinum*, suffering chronic undernutrition resulting from an intestinal intussusception. (Kevin Wright, Philadelphia Zoological Garden)

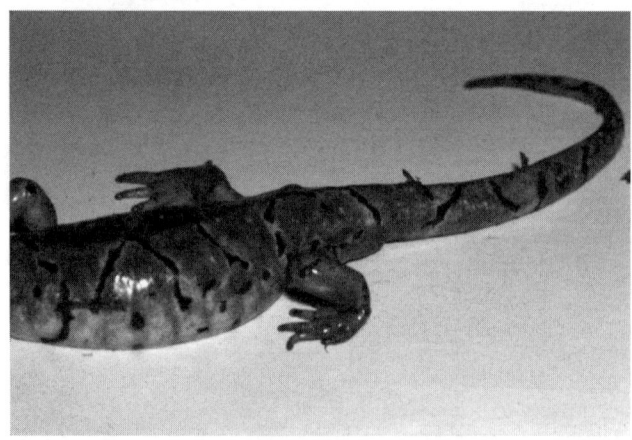

Figure 21.5. The tiger salamander from Figure 21.4. Note the poor muscle mass and tone, and an enlarged abdomen. (Kevin Wright, Philadelphia Zoological Garden)

Although rare, cystic calculi occur in amphibians. Cystotomy may be used to remove these calculi, as well as any other foreign objects such as monogenetic trematodes. Stay sutures should be used to secure the bladder prior to the cystotomy. The coelom may be packed with sterile gauze to minimize contamination by spilled bladder contents. Standard closure techniques are recommended using absorbable synthetic monofilament suture material. Urinary tract urate calculi have been removed successfully from a leaf frog, *Phyllomedusa* cf *tarsius* (see Plates 21.1–21.12), as well as from the uricotelic painted-belly monkey frog, *Phyllomedusa sauvagii*. Objects within the bladder, such as stones or trematodes, may often be diagnosed by transillumination or palpation. Catheterization may allow some objects to be flushed out of the bladder without surgery. If trematodes are suspected, a course of praziquantel therapy is recommended to treat the urinary bladder parasites, and the route of administration may be by direct inoculation into the bladder (see Chapter 24, Pharmacotherapeutics). If this treatment fails to eliminate the trematodes, a cystotomy may be considered.

21.5.5 Gonadectomy, Gonadal Biopsy

Gonadectomy has been used to study various physiological responses in amphibians. A single lateral incision was used to gain access to the testes in one study of nuptial pad development in the male northern leopard frog, *Rana pipiens* (Lynch & Blackburn, 1995). The testes were removed by electrocautery. The paramedian approach or ventral midline approach used for a celiotomy can be used to access the gonads of either sex for removal or biopsy (Ritke & Lessman, 1994; Saidapur & Hoque, 1996). Ovariectomy was performed on adult (300–500 g) females of the Indian bullfrog, *Rana tigrina*, via a 10–12-mm longitudinal midventral incision in the caudal abdomen (Saidapur & Hoque, 1996). Blood vessels were prominent in the mesenteries attaching the ovaries to the kidneys, and were ligated before cutting of the mesenteries. The frogs in this study were inappetent and lethargic for 3 days following surgery, but this may also have been a side effect of the ether used as anesthesia. In this study the ovariectomized frogs retained larger fat bodies and body mass compared to intact frogs undergoing the vitellogenic cycle. Fat bodies have been linked to reproductive cycles of females and/or males in several other species including the two-toed amphiuma, *Amphiuma means*, the red-spotted newt, *Notophthalmus viridescens*, the edible frog, *Rana esculenta*, and the six-fingered frog, *R. hexadactyla* (Saidapur & Hoque, 1996), so it is likely that gonadectomized amphibians have a tendency toward obesity.

21.5.6 Cloacal and Rectal Prolapse

Prolapse of either the cloacal or rectal tissue is a frequently encountered surgical emergency (Plates 21.14–21.17, Figure 21.6). This is most commonly encountered in anurans with nematodiasis, and impression smears of the exposed rectal tissue may reveal nematodes and their ova (Plate 21.18). Surprisingly, the anurans are generally bright and alert despite the prolapse. An anuran that is depressed is probably suffering from an underlying metabolic derangements such as hypocalcemia, gastric overload, or intoxication. Prolapse can be caused by other etiologies such as neo-

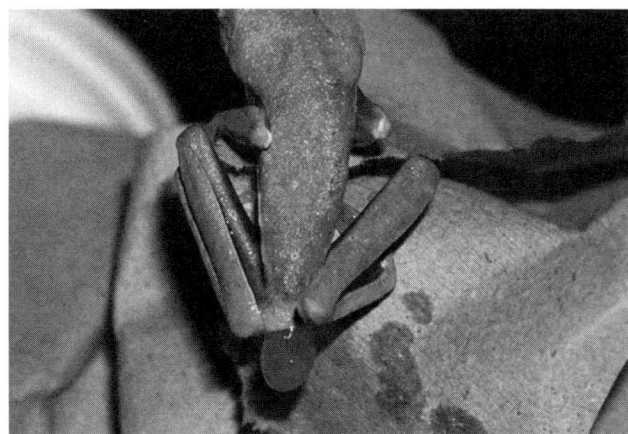

Figure 21.6. Red-eyed treefrog, *Agalychnis callidryas*, with cloacal prolapse. (Kevin Wright, Philadelphia Zoological Garden)

plasia (see Plates 21.15, 21.16), trauma, and the strain of passing impacted fecal matter, or gastrointestinal foreign objects, so care should be taken to rule out these etiologies concomitant with reduction of the prolapse. Reduction of the prolapse may be initiated by coating the tissue with hyperosmotic saline (i.e., 2–5%) ophthalmic solution (Plate 21.19). Hyperosmotic sugar solution can be used if the hyperosmotic saline is not available. The tissue should appear less edematous within a few minutes of contact with the hyperosmotic solution (Plate 21.20). A water-soluble lubricant can then be applied to the tissue prior to replacement. In some instances a lubricant containing an anti-inflammatory agent is recommended (Plate 21.21). Cotton tip applicators can be used to replace the tissue back through the cloacal opening (Plates 21.22, 21.23). A pursestring suture around the cloaca is recommended for severe prolapses or prolapses with a deeply erythematous appearance.

21.5.7 Enucleation

Enucleation is the last resort for a severely damaged optic globe, whether it is from infection, trauma, neoplasia, or any other etiology. Care must be taken to avoid damaging the membrane between the eye and the buccal cavity. Absorbable gelatin sponges (e.g., Gelfoam®, Upjohn, Kalamazoo, MI) may be used to pack the orbit to stop bleeding. In amphibians the surgical site may heal by second intention rather than attempt closure. Topical and systemic antibiotic treatment is warranted. In anurans that possess eyelids, the enucleation may be done either sparing the lids or removing the lids. If the lids are spared, the margins should be debrided prior to opposing the lids and suturing or gluing them together. Nonabsorbable synthetic suture material (e.g., nylon) is best used so that dissolution of the suture material is not a contributing factor for dehiscence. The dead space created behind the lids may serve as a nidus of infection, so topical and systemic antibiotic therapy is warranted for 14–21 days. Dehiscence is indicative of devitalized tissue or excessive tension on the lid margins.

21.6. POSTOPERATIVE ANALGESIA

Analgesia (antinociception) in amphibians has been studied purely from a research standpoint as amphibians are one of the most widely used nonmammalian models for pain (nociceptive) research (Brenner et al., 1994). Unfortunately the clinical usefulness of much of this research is limited as the pharmacologic agents investigated are primarily opioids (e.g., Pezalla, 1983; Pezalla & Stevens, 1984; Stevens, 1988; Stevens & Kirkendall, 1993; Stevens & Pezalla, 1983, 1984; Stevens et al., 1994, 1995). One recent study demonstrated the stress-induced analgesia by the endogenous production of endorphins in the northern leopard frog, *Rana pipiens* (Stevens et al., 1995), a physiological response that must be considered prior to the undertaking of prolonged procedures without general anesthesia. This stress-induced analgesia may be misinterpreted by the clinician unaware of this response.

Morphine sulfate administered at a dose of 38 mg/kg SQ to the northern leopard frog, *Rana pipiens*, produces significant analgesia for up to 8 hours (Stevens & Kirkendall, 1993). Higher dosages of morphine have profound adverse effects including immobilization with generalized muscular rigidity, explosive motor behavior, and death (Pezalla & Stevens, 1984). The appropriate dosages in other species of amphibians are unknown, and caution is advised in the use of morphine in other species due to possible variability in the opioid response. Nonetheless, at least one dose of morphine sulfate should be considered following a major surgical procedure on an amphibian.

The field of clinical analgesia in amphibians is in need of investigation. The acetic acid test methodology of assessing the nociceptive threshold in frogs has been described (Pezalla, 1983), and provides a standard by which analgesic compounds can be compared (Stevens, et al., 1994). Many of the more commonly used analgesics in domestic animal medicine await evaluation in amphibians. Flunixin meglumine at an empirical dose of 1 mg/kg IM q 24 h has been recommended for reptiles (Bennett, 1996) and diazepam (2.5 mg/kg PO SID) has proved effective in calming fractious and excitable specimens of the green iguana, *Iguana iguana* (Rossi, 1997), but their actions in amphibians are unknown. Topical administration might be an effective alternative route or administration. Either drug might be of use in managing nervous or delicate amphibians pre- and postoperatively.

REFERENCES

Ackerman, J. and E. Miller. 1992. Chromomycosis in an African bullfrog, *Pyxicephalus adspersus*. Bulletin of the Association of Reptilian and Amphibian Veterinarians 2(2):8–9.

Arntzen, J.W. 1994. Allometry and autotomy of the tail in the Golden-striped salamander, *Chioglossa lusitanica*. Amphibia-Reptilia 15:267–274.

Bennet, R.A. 1996. Anesthesia, *in* Mader, D.R. (Ed.): Reptile Medicine and Surgery. W.B. Saunders Co., Philadelphia, PA, pp. 241–247.

Bogert, C.M. 1947. A field study of homing in the Carolina toad. Am. Mus. Novit. 1355:1–24.

Borgens, R.B., J.W. Vanable, Jr., and L.F. Jaffe. 1977. Bioelectricity and regeneration: Large currents leave the stumps of regenerating newt limbs. Proc. Natl. Acad. Sci. USA 74:4528–4532.

Borgens, R.B., M. E. McGinnis, J.W. Vanable, Jr., and E.S. Miles. 1984. Stump currents in regenerating salamanders and newts. J. Exp. Zool. 231:249–256.

Brenner, G.M., A.J. Klopp, L.L. Deason, and C.W. Stevens. 1994. Analgesic potency of *alpha* adrenergic agents after systemic administration in amphibians. Journal of Pharmacology and Experimental Therapeutics 270(2):540–545.

Brown, C.S. 1995. Rear leg amputation and subsequent adaptive behavior during reintroduction of a green treefrog, *Hyla cinerea*. Bulletin of the Association of Reptilian and Amphibian Veterinarians 5(2):6–7.

Clarke, R.D. 1972. The effects of toe-clipping on survival in Fowler's toad (*Bufo woodhousei fowleri*). Copeia 1972(2):182–185.

Cooper, J.E. 1994. Biopsy techniques. Seminars in Avian and Exotic Pet Medicine 3(3):161–165.

Corn, P.S. 1992. Laboratory and field evaluation of effects of PIT tags. FROGLOG (December 1992) No. 4:2.

Emerson, 1983. Salamander biopsy. Proceedings of the American Association of Zoo Veterinarians 1983 Annual Meeting, pp. 194–195.

Fasola, M., F. Barbieri, and L. Canova. 1993. Test of an electronic individual tag for newts. Herpetological Journal 3:149–150.

Foley, G.L., L.E. Brown, R.R. Rosati, S.G. Diana, and V.R. Beasley. 1995. Subcutaneous abdominal mass in an African clawed frog (*Xenopus laevis*). Lab Animal May 1995, pp.21–22.

Frye, F.L. 1997. Percutaneous hepatic and renal biopsy employing the Anchor® soft tissue biopsy device. The North American Veterinary Conference 1997 Proceedings, p. 732.

Frye, F.L. and D.L. Williams. 1995. Self-Assessment Color Review of Reptiles and Amphibians. Iowa State University Press, Ames, IA, pp. 145–146.

Germano, D.J. and D.F. Williams. 1993. Field evaluation of using passive integrated transponder tags to permanently mark lizards. Herpetological Review 24(2):54–56.

Golay, N. and H. Durrer. 1994. Inflammation due to toe-clipping in natterjack toads (*Bufo calamita*). Amphibia-Reptilia 15:81–83.

Heusser, H. 1958. Markierungen an Amphibien. Vjschr Naturf. Ges. Zurich 103:304–321.

Honegger, R.E. 1979. Marking amphibians and reptiles for future identification. International Zoo Yearbook 19:4–22.

Jacobson, E. 1975. The effects of ACTH, glucagon, and norepinephrine on plasma glucose levels in the mud puppy, *Necturus maculosus*. PhD dissertation, Univeristy of Missouri.

Joly, P. and C. Miaud. 1989. Tattooing as an individual marking technique in urodeles. Alytes 8:11–16.

Kramer, L., B.L. Dresser, and E.J. Maruska. 1983. Sexing aquatic salamanders by laparoscopy. Proceedings of the 1983 American Association of Zoo Veterinarians Annual Meeting, pp. 193–194.

Lloyd, M. 1996. Chlorhexidine toxicosis from soaking in red-bellied short-necked turtles, *Emydura subglobosa*. Bulletin of the Association of Reptilian and Amphibian Veterinarians 6(4):6–7.

Lynch, L.C. and D.G. Blackburn. 1995. Effects of testosterone administration and gonadectomy on nuptial pad morphology in overwintering male leopard frogs, *Rana pipiens*. Amphibia-Reptilia 16:113–121.

Meier, J. 1982. Surgical repair of a ventral abdominal hernia in Madagascan tomato frog *Dyscophus antongili*. J. Zoo An. Med. 13:123–124.

Olson, M.E. and J. Bruce. 1987. Cyanoacrylate tissue adhesives. Lab Animal 16(2):27–30.

Parichy, D.M. and R.H. Kaplan. 1992. Developmental consequences of tail injury on larvae of the Oriental fire-bellied toad, *Bombina orientalis*. Copeia 1992(1):129–137.

Pezalla, P.D. 1983. Morphine-induced analgesia and explosive motor behavior in an amphibian. Brain Research 273:297–305.

Pezalla, P.D. and C.W. Stevens. 1984. Behavior effects of morphine, levorphanol, dextrorphan and naloxone in the frog *Rana pipiens*. Pharmacology Biochemistry & Behavior 21:213–217.

Reaser, J. 1995. Marking amphibians by toe-clipping: a response to Halliday. FROGLOG (March 1995) 12:1–2.

Ritke, M.E. and C.A. Lessman. 1994. Longitudinal study of ovarian dynamics in female gray treefrogs (*Hyla chrysoscelis*). Copeia 1994(4): 1014–1022.

Rossi, J.V. 1997. Quick tips for five common reptile problems. The North American Veterinary Conference 1997 Proceedings, p. 755.

Saidapur, S.K. and B. Hoque. 1996. Long-term effects of ovariectomy on abdominal fat body and body masses in the frog *Rana tigrina* during the recrudescent phase. Journal of Herpetology 30(1):70–73.

Sinsch, U. 1992a. Structure and dynamic of a natterjack toad metapopulation (*Bufo calamita*). Oecologia 90:489–499.

Sinsch, U. 1992b. Zwei neue Markierungsmethoden zur individuellen Identifikation von Amphibien in langfristigen Freilanduntersuchungen: Erste Erfahrungen bei Kreuzkroten. Salamandra 28:116–128.

Stevens, C.W. 1988. Opioid antinociception in amphibians. Brain Research Bulletin 21:959–962.

Stevens, C.W. and K. Kirkendall. 1993. Time course and magnitude of tolerance to the analgesic effects of systemic morphine in amphibians. Life Sciences 52:111–116.

Stevens, C.W. and P.D. Pezalla. 1983. A spinal site mediates opiate analgesia in frogs. Life Sciences 33:2097–2103.

Stevens, C.W. and P.D. Pezalla. 1984. Naloxone blocks the analgesic action of levorphanol but not dextrorphan in the leopard frog. Brain Research 301:171–174.

Stevens, C.W., A.J. Klopp, and J.A. Facello. 1994. Analgesic potency of *mu* and *kappa* opioids after systemic administration in amphibians. Journal of Pharmacology and Experimental Therapy 269(3):1086–1093.

Stevens, C.W., S. Sangha, and B.G. Ogg. 1995. Analgesia produced by immobilization stress and an enkephalinase inhibitor in amphibians. Pharmacology Biochemistry and Behvaior 51(4):675–679.

Van Gelder, J.J. and H. Strijbosch. 1996. Marking amphibians: effects of toe clipping on *Bufo bufo* (Anura: Bufonidae). Amphibia-Reptilia 17(2):169–174.

Vogelnest, L. 1994. Transponder implants for frog identification. Bulletin of the Association of Reptilian and Amphibian Veterinarians 4(1):4.

Woodward, S.C., J. B. Herrmann, J.L. Cameron, G. Brandes, E.J. Pulaski, and F. Lenoard. 1965. Histotoxicity of cyanoacrylate tissue adhesive in the rat. Ann. Surg. 162:113–122.

Wright, K.M. 1994. Amputation of the tail of a two-toed amphiuma, *Amphiuma means*. Bulletin of the Association of Reptilian and Amphibian Veterinarians 4(1):5.

CHAPTER 22
REPRODUCTION

Brent R. Whitaker, MS, DVM

22.1 INTRODUCTION

Due to great species diversity, we have only begun to appreciate the complexity of the behavioral and physiological mechanisms required for reproductive success in captive amphibians. Those who have attempted for the first time to breed an amphibian species in captivity know that it can be both challenging and frustrating. To accomplish this task efficiently and safely one must gain an understanding of the species' natural history and seek to recreate it in the captive environment. Social structure, identification of sex, nutritional requirements, environmental parameters, reproductive cycles, the need for parental care, and onset of sexual maturity should be fully evaluated and adjustments made where possible before considering the use of exogenous hormones to stimulate reproduction.

This chapter is intended as a brief overview of amphibian reproduction. Further investigation of the literature may be necessary to gain in-depth information on a particular species or subject. Table 22.1 summarizes the successful use of exogenous hormones in a few select species. Methods of artificial fertilization and a description of the most common reproductive disorders are presented. With this information, the clinician and herpetoculturist may be better able to address the reproductive challenges presented by captive amphibians.

22.2 REPRODUCTIVE STRATEGIES

Amphibians are found in a variety of environments from semi-arid climates to humid tropical rain forests. They may be totally aquatic, semiaquatic or terrestrial, living on or underneath the forest floor or high above in the canopy. A tremendous diversity of reproductive strategies must therefore exist with a mutual goal of producing as many surviving offspring as possible. Through natural selection each species has evolved a reproductive strategy that is successful in their habitat. A basic understanding of an amphibian's life history is essential in order to provide the necessary elements for a successful captive breeding program.

Many amphibians produce larvae that are dependent upon aquatic environments. In many cases, large numbers of young are produced in an effort to increase survivorship. Other amphibians produce a few offspring that are larger, and in some instances the larvae are cared for by their parents. Metamorphosis, the process associated with great physiological and morphological change, occurs within 90 days of hatching in most species, however, the bullfrog, *Rana catesbeiana,* may delay the transition for up to 2 years while some salamanders require almost 5 years. The majority of caecilians are viviparous while nearly all anurans and salamanders are oviparous. Internal fertilization occurs in most salamanders and all caecilians. After collecting sperm packets with the cloaca (Plate 22.2), female salamanders may store viable sperm in their spermotheca. This sperm may be used to fertilized eggs as they pass through the oviduct over a period of years. Most anurans rely predominately upon external fertilization with oviposition into water, however, some species may deposit their eggs next to or above water (Duellman & Trueb, 1994).

Seasonal breeding is another strategy used by many amphibians. Environmental cues such as temperature in temperate regions or rainfall where dry and wet seasons exist ensure the birth of young when conditions are favorable. Males of the Indian bullfrog, *Rana tigrina,* halt spermatogensis during the dry season despite near constant temperatures. Different populations of a species may also acquire alternative reproductive patterns as seen in the lowland alpine newt, *Triturus alpestris,* which breeds yearly in comparison to other amphibian inhabitants of the Alps which reproduce biennially (Jorgensen, 1992).

Reproductive success requires that spermiation, ovulation, oviposition, fertilization, embryonic development, and metamorphosis are accomplished. Environmental conditions, including lighting (spectrum and photoperiod), water quality, temperature, and humidity, are closely linked with reproductive success. Changes in rainfall, length of day, and temperature trigger endogenous cues placing the animal in a reproductive mode. Proper nutrition is equally important to the development and maintenance of vitellogenic oocytes. Preovulatory females of the bullfrog, *Rana catesbeiana*, can be brought into ovulatory condition within 8 weeks given a photoperiod of 12 h light and 12 h dark, and a heavy diet of live fish and/or crawfish. Deviation of photoperiod causes increased egg atresia (Culley, 1992). Amphibians subjected to stressful conditions for which they are unprepared are unlikely to be reproductive. Substrate may also play a role in the successful reproduction of some salamanders. The axolotl, *Ambystoma mexicanum*, must anchor its spermatophores, consisting of a gel-like substance capped with spermatozoa, to a substrate of course sand, fine gravel, or another suitably roughened surface. Glass and enamel do not allow proper binding and positioning of spermatophores which is necessary for insemination of the female (Subcommittee on Amphibian Standards, 1974).

Given a stable environment, reproductive success for an individual female is dependent upon several factors. In general, larger females tend to produce more eggs of larger size leading to increased fitness of larvae. Older reproductive females are apt to be larger and have more available energy for vitellogenesis, again increasing egg size. Where seasonal breeding occurs, larger females are able to draw upon greater body stores for egg production, while smaller animals with insufficient stores must delay reproductive efforts. By the time the required energy has been accumulated, the eggs or young may not survive if they are produced too late in the season to avoid unfavorable environmental change. If the breeding season is long enough, multiple clutches are possible giving larger females a distinct advantage over smaller ones. By delaying sexual maturation, females may increase body size and, therefore, reproductive success. In some species, breeding may not occur every season allowing the female to gain the energy stores required for successful reproduction in the future (Crump, 1995).

22.3 SEXUAL DIMORPHISM

Sexual dimorphism is present in many amphibians although lacking in most caecilians (see also Section 3.3.1, External Anatomy). Permanent or seasonal dimorphism may be seen. Permanent characteristics include size and coloration (Plate 22.3), and the presence of spines, tubercles, and tusks in males. In some dendrobatid frogs, the males have enlarged toe pads which are used to signal the female by tapping them on the ground (Plate 22.4A, B). The tympanic membrane may be larger in some male anurans as well. Seasonal dimorphism is dependent upon the presence of gonadotropic hormones.

Male salamanders develop the cloacal glands (Plate 22.5) necessary for production of the spermatophore (Adkins-Regan, 1987). In the male tiger salamander, *Ambystoma tigrinum*, a seasonal cycle has been correlated with circulating testosterone and dihydrotestosterone causing the cloacal gland to become enlarged during the breeding season (Norris, 1987). Other site-specific glands may also become hypertrophied over the head and body of male urodeles (Duellman & Trueb, 1994). Females may develop smooth skin seasonally in response to prolactin as seen in the roughskin newt, *Taricha torosa* (Halliday & Tejedo, 1995).

One of the most notable sexual characteristics in some male anurans and newts is the formation of nuptial pads as testicular hormones rise (Plate 22.6). In anurans these pads may be found on the digits, lower forearm, and mouth enabling the male to maintain contact with the female despite swift-moving water or the interference of other males. Male newts may develop black nuptial pads on their hind legs. Species that amplex in water tend to have better developed pads than those that do so on land. In addition, some breeding males form glands on their ventral abdomen that secrete an adhesive substance during amplexus. In some species, females may have similar glands on their dorsum (Duellman & Trueb, 1994).

Permanent or seasonal coloration in anurans is also an important dimorphic characteristic. The male crested newt, *Triturus cristatus*, for example, intensifies its coloration and develops a prominent dorsal crest during the breeding season (Dan, 1983). Pigmented vocal sacs are typically present during breeding season in some male anurans. Other amphibians show specific markings or more complete color changes allowing rapid differentiation of males and females independent of season (Plate 22.1) (Duellman & Trueb, 1994).

During the breeding season some male anurans may also be identified by their vocal abilities (Plate 22.7). Calling is thought to serve several purposes including attracting females to sites suitable for egg laying and announcing to other males that the territory is occupied. Duration and intensity of call, note repetition, and note addition are methods used by rival males competing in a chorus. Research has shown that calling in the African clawed frog, *Xenopus laevis*, is controlled by the hormone dihydrotestosterone which stimulates both laryngeal motor neurons and a midbrain nucleus that responds to auditory stimuli (Moore, 1987).

There are some species which do not show evident dimorphism based on a single trait. Some, such as the midwife toads, *Alytes obstetricans* and *A. cisternasii*, can only be confidently sexed following comparison of several morphological characteristics (Bosch & Marquez, 1996).

22.4 PARENTAL CARE

Parental care has been defined as any parental behavior towards its offspring that increases the likelihood of that offspring surviving (Trivers, 1972). Parental care is exhibited by amphibians and is more common with terrestrial forms. A few caecilians, approximately 10% of anurans, and most salamanders exhibit some form of parental care (Duellman & Trueb, 1994).

Anurans, the largest order, show the greatest reproductive diversity of the amphibians. In its simplest form, eggs are deposited directly into the water and the tadpoles, once hatched, are left to fend for themselves. Some aquatic and terrestrial anurans build foam nests that protect the developing young from desiccation and maintain a proper temperature for incubation. Others show advanced parental care of the young by carrying their eggs on their legs, carrying eggs or recently hatched young on their back (Plate 22.8), or carrying eggs in a dorsal or ventral pouch. In many cases, it is the male anuran that assumes this role, unlike caecilians and salamanders where the female typically cares for the eggs (Duellman & Trueb, 1994).

Parental care is well illustrated by the strawberry poison frog, *Dendrobates pumilio*. Soon after courtship up to five eggs are deposited into terrestrial leaf litter where the male fertilizes them and also urinates on them to keep them moist, protects them from predators, and removes dead and fungus-infected eggs. Approximately one week after hatching, the female returns, and the tadpoles wriggle onto her back. She then transports them to selected leaf axils containing water. Observations of wild *D. pumilio* (Brust, 1992) revealed that offspring are placed in different plants by the female, up to 4.5 m (15 feet) apart. The young received their first meal of unfertilized eggs within 2.7 ± 2.4 days. Subsequent meals were provided every 4.2 ± 1.6 days. Not all visits were made by genetic females, however, only genetic females fed their offspring. Younger tadpoles consumed only yolk while older animals ate the jelly as well. Orphaned tadpoles fed only ovarian eggs (that lacked the jelly capsule) grew no larger than tadpoles fed oviposited eggs by their mothers even though they received more food. It was therefore assumed that these eggs were not as nutritious as those oviposited from the parental mother (Brust, 1992).

22.5 REPRODUCTIVE CYCLE

Reproductive output varies with the species and the individual, ranging from one to greater than 80,000 offspring yearly (Duellman & Trueb, 1994). Frequency of reproduction is variable, with caecilians and salamanders reproducing annually, biennially or less often depending upon species and environmental factors. Temperate anurans and some high montane tropical species may reproduce once a year or every other year while lowland tropical species produce multiple clutches throughout the year. Some species, such as the North American spadefoot toads, *Spea* spp., may not reproduce yearly; they are dependent on intermittent heavy rains for the timing of reproductive activity, and these rains are not predictable on a year-by-year basis. Some cave-dwelling species are known to reproduce continuously throughout the year, presumably due to the constant environmental conditions present in these underground habitats (Duellman & Trueb, 1994).

The age of sexual maturity varies greatly among species of amphibians. Many anurans are capable of reproduction as early as 1 year of age while salamanders typically require at least 2 years or more to mature. Some amphibians however, do not reproduce until they are 6 years or older. In general, males mature before females (Duellman & Trueb, 1994).

Reproductive cycles are closely aligned with environmental cues in order to optimize survival of the offspring. Anurans in tropical or subtropical habitats typically reproduce throughout the year and are most dependent upon rainfall as a primary stimulus. The need for rain is obvious as most species of amphibians require the presence of water for their young. Other species that live in seasonally dry environments await the rainy season and the temporary bodies of water that are produced. Some populations of the fire salamander, *Salamandra salamandra*, give birth yearly when winter rains create temporary ponds while others of this species found in perennial streams give birth throughout the year (Degani & Warburg, 1995). In all cases, amphibians have evolved successfully to meet their requirement for water. As an environmental cue, temperature gains increasing importance in determining the amphibian's reproductive cycle as altitude and latitude increase. Both time of reproduction and length of breeding season are affected. The breeding activity of the European common toad, *Bufo bufo*, in a temperate climate for instance, occurs only after a certain amount of rainfall at or above a specific temperature (Duellman & Trueb, 1994).

The importance of controlling environmental parameters when breeding captive amphibians is well known. The National Aquarium in Baltimore has successfully spawned neotropical hylid frogs by first subjecting them to a period of low humidity and moisture followed by a period of high humidity and artificial rain. An increase in moisture is created by raining on the animals, covering the vivarium with plastic, raising humidity via an ultrasonic humidifier, and raising the water level in the pool. Broad leaves are provided for leaf spawners such as the red-eyed treefrog, *Agalychnis callidryas,* the orange-legged leaf frog, *Phyllomedusa hypochondrialis,* the brownbelly leaf frog, *P. tarsius,* and the black-legged poison frog, *Phyllobates bicolor* (Plate 22.9). Pool spawners (e.g., the New Granada cross-banded treefrog, *Smilisca phaeota*) deposit their eggs into shallow areas of the pool (Cover et al., 1994) (Plate 22.10). A drop in barometric pressure, such as that experienced by amphibians transported by air or produced by the arrival of rain storms, is also an important environmental cue that stimulates reproduction in a number of amphibian species including the tomato frog, *Dyscophus* spp. (personal communication, S. Hoegeman, 1996).

Many amphibians show a resting period in their reproductive cycle. During this time vitellogenesis does not occur ensuring that the female will rebuild her energy stores and reproduce offspring at a time of year when food will be abundant for her young (Jorgensen, 1992). In some animals this period is seasonal while in others, such as the green salamander, *Aneides aeneus,* follicular development proceeds slowly over a 2-year period (Canterbury & Pauley, 1994).

Successful reproduction is dependent upon a functioning central nervous hypophyseal-gonadal axis (King & Millar, 1979; Thornton & Geschwind, 1974). Appropriate environmental stimuli activate the hypophysiotropic area of the brain. Neurons carry the signal to capillaries located on the ventral surface of the median eminence of the hypothalamus causing neurotransmitters to be released into these capillaries which flow into the portal hypophyseal vessels. The signal is thus carried to capillaries of the anterior pituitary from which hormonal transmitters, including the gonadotropins, are released.

22.5.1 Oogenesis

The amphibian ovary contains two types of oocytes, small gonadotropin-independent oocytes and larger gonadotropin-dependent oocytes. Following metamorphosis the small, nonvitellogenic oocytes increase rapidly in number. As many as 30,000–40,000 nonvitellogenic oocytes may be present, a number that remains fairly constant throughout a female's life due to oogenesis. Environmental conditions do not influence this process (Jorgensen, 1992). Despite different reproductive strategies, the previtellogenic, vitellogenic, and postovulatory follicles are similar structurally in caecilians, anurans, and urodeles (Masood-Parveez & Nadkarni, 1993).

The production of healthy eggs begins with the synthesis of yolk and its incorporation into the growing oocyte, a process know as vitellogenesis. The presence of gonadotropin is essential for the growth and maintenance of vitellogenic oocytes in both anurans and urodeles. Synthesis of vitellogenin, a complex protein that is the precursor of yolk proteins, occurs in the liver and is induced by the presence of estrogens, especially estradiol (Carnevali & Mosconi, 1992). Evidence suggests that prolactin (PRL) may also play an important role in vitellogenin production (Mosconi et al., 1994a). Elevated levels of plasma growth hormone (GH) in the female edible frog, *Rana esculenta,* are also associated with vitellogenesis (Mosconi et al., 1994b). Photoperiod has a direct effect on vitellogenic growth. Amphibians exposed to inappropriate lighting regimes show greater egg atresia than those receiving an optimal photoperiod (Jorgensen, 1992). Laboratory frogs kept under constant environmental conditions do not produce healthy eggs (i.e., those capable of supporting development upon fertilization). This has been attributed to vitellogenic deficiencies as a result of low levels of estrogen production (Culley, 1992; Ho, 1987).

Once synthesized, blood carries vitellogenin from the liver to the developing oocytes. Protected by their follicular envelope, oocytes do not readily absorb vitellogenin. Gonadotropins are therefore necessary to induce follicular cells to have a high rate of vitellogenin uptake. Temperate anurans carry out this process only once a year, beginning just after spring spawning. Under natural conditions, vitellogenesis continues until winter hibernation begins (Ho, 1987).

In order to be fertilized, eggs must complete the first meiotic division. Falling temperatures may be of importance to hibernating amphibians as this is the period during which follicular maturation occurs and sensitivity to gonadotropins that will induce ovulation slowly increases. A preovulatory surge of a gonadotropin, luteinizing hormone (LH), plays a pivotal role as it induces the secretion of progesterone which binds receptors at or near the oocyte surface (Nagahama, 1987) thus initiating maturation of anuran and salamander oocytes (Licht, 1979; Nagahama, 1987).

Ovulation occurs as mature follicles burst, releasing eggs through an avascular region of the follicular wall called the stigma, into the peritoneal cavity before reaching the oviduct. Progesterone is suspected to be the most potent steroid capable of inducing ovulation in amphibians (Jorgensen, 1992). Once ovulated, the eggs move through the oviduct accumulating a thick jelly coat that will serve as protection for the egg or embryo. The eggs are maintained in the female's ovisac until conditions are appropriate for oviposition (Reichenbach-Klinke & Elkan, 1965).

22.5.2 Spermatogenesis

The testes of anurans and some salamanders are ovoid in shape while in other salamanders and all caecilians they are lobulated. In salamanders with lobulated testes, the number of lobes increases with age

(Lofts, 1987). Spermiation, like ovulation, requires a gonadotropin surge which may serve to coordinate ovulation and spermiation during breeding. Under the influence of gonadotropins, testicular tissue undergoes hypertrophy and hyperplasia, seminiferous tubules develop, and interstitial cells grow and increase in number (Jorgensen, 1992). Two chemically distinct gonadotropins similar to follicle-stimulating hormone (FSH) and luteinizing hormone (LH) have been identified in the pituitary gland of amphibians. While the actions of these hormones are not as specific as those in higher vertebrates, FSH stimulates spermatogenesis and LH causes androgenesis in many amphibians (Licht & Porter, 1987; Lofts, 1987). Males of the roughskin newt, *Taricha granulosa*, given exogenous corticosterone or exposed to acute stress show an inhibition of luteinizing hormone-releasing hormone (LH-RH) release from the hypothalamus resulting in a reduction of plasma androgen (Moore & Zoeller, 1985). In anurans, there is an obvious increase in testicular size and weight during spermatogenesis (Duellman & Trueb, 1994). Increased body weight has been associated with greater sperm production and reproductive success (Smith-Gill & Berven, 1980). Maturation of sperm in many anurans including the African clawed frog, *Xenopus laevis*, the European common toad, *Bufo bufo*, the edible frog, *Rana esculenta*, and the Japanese treefrog, *Hyla japonica*, requires 5–6 weeks (Jorgensen, 1992).

Spermatogenesis in amphibians is cystic, each containing cells in the same stage of development derived from a single spermatogonium. Follicular cells surround each primary (stem) spermatogonium to form the germinal cyst. Primary spermatogonia have irregularly shaped nuclei and are the largest of germ cells. Spermatogenetic activity begins with the repetitive division of primary spermatogonia into a cluster of daughter cells called secondary spermatogonia. The division of secondary spermatogonia represents the proliferative stage of spermatogenesis yielding large numbers of primary spermatocytes. After undergoing their first meiotic division these cells become secondary spermatocytes. A second meiotic division results in the formation of small globular cells called spermatids. As spermiogenesis begins, the spermatids undergo morphologic changes to form spermatozoa that are elongated and oriented against the wall of the cyst. Approximately 200 sperm are produced from each spermatogonia cell. Fish also utilize cystic spermatogenesis giving rise to the theory that this approach to fertilization is an adaptation which provides a large number of spermatozoa during external fertilization in an aquatic environment (Lofts, 1987; Saidapur, 1989).

Environmental changes appear to be the key in determining whether or not spermatogenesis is cyclical or continuous. Most tropical, subtropical, and some cave-dwelling species produce sperm throughout the year (Duellman & Trueb, 1994). In some subtropical species with seasonal production, germinal cysts develop no further than primary spermatocytes. If these animals are placed in an artificial environment and exposed to elevated temperatures, full spermatogenesis can be induced. Temperate anurans are unable to achieve this due to a true postnuptial testicular refractory phase (Lofts, 1987).

22.6 HORMONAL MANIPULATION

Exogenous hormones have long been used to induce reproduction in captive amphibians. Table 22.1 gives selected examples of hormones administered to amphibians with variable success. In some cases, they substitute for missing environmental, nutritional, or social cues needed to cause an endogenous release of natural hormones. Alternatively, laboratory work may necessitate the production of large numbers of eggs or larvae in a controlled setting. Hormones may also be administered to larval amphibians in an effort to produce specific numbers of males and females needed as breeding stock (Subcommittee on Amphibian Standards, 1974). Whatever the reason, the administration of exogenous hormones should be done judiciously, as an understanding of their effect is limited to a small number of amphibian species. Dosage, route of administration, and time of administration are all empirical. In addition, different analogues of hormones, such as those of luteinizing hormone-releasing hormone (LH-RH), induce varied responses when administered to amphibians. If used incorrectly, hormonal administration may exacerbate underlying disease or even cause death (Crawshaw, 1992). In other cases, death has occurred in apparently healthy anurans including White's treefrog, *Pelodryas caerulea*, horned frogs, *Ceratophrys* spp., Tschudi's African bullfrog, *Pyxicephalus adspersus*, and tomato frogs, *Dyscophus* spp. following the use of exogenous hormones. Mortality appears to be greater in males than females, however, the veracity of this observation has not been substantiated.

The effect of environment and nutrition on amphibian reproduction has been well documented. Photoperiod significantly affects spermatogenic cycles in salamanders and ovarian development in the frog (Easley et. al., 1979). Females of the bullfrog, *Rana catesbeiana*, require a photoperiod of 12 hours light to 12 hours dark for their ovary to reach its full reproductive potential. Increased egg atresia is seen when deviating in any way from this cycle. Inappropriate temperature also decreases gametogenesis. Nutritionally, the heavy feeding of live fish and/or crayfish

Table 22.1. Hormonal manipulation for artificial reproduction of select amphibian species.

Family/Species	Sex	Hormonal Regime	Result	Comments	Reference
Ascaphidae Hochstetter's New Zealand frog, *Leiopelma hochstetteri*	F, M	HCG 50 IU ICe over 2 days to gravid female; day 3 give LH-RH 5 µg ICe; give 50 IU ICe to male	induced amplexus and egg laying	no egg development achieved; female given additional 10 µg LH-RH died	Sharbel & Green, 1992
Bufonidae Puerto Rican crested toad, *Peltophryne lemur*	F, M	LH-RH (Sigma) Female, 0.1 µg/g SC; give male 0.05–0.1 µg/g SC 8–12 hours later	may induce reproductive behavior; egg laying and spermiation	greatest success in young toads; better results if amplexed before injection; if not amplexed, inject male first and then female once animals amplex; male may require more than one injection	Personal communication, G. Crawshaw, 1996
Hylidae Pacific treefrog, *Hyla regilla*	M	FSH/LH-RH in Holfreter's solution: 45–75 ng	spermiation within 5–30 min	higher doses gave more rapid response	Licht, 1974
Leptodactylidae Horned frog, *Ceratophrys* spp.	F, M	LH-RH (Sigma) 1 mg diluted in 10 ml sterile water: 0.1 ml/100 g weight ICe; give to female and male at the same time	ovulation and spermiation	injections given 10 pm–12 am; the following morning strip male and female	Personal communication, S. Hoegeman, 1996
Microhylidae Tomato frogs, *Dyscophus antongilli, D. guineti, D. insularis*	F, M	LH-RH (Sigma) 1 mg diluted in 10 ml sterile water: 0.1 ml/100 g weight ICe; give to female 10-24 hrs before injecting male	ovulation and spermiation	rain chamber used to induce amplexus before use of hormones; females can be injected 10 pm–12 am and males the following morning; *Dyscophus* spp. breed better with drop in barometric pressure such as that experienced after air travel or the arrival of a rain storm; species very sensitive to stress; if unsuccessful do not additional hormone	Personal communication, S. Hoegeman, 1996
Tomato frog, *Dyscophus guineti*	F	Gn-RH* (Cystorellin) 10 µg SQ given to two	ovulation and spermiation	rain chamber used to induce amplexus before use of	Personal communication, D. Harris and C.

	M	females; second dose of 20 µg SQ given to second female 18 h after first injection Gn-RH* (Cystorellin) 5 µg SQ to one male in tank		Cystorelin; fertile eggs from first female within 15 h; fertile eggs from second female within 24 h	Tabaka, 1997

Ranidae

Species	Sex	Treatment	Response	Comments	Reference
Tschudi's African bullfrog, *Pyxicephalus adspersus*	F, M	LH-RH (Sigma) 1 mg diluted in 10 ml sterile water: 0.1 ml/100 g weight ICe; give to female and male at the same time	ovulation and spermiation	animals injected 10 pm–12 am; the following morning strip male and female	Personal communication, S. Hoegeman, 1996
Bullfrog, *Rana catesbeiana*	M	FSH/LH-RH dissolved in distilled water: inject dorsal lymph sac with 10µg	spermiation	remove sperm within 30–45 min; injections given 1 h before onset of lights most effective on a 12L;12D photoperiod	Culley, 1992
Skipper frog, *Rana cyanophlyctis*	F	PDH (pituitary pars distalis homogenate) 4–5 homoplastic PDH	profuse spawning within 10–15 h		Saidapur, 1989
Northern leopard frog, *Rana pipiens* (Larval form)	L	Beta-Estradiol or Testosterone 50 µg/L	phenotype opposite of genotype	details of administration unspecified	Subcommittee on Amphibian Standards, 1974
Northern leopard frog, *Rana pipiens*	M	HCG 100 IU	sperm collected in 1–3 h by stimulating urination	route of injection unspecified	Subcommittee on Amphibian Standards, 1974
North American wood frog, *Rana sylvatica*	M	LH-RH (Calbiochem #438654) diluted in amphibian Ringer's to 100 µg/ml: 50 ng/g SC (0.05 ml solution/g)	spermiation in 15–30 min; max. output in larger males in 45–60 min	large male provided sperm for up to 8 in vitro fertilizations; multiple inj. in exhausted males failed to induce sperm	Smith-Gill & Berven, 1980

Pipidae

Species	Sex	Treatment	Response	Comments	Reference
Clawed frog, *Xenopus* sp.	F, M	LH-RH (Bachem Bioscience: H-7525) mix 1 mg in 100 ml 0.7% saline or Holtfreter's solution; give Female and male: 100 µl/10 g weight injected into dorsal lymph sac	ovulation within 24 h spermiation within 1 h	once injected, keep females in moist place but not water; in rare cases the female may require a second injection; once ovulated, best results occur if mated with male within 12–24 h	Berger et al., 1994

Table 22.1. Hormonal manipulation for artificial reproduction of select amphibian species. *(Continued)*

Family/Species	Sex	Hormonal Regime	Result	Comments	Reference
Clawed frog, *Xenopus* sp.	F, M	LH-RH (Sigma) 1 mg diluted in 10 ml sterile water: 0.1 ml/100g weight ICe Give to female 10–24 h before injecting male	ovulation and spermiation	females can be injected 10 pm–12 am and males the following morning; eggs and sperm produced in morning	Personal communication, S. Hoegeman, 1996
Clawed frog, *Xenopus* sp.	F, M	HCG dissolved in saline and injected in dorsal lymph sac: 500 IU to the female 250 IU to the male	spawning 12–24 h later	inject infrequently ovulated females with 100 IU primer dose 5 h in advance	Subcommittee on Amphibian Standards, 1974
Clawed frog, *Xenopus* sp.	F	HCG dissolved in saline and injected in dorsal lymph sac: 200–600 IU in frogs 100–165 g; 100–200 IU in frogs <100 g	ovulation 6–12 h later	higher HCG doses needed when stimulated outside of the breeding season	Wolf & Hendrick, 1971
Clawed frog, *Xenopus laevis*	F	PMSG is diluted in sterile water to give a concentration of 1000 IU/ml. Give 200 IU in the dorsal lymph sac 4–7 days prior to spawning. Give 800 IU HCG into the dorsal lymph sac 10-8 h before spawning		can strip eggs from frog every 30 min and store in Barth's modified high salt solution for several hours if needed	Personal communication M. Cranfield, 1996
Ambystomatidae Axolotl, *Ambystoma mexicanum*	F	FSH- 200–400 IU injected	spawning 18–48 h later	route of administration not given	Nelson & Humphrey, 1974
Axolotl, *Ambystoma mexicanum.*	F	FSH-180–200 IU given IM	spawning 18–24 h later		Subcommittee on Amphibian Standards, 1974
Plethodontidae Mountain dusky salamander, *Desmognathus ochraeophus*	F	LH-RH (Sigma) 5µg ICe	oviposition		Verrell, 1989
Salamandridae Crested newt, *Triturus cristatus*	F	LH-RH-24 µg ICe q 48 h for 8 treatments	spawning	greater effect by perfusion of pituitary in situ	Vellano et. al., 1974

Key:
IM-intramuscularly
SC-subcutaneously
ICe-intracoelomically
Gn-RH*—gonadorelin, Cystorelin, Rhone Merieux, Athens, GA

Bachem Bioscience Inc., King of Prussia, PA
Calbiochem-Novabiochem, San Diego, CA
Sigma, St. Louis, MO

to female bullfrogs kept at 25°C can induce reproductive condition within eight weeks despite the time of year the animals are collected (Culley, 1992). Every effort must therefore be made to provide amphibians with the proper environment and diet if reproduction is desired. The administration of exogenous hormones may be completely ineffective if conditions conducive to a successful reproductive effort have not been well established.

At least two forms of gonadotropin-releasing hormone (Gn-RH) have been identified in the brains of frogs and salamanders. One is very similar physiochemically and immunologically to that of mammals (Daniels & Licht, 1980). The second, found in small amounts, is a salmonidlike Gn-RH molecule (Sherwood et al., 1986). The specific role of each Gn-RH remains unclear.

The response of various species of amphibians to the administration of Gn-RH is highly variable and may reflect the animal's physiological state resulting from both intrinsic and extrinsic factors. In the adult bullfrog, *Rana catesbeiana*, a single injection of Gn-RH into the dorsal lymph sac causes an increase in LH and FSH within 15 minutes (Daniels & Licht, 1980; Licht & Porter, 1987). While ovarian and testicular growth, spermiation, and estrogen secretion appear to show little FSH or LH specificity, ovulation, testicular androgen and ovarian progesterone secretion are highly LH-dependent (Licht, 1979). Natural levels of LH begin to rise significantly during the last weeks of hibernation in the European common frog, *Rana temporaria*. Warming temperatures appear to stimulate LH release from the pituitary thus preparing animals such as *R. temporaria* for spawning shortly after estivation (Sotowaska-Brochocka et al., 1992).

Several factors appear to influence the response of amphibians given Gn-RH. First, the time of day or season that the Gn-RH is administered appears to be important in optimizing response (Daniels & Licht, 1980; Easley et al., 1979). A general rule however is not practical as one colony of amphibians is likely to be housed under different conditions than another, giving rise to altered diurnal rhythms in sensitivity to Gn-RH. Secondly, sex and age of the amphibian also influence response to exogenous Gn-RH. In general, female anurans do not respond to Gn-RH administration as reliably as do males. Males of the bullfrog, *Rana catesbeiana*, appear to be approximately 40-fold more sensitive to a Gn-RH agonist than females (McCreery et al., 1982). The primary effect of Gn-RH in a large number of male anurans is increased spermiation which typically occurs within 30–60 minutes of a single injection (Licht & Porter, 1987). In the Pacific treefrog, *Hyla regilla*, a graded response occurs with increasing doses of Gn-RH producing greater effect (Licht, 1974).

In contrast, female bullfrogs may require daily injections of a long-acting Gn-RH agonist over a period of three or more days in order to induce ovulation, presumably due to the need for prolonged pituitary stimulation by Gn-RH (McCreery & Licht, 1983). Unlike mammals in which the pituitary becomes refractory to continuous administration of low Gn-RH doses, male and female amphibians remain responsive resulting in spermatogenesis and ovulation (McCreery et al., 1982; McCreery & Licht, 1983). In the African clawed frog, *Xenopus laevis*, ovulation was induced in a few animals with Gn-RH injections, but only after extensive use of human chorionic gonadotropin (HCG) and pregnant mare serum gonadotropin (PMSG) (Thornton & Geschwind, 1974). Still, there are a number of species including Tschudi's African bullfrog, *Pyxicephalus adspersus*, the ornate horned frog, *Ceratophrys ornata*, the Western spadefoot toad, *Spea hammondi*, and White's treefrog, *Pelodryas caerulea*, where the female will ovulate within 24 hours following a single injection of long-acting Gn-RH (Licht & Porter, 1987). The age of the amphibian also plays an important role in ensuring reproductive success. Young postmetamorphic frogs are relatively unresponsive to Gn-RH stimulation (McCreery & Licht, 1983; Daniels & Licht, 1980). Finally, the route by which the Gn-RH is administered may influence the outcome and therefore, the practicality of its use. Female newts, *Triturus* spp., required daily injections of Gn-RH into the area of the in situ pituitary before ovulation was induced. Intracoelomic (ICe) injections were not nearly as effective (Vellano et al., 1974).

Synthetic LH-RH is another hormone that is frequently administered by those attempting to breed amphibians. This hormone effectively stimulates spermatogenesis or the recruitment of new oocytes in many amphibians (Crawshaw, 1992; Licht, 1979; Segal & Adejuwon, 1979; Vellano et al., 1974; Verrell, 1989). It may also induce sexual behavior as seen in the male roughskin newt, *Taricha granulosa*. When injected intracranially the ensuing increase in sexual behavior was reversible upon administration of an LH-RH antagonist (Moore et al., 1982). When injected intracoelomically, a synthetic LH-RH was used successfully to induce ovulation and oviposition in previously mated females of the mountain dusky salamander, *Desmognathus ochrophaeus* (Verrell, 1989). Despite the apparent success and popularity of this hormone among herpetoculturists, its effective use is not fully understood for every species. Mammalian LH-RH, for example, injected subcutaneously into wild-caught North American wood frogs, *Rana sylvatica*, can result in sperm production within 30 minutes with larger males yielding greater amounts of sperm. This regime, however, is only successful in frogs caught during the breeding season, and fertilization success declines when spermiation is repeatedly induced over several days (Smith-Gill & Berven, 1980).

Human chorionic gonadotropin (HCG), an LH analogue, has been used successfully to sustain vitellogenesis and, at higher doses, induce ovulation in toads (Jorgensen, 1992; Licht, 1979). Clawed frogs, *Xenopus* spp., and axolotls, *Ambystoma mexicanum*, can be induced to ovulate using HCG with or without pregnant mare serum gonadotropin (PMSG). It has been suggested that amphibians responding poorly to HCG and PMSG may do better with Gn-RH. The concurrent use of progesterone may increase success if attempting to induce ovulation outside the normal breeding season. Males treated with HCG may also require Gn-RH administration 8–24 hours later (Crawshaw, 1992).

22.7 ARTIFICIAL FERTILIZATION

Artificial fertilization is a useful technique when young of known genetic history or from synchronous fertilizations are required. In order to be successful with a given species its reproductive cycle must be fully understood. To prepare for artifical fertilization, both females and males must be appropriately conditioned using environmental (e.g., light, temperature, humidity) and nutritional enhancements. Synchronization of reproductive cycles is necessary so that ovulation and spermiation occur simultaneously. The use of exogenous hormones may be necessary to accomplish this (see Table 22.1). Reproductive maturity of females may be assessed by the presence of eggs at the cloaca, or in the coelom (see Plate 22.2). Visualization of egg masses using ultrasound or celioscopy (Kramer et al., 1983) if necessary, can be used in larger animals. In some species, eggs may be seen by transillumination of the coelomic cavity.

Once ovulation has occurred, sperm is collected from the male. This is easily accomplished in some species by administering Gn-RH (e.g., bullfrog, *Rana catesbeiana*, Culley, 1992) or HCG (e.g., northern leopard frog, *Rana pipiens*, Subcommittee on Amphibian Standards, 1974), and collecting the sperm from the cloaca with an eye dropper containing a small amount of 10% amphibian Ringer's solution (Table 22.2). In other cases where hormonal stimulation is not feasible, the surgical removal of one gonad or sacrifice of the animal is carried out so that the testes containing sperm can be obtained, macerated, and placed in a diluent (Subcommittee on Amphibian Standards, 1974). Sperm motility and concentration should be examined before eggs are collected, especially when a history of low fertility exists. The eggs are then gently stripped manually from the female, squeezing and stroking the abdomen in a craniocaudal direction, and directed into a petri dish containing the sperm suspension where they remain for up to an hour. If eggs are allowed to be laid naturally into fresh water the jelly will become hard after a short period of time preventing fertilization (personal communication, M. Cranfield, 1996). After fertilization has taken place, culture water is slowly added to the dish before gently scraping the eggs loose with a razor blade and transferring them to a larger container for incubation. Fertilized eggs can be identified as they will rotate showing the black animal hemisphere.

Artificial fertilization of eggs of the axolotl, *Ambystoma mexicanum*, has also been described (Subcommittee on Amphibian Standards, 1974; Nelson & Humphrey, 1974). The female is given FSH which stimulates ovulation within 18–24 hours. As spawning begins she is agitated for several hours by prodding her and shaking her enclosure in an effort to prevent deposition of the eggs accumulating in her oviduct. The eggs can then be stripped from the female into a covered watch glass. If additional eggs are needed, the female may then be pithed and decapitated in order to retrieve them from the oviduct. The ducti deferentes are quickly removed from a sacrificed male and placed into 10 ml of 10% Steinberg's or amphibian Ringer's solution. Tearing the tissue allows the sperm to be released into the solution which is then placed over the surface of the eggs. After 20 minutes, inseminated eggs are flooded with the physiological solution. Within the next 20–30 minutes the entire watch glass is placed into a larger bowl of the physiological solution. Eventually, eggs are scraped free using a sharp blade.

Maximizing success is dependent upon the knowledge and expertise of those carrying out the procedures. Difficulties encountered include the inability to induce ovulation or spermiation in a timely fashion, mechanical trauma to the eggs or female during stripping, poor sperm quality or quantity, and overripeness of eggs. Fertilization success is dependent upon the quality and quantity of sperm produced (Smith-Gill & Berven, 1980). Blunt forceps can be placed into the cloaca of some anurans during stripping, thus preventing the sphincter muscle from causing damage or retention of ovulated eggs. Once ovulated, the eggs should be fertilized within 12–24 hours as there is a decrease in viability of the progeny with increasing time between ovulation and fertilization (Berger et al., 1994). Should death occur following the use of hormonal therapy, the gonads may be surgically removed for evaluation of maturation and reproductive potential or used in attempts of artificial

Table 22.2. Physiological solutions used for diluting sperm or maintaining eggs.

Solution	Formulation	Final Concentration	Comments	References
Modified Barth's solution	For 1L, add the following to 800 ml of distilled H_2O: 5.1 g NaCl 0.075g KCl 0.045g $CaCl_2$ 0.056g $Ca(NO_3)_2$ 0.1g $MgSO_4$ 0.2g $NaHCO_3$ 10.0 ml 1M HEPES —Adjust to pH 7.4 with concentrated HCl or 5M NaOH —Add distilled H_2O to final volume of 1L	88 mM NaCl 1 mM KCl 0.41 mM $CaCl_2$ 0.34 mM $Ca(NO_3)_2$ 0.82 mM $MgSO_4$ 2.4 mM $NaHCO_3$ 10 mM HEPES	Used undiluted solution chilled to 4°C to store testes; culture fertilized eggs in 10% solution	Peng, 1991 Personal communication, R. Wagner, 1998
Modified Barth's solution—high salt	For 1L, add the following to 800 mL of distilled H_2O: 6.6 g NaCl 0.15g KCl 0.12 g $MgSO_4$ 0.17g $NaHCO_3$ 0.6 g $NaPO_4$ 1.8 g Trizma Base —Adjust to pH 7.6 with concentrated HCl —Add distilled H_2O to final volume of 1L	110 mM NaCl 2 mM KCl 1 mM $MgSO_4$ 2 mM $NaHCO_3$ 0.5 mM $NaPO_4$ 1 mM Tris	Use undiluted solution at room temperature to store eggs prior to fertilization	Peng, 1991; Personal communication, R. Wagner, 1998
Holtfreter's solution (with antibiotic)	Stock A—Mix into 500 ml distilled H_2O: 3.5 g NaCl 0.05 g KCl 0.1 g $CaCl_2$ Stock B—Mix into 500 ml distilled H_2O: 0.2 g $NaHCO_3$ —Sterilize stock solutions separately and mix 1:1 —Add 50–110 µg/ml gentamycin	60 mM NaCl 0.67 mM KCl 0.9 mM $CaCl_2$ 2.3 mM $NaHCO_3$	Use undiluted solution chilled to 4°C to maintain testes up to two weeks	Berger et al., 1994 Brothers, 1977
Artificial pond water	Stock A—Mix into 2L distilled H_2O: 175 g NaCl 35 g $CaCl_2$ Stock B—Mix into 2L distilled H_2O: 5g $NaHCO_3$ Add 20 ml of each solution to 5L of distilled H_2O	1.5 M NaCl 160 mM $CaCl_2$ 30 mM $NaHCO_3$	Use full strength to collect eggs or sperm	Maruska, 1994, Berger et al., 1994

Table 22.2. Physiological solutions used for diluting sperm or maintaining eggs. *(Continued)*

Solution	Formulation	Final Concentration	Comments	References
DeBoer's solution	For 1L, add the following to 800 ml of distilled H$_2$O: wash eggs in 5% 0.1 g KCl 0.049 g CaCl$_2$ —Adjust to pH 7.2 with 8.4% (1M) NaHCO$_3$ —Add distilled H$_2$O to final volume of 1L	110 mM NaCl 1.3 mM KCl 0.44 mM CaCl$_2$	*Eggs:* Strip into 100% DeBoer's solution; prior to insemination solution *Sperm:* collect in 100% solution; add suspension to eggs placed in 5% DeBoer's solution	Wolf & Hendrick, 1971 6.6 g NaCl
Steinberg's solution	Bring volume to 1L with distilled water 3.4 g NaCL 0.05g KCl 0.08g Ca(NO$_3$)$_2$ 0.205g MgSO$_4$ 4 mL 1N HCl 560 mg Trizma base, reagent grade	58 mM NaCl 0.67 mM KCl 0.34 mM Ca(NO$_3$)$_2$ 0.83 mM MgSO$_4$	Use a 10% solution; use HCL and Trizma base to buffer to a pH of 7.4	Brothers, 1977
Amphibian Ringer's solution	Mix into 1L of distilled H$_2$O: 6.6 g NaCl 0.15 g KCl 0.15 g CaCl$_2$ 0.2g NaHCO$_3$	110 mM NaCl 2 mM KCl 1.3 mM CaCl$_2$ 2.4 mH NaHCO$_3$	Use 10% solution for the collection of sperm or incubation of fertilized eggs	Humason, 1967

fertilization. It is highly recommended that animals be watched for several hours after receiving exogenous hormones so that the gonads can be salvaged promptly in the event of an animal's death.

22.8 REPRODUCTIVE DISORDERS

The list of amphibians bred in captivity continues to grow although many species still present a challenge. Successful reproduction involves ovulation in the female, spermiation in the male, fertilization, oviposition, embryonic development, and metamorphosis. With the exception of metamorphosis, the inability to successfully complete any one of these requirements may lead to reproductive failure. In most cases, the specific mechanisms are unknown and improper breeding conditions or stress is blamed.

True reproductive disorders in amphibians are not well documented. Only a handful of conditions have been recognized and described. Related health problems may arise, however, as attempts are made to prepare and then breed a group of amphibians. For example, territorial bouts between conspecific males, and sometimes females, can lead to serious trauma of combatants. A careful selection of tankmates with consideration given to the number of animals, sex ratio, animal size, and the species life history should help minimize this danger. Newly introduced animals must always be closely monitored for signs of incompatibility.

Preparing amphibians for reproduction often requires manipulation of environmental parameters to trigger hormonally induced events. Seasonal changes in temperature and/or moisture are well know cues for many amphibians. Hibernation or rain chambers are therefore used commonly to stimulate breeding activity in captive populations. For example, in preparation for breeding, temperate amphibians are often chilled and then warmed simulating a fall, winter, and spring cycle. Care must be taken by the herpetoculturist not to chill animals that have recently eaten, as digestion ceases at cooler temperatures. Undigested food in the gut becomes putrid with time as bacterial overgrowth occurs. In rain chambers, female tomato frogs, *Dyscophus* spp., may be drowned by ambitious males during amplexus if pools collecting water become too deep or lack an escape route (personal communication, S. Hoegeman, 1996). Water of inappropriate quality (temperature, hardness, pH, chlorine) used to rain upon amphibians, and inadequate ventilation may increase physiological stress resulting not only in reproductive failure, but poor health as well.

Once a strategy for breeding a species in an artificial environment has been successfully established, care must be taken not to completely exhaust the female's energy stores through repeated clutching. Doing so may predispose her to secondary infections and reproductive failure. Males may also become physically depleted through constant amplexus and the stress of repeated territorial defense. Frequent or prolonged amplexus can also cause dermal abrasions on the back of some species of female anurans such as the stubfoot toads, *Atelopus spumarius* and *A. varius,* and the crowned treefrog, *Anotheca spinosa* (personal communication, S. Barnett, 1996).

One of the most common reproductive problems observed in gravid females arises from a failure to lay some or all of her eggs. This has been attributed to sudden stress shortly preceding or during oviposition, lack of appropriate stimuli for release, or the onset of unrelated illness. In effect, any condition that causes blockage of the oviduct or cloaca will result in egg retention. This includes neoplastic, congenital, or infectious conditions. A detailed history is most valuable in identifying probable causes.

Egg retention occurs as maturing ova become lodged in the oviduct while the remainder of the egg mass is held within the ovisac. Adhesions begin to form resulting in an easily palpated, hard degenerative mass referred to as an "ovarian cyst." Liberated toxins and the displacement of internal organs can result in clinical depression, dehydration, septicemia, shock, and disseminated intravascular coagulation. Digital palpation, radiographs, and ultrasound may be used in combination to differentiate ovarian cysts from other coelomic masses such as bladder stones or neoplasia. Treatment requires stabilization of the animal using fluids, steroids and antibiotics followed by surgical removal of the mass. Preparations for cytology and culture should be obtained from blood and necrotic tissue to ensure that the best therapeutics have been selected.

Fungi have commonly been associated with immunosuppression and subsequent systemic disease in amphibians. Aquatic fungi, such as *Saprolegnia,* may ascend the oviduct causing infection. Saprophytic organisms are more likely to be found in the reproductive tissues of terrestrial animals as disseminated infections develop.

Microsporidia have on rare occasion been reported to infect the reproductive organs of amphibians. The pathogenicity of organisms, such as *Plistophora bufonis* found in the Bidder's organ of bufonids, is not known (Flynn, 1973). These or similar organisms have also been observed developing in the oocytes, but have not resulted in the formation of cysts (Canning et al., 1964). Microsporidia have also been found within the cytoplasm of discolored enlarged oocytes collected from the northern leopard frog, *Rana pipiens* (Schuetz et al., 1978). Despite ultrastructural changes, and increased potassium with decreased calcium concentrations, these oocytes are viable. Although the host appears unaffected by these organisms, it remains unclear whether or not these infections lead to diminished reproductive success.

On occasion, reproductively active female dendrobatid and hylid frogs have been found to accumulate large amounts of clear acellular fluid in their coelomic cavity and subcutaneous tissues (Plate 22.11). In its early stages, the condition may go unnoticed in frogs that normally have a large, rounded abdomen. The accumulation of fluid can become so severe that the animal can not maneuver its large abdomen in order to catch its prey. As fluid retention continues egg production slowly declines. In some cases, jelly continues to be produced with few or no eggs present. Affected amphibians never return to normal, although removing fluid with a needle and syringe returns mobility to the amphibian which will then readily catch and consume prey. We have successfully maintained amphibians with this condition for years by periodically withdrawing just enough fluid to allow the animal mobility. The etiology of this disorder remains unknown.

The premature hatching of a small percentage of dendrobatid eggs has been observed on rare occasion at the National Aquarium in Baltimore. Larvae from these eggs are easily identified as they maintain an intact external gill. If placed in an aquarium or deep bowl of water, these premature hatchlings usually do not survive. They can be successfully raised, however, by keeping them in a petri dish with just enough water to cover them. Evaporation is prevented by placing the entire petri dish into a bowl also containing a small amount of water and covered with plastic wrap. Care must be taken not to damage the external gill as this will result in death of the tadpole. When the external gills are no longer seen, the tadpoles can be safely moved from the dish and raised with the remainder of the clutch.

Neoplasia of reproductive organs is rare, but has been reported (Balls, 1962) (see also Section 26.8.1, Neoplasms of the Male Reproductive Tract, and Section 26.8.2, Neoplasms of the Female Reproductive Tract). In frogs, ovarian carcinoma and testicular teratocarcinoma have been observed. Lymphosarcoma, a common tumor of lymphoid tissue, may metastasize to many organs including the gonads.

REFERENCES

Adkins-Regan, E. 1987. Hormones and sexual differentiation, *in* Norris, D.O. and R.E. Jones (Eds.): Hormones and Reproduction in Fishes, Amphibians, and Reptiles. Plenum Press, New York, pp. 1–29.

Balls, M. 1962. Spontaneous neoplasms in amphibia: A review and descriptions of six new cases. Cancer Research 22:1142–1161.

Berger L., M. Rybacki, and H. Hotz, 1994. Artificial fertilization of water frogs. Amphibia-Reptilia 15:408–413.

Bosch, J. and R. Marquez. 1996. Discriminate functions for sex identification in two midwife toads (*Alyes obstetricans* and *A. cisternasii*). Herpetological Journal 6:105–109.

Brothers, A.J. 1977. Instructions for the care and feeding of axolotls. Axolotl Newsletter, Indiana Univ. 3:9–16.

Brust, D.G. 1992. Maternal brood care by *Dendrobates pumilio*: A frog that feeds its young. Journal of Herpetology 27:(1):96–98.

Canning, E.U., E. Elkan, and P.I. Tigg. 1964. *Plistophora myotrophica* spec. nv., causing high mortality in the common toad *Bufo bufo* L., with notes on the maintenance of *Bufo* and *Xenopus* in the laboratory. Journal Protozoology 11(2):157–166.

Canterbury, R.A. and T.K. Pauley. 1994. Time of mating and egg deposition of West Virginia populations of the salamander *Aneides aeneus*. Journal of Herpetology 28(4):431–434.

Carnevali, O. and G. Mosconi. 1992. In vitro induction of vitellogenin synthesis in *Rana esculenta*: Role of the pituitary. General and Comparative Endocrinology 86:352–358.

Cover, J.F., Jr., S.L. Barnett, and R.L. Saunders. 1994. Captive management and breeding of dendrobatid and neotropical hylid frogs at the National Aquarium in Baltimore, *in* Murphy J.B., K. Adler, and J.T. Collins (Eds.): Captive Management and Conservation of Amphibians and Reptiles, Society for the Study of Amphibians and Reptiles. Contributions to Herpetology, volume 11. Ithaca, NY, pp. 267–273.

Crawshaw, G.J. 1992. Amphibian medicine, *in* Fowler M.E. (Ed.): Zoo & Wild Animal Medicine Current Therapy 3. W.B. Saunders Company, Philadelphia, PA, pp. 131–139.

Crump, M.L. 1995. Parental care, *in* Heatwole H. and B.K. Sullivan (Eds.): Amphibian Biology, Volume 2. Surrey Beatty and Sons, New South Wales, Australia.

Culley, D.D. 1992. Managing a bullfrog research colony, *in* Schaeffer D.O., K.M. Kleinow and L. Krulisch (Eds.): The Care and Use of Amphibians, Reptiles and Fish in Research. Scientists Center for Animal Welfare, Bethesda, MD, pp. 30–40.

Dan, C. 1983. Reproduction twice a year of the crested nest in captivity, *in* Townson S. (Ed.): Breeding Reptiles and Amphibians. British Herpetological Society, London, Great Britain, UK, pp. 209–211.

Daniels, E. and P. Licht. 1980. Effects of gonadotropin-releasing hormone on the levels of plasma gonadotropins (FSH and LH) in the bullfrog, *Rana catesbeiana*. General and Comparative Endocrinology 42:455–463.

Degani, G. and M.R. Warburg. 1995. Variations in brood size and birth rates of *Salamandra salamandra* (Amphibia, Urodela) from different habitats in northern Israel. Amphibia-Reptilia 16:341–349.

Duellman, W.E. and L. Trueb. 1994. Biology of Amphibians. The Johns Hopkins University Press, Baltimore, MD, 670 pp.

Easley, K.A., D.D. Culley, N.D. Horseman, and J.E. Penkala. 1979. Environmental influences on hormonally induced spermiation of the bullfrog, *Rana catesbeiana*, Journal of Experimental Zoology 207:407–416.

Flynn, R.J. 1973. Parasites of Laboratory Animals. Iowa State University Press, Ames, IA, pp. 507–642.

Halliday, T.R. and M. Tejedo. 1995. Intersexual selection and alternative mating behavior, *in* Heatwole, H. and B.K. Sullivan (Eds.): Amphibian Biology, Volume 2. Surrey Beatty and Sons, NSW, Australia, pp. 5419–469.

Ho, S. 1987. Endocrinology of vitellogenesis, *in* Norris, D.O. and R.E. Jones (Eds.): Hormones and Reproduction in Fishes, Amphibians, and Reptiles. Plenum Press, New York, pp. 145–169.

Humason, G.L. 1967. Animal Tissue Techniques, Second edition. W.H. Freeman, San Francisco, CA, 569 pp.

Jorgensen, C.B. 1992. Growth and reproduction, *in* Feder, M.E. and W.W. Burggren (Eds.): Environmental Physiology of the Amphibians, University of Chicago Press, Chicago, pp. 439–466.

King, J.A. and R.P. Millar. 1979. Hypothalamic luteinizing hormone-releasing hormone content in relation to the seasonal reproductive cycle of *Xenopus laevis*. General and Comparative Endocrinology 39:309–312.

Kramer, L., B.L. Dresser, and E.J. Maruska. 1983. Sexing aquatic salamanders by laparoscopy. Proceedings American Association of Zoological Veterinarians, pp. 192–194.

Licht, P. 1974. Induction of sperm release in frogs by mammalian gonadotropin-releasing hormone. General and Comparative Endocrinology 23(3):352–354.

Licht, P. 1979. Reproductive endocrinology of reptiles and amphibians: Gonadotropins. Ann. Rev. Physiol. 41:337–51.

Licht, P. and D.A. Porter. 1987. Role of gonadotropin-releasing hormone, *in* Norris, D.O. and R.E. Jones (Eds.): Hormones and Reproduction in Fishes, Amphibians, and Reptiles. Plenum Press, New York, pp. 61–85.

Lofts, B. 1987. Testicular function, *in* Norris, D.O. and R.E. Jones (Eds.): Hormones and Reproduction in Fishes, Amphibians, and Reptiles. Plenum Press, New York, pp. 283–325.

Maruska, E.J. 1994. Procedures for setting up and maintaining a salamander colony, *in* Murphy, J.B., K. Adler and J.T. Collins (Eds.): Captive Management and Conservation of Amphibians and Reptiles. Society for the Study of Amphibians and Reptiles, Ithaca, NY. Contributions to Herpetology, volume 11, pp. 229–242.

Masood-Parveez, U. and V.B. Nadkarni. 1993. Morphological, histological and histochemical studies on the ovary of an oviparous caecilian, *Ichthyophis beddomei* (Peters). Journal of Herpetology 27(1):63–69.

McCreery, B.R. and P. Licht. 1983. Induced ovulation and changes in pituitary responsiveness to continuous infusion of gonadotropin-releasing hormone during the ovarian cycle in the bullfrog, *Rana catesbeiana*. Biol. of Reprod. 29:863–871.

McCreery, B.R., P. Licht, R. Barnes, J.E. Rivier, and W.W. Vale. 1982. Actions of agonistic and antagonistic analogs of gonadotropin-releasing hormone (Gn-RH) in the bullfrog *Rana catesbeiana*. General and Comparative Endocrinology 46:511–520.

Moore F.L. 1987. Regulation of reproductive behaviors, *in* Norris, D.O. and R.E. Jones (Eds.): Hormones and Reproduction in Fishes, Amphibians, and Reptiles. Plenum Press, New York, pp. 505–522.

Moore, F.L. and R.T. Zoeller. 1985. Stress-induced inhibition of reproduction: Evidence of suppressed secretion of LH-RH in an amphibian. General and Comparative Endocrinology 60:252–258.

Moore, F.L., L.J. Miler, S.P. Spielvogel, T. Kubiak, and K. Folkers. 1982. Luteinizing hormone-releasing hormone involvement in the reproductive behavior of a male amphibian. Neuroendocrinology 35:212–216.

Mosconi, G., K. Yamamoto, S. Kikuyama, O. Carnevali, A. Mancuso, and C. Vellano. 1994a. Seasonal changes of plasma prolactin concentration in the reproduction of the crested newt (*Triturus carnifex* Laur.). General and Comparative Endocrinology 95:342–349.

Mosconi, G., K. Yamamoto, O. Carnevali, M. Nabissi, A. Polzonetti-Magni, and S. Kikuyama. 1994b. Seasonal changes in plasma growth hormone and prolactin concentrations of the frog *Rana esculenta*. General and Comparative Endocrinology 93:380–387.

Nagahama Y. 1987. Endocrine control of oocyte maturation, *in* Norris, D.O. and R.E. Jones (Eds.): Hormones and Reproduction in Fishes, Amphibians, and Reptiles. Plenum Press, New York, pp. 171–202.

Nelson, C.E. and R.R. Humphrey. 1974. Artificial interspecific hybridization among Ambystoma. Herpetologica 28:27–32.

Norris, D.O. 1987. Regulation of male gonaducts and sex accessory structures, *in* Norris, D.O. and R.E. Jones (Eds.): Hormones and Reproduction in Fishes, Amphibians, and Reptiles. Plenum Press, New York, pp. 327–354.

Peng, H.B. 1991. Solutions and protocols, *in* Kay, B.K. and H.B. Peng (Eds.): Methods in Cell Biology; Volume 36 *Xenopus laevis*: Practical Uses in Cell and Molecular Biology. Academic Press, San Diego, CA, pp. 657–670.

Porter, D.A. and P. Licht. 1985. Pituitary responsiveness to superfused Gn-RH in two species of ranid frogs. General and Comparative Endocrinology 59:308–315.

Reichenbach-Klinke, H. and E. Elkan. 1965. The Principal Diseases of Lower Vertebrates: Book II Diseases of Amphibians. TFH Publications, Inc., Hong Kong.

Saidapur, S.K. 1989. Reproductive cycles of amphibians, *in* Saidapur, S.K. (Ed.): Reproductive Cycles of Indian Vertebrates. Allied Publishers Limited, Bombay, India, pp. 165–223.

Schuetz, A.W., K. Selman, and D. Samson. 1978. Alterations in growth, function and composition of *Rana pipiens* oocytes and follicles associated with microsporidian parasites. Journal of Experimental Zoology 204:81–94.

Segal, S.J. and C.A. Adejuwon. 1979. Direct effect of LHRH on testicular steroidogenesis in *Rana pipiens*. Biological Bulletin 157:393.

Sharbel, T.F. and D.M. Green. 1992. Captive maintenance of the primitive New Zealand frog, *Leiopelma hochstetteri*. Herpetology Review 23(3):77–79.

Sherwood, N.M., R.T. Zoeller, and F.L. Moore. 1986. Multiple forms of gonadotropin-releasing hormone on amphibian brains. General and Comparative Endocrinology 61:313–322.

Smith-Gill, S.J. and K.A. Berven. 1980. In vitro fertilization and assessment of male reproductive potential using mammalian gonadotropin-releasing hormone to induce spermiation in *Rana sylvatica*. Copeia 1980(4): 723–728.

Sotowaska-Brochocka, J., L. Martynska, and P. Licht. 1992. Changes of LH level in the pituitary gland and plasma in hibernating frogs, *Rana temporaria*. General and Comparative Endocrinology 87:286–291.

Subcommittee on Amphibian Standards. 1974. Committee on Standards, National Research Council, eds. Amphibians: Guidelines for the breeding, care, and management of laboratory animals. National Academy Press Inc., Washington, DC, 153 pp.

Thornton, V.F. and I.I. Geschwind. 1974. Hypothalamic control of gonadotropin release in amphibia: Evidence from studies of gonadotropin release in vitro and in vivo. General and Comparative Endocrinology 23:294–301.

Trivers, R.L. 1972. Parental investment and sexual selection, *in* Cambell, B.G. (Ed.): Sexual Selection and the Descent of Man. Aldine Press, Chicago, pp. 136–179.

Vellano, C., A. Bona, V. Mazzi, and D. Colucci. 1974. The effect of synthetic luteinizing hormone-releasing hormone on ovulation in the crested newt. General and Comparative Endocrinology 24:338–340.

Verrell, P.A. June 1989. Hormonal induction of ovulation and oviposition in the salamander *Desmognathis ochrophaeus* (Plethodontidae). Herpetological Review: 20(3):42–43.

Wolf, D.P. and J.L. Hendrick. 1971. A molecular approach to fertilization. II. Viability and artificial fertilization of *Xenopus laevis* gametes. Develelopmental Biology 25:348–359.

CHAPTER 23
QUARANTINE

Kevin M. Wright, DVM and Brent R. Whitaker, MS, DVM

23.1 SUGGESTED QUARANTINE PROTOCOLS

A relatively spartan enclosure suffices for the quarantine of many amphibians (Figure 23.1). Plastic shoe or sweater-boxes, polycarbonate vivaria, and glass aquariums serve as useful readily disinfected quarantine enclosures. Unbleached paper towels can serve as substrate, and crumpled balls of moistened paper towels will be used as retreats. Autoclaved cork bark pieces can be used as additional hiding spots, as well as plastic hide boxes and plastic aquarium plants. Sufficient visual barriers should exist to allow each individual the option of being out of sight from each other as well as from the caretaker (Figure 23.2). Individual inhabitants can be readily assessed on a daily basis for weight gain or loss, physical posture, and obvious changes in appearance such as abrasions or a change in skin texture or color. Feces are readily apparent and easily collected for parasite examination. This system has worked well even with many presumed delicate species such as mantellid frogs, *Mantella* spp., dendrobatid frogs, and plethodontid salamanders. If an individual appears to be doing poorly in this environment, additional furnishings can added such as plants, sterilized spaghnum moss, sheet moss, or pea gravel, although some individuals may need to be switched to a more complex environment such as the naturalistic enclosure intended for permanent housing (Figure 23.3). This can make monitoring of food intake and fecal output somewhat difficult and requires a higher degree of commitment from the caretaker. Diligent surveillance of the amphibian is essential for successful quarantine. Feeding time generally stimulates activity and allows one to assess the amphibian's vigor and appetite.

The tank should be covered with a lid that allows the option of keeping the relative humidity fairly high (>70% RH), which may be achieved with a plastic or tempered glass lid. Adequate ventilation is desirable, but avoid metal screening as rust and galvanized metals can be deleterious to amphibians. Frequent spray-misting with dechlorinated water may be needed to insure that the moisture remains sufficiently high. If there is a problem keeping the humidity elevated in the minimal quarantine tank, running an air stone into the tank's water source may overcome this problem. Alternatively, a room humidifier can be placed in

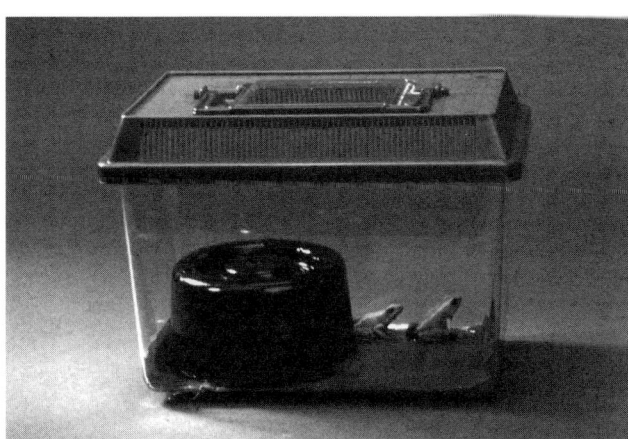

Figure 23.1. Spartan enclosures work well for the initial quarantine of many amphibians such as the black-legged poison frog, *Phyllobates bicolor*. (George Grall, National Aquarium in Baltimore)

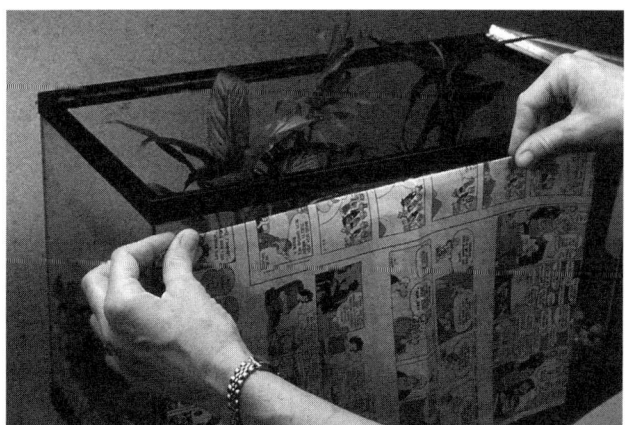

Figure 23.2. Patterned paper, such as the comics section of a newspaper, can be used to erect visual barriers. Some amphibians do not recognize clear glass barriers and will injure themselves as they explore the enclosure. This most frequently occurs during the initial acclimation to captivity. (George Grall, National Aquarium in Baltimore)

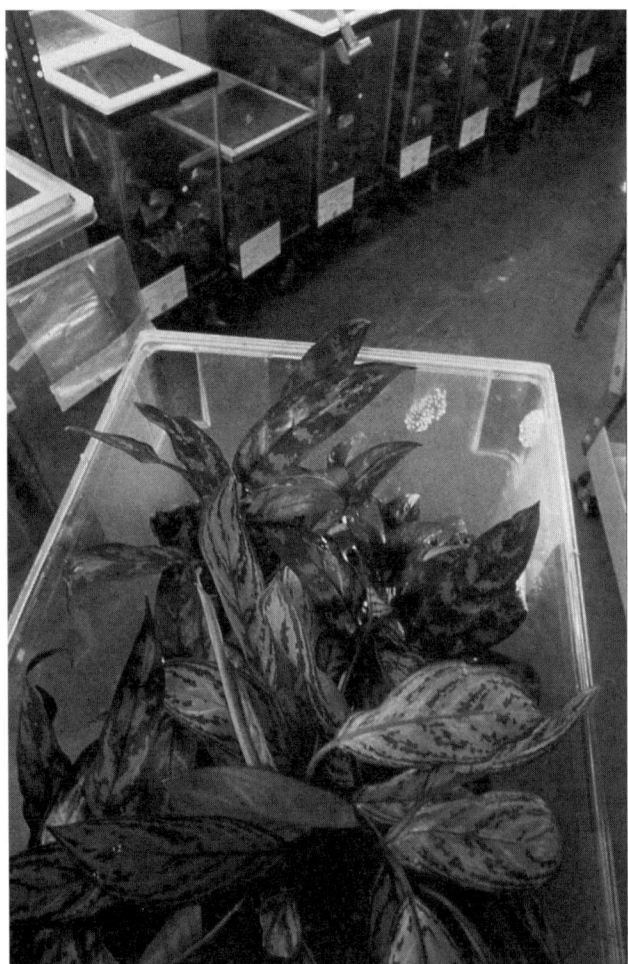

Figure 23.3. More naturalistic enclosures may be needed for delicate species of amphibians, or individuals that do not thrive in a spartan enclosure. (George Grall, National Aquarium in Baltimore)

be weighed and assessed. If this is not possible, an accurate weight should be obtained within 48 hours of arrival of an amphibian into the collection. With many specimens a milligram scale is essential to monitor weight fluctuations with precision. Careful examination of the amphibian may reveal skin discoloration, masses, or other lesions suggestive of parasitism or other infection. Any lesions should be sampled and evaluated.

Soon after arrival, a fecal sample should be submitted for parasite evaluation that includes acid-fast stain, direct examination, and flotation. Although rarely found in amphibians, the presence of *Cryptosporidium* spp. should be investigated. Until this organism is shown to be nonpathogenic for amphibians, every quarantined amphibian should be treated as if it is a confirmed shedder of *Cryptosporidium* spp. A solution of 5–10% ammonia should be used as one of the disinfectants. If *Cryptosporidium* spp. is detected in a fecal sample, the infected amphibian and its cagemates

the quarantine room so that the outside air is adequately humidified.

The quarantine cage should be placed in a room well separated from the room containing the permanent collection of amphibians to minimize the cross-transmission of airborne pathogens. If this is not practical every effort should be made to avoid cross contamination. The high stocking densities of amphibians at wholesale and retail dealers are stressful to the animals and expose them to large numbers of potential pathogens (Figure 23.4). Once the amphibians have been relocated, every effort should be made to reduce spread of pathogens between animals and enclosures. Tools should be disinfected for each quarantine enclosure, and a separate set of tools should be used for the permanent collection. Disposable gloves should be worn and discarded after servicing a quarantine cage. Quarantine cages should be serviced last, after all of the other enclosures have been serviced.

Immediately upon arrival each amphibian should

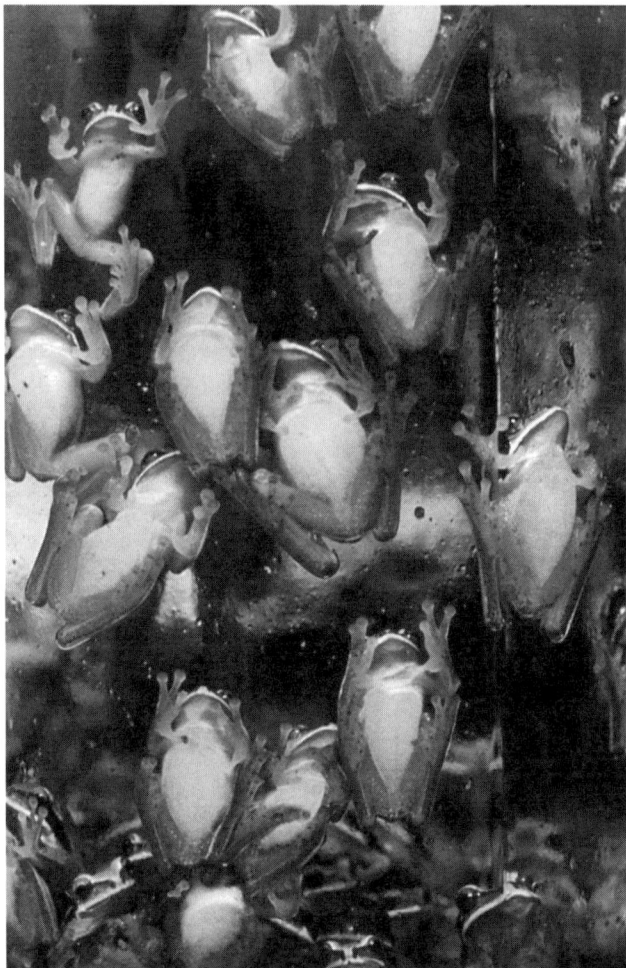

Figure 23.4. The abnormally high stocking density that occurs at many wholesale and retail dealers facilitates the spread of potential pathogens. (George Grall, National Aquarium in Baltimore)

should not be incorporated into the permanent collection. If the amphibians are of particular value, they may be maintained under quarantine for *Cryptosporidium* spp. with fecal samples submitted monthly to be evaluated for oocysts. A recent report suggests that a commercially available monoclonal antibody test is more sensitive at detecting *Cryptosporidium serpentes* and *C. parvum* than examination of an acid-fast stained slide (Graczyk et al., 1995), so at least one fecal sample should be screened in this way as an added precaution. *Cryptosporidium*-infected quarantine enclosures should be labeled with prominent warning signs, and the tools used to service this cage should be used nowhere else. If cleared fecal samples are obtained for 6 consecutive months, "recovered" individuals should be subjected to an assumed immunosuppressive dosage of dexamethasone (e.g., 1–2 mg/kg IM once), and weekly fecal samples evaluated for a minimum of 3 weeks. If these are negative, the quarantine for cryptosporidiosis may be lifted at the discretion of the client.

Appropriate antiparasitic treatment for the quarantined amphibian is contextual (see Chapter 15, Protozoa and Metazoa Infecting Amphibians, and Chapter 24, Pharmacotherapeutics, for further discussion). There is some concern that the amphibian's reaction to the death of large numbers of protozoans and metazoans could be more deleterious to the amphibian than the continued presence of these organisms, but often this concern is outweighed by the fact that the stress of transport and acclimation to a new environment can immunosuppress the amphibian making it more prone to disease from parasites. The risk and benefit of treatment should be clearly explained to the client. Treatment with fenbendazole is recommended as prophylaxis for nonaquatic amphibians due to the prevalence of nematode-related disease in captive amphibians. A suggested prophylactic anthelmintic regimen is immediate treatment with fenbendazole, followed on a subsequent day by ivermectin. Treatment with praziquantel should also be considered especially where the presence of trematodes or cestodes has been confirmed. Although protozoa may be found in the gastrointestinal tract of apparently healthy amphibians, metronidazole is indicated for recent arrivals that fail to thrive and show an abundance of protozoans in their feces (Poynton & Whitaker, 1994). Aquatic amphibians should receive immediate treatment with oral fenbendazole where possible, followed by a levamisole bath, and a praziquantel bath on the following day.

A more conservative approach to the treatment of quarantined amphibians is to provide therapeutics based upon the results of examining at least three fecal samples collected during the quarantine period. These samples may be obtained from individuals every 5 days or from a group every 3 days. If found positive for an organism of concern, the individual and other animals in contact with the infected individual should be treated appropriately. At least three fecal samples should be submitted over the next 2-week period to confirm successful elimination or control of the targeted organism. Fecal collection can be assisted by tube-feeding a small amount of a slurry containing Repto-Min® (Tetra Terrafauna Products, Morris Plains, NJ) as many amphibians will defecate within a few hours of ingesting this product. Amphibians that have diarrhea should be fully evaluated by collecting a sample for cytology and culture. Treatment with oral trimethoprim-sulfa should be considered as these amphibians frequently have a bacterial gastroenteritis that may or may not be associated with gastrointestinal coccidia.

Transfer to a new enclosure should occur at the end of the first week to remove the amphibians from possible sources of reinfection. All contaminated case furnishings such as cork and plants should be disposed of. No more than 3 weeks later the antiparasitic regimen chosen should be repeated, and again the amphibians placed in a new enclosure. A fecal sample should again be evaluated. If no parasites are detected, a fecal sample should be evaluated every 5 days until three negative samples are obtained. In many instances an anthelmintic must be administered a minimum of three separate treatments in order to successfuly eliminate parasites. A followup fecal examination should be performed within 60 days of release from quarantine, and a regular program of fecal sample monitoring and deparasitization begun as deemed appropriate. If parasites continue to be shed from an amphibian despite numerous anthelmintic/antiprotozoal treatments, release from quarantine is problematical. Continuous exposure to antiparasitic baths (e.g., levamisole, praziquantel, metronidazole) for over 24 h may eliminate certain resistant infections, but there is an increasing risk of toxicity developing in the amphibian patient with each successive day of exposure. If the amphibian is in good flesh, eating well, and passing normal stool, a release from quarantine with a more rigorous monitoring and deparasitization program is suggested. Care should be taken to avoid cross-contamination of other amphibian enclosures from the one containing resistant parasites. Amphibians with questionable health should be held in a permanent quarantine with strict anticontamination measures undertaken. These quarantined amphibians may be released into their final enclosure, but it should be serviced only after all other amphibians have been serviced or handled, and designated quarantine tools be assigned only for use with that particular enclosure. Sometimes the parasite ova will cease to be found once the amphibians have adapted to their new enclosure. Additionally, metazoans and protozoans with indirect life cycles will eventually disappear if the intermediate or final host is not present.

Even with stringent quarantine efforts, problems may follow. Larval helminths may be resistant to anthelmintic treatments, and may not be detectable by fecal parasite examinations. Encysted helminths can compromise organ function as is, or upon awakening from the abiotic state can resume their parasitic relationship. Transillumination may detect parasitic cysts in the muscle and viscera of some amphibians, but little can be done to effect a cure.

A microbial culture of the oropharynx and cloaca of the quarantined amphibian may be warranted as a screening tool during quarantine. At the very least this will provide a database of the amphibian's bacterial flora when it is clinically healthy, information that may help one identify the pathogenic organisms should the amphibian become sick.

A minimum length of 30 days is recommended for the quarantine period of any amphibian that arrived with a clean fecal sample, but often a 60-day quarantine period is a more reasonable length of time needed to process an amphibian through a prophylactic anthelmintic program and subsequent fecal examinations. Wild-caught amphibians, whether obtained directly or indirectly, should be held for an extended quarantine of 90 days or more. This is also recommended for amphibians of unknown origin and those that have been exposed to especially stressful conditions during shipment or prior to shipment. Amphibians purchased from commercial suppliers for biomedical research have often been held at two or more facilities, and the conditions at each facility may vary markedly. If there is any suspicion of adverse circumstances accompanying a shipment, a 90-day quarantine is recommended. If any signs of ill health are detected, the quarantine should be extended an additional 14 days beyond the animal's return to normal health or the quarantine may be restarted at day one. If individuals die during quarantine, the rest of the animals in quarantine should not be released until a final histopathologic diagnosis has been rendered. If viral disease is implicated or confirmed as a cause of death, the client should be cautioned against releasing exposed amphibians into their established collection.

Detailed husbandry records in conjunction with detailed medical records are essential if the clinician is to evaluate the effectiveness of a quarantine process. Clients should be given a written protocol to assist them in following all aspects of the quarantine. If a problem is encountered in a collection after a quarantine release, it can be objectively analyzed to determine if the quarantine process was at fault. The clinician may further refine the quarantine process on a species by species basis. If a particular supplier consistently supplies amphibians with abrasions, prophylactic antibiotic baths can be prepared and ready for the arrival of the next shipment of amphibians.

Unfortunately, an occasional amphibian will die during the quarantine process. It is extremely important to perform a necropsy on such specimens. Clients should be instructed to place the amphibian in a tightly sealed small container (e.g., sandwich bag) and deliver it for immediate assessment. A complete gross examination followed by a survey of all major organs including skin and muscle can be done in a short amount of time (see Chapter 25, Necropsy). Squash preparations are made by taking a small piece of tissue and gently flattening it between a glass slide with a drop of saline and coverslip for viewing under a light microscope. A small amount of contents from the stomach, large, and small intestine should also be examined. Any abnormalities such as whitish foci or discolored tissues should be scrutinized. If the amphibian is relatively fresh, samples for histopathology should be preserved in 10% buffered formalin. Immediate findings from the necropsy may be pertinent in the treatment of cagemates or other amphibians remaining in quarantine.

23.2 ACCLIMATION AND MALADAPTATION SYNDROME

Acclimation and maladaptation syndrome (AMS) is commonly observed in newly acquired amphibians, especially in those amphibians that were wild-caught and imported. AMS is a complex of clinical signs associated with the failure of an amphibian to adapt to its new (captive) environment even when that environment is an enriched enclosure that closely simulates the natural habitat of the amphibian. AMS can be minimized or avoided by proper research of the amphibian's needs prior to acquisition of any specimens, thus appropriate care can be given to vivarium design and construction. Furthermore, early recognition of AMS is the most important factor influencing the outcome of any corrective therapy thereafter instituted for the afflicted amphibian.

Some anurans suffering AMS may develop rostral lesions, usually the result of explosive escape jumping in the "fight or flight" mode. A cursorial anuran such as a dendrobatid frog may also develop a rostral lesion as it explores its enclosure. Prevention of this injury relies on providing a secure environment for the new anuran. This can be achieved by minimizing the visual stimulation of the anuran. One method is to cover the glass or clear plastic walls with an opaque substance (e.g., tape a piece of paper to the outside of the window) while the anuran is adjusting to the new enclosure. Hiding spots must be provided but the appropriate cage furniture depends on the species involved. Sudden loud noises can startle an anuran and cause it to jump into the walls of the vivarium, so excitable species may need to be kept in a quiet room with a minimum of human traffic until well adjusted to captivity. Ranid frogs and other anurans that are explosive jumpers may benefit from a cushion layer of plastic or plastic bubble wrap on the interior wall of the vivarium. The plastic drape absorbs some of the shock of impact, and the anuran will slide to the bottom of the enclosure with less damage than if it had hit an unyielding solid wall. Metal mesh screens should be avoided in the vivarium as the rough surface is more likely to be a source of rostral injuries than a soft plastic mesh. Finally, the cagemate may be the main source of stress promoting the anuran's injuries, so any frog or toad that develops a rostral lesion may need to be kept in a vivarium free of other inhabitants, and future reintroductions should be closely monitored for aggressive interactions. Any amphibian that develops a skin lesion should be closely monitored, and appropriate changes to the enclosure instituted. Topical and parenteral antibacterial, antifungal or antiparasitic therapy may be necessary if the lesion continues to enlarge, or if the amphibian displays other signs of generalized illness. (See also Section 17.1, Abrasions, Chapter 13, Bacterial Diseases, Chapter 14, Fungal Diseases, and Chapter 15, Protozoa and Metazoa Infecting Amphibians.)

Weight loss in the face of good appetite can be another clinical sign of acclimation and maladaptation syndrome. The difficulty lies in determining if this sign is the result of other correctable conditions such as parasitism, malnutrition, an imbalance of the gastrointestinal flora, or whether it is associated with a terminal illness such as gastrointestinal mycobacteriosis. If the amphibian has received appropriate anthelmintic therapy and is passing stools free of parasites or parasite ova, then parasitism may not be the cause of the weight loss. Temperatures above its preferred body temperature can cause weight loss as its metabolic rate may exceed its ability to assimilate calories. If the diet is appropriate in content and condition, and has a proven track record (either from published husbandry reports or supporting statements from other herpetoculturists maintaining that species), then malnutrition is unlikely to be the inciting culprit. However, the stress associated with inappropriate conditions may in turn place a higher than usual demand on certain key nutrients by the amphibian, and supplementation with vitamins, minerals, and certain amino acids may prove an essential aspect of corrective therapy for this condition. Additionally, many amphibians are not fed while in holding cages prior to export from the country of origin, and as a result the villous lining of the intestinal tract may atrophy. Without the absorptive surface of the intestine operating, ingested food will not be utilized by the animal. The natural balance of intestinal flora may also be affected causing diarrhea and the loss of nutrients. Frequent feedings of small amounts of increasing concentration is recommended to "jump start" the gastrointestinal tract, and it may be necessary to tube-feed the amphibian initially (see Section 7.13, Nutritional Support for the Ill and Inappetent Amphibian). In some cases, a broad spectrum oral antibiotic may be required. Once the amphibian is able to digest and assimilate the nutrients, assist feeding high fat items, such as waxworms, butterworms, recently nursed pinkie mice, and gravid crickets, may be necessary for the amphibian to regain its weight. Surveillance for *Mycobacterium* spp. is recommended whenever an amphibian is showing inexplicable weight loss. If an amphibian has been exposed to inappropriately high temperatures, even for brief periods, this may profoundly affect its metabolism afterward. Amphibians from cool environments often cannot reestablish homeostasis after a hyperthermic episode, and often become emaciated before death. This is an unfortunately common occurrence for many European newts, *Triturus* spp., imported for the pet trade.

Poor appetite is another distinct clinical sign of acclimation and maladaptation syndrome in amphibians. As mentioned previously, parasitism can also cause this sign and needs to be ruled out. An overabundance of flagellated protozoans has been associated with AMS and treatment with metronidazole may be effective in regaining normal homeostasis (Poynton & Whitaker, 1994). Another factor that may be involved in this clinical sign of poor appetite is the fact that the prey items offered in captivity may not match the search image of the amphibian, and therefore may not stimulate the feeding reflex. This is most likely to be a factor in species with highly specialized diets (e.g., narrow mouthed toads, *Gastrophryne* spp.), but poor appetite also has been noted in generalist predators that have become imprinted on a particular item (e.g., Surinam horn frog, *Ceratophrys cornuta*). Recognition of prey may be enhanced by proper illumination (e.g., ultraviolet radiation may reveal otherwise "invisible" patterns on the prey item). Thus a range of prey items (e.g., sweepings of meadow insects, small frogs, small lizards, earthworms, slugs, etc.) should be offered under appropriate lighting regimes (e.g., 12 h light photoperiod with near full-spectrum illumination for a tropical diurnal species, or 10 h light photoperiod with moonlight-equivalent fluorescent bulbs for a temperate crepuscular species). The temperature of the enclosure should be evaluated as temperatures below or above the preferred body temperature can be the cause of inappetence. Atrophy of the gastrointestinal tract lining may also decrease appetite, and should be approached as described previously.

Amphibians with AMS often do not display a normal hue to their skin. Greens and yellows are often muted or become entirely brown. Reds and blues become faded. Skin that should be glossy black may appear gray or mottled. Cutaneous infections can cause skin discoloration, but are more prone to local lesions than a bodywide color change. Malnutrition may play a role in the epidermal coloration of long-term captives, but certainly can affect the coloration of improperly handled recently caught specimens.

23.3 SUGGESTED DISINFECTION PROCEDURES

Cleaning and disinfection are aspects of amphibian husbandry that should be practiced diligently, and with careful attention paid to the thoroughness of the cleaning and the appropriate choice of a disinfectant.

The distinction between cleaning, disinfecting, and sterilizing should be made. Cleaning refers to the action of physically removing organic and inorganic debris from an item such as a feeding tong. Cleaning does little to reduce the load of bacteria and other potentially pathogenic organisms on an item. It is noted that complex naturalistic vivaria may be set up for years and require little attention other than spot-cleaning to remove uneaten food and feces. If the biological filtration is in order, it is rare for pathogens to become problematic in such a system.

It is extremely important to thoroughly clean an item prior to making an attempt to disinfect or sterilize it since most disinfectants are inactivated by organic debris. The overlying layer of material must be removed so that the disinfectant can contact the actual working surfaces of an item. It is a waste of time and money to start squirting disinfecting solutions into an enclosure until the dirt has been removed. Hot or warm water is more effective than cold water to quickly loosen encrusted debris.

There is also a level of difference between disinfection and sterilization. Disinfecting an item reduces the load of contaminating organisms to a large extent, but not completely. A disinfected cage will still harbor a low level of bacteria, fungi, and even viruses, but these organisms should be at a low enough level that they are not serving as a source of infection. Sterilizing an item renders that item devoid of all life. Once an item has been cleaned, the question arises as to what level of sterility is required for the cage, water bowl, or feeding tools. It is difficult and time consuming to completely sterilize anything, especially in a home setting. For a well established amphibian collection, one that has had no infectious diseases within a year and no new specimens added within a year, there is little need to attempt to sterilize cages and tools. However, if a collection is experiencing disease, and/or is adding new animals frequently, a higher level of care is needed so that items are sterilized and do not serve as a source of contamination within the collection. Since the two types of collection require different approaches, they will be individually discussed.

23.3.1 The Established Collection

The routine for an established collection should involve two separate disinfectants. Any tool that is used in a cage should be cleaned first, and then placed in the first disinfectant (e.g., chlorine bleach or ammonia) for a minimum of 5 minutes. It should be water rinsed, and then placed in the second disinfectant (e.g., ammonia or chlorine bleach) for a minimum of 5 minutes, and water rinsed before being used to service the next cage. The water rinsing between disinfectants is very important as some chemicals may combine to form toxic gases (e.g., bleach and ammonia). Some individuals have a tendency to hasten the soaking portion of this cycle because they are trying to rush through the cage servicing. This is dangerous since quick exposure to a disinfectant will not kill a pathogen. Prolonged exposure (greater than 15 min) to a disinfectant is recommended for greater levels of disinfection. Even with an established collection with a known minimal infectious disease risk, it is unwise to shorten the disinfectant exposure time to less than 5 minutes. Given this limiting factor, a way to expedite cage servicing is to have a second set of tools to be used while the primary set is being disinfected.

If a cage needs to be disinfected remember that plastics tend to retain disinfectants. These disinfectants can leach out into the cage substrate or water, with lethal effects to the inhabitants. Povidone-iodine, for example, was implicated in a rapid die-off of dendrobatids placed into a plastic container that had previously held a solution of this disinfectant (Stoskopf et al., 1985) (see Section 16.8, Halogens). Ammonia or chlorine bleach are excellent choices for disinfecting amphibian enclosures and tools, but thorough rinsing is essential. A useful dilution of household bleach (approximately 5% sodium hpyochlorite) is to add 50 ml of household bleach to each liter of water (or an 8-ounce cup of bleach to each gallon of water), while household ammonia (approximately 5 to 10% ammonia) can be used at full strength. Either solution is adequate to kill most pathogens. If chlorine bleach is used, a dechlorinating agent such as sodium thiosulfate may be used in the rinse water. If household ammonia is used, the brand chosen should not contain any additives such as detergents or deodorants. The rinse water of the disinfected tank should be checked with an ammonia test kit to ensure that ammonia levels remaining in the cage are not significantly elevated. Once again, the disinfectant used must remain on cage surfaces for a minimum of 5 minutes. A spray bottle containing the appropriate dilution of disinfectant is a quick and economical way to apply the disinfectant.

23.3.2 The Quarantined Collection

The collection with known infectious diseases, or with new amphibians, is at more of a risk for disease outbreaks than the established collection. While many pathogens can be killed by the disinfectants already discussed (i.e., ammonia and chlorine), *Mycobacterium* spp. and the ova of some metazoan parasites are resistant to the majority of available disinfectants. Prolonged exposure to steam appears to be an effective method of sterilization for these problematical pathogens, but this type of sterilization is not a practical solution. Formalized saline (>500 ppm formalin) is another disinfectant option, but should not be used without adequate ventilation and respiratory protection. Formalin dilutions also should not be used with wood or other permeable substances; these items should be discarded rather than reused. Tuberculocidal disinfectants are commercially available, but many of the formerly available products are no longer rated as active against *Mycobacterium* spp. A quarantine collection should have more than one set of tools so that adequate exposure time to the disinfectant is maintained.

When using disinfectants on tools or materials used with quarantined amphibians, it is important to maintain contact with the chemical for a minimum of 30 min and preferably longer. It is imperative that the quarantine tools and cages be maintained well separated from established amphibians, and that the new and ill amphibians be serviced after the healthy and established members of a collection. Disposable latex or vinyl gloves are recommended when working with the quarantined amphibians, and disinfectant solutions should be poured out and the buckets rinsed in an area distinct from the sink where water bowls and items from the established collection are rinsed. If an amphibian dies from a disease such as a mycobacteriosis, all organic items (e.g., wood) and permeable inorganic items (e.g., lava rock) should be discarded. It is extremely difficult to disinfect these items, and the best way to ensure that these resistant pathogens do not spread through a collection is to avoid recycling cage furniture.

The cleaning and disinfection routine for a collection is not something that follows any prescribed formula, but rather should evolve out of consideration for the makeup of the amphibian collection, the health and disease risk of the collection, and of course the budget of the client. The veterinarian who works with a particular collection is best able to recommend the disinfectants and exposure times. It is the client's responsibility to follow those guidelines, and to avoid making changes without first double-checking that the changes are compatible with an adequate level of cleaning and disinfection.

REFERENCES

Grazyk, T.D., M.R. Cranfield, and R. Fayer. 1995. A comparative assessment of direct fluorescence antibody, modified acid-fast stain, and sucrose flotation techniques for detection of *Cryptosporidium serpentes* oocyst in snake fecal specimens. Journal of Zoo and Wildlife Medicine 26(3):396–402.

Poynton, S.L. and B.R. Whitaker. 1994. Protozoa in poison dart frogs (Dendrobatidae): clinical assessment and identification. Journal of Zoo and Wildlife Medicine 25(1):29–39.

Stoskopf, M.K., A. Wisnieski, and L. Pieper. 1985. Iodine toxicity in poison arrow frogs. Proceedings of the American Association of Zoo Veterinarians, pp. 86–88.

CHAPTER 24
PHARMACOTHERAPEUTICS

Kevin M. Wright, DVM and Brent R. Whitaker, MS, DVM

24.1 INTRODUCTION

Many of the bacterial, fungal, viral, and parasitic diseases observed in captive larval and adult amphibians are the result of improper husbandry. A captive management plan that works well for one species may be inappropriate for another species and these inappropriate conditions can cause chronic stress. The physiological changes that result are an attempt by the animal to adapt to the stressor(s). Energetically this is expensive and over time can have detrimental consequences such as reduced immune function, decreased growth, and inability to reproduce. Most commonly, amphibians become sick with the opportunistic pathogens that are ubiquitous in their environment. The clinician's responsibilities to the client include identification of the inciting cause of the illness, assignment of a clinical diagnosis, provision of an appropriate therapeutic regime, and reevaluation of the case (from husbandry to diagnostics) as necessary. Simply administering antibiotics for a confirmed bacterial infection will not ultimately solve the client's problem if basic husbandry issues are neglected.

There are few published pharmacokinetic studies of therapeutic agents used in amphibians. Significant data has been accumulated for fishes in recent years which may provide guidance in many cases. With most amphibian patients, the clinician makes choices of drug selection, dose rate, route of administration, and duration of treatment based upon empirically derived information and previously experienced successes rather than definitive pharmacokinetic data. All Tables mentioned are presented at the end of this chapter.

24.2 ANTIVIRAL AGENTS

It is often difficult to diagnose a viral disease in a collection of amphibians before significant morbidity and mortality result. The rapid invasion by bacteria and fungi limit the window of opportunity in which a specific antiviral agent would prove beneficial, as does the delay involved in confirming an outbreak of viral disease. In all cases of viral disease, antimicrobial therapy aimed at the secondary bacterial and fungal invaders is appropriate.

Antiviral agents have rarely been used to treat disease in amphibians. Oral administration of acyclovir (80 mg/kg PO SID) has been recommended for reptiles (Frye, 1991), and may be useful as a prophylactic treatment of asymptomatic anurans exposed to a clinical case of herpesvirus, such as Lucke's virus, but its efficacy in amphibians is unknown. Acyclovir is available as a 5% ointment which might have systemic effects in amphibians. Anti-inflammatory agents such as systemic corticosteroids (e.g., dexamethasone sodium phosphate 0.1–0.5 mg/kg TO, IM or ICe SID × 3–5 days, then taper the dose downward) may prove useful in mediating the damage caused by a viral agent, but these should be used in conjunction with concomitant antimicrobials targeted for bacteria and fungi.

24.3 ANTIBACTERIAL AGENTS

When used appropriately, antibiotics provide the clinician with an important tool to fight bacterial disease. If the illness is not immediately life-threatening, selection of an antibiotic should be made via culture and sensitivity of the isolates with the most powerful antibiotics held in reserve when other drugs appear ineffective. It is important to remember the "four quadrant" approach to antibiotic therapy since the majority of amphibian infections will be comprised of a mixed bacterial fauna. No single antibiotic is effective against all four "quadrants" of bacteria (G− aerobes, G− anaerobes, G+ aerobes, G+ anaerobes), so the clinician must often administer combinations of antibiotics in order to eliminate all the taxa of bacteria which may be causing disease in an amphibian.

An impediment to the scientific treatment of infectious diseases in amphibians is the paucity of pharmacokinetic data. The research that has been published focuses primarily on a few North American species (e.g., bullfrog, *Rana catesbeiana*, northern leopard frog, *Rana pipiens*, mudpuppy, *Necturus maculosa*), and the strict application of this data to other species is questionable given the divergence in physiologic processes documented within the class Amphibia. Thus the majority of the recommendations for antibiotic therapy in this section are made in the absence of pharmacokinetic data and the clinician is advised to apply these recommendations with caution. It may be dangerous to extrapolate any one study too broadly based on the variation in data resulting from pharmacokinetic studies of gentamicin in a salamander and an anuran (Stoskopf et al., 1987; Teare et al., 1991). It is important to explain to clients the limits of pharmacological knowledge in amphibians and to obtain their express permission prior to administration of any drug to their animals.

Many infected amphibians will die despite seemingly appropriate drug choices. Although a resistant strain of the pathogen is an obvious conclusion, there are several other possible factors that contribute to this apparent treatment failure including, but not limited to, "silent" pathogens not recognized in the therapeutic plan, inappropriate drug dosage, inappropriate dosing frequency, early cessation of treatment, inappropriate route of administration, inappropriate sanitation efforts (failure to remove and eliminate pathogens from the environment), immunosuppression of the host amphibian, and inappropriate supportive care.

Although attention has been focused on behavioral fever in reptiles and its role in combatting bacterial infections (Kluger, 1979; Vaughn et al., 1974), thermoregulation and its link to immunocompetence in reptiles or amphibians is poorly understood (Evans, 1963; Green & Cohen, 1977; Hutchison & Dupré, 1992; Kollias, 1984; Wright & Cooper, 1981). The ill amphibian should be provided with an optimal thermal environment to enhance physiological processes and immunocompetence. A thermal mosaic which incorporates a vertical as well as horizontal variation in temperature should be provided in the enclosure to allow the amphibian the ability to thermoregulate independent of light and moisture levels. A mosaic provides a "checkerboard" of choices for the amphibian. For example, the enclosure should contain dark spots that are warm and dry or warm and moist, and normally illuminated spots (during the day cycle) that are warm and dry or warm and moist. A similar arrangement of cool spots and moderate-temperature (i.e., the preferred body temperature) spots are needed also. The effectiveness of any treatments may be enhanced in such an environment, and research into this aspect of amphibian medicine is needed. A suggested range of temperatures would include the warm spots in the enclosure that exceed the amphibian's preferred body temperature by at least 4°C (8°F) while the cool spots range to more than 4°C (8°F) below the preferred body temperature. In most instances the thermal mosaic is accomplished by establishing a thermocline within the cage wherein one end is warm and the opposite end is cool. A thermal mosaic can be established in an aquatic system by decreasing the temperature of the water (e.g., cooling the entire room with an air conditioner) and distributing one or more focused heating elements in the tank.

Additional furnishings may be needed to accommodate other behavioral needs of some species in order to promote behavioral thermoregulation. Since arboreal frogs tend to perch on the side of an enclosure or near the top, additional heat may be provided by attaching a heat pad to the side of the tank or to focus a basking light near the top of the enclosure. Strips of black plastic or some other cover may be draped over the area warmed by the heat pad or basking light, and similar cover should be provided over the cool end of the enclosure, so that lack of cover does not dissuade the frogs from movement to warm or cool areas as desired. Terrestrial amphibians may need undertank heating or cooling to promote a thermal mosaic.

Cooling to 8–10°C (46–50°F) has been used as an adjunct therapy for treating "*Salmonella-Shigella*" infections in the axolotl, *Ambystoma mexicanum* (Maruska, 1994) (The authors have placed quotation marks to indicate lack of additional published supporting evidence for this etiologic diagnosis). In theory, the lowered temperature of the amphibian inhibits reproduction of the bacteria and allows the host's immune system time to mount a more effective response to the infection. This adjunct therapy is most applicable to large scale operations, such as research vivariums and holding facilities, and other situations wherein it is not practical to provide an enriched environment with thermal mosaics. The temperature for which a particular species can be cooled without adverse effects varies. A general guideline for therapeutic cooling is that temperate and tropical montane species can be cooled to 8–10°C (46–50°F) and tropical lowland and subtropical species can be cooled to 15–18°C (60–64°F). Cooling may be considered for the obviously septic amphibian as an adjunct therapy while antibiotics distribute through the body.

Amphibians may combat some infections more effectively when they are maintained at a consistently elevated temperature. Several specimens of the crocodile newt, *Tylototriton shanjing*, were received by the Philadelphia Zoo with ulcerating skin lesions on the mandible. Specimens that were maintained at temperatures of 23–26°C (75–80°F) showed improved healing times compared to those maintained at 10–15°C (50–60°F). When the cool-habituated salamanders were transferred to the warmer environment, the lesions resolved quickly. This may reflect the increased epithelialization activity at the higher temperature rather than a direct antibacterial effect. A change in the patient's thermal environment should be considered if lesions fail to resolve or show progress toward resolution.

Saprolegniasis often occurs at temperatures below 20°C (68°F) and adjunct therapy should include elevating the enclosure temperature above this if the amphibian can tolerate the higher temperatures. Some external protozoal infections may be better managed with a warmer than normal thermal environment. *Dermocystidium* and *Dermosporidium* infections purportedly have been eliminated when temperate amphibians are maintained at 25°C (77°F) (Raphael, 1993).

One study documented the pharmacokinetics of a single intramuscular injection of three different antibiotics in the North American bullfrog, *Rana catesbeiana* (Letcher & Papich, 1994). In this study amikacin remained at an effective level for many Gram-negative pathogens 38 h after a single injection at a dosage of 5 mg/kg. Enrofloxacin was maintained above therapeutic levels at dosages of either 5 or 10 mg/kg IM once daily, and oxytetracycline remained at an effective concentration at the dosages of 50 or 100 mg/kg IM once every 48 h. Interestingly, these levels are in keeping with empiric dosages published for amphibians. Amikacin (5 mg/kg SQ, IM or ICe q 24–48 h for a minimum of seven treatments) and enrofloxacin (5–10 mg/kg SQ, IM, ICe, or PO q 24 h for a minimum of ten treatments) are the therapies of choice for the initial treatment of most Gram-negative bacterial infections in amphibians, and as adjunct therapy for most clinically ill amphibians.

The availability of advanced quinilones such as enrofloxacin and ciprofloxacin has provided clinicians with a powerful arsenal with which to combat serious bacterial infections. The advantages of using these drugs include rapid assimilation, ease of administration, and minimal potential for toxicity. Enrofloxacin has been used with great success at the National Aquarium in Baltimore, especially where organisms were resistant to other agents. In addition to the parenteral routes (SQ, IM, ICe), the injectable preparation of enrofloxacin is easily given orally to even the smallest of patients using a microliter syringe with disposable tips (see Chapter 8, Clinical Techniques). Although it may be difficult to administer enrofloxacin orally, this is the preferred route for many amphibians. Skin discoloration and sloughing have been noted in some amphibians at the site of an enrofloxacin injection. Data from reptiles suggest that uptake and distribution of the injectable preparation of enrofloxacin is similar whether orally or parenterally administered (Klingenberg, 1996). In cases where there is concern that the n-butyl alcohol carrier of the injectable enrofloxacin is irritating, a suspension may be made by grinding tablets into a fine powder and using a water-soluble gel (e.g., KY Jelly) to suspend it before administering it orally. This suspension may be too thick to be dispensed via microliter syringe. Injectable enrofloxacin has been used topically in small amphibians, but there is a risk of irritation caused by the carrier vehicle. If irritation is noted, usually indicated by agitated movements of the amphibian, the medication should be rinsed off with water and an alternate route or agent used.

Ciprofloxacin has been used successfully as a bath, 500 mg per 75 l (20 gallons) for 6–8 h SID for 7 days, for septicemic fishes and is also of use in treating amphibians. Ciprofloxacin baths should be considered where large numbers of aquatic amphibians require treatment such as in a laboratory vivarium or holding facility. Ciprofloxacin also may be used orally as described for enrofloxacin. Although the reptilian dosage is 10 mg/kg PO q 48 h (Klingenberg, 1996), given the pharmacokinetic data of enrofloxacin in the bullfrog, *Rana catesbeiana*, a dosing frequency of every 24 h is a reasonable empiric dosage in amphibians.

Gentamicin has been the subject of a few pharmacokinetic studies in amphibians. At 22.2°C (72°F), the recommended dosing schedule was 3 mg/kg IM q 24 h intramuscular injection in the northern leopard frog, *Rana pipiens* (Teare et al., 1991). This is a marked contrast to the dosing schedule recommended for the mudpuppy, *Necturus maculosa*, 2.5 mg/kg IM q 72 h at 3°C (37°F) (Stoskopf et al., 1987), but whether the difference is a species-specific difference or the result of the environmental temperature difference between the two studies is unknown. Until further pharmacokinetic information becomes available at different temperatures or documenting species-specific difference, it is recommended that the frog data be the basis for the gentamicin dose for all amphibians except for coldwater aquatic salamanders, which should be dosed according to the mudpuppy study. A higher dosage of 13 mg/kg IM q 48 h has been used in the axolotl, *Ambystoma mexicanum* (Maruska, 1994), suggesting that higher dosages of gentamicin may be used in some aquatic amphibians. The point has previously been mentioned in regard to all pharmaceuticals used in amphibians, but is re-emphasized here since fatalities have been associated with inappropriately high serum levels of gentamicin (Teare et al., 1991). The clinician should exercise caution when prescribing any antibiotic, such as gentamicin, for an unfamiliar species of amphibian, and the client should be appropriately informed of the risks associated with the therapeutic plan.

Trimethoprim and sulfa drug combinations have been recommended for the treatment of bacterial infections at a dosage of 3 mg/kg SQ or PO q 24 h (Crawshaw, 1992; Raphael, 1993), and a proprietary sulfa drug has been used as a continuous bath to treat suspected columnaris (possibly *Cytophaga colmunaris*) in the axolotl, *Ambystoma mexicanum*. Trimethoprim and sulfamethoxazole (20 μg/ml and 80 μg/ml respectively in 0.5% saline) has been used as a bath to treat bacterial disease in laboratory-maintained frogs

(Menard, 1984). At the National Aquarium in Baltimore there has been excellent clinical response to trimethoprim and sulfamethoxazole (Biocraft Laboratories, Elmwood Park, NJ) given at doses of 15 mg/kg PO q 24 h for up to 21 days. In many cases this broad spectrum antibiotic was used to treat thin animals showing chronic diarrhea. The goal is twofold, first to treat bacterial enteritis and second to treat potential coccidiosis which in our experience has been difficult to diagnose antemortem. Although clinical improvement has been evident in many animals, postmortem examination of recovered anurans has shown that coccidia are not eliminated by this regime.

Topical antibiotics are commonly used in amphibians given the small body size of some patients or the sheer numbers of patients utilized in research laboratories. One study demonstrated that the use of antibiotics in saline baths (0.5% saline was reportedly more effective than 0.15% saline) markedly increased the survival rates of the northern leopard frog, *Rana pipiens,* as well as the green frog, *Rana clamitans,* and the European common frog, *Rana temporaria,* over treatment with antibiotics alone (Menard, 1984), thus helping to establish the importance of maintaining electrolyte balance in the ill amphibian (see also Section 24.9, Maintaining the Electrolyte Balance of the Ill Amphibian). The antibiotics that were effective were tetracycline hydrochloride (10 μg/ml 0.5% saline), chloramphenicol (10 μg/ml 0.5% saline), nalidixic acid (10 μg/ml 0.5% saline), gentamicin sulfate (8 μg/ml 0.5% saline), nitrofurantoin (50 μg/ml 0.5% saline), and trimethoprim and sulfamethoxazole (20 μg/ml and 80 μg/ml 0.5% saline respectively). The solutions were made fresh daily. The treatment regimen described included isolation of affected frogs and antibiotics were chosen in response to sensitivity patterns of Gram-negative, nonlactose-fermenting, oxidase-positive isolates cultured from skin lesions of the ill frogs. Chloramphenicol was the drug of choice unless resistance to it was noted in the sensitivity patterns of the isolates. This study did not document the tissue or plasma levels of the antibiotics used in the course of treatment nor did it confirm that skin isolates were the true etiologic agents impacting survival of the frogs.

Percutaneous absorption of metronidazole was studied in the firebelly toad, *Bombina orientalis* (Mombarg & Zwart, 1991). In this study, 50 μl of 1.008 mg/ml metronidazole solution was administered to frogs with an average body weight of 1.8 g (a dosage of 28 mg/kg). The metronidazole dose was left on the frog for one hour before the frog was rinsed in fresh water. The total metronidazole absorbed was 21 mg/kg, 75% of the applied dose, but 15% below the oral dose of 25 mg/kg considered appropriate by Mombarg and Zwart (1991). Human absorption studies indicate that 6–15% of the metronidazole administered orally is excreted in feces (Package insert, Flagyl® Tablets, G.D. Searle and Company, Chicago, IL). The oral absorption, distribution and excretion of metronidazole in amphibians is undocumented, but a variety of empirical dosages have been used successfully: 10 mg/kg PO q 24 h for 5–10 days for the treatment of chronic diarrhea (Poynton & Whitaker, 1994); 50 mg/kg PO q 24 h for 3 days for the initial treatment of anaerobic infections or severe amoebiasis (Wright, 1996); 100–150 mg/kg PO q 14 days for mild amoebic infections (Wright, 1996). Extrapolating from the absorption study (Mombarg & Zwart, 1991) and the assumption that approximately 90% of the oral metronidazole is absorbed (a value consistent with human studies), metronidazole may be applied topically at a dosage around 20% higher than the oral dosage to achieve the same absorption. Thus a topical dosage of 12 mg/kg may yield an absorption similar to what can be expected for an oral dosage of 10 mg/kg. With aquatic amphibians it may be difficult to dose metronidazole precisely. A topical bath of 50 mg/L for up to 24 h has been used empirically.

Other forms of metronidazole and related chemicals are available. Intravenous forms of metronidazole (Flagyl® I.V. RTU, Schiapparelli Searle, Chicago, IL; Metronidazole Redi-Infusion™, Elkins-Sinn, Inc., Cherry Hill, NJ) and metronidazole hydrochloride (Flagyl® I.V., Schiapparelli Searle, Chicago, IL) are available. Metronidazole hydrochloride is extremely acidic (pH 0.5–2.0) and was designed to be administered intravenously. As with other drugs that are extremely acidic, administration by extra-label routes should be done after due consideration is given to the consequences. If an intravenous solution of metronidazole is buffered to a neutral or near neutral pH (e.g., Flagyl® I.V. RTU), there is less concern when it is used orally, topically, intravenously, or intracoelomically in amphibians. A dosage of 10 mg/kg SID for 2 days is suggested for either intravenous or intracoelomic administration of metronidazole. Metronidazole is the major component appearing in human plasma, and does not appear irritating if used infrequently by parenteral routes.

A 0.75% topical gel form of metronidazole is available (Metrogel®, Curatek Pharmaceuticals, Elk Grove Village, IL), and may prove a more practical form for topical administration of metronidazole to amphibians. The percutaneous absorption of metronidazole from the carrier vehicle is unknown but the total dose of metronidazole should not exceed that recommended topically.

Metronidazole is an excellent choice for treating anaerobic infections as it distributes well reaching bacteriocidal levels in humans even in hepatic abscesses. It should not be used in isolation as aerobic bacteria are concomitant with anaerobic bacteria in most septic amphibians.

One pharmacokinetic study reported that continuous soaking of a northern leopard frog, *Rana pipiens,* in a 1 mg/ml solution of gentamicin produced therapeutic serum gentamicin levels (>4 μg/ml) within 12 hours (Riveiere et al., 1979). The serum gentamicin levels reported in that study were reported as unchanged over 12 days of exposure to this concentration of gentamicin. A more recent report suggested caution when applying gentamicin cutaneously since serum gentamicin levels continued to elevate beyond the therapeutic level obtained at 8 hours, and continued to elevate beyond the 24 h sampling, with levels as high as 69.7 μg/ml reported at day 6, and fatalities occuring from day 5 onward (Teare et al., 1991). The concentration of gentamicin used in these two studies is markedly increased over the 8 μg/ml level reported effective in increasing survival in a laboratory situation (Menard, 1984). Given the toxic potential of gentamicin, long-term baths should be used with caution. Pending further pharmacokinetic studies, if topical gentamicin is the drug and route of choice for a given bacterial infection, a potential course of treatment would be an 8 h bath in 1 mg/ml gentamicin solution every 24–48 h. A more practical regimen is a continuous bath in the more dilute solution of 8 μg/ml gentamicin in 0.5% saline used for no more than 5 days in a row.

A proprietary combination of methylene blue, furazolidone, and monofuracin (Furazone Green®, DYNA-PET, Campbell, CA), a broad spectrum antibacterial agent developed for fishes, has been used to successfully treat bacterial disease in tadpoles. This powder, dissolved directly into the water per manufacturer's instructions, approximately 0.65 g/38 L (10 gal), has treated successfully Gram-negative bacterial infections including *Aeromonas hydrophila*. Unfortunately, "shotgun" therapy such as this abounds in the literature on amphibian husbandry and medicine and there is no way of knowing what was the important point of the treatment due to the number of drugs used. A complex cocktail of antibiotics has been reported for the treatment of advanced "red leg" in larvae of some European newts, *Pleurodeles* spp. (Read, 1994). The recipe for Read's solution is as follows: 6 g NaCl, 12 mg ciprofloxacin, 20 mg gentamicin, 10,000 iu nystatin, 3.84% amprolium at 1 part per 100, 1 mg vitamin K, 1000 ml water. The bath was administered at a volume of 10 times the volume of larvae to be treated, and the larvae were kept in pure oxygen at 30°C (86°F). There is no way to know which of the agents involved, if any, resolved the disease, nor what, if any, was the causative infectious agent. The cocktail included drugs to treat bacterial infection (ciprofloxacin, gentamicin), fungal infection (nystatin), coccidial infection (amprolium), electrolyte imbalance (NaCl), clotting abnormalities (vitamin K), and hypoxemia (O_2), without ever a clear diagnosis for the underlying etiology. There is certainly the temptation to take such an approach, especially when a massive die-off is occurring in the collection. A systematic work up of the collection that includes a thorough necropsy on dead, freshly euthanized, clinically ill specimens, and freshly euthanized but clinically healthy specimens, is to be encouraged over shotgun therapy, and should occur concomitant with a direct and focused pharmaceutical plan.

The importance of supplemental oxygen cannot be understated as many amphibians respire in part through their skin thus any damage to the skin might impair exchange of respiratory gases. In addition, many bacterial pathogens show inhibited growth if exposed to oxygen levels above that found in room air.

Other antibiotics that have been used in amphibians may be found in Table 24.1.

24.4 ANTIFUNGAL AGENTS

The authors are unaware of any published pharmacokinetic studies of antifungal agents in amphibians, although an inconclusive itraconazole study has been performed (personal communication, W.K. Suedemyer, 1997). Specific parenteral antifungal drugs that are commonly used in mammals include amphotericin-B, ketoconazole, itraconazole, and fluconazole, and topical antifungals include tolnaftate, clotrimazole, miconazole, and ketoconazole. Most of these drugs have been used in amphibians, but their efficacy and toxicity remain inconclusive.

Topical antifungal therapy for aquatic amphibians is based upon those regimens that have proved effective in the management of disease in cold and tropical freshwater fish. Benzalkonium chloride is probably the topical of choice for the treatment of diffuse fungal disease in aquatic amphibians, and has been used at a level of 2 mg/L as a 60 min bath daily. One author recommends 0.25 mg/L bath continuously for 72 h or a 1:4,000,000 dilution for longer periods of time (Raphael, 1993). Hypertonic electrolyte (salt) baths lasting 5–30 min, either using sodium chloride or artifical sea salts at 10–25 g/L, daily are sometimes effective. A 10–100% Whitaker-Wright solution may also be effective. Topical application of potassium permanganate (1 g/100 ml water) to lesions followed by maintenance in 100% modified Holtfreter's solution has been effective at an institution with a large amphibian collection (Maruska, 1994). The Shedd Aquarium has used the oxidant sodium chlorite ($NaOCl_2$) at a level of 20 mg/L for a 6–8 h bath to treat external fungal infections (saprolegniasis) of anuran tadpoles (personal communication, M. Greenwell, 1997). Malachite green solutions appear to be effective in combatting some fungal infections in tadpoles, but trials at the National Aquarium in Baltimore demonstrated a marked reduction in growth rate for healthy tadpoles treated with malachite green. Other treatments effective in fish may be tried (e.g., methylene blue), but generally any fungal agent that is resistant to benzalkonium chloride or salt baths may require concomitant use of parenteral agents such as itraconazole, ketoconazole or amphotericin-B. Any treatment should be closely monitored so that the patient may be removed if showing signs of distress (e.g., extreme agitation, excessive mucus production). Rinse the distressed amphibian thoroughly with fresh water. If exfoliation occurs, as may occur with malachite green, benzalkonium chloride, formalin, and other medicated baths, the amphibian may need additional supportive care to maintain electrolyte balance and combat secondary infection.

Terrestrial amphibians provide a wider range of treatment options for topical fungal infections. Antiseptic solutions, such as benzalkonium chloride, salt solutions, or potassium permanganate, may be applied directly to isolated lesions and rinsed off after an appropriate time. Daily applications of a topical antifungal solution or cream of miconazole or ketoconazole may prove effective in managing certain fungal lesions. Ketoconazole and miconazole appear to be less irritating than tolnaftate or clotrimazole. Since dermatitis is the prevalent disease noted with amphibian fungal infections, topical treatment may affect the invading organism better and faster than if the drug is administered orally or intracoelomically. Liquid itraconozole is designed for oral use in mammals but it may prove effective if used topically in amphibians. Topical itraconazole (0.01% SID for 5 min x 11 days) has been effective in treating chytridiomycosis (Nichols & Lamirande, 2000). If parenteral therapy is combined with topical therapy, the clinician is well advised to calculate the maximum possible amount of drug contained in each topical treatment and be aware when the total dose is above the recommended range. Maintenance of the amphibian's water and electrolyte balance is an essential adjunct therapy, especially in anurans with an affected drink patch or other serious skin lesions.

Parenteral antifungals have been used on occasion. A reasonable starting dosage for ketoconazole is 10–20 mg/kg PO q 24 h for 14–28 days. Fluconazole has been used in several amphibians with confirmed fungal infections at the National Aquarium in Baltimore. A confirmed fungal uveitis in a harlequin poison frog, *Dendrobates histrionicus,* resolved when given fluconazole at a seemingly high dose of 1 mg to a 1.8-g frog PO q 24 h for 7 days (a daily dose of approximately 556 mg/kg). Despite the tolerance for this high dosage, a suggested dosage for fluconazole is between 10–100 mg/kg PO q 24 h × 14–28 d. Other options include amphotericin-B at 1 mg/kg ICe SID or miconazole at 5 mg/kg ICe SID × 14–28 days.

Itraconazole has been used at a dosage of 2 mg/kg PO SID in several species. However a study of itraconazole pharmacokinetics in the giant toad, *Bufo marinus,* failed to demonstrate therapeutic blood levels (i.e., 0.1–1.0 µg/ml) in the 24 h following a single oral administration of either 5 or 10 mg/kg (personal communciation, W.K. Suedemyer, 1997). No harmful side effects were noted at these dosages, although one toad voided greenish urine. In this study the itraconazole was dissolved in weakly acidic solutions to form a solution rather than a suspension. The solution used was 100 mg itraconazole in 10 ml orange juice and 10 ml white vinegar which took several hours to dissolve. Itraconazole can be dissolved in 10% citric acid, but it may take over 24 h for the medication to dissolve fully. The stability of these solutions is unknown. A commericial liquid form of itraconazole (Sporanox, 10 mg/ml, Janssen Pharmaceuticals, Titusville, NJ) became available recently. Itraconazole may be used at 2–10 mg/kg PO q 24 h.

Other antifungal agents that have been used in amphibians are listed in Table 24.1.

24.5 EMERGENCY TREATMENT FOR THE SEPTIC AMPHIBIAN

The practical approach to the septic amphibian is dependent on the degree of client cooperation that can be expected. If at all possible, a sample of the blood, coelomic fluid, subcutaneous fluid, cloacal swab, tracheal swab, and/or skin lesions should be obtained and submitted for culture and sensitivity prior to instituting antibiotic therapy. This is not always practical, but in the absence of complete diagnostic testing it is difficult to determine an appropriate course of action should the initial therapeutic regimen prove unsuccessful. If at all possible, every amphibian in an infected enclosure should be sampled for comparison. In the event of large groups, a representative sample of clinically ill and clinically healthy individuals should be sampled. Initial therapy should include maintenance in a bath of an isotonic or near-isotonic electrolyte solution (e.g., amphibian Ringer's solution, 0.6–0.8% saline, 5% Whitaker-Wright solution, 100% Holtfreter's or modified Holtfreter's solution) to help stabilize the patient's electrolytes. Daily treatment with itraconazole topically is suggested whenever chytridiomycosis is suspected. If an amphibian appears to be suffering from fluid overload (hydrocoelom, edema), a hypertonic electrolyte solution may be used instead (e.g., hypertonic amphibian Ringer's solution, 0.9% saline, or 10–100% Whitaker-Wright solution). Supplemental oxygen is suggested. Poorly responsive amphibians may be cooled below their preferred body temperature (e.g., maintain at 8–10°C) for the first 72–120 h of treatment (Maruska, 1994). This may allow the antibiotic to distribute throughout the body at a faster rate than the bacterial dissemination and growth. Antibiotic therapy should include broad-spectrum antibiotics with emphasis on anaerobic and Gram-negative bacteria. Chlamydiosis must be considered as an underlying etiology (Wright, 1996), and appropriate antibiotics (e.g., doxycycline or other tetracyclines) should be used if this is highly ranked on the differential diagnosis or if its presence is confirmed.

Individual amphibians may be started on a combination of piperacillin (although this drug is well known for its effectiveness on specific *Pseudomonas* spp., it is effective against many anaerobes, most Gram-positive bacteria and many Gram-negative bacteria) and amikacin (effective against most aerobic Gram-negative bacteria) therapy. In the case of recently acquired animals, parenteral oxytetracycline may be used in place of piperacillin due to its effectiveness against chlamydiosis, Gram-positive bacteria, and many anaerobes, but it is rarely effective on amikacin-resistant Gram-negative pathogens. Metronidazole (25–50 mg/kg PO SID for 3 days, 10 mg/kg IV or ICe SID for 2 days, or 60 mg/kg TO SID for 3 days) may be used if anaerobic infection is confirmed. Metronidazole should be considered in addition to amikacin if piperacillin is unavailable. Enrofloxacin or ciprofloxacin are good single drug choices with a broad spectrum of Gram-negative activity. If at all possible, it is desirable to give individual treatments with measured dosages over topical treatments such as baths.

Large-scale treatments, such as for laboratory vivariums or holding facilities, often must be managed by group treatments. Ciprofloxacin, 500 to 750 mg per 75 L (20 gallons) for 6–8 h SID × 7 days, may be considered where large numbers of aquatic amphibians require treatment. It is helpful to provide gentle circulation with medicated baths to ensure that the drug is distributed equally throughout the enclosure, but do not use chemical filtration as this may remove the drug from the water. An option other than ciprofloxacin is to start the amphibians on a 16-h 100 mg/L oxytetracycline bath dissolved in an isotonic or near isotonic electrolyte solution (e.g., amphibian Ringer's solution) alternated with an 8-h 1 mg/ml gentamicin bath in 0.5% saline. If this is impractical, a 12-h bath of tetracycline hydrochloride (10 μg/ml in 0.5% saline) alternated with a 12-h bath of gentamicin sulfate (8 μg/ml in 0.5% saline) may be used. Supplemental oxygen is recommended. Fresh water may be used as a rinse solution between antibiotic baths. Metronidazole (50 mg/L as a 24-h bath) may be administered concurrently if anaerobic infections are suspected, but the amphibians should be closely monitored for neurologic signs which may suggest metronidazole intoxication. If the caretakers have been trained to handle chloramphenicol in an appropriate and safe manner, and the facility makes readily available sufficient protective equipment to eliminate employee contact with the drug, then a bath of 10 μg/ml chloramphenicol in 0.5% saline (Menard, 1984) is the drug of choice pending culture and sensitivity results (The authors advise caution when dispensing chloramphenicol to private clients given the health risk associated with human contact with the drug). Careful records should be maintained in such a facility as analysis of the isolates recovered and their antibiotic sensitivity patterns may suggest a different initial drug of choice. Obviously septic amphibians should be isolated from unaffected individuals, but all groups should receive treatments until the problem is under control.

24.6 ANTIPROTOZOAL AGENTS

Metronidazole may be of use in treating amphibians that are anorectic, thin, and show large numbers of flagellates in their feces. This is most commonly seen in recent arrivals that fail to adapt to their new environment. Doses for this purpose are 10 mg/kg PO q 24 h for 5–10 days concurrent with assisted feedings (e.g., Feline Clinical Care Liquid®). The goal of this therapy is not to eliminate the flagellates, but rather reduce them (and any harmful gastrointestinal bacteria) to acceptable levels. If the amphibian is anorectic, concomitant nutritional support is essential to establish normal gastrointestinal fauna.

In the event of suspected or confirmed amoebiasis, metronidazole is the drug of choice. A course of metronidazole also may be given to reduce the populations of gastrointestinal flagellates and ciliates. Metronidazole may be administered orally at 100–150 mg/kg q 14–21 days for suspected cases of amoebiasis. Confirmed cases (i.e., leukocytes were found in the fecal sample in addition to amoebic trophozoites) warrant more aggressive metronidazole therapy (i.e., 50 mg/kg PO SID for a minimum of 3 d) as well as concomitant antibiotic therapy aimed at aerobic bacteria. In small amphibians and aquatic amphibians, a 24-h bath in a metronidazole solution of 50 mg/L is generally effective. Metronidazole-impregnated food (5 gm/kg food) has been suggested for 3–4 daily feedings to treat protozoal infections (Crawshaw, 1992). In some cases of amoebiasis, higher dosages or a more prolonged treatment may be required for a cure. It is likely that some species may experience adverse effects at the higher dosages of metronidazole recommended for treating amoebiasis, so the dosage recommended for reducing flagellate populations (i.e., 10 mg/kg PO q 24 h for 5–10 d) may need to be used instead.

Paromomycin (50–75 mg/kg PO q 24 h) may be used if an amoebic infection does not respond to metronidazole, and also may be used to control levels of ciliated protozoans.

Various forms of sulfa drugs, alone or in combination

with trimethoprim, may prove useful to eliminate or decrease the shedding of coccidial organisms. At the National Aquarium in Baltimore there has been excellent clinical response to trimethoprim/sulfamethoxazole (Biocraft Laboratories, Elmwood Park, NJ) given at doses of 15 mg/kg PO q 24 h for up to 21 days, however coccidia were still apparent in the gastrointestinal tracts despite this extensive treatment. No treatment has proven effective against cryptosporidiosis, although oral hyperimmunized bovine colostrum has been effective in experimental trials in snakes infected with *Cryptosporidium serpents* (personal communication, M. Cranfield, 1997).

External protozoans can be reduced or eliminated in a variety of ways depending on species. Acriflavin, copper sulfate, distilled water, formalin, salt solutions (e.g., 1.0–2.5% saline or sea salts, 10–100% Whitaker-Wright solution, 40–100% Holtfreter's and modified Holtfreter's solutions), acidic solutions (Steinberg's solution), malachite green, methylene blue, potassium permanganate, and temperature elevation have all been described as useful in treating various protozoal infections. Recommended uses and dosages of antiprotozoal drugs may be found in Table 24.2.

Caution should be exercized when using any of these baths. Formalin should be used with extreme caution as it can cause mortality in some amphibians, especially in those with epithelial defects. The amphibian should be closely monitored for signs of distress, and if distressed should be removed immediately and thoroughly rinsed with well-oxygenated fresh water. Artificial slime may be added to the water to soothe skin irritated by the chemical agents, and it may be prudent afterwards to maintain the amphibian in an isotonic or near-isotonic electrolyte solution such as amphibian Ringer's solution. Copper may prove immunosuppressive, and should not be used when concomitant bacterial or fungal systemic infections are present or suspected.

24.7 ANTHELMINTICS

Percutaneous absorption of levamisole has been demonstrated in the firebelly toad, *Bombina orientalis* (Mombarg & Zwart, 1991). In this study, 50 µl of a 3.767 mg/ml levamisole solution was administered to frogs with an average body weight of 1.8 g (a dosage of 105 mg/kg) and left on the frog for 1 h before the frog was rinsed in fresh water. The total levamisole absorbed was 94 mg/kg, 90% of the applied dose.

Levamisole is useful in the treatment of cutaneous infestation of nematodes in aquatic amphibians. A levamisole bath (100–300 mg/L × 24 h) using aquaculture grade levamisole powder should be repeated every 7–14 days for a minimum of 3 treatments, and at least one additional treatment after the elimination of cutaneous lesions. This treatment can be used for an entire tank provided that chemical filtration with activated carbon is not used during the levamisole bath. Chemical filtration can be resumed the following day, and at least a 100% water change is recommended at that time. Fresh levamisole baths should be prepared daily if prolonged treatment (e.g., over 24 h) is pursued to eliminate resistant infections.

Levamisole baths have proven useful in eliminating nematode infections in terrestrial amphibians, and have been used at concentrations ranging from 10–100 mg/L as a continuous bath for 3–5 days. Levamisole has been used in enclosures with recirculating rain systems in attempts to eliminate resistant infections and to treat the substrate, but its efficacy has been difficult to evaluate.

Caution is warranted when using levamisole as the risk of toxicity increases with length of exposure or at higher concentrations. Flaccid paralysis has been noted in aquatic caecilians, *Typhlonectes* spp., and specimens of the Surinam toad, *Pipa pipa,* exposed to 200–300 mg/L of levamisole for more than 24 h. In some specimens of the Rio Cauca caecilian, *Typhlonectes natans,* tolerance for levamisole treatments decreased with each subsequent treatment, so levamisole baths are limited to 50–100 mg/L for 1–8 h q 7 days in this species.

If an amphibian is paralyzed by levamisole treatments it may drown. Any amphibian undergoing treatment with levamisole should be monitored regularly, typically every 1–8 h. No specific treatment is indicated for levamisole toxicity other than to maintain respiration. A common cause of levamisole intoxication is failure to remove all the levamisole from a system after treatment; chemical filtration with activated carbon and a complete water change will minimize this risk, but sometimes two or more water changes are needed to flush the levamisole out of the system. Modified Nessler's reagent (a combination of potassium iodide, mercuric chloride, and potassium hydroxide), often used as the ammonia test agent in water quality test kits, precipitates with levamisole. White flocculent material will form even at very low levamisole concentrations (less than 10 mg/L levamisole), and may help confirm a case of levamisole toxicosis.

Injectable grade levamisole may be given as a sole or concomitant agent in the elimination of endoparasitic nematodes including *Rhabdias* spp. Topical administration of 8–10 mg/kg is recommended for small amphibians (e.g., *Mantella* spp.), and the oral, subcutaneous or intracoelomic route is recommended for larger specimens. Intratracheal or intrapneumonic injections may be used for confirmed cases of lungworm (e.g., *Rhabdias* spp.). Nebulization may work for some amphibians, but this has proved immediately lethal to some small anurans (personal communication, C. Tabaka, 1998). The exact cause of the nebulization deaths is unknown, but it is difficult to gauge the dosage using this route and the nebulized mist is often warmer than surrounding air. Levamisole does appear to be irritating to some individual amphibians by any route, so the patient should be observed for several minutes following administration. If the topical route appears irritating, it should be rinsed with water and the aquaculture grade levamisole used instead.

Avermectins have proved useful in managing nematodiasis in amphibians, as well as acariasis and tick infestation. Ivermectin has been the subject of at least one study in anurans (Letcher & Glade, 1992). Up to 20 mg/kg was used topically without ill effect in the northern leopard frog, *Rana pipiens*, (Letcher & Glade, 1992); topical use of injectable grade ivermectin is recommended at a dosage between 0.2–2.0 mg/kg, and the dilution made if necessary with propylene glycol or water. Additives in the propylene glycol may cause irritation of the amphibian. Color changes, flaccid paralysis and death have occurred at dosages approaching 0.2 mg/kg in some frogs (personal communication, G. Crawshaw, 1997) suggesting species-specific reactions. Supportive care in the form of maintenance in electrolyte solutions and supplemental oxygen is suggested should this occur. The veterinarian is cautioned to advise the client of potential adverse affects prior to use of this drug in any amphibian.

Injectable ivermectin may be used for a bath to reduce or eliminate nematode infections. Many amphibians tolerate an ivermectin bath (10 mg/L) for 60 min q 7 d, and this regimen has proven effective in managing even *Rhabdias* spp. infections. In the event of a resistant infection, the concentration of the bath may be increased (e.g., 20 mg/L) or the length of a bath may be extended beyond 60 min for resistant infections. The risk of ivermectin toxicosis is increased at higher concentrations or longer exposure times.

Injectable ivermectin can be administered at a dose of 0.2 mg/kg IM without ill effect in most amphibians. One study documented its efficaciousness in clearing nematodes from the northern leopard frog, *Rana pipiens* (Letcher & Glade, 1992). Some amphibians may be able to tolerate higher dosages, up to 0.4 mg/kg, but this is not recommended unless the clinician is confident of the tolerance of a particular species for this higher dose and that no other anthelmintic modalities have eliminated the parasite. If two treatments of ivermectin at 0.2 mg/kg PO q 14 days apart fail to reduce the number of ova detected in the feces, consider extending the treatment a total of 12 treatments. If this fails, consider trying ivermectin at 0.4 mg/kg PO q 14 days or switch to a different anthelmintic.

Fenbendazole is effective in reducing or eliminating many nematode infections in amphibians. Fenbendazole (100 mg/kg PO q 7–14 d) is used often for prophylaxis during quarantine or as therapy for confirmed gastrointestinal nematodiasis in amphibians. Granular fenbendazole may be used to dust insects for administration to small amphibians, but this modality renders it impractical to quantify the amount of drug ingested by an amphibian. No adverse reactions have been noted at this dosage. In resistant cases, fenbendazole may be administered at a lower dose on a more frequent basis to effect a cure (e.g., 50 mg/kg PO q 24 h for 3–5 days, repeated every 2–3 weeks).

Praziquantel (8–24 mg/kg PO, SQ, ICe, or topically q 7–21 d) has been used with variable success to treat trematode and cestode infections in amphibians. Local reactions to praziquantel injections have been noted in aquatic caecialians, *Typhlonectes* spp. (personal communication, G. Crawshaw, 1997). If the appropriate form is available from a chemical supply house, praziquantel can also be used as a bath (10 mg/L for 3 h). It appears effective against adult trematodes and cestodes, but immature and encysted forms are resistant and may require surgical removal. Monogenic trematodes may be eliminated from the bladder via infusion of praziquantel. A reported treatment of monogenic trematodes in amphibians was 0.5–1.0% formalin for an unspecified length of time (Raphael, 1993). Brief exposure is advised if this is attempted. Since formalin is toxic to many amphibians, it should be used only if praziquantel is not available and the parasite appears to be causing distress to its amphibian host.

Recommended uses and dosages for anthelmintics are included in Table 24.2.

With any diagnosis of helminth infestation, and especially with certain types of nematodes (e.g. *Rhabdias* spp.), attention to hygiene is a very important component of therapy. The original enclosure should be broken down and all material to be reused should be cleaned and sterilized, preferably by heat treatment as many ova are resistant to standard disinfectants. Plants and porous organic material should not be reused as they may provide refugia for nematode ova and larvae. Placing organic material in levamisole or ivermectin baths may reduce its level of contamination, but these baths are unlikely to render plants, wood and other organic objects completely safe for reuse. (Unfortunately, since *Rhabdias* spp. may have a free-living (nonparasitic) generation in soil, all amphibians are at risk of infection if live plants are used in their enclosures.) The amphibian should be moved to a quarantine-style tank with minimal furnishings, and all fecal matter should be removed immediately. Repeated sterilization of the enclosure should follow each anthelmintic treatment. Provision of a thermal mosaic with temperatures above and below the preferred body temperature is recommended.

24.8 ELIMINATING OTHER PARASITES

For some parasites (e.g., subcutaneous leeches, subcutaneous fly larvae or bots) surgical removal is the recommended treatment modality (Raphael, 1993; Vogelnest, 1994; Wright, 1996). Removal of external leeches may be facilitated by immersing the leech-bearing amphibian in hypertonic solutions (e.g., 25 g salt/L, 10–100% Whitaker-Wright solution). Larvae of the toadfly, *Bufolucilla* spp., may infest the nasal passage of anurans. Parenteral levamisole in conjunction with oronasal flushes of levamisole (100 mg/L) may have some impact on small larvae. Ivermectin flushes (10 mg/L) also may paralyze fly larvae and facilitate their removal. Short-term exposure to volatile organophosphate products (e.g., dichlorvos) may kill larvae, but toxicity of the patient is an obvious concern. No matter what medical treatment is used, removal of the dead or paralyzed parasites is essential as decomposition of fly larvae or leeches in situ may kill an amphibian.

Trombiculid mites may be treated with parenteral ivermectin or high dose topical ivermectin (i.e., 2 mg/kg, possibly up to 20 mg/kg). A weekly 60-min bath in a dilute ivermectin solution (10 mg ivermectin in one liter of water) may be effective if high dose topical ivermectin fails. It may take 12 treatments or more to eliminate mites. Hypertonic salt (electrolyte) solutions may have some effect, but may not be as well tolerated by the amphibian as the ivermectin baths.

Aquatic amphibians may occasionally be found with copepod infestation. Hypertonic salt baths (25 g/L NaCl, 10–100% Whitaker-Wright solution) or dilute ivermectin baths (10 mg/L × 60 min q 7 d) are the suggested treatment.

24.9 MAINTAINING THE ELECTROLYTE BALANCE OF THE ILL AMPHIBIAN

The importance of maintaining the electrolyte balance of ill amphibians cannot be overstated, as mentioned in Section 24.3, Antibacterial Agents. This importance was well demonstrated when the the use of antibiotics in saline baths markedly increased the survival rates of laboratory frogs over treatment with antibiotics alone (Menard, 1984). A healthy amphibian typically maintains a plasma osmolality in excess of 200 mOsm, and usually at least 250 mOsm (Boutilier et al., 1992). In contrast, "fresh" water has an osmolality 20–40 mOsm/kg H_2O, and distilled water has an osmolality of 0 mOsm/kg H_2O. Aquatic and semiaquatic amphibians are expending considerable effort to conserve their electrolytes in the freshwater medium they inhabit; they are at risk of developing fatal electrolyte imbalances when their skin, gills, or kidneys are damaged, as occurs with many infectious diseases. Aquatic amphibians generally present with a fluid overload due to the influx of water into their systems occurring at a faster rate than its excretion, and the loss of their electrolytes to the environment through damaged epithelial surfaces. Terrestrial amphibians may present with a fluid overload, as happens with aquatic amphibians, if they have ready access to shallow water or a moist environment. Conversely, terrestrial amphibians may be undergoing dehydration stress, losing both water and electrolytes, if they are kept under drier conditions. In addition to the consequences of damaged epithelia on maintaining fluid and electrolyte balance, diarrhea or emesis may further alter the fluid and electrolyte balance.

Various electrolyte baths may be used at differing concentrations to maintain or treat ill amphibians (Tables 24.3, 24.4, 24.5, 24.6A, B, 24.7, 24.8). Holtfreter's and Steinberg's solutions were developed to increase the survival of surgically manipulated axolotl embryos; permutations of the original formulas were developed to increase the chances of success for specific surgical procedures. For example, calcium-free solutions may promote healing in certain tissue-transplant surgeries while extra calcium and magnesium may aid healing with other surgeries (Asashima et al., 1989). Maruska (1994) reports using different solutions to increase the osmolality of the water for aquatic amphibians undergoing antibiotic treatment to offset the electrolyte losses experienced by these amphibians. Maruska (1994) reports increased survival when aquatic amphibians are immediately placed in 10–20% amphibian Ringer's solution rather than left in fresh water. Electrolyte solutions should be used routinely to complement antibiotic and antifungal agents, and are an essential therapy whenever there are obvious skin or gill lesions or suspected renal disease.

Since ill aquatic amphibians are typically at risk of fluid overload, they should be maintained in an electrolyte solution rather than "fresh" water. In many cases, it is appropriate to use near-isotonic or isotonic electrolyte solutions during treatment for an infectious disease. A continuous bath of 10–100% amphibian Ringer's solution is an excellent first choice for an ill aquatic amphibian. If the amphibian is not showing signs of fluid overload, other more hypotonic solutions may be used, such as 100% Holtfreter's or modified Holtfreter's solution, 5% Whitaker-Wright solution, or 0.5–0.7% saline (5–7 g NaCl/L water). Hypertonic amphibian Ringer's solution may be used as a continuous bath to treat mild cases of fluid overload (as evidenced by hydrocoelom or edema) (see Table 24.6B). Whitaker-Wright solution may be used at 10% or higher concentrations to combat serious fluid overload. Hypertonic saline, 0.8–2.5%, may be used if the other solutions are not available. Hypertonic solutions should not be used for more than 4 h without reassessment of the patient. Once the hydrocoelom or subcutaneous edema shows a substantial reduction in volume, a lower osmolality (isotonic or hypotonic) electrolyte solution can be used for maintenance of the aquatic amphibian.

Terrestrial amphibians should have access to a pool of fresh water and a pool containing either full strength amphibian Ringer's solution, 5–7.5% Whitaker-Wright solution, 100% Holtfreter's solution or modified Holtfreter's solution, or 0.5–0.8% saline during treatment for an infectious disease. In the event of serious fluid overload, the terrestrial amphibian should be placed into a continuous shallow bath of higher osmolality (hypertonic) solutions. As with aquatic amphibians, baths in hypertonic solutions should not be used for more than 4 h without reassessment of the patient.

Many electrolyte solutions, such as 100% Steinberg's solution, 100% Holtfreter's solution, hypertonic amphibian Ringer's solution, hypertonic saline, or hypertonic Whitaker-Wright solution, may be effective against pathogens such as external protozoa in and of themselves in addition to their therapeutic effects on the amphibian's fluid balance. However, the osmolality is not the sole factor determining a solution's effectiveness. A solution's effectiveness depends in part on a protozoa's sensitivity to the balance of electrolytes and the pH of the solution.

In most cases, diluted or full strength amphibian Ringer's solution is the first choice as the maintenance fluid for ill amphibians, even those with mild hydrocoelom or edema. Hypertonic solutions should be used if the hydrocoelom or subcutaneous edema is unchanged or increasing within 24 h of treatment or if the fluid overload is life-threatening.

It is worth reemphasizing that it is important to also provide access to "regular" water on a daily basis for terrestrial amphibians to avoid iatrogenic dehydration of the patient.

Ideally the clinic should carry stocks of the dry chemicals to create the baths which are more tailored to the amphibian physiology. Compounding pharmacies may produce stock formulas of various amphibian electrolyte solutions. The external use of the appropriate fluid, whether it is artifical pondwater, reconstituted soft water, amphibian Ringer's solution, Whitaker-Wright solution, Holtfreter's solutions, or saline solution, is a vital part of therapy. The use of artificial slime (e.g., Shield-X®, Polyaqua®) may help stabilize the protective mucous coat of the skin and reduce electrolyte loss.

Intracoelomic administration of balanced electrolyte solutions may be administered to the depressed and dehydrated amphibian, or as concomitant therapy with antibiotics, or following blood loss (Table 24.9). The use of lactated Ringer's solution as fluid therapy in reptiles has been questioned (Prezant & Jarchow, 1997), and many of the same concerns voiced for reptiles are appropriate for intracoelomic, intravenous, or subcutaneous fluid therapy in amphibians. Lactated Ringer's solution (273 mOsm/kg H_2O) is hypertonic for amphibians. Lactic acid is a by-product of muscle metabolism in amphibians, and is the main chemical that elicits fatigue in the muscles of amphibians, as well as mammals, birds and reptiles. Amphibian clearance of lactic acid is slow, and can take hours to days to be eliminated following a brief bout of vigorous activity (Gatten et al., 1992). Lactated Ringer's solution contains sodium lactate as a buffer, and this may contribute to the lactic acid load of an amphibian. Furthermore, standard nonlactate electrolyte solutions for intravenous use (e.g., Plasmalyte-A, Plasmalyte-148, Baxter Pharmaceuticals) are hypertonic for amphibians, and are not balanced for restoring either their extracellular or intracellular fluid compartments. However, a recipe consisting of one or two parts balanced electrolyte intravenous solution added to one part 5% dextrose provides a more suitable intracoelomically administered electrolyte solution for amphibians that are dehydrated. The choice of the fluid used is predicated on the amphibian's suspected state of dehydration or confirmed plasma osmolality. Generally, the more dehydrated an amphibian (the higher the plasma osmolality), the more water is needed to restore fluid balance. Consequently, the fluid used in a severely dehydrated amphibian should have a lower ratio of electrolyte solution to dextrose (i.e., 1:1 versus 2:1) than the fluid used in a well hydrated amphibian.

There are few circumstances where the use of intracoelomic, intravenous, or subcutaneous fluid therapy is indicated over topical (bath) therapy. Life-threatening dehydration, paralytic conditions or extreme weakness (since these conditions put the amphibian at risk of drowning), thermal trauma, and blood loss are the main disorders in amphibians that call for systemic fluid therapy.

On a final note, the preservatives in the readily available intravenous electrolyte solutions might prove irritating to some amphibians.

24.10 MISCELLANEOUS DRUGS AND PRODUCTS USED IN AMPHIBIANS

A variety of other products have been used in the supportive care and specific treatment of disease in amphibians, ranging from vitamin supplements to analgesics such as morphine (Stevens & Kirkendall, 1993) (see Table 24.9).

Table 24.1. Antibacterial and antifungal agents used in amphibians.

Drug	Dosage	Comments
Acriflavin	500 mg/L as a 30-min bath q 24 h	
Acriflavin-methylene blue	0.5 ml of stock solution of 0.045% acriflavin and 0.0075% methylene blue added to 1 liter of modified Holtfreter's solution. Use as 24-h bath for 2–5 days	Maruska, 1994
Amikacin	5 mg/kg q 48 h IM × 5–14 Tx	Pharmacokinetic data from Letcher & Papich, 1994
Amikacin	5 mg/kg SQ, IM, ICe q 24–48 h	Raphael, 1993
Amphotericin-B	1 mg/kg ICe q 24 hrs × 14–28 Tx	
Benzalkonium chloride	2 mg/L as a 60-min bath q 24 h	Saprolegniasis
Benzalkonium chloride	0.25 mg/L bath for 72 h	Saprolegniasis. Crawshaw, 1992
Benzalkonium chloride	1:4,000,000 as a continuous soak, change water 3 × week	Saprolegniasis. Raphael, 1993
Carbenicillin	200 mg/kg SQ, IM, ICe q 24 h	Crawshaw, 1992
Ceftazadime	20 mg/kg IM q 48–72 h	
Chloramphenicol	50 mg/kg SQ, IM or ICe q 24 h	Crawshaw, 1992
Chloramphenicol	20 mg/L bath	Crawshaw, 1992
Chloramphenicol	10 µg/ml in 0.5% or 0.15% saline as 24-h bath made fresh daily	Menard, 1984
Chlorinated water	not to exceed 5 ppm as a bath for up to 2 h daily	
Ciprofloxacin	10 mg/kg PO q 24 to 48 h × 7 Tx minimum	
Ciprofloxacin	500–750mg /75 liters (500–750 mg/20 gallons) as a 6–8-h bath q 24 h for 7 days	
Copper sulfate	500 mg/L 2 min q 24 h × 5 days, then q 7 days until healed	Saprolegniasis
Doxycycline	10–50 mg/kg PO q 24 h	
Enrofloxacin	5–10 mg/kg IM q 24 h × 7 Tx minimum	Pharmacokinetic data from Letcher & Papich, 1994
Enrofloxacin	5–10 mg/kg SQ, ICe, TO, or PO q 24 h × 7 Tx minimum	Distribution via these routes undocumented
Fluconazole	60 mg/kg PO q 24 h × 7 days	
Furazone Green	0.65 g/38 L (0.65 g/10 gal)	Proprietary combination of methylene blue, furazolidone, and monofuracin
Gentamicin (cold-water aquatic salamanders)	2.5 mg/kg IM q 72 h @ 3°C (37°F)	Pharmacokinetic data from Stoskopf et al, 1987
Gentamicin (axolotl, *Ambystoma mexicanum*, and aquatic amphibians)	1.8 mg q 48 h for 140-g adult (i.e., 13 mg/kg)	Maruska, 1994

Table 24.1. Antibacterial and antifungal agents used in amphibians. *(Continued)*

Drug	Dosage	Comments
Gentamicin (anuran)	3 mg/kg IM q 24 h at 22.2°C (72°F)	Pharmacokinetic data from Teare et al, 1991
Gentamicin	8 μg/ml in 0.5% or 0.15% saline as 24-h bath × 5 days made fresh daily	Menard, 1984
Gentamicin	1 mg/ml solution as an 8-h bath q 24-48 h	Modified from Riveiere et al, 1979 based on pharmacokinetic data from Teare et al, 1991
Isoniazid	12.5 mg/L as a 24-h bath	Fox, 1980
Itraconazole	2–10 mg/kg PO q 24 h × 14–28 days dissolve in weakly acidic solution overnight (see text) or use liquid form (Sporanox 10 mg/ml, Janssen Pharmaceutica, Titusville, NJ) 0.01% in 0.6% saline as a soak 5 min daily for 11 days	Nichols & Lamirande, 2000
Ketoconazole	10 mg/kg PO q 24 h	Crawshaw, 1992
Ketoconazole	10–20 mg/kg PO q 24 h × 14–28 days	Wright, 1996
Malachite green	0.2 mg/L as a bath for 1 h daily	Saprolegniasis. Wright, 1996
Malachite green	67 mg/L as a 15-sec dip q 24 h × 2–3 days	Saprolegniasis. Longer exposure may cause exfoliation.
Methylene blue	50 mg/ml as a 10-sec dip	Saprolegniasis. Wright, 1996. Tadpoles should not exceed 2 mg/ml.
Methylene blue	4 mg/L as a continuous bath	Saprolegniasis. Crawshaw, 1992
Methylene blue	3 mg/L as a continuous bath for up to 5 days	Saprolegniasis. Wright, 1996. Tadpoles should not exceed 2 mg/ml.
Methylene blue	2 mg/L as a continuous bath	Saprolegniasis. Raphael, 1993
Methylene blue-acriflavin	0.5 ml of stock solution of 0.0075% methylene blue and 0.045% acriflavin added to 1 liter of modified Holtfreter's solution Use as 24-h bath for 2–5 days	Maruska, 1994
Metronidazole	10 mg/kg PO q 24 h for 5 to 10 days	Chronic diarrhea. Poynton and Whitaker, 1994. Increase dose by 20% if used topically.
Metronidazole	50 mg/kg PO q 24 h × 3 days	For anaerobic infections and confirmed amoebic infections. Increase dose by 20% if used topically.
Metronidazole	50 mg/L bath for up to 24 h	For anaerobic infections
Miconazole	5 mg/kg ICe, to q 24 h × 14–28 days	Wright, 1996
Nalidixic acid	10 mg/L bath to effect	Crawshaw, 1992
Nalidixic acid	10 μg/ml in 0.5% or 0.15% saline as 24-h bath made fresh daily	Menard, 1984
Nitrofurantoin	50 μg/ml in 0.5% or 0.15% saline as 24-h bath made fresh daily	Menard, 1984

Table 24.1. Antibacterial and antifungal agents used in amphibians. *(Continued)*

Drug	Dosage	Comments
Nitrofurazone	10–20 mg/L as 24-h bath made fresh daily	Crawshaw, 1992
Nitrofurazone	100 mg/L as a 24-h bath made fresh daily for up to 2 days	May cause diarrhea. Maruska, 1994
Oxytetracycline	50–100 mg/kg IM q 48 h	Pharmacokinetic data from Letcher & Papich, 1994
Oxytetracycline	25 mg/kg SQ, IM q 24 h	Crawshaw, 1992
Oxytetracycline	50 mg/kg PO q 24 h	Wright, 1996
Oxytetracycline	50 mg PO q 12 h	Crawshaw, 1992
Oxytetracycline	1 g/kg diet for 7 days	Presumably for tadpoles and larvae. Crawshaw, 1992
Oxytetracycline	100 mg/L as a bath 1 h daily	Wright, 1996
Oxytetracycline	125 mg/L as a 24-h bath made fresh q 12–24 h for up to 3 days	Maruska, 1994
Penicillin (axolotl *Ambystoma mexicanum*)	25,000 iu 140-g adult (combination of benzathine penicillin G 150,000 iu/ml and procaine penicillin G 150,000 iu/ml)	Maruska, 1994
Piperacillin	100 mg/kg IM or SQ q 24 h	Wright, 1996
Potassium permanganate	200 mg/L as a 5-minute bath daily	Saprolegniasis. Raphael, 1993
Potassium permanganate	1 g/100 ml distilled water as topical solution. Place animal in 50% or 100 % modified Holtfreter's solution afterward. Repeat q 48–72 h	Saprolegniasis. Maruska, 1994
Rifampin	25 mg/L as a 24 h bath	Fox, 1980
Sea salts	10–25 g/L as a bath for 5–30 min	Saprolegniasis. Wright, 1996
Sodium chloride	4–6 g/L as a bath for 72 h	Crawshaw, 1992
Sodium chloride	10–25 g/L as a bath for 5–30 min	Saprolegniasis. Wright, 1996. Raphael, 1993 does not recommend 25 g/L for more than 10 min.
Sodium chlorite ($NaOCl_2$)	20 mg/L as a 6–8-h bath (sodium chlorite, Alfa Aesur, Ward Hill, MA)	External fungal infections of tadpoles. Personal communication, M. Greenwell, 1997
Sulfadiazine	132 mg/kg q 24 h	No route specified. Raphael, 1993
Sulfamethazine	1 g/L bath made fresh daily	Crawshaw, 1992
Temperature elevation	elevate enclosure temperature to 25°C (77°F)	*Dermocystidium, Dermosporidium.* In temperate amphibians. Raphael, 1993
Tetracycline	50 mg/kg PO q 12 h	Raphael, 1993
Tetracycline	10 µg/ml in 0.5% saline as 24-h bath made fresh daily	Menard, 1984

Table 24.1. Antibacterial and antifungal agents used in amphibians. *(Continued)*

Drug	Dosage	Comments
Trimethoprim/ sulfamethoxazole	15 mg/kg PO q 24 h for up to 21 days	Biocraft Laboratories, Elmwood Park, NJ. For chronic diarrhea.
Trimethoprim/ sulfamethoxazole	20 μg/ml and 80 μg/ml respectively in 0.5% or 0.15% saline as 24-h bath made fresh daily	Menard, 1984
Trimethoprim/sulfa (unspecified form)	3 mg/kg SQ, PO q 24 h	Crawshaw, 1992
Trimethoprim/sulfadiazine	15–20 mg/kg IM q 48 h × 5–7 Tx	Maruska, 1994

Table 24.2. Antiparasitic agents used in amphibians.

Drug	Dosage	Comments
Acriflavin	0.025% as 24-h bath for 5 days	Presumably for external protozoans. Raphael, 1993
Copper sulfate	0.0001 mg/L as a continuous bath to effect	External protozoans. May be toxic to some species. Wright, 1996
Copper sulfate	500 mg/L as a 2-min dip q 24 h to effect	External protozoans: *Charcesium, Vorticella, Oodinium, Trichodina*. May be toxic to some species. Raphael, 1993; Crawshaw, 1992
Distilled water	2–3-h bath	External protozoa: *Charcesium, Vorticella, Oodinium, Trichodina*. Raphael, 1993
Fenbendazole	100 mg/kg PO q 10 days	Nematodes. Poynton and Whitaker, 1994
Fenbendazole	100 mg/kg PO q 14–21 days	Nematodes. Wright, 1996
Fenbendazole	100 mg/kg PO q 10–14 days	Nematodes. Maruska, 1994
Fenbendazole	50 mg/kg PO SID × 3–5 days	For resistant nematode infections
Fenbendazole	10 mg/kg PO once	Nematodes. Raphael, 1993
Formalin 10%	1.5 ml/L dip for 10 min q 48 h to effect	External protozoans. Avoid using in amphibians with ulcerated skin lesions and provide adequate oxygenation. Crawshaw, 1992. MAY BE TOXIC!
Formalin 0.5–1.0%	unspecified	Monogenic trematodes: *Polystoma, Gyrodactylus*. Raphael, 1993. MAY BE TOXIC!
Ivermectin	2 mg/kg cutaneously	Nematodes and arthropods. From efficacy trials of Letcher & Glade, 1992. Ivermectin was not toxic at levels of 20.0 mg/kg cutaneously in the leopard frog, *Rana pipiens*.
Ivermectin	0.2–0.4 mg/kg IM or PO q 14 days	Nematodes and arthropods. From efficacy trials of Letcher & Glade, 1992.
Ivermectin	0.2–0.4 mg/kg PO	Nematodes and arthropods. Wright, 1996

Table 24.2. Antiparasitic agents used in amphibians. *(Continued)*

Drug	Dosage	Comments
Levamisole	8–10 mg/kg ICe or topically q 14–21 days	Nematodes. Wright, 1996. Dosages as high as 24 mg/kg ICe have been used without ill effect in some species.
Levamisole	50–100 mg/L as a 1–8-h bath q 7 days	Lower dose used for sensitive species such as *Typhlonectes natans*
Levamisole	10 mg/kg IM q 14 days	Nematodes. Raphael, 1993
Levamisole	100–300 mg/L as a 24-h bath q 7–14 days for a minimum of 3 treatments	Nematodes.
Levamisole	100–300 mg/L as a bath for 72 h made fresh daily q 14–21 days for a minimum of 3 treatments.	Useful for resistant infections of nematodes. Can be used in rain systems for arboreal amphibians.
Malachite green	0.15 mg/L bath 1 h/day to effect	External protozoans. Raphael, 1993
Mebendazole	20 mg/kg PO q 14 days	Nematodes. Raphael, 1993
Methylene blue	2 mg/L as a continuous bath	External protozoans. Raphael, 1993
Metronidazole	10 mg/kg PO q 24 h for 5–10 days	Flagellates. Poynton and Whitaker, 1994
Metronidazole	100–150 mg/kg PO q 14–21 days	For suspected amoebiasis and low levels of flagellates. Wright, 1996
Metronidazole	50 mg/kg PO q 24 h × 3–5 days	For confirmed amoebiasis and high levels of flagellates. Wright, 1996
Metronidazole	10 mg/kg PO once	For amoebiasis and flagellates. Maruska, 1994
Metronidazole	5 gm/kg food for 3–4 feedings	Presumably for tadpoles and larvae. Crawshaw, 1992
Metronidazole	50 mg/L bath for up to 24 h	For aquatic amphibians. Wright, 1996
Modified Holtfreter's solution	100% solution as 24-h bath for 3–5 days	External protozoa: *Vorticella*. Cover container to prevent evaporation. Maruska, 1994
Paramomycin	50–75 mg/kg PO q 24 h	Amoebiasis. Wright, 1996
Potassium permanganate	7 mg/L up to 5 min q 24 h to effect	External protozoans. Raphael, 1993
Praziquantel	8–24 mg/kg PO, SQ, ICe, or cutaneously q 7–21 days	Trematodes and cestodes. Wright, 1996
Praziquantel	10 mg/L bath for up to 3 h q 7–21 days	Trematodes and cestodes. Wright, 1996
Quinine sulfate	30 mg/L bath for up to 1 h	Hemoprotozoans. Wright, 1996
Sea salts	10–25 g/L as a bath for 5–30 min	External parasites. Wright, 1996
Sodium chloride	10–25 g/L as a bath for 5–30 min	External parasites. Wright, 1996. Note that Crawshaw, 1992, does not recommend more than 10 min when using for 25 g/L.
Sodium chloride	4–6 g/L as a 24-h bath for up to 72 h	External parasites. Crawshaw, 1992
Sodium chloride	6 g/L as a 24 h bath for 3–5 days	External protozoa: *Charcesium, Vorticella, Oodinium, richodina*. Raphael, 1993
Sodium hydroxide	10 ggt of 0.1 M NaOH/L as a bath for 10 min	External protozoans. Maruska, 1994

Table 24.2. Antiparasitic agents used in amphibians. *(Continued)*

Drug	Dosage	Comments
Steinberg's solution	100% as a 24-h bath for 3–5 days	External protozoa: *Vorticella*. Cover container to prevent evaporation. Maruska, 1994
Sulfadiazine	132 mg/kg q 24 h. No route specified	Potentially useful for coccidia
Sulfamethazine	1 g/L bath made fresh daily	Potentially useful for coccidia
Thiabendazole	50–100 mg/kg PO q 2 weeks	Cutaneous nematodes. Cosgrove & Jared, 1977
Trimethoprim/ sulfamethoxazole	15 mg/kg PO q 24 h for 5–10 days	Chronic diarrhea. May not eliminate coccidia.
Trimethoprim/ sulfamethoxazole	20 µg/ml and 80 µg/ml respectively in 0.5% or 0.15% saline as 24-h bath made fresh daily	Probably not useful for coccidia
Trimethoprim/sulfa (unspecified form)	3 mg/kg PO q 24 h	Probably not useful for coccidia. Crawshaw, 1992
Temperature elevation	elevate temperature in enclosure to 25°C (77°F)	*Dermocystidium, Dermosporidium.* In temperate amphibians. Raphael, 1993

Table 24.3. Two formulas for the production of water suitable for amphibian husbandry.

Artificial pond water (Mattison, 1982).
Add 20 ml of solution A and 20 ml solution B to 5 L distilled water to make artificial pond water. Note: This formula has been associated with spindly leg development in the dyeing poison frog, *Dendrobates tinctorius*, at the Philadelphia Zoo perhaps due to insufficient levels of magnesium or potassium.

STOCK SOLUTION A	STOCK SOLUTION B
175 g NaCl 35 g $CaCl_2$ 2 L water (distilled) Mix solution thoroughly to ensure that all crystals are dissolved. Agitate thoroughly before use. Keep in a closed container to reduce evaporation.	5 g $NaHCO_3$ 2 L distilled water Mix solution thoroughly to ensure that all crystals are dissolved. Agitate thoroughly before use. Keep in a closed container to reduce evaporation.

Reconstituted soft water (Stephens, 1975).
This is a standard water formula used to minimize water quality effects on acute toxicity tests for fish and amphibians.

48 mg $NaHCO_3$ 30 mg $CaSO_4 \cdot 2H_2O$ 30 mg $MgSO_4$ 2 mg KCl 1 L H_2O	Mix solution thoroughly to ensure that all crystals are dissolved. Agitate thoroughly before use to ensure oxygenation. Final pH should range from 7.2–7.6. Keep in a closed container to reduce evaporation.

Table 24.4. Holtfreter's and modified Holtfreter's solutions (Asashima et al., 1989).

Holtfreter's solution

NaCl, 3.46 g
KCl, 0.05 g
$CaCl_2$, 0.1 g
$NaHCO_3$, 0.2 g (buffer) in 1 liter of distilled water
pH adjusted to 7.4

    Holtfreter's solution is adjusted to pH 7.7 for the axolotl (*Ambystoma mexicanum*) by some investigators. A 40–50% solution is used for maintaining adult axolotls and a 20–25% solution is used for maintaining embryos.

Modified Holtfreter's solution

Add 0.2 g $MgSO_4 \cdot 7H_2O$ to the recipe.

40% modified Holtfreter's, Indiana Univesrity Axolotl Colony Formula (personal communication, S. Duhon, 1998)

1 teaspoon KCl
2.5 teaspoons $CaCl_2$
2 tablespoons $MgSO_4 \cdot 7H_2O$
240 cubic centimeters (dry volume) NaCl
44 gal "purified" water

Table 24.6A. Amphibian Ringer's solution (Humason, 1967 as cited in Maruska, 1994).

Distilled Water	1 Liter	1 Gallon
NaCl	6.6 g	25 g
KCl	0.15 g	0.57 g
$CaCl_2$	0.15 g	0.57 g
$NaHCO_3$	0.2 g	0.76 g

Mix solution thoroughly to ensure that all crystals are dissolved. Agitate thoroughly before use. Keep in a closed container to reduce evaporation.

Table 24.6B. 110% Hypertonic amphibian Ringer's solution.

Distilled Water	1 Liter	1 Gallon
NaCl	7.3 g	27.6 g
KCl	0.17 g	0.64 g
$CaCl_2$	0.17 g	0.64 g
$NaHCO_3$	0.22 g	0.83 g

Mix solution thoroughly to ensure that all crystals are dissolved. Agitate thoroughly before use. Keep in a closed container to reduce evaporation.

Table 24.5. Steinberg's solutions.

Steinberg's solution was developed for surgical manipulation and initial postoperative culturing of axolotl embryos. It is typically used at full strength preoperatively and for up to 10 h postoperatively. 20% Steinberg's solution with antibiotics is used for culturing healed embryos.

Steinberg's solution (Asashima et al., 1989)

NaCl, 3.4 g
KCl, 0.05 g
$Ca(NO_3)_2 \cdot 4H_2O$, 0.08 g or $CaCl_2$, 0.05 g
$MgSO_4 \cdot 7H_2O$, 0.205 g
Tris, 0.56 g
1 liter distilled water
HCl to pH 7.4

    An alternative formula substitutes HEPES buffer 1.10 g for Tris 0.56 g. NaOH is used to adjust pH to 7.4
    500 mg kanamycin sulfate may be added per liter. This antibiotic is often chosen since it can be autoclaved and retain its activity. Other antibiotics are used in combination (400 mg sodium penicillin-G, 400 mg streptomycin sulfate and 25 mg gentamicin sulfate) but these antibiotics are heat-sensitive and the solution must be filtered for sterilization. Some researchers perform transplants in the above solution but do not add calcium-containing compounds.

Calcium and magnesium-enriched Steinberg's solution

Substitute 0.16 g $Ca(NO_3)_2 \cdot 4H_2O$ and 0.4 g $MgSO_4 \cdot 7H_2O$ for the amounts listed above.

Steinberg's solution (Brothers, 1977)

20 ml 17.0% NaCl
10 ml 0.5% KCl
10 ml 0.8% $Ca(NO_3)_2 \cdot 4H_2O$
10 ml 2.05% $MgSO_4 \cdot 7H_2O$
4 ml 1 N HCl
560 mg Tris buffer (Trizma Base, reagent grade)
946 ml distilled water

Mix solution thoroughly to ensure that all crystals are dissolved. Agitate thoroughly before use. Keep in a closed container to reduce evaporation.

Table 24.7. Whitaker-Wright solution.

Distilled Water	1 Liter	1 Gallon
NaCl	113.0 g	428.0 g
$MgSO_4 \cdot 7H_2O$	8.6 g	32.6 g
$CaCl_2$	4.2 g	15.9 g
KCl	1.7 g	6.4 g

Dissolve crystals thoroughly in distilled water. Keep container covered to prevent evaporation. Add Trizma (7.4) base, fish grade, as needed to stabilize pH of solution between 7.0–7.3. This is 100% stock solution from which serial dilutions may be made. For example, 5% Whitaker-Wright solution may be made by adding 5 ml stock solution to 95 ml distilled water.

Table 24.8. Measured osmolality and pH of various solutions used in managing amphibians. All measurements performed in the Water Quality Laboratory of the National Aquarium in Baltimore. Note that calculated osmolality may vary from measured osmolality.

Fluid type	Temperature (°C)	pH	Osmolality (mmol/kg)
"Fresh" Water			
Reconstituted soft water	21.5	7.66	29
Artificial pond water	21.4	7.31	37
Electrolyte Solutions			
Steinberg's solution	21.9	6.97	130
0.6% saline	–	–	190
0.9 % saline	21.1	5.28	277
Ringer's solution, amphibian, isotonic	21.7	7.99	229
Ringer's solution, reptile	21.8	6.19	255
Ringer's solution, lactated (mammal)	21.0	6.5	273
Whitaker-Wright solutions			
5% Whitaker-Wright solution	21.7	7.0	206
10% Whitaker-Wright solution	21.3	7.17	357
20% Whitaker-Wright solution	21.1	7.24	705
30% Whitaker-Wright solution	21.2	7.26	1077
40% Whitaker-Wright solution	21.0	7.26	1341
50% Whitaker-Wright solution	21.2	7.27	1753
60% Whitaker-Wright solution	21.4	7.27	2129
70% Whitaker-Wright solution	21.5	7.26	2538
80% Whitaker-Wright solution	21.7	7.26	2935
90% Whitaker-Wright solution	21.9	7.25	3376
100% Whitaker-Wright solution	20.5	7.3	3815
Holtfreter's solutions			
40% modified Holtfreter's solution (Indiana University Axolotl Colony's formula)	20.9	6.55	76
100% Holtfreter's solution	22.0	8.06	122
100% modified Holtfreter's solution	22.1	8.12	130

Osmolality data obtained using a Westcor Vapor Pressure Osmometer. This table developed by Michele Martin and Christine Steinert.

Table 24.9. Miscellaneous drugs and other products used in amphibians.

Drug or product name	Dosage	Comments
Allopurinol	10 mg/kg PO q 24 h	Gout. (Reptile dose.)
Atropine	0.1 mg/kg SQ or IM prn	Starting dose used to treat organophosphate toxicoses
Calcitonin	50 iu/kg q 7 days	Reptile dose. Questionable efficacy for metabolic bone disease in amphibians.
Calcium glubionate	1 ml/kg PO q 24 h	Metabolic bone disease. Neo-Calglucon®.
Calcium gluconate, 10%	100 mg/kg IM, IV, ICe	For hypocalcemic tetany
Dexamethasone	1 mg/kg IM or IV	High dose for shock
Doxapram	2 ggt/100 g	Respiratory arrest
Epinephrine 1:1000	1 ggt/100 g	Respiratory and cardiac arrest
Fluids—nonlactated replacement solutions (e.g., Plasmalyte-A, Plasmalyte 148, Normosol-R)	volume not to exceed 2–5% of amphibian's body weight ICe in a 12-h period	May be hypertonic to an amphibian. May be of use for freshwater drowning victim.
Fluids—1 or 2 parts nonlactated replacement solution and 1 part 5% Dextrose	volume not to exceed 2–5% of amphibian's body weight ICe in a 12-h period	Rehydration. Lower ratio of electrolyte solution for severely dehydrated amphibians, higher ratio for minimally dehydrated amphibians or as a maintenance solution.
Fluids—9 parts non-lactated replacement solutions to 1 part sterile water	volume not to exceed 2–5% of amphibian's body weight ICe in a 12-h period	Rehydration of minimally dehydrated amphibians, or use as a maintenance solution
Fluids—1 or 2 parts saline and 1 part 5% Dextrose	volume not to exceed 2–5% of amphibian's body weight ICe in a 12-h period	Emergency rehydration only if no other fluids available. Not a balanced electrolyte solution.
Fluids—9 parts saline and 1 part sterile water	volume not to exceed 2–5% of amphibian's body weight ICe 12-h period, or may be used as a bath	Emergency rehydration only if no other fluids available. Not a balanced electrolyte solution.
Fluids—Amphibian Ringer's solution	volume not to exceed 2–5% of amphibian's body weight ICe in a 12-h period, and must be sterilized in autoclave first. May be used as a bath.	Hydration maintenance. See Chapter 26 for formula.
Flunixin meglumine	1 mg/kg SQ or IM q 24 h	Analgesia. (Reptile dose.)
Methylene blue	2 mg/ml bath	For nitrite/nitrate toxicity
Morphine	38 mg/kg SQ once	Analgesia in the northern leopard frog, *Rana pipiens*. Stephens & Kirkendall, 1993
Polyaqua®	continuous bath	Kordon Division of Novalek Corp., Hayward, CA. Artificial slime product.
Prednisolone sodium succinate	5–10 mg/kg IM	High dose for shock

Table 24.9. Miscellaneous drugs and other products used in amphibians. *(Continued)*

Drug or product name	Dosage	Comments
Reptomin®	soaked in water and given PO	Tetra Products. Used as a purgative to obtain fecal samples.
Shield-X®	continuous bath	Aquatronics, Malibu, CA. Artificial slime product with vitamin E.
Sodium thiosulfate	1% solution as a bath	Halogen toxicoses
Thiamine	50–100 mg/kg IM prn	Neurologic signs
Vitamin B complex	0.5–1.0 ml/gal water	Spindly leg syndrome, paralysis. B complex, VEDCO Inc., St. Joseph, MO.
Vitamin D_3	1000 iu/kg IM once 24 h after resolution of tetany 100–400 iu/kg PO q 24 h 2–3 iu/ml continuous bath	Following calcium treatment of hypocalcemic tetany For treatment of metabolic bone disease, High-D 2× Dispersible Vitamin D_3 Liquid Concentrate, I.D. Russell Company, Laboratories, Longmont, CO.
Vitamin E	1 mg/kg IM or PO q 7 days	Steatitis

REFERENCES

Asashima, M., G.M. Malacinski, and S.C. Smith. 1989. Surgical manipulation of embryos, *in* J.B. Armstrong and G.M. Malacinski (Eds.), Developmental Biology of the Axolotl. Oxford University Press, New York, pp. 255–263.

Boutilier, R.G., D.F. Stiffler, and D.P. Toews. 1992. Exchange of respiratory gases, ions, and water in amphibious and aquatic amphibians, *in* Feder, M.E. and W.W. Burggren: Environmental Physiology of the Amphibians. University of Chicago Press, Chicago, pp. 81–124

Brothers, A.J. 1977. Instructions for the care and feeding of axolotls. Axolotl Newsletter 3:9–16.

Cosgrove, G.E. and D.W. Jared. 1977. Treatment of skin-invading capillarid nematodes in a colony of South African clawed frogs. Laboratory Animal Science 27(4):526.

Crawshaw, G.J. 1992. Amphibian medicine, *in* Kirk, R.W. and J.D. Bonagura (Eds.): Kirk's Current Veterinary Therapy XI. Small Animal Practice. W.B. Saunders Co., Philadelphia, PA, pp. 1219–1230.

Evans, E.E. 1963. Comparative immunology: antibody response in *Dipsosaurus dorsalis* at different temperatures. Proceedings of the Society Experimental Biology and Medicine 112:531

Fox, W.F. 1980. Treatments and dosages. Axolotl Newsletter 9:6.

Frye, F.L. 1991. Fungal, actinomycete, bacterial, rickettsial, and viral diseases, *in* Frye, F.L. (Ed.): Biomedical and Surgical Aspects of Captive Reptile Husbandry. Krieger Publishing Co., Malabar, FL, pp. 101–160.

Gatten, R.E., K. Miller, and R.J. Full. 1992. Energetics at Rest and During Locomotion, *in* Feder, M.E. and W.W. Burggren: Environmental Physiology of the Amphibians. University of Chicago Press, Chicago, pp. 314–377.

Green, N. and N. Cohen. 1977. Effect of temperature on serum complement levels in the leopard frog *Rana pipiens*. Developmental and Comparative Pathology 1:59–64.

Hutchison, V.H. and R.K. Dupré. 1992. Thermoregulation, *in* Feder, M.E. and W.W. Burggren: Environmental Physiology of the Amphibians. University of Chicago Press, Chicago, pp. 206–249.

Klingenberg, R.J. 1996. Therapeutics, *in* Mader, D.R. (Ed.): Reptile Medicine and Surgery. W.B. Saunders Co., Philadelphia, PA, pp. 299–321.

Kluger, M.J. 1979. Fever in ectotherms: evolutionary implications. American Zoologist 19:295

Kollias, G.V. 1984. Immunologic aspects of infectious disease. *in* Hoff, G.L., Frye, F.L., and E.R. Jacobson. Diseases of Amphibians and Reptiles. Plenum Press, New York, pp. 661–692.

Letcher, J. and M. Papich. 1994. Pharmacokinetics of intramuscular administration of three antibiotics in bullfrogs (*Rana catesbeiana*). 1994 Proceedings American Association of Zoo Veterinarians, pp. 79–93.

Letcher, J. and M. Glade. 1992. Efficacy of ivermectin as an anthelmintic in leopard frogs. Journal of the American Veterinary Medical Association 200(4):537–538.

Maruska, E.J. 1994. Procedures for setting up and maintaining a salamander colony, *in* Murphy, J.B., K. Adler, and J.T. Collins (Eds.): Captive Management and Conservation of Amphibians and Reptiles. Society for the Study of Amphibians and Reptiles, Ithaca, NY. Contributions to Herpetology, volume 11, pp. 229–242.

Mattison, C. 1982. Order Anura—frogs and toads, *in* The Care of Reptiles and Amphibians in Captivity. Blanford Press, Poole Dorset, UK, pp. 121–157.

Menard, M.R. 1984. External application of antibiotic to improve survival of adult laboratory frogs (*Rana pipiens*). Laboratory Animal Science 34(1):94–96.

Mombarg, M. and P. Zwart. 1991. Percutaneous absorption of metronidazole and levamisole in *Bombina orientalis*. Proceedings of the Fourth International Colloquium on Pathology and Medicine of Reptiles and Amphibians, pp. 318–322.

Nichols, D.K. and E.W. Lamirande. 2000. POSTER—Treatment of cutaneous chytridiomycosis in blue-and-yellow poison dart frogs (*Dendrobates tinctorius*). Getting the Jump! on Amphibian Diseases Conference.

Poynton, S.L. and B.R. Whitaker. 1994. Protozoa in poison dart frogs (Dendrobatidae): clinical assessment and identification. Journal of Zoo and Wildlife Medicine 25(1):29–39.

Prezant, R. and J. Jarchow. 1997. Lactated fluid use in reptiles: Is there a better solution? Proceedings of the Association of Reptilian and Amphibian Veterinarians, pp. 83–87.

Raphael, B.L. Amphibians. 1993. Veterinary Clinics of North America: Small Animal Practice 23(6):1271–1286.

Read, A.W. 1994. Treatment of redleg in tadpoles of *Pleurodeles*. British Herpetological Society Bulletin 49:7.

Riveiere, J.E., D.P. Shapiro, and G.L. Coppoc. 1979. Percutaneous absorption of gentamicin by the leopard frog *Rana pipiens*. Journal of Veterinary Pharmacologic Therapy 2:235–239.

Stephens, C.E. 1975. Methods for acute toxicity tests with fish, macroinvertebrates, and amphibians. EPA-660/3-75-009. National Environmental Research Center, Environmental Protection Agency, Corvallis, OR.

Stevens, C.W. and K. Kirkendall. 1993. Time course and magnitude of tolerance to the analgesic effects of systemic morphone in amphibians. Life Sciences 52:111–116.

Stoskopf, M.S., B.S. Arnold, and M. Mason. 1987. Aminoglycoside antibiotic levels in the aquatic salamander *Necturus necturus*. Journal of Zoo and Wildlife Medicine 18:81–85.

Teare, J.A., R.S. Wallace, and M. Bush. 1991. Pharmacology of gentamicin in the leopard frog *Rana pipiens*. Proceedings of the American Association of Zoo Veterinarians, pp. 128–131.

Vaughn, L.K., H.A. Bernheim, and M. Kluger. 1974. Fever in the lizard *Dipsosaurus dorsalis*. Nature 252:473.

Vogelnest, L. 1994. Myiasis in a green treefrog *Litoria caerulea*. Bulletin of the Association of Reptile and Amphibian Veterinarians 4(1):4.

Wright, K.M. 1996. Amphibian husbandry and medicine, *in* Mader, D.R. (Ed.): Reptile Medicine and Surgery. W.B. Saunders Co., Philadelphia, PA, pp. 436–459.

Wright, R.K. and E.L. Cooper. 1981. Temperature effects on ectotherm immune responses. Developmental and Comparative Immunology 5 (Suppl.) 1:117.

CHAPTER 25
NECROPSY

Donald K. Nichols, DVM, Diplomate ACVP

25.1 ANAMNESIS

Before performing the postmortem examination of an amphibian, a thorough history of the animal should be obtained and recorded. In addition to information about the clinical disease leading to the animal's death, data should be collected regarding the source of the animal, past and current husbandry practices, possible changes in the external environment, and the number and types of other animals housed in proximity to the deceased animal. By thorough questioning of the client, information can usually be discovered that proves to be crucial to understanding why a particular animal died, what factors led to the development of the fatal disease, and how to prevent similar cases in the future. A sample list of questions that one might ask a client has been compiled in an Amphibian pathology questionnaire (Table 25.1).

25.2 EQUIPMENT

The equipment and materials needed to conduct complete examinations of dead amphibians should be readily available in any well-equipped veterinary hospital or laboratory. The basic instruments needed to perform a necropsy are scalpels, surgical and/or dissecting scissors of various sizes, and forceps. Other supplies should include gloves, alcohol or iodine swabs, sterile syringes and needles, tissue bags or other containers suitable for freezing samples, microscope slides and cover slips, sterile culture swabs, and containers with 10% buffered formalin. Some method to sterilize instruments is also necessary, either by heat (alcohol lamp, Bunsen burner, or autoclave) or chemical/liquid sterilization. In addition to a standard light microscope, it is useful to have a dissecting microscope or magnifying glass available, especially when looking for parasites.

25.3 CULTURE

Samples from amphibians submitted for routine aerobic and/or anaerobic bacterial culture should be inoculated into/onto the standard culture media used for culturing specimens from mammalian species. Because some bacterial pathogens of ectothermic animals may grow best at "room temperature", replicates of each culture can be incubated at 20–25°C (68–77°F), as well as 37°C (98.6°F). However, in the author's experience this may not be necessary because pathogenic bacteria of amphibians appear to grow well and usually more quickly at 37°C.

Specimens for fungal, mycobacterial, viral, or other special cultures should be placed in sterile containers and refrigerated (short-term storage) or frozen (long-term storage) until sent to the appropriate laboratory. If the need for special cultures is anticipated, the proper laboratory should be contacted *before* the necropsy is performed to determine the best specimen collection and handling procedures.

25.4 CYTOLOGY

The usefulness of lesion impression cytology and wet mounts of skin scrapings and/or gill clippings cannot be overstated. These can quickly indicate the presence of infectious organisms such as fungi, mycobacteria, or parasites so that the proper samples can be collected and sent to the appropriate reference laboratory. This is particularly important when other animals in a collection are at risk.

When making cytologic impressions of a lesion, *a minimum* of three slides should be prepared. The first slide is stained with a Romanowsky's stain (e.g., Wright's stain or "Dif Quick" stain). Depending on the results of the examination of that slide, the other slides are then available for staining with a Gram, acid-fast, or other special stains.

Wet mounts of skin scrapings and gill samples are prepared by first placing the specimens on a microscope slide. These are then moistened with one or two drops of water or a physiologic saline solution, coverslipped, and examined microscopically for the presence of fungi or ectoparasites.

Table 25.1. Amphibian pathology questionnaire.

Client/Owner: _____
Address: _____
Species: _____ Sex _____
ID: _____ Age: ___Yr ___Mo ___Day (Actual/Estimate)

Captive-Born: Yes   No   If captive-born, where was it born and what were the dates of hatching/ metamorphosis:
_____

Wild-Caught: Yes   No

Where did you obtain the animal and how long have you had it:

How was this animal housed?

    Cage size and type:

    Substrate used and types of plants present:

    Sources of water: Tap water   Filtered tap water   Bottled water

      Other (describe):

    Sources of moisture in cage: Bowl   Misting   Humidifier

      Other (describe):

    Types of cage furniture present:

    Cage temperature and method of temperature control:

    Cage lighting and approximate light/dark cycle:

    Number and species of cage mates, if present:

    Number and species of other animals housed in nearby enclosures:

    Frequency of cage cleaning:

    Method of cage cleaning and any cleaning agents or disinfectants used:

How frequently was food offered and how frequently did the animal eat:

What was the exact diet offered to this animal, and what was it observed to consume:

What was the source of the diet:

Have there been *any* changes in the diet, water or housing?   Yes   No

    If so, what are these changes and when did they occur:

Types and duration of clinical signs noted prior to death:

Please list any other information you believe is important:

25.5 NECROPSY PROCEDURES

Once a complete history has been recorded (Table 25.1) and evaluated, the gross necropsy can begin. To assist in recording the gross necropsy findings and those specimens collected for potential histopathologic examination, examples of a "Gross necropsy worksheet" and a "Necropsy tissue checklist" have been included (Tables 25.2, 25.3). To begin the necropsy, the carcass should be evaluated for overall condition, state of hydration, and degree of autolysis. Then the external surfaces and body orifices should be carefully examined for signs of trauma or infection. Because amphibians rely heavily on their skin for maintenance of metabolic homeostasis and many species conduct some or all of their respiration cutaneously, skin lesions that would be considered to be relatively minor in other vertebrate species can have significant effects on an amphibian's health. Therefore, it is important to examine the entire skin closely for abnormalities such as ulceration, thickening or roughening, unusual dryness, or excess mucus production. A magnifying glass or dissecting microscope can aid in this examination. Abnormal areas seen at this time should be sampled for histopathology. Lesions should be scraped with a scalpel blade or im-

Table 25.2. Gross necropsy worksheet.

GROSS NECROPSY WORKSHEET

Client/Owner: _____
Species: _____ ID: _____
Sex: _____ Age: _____ Weight: _____ Snout-Vent Length: _____
Death Date: _____ Necropsy Date: _____

GROSS NECROPSY FINDINGS

Use the space provided to record any gross observations for each of the following:

General Exam (physical condition, skin, fat stores, body orifices)

Musculoskeletal System (bones, joints, muscles)

Respiratory System (nasal passages, pharynx, larynx, trachea, lungs, gills)

Cardiovascular System (heart, great vessels)

Digestive System (mouth, tongue, esophagus, stomach, intestines, cloaca, liver and gall bladder, pancreas)

Spleen

Urinary System (kidneys, ureters, urinary bladder)

Reproductive System (gonads, oviducts)

Endocrine System (thyroid, parathyroids, pituitary)

Nervous System (nerves, brain, spinal cord, eyes)

Additional Comments or Observations

---

pressions can be made of the lesions for cytologic evaluation. Samples of the lesion(s) may also be taken for potential bacterial, fungal, or viral culture. Even if no cutaneous lesions are detected grossly, samples of skin from several parts of the body should be collected for histopathology.

In aquatic forms with external gills, the gills should be inspected in a manner similar to the skin and samples taken for histopathology. Wet mounts of gill clippings can be made and examined for the presence of fungi or ectoparasites.

Once the external examination is completed, the carcass is placed in dorsal recumbency and its ventral surface disinfected with 70% ethanol or an iodine solution (Plate 25.1). A ventral midline incision is then made in the skin from the mandibular symphysis to the external cloacal opening.

In anurans, the skin is loosely attached to the underlying musculature and a large potential subcutaneous space exists; this allows for the skin to be easily reflected back from the midline incision without incising the abdominal muscles (Plate 25.2). The

Table 25.3. Necropsy tissue checklist.

> **NECROPSY TISSUE CHECKLIST**
>
> Tissue samples collected for histopathology should be placed in buffered 10% formalin at a ratio of approximately 1 part tissue to 10 parts solution. Samples should be no thicker than 1 cm.
>
> **Circle or check each organ that was sampled** (include any additional notations such as the number or location of samples):
>
> | | | |
> |---|---|---|
> | SKIN | MUSCLE | NERVE |
> | TONGUE | ESOPHAGUS | STOMACH |
> | SMALL INTESTINE | COLON | CLOACA |
> | LIVER | GALL BLADDER | PANCREAS |
> | SPLEEN | HEART | AORTA |
> | LARYNX/ TRACHEA | LUNGS | GILLS |
> | KIDNEYS | URINARY BLADDER | GONAD |
> | OVIDUCT | BRAIN | EYE |
> | BONE/JOINT | OTHER | |

quantity and characteristics of any subcutaneous fluid present should be noted and samples of this can be taken for culture and/or cytology using a sterile syringe and needle. The ventral and limb musculature are then inspected for the presence of lesions. The instruments used to make the skin incision should then be sterilized or a separate set of instruments obtained before making a midline incision in the abdominal musculature and reflecting the muscles to expose the coelomic viscera (Plate 25.3).

In salamanders and caecelians, the skin is much more closely adhered to the underlying soft tissues and separating them is very difficult. Therefore, after making the ventral midline incision, the abdominal skin and musculature are reflected to expose the coelomic contents (Plates 25.4, 25.5).

At this point, the coelomic contents are quickly examined in situ. Any lesions noted can be sampled for culture and/or cytologic evaluation. In cases where bacterial septicemia is suspected and little autolysis is present, a sample of heart blood may be collected for culture using a sterile syringe and needle (Plates 25.6, 25.7) (Note: To obtain a sample of heart blood, it may be necessary to incise and/or remove the xiphoid cartilage and sternum). If heart blood is not available, a carefully selected piece of liver is the next best choice for bacterial culture. If coelomic fluid is present, this is another good choice for bacterial culture.

Once specimens have been collected for culture, the viscera should be removed and examined more closely. This is most easily accomplished by first freeing the tongue, glottis, and pharynx from their surrounding soft tissue attachments. While holding firmly to the tongue and pulling it in a ventrocaudal direction, the entire digestive system, heart, and respiratory tract can be removed by cutting their dorsal attachments to the body wall (see Plate 25.7). In most animals, the urogenital tract is also easily removed at this time. After the viscera have been removed, the organ systems should be separated and individually examined. Samples for cytology and histopathology are then collected. Lesions not detected previously can be cultured if care is taken to minimize contamination. If gastrointestinal or pulmonary parasitism is suspected, parasitology can be performed on samples of colonic contents or scrapings of the lung.

The brain can be examined and collected at the time of necropsy by carefully using scissors and/or forceps to chip away the skull and overlying soft tissues, beginning at the foramen magnum and working rostrally. This can be accomplished using either a dorsal (Plate 25.8A–C) or a ventral approach (Plate 25.9A, B). In small amphibians, this is often very difficult to accomplish without severely damaging the brain. Another method that can be used for these animals is to remove the head at the atlanto-occipital joint and place it in formalin for 48–72 h to fix the brain in situ before attempting to remove it.

Sampling for histopathology should be done liberally; all of the specimens collected do not necessarily have to be submitted for histopathologic examination. Tissue samples can be discarded after fixation which is much preferable to later realizing that an important sample was not collected. It is often useful to keep these extra tissue samples until the histopathology report is received because initial histology results may indicate the need for further sample submission.

CHAPTER 26
SPONTANEOUS NEOPLASIA IN AMPHIBIA

D. Earl Green, DVM, Diplomate ACVP and John C. Harshbarger, PhD

26.1 INTRODUCTION

Neoplasms have been observed in amphibians for more than a hundred years (Eberth, 1868). The best studied neoplasm of amphibians is the Lucke carcinoma of the mesonephros of the northern leopard frog, *Rana pipiens*. Other virus-induced or virus-associated proliferative diseases have been reported in the Japanese firebelly newt, *Cynops pyrrhogaster*, the African clawed frog, *Xenopus laevis*, and various laboratory-produced hybrid ranids. The vast majority of reported neoplasms in amphibians have been Lucke renal carcinomata in the northern leopard frog, and epidermal papillomata in the Japanese firebelly newt, *Cynops pyrrhogaster*. Other reported neoplasms have been from a variety of amphibian taxa, most notably from laboratory colonies of leopard frogs, *Rana* spp., the axolotl, *Ambystoma mexicanum*, clawed frogs, *Xenopus* spp., and from zoological specimens. In recent years, there are greater numbers of case reports in amphibians that have been kept as pets and in zoos (Frye et al., 1989a; Kabisch et al., 1991). Epidemics of neoplasms have been reported in at least four instances, in two species of ranids near Leningrad, Russia, in one population of the tiger salamander, *Ambystoma tigrinum*, in a sewage pond in Texas, in captive-bred hybrid Asian frogs, and in populations of the crested newt, *Triturus cristatus*, in Italy. As in other classes of vertebrates, neoplasms (other than Lucke's renal carcinoma and newt epidermal papillomata) are seldom encountered in wild amphibians, but are more likely to be discovered and reported in captive laboratory and zoo animals and pets that are free of the threats of predation and natural catastrophes. As amphibian husbandry improves, so will the life-span of captive amphibians. Older captive amphibians may be prone to a variety of disease processes (e.g., atherosclerosis, lipid keratopathy) as well as neoplasia.

26.1.1 Tumors vs. Neoplasms

The literature on amphibian neoplasms is unlike that of any other class of vertebrates, for granulomata and granulomatous disease have been reported mistakenly as neoplasms by numerous authors. In many cases, gross and histologic descriptions inadequately document the suspected neoplasm, and illustrations are lacking or equivocal. Consequently, interpretation by the reader of suspected neoplasms is impossible. However, such inadequately described swellings, often in the liver, spleen, and kidneys, may be considered tumors in the broadest sense of the word. A tumor is a swelling and is not synonymous with neoplasia. A tumor may be inflammatory in nature (granulomata), parasitic (e.g., "encysted" immature trematodes), hyperplastic (e.g., possibly some newt papillomata), or neoplastic. The term pseudotumor is nonsense. This chapter will be limited to spontaneous neoplastic and hyperplastic diseases of wild and captive amphibians.

Reports of spontaneous neoplasms in amphibians are widely scattered in the literature. Most of the cases illustrated in this chapter come from material donated to the Registry of Tumors in Lower Animals and the Registry of Comparative Pathology at the Armed Forces Institute of Pathology, some of which have not been published or previously described.

26.1.2 Experimental Carcinogenesis

Some researchers report that neoplasms are so readily induced in amphibians that they may be used in screening tests for carcinogens (Breedis, 1952; Khudoley, 1977; Khudoley & Picard, 1980), while others have found amphibians comparatively resistant to chemical carcinogenesis (Balls & Ruben, 1964; Balls et al., 1983; Ingram, 1972). Many chemicals that are known to be potent carcinogens in laboratory rodents and humans will induce neoplasms in amphibians, but not necessarily at the same high rates (Clothier, 1983). Many early studies of amphibian carcinogenesis used polycyclic hydrocarbons and N-dimethylnitrosamine (DMN) with limited success. Much greater success was obtained using N-methyl-N-nitrosourea (MNU) and methylcholanthrene (Afifi et al., 1991; Balls et al., 1983; Clothier et al., 1989; Matz, 1982). However, not all suspected carcinogens are confined to laboratory conditions, as demonstrated by a wild population of the barred tiger salamander, *Ambystoma tigrinum mavortium*, in a sewage lagoon in Texas (Rose, 1976, 1981). Many neoplasms that develop in amphibians subsequent to carcinogen exposure are poorly differentiated and difficult to categorize. Some chemically induced lesions may be hyperplasias, metaplasias, benign neoplasms, or malignant neoplasms. The criteria for distinguishing experimental chemically induced hyperplasia from benign neoplasia in amphibians has scarcely been addressed (Balls & Clothier, 1989). There is a tendency to assume most chemically induced tumors (tumors used in the broadest sense) are malignancies (Balls et al., 1989), when it is probable that many are hyperplasia or metaplastic changes, or benign neoplasms. Occasionally, ultrastructural examinations are helpful in identifying the cell of origin of some neoplasms.

The literature on experimental amphibian oncology, especially lymphoproliferative and hepatosplenic disorders, contains much misinformation and incorrect diagnoses. Most of the published literature concerning experimental transmission studies of lymphoproliferative disorders in newts, clawed frogs, *Xenopus* spp., the axolotl *Ambystoma mexicanum*, and the square-marked toad, *Bufo regularis,* are not experiments on lymphosarcomata or reticulum cell sarcomata (Ruben & Stevens, 1970), but mycobacterial transmission studies. Any transmission studies in which lymphosarcomalike disease was transmitted from one amphibian genus to another are most likely studies of granulomatous disease induced by experimental transmission of mycobacteria, not the transmission (or transplantation) of lymphoproliferative neoplasms. The problem was addressed as long ago as the 1960s, but published articles claiming to be studies of lymphosarcomata continued to be published into the 1990s. Clearly, any study of lymphoproliferative and myeloproliferative disorders in amphibians must, as a preliminary basic verification, report the results of acid-fast stains or mycobacterial cultures of the suspected neoplasm. Because of the confusion over lymphoproliferative disorders and granulomatous mycobacteriosis in amphibians, it should be required for the next decade or two that all manuscripts concerning lymphohematopoietic neoplasia in amphibians have a statement reporting the results of examinations of acid-fast-stained slides of the purported neoplasm or mycobacterial cultures of the suspected neoplastic cells. Furthermore, until clear and decisive research proves otherwise, claims that neoplasms or neoplastic cell lines of amphibian origin are secondarily or opportunistically infected with mycobacteria (Ruben & Stevens, 1970) remain suspect.

Reports of neoplasms in amphibians must be viewed cautiously. The two principal reasons for this critical evaluation of many published reports of spontaneous neoplasms are that some superficially excellent reports consist solely of camera lucida drawings (and original material has never been deposited in tumor registries nor seen by any colleagues or other independent researchers) and that considerable confusion exists concerning mycobacterial granulomata versus lymphoproliferative disorders, as discussed in the previous paragraph (Asfari, 1988; Dawe, 1969b; El-Mofty et al., 1991a, b, 1992, 1993; Hadji-Azimi, 1970; Inoue et al., 1965; Ruben & Stevens, 1970). For these reasons, several published reports of spontaneous neoplasms in amphibians by Stolk have not been included in this chapter, and probably should be forgotten unless or until the original material becomes available for independent review and verification of diagnoses. The situation concerning published literature on purported lymphoproliferative and myeloproliferative diseases, hepatosplenic nodules, and possibly some gastric nodules, remains very difficult to evaluate. Many of these purported neoplasms probably were verminous or mycobacterial granulomata, but it certainly is possible that some tumors in these groups of experimental amphibians were legitimate neoplasms. In many cases, the involved organs, histologic descriptions, photomicrographs, and ultrastructural studies did not convince these authors that the case in question was neoplastic disease. In 1988 it was stated by Asfari that, of all the published reports of lymphosarcomata in *Xenopus* spp., only one case may be a true lymphosarcoma. Fortunately, a few more cases of lymphoproliferative disease have been donated to the Registry of Tumors in Lower Animals.

All neoplasms mentioned in this chapter were either examined by the authors at the Registry of Tumors in Lower Animals and archives of the Armed Forces Institute of Pathology (both in Washington, DC), or were taken from published articles in which photomicrographs were considered clearly diagnostic of the purported neoplasm.

26.2 INTEGUMENT

Approximately half of all reported spontaneous hyperplastic and neoplastic lesions of amphibians are integumentary in origin (Asashima et al., 1987).

The skin of amphibians has a diverse array of cell types that may potentially give rise to neoplasms and hyperplastic lesions. Neoplasms originating from epidermal cells, melanophores, dermal glands, and neuromast cells (i.e., lateral line cells) have been reported. Neoplasms of many amphibian cell types have not been encountered or described, including Merkel cells, Leydig cells, flask cells, and others. Probably due to the brevity of the larval stage in most species, neoplasms of aquatic larvae are exceptionally rare, except those inadequately described "tumors" that occur in experimentally manipulated embryos derived from "overripe" and haploid eggs, and unnatural hybrids produced in the laboratory.

26.2.1 Epithelial Cell Neoplasms

Hyperplasia of epidermis (Pseudo-epitheliomatous hyperplasia). Hyperplasia of the epidermis in the barred tiger salamander, *Ambystoma tigrinum mavortium,* probably is a chemical-induced lesion, but the lesion was noted in a wild population (Harshbarger & Snyder, 1989; Rose, 1981). The epidermis is markedly hyperplastic but only slightly elevated. Mostly there is proliferation of cells in the stratum spinosum and stratum granulosum with loss of specialized epidermal cells such as Leydig cells. The hyperplastic epidermis does not form folds or projections above the surface of the skin but remains more or less flat or mildly elevated. Pegs of epidermal cells project deeply into the dermis, with some pegs of cells appearing to invade or replace dermal glands, and some pegs projecting below dermal glands to the stratum compactum (Harshbarger & Snyder, 1989). The dermis is hypocellular and may be edematous. Dermal glands and chromatophores may be greatly reduced in numbers or absent (Figure 26.1). Following transfer of affected neotenic salamanders to clean water, these lesions regress spontaneously after 4 months in laboratory conditions, suggesting continued exposure to one or more chemicals is necessary for persistence of the hyperplastic lesions (Rose, 1981).

Squamous cell papilloma (infectious wart). Squamous cell papilloma is a proliferation of cells in the stratum spinosum or stratum granulosum that has been reported in the Japanese firebelly newt, *Cynops pyrrhogaster* (Figure 26.2) (Asashima et al., 1982), a population of the barred tiger salamander, *Ambystoma tigrinum mavortium* (Figure 26.3) in Texas (Harshbarger & Snyder, 1989), a population of the Aomori salamander, *Hynobius lichenatus* (Asashima & Meyer-Rochow, 1988), and other species (Figure 26.4).

In the Japanese firebelly newt, *C. pyrrhogaster,* most papillomata regressed spontaneously within 2–12 months. In about 30% of newts, the disease is progressive, deforming, and probably directly or indirectly fatal (Asashima & Komazaki, 1980; Pfeiffer et al., 1979). Papilloma growth also is sensitive to ultraviolet radiation and is temperature-dependent (Asashima et al., 1985; Oka et al., 1992).

In one large pond containing neotenes of the barred tiger salamander, *A. tigrinum mavortium,* no skin neoplasms were observed in over 2500 salamanders examined in 1970. In 1971, 25% of salamanders had a variety of skin neoplasms and in 1975, 55% had neoplasms. Since 1975, the prevalance has declined steadily (Harshbarger & Snyder 1989).

The squamous cell papilloma of newts is benign, and consistently sessile. Pedunculated forms and metastases have not been reported. Papillomata in the Japanese firebelly newt, *Cynops pyrrhogaster,* and the Aomori salamander, *Hynobius lichenatus,* may be found anywhere on the body, head or appendages. Most are hypopigmented and solitary, although occasional specimens may have multiple papillomata. Papillomata are raised, have a finely nodular surface, are glistening, and, grossly, may resemble minute cysts. In an occasional specimen, the papillomata may be progressive, and cause marked superficial deformities of the head or limbs (Asashima & Komazaki, 1980). The diameter of the papilloma is usually 1–2 mm, but may be 10 mm or greater. The normal epidermis of the newt is one to five cells thick. The papilloma is continuous with normal epidermis, but is up to 17 cells thick. The hyperplastic epidermis consists of proliferating epidermal

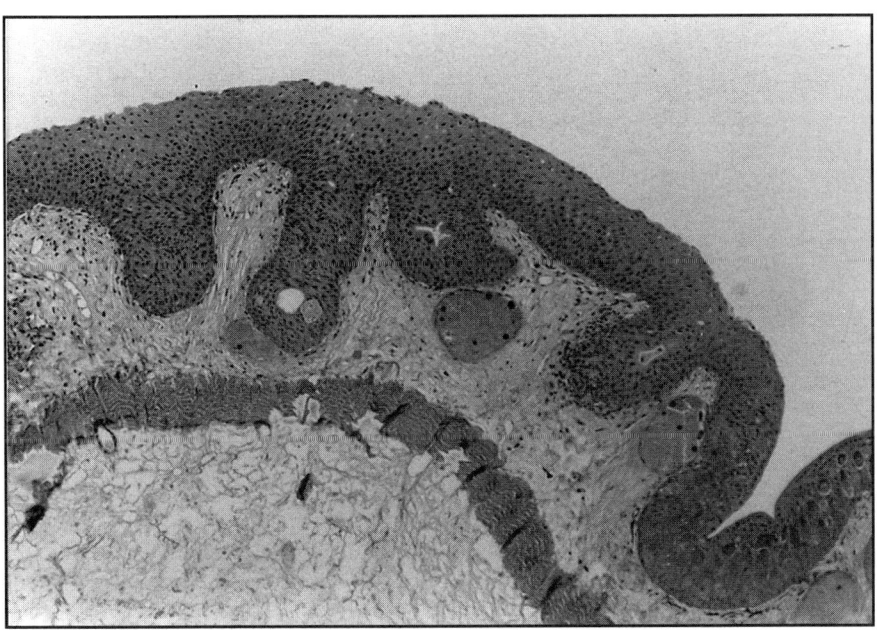

Figure 26.1. Pseudo-epitheliomatous hyperplasia of the skin of a neotenic barred tiger salamander, *Ambystoma tigrinum mavortium.* Note prominently hypercellular and thickened epidermis with pegs of epidermal cells projecting into the dermis but not penetrating the stratum compactum. Note the lack of intra-epidermal Leydig cells in the hyperplastic epidermis compared to a segment of normal skin in the lower right corner. (F.L. Rose, RTLA 908)

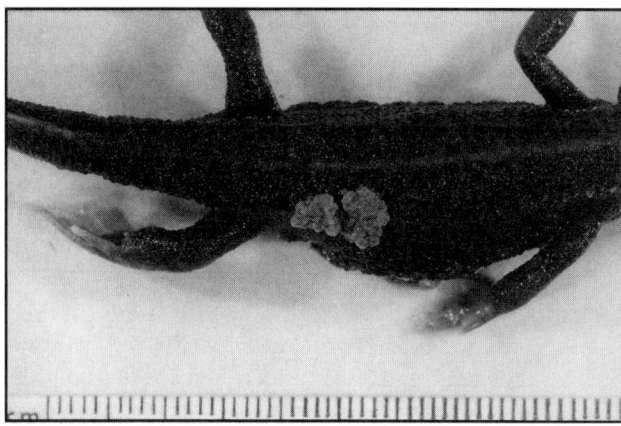

Figure 26.2. Squamous cell papilloma in a Japanese firebelly newt *Cynops pyrrhogaster*. (W.R. Duryee, RTLA 539)

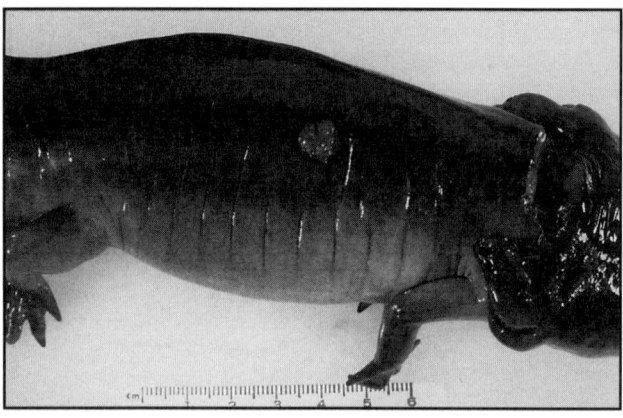

Figure 26.3. Squamous cell papilloma in a wild neotenic barred tiger salamander, *Ambystoma tigrinum mavortium*. (F.L. Rose, RTLA 945)

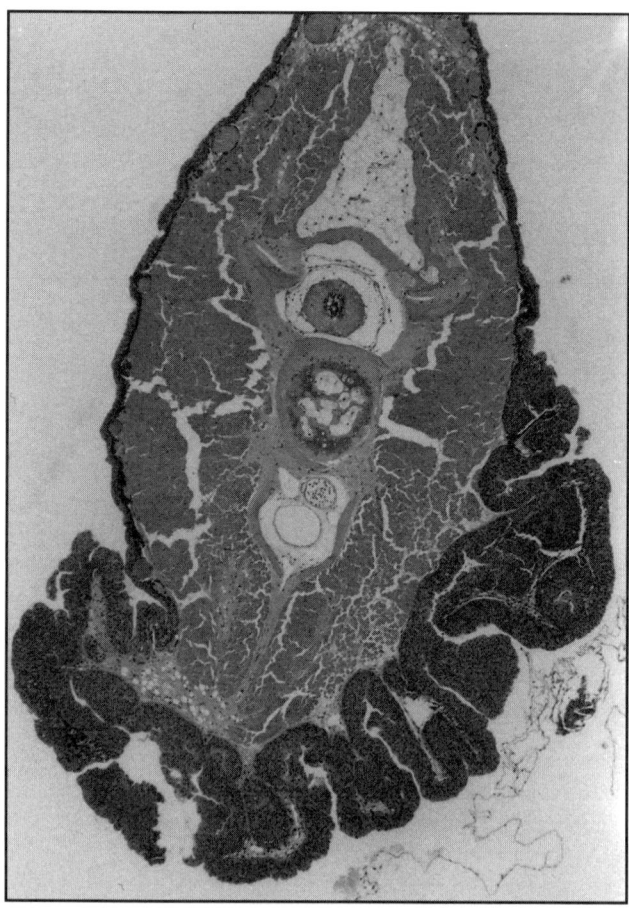

Figure 26.4. Squamous cell papilloma on the tail of a redbelly newt, *Taricha rivularis*. Note the markedly thickened epidermis which forms folds and simple papillary projections. Dermal fibrovascular stroma is scant. (F.L. Rose, RTLA 4227)

cells with few or no Leydig cells, which forms discrete, unbranched, foldlike projections on mildly to moderately prominent fibrovascular dermal stroma (Figures 26.5, 26.6). The dermis in the papillary projections may be edematous and usually has much fewer or no dermal glands and chromatophores (Rose & Harshbarger, 1977). There is no obvious proliferation of the connective tissue stroma, as occurs in a fibropapilloma. Rarely, the proliferating epidermal cells may appear to penetrate the basement membrane to form nodules in the dermis. Such nodules may be metaplastic or replaced dermal glands (Figures 26.7, 26.8) (Asashima & Komazaki, 1980; Rose & Harshbarger, 1977). The

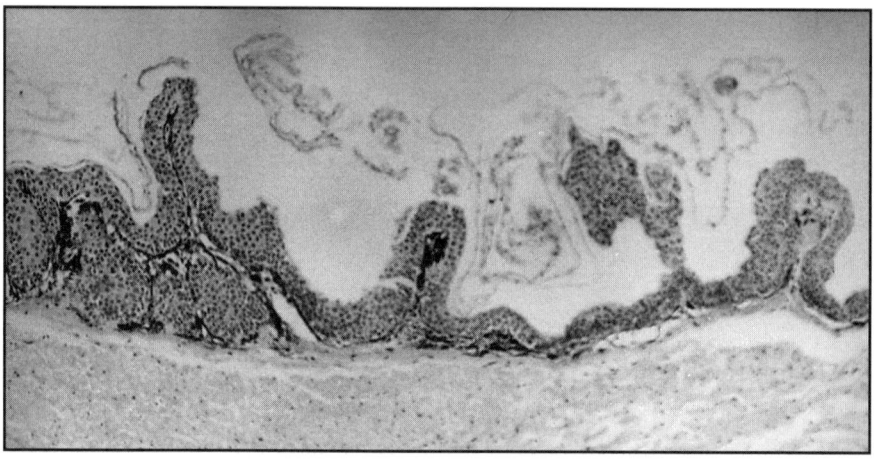

Figure 26.5. Squamous cell papilloma of a Japanese firebelly newt, *Cynops pyrrhogaster*. Note the distinct perpendicular papillary projections covered by a thickened layer of epithelial cells on a thin dermal stroma that lacks dermal glands. The cornified layer (stratum corneum) is artifactually detached, but has a multilayered appearance as if it had been retained through multiple molts. (W.R. Duryee, RTLA 513)

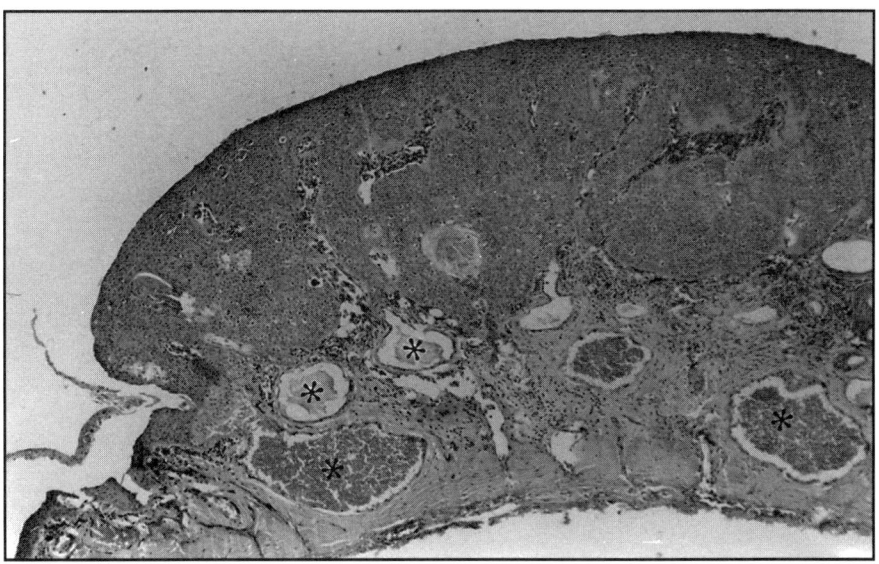

Figure 26.6. Squamous cell papilloma of a northern leopard frog, *Rana pipiens*. This prominently elevated, hypercellular epidermal plaque lacks the distinctive papillary projections common to papillomata of salamanders (see Figures 26.4, 26.5). Thin dermal fibrovascular septae project into the cellular plaque. Dermal glands are dilated and cystlike, suggesting they are unable to discharge secretory products. (B.J. Cohen, RTLA 656)

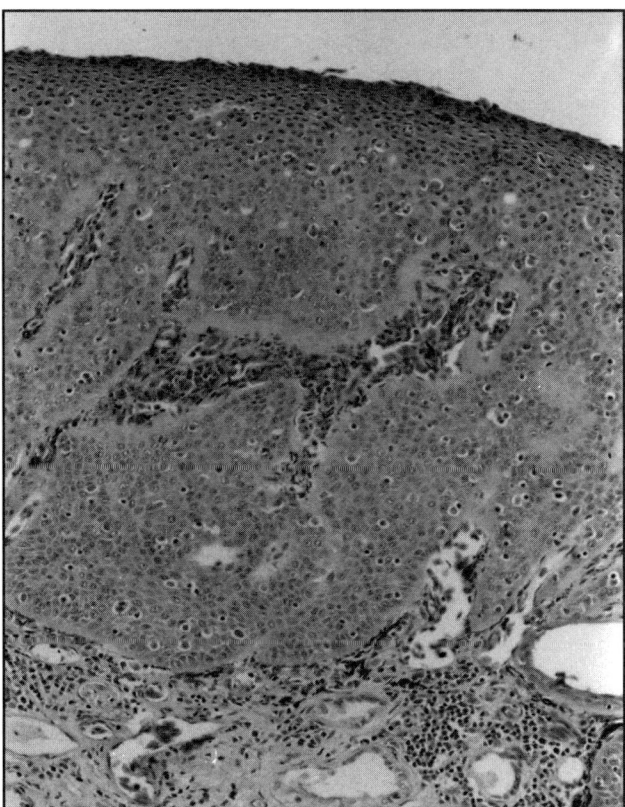

Figure 26.7. Squamous cell papilloma of a northern leopard frog, *Rana pipiens*, higher magnification of Figure 26.6. Note the columnar basal cells, hyperplastic stratum intermedium, and thin fibrovascular stroma. Mild infiltrates of lymphocytes and macrophages are present in the subjacent dermis. (B.J. Cohen, RTLA 656)

stratum corneum may appear normal, eroded, frayed, absent, or multilaminated as if the corneum had not been shed through repeated molts. Cells in the stratum spinosum and stratum granulosum may have subtle to mild increased intercellular space. Nuclei are irregular in density and pleomorphic. Intranuclear and intracytoplasmic inclusions have not been reported. Scattered necrotic cells in the stratum spinosum may be found (Pfeiffer et al., 1989). Mitotic rate is low, but mitoses may be detected in the stratum spinosum as well as the stratum basale. In the epidermis of the normal Japanese firebelly newt, *Cynops pyrrhogaster*, 0.1–0.5% of basal cells are mitotic, while in the papilloma the mitotic index is 1.0–3.5% (Asashima and Komazaki, 1980). The papillomata of the Japanese firebelly newt, *C. pyrrhogaster*, have been described ultrastructurally (Asashima & Komazaki, 1980; Asashima et al., 1982; Pfeiffer et al., 1979). In the Japanese firebelly newt, *C. pyrrhogaster*, the papillomata have been associated with an hexagonal, cytoplasmic, 50–200 nm diameter virus particle. It has been suggested the virus was herpes (Asashima et al., 1982), but the localization of particles to the cytoplasm of infected cells is more consistent with an iridiovirus. It seems likely that the squamous papillomata of the Japanese firebelly newt, *C. pyrrhogaster*, has an viral etiology. Histologic features of regressing newt papillomata have not been reported.

In the northern leopard frog, *Rana pipiens*, the squamous cell papilloma shows marked thickening of the epidermis, but does not form distinct folds or papillary projections as in the Japanese firebelly newt, *Cynops pyrrhogaster* (see Figures 26.5, 26.6) (Van Der Steen et al., 1972). Pegs of dermal fibrovascular tissue may project into the epidermis (see Figure 26.6), but these are usually very thin. Subjacent glands may be normal or mildly reduced in numbers, and some may have dilated lumina as if secretory products are not escaping through ducts in the thickened epidermis.

A large persistant papilloma was reported in one of three 18-month-old captive specimens of the black-spotted frog, *Rana nigromaculata*, from far eastern Russia. Grossly, the neoplasm was pinkish, markedly raised, multinodular, and located over the right tympanum extending to the eye, oral commissure, and axilla. The nodules were composed of very thick layers of epidermal cells (>20) on a prominent, edematous and arborizing connective tissue stroma. The papilloma grew progressively for 9 months, but two cagemates remained unaffected (Kabisch et al., 1991).

Fibropapilloma (Polypoid Dermal Fibroma). The fibropapilloma is characterized by proliferation of dermal fibrocytes far greater than the epithelial cells (Figure 26.9). At present, the distinction between a fibropapilloma and a fibroma of the amphibian skin is vague in the published literature and is worthy of additional study, but a fibropapilloma, by definition, should be confined to the dermis. Fibropapillomalike nodules have been described in one free-ranging population of the barred tiger salamander, *Ambystoma tigrinum mavortium*, in a sewage lagoon in Texas (Rose & Harshbarger, 1977). Affected individuals were neotenes which suggests the aquatic individuals had been in direct contact with chemicals in the lagoon for many months or years. Analysis of the sludge revealed high levels of perylene (300 ppb) and a variety of polycyclic aromatic hydrocarbons (Rose, 1981). A variety of other dermoepidermal neoplasms also were found in these salamanders. The fibropapilloma may appear grossly as a smooth, single or multilobular nodule with mild or marked hypopigmentation. Microscopically, the nodule consists of proliferating fibrocytes in the dermis that are numerous, and arranged in randomly oriented bundles and whorls (see Figure 26.9). Segments of the overlying epidermis may be normal, thin, eroded, ulcerated, and mildly hyperplastic. Cords or pegs of epithelial cells may appear to penetrate into the mass of proliferating fibrocytes.

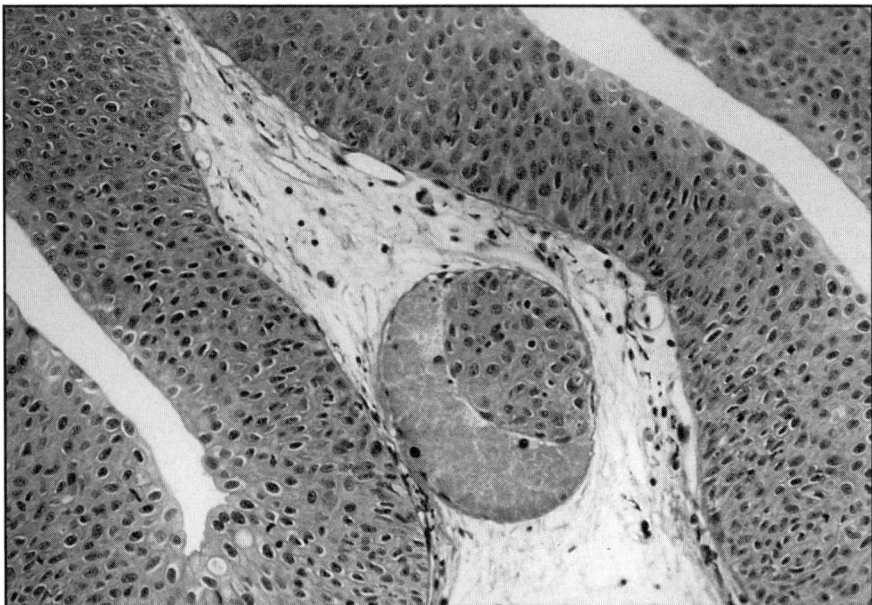

Figure 26.8. Squamous cell papilloma in a wild neotenic barred tiger salamander, *Ambystoma tigrinum mavortium*. Within the dermal stroma, one dermal gland is about half replaced by hyperplastic epidermal cells. Note monotypic nature of epidermal cells in the hyperplastic epidermis, and absence of other epidermal cells (e.g., Leydig cells). (F.L. Rose, RTLA 913)

Intracutaneous Cornifying Epithelioma (Keratoacanthoma). Although there are no published reports of intracutaneous cornifying epithelium (ICE) in amphibians, there are two anuran cases at the Registry of Tumors in Lower Animals. This benign, discrete neoplasm is composed of a single cavity lined by abruptly cornifying epithelium and is filled with concentric layers of keratinized cells (Figures 26.10, 26.11). Melanin pigment, calcification, and inflammatory cells are scanty or absent (Weiss & Frese, 1974). The keratin-filled cavity impinges into the dermis and may cause mild eleva-

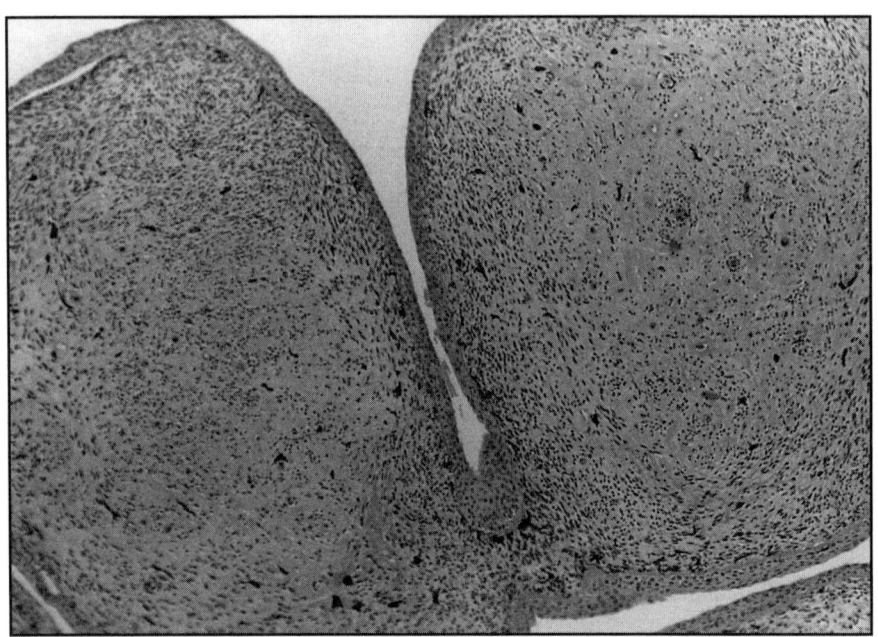

Figure 26.9. Fibropapilloma in a wild neotenic barred tiger salamander, *Ambystoma tigrinum mavortium*. Nodular proliferation of dermal fibrocytes far exceeds proliferation of epidermal cells. (F.L. Rose, RTLA 909)

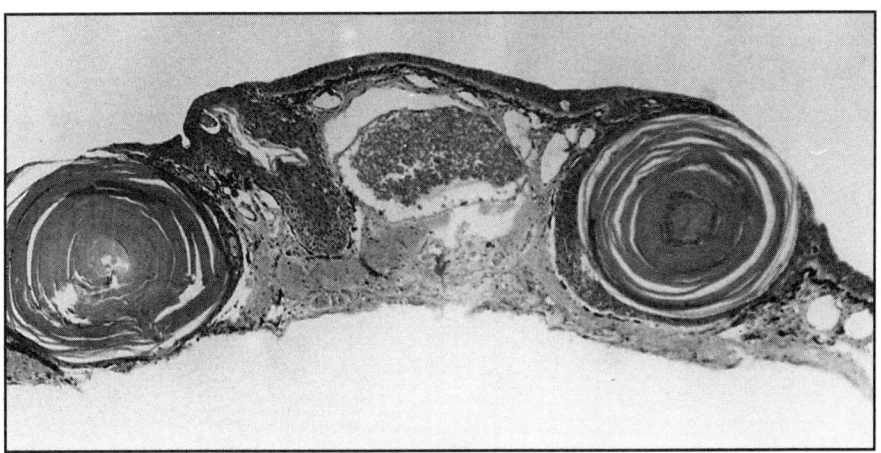

Figure 26.10. Intracutaneous cornifying epithelioma (ICE) in a northern leopard frog, *Rana pipiens*. This lesion of possible dermal gland origin is well demarcated, intradermal, and filled with laminated, concentrically arranged keratin-like material. Two ICE are present in the figure. (B.J. Cohen, RTLA 658)

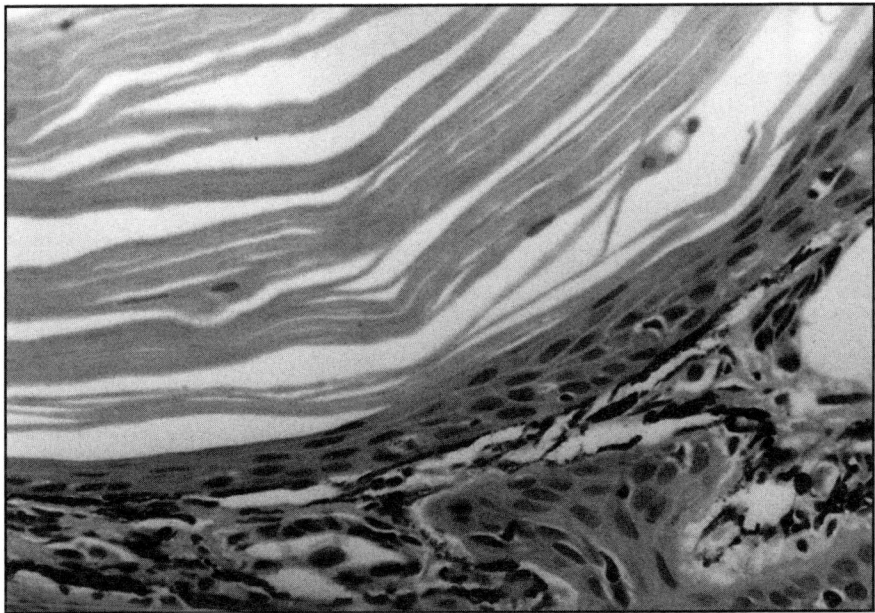

Figure 26.11. Intracutaneous cornifying epithelioma (ICE); higher magnification of Figure 26.10. The wall of the nodule is lined by thin epidermis showing abrupt keratinization (B.J. Cohen, RTLA 658)

tion of the epidermis. Multiloculated cavities and papillary projections into the cavity have not been observed but multicentric ICE have been seen. The epidermis adjacent to and overlying the ICE may appear mildly hyperplastic.

Basal Cell Tumor (Basal Cell Carcinoma, Trichoblastoma). There is one report of a basal cell tumor in a wild marbled salamander, *Ambystoma opacum* (Counts et al., 1975). This diagnosis is unlikely since this tumor is presently believed to derive from primitive hair germ cells, or the primitive cells of the hair and sebaceous gland unit of mammals (Walder & Gross, 1992). Since amphibians lack sebaceous glands, hair, and any structure resembling a hair follicle, the occurrence of a basal cell tumor in any amphibian seems highly improbable. The neoplasm in this marbled salamander, *A. opacum*, has been examined by the authors of this chapter and reclassified as a mixed cell adenoma (see below).

Squamous Cell Carcinoma ("Epithelioma"). The squamous cell carcinoma (SCC) is an aggressive invasive malignancy arising from epidermal cells. All reported amphibian squamous cell carcinomata have been well differentiated. In the northern leopard frog, *Rana pipiens,* the neoplasm was found only in aged animals, from 3.5 to over 5 years of age (Van Der Steen et al., 1972). Grossly, SCC have been described as buttonlike or slightly pedunculated, discrete, raised, and hypopigmented (Figures 26.12, 26.13). Neoplastic squamous cells form solid cords and nests that invade the dermis and may invade the subcutis (Figures 26.14, 26.15), skeletal muscle, and bone. Occasionally, nests and cords of squamous cells may appear to form central cavities that at low magnifications give a glandular (tubular) appearance. These tubulelike cords of cells may be diagnostically confusing (Murray, 1908). At the periphery of each nest, cells are smaller, more basophilic and cuboidal. Moving centrally, cells become larger, polygonal, with abundant eosinophilic cytoplasm that shows keratin formation. Cell borders are consistently distinct. Intercellular bridges are easily demonstrated, and are considered a hallmark of the squamous cell carcinoma (see Figure 26.15). Larger central cells may have nuclear-cytoplasmic ratios of 1:5 to 1:10. Centrally, keratinization may progress into nodules of concentric lamination called keratin pearls. Numerous necrotic cells are often scattered throughout the nests. Mitotic rates are highly variable, but, in those examined to date, have ranged from one per five high power fields to one per one high power field. Metastases have not been reported, although multicentric neoplasms have oc-

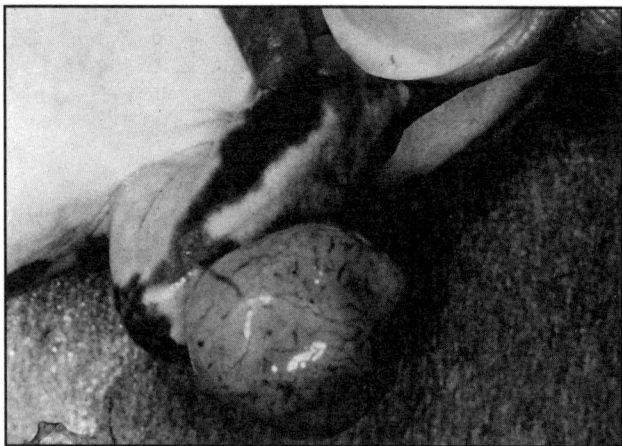

Figure 26.12. Squamous cell carcinoma of northern leopard frog, *Rana pipiens*. This fleshy pedunculated mass occurred on a forelimb at the humero-radioulnar joint. A second, possibly metastatic, smaller nodule was present in the skin over the sternum. (D.H. Ringler, University of Michigan, taken from Van Der Steen et al., 1972, with permission)

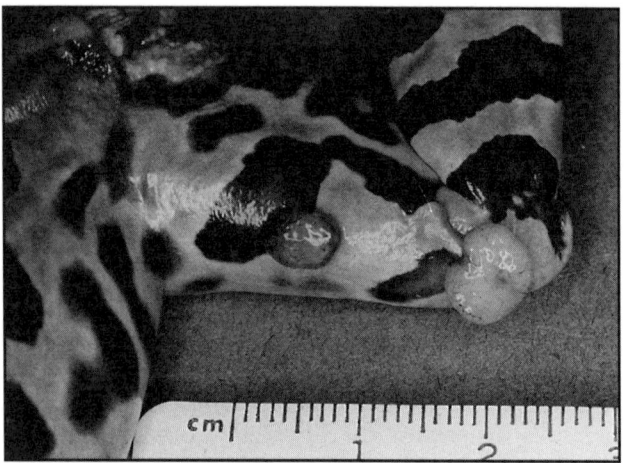

Figure 26.13. Squamous cell carcinomata on the hindlimb of a northern leopard frog, *Rana pipiens*. The smaller midthigh mass may be metastic from the larger fleshy mass at the stifle. (D.H. Ringler, University of Michigan, taken from Van Der Steen et al., 1972, with permission)

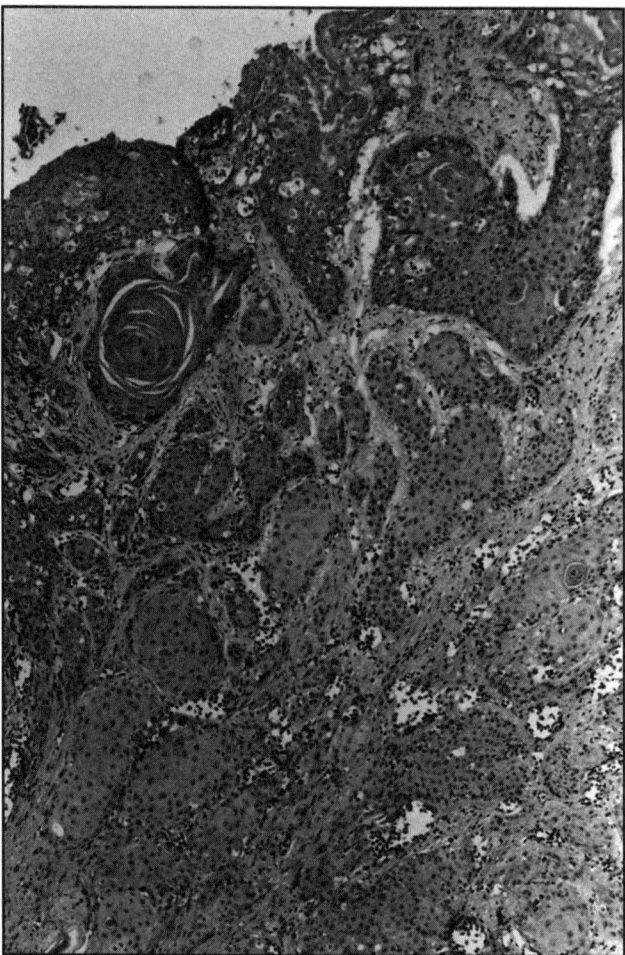

Figure 26.14. Squamous cell carcinoma in a northern leopard frog, *Rana pipiens*. The digital skin has cords of neoplastic cells invading dermis and subcutis. Smaller, basal-like epithelial cells are present at the periphery with larger plump cells centrally in each cord. Occasional concentrically lamellated nodules of keratin ("keratin pearls") occur centrally in some cords. (B.J. Cohen, RTLA 660)

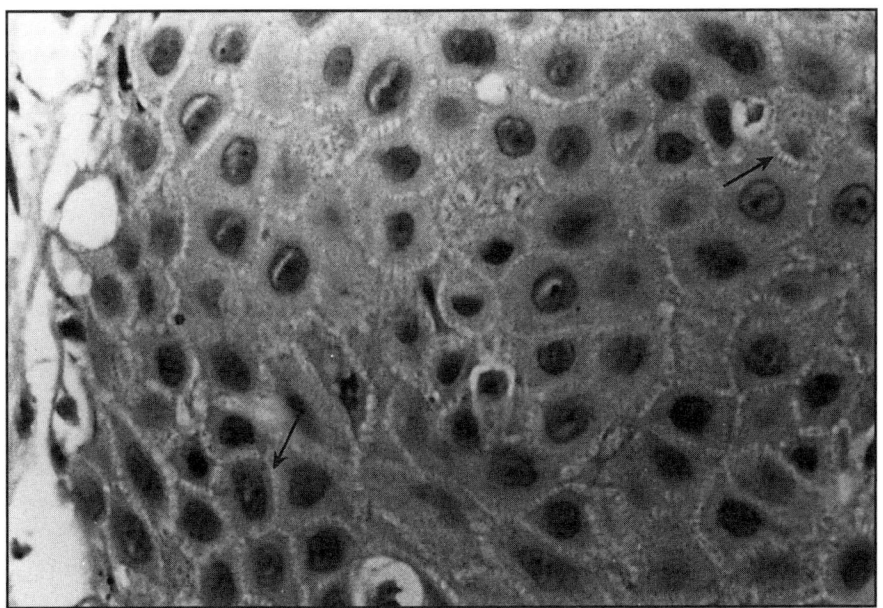

Figure 26.15. Squamous cell carcinoma in a northern leopard frog, *Rana pipiens;* higher magnification of Figure 26.14. This portion of one cord of neoplastic cells shows characteristic prominent intercellular bridges (arrows). (B.J. Cohen, RTLA 660)

curred and local deep invasion of skeletal muscles and bone may be extensive (Murray, 1908; Van Der Steen et al., 1972).

26.2.2 Dermal Gland Neoplasms

The skin of anurans and salmanders is rich in glandular tissue. Glands are distributed over most of the body and may coalesce into distinct grossly recognizable skin glands such as the parotid gland, mental gland, and others. A complex mix of glands also is present in the cloaca. Although these cloacal glands resemble highly specialized dermal glands and could be discussed in this section on integument, these cloacal neoplasms are for convenience described in Section 26.7, Neoplasms of the Alimentary Tract.

The normal dermal gland may consist of three or more cell types, depending on how many types of duct cells are counted. There are the basic secretory epithelial gland cells, surrounding myoepithelial cells, and duct cells. In mammals the neoplastic myoepithelial cell is a pleuripotential mesenchymal cell that may form bundles and streams of fibroblastic or leiomyocytelike cells as well as myxoid material, cartilage and bone. Benign and malignant tumors composed only of the duct cells or myoepithelial cells have not been published in amphibians, however, three reports (Broz, 1947; Counts et al., 1975; Pirlot & Welsch, 1934) of skin tumors that contained cartilage have been reinterpreted as skin tumors containing neoplastic myoepithelial cells.

In studies of large numbers of Russian and North American ranids, neoplasms of dermal glands were found. Among 1300 Russian ranids, neoplasms were papillary cystadenomata and cystadenocarcinomata; one to seven neoplasms per frog were found. A spontaneous dermal gland adenocarcinoma was reported on the hindlimb of a leopard frog (possibly *Rana berlandieri*) from Mexico (Van Der Steen et al., 1974). Most of the neoplasms in the Russian frogs also were found on the limbs or ventral body skin (Khudoley & Mizgireuv, 1980).

Papillary Cystadenoma (Cystadenopapilloma). Papillary cystadenoma has been reported only in European frogs, mostly the European common frog, *Rana temporaria,* and the marsh frog, *R. ridibunda.* The vast majority of cases come from frogs in Russia near Leningrad (Khudoley & Mizgireuv, 1980). This same population of frogs had several cystic adenocarcinomata of dermal mucous glands, suggesting the suspected benign neoplasms may transform into malignancies (Khudoley & Mizgireuv, 1980). Each frog had one to seven neoplasms in the skin, but the authors were not clear how many frogs had benign neoplasms and how many had malignancies. In another frog (*Rana* sp.), 24 separate tumors were found in the skin, all of which were confined to the dermis (Pentimalli, 1914). Also, it was noted that the tumors were highly vascular and bled freely when abraded or cut (Pentimalli, 1914). Histologically, one or multiple adjacent dermal glands have markedly dilated central lumina and stratified cellular walls that often produce simple papillary projections into the lumen (Figures 26.16, 26.17). Instead of the normal one cell thickness in the gland, cells are stacked three to ten cells deep. Cells are cuboidal or polygonal, with dense round central nuclei and a nuclear to cytoplasmic ratio of 1:1 to 1:3. Cytoplasm is pale-staining, and often contains clear vacuoles. Variable numbers of necrotic gland cells are present in the wall and lumen. Although blood vessels may be numerous, fibrous stroma is scant.

Mixed Cell Adenoma (Compound Adenoma). Normal dermal glands of amphibians are composed of two (three, if ductal cells are included) major cell types: the secretory cells and the myoepithelial cells, that are flattened and very thin. The myoepithelial cell is an epithelial cell containing myofilaments. Both cells may give rise to neoplasms, either independently or in combination. The combined (or compound) neoplasm is referred to as a mixed (or compound)

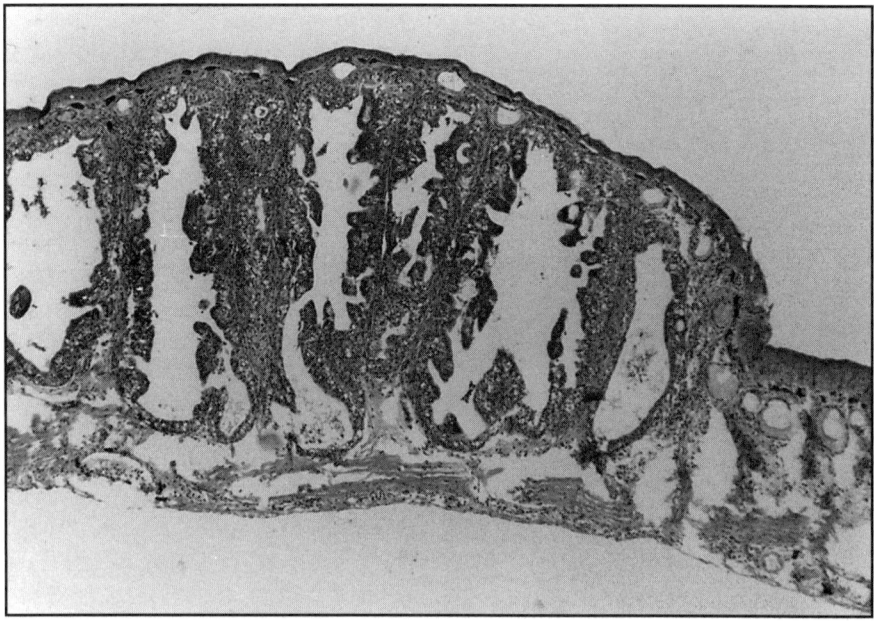

Figure 26.16. Papillary cystadenoma of dermal glands in a European common frog, *Rana temporaria*. Multiple dilated dermal glands show cellular papillary projections into lumina but no perforation of basement membranes. (V.V. Khudoley, RTLA 2127)

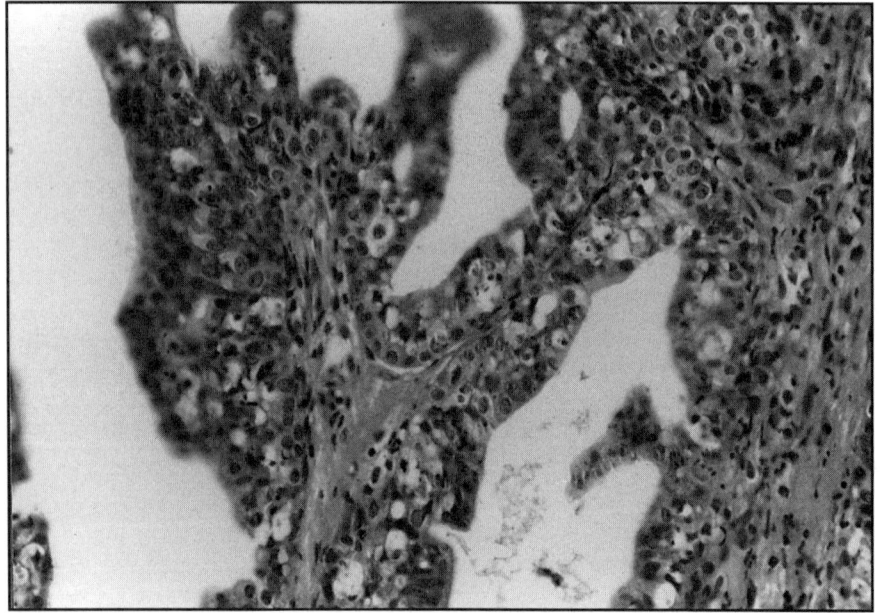

Figure 26.17. Papillary cystadenoma of dermal glands in a European common frog, *Rana temporaria*; higher magnification of Figure 26.16. (V.V. Khudoley, RTLA 2127)

by myoepithelial cells is often well differentiated and resembles mature cartilage (Figures 26.18, 26.19). One neoplasm composed of proliferating glandular cells and myoepithelial cells has been described in the neck region of a wild adult male marbled salamander, *Ambystoma opacum,* from West Virginia, U.S.A. (Counts et al., 1975). The authors considered the neoplasm to be a basal cell tumor, and the myoepithelial component of the neoplasm was misinterpreted as simple stroma. Grossly, the neoplasm was encapsulated, markedly domed or hemispherical, and had grayishly discolored, nonulcerated overlying skin. Histologically, the mixed cell neoplasm contains two cell types: nests of basophilic glandular cells forming tubules, and myoepithelial cells. The latter are pale spindle cells forming concentric layers around proliferating glands and bundles and streams of cells which differentiate into irregularly shaped nodules of cartilage (see Figure 26.18). In the neoplasm of the marbled salamander, the glandular nests are composed of tubules lined by cuboidal and columnar epithelium. Occasional tubules appear to have a double layer of epithelial cells, suggestive of duct cell origin (see Figure 26.18).

Myoepithelial Adenoma (Myoepithelioma). Adenomas and adenocarcinomas composed solely of myoepithelial cells have not been recognized or reported in amphibians. However, there are two reports (Broz, 1947; Pirlot & Welsch, 1934) of multiple "chondromas" in the skin of amphibians that can be reinterpreted as myoepithelial adenomata (myoepithelioma). In the two amphibians, a smooth newt, *Triturus vulgaris* (formerly *Triton taeniatus*) and a frog, *Rana fusca*, nodules of well-differentiated cartilage were present in the dermis. At the time both neoplasms were reported, the existence or appearance of neoplastic myoepithelial cells was probably unknown, as was the propensity for myoepithelial cells to produce chondroid stroma.

tumor, while the neoplasm composed only of myoepithelium is called a myoepithelioma. Proliferative myoepithelium resembles fibrous stroma, but often produces a myxoid or chondroid component. In mammals, bone also may be produced by proliferating myoepithelial cells, but bone has not been reported in association with any amphibian dermal neoplasms. The chondroid stroma (cartilage) produced

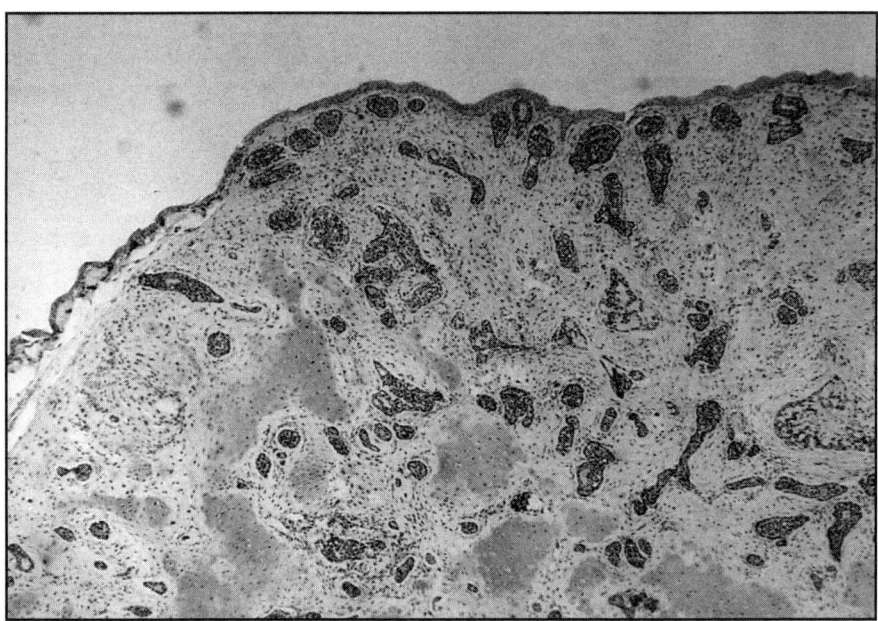

Figure 26.18. Mixed cell adenoma of dermal gland in a marbled salamander, *Ambystoma opacum*. This neoplasm is composed of two cell types: secretory gland cells and nonsecretory myoepithelial cells. Irregular nests of dark glandular cells are surrounded by loose fusiform cells (myoepithelial cells). Myoepithelial cells also have differentiated into irregular islands of cartilage. (C.L. Counts, RTLA 820)

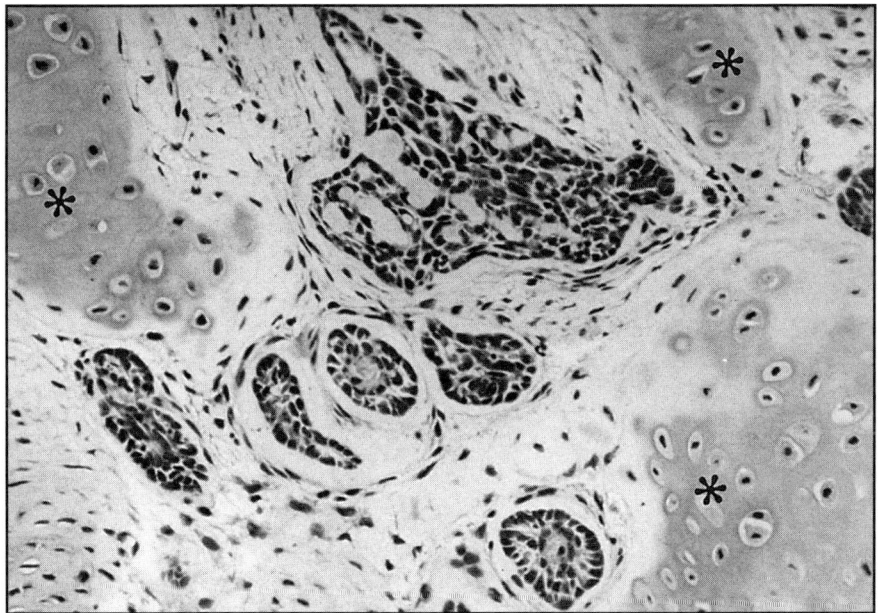

Figure 26.19. Mixed cell adenoma of dermal gland in a marbled salamander, *Ambystoma opacum*; higher magnification of Figure 26.18. The secretory epithelial cells form tubules, some of which appear to have a double layer of cuboidal cells. Neoplastic tubules are surrounded and separated by fusiform myoepithelial cells with islands of cartilage (asterisks). (C.L. Counts, RTLA 820)

A case of multiple "chondromata" in the skin of a smooth newt, *Triturus vulgaris,* one published photomicrograph shows a nodule of well-differentiated dermal cartilage clearly arising from the capsule (and therefore the myoepithelial region) of a dermal gland. This physical connection between a dermal gland and the nodule of cartilage is sufficiently well illustrated (Broz, 1947) to permit a revised morphologic diagnosis of multiple myoepithelial adenomata (myoepitheliomata).

Cystadenocarcinoma. Cystadenocarcinomas have been reported only in wild specimens of the European common frog, *Rana temporaria,* and the marsh frog, *R. ridibunda,* near Leningrad. These malignancies occurred in conjunction with a number of benign counterparts, cystadenomas. The precise number of malignant neoplasms in these Russian frogs was not clear for benign and malignant neoplasms were listed as a single group. Among 320 specimens of the European common frog, *R. temporaria,* collected in the autumns of 1976–1978, seven (2.2%) had 31 dermal gland neoplasms. Among 978 specimens of the marsh frog, *R. ridibunda,* collected in the same time period, 16 (1.6%) had 47 skin neoplasms. It was not clear if any frogs with multiple neoplasms had both benign and malignant tumors. The malignant neoplasms resembled the benign tumors (see above), except there was invasion of the basement membrane of the gland, and of the dermis and subcutis. Only one mucous gland neoplasm among 23 affected frogs (or 1.3% of all 78 detected neoplasms) from Leningrad demonstrated metastasis, although many others were locally aggressive (Khudoley & Mizgireuv, 1980).

Adenocarcinoma, Tubular Type. The few reports of dermal gland malignancies usually do not specify whether the neoplasm arose from mucous or serous (granular) dermal glands. Adenocarcinomata with solid or signet-ring patterns have not been reported in amphibians. A dermal gland adenocarcinoma occurred on the hindlimb of a leopard frog recently imported from Mexico (probably the Rio Grande leopard frog, *Rana berlandieri*) (Figure 26.20). Grossly, the frog had a single dermal nodule that was distinctly dome-shaped, almost pedunculated, and well demarcated. The overlying epidermis was "stretched" (Van Der Steen et al., 1972). Histologically, numerous small glandlike cellular nests have a prominent or indistinct central lumen (Figures 26.21, 26.22). The glandlike nests contain about 5–100 cells. Smaller acini have a single cell layer of cuboidal cells, while more cellular nests may have an indistinct or no central lumen. Thin cords of cells also are evident. Cells are cuboidal or polygonal with mostly round nuclei, often with indistinct cytoplasmic

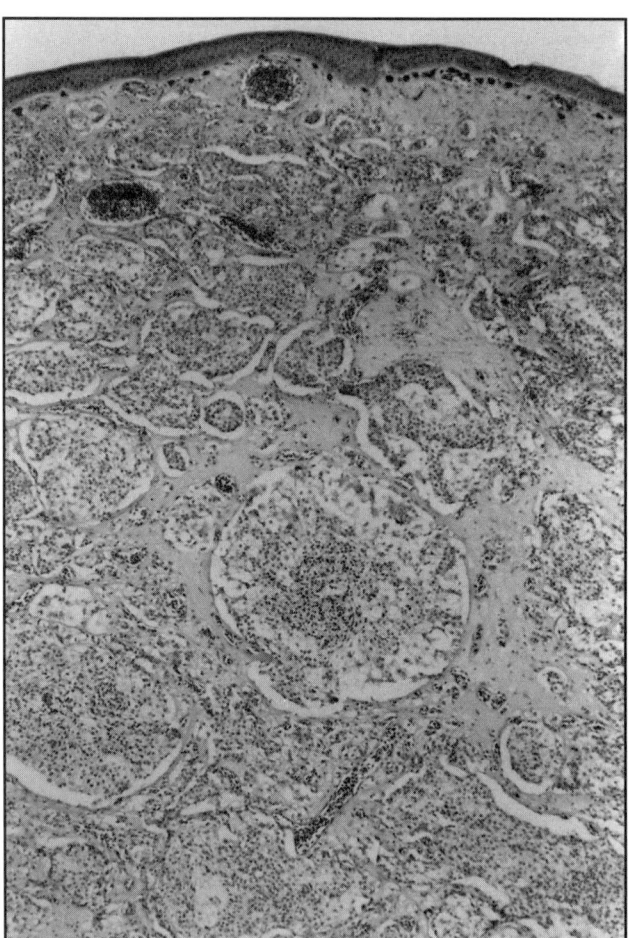

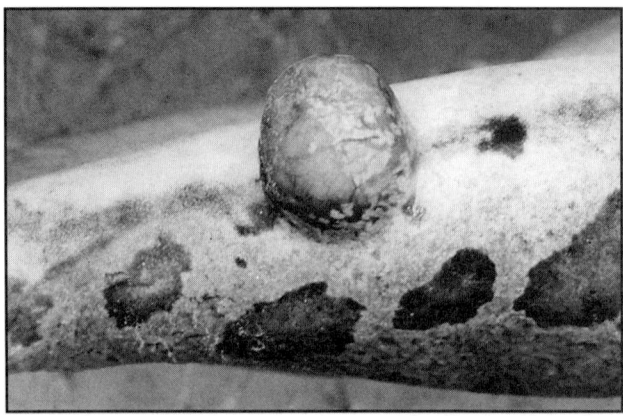

Figure 26.20. Adenocarcinoma of dermal gland in a leopard frog from Mexico (possibly *Rana berlandieri* or *Rana chiricahuensis*). The intradermal mass of the left hindlimb elevates and stretches the epidermis (D.H. Ringler, University of Michigan, taken from Van Der Steen et al., 1972, with permission)

Figure 26.21. Adenocarcinoma of dermal gland, tubular type, histology of Figure 26.20. The irregular sizes and shapes of nests of neoplastic dermal glands are separated by moderate amounts of edematous fibrovascular stroma. (B.J. Cohen, RTLA 659)

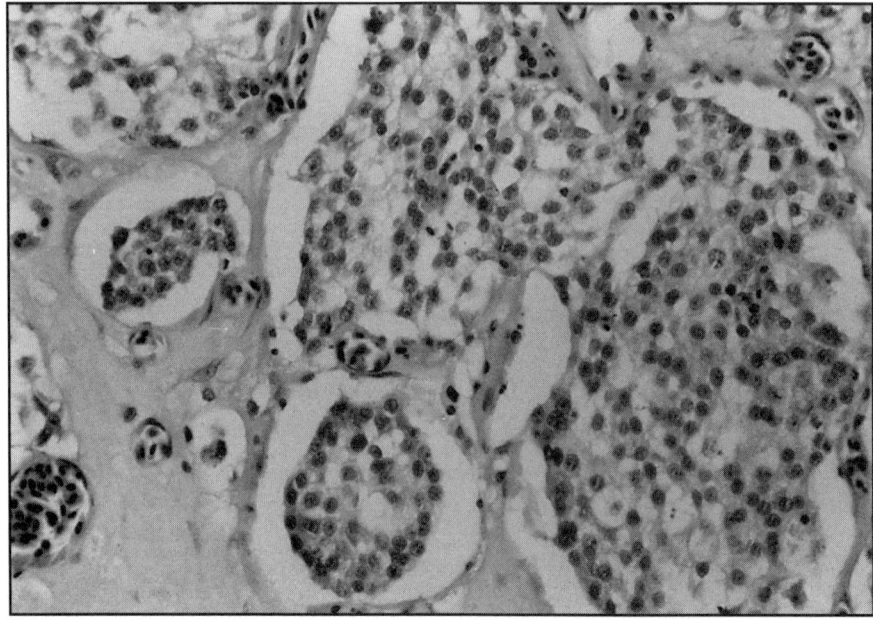

Figure 26.22. Adenocarcinoma of dermal gland, tubular type; higher magnification of Figure 26.21. Neoplastic cells have irregular subtle tubular lumina. The clear spaces separating clusters of neoplastic cells from the basement membrane are due to mild autolysis and artifacts of processing. (B.J. Cohen, RTLA 659)

borders. Nucleoli are single and variable in size. Some stain distinctly magenta. Mitotic rate is low, about one per five high power fields (400×). Scattered necrotic cells and multinucleated cells may be evident. Fibrovascular stroma is moderate and often edematous. Invasion of the stratum compactum and subcutis may occur.

26.2.3 Neoplasms of Chromatophores

Amphibians have at least five types of pigment cells: melanophores, xanthophores, iridophores, erythrophores, and laminophores. The only reported neoplasms of amphibian chromatophores have arisen from melanophores.

Terminology surrounding neoplasms of pigment cells, especially melanophores (called melanocytes in birds and mammals), is confusing and shifting. The authors of this chapter prefer the term melanophoroma over other terms, such as melanophoma, melanocytoma, melanoma, and melanosarcoma (Khudoley & Elisiev, 1979).

Most reports of melanophoromata in amphibians are one or a few cases among hundreds or thousands of amphibians or in collections of many types of neoplasia. However, abnormally high prevalences of melanophoromata have been reported in two populations of wild caudates: neotenic specimens of the barred tiger salamander, *Ambystoma tigrinum mavortium*, from a sewage lagoon in Texas (Figures 26.23, 26.24, 26.25), and specimens of the northern crested newt, *Triturus cristatus*, associated with rice paddy agriculture in Italy (Rose, 1981; Rose & Harshbarger, 1977; Zavanella, 1974, 1975). Both amphibian populations appear to have been chronically exposed to potentially carcinogenic chemical pollutants. When some neotenes of the barred tiger salamander, *Ambystoma tigrinum mavortium*, were placed in clean water, regression of small melanophoromata occurred (Rose, 1981).

Melanophoromata of the axolotl, *Ambystoma mexicanum*, and the African clawed frog, *Xenopus laevis*, have two interesting additional biological features: an inherited predisposition to dermal melanophoromata

Figure 26.23. Melanophoroma, intradermal type, in a wild neotenic barred tiger salamander, *Ambystoma tigrinum mavortium*. (F.L. Rose, RTLA 954)

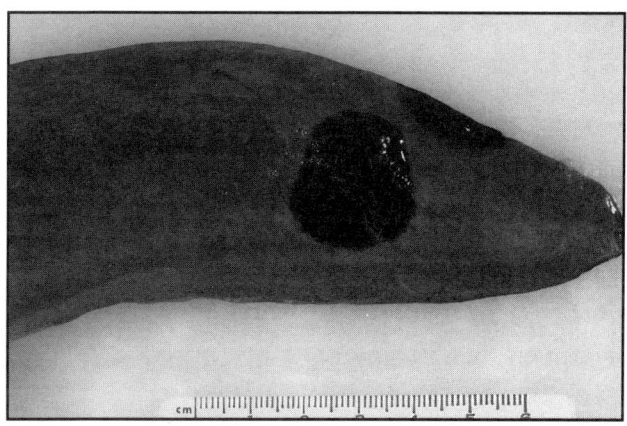

Figure 26.24. Melanophoromata, intradermal type, in a wild neotenic barred tiger salamander, *Ambystoma tigrinum mavortium*. (F.L. Rose, RTLA 950)

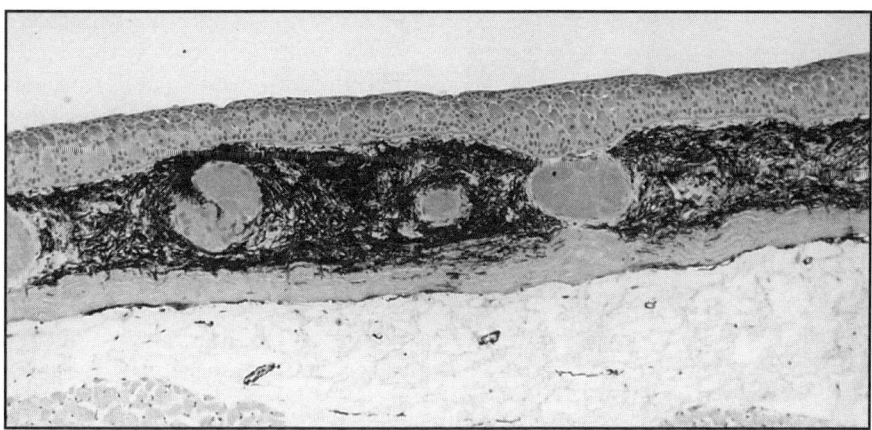

Figure 26.25. Benign melanophoroma, dendritic and intradermal type, in a neotenic barred tiger salamander, *Ambystoma tigrinum mavortium*. Dendritic melanophores are prominent within the dermis but have not invaded the epidermis and subcutis. Some intradermal proliferations of melanophores regressed in salamanders that were placed in clean water for several months. (F.L. Rose, RTLA 916)

was observed in an axolotl colony in Germany (Sheremetieva-Brunst & Brunst, 1948), and herpesvirus-like particles have been detected ultrastructurally in the nuclei of melanophoroma cells in a colony of African clawed frogs in Japan (Asashima et al., 1989; Oinuma et al., 1984). The colony of axolotls with inherited melanophoromas was lost in World War II.

Melanophoroma, Dendritic Type. Most (presumably) benign melanophoromas have occurred in captive specimens of the axolotl, *Ambystoma mexicanum* (Figure 26.26), and wild neotenic specimens of the tiger salamander, *A. tigrinum* (see Figure 26.25), and the northern crested newt, *Triturus cristattus*. Excluding clawed frogs, *Xenopus* spp., only two melanophoromas have been reported in anurans (see Table 26.1 appearing at the end of this chapter). This usually benign neoplasm in amphibians arises in the dermis. Grossly, the tumor is small (<1 cm), very darkly pigmented on natural and cut surfaces, and causes minimal to marked swelling of the epidermis. Most are poorly or not at all encapsulated. Melanophores are consistently laden with melanin. Cell bodies are black globules with the nuclei usually obscured, hence, studies of mitotic rates are seldom reported. In one report in which a melanin bleach technique was used (Khudoley & Elisiev, 1979), the nuclei were pleomorphic, lacked mitotic figures, and frequent multinucleated cells were evident. In less densely cellular regions, melanophores have numerous, irregularly branching cytoplasmic projections, diagnostic of the dendritic cell type.

Melanophoroma, Fibromatous Type. Fibromatous melanophoromas probably are benign. Neoplasms of this type occurred in neotenes of the barred tiger salamander, *Ambystoma tigrinum mavortium*, in a sewage lagoon in Texas (Rose & Harshbarger, 1977) (Figures 26.27, 26.28). Many other salamanders in the lagoon had a variety of other neoplastic and hyperplastic (and possibly metaplastic) diseases of the skin. In one specimen, a marked cellular thickening of the dermis caused a domelike elevation of the overlying epidermis. Histologically, the neoplastic spindle-shaped melanophores are hypomelanotic, but a few scattered single or clustered melanin-laden melanophages are evident. Tumor cells are spindle-shaped, and form streaming and interweaving bundles (see Figure 26.27). Cytoplasm is pale, eosinophilic, fibrous, and abundant, but cell borders are indistinct. Nuclei are variable in size, mostly elongate, have thin but prominent chromatinic rims, fine to coarse euchromatin, and small single or double nucleoli. Mitotic rate is less than one per ten high power fields. No invasion of the subcutis or deeper structures occurs.

Melanophoroma, Epithelioid Type. Epithelioid melanophoromas probably are malignant. At least two of eight specimens of the African clawed frog, *Xenopus laevis*, with melanophoromas had neoplastic cell features consistent with this type (Asashima et al., 1989; Oinuma et al., 1984) (It appears that four of the eight neoplasms reported by Asashima et al., 1989, were previously reported by Oinuma et al., 1984). In a 1-year period, four melanophoromas were detected grossly in a population of about 20,000 clawed frogs (Oinuma et al., 1984). The neoplasms were distinct masses in the dermis of the back (n = 5), on the legs (n = 2) or the ventral abdomen (n = 1). Dorsal neoplasms often projected caudally from the scapular region to the proximal hindlimbs (Asashima et al., 1989). The tumors were 5–18 mm in diameter, firm to hard, often had a central necrotic cavity, and cut surfaces were whitish with "several black spots" (Oinuma et al., 1984). Neoplastic cells in the dermis are plump, polygonal, epithelial-shaped, have relatively abundant cytoplasm, distinct cell borders, and form solid sheets of cells with scant fibrovascular

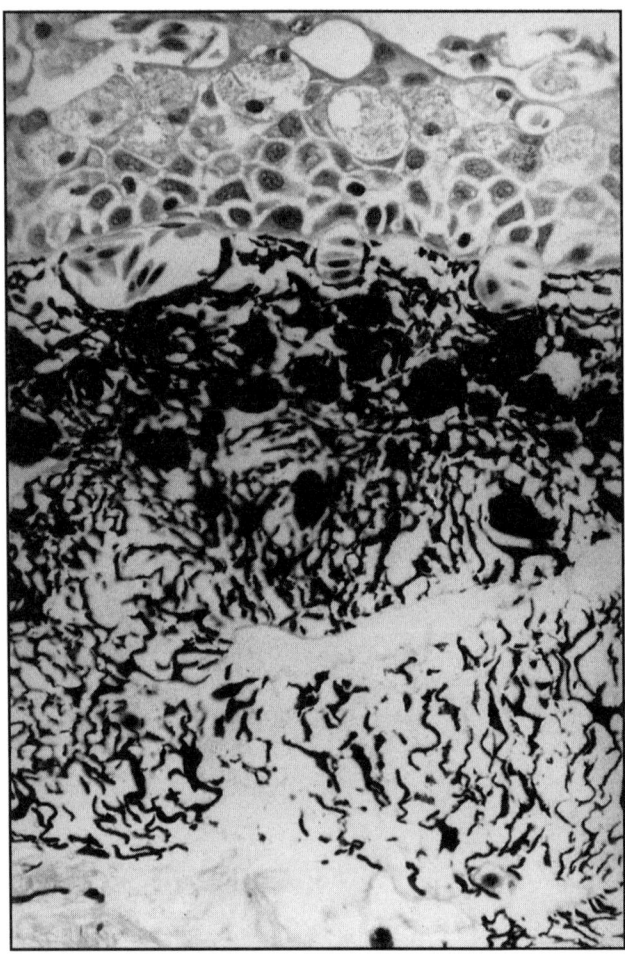

Figure 26.26. Melanophoroma, dendritic type, in an axolotl, *Ambystoma mexicanum*. The dermis is nearly completely replaced by dendritic melanophores. Dendritic melanophoroma cells nearly always are heavily laden with melanin, thus obscuring nuclear morphology and mitotic rate. (L.E. Delanney, RTLA 2803)

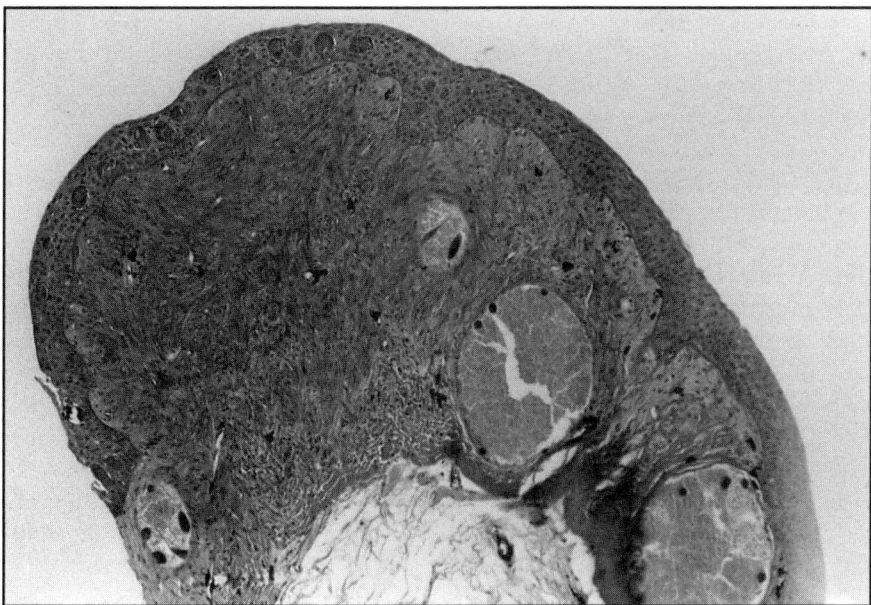

Figure 26.27. Benign melanophoroma, fibromatous and hypomelanotic type, in a neotenic barred tiger salamander, *Ambystoma tigrinum mavortium*. Note the streaming fibromatous character of neoplastic cells, and absence of invasion of the stratum compactum. (F.L. Rose, RTLA 791)

stroma. Cells near the necrotic core tend to be larger and have more cytoplasm, while those at the periphery that may be involved in active invasion of dermal and muscular tissue are smaller and more fibroblastic, or even dendritic in shape. Nearly all neoplastic cells are hypomelanotic. Neoplastic cells have a fine dusting of melanin granules, and a few scattered distinct globular melanophages (melanin-laden macrophages) are present. Nuclei are pleomorphic, anisokaryosis is usually evident, and mitoses are infrequent (six of 1926 nuclei, 0.31%) (Oinuma et al., 1984). Nucleoli were not described, but in epithelioid malignant melanomas of domestic mammals, nucleoli are often large and very prominent. The neoplasms were considered malignant because invasion of skeletal musculature and spread (or metastasis) via the caudally

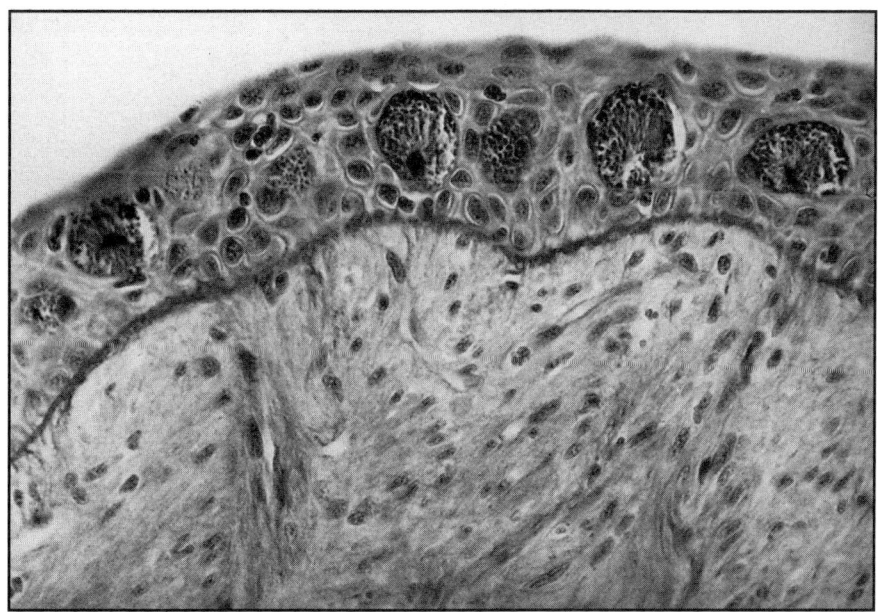

Figure 26.28. Benign melanophoroma, fibromatous and hypomelanotic type; higher magnification of Figure 26.27. Note the fibrocyte-like appearance of the neoplastic melanophores. Basement membrane is not invaded and melanin and mitotic figures are sparse. (F.L. Rose, RTLA 791)

draining lymphatic sacs was evident (Asashima et al., 1989; Carter, 1979). As previously noted, one potentially very significant ultrastructural feature of melanophoromas in the African clawed frog, *Xenopus laevis,* is the presence, in an unspecified number of neoplasm-bearing frogs, of intranuclear and cytoplasmic icosohedral virus particles, highly suggestive of a herpevirus (Asashima et al., 1989).

Malignant Melanophoroma. Malignant melanophoromas may be heavily pigmented or hypomelanotic tumors, but show clear invasion of the subcutis (subcutaneous lymph sacs), infiltration of underlying skeletal muscle, or metastasis to internal organs (Harshbarger & Snyder, 1989). Cellular morphology usually is dendritic in the pigmented neoplasms (Figure 26.29), and epithelioid in the hypopigmented malignancies (Figures 26.30, 26.31, 26.32). Amphibians with multiple melanophoromata have been reported but in some cases it has been suggested that the neoplasms arose independently, rather than being metastatic.

26.2.4 Neoplasms of Epidermal Neurosensory Cells (Lateral Line and Ampullary Organ Cells)

Sensory cells of the lateral line system on the head, body, and tail of larval and other aquatic amphibians are called neuromast cells, thus a neoplasm of these cells should be called a neuromastoma. Reports in the literature usually refer to this tumor as a neuroepithelioma. Early reports, especially of those neoplasms arising on the head, may have referred to this neoplasm as an epithelioma (Champy & Champy, 1935) or as having arisen from olfactory neuroepithelial cells, however, presence of these neoplasms on the body and tail makes the latter origin unlikely. Recently recognized ampullary organs, restricted to the head of some caudate taxa (e.g., the axolotl, *Ambystoma mexicanum*),

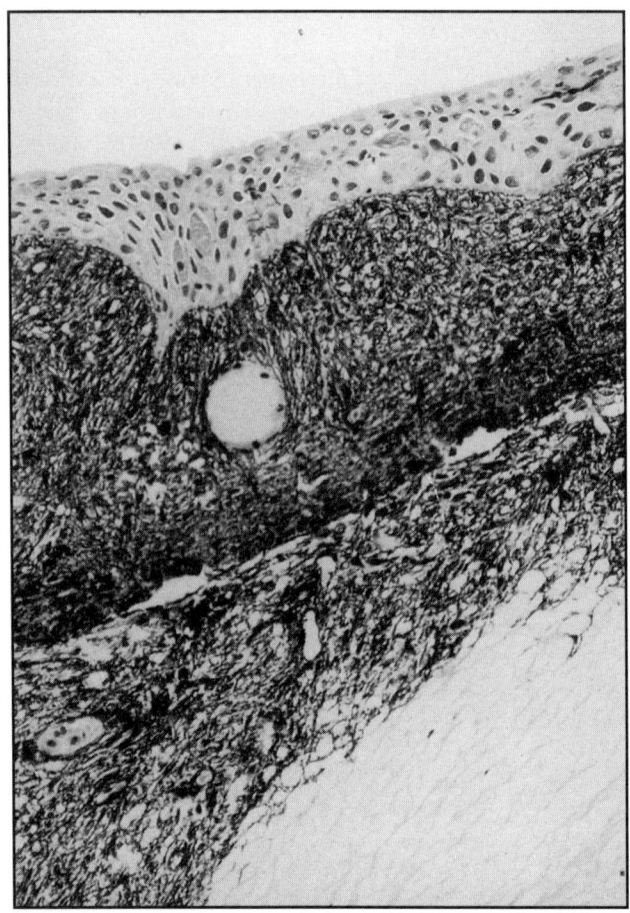

Figure 26.29. Malignant melanophoroma, dendritic type, in a neotenic barred tiger salamander, *Ambystoma tigrinum mavortium*. The stratum compactum and subcutis have been invaded by dendritic-shaped melanophores; invasion of skeletal muscles also was present (not shown). Neoplastic cells are infiltrating laterally in the dermis. (C.E. Smith, RTLA 3286)

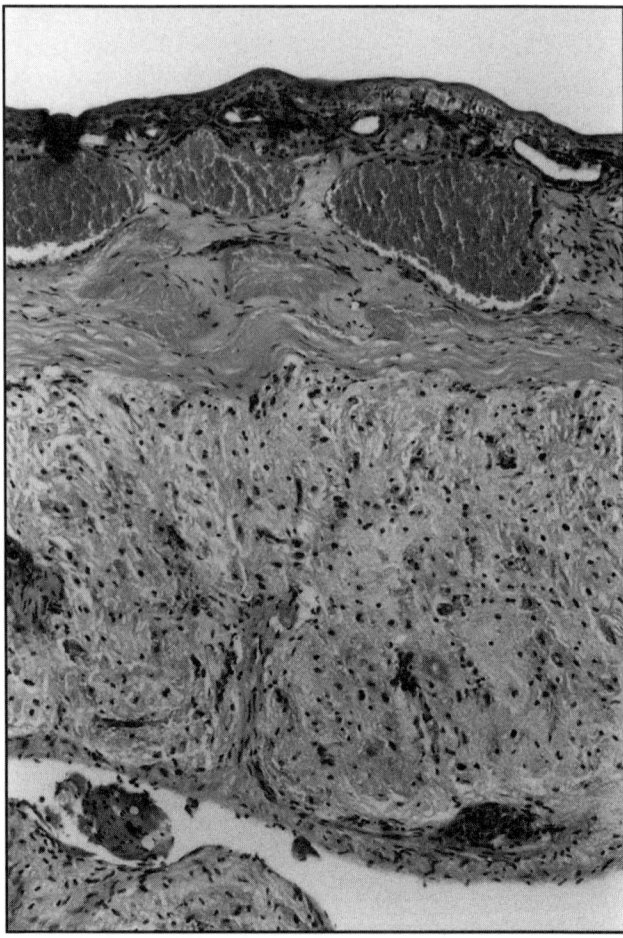

Figure 26.30. Malignant melanophoroma, epithelioid type, in a veined (golden-eyed) treefrog, *Phrynohyas venulosa*. Malignant melanophores have abundant cytoplasm but indistinct cell borders and scant amounts of melanin granules. (M.D. McGavin, AFIP 1761009)

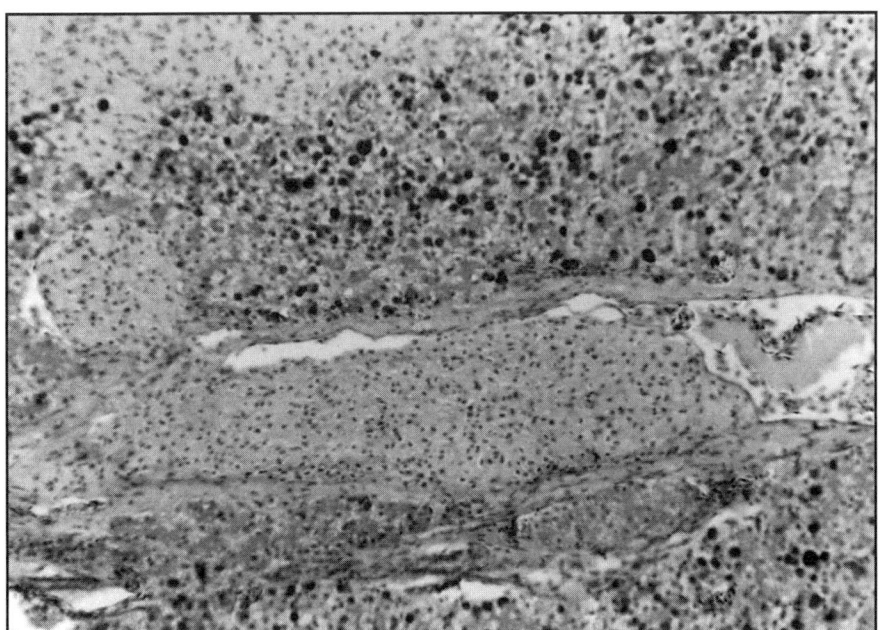

Figure 26.31. Malignant melanophoroma, epithelioid type, same as Figure 26.30. Metastatic nodules of tumor cells are present in this section of liver, and were present in many other organs. Centrally, note the intravascular invasion by metastatic cells. (M.D. McGavin, AFIP 1761009)

are composed of similar cells that are called electroreceptors. At present, it is not possible to determine whether a neuromastoma on the head arose from cells of the lateral line system, pit organs, ampullary organs, or the olfactory epithelium. However, since only lateral line neuromasts occur caudal to the neck, a neuroepithelial neoplasm on the body or tail almost certainly arose from lateral line neuromasts. Oral neuroepitheliomas have been reported in the axolotl, *A. mexicanum* (Brunst & Roque, 1967; Humphrey, 1969), but distinguishing the neoplasms of possible olfactory cell origin from neuromasts (or electroreceptor cells), is not possible at this time.

Neuromastoma (Neuroepithelioma). Three, possibly four, neoplasms of neuromasts have been reported: two (or three) from Laurenti's alpine newt, *Triturus alpestris,* and one from the tail of an axolotl, *Ambystoma mexicanum*. One neoplasm on the head of a newt was centered dorsally between the eyes, occupied most of the space between the upper lids, was distinctly domed, and was covered by glistening epithelium. Histologically, cells form well-delineated nests, lobes, and rosettes of varying size, often with a distinct central lumen (Figure 26.33). The lumen of the rosette usually is empty but may contain coagulated material, occasional sloughed tumor cells, other cellular debris, and rarely erythrocytes. Fibrovascular stroma prominently separates lobes. The cells are columnar to elongate, are arranged perpendicularly to the peripheral edge of the lobe, and may be one layer thick or stratified (see Figure 26.33). In rosettes that are one or two cell layers thick, the nuclei are often basally (peripherally) located, leaving only prominent segments of cytoplasm in the region adjacent to the central lumen. Nuclei are ovoid to spindaloid, dense and dark, or heavily stippled with heterochromatin. Mitotic rate is low, usually less than 1% of neoplastic cells. Special stains may demonstrate neurite-like neurofibrils (Brunst & Roque, 1967). Invasion of the dermis and subcutis occurs, but distant metastases have not been reported. One of the three spontaneous neoplasms reported in Laurenti's alpine newt, *T. alpestris,* appears to have had several features of a neuromastoma (Champy & Champy, 1935). Neuromastomata

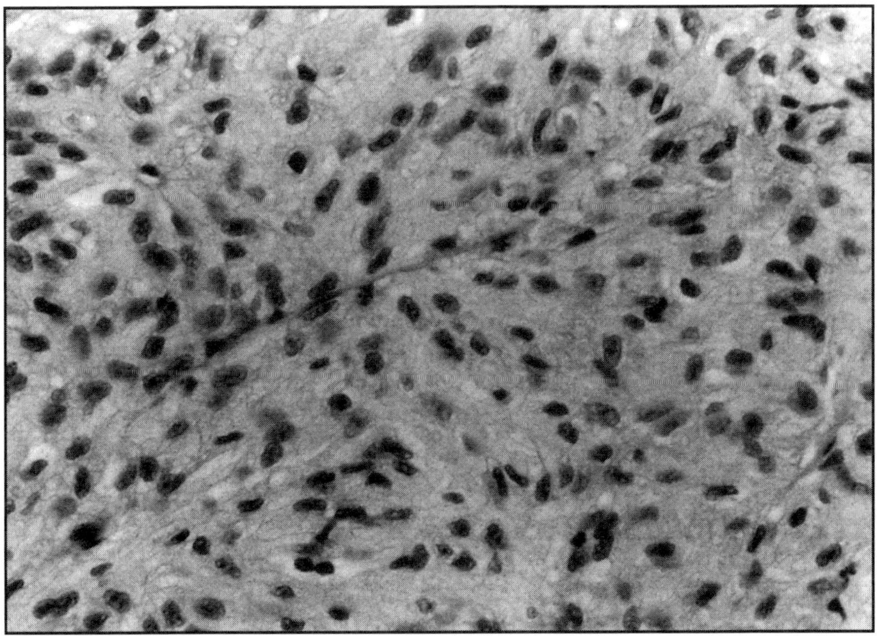

Figure 26.32. Malignant melanophoroma, epithelioid type; higher magnification of Figure 26.31. Anisokaryosis and karyomegaly are evident. Occasionally, large prominent nucleoli are present in karyomegalic malignant cells. (M.D. McGavin, AFIP 1761009)

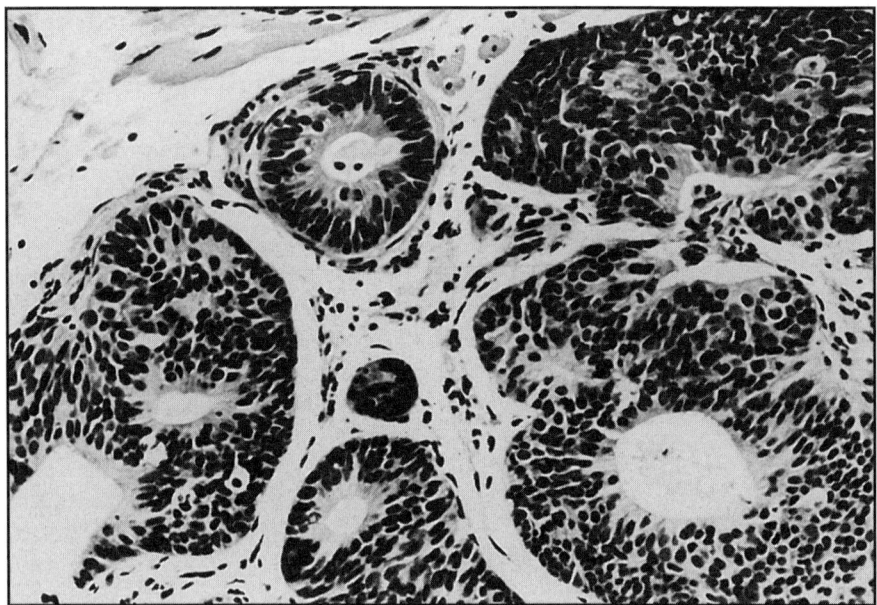

Figure 26.33. Neuromastoma in the pelvic subcutis of an axolotl, *Ambystoma mexicanum*. Note the discrete nests of cells separated by prominent stroma. Cords of columnar cells usually form rosettes; cells have a stratified appearance with uniformly dark, ovoid to elongate nuclei located peripherally. (L.E. Delanney, RTLA 1674)

have been successfully transplanted and have been experimentally induced by various carcinogens (Darquenne, 1972; Matz, 1982).

26.3 NEOPLASMS OF THE MESENCHYMAL TISSUES

26.3.1 Neoplasms of Fibrous Tissue

Fibroma. Fibromas of the oral cavity, coelom, limb, and skin have been reported (Elkan 1960; Rose 1981; Schwarz 1923; Vaillant & Pettit, 1902 as cited by Balls & Clothier, 1974). It is possible some fibrocytic neoplasms that were reported as dermal fibromas were actually fibropapillomas. The first reported fibroma in an amphibian is a remarkable case. A giant Japanese salamander, *Andrias japonicus*, in Paris, was in captivity from 1859 until its death in 1897. The salamander had a tumor on the palmar surface of the right forelimb that persisted for 25 years. At death, the tumor measured 10 cm in diameter, had a multinodular surface, and intact overlying epidermis. Histologically, the mass consisted of interweaving bundles and whorls of spindle cells with prominent vascularity. Nuclei of the cells varied greatly in size; some were small with abundant chromatin and others were large and vesicular (Vaillant & Pettit, 1902, as cited by Schlumberger & Lucke, 1948). A second case of fibroma in the same salamander species was reported two decades later. This tumor also occurred on a forelimb, was 2 cm in diameter, and had histologic features similar to the previous case (Schwarz, 1923 as cited by Schlumberger & Lucke, 1948).

More recent reports of fibromata in amphibians have less certain diagnoses. Some dermal neoplasms found on neotenes of the barred tiger salamander, *Ambystoma tigrinum mavortium,* from a polluted sewage lagoon in Texas, have been reported as fibromas (Rose 1981; Rose & Harshbarger 1977), but a few were, instead, fibropapillomata or mast cell tumors. Grossly the fibromata were gray, smooth-surfaced, and occasionally had multilobular protuberances. Histologically, the neoplasms consisted of randomly oriented bundles of fibrocytes (Rose & Harshbarger, 1977).

Two fibromata reported in the African clawed frog, *Xenopus laevis,* were located in the pelvic canal and around the nares (Elkan, 1960). The pelvic mass was more likely a chronic inflammatory polyp, while the other around the nares was reported as facial fibromata although the author clearly notes the facial tumors had "completely disappeared" when the frog was examined histologically 9 months later.

Myxoma and Fibromyxoma. These benign neoplasms are relatively hypocellular, edematous masses with a matrix of sparse collagen and fine reticulin fibers, but with an abundance of mucopolysaccharides. The cell of origin is probably a primitive mesenchymal cell. All cases have been reported in neotenes of the barred tiger salamander, *Ambystoma tigrinum mavortium,* from a polluted sewage lagoon in Texas (Rose & Harshbarger, 1977). Histologically, these authors distinguished this neoplasm from fibromata by their less cellular density. All fibromyxomata in these salamanders were dermal, and grossly were indistinguishable from fibromata (Rose & Harshbarger 1977).

Histologically, the cells of a myxoma are chiefly and characteristically stellate and are surrounded by a very loose, poorly staining matrix of mucopolysaccharides (mucinous material) that should be hyaluronidase-sensitive (Lattes, 1982; Weiss, 1974). However, there are no reports of the use of special stains (with and without pretreatment with hyaluronidase) that demonstrate the presence of mucopolysaccharides in amphibian myxomata. True myxomata of humans show a striking paucity of blood vessels (Lattes, 1982), but it is unclear if this also is a feature of amphibian myxomata.

Not all myxoid proliferations are neoplastic. Several

suspected and reported myxomata of amphibians may be myxedema. In addition, many neoplasms and hyperplastic lesions may have myxoid areas in them, but this does not warrant calling them a myxoma. In human medicine, some pathologists consider it inappropriate to label neoplasms with a myxoid component with the preface "myxo-", as in myxochondroma or myxolipoma (Lattes, 1982). For the most part, the myxoid component should be ignored and not used in the morphological diagnosis of a neoplasm.

Fibrosarcoma. Malignant neoplasms of fibrocytes, i.e., fibrosarcomas, have been reported in many neotenes of the barred tiger salamanders, *Ambystoma tigrinum mavortium,* from one locality in Texas (Harshbarger & Snyder, 1989), and as isolated spontaneous cases in a goliath frog, *Conraua goliath* (Frye et al., 1991) (Figure 26.34), and an ornate horned frog, *Ceratophrys ornata* (Volterra, 1928). Grossly, this tumor may be solitary or multicentric, and appear as firm whitish or gray masses up to 2 cm in diameter on the limbs, mandible, or body. Histologically, the elongate neoplastic cells form parallel bundles of streaming cells, interweaving bundles, subtle to marked whorls, and occasional herringbone patterns (Harshbarger et al., 1989). Vascular stroma is usually minimal, as is collagen production. Cells may be separated by elongate or elliptical clear spaces, especially at the periphery of the mass. Nuclei are hyperchromatic, large, elongate, and have one or two prominent nucleoli. Mitoses are usually evident but are "not particularly numerous" (Frye et al., 1991), or may be numerous and atypical (Volterra, 1928). No metastases were reported among specimens of the barred tiger salamander, *A. tigrinum mavortium,* although several neoplasms were deeply invasive locally (Harshbarger et al., 1989), while the neoplasm in the goliath frog, *C. goliath* (Frye et al., 1991), appeared multicentric, and the fibrosarcoma in the ornate horned frog, *C. ornata* (Volterra, 1928), was highly infiltrative and destructive of muscles, cartilage and bone of the limb as well as being metastatic to the liver.

Myxosarcoma. One of only two neoplasms of larval amphibians was diagnosed as a myxosarcoma in a tadpole of the green frog, *Rana clamitans* (Lucke, 1937). The neoplasm was only briefly described as located dorsally on the tail and was approximately as large as the tadpole's head. Cellular features were not described, but the neoplasm had invaded and destroyed dorsal muscles of the tail.

26.3.2 Neoplasms of Fat Tissue

Unlike endothermic animals, lipocytes in amphibians are localized principally in the paired intra-abdominal fat bodies and bone marrow. Consequently, neoplasms of fat cells are rarely detected and reported, nor would they be expected to arise in the subcutis as is so often the case in birds and mammals.

Lipoma. One lipoma has been reported in an adult female South African clawed frog, *Xenopus laevis.* Although encapsulated, the mass appears to have arisen in the right fat body and projected through the dorsolateral body wall to form a 2-cm mass in the subcutis of the back (Balls, 1962). The cells were not described microscopically other than a mention that they resembled fat body cells.

Liposarcoma. Two malignant tumors of lipocyte origin were reported in the northern leopard frog, *Rana pipiens* (Duryee, 1965). The neoplasms consisted of irregular masses within the coelomic cavity that were attached to the spleen, urinary bladder, and parietal mesothelium.

26.3.3 Neoplasms of Muscle Tissue

Leiomyoma and Leiomyosarcoma. In the opinion of the authors of this chapter, no convincing neoplasms of smooth muscle cells (i.e., leiomyoma and leiomyosarcoma) have been reported in amphibians.

Purported benign neoplasms of smooth muscle cells have been

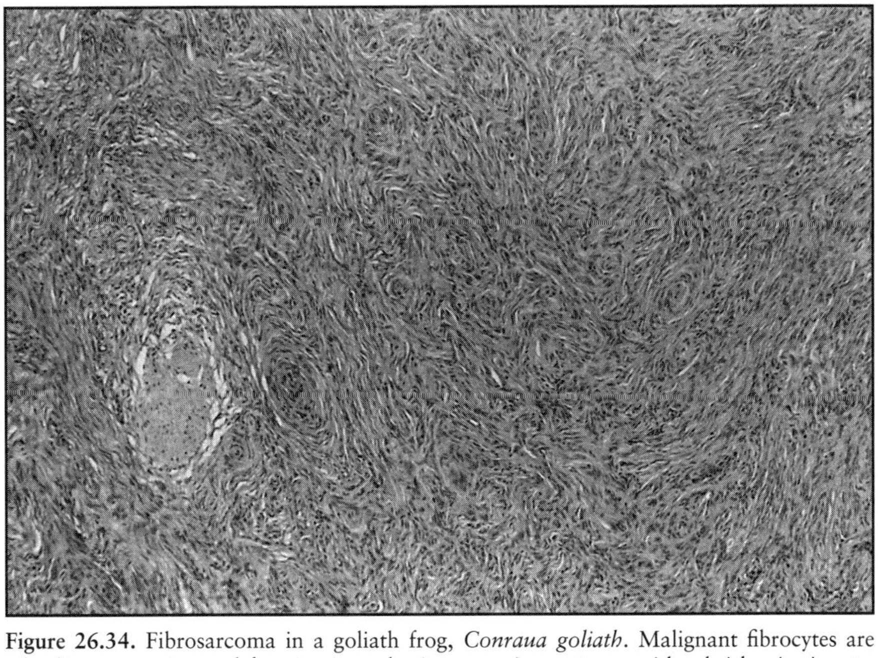

Figure 26.34. Fibrosarcoma in a goliath frog, *Conraua goliath*. Malignant fibrocytes are whorling, streaming and forming irregular interweaving patterns with a brisk mitotic rate. Necrotic neoplastic cells are present on the left. (F.L. Frye, RTLA 4908)

reported only in the Japanese firebelly newt, *Cynops pyrrhogaster*, and have been studied ultrastructurally (Asashima & Meyer-Rochow, 1989; Pfeiffer & Asashima, 1990). The initial report of leiomyomata in the stomachs of seven (3.5% of 200) newts (Asashima & Meyer-Rochow, 1989) is not convincing based on the authors' descriptions and illustrations. The purported illustrated neoplasms more closely resemble granulomata than any previously described vertebrate leiomyomata. A second report on an additional 19 (2.7% of 700) newts with gastric leiomyomata (Pfeiffer & Asashima, 1990) is no more convincing, despite ultrastructural examinations. Although semithin sections (1 micron thick) were prepared (Pfeiffer & Asashima, 1990), the histologic features were very briefly described. It was noted the purported neoplasms were without vascularization, a feature consistent with granulomata rather than neoplasia. Other ultrastructural features, such as the presence of only concentric whorls of cells without any interweaving cellular patterns, the paucity of characteristic myocytic mitochondria, and statements such as the neoplasms had variable stages of development, and neoplastic cells were markedly distinct from normal smooth muscle cells, suggest the cells of the nodules consisted of epithelioid macrophages (i.e., granulomata), not neoplastic smooth muscle cells. Failure of the authors to discuss the possibility that the tumors were granulomata, and their failure to state that nodules that were clearly granulomata were excluded from the studies, further suggests the tumors were inflammatory rather than neoplastic. It is distinctly possible some of the many observed gastric nodules were neoplasms, but the published illustrations and descriptions do not support such a diagnosis.

Rhabdomyoma and Rhabdomyosarcoma. One rhabdomyosarcoma of the left hindlimb has been reported in a northern leopard frog, *Rana pipiens*, that had experimentally received an intraocular transplant of Lucke renal carcinoma (Mizell et al., 1966a, b). The muscle neoplasm was first detected about 2.5 months following the intraocular transplantation, and it grew rapidly, approximately doubling in size in 30 days. Grossly, it was grayish white, and invasive of femoral musculature. Histologically, the neoplasm was characterized as highly cellular, infiltrative, and showed necrosis. Neoplastic cells were best preserved around blood vessels where they showed moderately abundant eosinophilic cytoplasm with infrequent cross-striations suggestive of abortive myofibril formation. Nuclei were variable in size, ovoid, and indented, with prominent nucleoli. Mitotic rate was not assessed histologically, but was considered high by autoradiography following tritiated thymidine labeling.

Granular Cell Tumor ("Myoblastoma," Granular Cell Myoblastoma). The cell of origin of this tumor is uncertain in higher vertebrates, and was not determined in the one reported case of granular cell tumor in a 2-year-old African clawed frog, *Xenopus laevis*. The origin of the mammalian neoplasms has been attributed to striated myocytes, fibroblasts, undifferentiated mesenchymal cells, Schwann cells, an undifferentiated neural crest cell, or a primitive, neuroectodermal cell (Bouchard et al., 1995; Sanford et al., 1984).

The neoplasm in the frog arose on the head following experimental treatment with the carcinogen, methyl-nitroso-urea (Figures 26.35, 26.36), but in other vertebrates it may arise in many other organs. Histologically, the granular cell tumor has characteristic features. Cells at the periphery of the nonencapsulated neoplasm are usually plump, polygonal, with moderate to abundant amounts of granular eosinophilic cytoplasm. The granules are distinctly and characteristically PAS-positive. In central regions of the neoplasm, cells are more spindaloid, fibrous, and

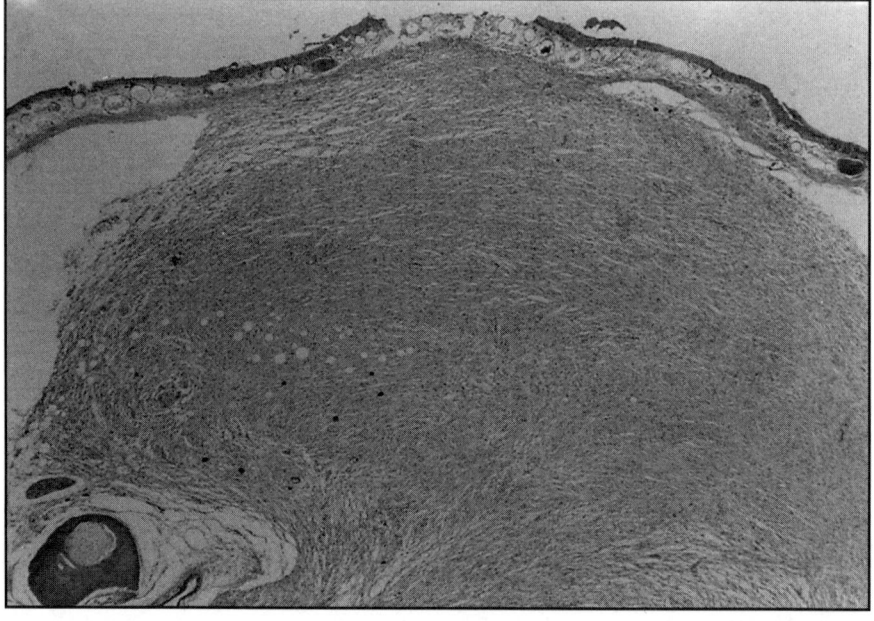

Figure 26.35. Granular cell tumor (formerly granular cell myoblastoma) in an African clawed frog, *Xenopus laevis*. This neoplasm was experimentally induced with the carcinogen, methylnitrosourea (MNU). Most of the neoplasm consists of fibroblast-like cells, but at the periphery, some cells become plump, polygonal, and have granular cytoplasm (see Figure 26.36). Cytoplasmic granules in plump peripheral cells are characteristically PAS-positive. (W. Janisch & T. Schmidt, RTLA 2219)

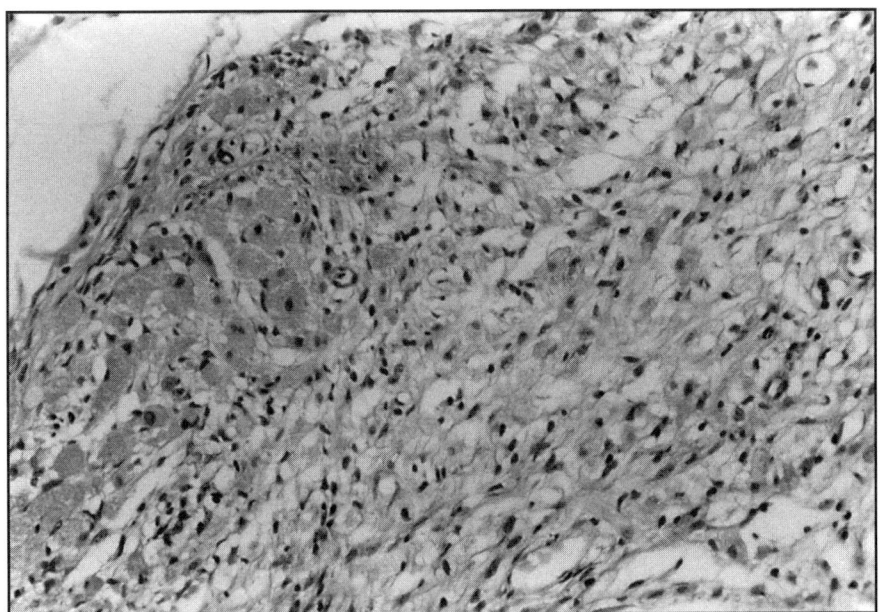

Figure 26.36. Granular cell tumor in an African clawed frog, *Xenopus laevis;* higher magnification of peripheral cells from Figure 26.35. Plump polygonal cells (on the left) at the periphery of the neoplasm contain eosinophilic granules that are PAS-positive. (W. Janisch & T. Schmidt, RTLA 2219)

have less cytoplasm and few or no PAS-positive granules. The original term, myoblastoma, for this neoplasm arose from the presence of a few elongate or straplike cells with cytoplasmic cross-striations that were thought to resemble primitive myocytes. Such cells were not evident in the one experimentally induced amphibian neoplasm.

26.3.4 Neoplasms of Blood and Lymph Vessels

Hemangioma (Cavernous Hemangioma). No spontaneous benign neoplasms of endothelial cell origin (i.e., hemangioma) have been described in amphibians.

Hemangiosarcoma (Angiosarcoma, Malignant Hemangioendothelioma). No spontaneous malignancies of endothelial cells (i.e., hemangiosarcoma) have been reported in amphibians. Multiple experimentally induced hemangiosarcomata were reported in the Spanish ribbed newt, *Pleurodeles waltl* (Janisch & Schmidt, 1980) (Figures 26.37, 26.38). Among 50 ribbed newts exposed to ethyl- and methyl-nitrosourea, 10 animals developed neoplasms. Nonvascular neoplasms included fibrosarcomata and nephroblastomata (Janisch & Schmidt, 1980).

Lymphangioma. No benign or malignant neoplasms originating from lymphatic vessels or sacs have been reported, although one dermal neoplasm in a 2.5-year-old albino axolotl, *Ambystoma mexicanum,* that was diagnosed as both a teratoma and carcinoma bears striking resemblence to a lymphangioma (Koyama et al., 1989). Grossly, the neoplasm was circular, dome-shaped, and covered by normal epidermis. Histologically, the neoplasm consisted of large irregularly shaped cavities (or cisternae) containing lymphatic fluids but no erythrocytes. Endothelial-like cells lining the cavities were thin, flattened, and had darkly stained nuclei with scant cytoplasm. Microvilli were occasionally prominent on the cells. Between the cystic cavities the stroma consists of "seemingly normal layers and muscular tissue" (Koyama et al., 1989). Mitotic rate was not reported.

26.3.5 Miscellaneous, Undifferentiated, and Mesenchymal Cell Neoplasms

Mesenchymal Cell Neoplasm. A poorly differentiated subcutaneous neoplasm was reported in one wild red-spotted newt, *Notophthalmus viridescens.* The neoplasm was examined by many physician pathologists and given many different diagnoses, such as granular cell tumor, mesenchymal cell tumor, rhabdomyoma, histiocytoma, fibrosarcoma, and sarcoma. Stains for demonstrating mast cell granules were not attempted. The morphology of the tumor cells resembled a mast cell tumor, a neoplasm that had not been recognized in amphibians at the time of the published report (Burns & White, 1971), and which was a neoplasm rarely observed in human medicine. The newt neoplasm was remarkably similar to mast cell tumor of the axolotl, *Ambystoma mexicanum* (see Section 26.4, Neoplasms of Hematopoietic and Lymphoid Cells and Organs).

The newt's mesenchymal neoplasm was a prominent raised nodule, 14 × 11 mm, located laterally in the proximal half of the body. The cut surface was solidly cellular. Histologically, the tumor consisted of pleomorphic small and large cells, varying cell density with edema, and infiltrates into the skeletal muscle. Degenerating and, possibly, regenerating rhabdomyocytes were evident. Neoplastic cells had moderate to abundant cytoplasm containing fine and coarse acidophilic granules. Some granules were periodic acid-Schiff-positive, very dark in toluidine blue, and stained by alcian blue. These special stain features are consistent with a mast cell tumor. Results of Giemsa stain for metachromatic granules were not reported, nor was the presence or absence of eosinophils mentioned. Nuclei were exceptionally variable in size, shape, and density. A few multinucleated cells were evident, but mitoses were not. Elongate or "strap" cells were occasionally found,

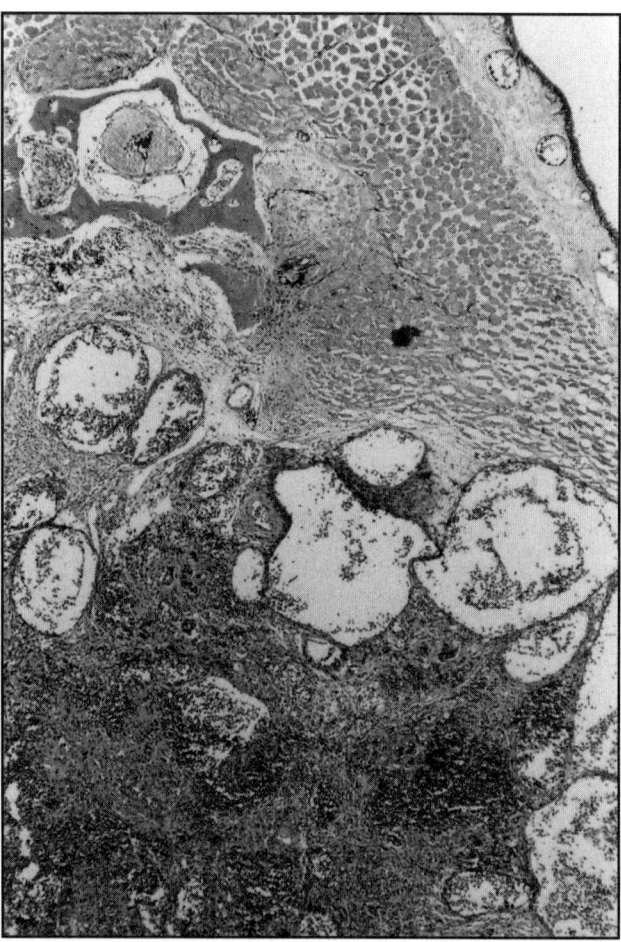

Figure 26.37. Hemangiosarcoma associated with experimental exposure to the carcinogen, methylnitrosourea (MNU), in a Spanish ribbed newt, *Pleurodeles waltl*. Numerous endothelial-lined cavities of varying diameters are partially or fully filled with erythrocytes. Compression of adjacent musculature is evident. Caudal vertebra and spinal cord at upper left. (W. Janisch & T. Schmidt, RTLA 1959)

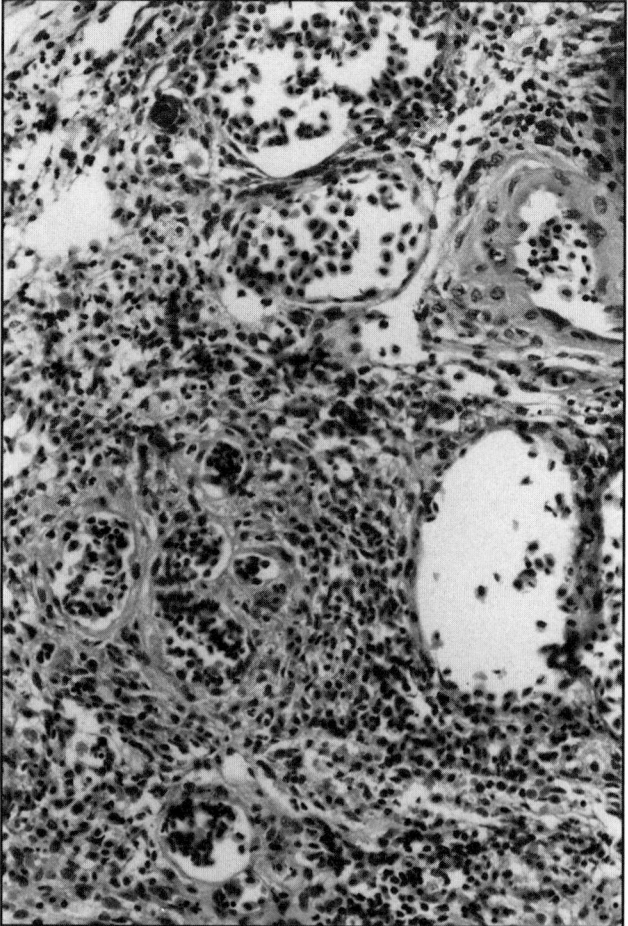

Figure 26.38. Hemangiosarcoma in a Spanish ribbed newt, *Pleurodeles waltl*; higher magnification of Figure 26.37. Pale fibrinoid material around some neoplastic vessels is often observed in neoplasms of endothelial cells. (W. Janisch & T. Schmidt, RTLA 1959)

but it was unclear whether these cells were degenerating rhabdomyocytes or neoplastic myocytes. The pleomorphic nature of the neoplastic cells resulted in a diagnosis of mesenchymal cell neoplasm (Burns & White, 1971), but in the opinion of the authors of this chapter, a diagnosis of mast cell tumor is more plausible (see Section 26.4.4, Neoplasms of Mast Cells).

"Sarcomas" of Soft Tissues. Undifferentiated or poorly described tumors (in the broadest sense of the word) have been reported as neoplasms from a variety of amphibian hosts (El-Mofty et al., 1991a, b, 1992; Gheorghiu, 1930; Inoue & Singer, 1970). Some were successfully transplanted (Gheorghiu, 1930; Inoue & Singer, 1970) to the same host species or other taxa. However, most of these poorly described "sarcomas" are infectious granulomata (Sheremetieva-Brunst & Brunst, 1948). Some of these granulomata may be due to mycobacterial or filarial infections (Asfari, 1988; Dawe, 1969c; Gheorghiu, 1930; Sheremetieva-Brunst & Brunst, 1948). However, legitimate undifferentiated sarcomas of unknown cell origin may occur.

26.4 NEOPLASMS OF HEMATOPOIETIC AND LYMPHOID CELLS AND ORGANS

26.4.1 Lymphoproliferative Diseases

Nodular Hyperplasia. Nodular hyperplasia is a non-neoplastic condition of the lymphocytes that has not been described in the literature in amphibians. In the files of the Registry of Tumors in Lower Animals, one suspected case occurred in the mesonephroi of a mudpuppy, *Necturus maculosus*. However, this salamander had received whole body radiation for about 72 hours before death, and cellular morphology was altered. Grossly, the animal had multiple 2–4 mm diameter, raised capsular nodules in the mesonephroi. Histologically, the nodules consisted mostly of small and medium sized lymphocytes cells with open-faced (degenerate) nuclei and rare mitoses. Confirmation of this disease in additional amphibians is needed.

Lymphosarcoma (Malignant Lymphoma, Lymphoid Leukemia). Malignancies of lymphocytes have been reported in several amphibian taxa, however, infectious granulomata have been commonly misdiagnosed and reported as lymphosarcomata (Asfari, 1988; Dawe, 1969a), hence, the precise number of true lymphocytic neoplasms and number of host taxa are uncertain. The situation is especially confusing in the African clawed frog, *Xenopus laevis,* Japanese firebelly newt, *Cynops pyrrhogaster,* and a few other amphibian taxa that have received transplanted cells from them. Historically, presumptive lymphosarcomata in the African clawed frog, *X. laevis,* were categorized as either types L-1 or L-2 (Balls & Ruben, 1968; Ruben & Stevens, 1970). At present, it is probable both were granulomata (Asfari, 1988; Dawe, 1969b). As late as 1988, only one acceptable case of spontaneous lymphosarcoma in the African clawed frog, *X. laevis,* was on file at the Registry of Tumors in Lower Animals (RTLA #238) despite many submissions that were claimed to be, and published as, lymphocytic neoplasms (Asfari, 1988). Three additional cases in African clawed toads were suspected (see Table 26.1), but due to autolysis, the diagnosis in all three animals remains uncertain.

Although the infectious nature of many reported lymphoid neoplasms was suspected in the 1960s (Dawe, 1969a; Inoue et al., 1965), acceptance among researchers was slow. There was considerable interest in documenting a viral etiology for many forms of cancer, difficulty in resolving whether "tumors" induced in amphibians receiving putative neoplastic cells (and supernatants) were actually transplant or transmission effects, and suggestions that the observed bacilli in "tumors" were secondary or opportunistic infections of neoplastic cells (Balls, 1965; Ruben & Stevens, 1970), or actually induced the suspected neoplasms. The infectious nature, rather than neoplastic nature, has been documented for most reported amphibian "lymphosarcomas" (Asfari, 1988; Asfari & Thiebaud, 1988; Inoue et al., 1965). It was observed that the acid-fast bacillus (which was not culturally identified to the species level) from Japanese firebelly newt, *C. pyrrhogaster,* with "lymphosarcomatous disease," when injected into clawed frog, *Xenopus* spp., produced disease in the clawed toads that was histologically identical to "lymphosarcoma" (L-1 type) (Inoue & Singer, 1970). The acid-fast bacillus in clawed frog, *Xenopus* spp., with putative lymphosarcomas has been identified as *Mycobacterium marinum* (Asfari, 1988;

Clothier & Balls, 1973). The spontaneous and transmissable abnormal growths of the clawed frog, *Xenopus* spp., that for years had been considered lymphosarcomas, were actually infectious mycobacterial granulomata (Asfari, 1988). The authors of this chapter concur with her interpretations and conclusions.

Due to the confusion over granulomata and true neoplastic disease, there has been little or no attempt to further characterize the lymphosarcomata of amphibians. No groupings have been reported as occur in human and domestic animal medicine, hence, amphibian lymphosarcomata have not been typed as B-cell or T-cell, lymphocytic, prolymphocytic, lymphoblastic or histio-lymphocytic, large cell or medium cell, acute or chronic, and other categories. Larger collections of undisputed lymphosarcomata in amphibians need to be documented before such categories may be applied, or discarded as inappropriate to amphibians.

Site of origin of amphibian lymphosarcomata has scarcely been addressed in the literature. It is well to remember that most aquatic amphibians lack bone marrow. Lymphopoiesis occurs in the thymus, spleen, lymphomyeloid organs (in anurans only), subcapsular regions of the liver and mesonephroi, and in gut-associated lymphoid tissue (GALT). In terrestrial amphibians, lymphohematopoietic bone marrow is usually present. The vast majority of lymphosarcoma cases in amphibians have been diagnosed at necropsy, hence it is unknown what percentage may become leukemic and amendable to antemortem clinicopathological diagnosis. At present, most legitimate lymphoproliferative disease appears to affect the mesonephroi, spleen, and liver, however, by the time the amphibian succumbs to the neoplasia and is necropsied, most lymphosarcomata are generalized and the organ of origin is uncertain.

Well-documented neoplasms of lymphocytic cells occur in the thymus of captive African clawed frogs, *Xenopus laevis*. These neoplasms are sporadic, have been documented in five individuals (Robert et al., 1994; Robert & Du Pasquier, 1995, 1996), are lymphoblastic in morphology, and have molecular markers of the T-cell lineage (Du Pasquier & Robert, 1992). Grossly, the neoplasm presents in adult frogs as a unilateral swelling in the lateral neck region overlying the thymus (Du Pasquier & Robert, 1992; Robert & Du Pasquier, 1995). The lymphosarcomas have not been described histologically, but one was illustrated (Du Pasquier & Robert, 1992). The neoplasm consists of a monomorphic population of large polygonal cells with mild to moderate amounts of cytoplasm; a mild moth-eaten appearance is evident. Metastases to the skin occurred in one spontaneous case, and metastases to the liver, spleen, thymus, and dorsal musculature (near the site of injection) occur in histocompatible experimental froglets receiving transplants soon after metamorphosis. The etiology of the five spontaneous neoplasms does not appear to be viral (Robert & Du Pasquier, 1995). The five spontaneous thymic lymphosarcomas have been successfully transplanted into histocompatible froglets, the tumor cells have been studied molecularly, and cell lines have been established (Du Pasquier & Robert, 1992; Robert & Du Pasquier, 1995, 1996).

Five lymphosarcomata from clawed frogs, *Xenopus* spp., were found in the files of the Registry of Tumors in Lower Animals. Three cases showed marked autolysis, hence, the diagnosis of lymphosarcoma is equivocal. One case had been previously reported as an anaplastic renal cell carcinoma (Elkan, 1970), and others (Masahito et al.,1995) suggested a diagnosis of pancreatic carcinoma, hence the diagnosis on this fourth case is also uncertain. All five lymphosarcomata and suspected lymphosarcomata of clawed frogs, *Xenopus* spp., were generalized, one was leukemic, and the sites of origin could not be determined. At low magnification, the neoplasm is is hypercellular and basophilic. The cells freely infiltrate the parenchyma and usually do not form distinct nodules (Figures 26.39, 26.40, 26.41). Most neoplasms have a distinct moth-eaten appearance at low magnification due to apoptosis and drop-out of scattered neoplastic cells. Cells form no distinct patterns, but have distinct cell borders, and are round to ovoid, although in densely cellular regions their shape may be compressed on several surfaces to become polygonal. Nuclear to cytoplasmic ratios vary from 1:1 to 3:1. Cytoplasm is faintly basophilic. Nuclei are round or ovoid, and occasionally have a prominent central eosinophilic nucleolus. Mitotic rate is highly variable, but may be as high as 5 mitotic cells/high power field (see axolotl lymphosarcoma, Figure 26.42). Bizarre mitotic figures may be evident (see axolotl lymphosarcoma, Figure 26.43). No fibrovascular stroma forms with infiltrating neoplastic cells, although loss of parenchymal cells may leave remnants of preexisting stroma among the neoplastic lymphocytes.

Lymphosarcomata have been reported in the axolotl, *Ambystoma mexicanum* (Delanney, 1969) (see Figures 26.42, 26.43). Unlike the disproven transmissible "lymphosarcomata" of the clawed frog,

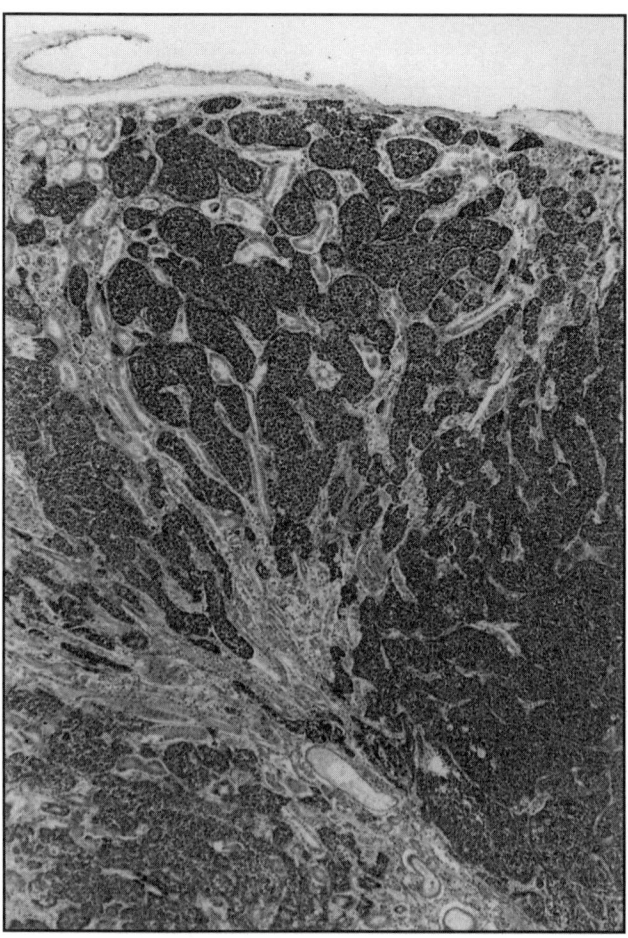

Figure 26.39. Lymphosarcoma in the mesonephros of an African clawed frog, *Xenopus laevis*. Note the infiltrative character of neoplastic cells in the renal interstitium with isolation, necrosis, and disappearance of renal tubules. (E. Elkan, RTLA 238)

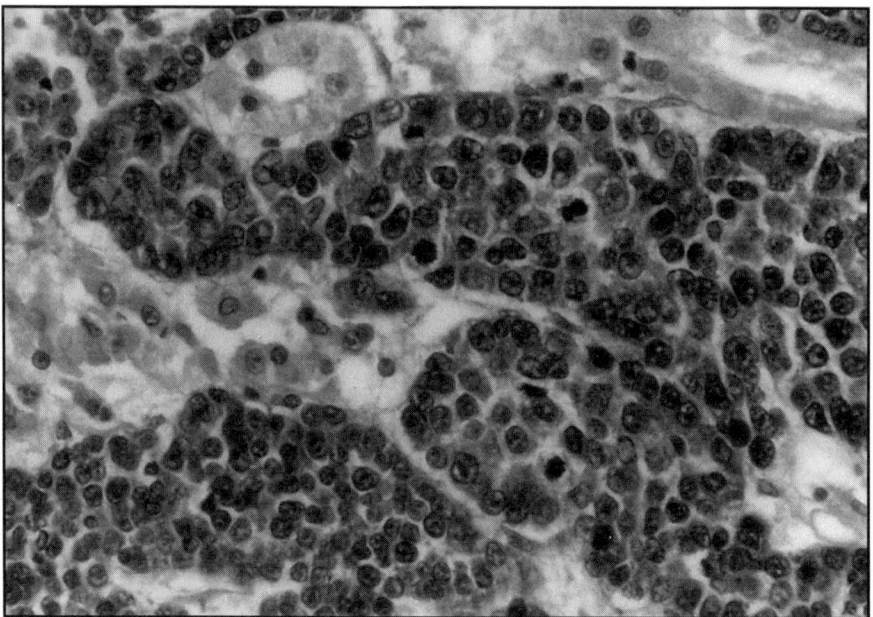

Figure 26.40. Lymphosarcoma of an African clawed frog, *Xenopus laevis*; higher magnification of Figure 26.39. Mitotic rate is high. (E. Elkan, RTLA 238)

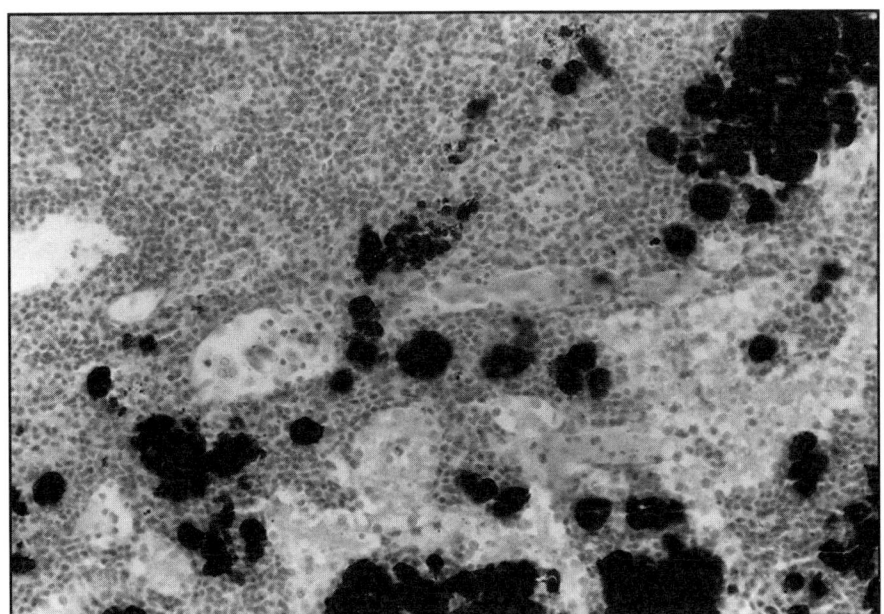

Figure 26.41. Lymphosarcoma in the liver of an African clawed frog, *Xenopus laevis*. A mass of neoplastic lymphocytes is present in the upper left corner, and tumor cells are freely infiltrating sinusoids and separating pale-staining hepatic cords and some black melanomacrophage aggregates. No capsule, distinct nodules, or compression of normal tissue are found. (G.E. Cosgrove, RTLA 1665)

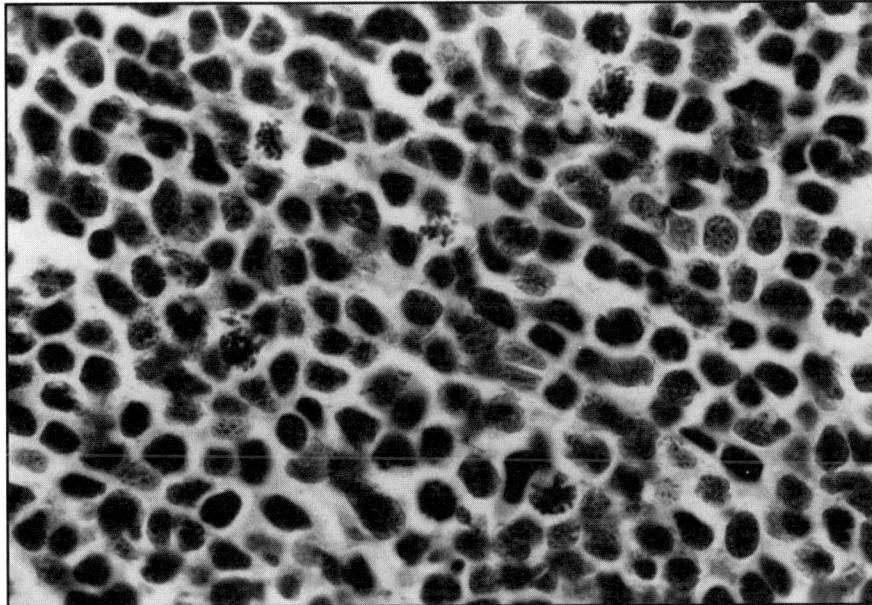

Figure 26.42. Lymphosarcoma in the intestine of an axolotl, *Ambystoma mexicanum*. Note the high mitotic rate, scant amounts of cytoplasm, and individualization of most cells. (D.L. Graham, RTLA 4920)

found in the skin at the site of multiple allografts (Delanney et al., 1964, 1967). In successful transplant recipients, the neoplasm readily progresses to terminal leukemia (Delanney, 1969, 1974).

Plasmacytoma (Myeloma). One plasmacytoma has been described grossly, histologically, and ultrastructurally in an adult female northern leopard frog, *Rana pipiens*, that, 2.5 months before appearance of the neoplasm, had received an intraocular transplantation of cells of a Lucke renal carcinoma (Schochet & Lampert, 1969). The neoplasm arose in the femoral musculature, grew rapidly, and approximately doubled in volume in 30 days. The tumor was grayish white, infiltrated the thigh muscles, but did not involve the skin or femur. Histologically, the mass was cellular and composed of plasmacyte-like cells in varying stages of maturity. Some cells resembled mature plasmacytes. They had amphophilic cytoplasm, a perinuclear clear zone, and a large eccentric nucleus with peripheralized chromatin. The majority of tumor cells were immature-appearing plasmacytes that were smaller, had finely granular amphophilic cytoplasm, and a large nucleus with a prominent nucleolus. Mitosis was common. Throughout the mass there were infrequent but highly characteristic cells containing a few large cytoplasmic droplets or inclusions ("Russell bodies") or multiple small intracytoplasmic inclusions ("Mott cells"). The large inclusions in Russell bodies are eosinophilic but unstained by the PAS reaction. Ultrastructurally, the majority of cells resembled plasmacytes by having varying sized, granular, weakly osmiophilic, proteinaceous cisterns (vesicles). Some cisterns contained more densely osmiophilic material, and coalesced cisterns formed Russell bodies. An additional striking feature was the presence of intracytoplasmic tubular inclusions that were frequently oriented parallel to each other and formed interweaving fascicles.

Xenopus laevis, the suspected lymphosarcomata of the axolotl, *A. mexicanum*, cannot be transmitted or transplanted into other amphibian species (Delanney & Blackler, 1969), but can be successfully transplanted into axolotls of the same histocompatiibility group, C(H^C). One lymphosarcoma was initially

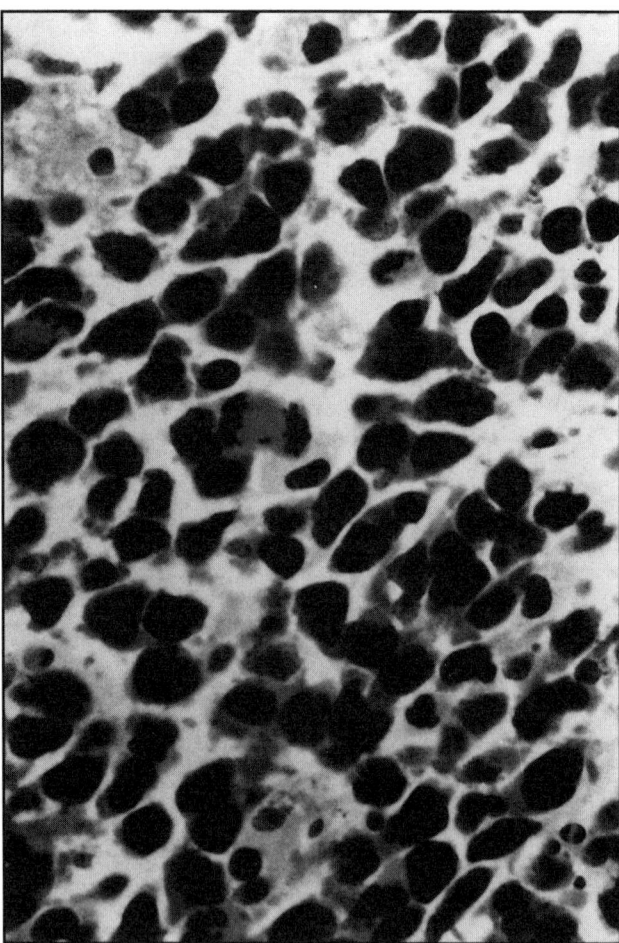

Figure 26.43. Lymphosarcoma in the skin of an axolotl, *Ambystoma mexicanum*. Note scant cytoplasm and individualization of most neoplastic lymphocytes. Centrally, note the bizarre mitotic figure with a lagging (detached) chromosome. (L.E. Delanney, RTLA 506)

These tubules were approximately 40 millimicrons in diameter, and possessed a double wall formed of two concentric shells. In fortuitous longitudinal sections, the outer shell of the tubules was found to be contiguous with rough endoplasmic reticulum. Such tubules have been detected in a variety of neoplasms and viral infections of vertebrates, including various herpesviral infections such as cells of Lucke renal carcinoma and human Burkitt lymphoma. It is unclear whether this plasmacytoma was spontaneous or secondary to the intraocularly transplanted Lucke herpesviral tumor. It is worth noting that other cases of "spontaneous" neoplasms have occurred in leopard frogs within 6 months of receipt of an intraocular transplant of Lucke renal carcinoma (e.g., an embryonal rhabdomyosarcoma) (Mizell et al., 1966a, b).

26.4.2 Neoplasms of Granulocytic Cells

Nodular Hyperplasia of Hematopoietic Tissue. As a general rule, hematopoietic tissue is found in the bone marrow of only terrestrial amphibians; in aquatic amphibians, hematopoietic cells are found mostly in the subcapsular regions of the liver and mesonephroi. Occasionally, 1–5 mm diameter nodules of proliferating, non-neoplastic hematopoietic cells are found during necropsy or histologically in the liver or mesonephroi of aquatic amphibians. Such nodules may be yellowish, roughly spherical, and may bulge from the capsular surface, but have not been described as pedunculated. Histologically, nodules of hyperplastic hematopoietic tissue consist mostly of normal-appearing granulocytes in all stages of maturation, but also may contain distinct clusters of mature lipocytes. Mitotic activity among myeloblastic cells within the nodule is as common as it is in the normal subcapsular hematopoietic zone. Unusually large foci of normal-appearing hematopoietic cells were observed in the liver of one barred tiger salamander, *Ambystoma tigrinum mavortium* (RTLA #2468), from a polluted sewage lagoon in Texas. Experimentally, benign hematopoietic proliferations in the liver and mesonephroi were induced in specimens of the Marsabit clawed frog, *Xenopus borealis*, exposed to N-nitrosodimethylamine (NDMA) (Afifi et al., 1991). At present, it is not known whether nodular hyperplasia of hematopoietic tissue in the liver and mesonephroi is a geriatric condition analogous to nodular lymphocytic hyperplasia in the spleen of aged domestic dogs (Jarrett & Mackey, 1974), or whether it occurs in response to chronic inflammatory disease, anemia, abnormalities of hematopoietin production in the mesonephroi, or other conditions.

Granulocytic (Myeloid) Leukemia (Chloroma). Two cases of spontaneous neoplasia of granulocytes are present in the files of the Registry of Tumors in Lower Animals. Both amphibians were toads, *Bufo* spp. Gross lesions were not described, hence, it is unknown whether this neoplasm caused hepatomegaly or a greenish discoloration (hence the older term, chloroma) of the liver. A possible third case in an African clawed frog, *Xenopus laevis*, is present in the files, but this animal had concurrent chlamydiosis, hence, the extensive infiltrates of mature and immature granulocytes in the liver may have been a leukemoid reaction to the infectious agent. In both toads, blood smears were not available, so the existence of antemortem leukemia cannot be assessed.

Both toads, *Bufo* spp., had extensive infiltrates of neoplastic cells in the sinusoids of the liver. Hepatic chords show atrophy, and degenerate and necrotic hepatocytes are common. Neoplastic cells are mostly round but may be polygonal in densely cellular regions. Most cells have a nuclear to cytoplasmic ratio of 2:1 to 1:1. Cytoplasm is mostly clear or faintly eosinophilic, but a few cells may contain faint granules.

Nuclei are pleomorphic, but most are roughly round and typical of blastic cells. A few cells show greater differentiation or maturation, and these have characteristic dumbbell-shaped, horseshoe-shaped or bilobed nuclei. Mitotic rate is usually marked. Use of special stains, such as perioxidase, Sudan black, and esterases, may be necessary for accurate recognition of the cell series in blood smears and histologic sections (Hruban et al., 1989; Jarrett & Mackey, 1974).

Eosinophilic Myeloid Leukemia. Spontaneous neoplasia of eosinophils has not been reported in amphibians.

Basophilic Myeloid Leukemia. Spontaneous neoplasia of basophils has not been reported. Leukemic basophilic neoplasia would be difficult to distinguish from leukemic mast cell tumor. See Section 26.4.4, Neoplasms of Mast Cells.

Unclassified Myeloproliferative Disease. Unclassified myeloproliferative disease refers to hyperplastic and neoplastic disease of uncertain cell origin or multiple cell types. No cases of this type have been reported in amphibians.

26.4.3 Neoplasms of Suspected Histiocytic Cells

Reticulum Cell Sarcoma. No spontaneous reticulum cell sarcoma have been reported in amphibians. Experimentally, some authors have suggested the "lymphosarcomas" associated with mycobacterial infections had more resemblance to reticulum cell sarcomata, but all these experimental cases can be considered mycobacterial granulomata.

Monocytoid Leukemia. No cases of spontaneous monocytoid leukemia have been reported in amphibians. Suspected monocytic leukemia occurred in 15 specimens of the square-marked toad, *Bufo regularis*, treated with the antifungal drug griseofulvin, and 13 cases in the same toad species treated with the carcinogen, 7,10-dimethyl-benz(a)anthracene (DMBA) (El-Mofty et al., 1995). These 28 cases were based on ultrastructural studies of buffy coats only; gross, cytological, and histological findings were not reported. Description of these suspected neoplasms from histological and histochemical examinations are needed.

26.4.4 Neoplasms of Mast Cells

Mast Cell Tumor. Numerous cases of mast cell tumor have been detected in the axolotl, *Ambystoma mexicanum*, from only one colony (Delanney et al., 1981). This neoplasm is rare in human medicine, but fairly common in many domestic mammals, hence, veterinary pathologists are more likely to readily recognize this neoplasm than physicians, as may have been the case with a newt neoplasm (Counts, 1980). In the files of RTLA, 18 mast cell tumors are from aged axolotls, 10–17 years old. Additional mast cell tumors were found in neotenes of the barred tiger salamander, *Ambystoma tigrinum mavortium*, from a polluted sewage lagoon in Texas. These neoplasms were misdiagnosed and reported years before mast cell tumors were recognized in axolotls and amphibians in general. The mast cell tumors of these salamanders were variously misdiagnosed as dermal fibromata, fibrosarcomata, and a myxosarcoma (Rose 1981; Rose & Harshbarger, 1977).

Grossly, mast cell tumors of the axolotl, *Ambystoma mexicanum*, occur in the dermis only of the head (n = 4), lateral body (n = 5), pelvic region (n = 3), tail (n = 6), and elsewhere. Axolotl mast cell tumors were elevated to domed, firm, glistening, and often were bright red with ulceration of the overlying epidermis (Figure 26.44). Single tumors were most common, but multiple neoplasms were found. Size at initial detection ranged 2–8 mm in maximum diameter (Delanney et al., 1981). The mast cell tumor has distinctive histological, histochemical, and ultrastructural features, but these may be altered rapidly by degranulation of mast cells and infiltrating degranulating eosinophils, and imbibition of water if the overlying skin is ulcerated. Mast cell tumors may be discrete dermal nodules, or have indistinct infiltrative borders. Well-differentiated mast cells are usually plump and have moderate to extensive amounts of cytoplasm. Mast cells may also be polygonal, spindle-shaped, stellate, and dendritic. Small mast cells with scant cytoplasm also are present. Cytoplasmic borders may quickly become indistinct in specimens that are not fixed promptly. Intercellular

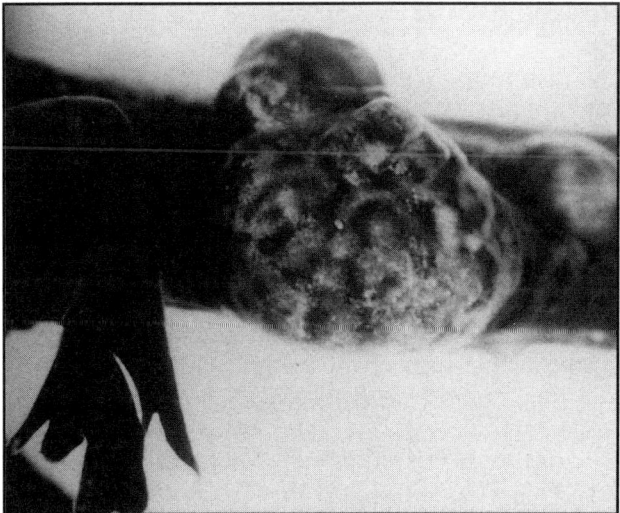

Figure 26.44. Mast cell tumor in the skin of an axolotl, *Ambystoma mexicanum*. This well-circumscribed, distinctly dome-shaped tumor had extensive epidermal ulceration. (F.L. Rose, RTLA 1678)

edema may be a striking feature of these neoplasms. Mild to extensive edema may separate tumor cells. The cytoplasm contains fine granules that may be detectable in only a few cells in standard H&E stains. Granules are distinctly and characteristically metachromatic in the Giemsa, azure A and toluidine blue stains, and some are periodic acid-Schiff-positive (Kapa et al., 1970). Other special stains as applied to mammalian mast cells have not been attempted but are worthy of investigation. Metachromatic granules may be detected in 5–25% of neoplastic mast cells using the Giemsa stain. Nuclei show marked pleomorphism and anisokaryosis but usually have homogenously distributed euchromatin and indistinct nucleoli. Karyomegaly may be rare or marked, and large nuclei may have exceptionally large nucleoli. Mitotic rate varies from 0–2 cells per high power field. Eosinophils infiltrate all axolotl and tiger salmander mast cell tumors; their numbers are mild to moderate, and their presence is a helpful clue in recognition of this neoplasm. Neoplastic cells may abutt the basement membrane of the epidermis and freely infiltrate the stratum compactum, subcutis, and skeletal muscles. The overlying epidermis may be intact, eroded, or ulcerated (Figures 26.45, 26.46, 26.47). Ultrastructurally, neoplastic cells have abundant numbers of characteristic electron-dense, 150 nm, cytoplasmic granules, and the pleomorphic nuclei show numerous folds, clefts, and notches.

At the Registry of Tumors in Lower Animals, at least three mast cell tumors were present among a large group of spontaneous neoplasms in neotenes of the barred tiger salamander, *Ambystoma tigrinum mavortium,* from a polluted sewage lagoon in Texas (Rose & Harshbarger, 1977). All were misidentified as other mesenchymal neoplasms (see Table 26.1). Three neoplasms were nonulcerated dermal or subcutaneous nodules composed of pleomorphic polygonal, spindled, and stellate cells with mostly indistinct cell borders and moderate intercellular (edema) (see Figure 26.47; Figure 26.48). Cytoplasm may be clear, diffusely eosinophilic, or contain eosinophilic granules. Eosinophils were present in mild to extensive numbers. Metachromatic cytoplasmic granules were demonstrated in the Giemsa stain.

Finally, two spontaneous neoplasms in the red-spotted

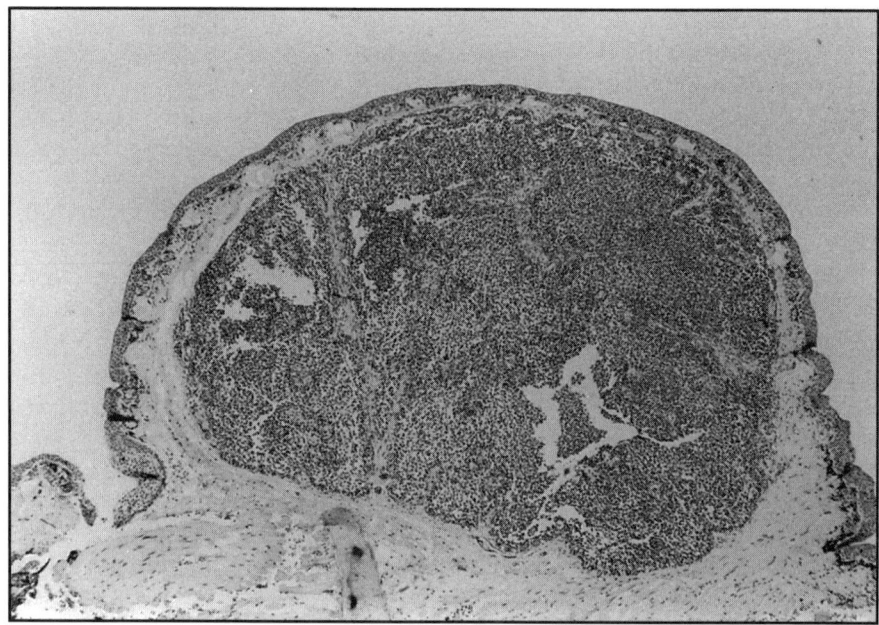

Figure 26.45. Mast cell tumor in the dermis of a wild red-spotted newt, *Notophthalmus viridescens viridescens*. This discrete, nonulcerated mast cell tumor was initially misidentified and reported as a neuroblastoma (Counts, 1980). A Giemsa stain performed many years later demonstrated faint metachromatic cytoplasmic granules and mild infiltrates of eosinophils which are characteristic features of mast cell tumors. (C.L. Counts & F. Hissom, RTLA 1135)

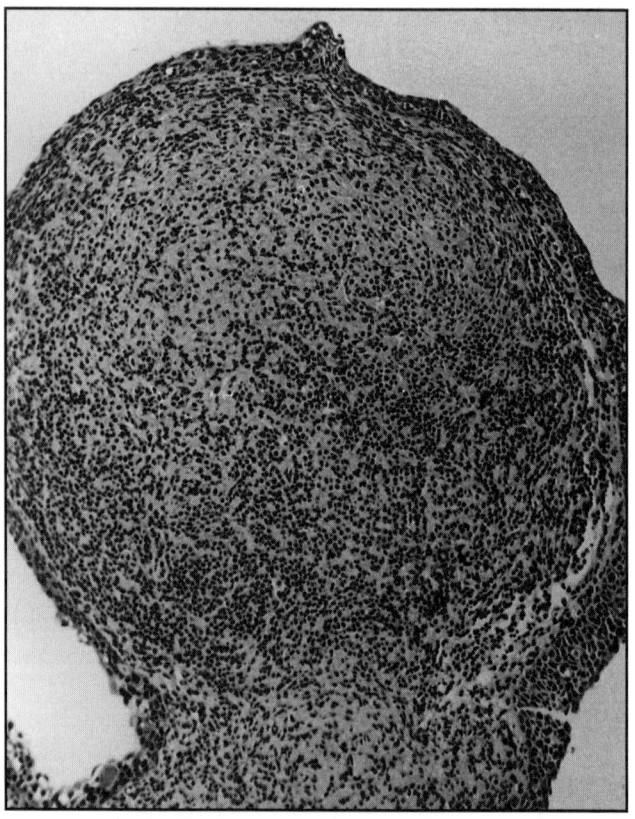

Figure 26.46. Mast cell tumor in the dermis of an axolotl, *Ambystoma mexicanum*. This neoplasm shows minimal intercellular edema and no evidence of epidermal ulceration. Compare to Figure 26.47. (L.E. Delanney, RTLA 1688)

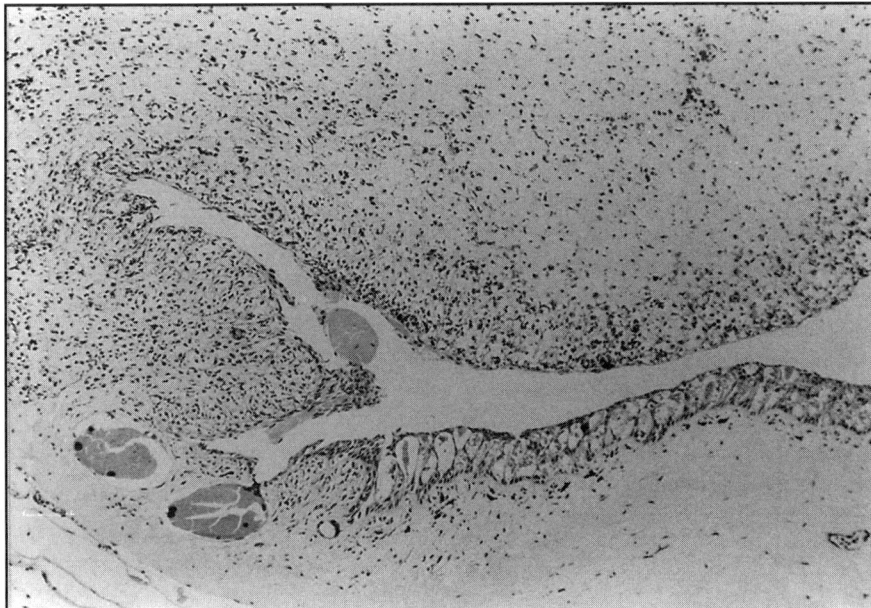

Figure 26.47. Mast cell tumor in the dermis of a wild neotenic barred tiger salamander, *Ambystoma tigrinum mavortium*. Intact normal epidermis with an edematous dermis is in the lower center and lower right corner; mast cell tumor with marked intercellular edema is at top and left. Note the extensive ulceration of epidermis overlying the nodular neoplasm. (F.L. Rose, RTLA 999)

newt, *Notophthalmus viridescens*, have been reported as a neuroblastoma and a mesenchymal cell neoplasm (Burns & White, 1971; Counts, 1980). Both tumors were located in the lateral neck region, were prominently domed (see Figure 26.45), and were composed of pleomorphic cells with highly variable nuclear sizes, and pale eosinophilic cytoplasmic granules. In 1996, the reported neuroblastoma was reexamined with a Giemsa stain, and metachromatic granules were found in the cytoplasm of neoplastic cells (Figure 26.49); the diagnosis in this case is revised from neuroblastoma to mast cell tumor. The Giemsa stain also demonstrated eosinophils that were not readily apparent in a hematoxylin and eosin stain. In the second newt, the

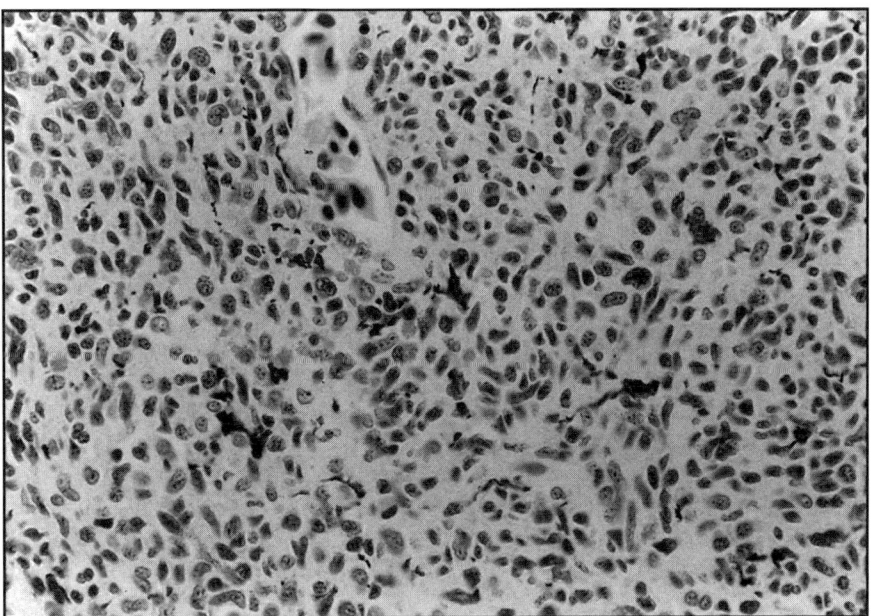

Figure 26.48. Mast cell tumor in the dermis of a wild neotenic barred tiger salamander, *Ambystoma tigrinum mavortium*. Nuclei show pleomorphism, anisokaryosis, karyomegaly, and occasional prominent nucleoli. Dark irregular cytoplasmic material is metachromatic granules. Giemsa stain. (F.L. Rose, RTLA 991)

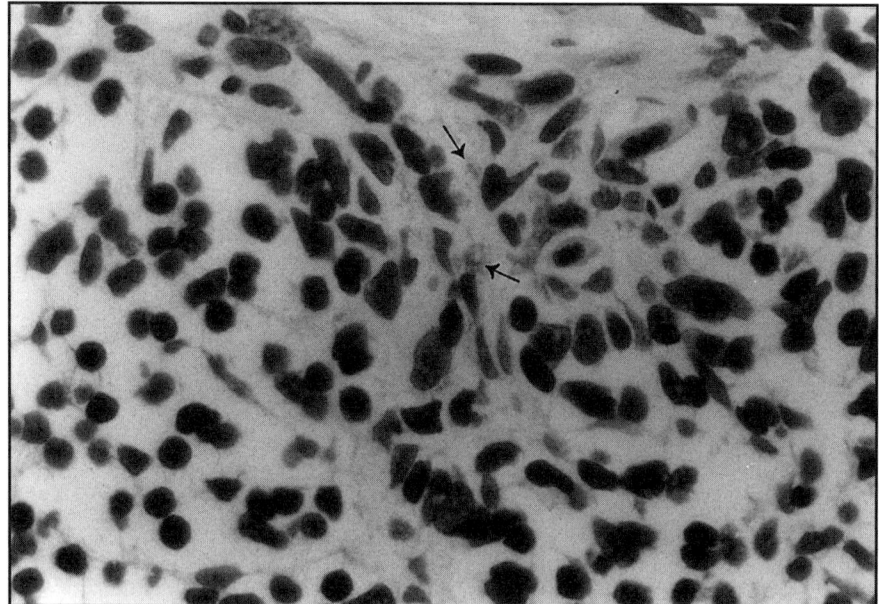

Figure 26.49. Mast cell tumor in the dermis of a wild red-spotted newt, *Notophthalmus viridescens viridescens*; higher magnification of Figure 26.45. Note the nuclear pleomorphism. Faint cytoplasmic granules (arrows) show weak metachromasia. This mast cell tumor was considered poorly differentiated (anaplastic). Giemsa stain. (C.L. Counts & F. Hissom, RTLA 1135)

neoplasm was diagnosed and published as a mesenchymoma, which was a reasonable diagnosis if mast cell tumor had not been considered. In this chapter, the diagnoses of both newt neoplasms have been revised to that of mast cell tumor, although this diagnosis has not been confirmed by demonstration of metachromatic mast cell granules in the reported mesenchymoma.

26.4.5 Neoplasms of the Thymus

Thymoma. Spontaneous and experimental neoplasms of thymic reticuloepithelial cells have not been reported.

26.5 NEOPLASMS OF THE KIDNEYS AND URINARY BLADDER

26.5.1 Neoplasms of the Kidney

Nephroblastoma (Embyronal Nephroma). Nephroblastomas are true embryonal tumors arising from primitive mesonephric blastema (as opposed to the metanephric blastema in reptiles, birds, and mammals). This tumor has not been documented in the pronephric blastema of larvae. Two spontaneous nephroblastomas have been reported in a captive Japanese firebelly newt, *Cynops pyrrhogaster*, and an African clawed frog, *Xenopus laevis*. In mammals, these neoplasms may become huge before they are detected. Histologically, the tumor consists of two distinct cell types, primitive mesenchymal cells and epithelial cells that form primitive glomeruli and tubules (Figures 26.50, 26.51). One or the other cell type may predominate in different regions of the tumor. Mesenchymal cells are spindaloid or stellate, may be densely packed, or very myxedematous. Epithelial cells are cuboidal or columnar, have ony mild amounts of basophilic cytoplasm, and may form tubules and small papillary structures resembling primitive (embryonic) glomeruli (Elkan, 1976, 1983; Zwart, 1970). Few nephroblastomata have been reported in fish, but one, in a striped bass, *Morone saxatilis*, had striking amounts of cartilage in the mesenchymal component (Helmboldt & Wyand, 1971).

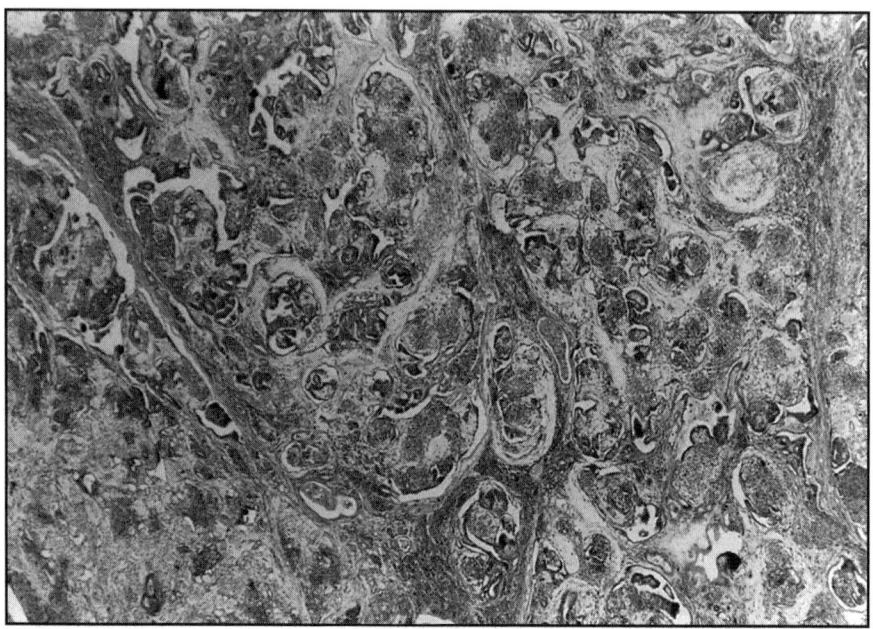

Figure 26.50. Nephroblastoma (embryonal nephroma) in the mesonephros of an African clawed frog, *Xenopus laevis*. These neoplasms have two distinct cell types: spindle-shaped mesenchymal cells, and epithelial cells that form tubules and abortive glomeruli. One or the other cell type may predominate in some neoplasms, and great variations in cell composition may be evident in different regions of the same neoplasm. (E. Elkan, RTLA 32)

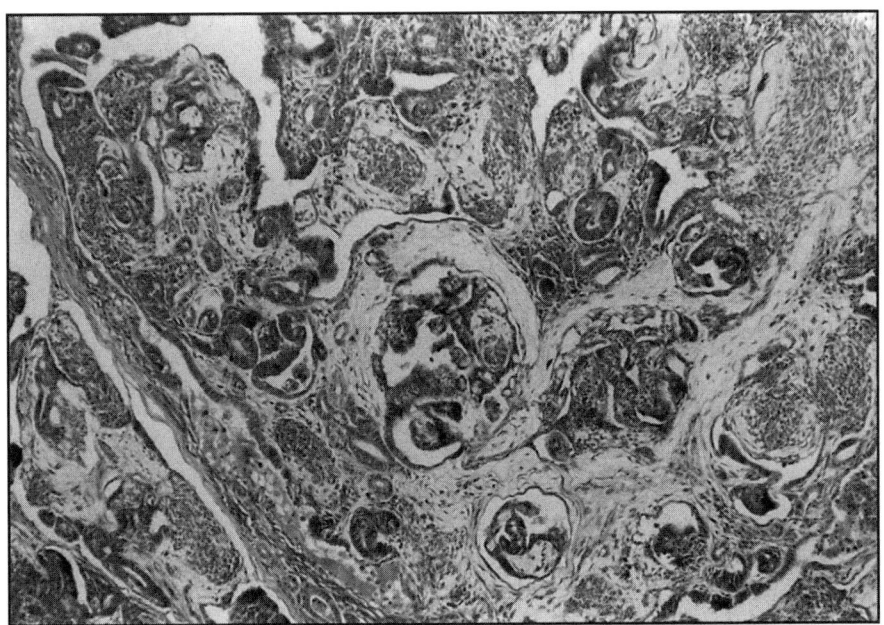

Figure 26.51. Nephroblastoma (embryonal nephroma) in the mesonephros of an African clawed frog, *Xenopus laevis*; higher magnification of Figure 26.50. Epithelial cells are forming tubules and abortive glomeruli. (E. Elkan, RTLA 32)

Differentiation of the neoplastic mesenchymal cells into bone, muscle, cartilage or other tissues has not been reported in amphibians, but may be expected to occur.

Experimentally, nephroblastomata have been induced in the Spanish ribbed newt, *Pleurodeles waltl*, exposed to N-methyl-N-nitrosourea (MNU) (Janisch & Schmidt, 1980). These neoplasms tend to be anaplastic, with a predominance of stromal cells, and few glomeruluslike formations. Multiple (multicentric?) "carcinosarcoma" were reported in an adult northern leopard frog, *Rana pipiens*, that had received an intraocular transplant of a Lucke renal carcinoma (Mizell et al., 1966a). The neoplasm was composed of two cell types: fusiform cells forming irregular masses and whorling patterns, and tubules lined by cuboidal and columnar epithelial cells. This description is suggestive of a nephroblastoma.

Lucke's Renal Carcinoma (Lucke's Renal "Adenocarcinoma"). Lucke's renal carcinoma occurs spontaneously only in the northern leopard frog, *Rana pipiens*, which was a source of mild confusion before it was realized that leopard frogs from the southern United States were multiple distinct species. Experimentally, pronephric renal carcinomata may be induced (McKinnell et al., 1989; McKinnell & John, 1995), but all spontaneous Lucke renal carcinomata develop in the mesonephros. The spontaneous neoplasm is caused by a herpesvirus (Lucke tumor herpesvirus [LTV]), which is transmitted to eggs, embryos, or larvae during spring breeding. Leopard frogs are not susceptible to renal carcinomas if first exposed to Lucke herpesvirus as adults (McKinnell et al., 1989). The Lucke herpesvirus, like many other vertebrate herpesviruses, is host-specific. However, experimental transmission of the Lucke tumor herpesvirus to various other North American ranids (southern leopard frog, *Rana utricularia*, pickerel frog, *R. palustris*, green frog, *R. clamitans*, and various interspecific hybrids with *R. pipiens*) may result in the development of renal carcinomata (McKinnell & DuPlantier, 1970; Mulcare, 1969). The Burnsi mutant of the northern leopard frog, *R. pipiens*, which for a few years was elevated to the status of a species, is susceptible to this neoplasm (McKinnell, 1965, 1969).

Prevalence of the neoplasm in wild populations varies greatly by region and year. In 1933 in Vermont and adjacent areas of Canada, 2.1% of frogs were infected, but none of the frogs from Michigan had the neoplasm (Lucke, 1934). In 1994, adult wild frogs from northern Vermont had a prevalence of 24%, after being held in captivity for 14 months (McKinnell & John, 1995). For several decades, Dr. McKinnell has extensively studied Lucke renal carcinoma, and has noted considerable fluctuation in tumor prevalence in leopard frogs from Minnesota (McKinnell & McKinnell, 1968). Prevalence in 1963 in Minnesotan leopard frogs was 8.5%, while in 1966–1968 it was about 6% (McKinnell et al., 1979). In the years between 1977 and 1987 the prevalence was almost zero, but into the 1990s, the neoplasm appeared to rise steadily. Many reports on the prevalence of Lucke renal carcinoma are based on gross examinations only; under certain circumstances, when kidneys are examined histologically, the prevalence approaches 100% (Marlow & Mizell, 1972).

Several biological features of the Lucke renal carcinoma are temperature-dependent, including virus formation, development of characteristic intranuclear herpesviral inclusion bodies, detachment of cells from the neoplastic mass, invasion and metastasis. Inclusion bodies and virus formation occur in the algid phase ("winter tumors"), while tumor growth, invasion and metastasis occur principally in the calid phase at warmer (summer) temperatures (Anver & Pond 1984; McKinnell et al., 1989).

Early studies suggested this neoplasm was more prevalent in male leopard frogs, but more recent studies have found no sexual predisposition (McKinnell,

1965). In frogs with one neoplastic nodule, the right mesonephros may be slightly more affected than the left (Lucke, 1934). No favored location within the mesonephros has been found.

Grossly, the neoplasm may affect one or both mesonephroi, and may be so small as to be barely detectable at necropsy, or may fill much of the body cavity and be readily palpable in the live frog (McKinnell, 1965). About half of affected frogs are found to have tumor nodules in both mesonephroi (Lucke, 1934). Multicentric neoplasms are common with up to 12 masses occurring in the mesonephroi of each frog. At necropsy, the small neoplasms are difficult to distinguish from encysted trematodes (McKinnell, 1965). Most Lucke neoplasms initially are spherical, and ivory-white (Lucke, 1934) to light yellow (McKinnell, 1965). Tumor nodules are rubbery, homogenous in texture, solid or partially cystic on cut surface, and rarely bloody or necrotic (Lucke, 1934). In about half of frogs with this neoplasm, the tumor nodules were 4–6 mm in greatest diameter; the normal leopard frog kidney averages 16 mm in length (Lucke, 1934, 1938).

Histologically, the Lucke renal carcinoma forms tubules that may be small in diameter or large and cystlike (Figure 26.52). Neoplastic tubules are very irregular in outline and bizarre in shape, and may have varying numbers of mostly simple papillary projections. Some carcinomata may have prominent branching papillary projections (Figures 26.53, 26.54). Cells lining the tubule are usually much larger and more basophilic than normal tubule cells (Lucke, 1938). The neoplastic tubular cells are cuboidal or columnar, 1–5 cells thick, and often irregularly pseudostratified. Neoplastic tubular lumina are usually empty, but may contain sloughed and necrotic cells. Some neoplastic nodules may have regions of solid cellularity, composed of small tubules that lack lumina, or closely packed papillary projections. The fibrovascular stroma is highly variable from tumor to tumor and from region to region within a carcinoma. Some carcinomata have scant stroma separating neoplastic tubules, while other regions have moderate to abundant fibrovascular stroma that typically shows marked edema. Fibrous capsules around the neoplasms are absent or very thin. Normal renal tissue at the edges of the neoplasm commonly shows marked

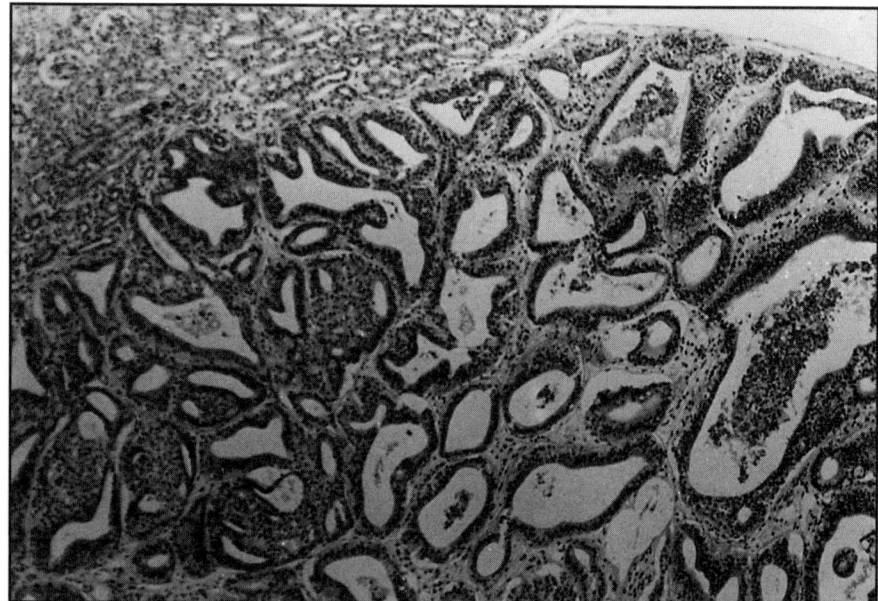

Figure 26.52. Lucke renal carcinoma in the mesonephros of a northern leopard frog, *Rana pipiens*. This summer (calid) phase carcinoma is characterized by the paucity or absence of intranuclear inclusion bodies. This neoplasm shows principally a tubular pattern. (W.R. Duryee, RTLA 577A)

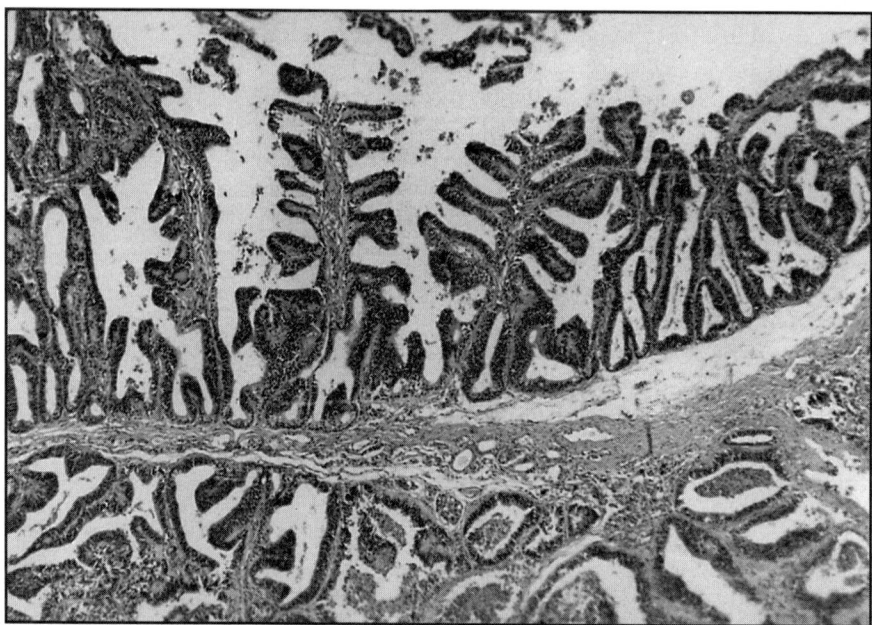

Figure 26.53. Lucke renal carcinoma in the mesonephros of a northern leopard frog, *Rana pipiens*. This calid phase neoplasm shows a prominent papillary pattern (J.S. Waterhouse, RTLA 41)

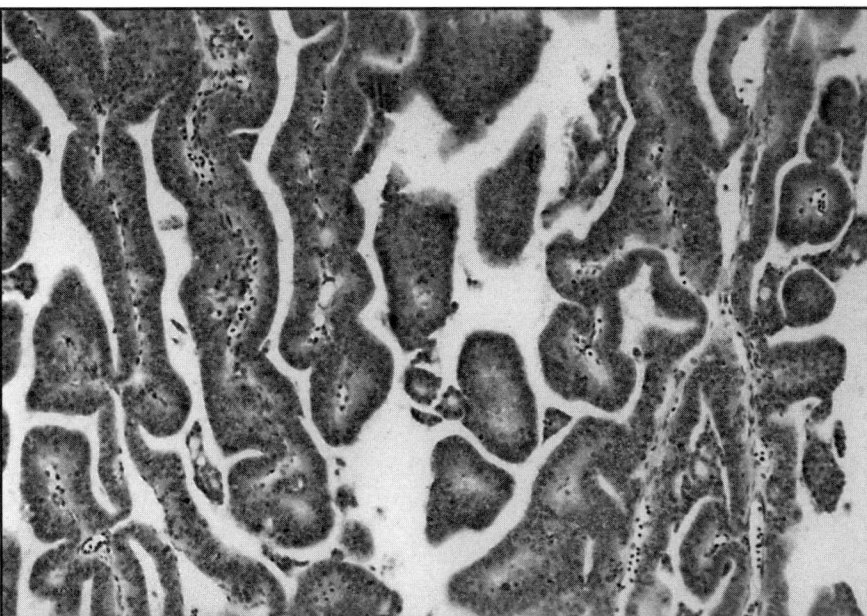

Figure 26.54. Experimental Lucke renal carcinoma in the mesonephros of a green frog tadpole, *Rana clamitans*. This amphibian was injected with Lucke herpesvirus as an embryo and was sacrificed at 4 months of age while still a tadpole. A papillary pattern predominates in this calid phase carcinoma. (D.J. Mulcare, RTLA 1058)

compression and atrophy of the tubules. Inflammatory cell reaction occurs in about 70% of cases, usually at the periphery of the neoplasm (Lucke, 1934). Lymphocytes predominate, but macrophages, neutrophils and eosinophils may be present in much fewer numbers. This neoplasm may resemble a benign adenoma, a cystadenoma, a papillary cystadenoma, or a "frankly malignant, invasive, and destructive" carcinoma (Lucke, 1938).

Nuclear to cytoplasmic ratio is usually 1:1 to 1:2. Nuclei are usually round or ovoid, but may be elongate or have notches. Each nucleus usually has a single prominent acidophilic central nucleolus, but occasionally two are present. In those neoplasms obtained from frogs during the summer, acidophilic intranuclear inclusion bodies typical of herpesviruses (socalled Cowdry type A inclusion body) are rare or absent. Neoplasms taken from frogs during the winter and at breeding time have numerous nuclear inclusions in the neoplastic cells (Rafferty, 1964). Up to 75% of neoplastic cells from algid (winter) tumors contained nuclear inclusions (Lucke, 1938).

The inclusions fill about 75% of the nuclear core, are roughly round, and stain red to magenta in most acidophilic stains. Nuclei with inclusions are slightly swollen, and have prominent nuclear rims thickened by marginated chromatin (Figure 26.55). Nuclear inclusions do not occur in preexisting normal renal tubule cells, in stromal cells, or cells of any other organ (Lucke, 1934, 1938, 1952). Mitotic figures are more common in calid (summer) tumors.

Metastases occur principally in summer stage neoplasms. Metastases may be distant, probably via the venous or lymphatic circulation, or transcoelomic. Among 362 cases of Lucke renal carcinoma, metastases were found in 22 (6%) (Lucke & Schlumberger, 1949). Lungs and liver are the most frequent sites of distinct metastasis.

Lucke renal carcinomata have been studied ultrastructurally (Barch et al., 1965; Zambernard et al., 1966). In calid neoplasms, herpesvirus particles are rare or undetectable. In these "summer phase" tumors, the viral genome is incorporated into

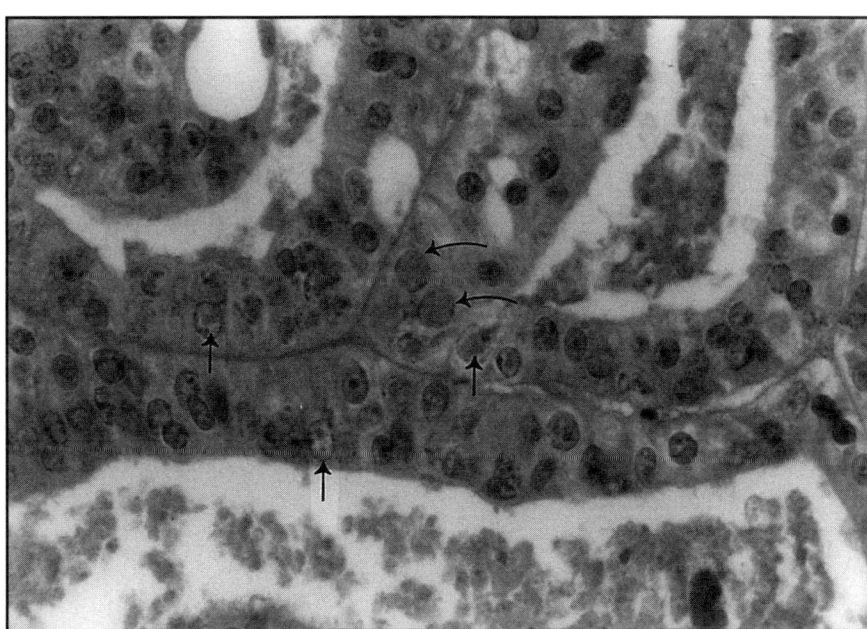

Figure 26.55. Lucke renal carcinoma in the mesonephros of a northern leopard frog *Rana pipiens*. This winter (algid) phase neoplasm shows intranuclear inclusion bodies in many tumor cells. Some inclusions (straight arrows) are Cowdry type A (dense core, clear halo, and thin nuclear rim) while others are more smudgy, lack a clear halo, and nearly fill the nucleus (curved arrows). Both types of inclusions are characteristic of herpesviruses. (W.R. Duryee, RTLA 492)

the host nucleus. In the algid phase, characterized histologically by acidophilic intranuclear inclusions, many typical herpesvirus particles are present in the nuclei and cytoplasm of neoplastic cells. These particles are icosohedral, 95–110 nm, have 162 capsomers, and, when present in the host cytoplasm, usually have an envelope (Anver & Pond, 1984; Barch et al., 1965).

In studies of transplantation of cells of the Lucke renal carcinoma, it has been found that the vast majority of transplants are quickly rejected by the amphibian host, except when transplanted into immunologically privileged sites such as the globe of the eye. Transplanted carcinomata usually flourish within the eye. One curious side effect of intraocular carcinoma transplantation in a low percentage of animals is the occurrence of other malignancies in the host-recipient frog, invariably at sites distant from the eye. These unrelated distinct neoplasms include a plasmacytoma in the femoral musculature (Schochet & Lampert, 1969), carcinosarcomas (possibly nephroblastomas) in the kidney (Mizell et al., 1966a), and a rhabdomyosarcoma of the femoral muscles (Mizell et al., 1966a, b). These neoplasms arose 2.5–6 months following receipt of the intraocular Lucke carcinoma. Whether these neoplasms were purely spontaneous and coincidental to the Lucke carcinoma transplants, or whether there is a pattern of induced additional malignancies secondary to the Lucke carcinoma requires further study.

Renal Cell Carcinoma in Other Amphibians. Few spontaneous primary neoplasms of the mesonephros have been described in amphibians, and the literature contains no reports of benign renal cell tumors (renal cell adenoma). Even in human medicine, renal cell tumors are a diagnostic problem because no criteria for distinguishing benign and malignant tumors have been defined. No histologic or ultrastructural features distinguish the renal cortical adenoma from a carcinoma (Gatalica et al., 1996). In higher vertebrates, the malignant neoplasms usually have one of three patterns: tubular, papillary, or solid. Occasionally in endotherms, more than one pattern may be evident in a single neoplasm (Nielsen et al., 1976). Two renal cell carcinomata were reported in captive specimens of the African clawed frog, *Xenopus laevis* (Elkan, 1960), an ornate horned frog, *Ceratophrys ornata* (RTLA #3982) (Figures

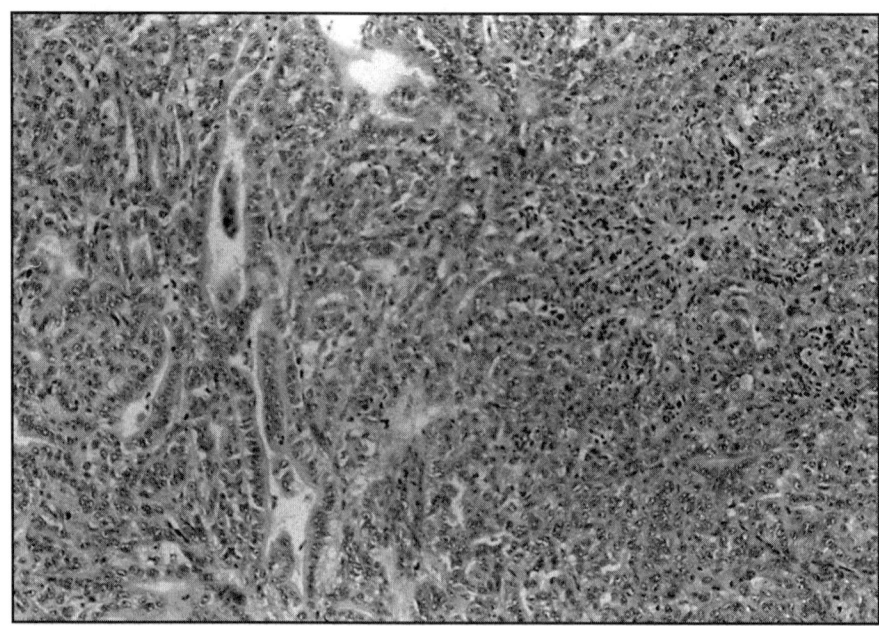

Figure 26.56. Renal cell carcinoma, tubular and solid patterns, in an ornate horned frog, *Ceratophrys ornata.* (F.L. Frye, RTLA 3982)

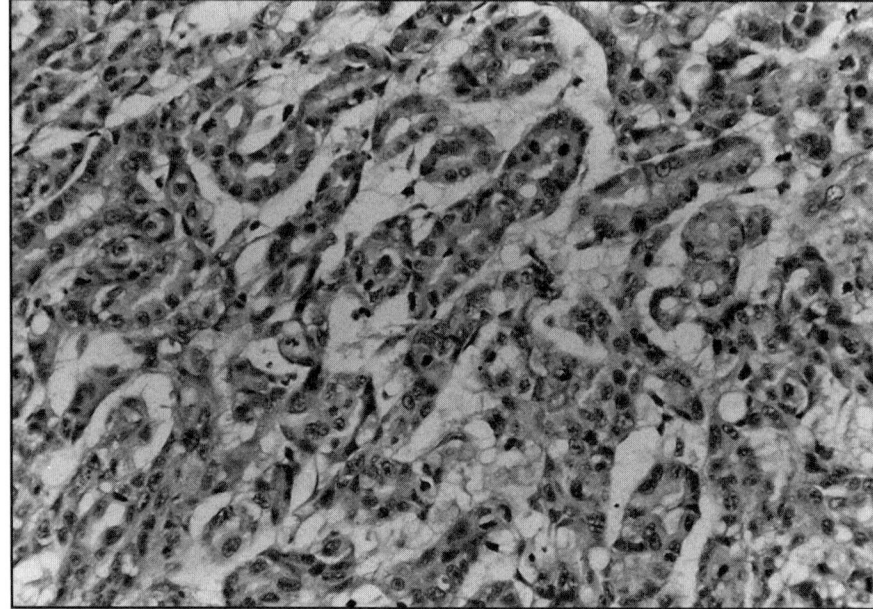

Figure 26.57. Renal cell carcinoma, tubular pattern in an ornate horned frog, *Ceratophrys ornata;* higher magnification of Figure 26.56. Neoplastic tubules are lined by cuboidal cells and separated by mild amounts of edematous fibrovascular stroma. The amounts of fibrovascular stroma may vary greatly within a tumor and between tumors. (F.L. Frye, RTLA 3982)

26.56, 26.57), and a mudpuppy, *Necturus maculosus* (Schlumberger, 1958, as cited by Balls & Clothier, 1974). Unfortunately, one of the two renal carcinomata described by Elkan and which is on file at the Registry of Tumors in Lower Animals (#238) appears to be a primary lymphosarcoma of the mesonephros. The other carcinoma in a clawed frog had moderate amounts of fibrovascular stroma separating well-differentiated neoplastic tubules (tubular type renal cell carcinoma).

Twenty-two fatal renal cell carcinomata in laboratory-bred and raised hybrid toads (*Bufo japonicus* × *B. raddei*) in Japan were briefly reported, but histological findings were not given (Nishioka & Kondo, 1987; Nishioka et al., 1994).

Transitional Cell Carcinoma. There are no published reports of this neoplasm which originates from the transitional epithelium of the mesonephric tubules ("ureters") and urinary bladder, however, a single case from a captive barred tiger salamander, *Ambystoma tigrinum mavortium,* had a resemblance to the mammalian form of this neoplasm. Grossly, a single 1.5-cm diameter yellowish white spherical mass was present in the proximodorsal cloacal region. It displaced the cloaca ventrally and produced external bilateral swellings of the cloaca. Histologically, the neoplasm consists of numerous nests of cells forming tubulelike structures. The tubules are loosely stratified by large polygonal cells having abundant eosinophilic cytoplasm and distinct cell borders (Figures 26.58, 26.59). The size of cells and abundance of cytoplasm is reminiscent of a squamous cell carcinoma, but intercellular bridging is absent. Nuclei are large and pleomorphic. Occasional binucleated and multinucleated cells are present (see Figures 26.58, 26.59).

26.5.2 Neoplasms of the Urinary Bladder

No spontaneous neoplasms of the urinary bladder have been reported, although metastatic disease and

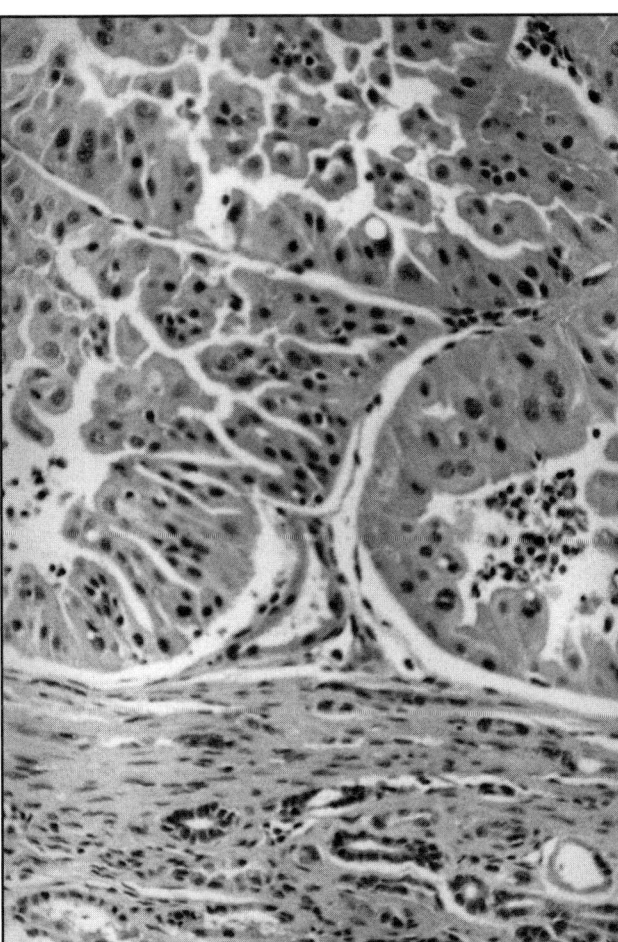

Figure 26.58. Transitional cell carcinoma in pelvic and cloacal region of a barred tiger salamander, *Ambystoma tigrinum mavortium.* Note the large cuboidal and columnar cells with abundant (eosinophilic) cytoplasm and marked anisokaryosis. (R.E. Miller, RTLA 3238)

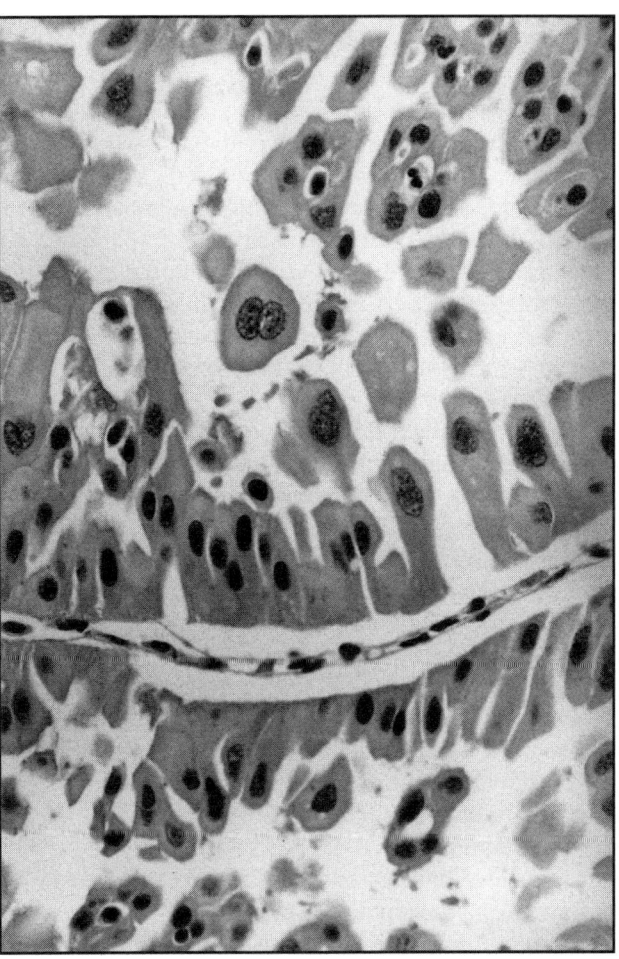

Figure 26.59. Transitional cell carcinoma in pelvic and cloacal region of a barred tiger salamander, *Ambystoma tigrinum mavortium;* higher magnification of Figure 26.58. Note the thin stroma, abundant cytoplasm, nuclear pleomorphism and anisokaryosis, and occasional binucleate cells. Such large neoplastic cells could be mistaken for a squamous cell carcinoma, but there is no keratinization of cells and no intercellular bridges. (R.E. Miller, RTLA 3238)

various granulomata have been recorded. A papillary adenocarcinoma of the urinary bladder in an African clawed frog, *Xenopus laevis,* was found following experimental treatment with an estrogen compound (Mizgireuv & Khudoley, RTLA #3078). One suspected transitional cell carcinoma in a tiger salamander (see previous paragraph) may have originated from the urinary bladder.

26.6 NEOPLASMS OF THE LIVER, BILIARY SYSTEM, AND PANCREAS

26.6.1 Hepatic Neoplasms

Four types of spontaneous primary neoplasms of the liver have been reported (Abrams 1969; Harshbarger & Snyder, 1989; Reichenbach-Klinke & Elkan, 1965; Willis 1964). These tumors represent hepatocellular neoplasms and one potential biliary duct neoplasm. In addition, two unclassified "sarcomas" were reported from the Japanese firebelly newt, *Cynops pyrrhogaster* (Mori, 1954), but in view of the susceptibility of this amphibian to spontaneous and experimental mycobacteriosis (Inoue et al., 1965), it is probable the two hepatic sarcomas were mycobacterial granulomata (Balls & Clothier, 1974). As is the situation with suspected lymphoproliferative disorders in amphibians, it would be prudent to routinely examine all dubious or poorly differentiated hepatic neoplasms with a variety of special stains for microorganisms, but especially an acid-fast stain.

A series of subacute carcinogenicity studies induced over 80 hepatocellular carcinomata and a few lymphosarcomata and fibrosarcomata in wild-caught specimens of the square-marked toad, *Bufo regularis,* using a variety of chemicals, such as adriamycin, aflatoxin-B1, griseofulvin, and an extract of black pepper (El-Mofty & Sakr, 1988; El-Mofty et al., 1980, 1983, 1991a, b, 1992, 1993). However, most of the illustrated tumors (El-Mofty et al., 1991a, b) resemble granulomata and granulomatous inflammation. Unfortunately, all suspected neoplasms from these studies that were donated to the Registry of Tumors in Lower Animals appeared to be granulomata. Use of acid-fast stains were not reported by the authors, and it is conceivable that epithelioid macrophages could be mistaken for neoplastic hepatocytes because both cell types may have generous amounts of pale to eosinophilic cytoplasm with central nuclei. The multinucleated cells (El-Mofty et al., 1991a) in some tumors probably were multinucleated giant cells of granulomatous inflammation rather than neoplastic multinucleated cells. The hepatocellular neoplasms were reported to metastasize to the mesonephroi, fat bodies, ovaries, and spleens. In mammals hepatocellular neoplasms typically metastasize to the lung but rarely any other organ (Ponomarkov & Mackey, 1976). Mycobacterial infections are commonly detected first in the liver (although the first site of infection is often the skin or intestine), and then disseminate to the mesonephroi, spleen, lungs, fat bodies, and other organs. In addition to the gross, histologic, and "metastatic" features of the hepatic nodules in the experimental toads, the rather short length of time for tumor development (4–12 weeks), suggests an infectious etiology for many of the suspected experimental "neoplasms" (El-Mofty et al., 1991a, b, 1992, 1993). It remains distinctly possible that some of the many reported tumors were neoplasms, but confirmation of the carcinogenicity of these chemicals to amphibians is needed.

Regenerative (hyperplastic) nodules of hepatocytes may be mistaken for benign hepatocellular adenomata. Usually, the hepatoma is single and large, while regenerative nodules are multiple. Often, evidence of damage to the remaining liver is found between the regenerative nodules. Hepatic acini may appear to have greatly reduced numbers of hepatocytes (as judged by the proximity of triads and central veins), or evidence of fibrosis, bile duct hyperplasia, and increased amounts of melanin and melanomacrophage aggregates. In experimental studies in which the administered chemical is known to be hepatotoxic (e.g., dimethylnitrosamine), animals that survive for 2 or more months may be anticipated to demonstrate multiple regenerative nodules with interspersed segments of coalesced bile ducts in a fibrous stroma. It appears that in some published studies using hepatotoxic chemicals (Ingram, 1972), the reparative process (regenerative nodules) in the liver was not considered or understood prior to making diagnoses of hepatocellular and cholangial neoplasms.

Hepatoma (Hepatocellular Adenoma). The hepatoma, a benign hepatocellular tumor, has been detected as spontaneous neoplasms in an edible frog, *Rana esculenta* (Willis, 1964), a northern leopard frog, *Rana pipiens* (Abrams, 1969), a barking treefrog, *Hyla gratiosa* (Harshbarger & Snyder, 1989), and a hybrid Chinese-Japanese frog (Masahito et al., 1995). All neoplasms are composed of plump, well-differentiated hepatocytes that form irregular cords. The neoplasms cause marked compression of surrounding parenchyma, and lack a true capsule, although subtle compression capsules may be evident segmentally. The neoplasms are noteworthy for the absence of biliary structures and melanomacrophage aggregates (Harshbarger & Snyder, 1989) although Willis (1964) showed a scattered melanophages in a ranid hepatoma (Figures 26.60, 26.61).

Hepatocellular Carcinoma. The distinction between a well-differentiated hepatocellular carcinoma and a

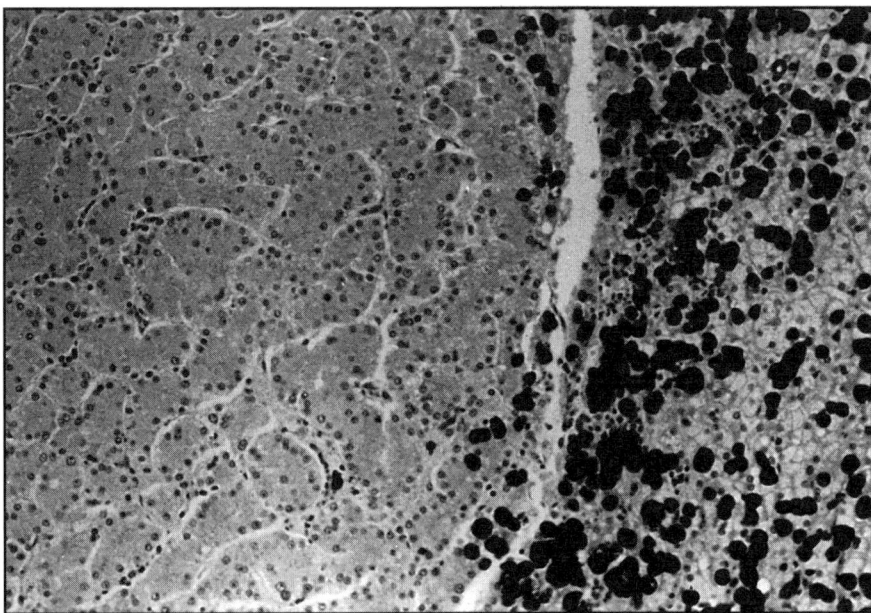

Figure 26.60. Hepatocellular adenoma (hepatoma) in a barking treefrog, *Hyla gratiosa*. Neoplasm (left) is forming cords of well-differentiated hepatocytes. Note the lack of biliary structures, triads, and melanomacrophage aggregates in the tumor (R.L. Snyder, RTLA 3579)

hepatoma is not precise. In endothermic animals, the distinction can be made when metastatic foci are found in the lungs, or if there is evidence of vascular invasion in the liver. Mitotic rates generally are not helpful, unless bizarre mitoses are found. One hepatocellular carcinoma has been described in a neotenic barred tiger salamander, *Ambystoma tigrinum mavortium*, that had been experimentally injected with perylene (a polycyclic aromatic hydrocarbon) (Harshbarger & Snyder, 1989), and it is possible the hepatoma in a barking treefrog, *Hyla gratiosa*, as described above was a well-differentiated hepatocellular carcinoma. Other hepatocellular carcinomas (n = 13) have been induced experimentally with the carcino-

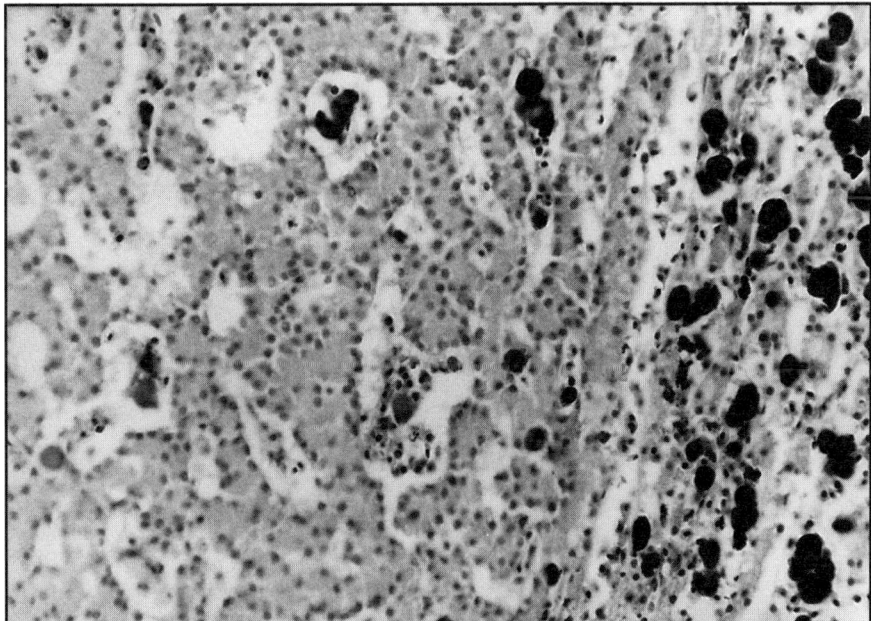

Figure 26.61. Hepatocellular adenoma (hepatoma) in a South American bullfrog, *Leptodactylus pentadactylus*. Compressed normal hepatocytes and melanomacrophage aggregates are on the right. Well-differentiated neoplastic cells (left) form irregular chords, and nuclei are oriented in rows at the sinusoidal (vascular) surface. (National Zoological Park, AFIP 1403734)

gen, N-nitroso-dimethylamine, in the Marsabit clawed frog, *Xenopus borealis* (Khudoley & Picard, 1980). These chemically induced carcinomas contained enlarged, polygonal, basophilic cells with small nuclei forming irregular cords. Occasional multinucleated neoplastic cells were present, invasive growth was consistently evident, but distant metastases have not been reported.

Hepatoblastoma. One suspected hepatoblastoma was reported in an aged African clawed frog, *Xenopus laevis* (Harshbarger & Snyder, 1989). In mammals, cells of this neoplasm resemble fetal hepatocytes in that they are small and have granular or vacuolated cytoplasm. The cells form orderly trabecular and microacinar patterns with sinusoids and prominent amounts of intrasinusoidal hematopoietic cells (Ponomarlov & Mackey, 1976). Grossly, the frog had a 7-mm encapsulated and sclerotic mass with several additional nonencapsulated scattered foci in the liver. Neoplastic liver cells had ill-defined sinusoids, and formed clusters resembling hepatic cords and embryonic rosettelike (acini-like) structures. This one example of an amphibian hepatoblastoma is noteworthy for the paucity of sinusoidal hematopoiesis (Figure 26.62).

26.6.2 Bile Duct Neoplasms

Cholangioma and Cholangiocarcinoma. Spontaneous cholangiomas and cholangiocarcinomas are very rare in amphibians, although they may develop secondary to experimental treatments with various carcinogens. As in many classes of vertebrates, the distinction between severe hyperplasia and neoplasia of bile ducts is indistinct. Hepatotoxic chemicals may destroy entire hepatic acini, but spare the bile ducts. In such situations, bile ducts may coalesce, and then may undergo hypertrophy and hyperplasia to the extent that over 50% of the liver section may appear to be composed of bile ducts histologically.

Two spontaneous bile duct adenomata have been reported in a clawed frog, *Xenopus* sp., and a hybrid Chinese-Japanese frog, *Rana* sp. (Reichenbach-Klinke & Elkan 1965; Masahito et al., 1995), but no gross or histologic descriptions were provided. Apparently, only one spontaneous malignancy of bile ducts (cholangiocarcinoma) has been reported in an amphibian—a neotenic barred tiger salamander, *Ambystoma tigrinum mavortium*, that had been exposed to high levels of perylene (Rose & Harshbarger, 1977). However, even in this latter case, there remains a possibility the lesion was not neoplastic but rather a case of severe diffuse bile duct hyperplasia.

One spontaneous sclerosing cholangiocarcinoma was found in the files at the RTLA. This individual, an African clawed frog, *Xenopus laevis*, also had a large hepatoblastoma (see above). The subcapsular nodule had marked edematous fibroplasia (sclerosis) in which scattered, irregularly shaped neoplastic bile ducts were lined by flattened or cuboidal epithelium. Mitotic rate was minimal, but cells and nuclei were pleomorphic (Figure 26.63). Fibroplasia between and around neoplastic ducts may be extensive.

Experimentally, the carcinogen, N-nitroso-dimethylamine (at 400 ppm in aquarium water), induced 32 cholangiocarcinomata in the Marsabit clawed frog, *Xenopus borealis* (Khudoley & Picard, 1980). These neoplasms were described as consisting of "enlarged, atypical cells with irregular, polygonal or rounded forms. Enlarged nuclei occupied a large proportion of the . . . cells. Pathological mitoses were frequent and invasive growth was observed in each case. Stromal fibrosis was prominent . . . As a rule, these tumors developed on a background of hyperplastic processes and disorganization of the liver structure" (Khudoley & Picard, 1980). It should be noted that the carcinogen initially caused marked hep-

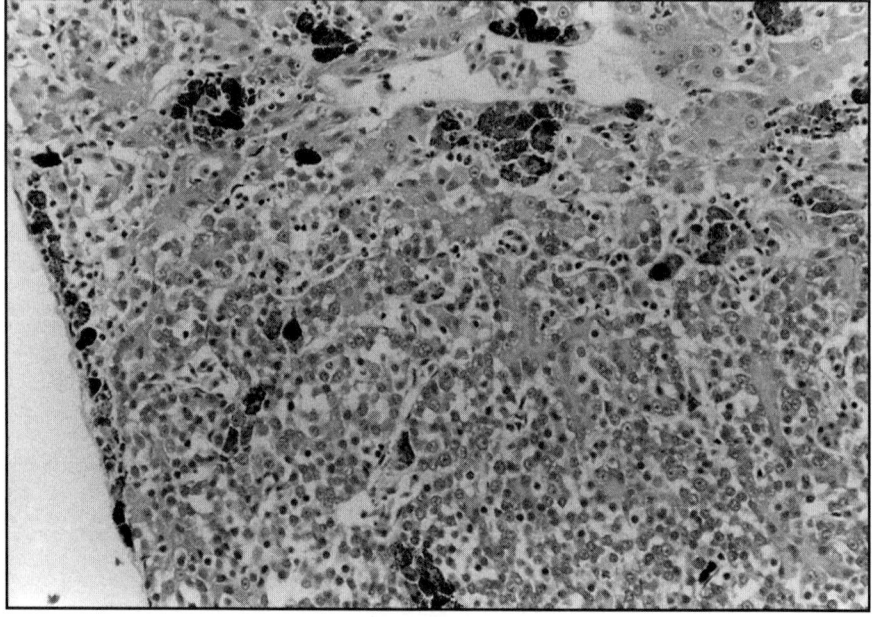

Figure 26.62. Hepatoblastoma in an African clawed frog, *Xenopus laevis*. Normal hepatocytes are in the upper right corner. Neoplastic hepatoblasts are smaller cells with mild amounts of eosinophilic cytoplasm that form irregular cords. Mild numbers of erythrocytes, hematopoietic cells, and melanomacrophage aggregates are present in the "sinusoids" between neoplastic cells. (R.L. Snyder, RTLA 3577)

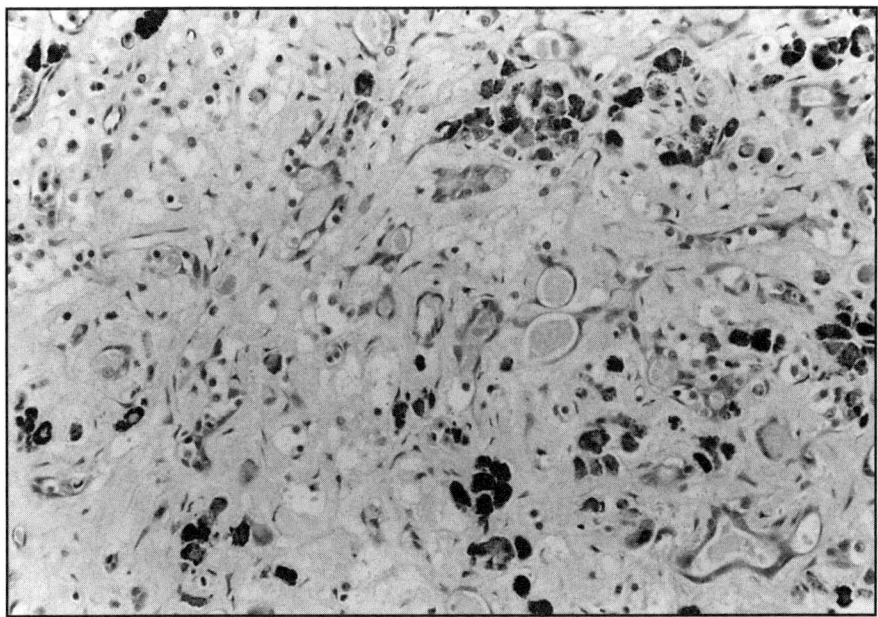

Figure 26.63. Cholangiocarcinoma in an African clawed frog, *Xenopus laevis*. Irregular neoplastic bile ducts are lined by flattened and cuboidal cells. Acellular fluid is present within neoplastic ducts. Fibroplasia (sclerosis) is marked. (R.L. Snyder, RTLA 3577)

atocellular vacuolation and necrosis followed by nodular hepatocellular regeneration and biliary hyperplasia before neoplasms were found.

26.6.3 Pancreatic Neoplasms

The pancreas of amphibians consists of two principal parenchymal cells: exocrine acinar cells and endocrine cells of the islets of Langerhans. Prior to 1987, only two spontaneous neoplasms of the pancreas had been reported in amphibians. More recently from the Laboratory of Amphibian Biology in Japan, over 100 pancreatic neoplasms have been detected mostly in captive-bred, hybrid frogs and toads (Masahito et al., 1995; Nishioka & Kondo, 1987; Nishioka & Ueda, 1987). It is likely that the 57 pancreatic neoplasms reported by Nishioka and Ueda (1987) were included in the 99 neoplasms reported by Masahito et al. (1995). Of the 99 pancreatic neoplasms detected at necropsy, 29 were studied histologically, immunohistochemically, or ultrastructurally (Masahito et al., 1995). These studies suggest most of the 99 neoplasms were of endocrine (islet cell) origin, but the precise number of endocrine and exocrine neoplasms was not stated (Masahito et al., 1995).

Grossly, pancreatic neoplasms are 5–37 mm in greatest diameter and are located between the liver and duodenum. Cut surfaces are yellowish white, solid or polycystic. Histologically, the neoplasms in hybrid frogs are characteristic of endocrine neoplasms. They are composed of solid nests of cells separated by fine trabeculae or fibrovascular stroma. These features are often referred to as a medullary pattern. Cells are rather uniform in size and shape and have round nuclei. There may be a tendency for cells at the periphery of each nest or lobule to form rows of cells on the vascular trabeculae. Some lobules have irregularly shaped cavities or spaces that contain protein-rich fluid and few cells. Metastases to the lung, heart, liver, kidney, stomach, and ovary were detected in seven hybrid frogs (Masahito et al., 1995). Immunohistochemically, somatostatin, insulin, or both, may be demonstrated, but glucagon-positive cells have not been found (Masahito et al., 1995). Ultrastructurally, three pancreatic neoplasms, as well as islet cells from normal frogs, have endocrine secretory granules measuring up to 350 nm. All three neoplasms, but not control pancreases, had mature extracellular C-type retrovirus particles measuring 100 nm, and some "particles appeared to be budding from cytoplasmic membranes" (Masahito et al., 1995).

Only a few of the scores of pancreatic neoplasms in hybrid frogs may have been exocrine in origin, as evidenced histologically by "quasinormal acinar or tubular cell differentiation" (Masahito et al., 1995). In the suspected exocrine neoplasms, the cells are larger, have greater amounts of cytoplasm, and tend to form acinar- and tubular-like structures lined by cuboidal, high cuboidal, or columnar cells.

Epidemiologically, the spontaneous neoplasms in the experimentally produced hybrid frogs at the Laboratory for Amphibian Biology (Hiroshima University, Japan) did not appear until wild specimens of the Peking frog, *Rana p. plancyi*, and the black-spotted frog, *R. nigromaculata*, from the vicinity of Beijing were introduced into the laboratory and crossbred with frogs native to Korea, Japan, and Formosa. No pancreatic tumors were observed in numerous non-Chinese crossbred frogs during 1975–1987, but, following introduction of Chinese frogs into the laboratory, "tumors began to appear . . . , although very rarely, in Japanese and [non-Chinese] hybrid frogs" (Masahito et al., 1995). However, it is not clear whether hybrid amphibians are more prone to develop spontaneous neoplasms and whether the observed retroviruses were the causative agent or merely passengers (Masahito et al., 1995). An encapsulated, ovoid tumor was noted on the pancreas of an unidentified frog (Pawlowski, 1912). The nodule had prominent fibrovascular stroma separating nests of glandlike cells that had eosinophilic granular cytoplasm. This brief description is consistent with an exocrine pancreatic carcinoma.

26.7 NEOPLASMS OF THE ALIMENTARY TRACT

26.7.1 Neuroepithelioma of the Mouth

This neoplasm presumably originates from the olfactory epithelium, and has marked resemblance to the previously described skin neoplasms of lateral line (neuromast) origin. Four neuroepitheliomata have been reported from the roof of the mouth in captive specimens of the axolotl, *Ambystoma mexicanum* (Brunst & Roque, 1967; Humphrey, 1969), but only two have been described (Brunst & Roque, 1967). An additional three neoplasms of the mouth (or nasal cavity), that were characterized as "adenocarcinomas", were detected in axolotls (Sheremetieva-Brunst, 1961), but it is not clear if these cases were included in the report by Brunst and Roque (1967). Histologically, this neoplasm is composed of many discrete, well-formed lobes separated by markedly varying amounts of fibrovascular stroma. Lobes usually have a distinct tubular structure with a central lumen that is generally clear but occasionally contains coagulated material, and a cellular wall composed of columnar or elongate cells oriented perpendicularly to the central lumen and peripheral margin. Tumor cells are usually bipolar, with large abluminal, ovoid to elongate nuclei and prominent nucleoli. In H&E stains, fibrils may be detected in some elongate cells, but with special stains many more fibrils are evident. Fibrils are red in the aniline blue stain and blue and black in various silver stains. These fibrils were considered to be neurofibrils (Brunst & Roque, 1967). Mitotic rate is variable from lobe to lobe, but usually 1–5%. These neoplasms were successfully transplanted into the subcutis of other axolotls (Brunst & Roque, 1967).

26.7.2 Hyperkeratosis of the Tongue

One case of hyperkeratosis (i.e., "warty" proliferations) on the free margin of the tongue was reported in a >7-year-old, emaciated, captive pig frog, *Rana grylio* (Elkan, 1968). The free margin of the tongue had an irregular outline and was indurated and solid upon palpation. The fat bodies were completely atrophied, suggesting the frog starved due to inability to capture feed with the diseased tongue. Histologically, the tongue showed extensive infolding of the epithelium, and an increase in epithelial cell numbers from a normal of 1–2 cell layers to as many as 10 cells deep. There was extensive thickening of the keratinized layer. In addition, the author (Elkan, 1968) used the terms "hyperkeratosis," "parakeratosis," "keratoprecancerosis," and "warty" to describe the lesion. There was no evidence of penetration of the basement membrane, although from photomicrographs it was not clear whether there was squamous metaplasia of submucosal glands, or actual infolding of the keratinized epithelium. The lesion was considered hyperplastic and possibly precancerous by the author, but the possibility of squamous metaplasia secondary to chronic vitamin A deficiency must be considered a possible alternative diagnosis.

26.7.3 Adenocarcinoma of the Stomach

One gastric adenocarcinoma with metastatic disease has been reported in a captive African clawed frog, *Xenopus laevis* (Elkan, 1983). Minimal details were given, but the neoplasm formed distinct nests and cords of pleomorphic epithelial cells that were actively invading submucosal, muscular and serosal tunics, and had metastasized to the pancreas and urinary bladder possibly transcoelomically. Moderate amounts of fibrovascular stroma separated the nests of neoplastic cells in this neoplasm, but in other gastrointestinal adenocarcinomata of vertebrates the fibrous stroma may be abundant (sclerosing adenocarcinoma). Adenomas and carcinoids of the gastric mucosa have not been reported in amphibians. Neoplasms of connective tissues (blood vessels, smooth muscle cells, mesothelium, etc.) are discussed in Section 26.3, Neoplasms of the Mesenchymal Tissues. Published reports of leiomyomata in the stomachs of the Japanese firebelly newt, *Cynops pyrrhogaster*, are questionable (Asashima & Meyer-Rochow, 1989; Pfeiffer & Asashima, 1990) for the illustrated tumors are suggestive of granulomata. The stomach may be involved in metastatic disease (Elkan, 1970), such as lymphosarcomas.

26.7.4 Intestinal Neoplasms

Four neoplasms, all malignant, have been reported in the intestines of amphibians. These include an African clawed frog, *Xenopus laevis* (Elkan, 1970), a leopard frog, *Rana pipiens* (Downs, 1932), a giant toad, *Bufo marinus* (RTLA #1921), and an Oriental firebelly toad, *Bombina orientalis* (RTLA #5850). The precise nature of the neoplasm in the northern leopard frog, *R. pipiens*, is not certain. Grossly, the neoplasm nearly filled the body cavity, was roughly cubical, and yellowish brown. Histologically, the neoplasm was briefly described as "cells . . . arranged in irregular acini suggesting a tumor arising from the intestine" and was diagnosed simply as an "epithelial tumour" (Downs, 1932). This description is considered insufficient to determine whether the neoplasm originated from intestinal mucosal epithelium, intestinal neuroendocrine cells, the exocrine pancreas, or some other adjacent organ.

An anaplastic and metastatic neoplasm of possible intestinal epithelial cell origin was reported in an African clawed frog, *Xenopus laevis*. There was extensive metastatic disease involving the stomach, intestines, pancreas, kidneys, urinary bladder, and blood vessels (Elkan, 1970). In the opinion of the authors of this chapter, the neoplasm probably was not a carcinoma of intestinal origin. The histologic features of the cells were scarcely described, but the widespread infiltrative features, and presence of neoplastic cells in multiple blood and lymphatic vessels, suggests the neoplasm was a lymphosarcoma or myeloid neoplasm. Others (Masahito et al., 1995) have suggested the neoplasm was of pancreatic origin.

Adenocarcinoma of the Intestine. One clear example of a primary intestinal neoplasm in an amphibian is that of an unpublished sclerosing adenocarcinoma in a giant toad, *Bufo marinus* (RTLA #1921). Subgrossly, the neoplasm caused very marked thickening of the intestinal wall. Neoplastic intestinal epithelial cells invaded all three tunics, forming very small nests, islands, and tubules of pleomorphic cells separated by large amounts of reactive fibrocytes and edema. The intestinal mucosa was ulcerated in numerous large segments (Figures 26.64, 26.65). The neoplastic epithelial cells are pleomorphic: some nests of cells have a small irregular central lumen and the cells are squamous, cuboidal and, occasionally columnar. Cytoplasm varies in amount, but is usually clear, light blue or dark blue. Lumina may appear empty, indistinct, or contain mild amounts of mucuslike material and necrotic cells. Nuclei also are pleomorphic; some are small, dense and round, while others are elongate and have course clumps of heterochromatin. Mitotic rate is usually high, but due to the

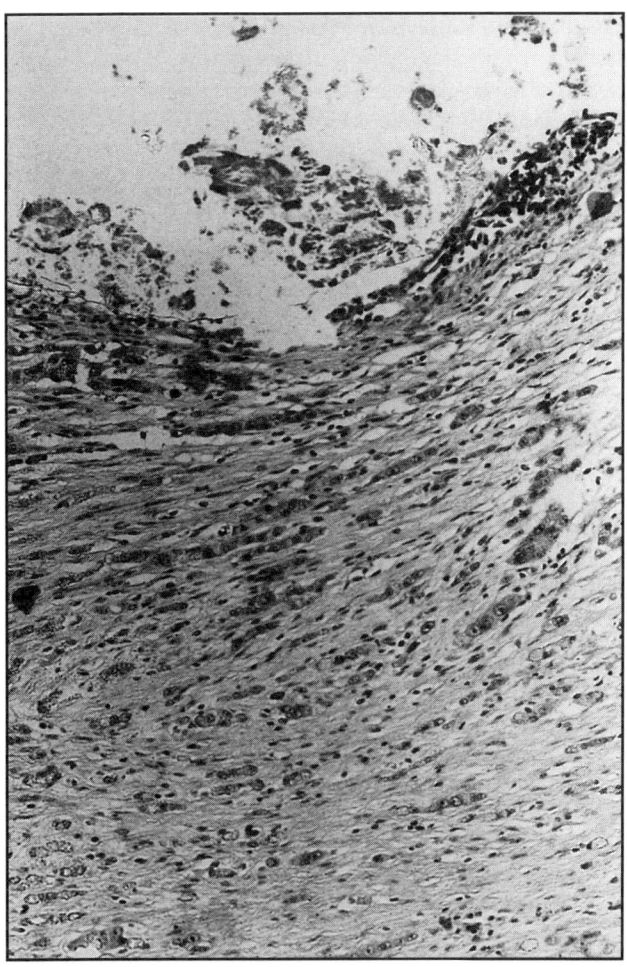

Figure 26.64. Intestinal adenocarcinoma in a giant toad, *Bufo marinus*. Nests and tubules of neoplastic epithelial cells are invading the submucosal and muscular tunics (center and bottom) while the mucosal epithelium (top) shows marked necrosis and ulceration. (A.J. Herron, RTLA 1921)

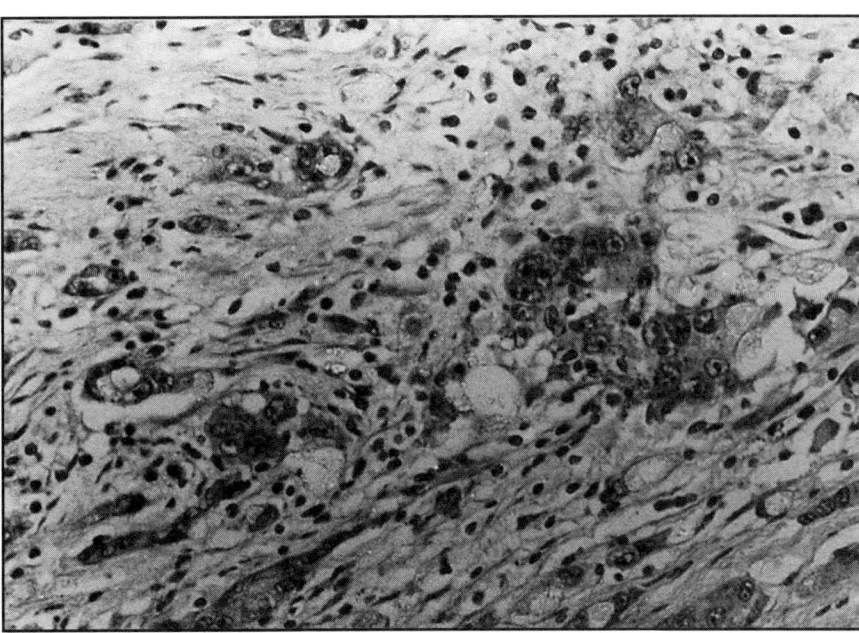

Figure 26.65. Intestinal adenocarcinoma in a giant toad, *Bufo marinus;* higher magnification of Figure 26.64. Highly irregular nests and tubules of pleomorphic neoplastic mucosal epithelial cells are separated by edematous fibrous stroma. Some neoplastic cells contain large pale-staining mucus-filled cytoplasmic vacuoles. (A.J. Herron, RTLA 1921)

extensive amounts of edema and sclerosis, few neoplastic cells are observed per high power field. Metastatic potential of this neoplasm is unknown, but is probably high.

Cloacal Adenocarcinoma. One unpublished cloacal adenocarcinoma of probable cloacal gland origin is present in the files of the Registry of Tumors in Lower Animals. At present, it is not clear whether this neoplasm originated from the dermally related cloacal glands or the cloacal mucosal epithelium (Figures 26.66, 26.67).

Squamous Cell Carcinoma of the Colo-Cloacal Region. One unpublished polypoid squamous cell carcinoma of the distal colon is present in the Registry of Tumors in Lower Animals (RTLA #5850). The neoplasm was an incidental histologic finding in an aged Oriental firebelly toad, *Bombina* sp. (presumably *B. orientalis*), from Korea that had been in captivity for many years in the U.S. Histologically, the neoplasm was about 2 × 3 mm and had a thin fibrous stalk attaching

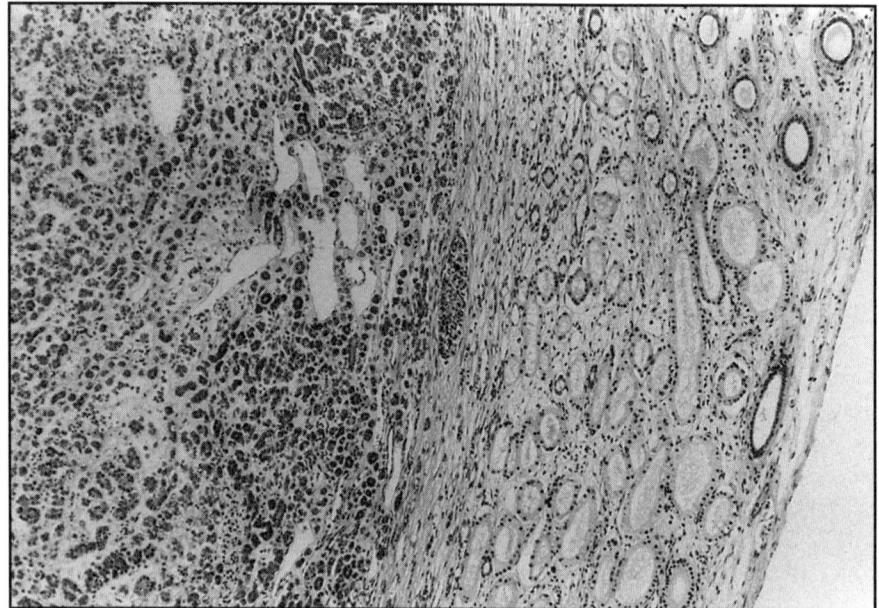

Figure 26.66. Cloacal gland adenocarcinoma, tubular type, in an axolotl, *Ambystoma mexicanum*. Dilated, atrophied and compressed pre-existing cloacal glands are at the right, and neoplastic glands and tubules are on the left. (R. Verhoeff-DeFremery, RTLA 2847)

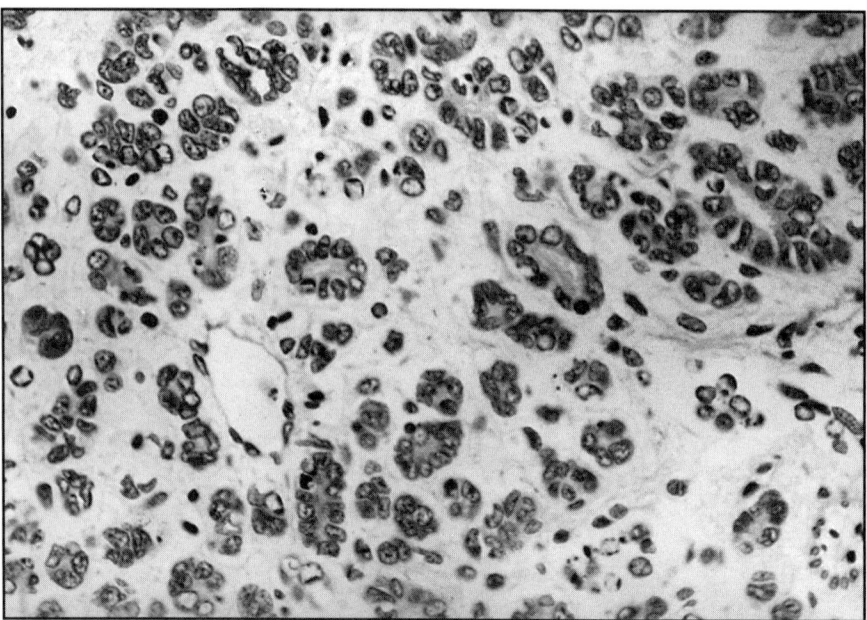

Figure 26.67. Cloacal gland adenocarcinoma in an axolotl, *Ambystoma mexicanum*, tubular type; higher magnification of Figure 26.66. Neoplastic glandular tubulo-alveoli are lined by cuboidal cells with mostly round nuclei. Fibrovascular stroma is prominent and edematous. (R. Verhoeff-DeFremery, RTLA 2847)

it to the colonic mucosa (Figure 26.68). The cells consisted of polygonal, plump epithelioid cells with moderate amounts of eosinophilic cytoplasm (Figure 26.69) and prominent intercellular bridges. Although a colonic location for a squamous cell carcinoma is unusual, it is well documented in human medicine (Wood, 1967).

Leiomyoma and Leiomyosarcoma. See Section 26.3, Neoplasms of Mesenchymal Tissues.

26.8 NEOPLASMS OF THE REPRODUCTIVE SYSTEMS

26.8.1 Neoplasms of the Male Reproductive Tract

Testicular Neoplasms. There are four reports of spontaneous testicular neoplasms in amphibians: the axolotl, *Ambystoma mexicanum,* a Japanese giant salamander, *Andrias japonicus,* a hybrid mole salamander, *Ambystoma mexicanum* × *A. opacum,* a hellbender, *Cryptobranchus alleganiensis,* and a wild hybrid ranid (Cosgrove & Harshbarger, 1971; Hardy & Gillespie, 1976; Humphrey, 1969; Pick & Poll, 1903, as cited by Balls & Clothier, 1974). A total of 15 testicular neoplasms were reported in mature specimens of the axolotl, *A. mexicanum,* but were not accompanied by a diagnosis (Humphrey, 1969). In the opinion of the authors, the tumors were most likely tubular (or intratubular) Sertoli cell tumors. The one testicular neoplasm in a Japanese giant salamander, *A. japonicus,* was diagnosed as a cystic carcinoma in 1903 but, based on current veterinary classification schemes (Nielsen & Lein, 1974), this neoplasm also may have been a tubular Sertoli cell tumor. The neoplasm in the hellbender was diagnosed as an adenoma of seminiferous epithelium (Sertoli cell adenoma).

Sertoli Cell Tumor. Among 497 male specimens of the axolotl, *Ambystoma mexicanum,* submitted for necropsy, 16 (3.2%) had testicular neoplasms. The majority of specimens were less than 3 years old. Fourteen of 16 specimens were "white axolotls," and

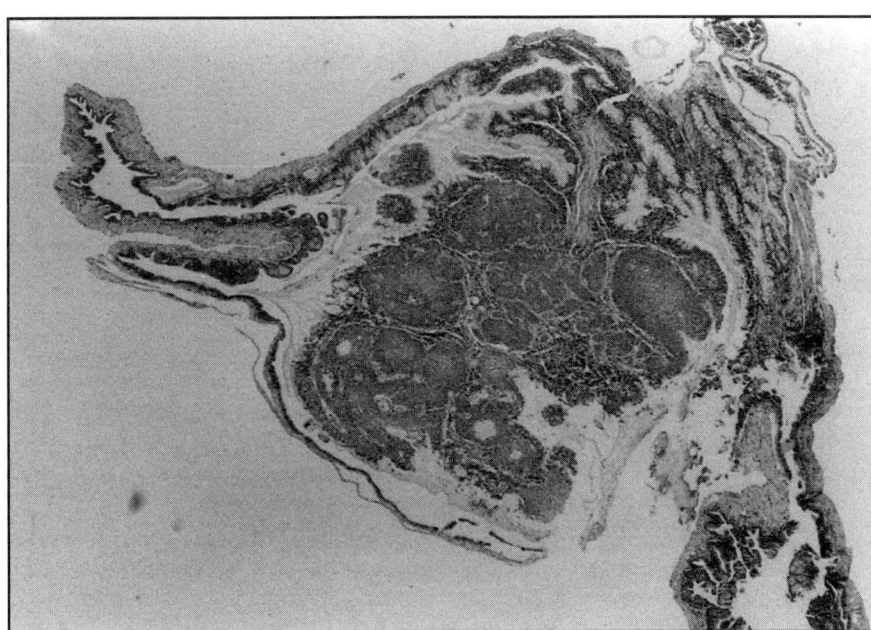

Figure 26.68. Polypoid squamous cell carcinoma of colo-cloacal region in a captive Oriental firebelly toad, *Bombina orientalis*. This carcinoma had a prominent fibrovascular stalk, but no evidence of invasion of the intestinal wall. (D.E. Green, RTLA 5850)

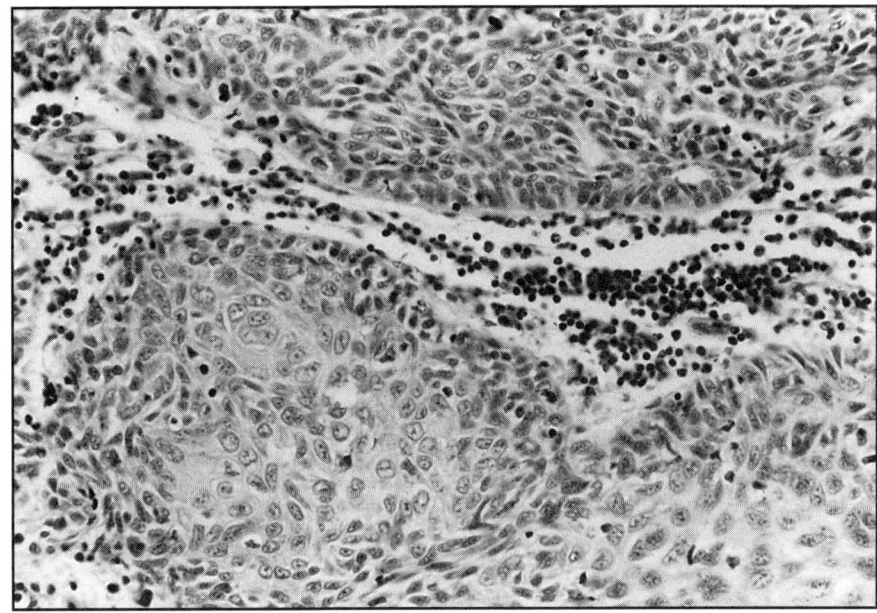

Figure 26.69. Squamous cell carcinoma of colo-cloacal region in a captive Oriental firebelly toad, *Bombina orientalis;* higher magnification of Figure 26.68. Squamous cells show cytoplasmic keratinization, intercellular bridges, and a mild mitotic rate. (D.E. Green, RTLA 5850)

13 of 16 specimens were descendants of one female. Grossly, the testicular neoplasms were pedunculated, 0.8–4.5 cm in diameter, whitish, had deep fissures forming multiple lobes, and had a "pebbled" surface. Most were rather solid on cut surface, but some were spongy or polycystic (Humphrey, 1969).

Histologically, Sertoli cell tumors of the axolotl, *Ambystoma mexicanum,* are composed of elongate, branching tubules lined by simple or stratified columnar cells (e.g., Figures 26.70, 26.71). At the periphery (subcapsular region), the tubules are numerous, compact, and have indistinct lumina although centrally the tubules become progressively larger with distinct large lumina. Most tubules lack spermatogonia, but smaller (<1 cm diameter) tumors may contain degenerating germ cells, or germ cells showing abnormal multiple stages of development (spermatogonia, spermatocytes, spermatids) within the same tubule. Neoplastic Sertoli cells are usually columnar or elongate, but in smaller tubules may be cuboidal, and in large densely cellular tubules, cells may appear polygonal. Neoplastic cells may appear stratified within tubules and lining the papillary projections (see Figures 26.70, 26.71). Fibrovascular stroma at the periphery of the tumor is scanty to mild in amount, but increases markedly centrally. Cytoplasmic borders are indistinct, and the cytoplasm is pale, poorly stained, clear, or vacuolated.

Nuclei are pleomorphic, have prominent chromatinic rims, and abundant heterochromatin. Mitotic rate may be brisk, especially in subcapsular regions. Solid cords of Sertoli cells and metastases were not reported in the axolotls. However, remaining testicular tissue and the contralateral testis often show marked atrophy. Secondary sexual glands, such as male cloacal glands, and the ductus deferens appear normal. In castrated specimens of the axolotl, *A. mexicanum,* the cloacal glands and ductus deferens undergo marked atrophy (Humphrey, 1969).

Sertoli cell tumors may also have a solid cellularity called a diffuse type tumor. One diffuse Sertoli cell tumor in a hybrid ranid frog, (*Rana pipiens* × *R. palustris*) was present in the files of the Registry of Tumors in Lower Animals (Figure 26.72). This neoplasm was bilateral. There is marked destruction of the tubular architecture by masses of polygonal and fusiform cells that often contain clear (lipid) vacuoles. Cytoplasmic

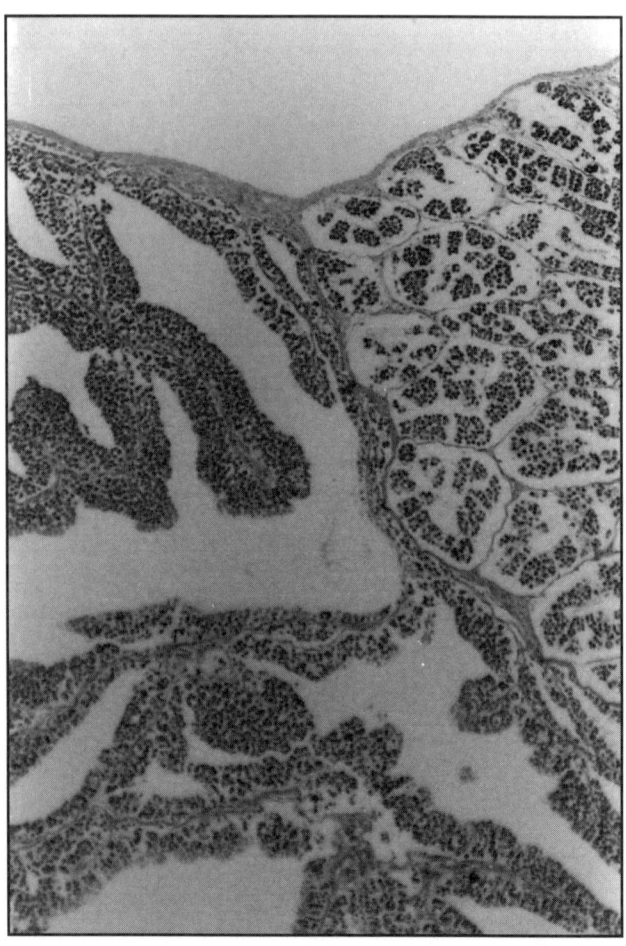

Figure 26.70. Sertoli cell tumor, intratubular type, in a hellbender, *Cryptobranchus alleganiensis*. Normal testis is at right and neoplastic Sertoli cells at bottom and left. (G.E. Cosgrove, RTLA 233)

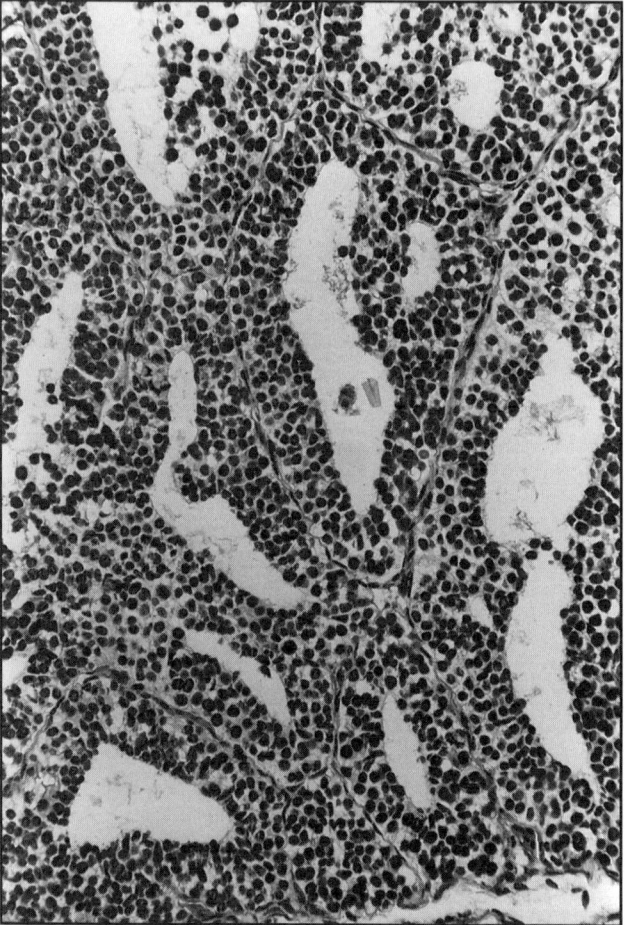

Figure 26.71. Sertoli cell tumor, intratubular type, in a hellbender, *Cryptobranchus alleganiensis;* higher magnification of Figure 26.70. Neoplastic cells line the tubules, and there is uniformity of nuclear size. No germ cells remain. (G.E. Cosgrove, RTLA 233)

borders are indistinct, and nuclei are elongate (in fusiform cells), round or ovoid, and consistently dense and dark. Mitotic rate is very low. Fibrovascular stroma is scant, but occasionally, neoplastic cells appear oriented around vessels.

Neoplasms of Bidder's Organ. In 1987, Nishioka and Kondo, and Nishioka and Ueda briefly mentioned the occurrence of tumors of Bidder's organs in about 10 laboratory-bred hybrid toads. No specific details, descriptions or diagnoses were given.

Seminoma, Teratoma, and Leydig Cell Tumors. These neoplasms have not been detected or reported in the amphibian testis.

26.8.2 Neoplasms of the Female Reproductive Tract

Granulosa Cell Tumor. There are no published reports or descriptions of granulosa cell tumors in amphibians, but one case of this ovarian neoplasm is present in the files of the Registry of Tumors in Lower Animals (RTLA #3575). This single case in an 11-year-old, captive ornate horned frog, *Ceratophrys ornata,* involved one ovary. Histologically, the neoplasm consists of a uniform cellular population resembling normal granulosa cells that form large cords or nests separated by mildly prominent fibrovascular stroma and may contain irregular large clefts and clear spaces (Figures 26.73, 26.74). Cells are plump, polygonal or fusiform, and have abundant pale eosinophilic cytoplasm. Cell borders vary from distinct among polygonal cells to indistinct among fusiform cells. Nuclei are central, round or ovoid in polygonal cells, but more elongate in fusiform cells. Chromatin is usually coarse, clumped and prominent, but seldom vesicular. Mitoses are few or absent. Small foci of prominent basophilic necrosis are present, but Call-Exner bodies and follicular patterns were not observed.

Ovarian Adenocarcinoma. Ovarian adenocarcinomas are often referred to as "epithelial" neoplasms although it is likely that they are derived from the ovarian surface "epithelium," which is coelomic mesothelium. Insufficient numbers of amphibian ovarian "epithelial" neoplasms have been reported and described to determine whether any are benign (adenoma) or malignant

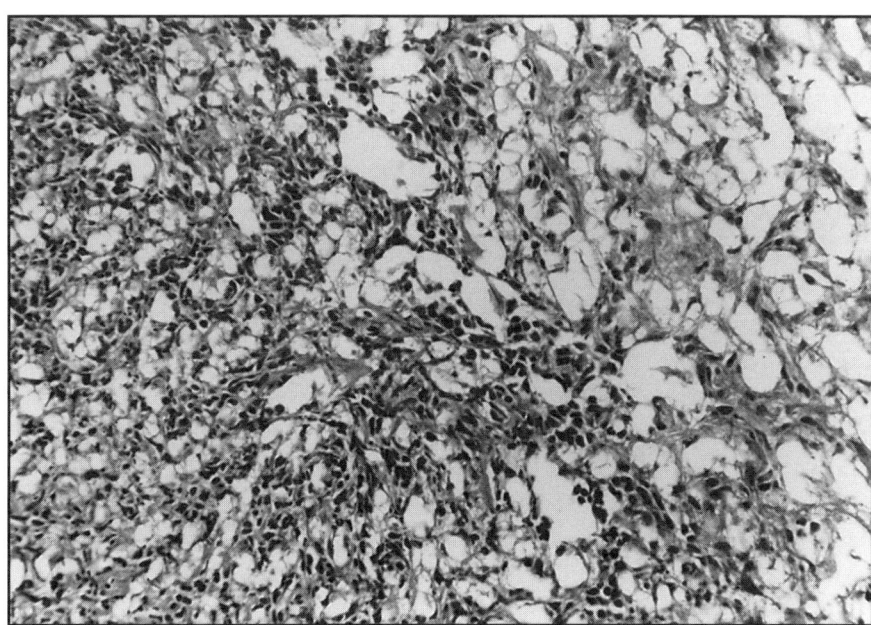

Figure 26.72. Sertoli cell tumor, diffuse type, in a wild hybrid frog, *Rana pipiens* × *R. palustris.* Note destruction of tubules and abundance of cytoplasmic lipids. Nuclei are pleomorphic. (J.D. Hardy, RTLA 403)

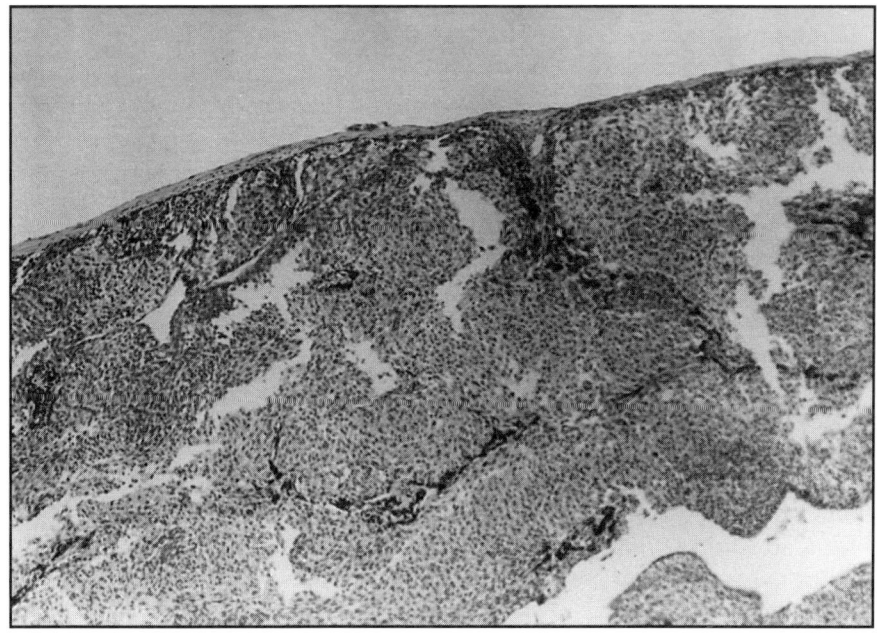

Figure 26.73. Granulosa cell tumor in an ornate horned frog, *Ceratophrys ornata.* This ovarian tumor has solidly cellular lobules, and cells have abundant eosinophilic cytoplasm. (F.L. Frye, RTLA 3575)

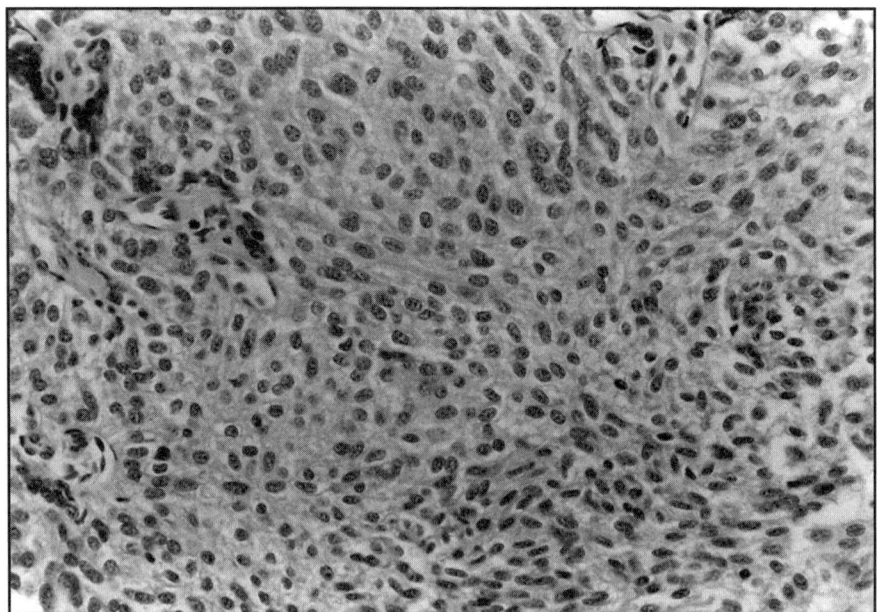

Figure 26.74. Granulosa cell tumor in an ornate horned frog, *Ceratophrys ornata*; higher magnification of Figure 26.73. Cells are polygonal with abundant lightly staining eosinophilic cytoplasm, but fusiform cells also are evident. Nuclei are mostly ovoid with few or no cells undergoing mitosis. (F.L. Frye, RTLA 3575)

the three major germ layers: endoderm, mesoderm, and ectoderm. Most contain the latter two germ cells that have differentiated into skin, bone, cartilage, fat, muscle, skin, or teeth. Nervous tissue may also be present. One teratoma has been reported from a northern leopard frog, *Rana pipiens* (Streett, 1964). Histologically, the 12 × 8 × 8-mm neoplasm in the right ovary contained cartilage, bone, bone marrow, intestine, and skin (Figure 26.75) (A teratoma in the dermis and muscles of a mature axolotl, *Ambystoma mexicanum*, has also been reported. See Section 26.14, Miscellaneous Neoplasms).

(adenocarcinoma). In similar neoplasms of domestic animals, division into benign and malignant categories is considered arbitrary in most cases (Nielsen & Lein, 1974). In other vertebrates, these ovarian neoplasms usually have one of two forms, either papillary or cystic. Epithelial ovarian neoplasms have been reported in a northern leopard frog, *Rana pipiens* (Abrams, 1969), an edible frog, *Rana esculenta* (Plehn, 1906, as cited by Balls & Clothier, 1974), and 46 captive toad hybrids (*Bufo bufo* × *Bufo gargarizans*) (Nishioka & Ueda, 1987).

The neoplasm in the edible frog, *Rana esculenta*, was characterized as a possible multicentric bilateral carcinoma. The neoplasm in the northern leopard frog, *Rana pipiens*, was a cystadenocarcinoma that occupied about 25–33% of the caudal body cavity. It was multilobulated and multicystic grossly. Histologically, the neoplasm consisted of numerous, variably sized and shaped cavities lined by cuboidal epithelial cells that were one to three cells thick and, in larger cavities, formed short simple mounds of cells, and occasional short papillary projections. Most cavities contain a light proteinous fluid and very few sloughed cells. One neoplasm in a hybrid toad (*Bufo bufo* × *B. gargarizans*) occupied over half of the body cavity and was diagnosed as an ovarian carcinoma. Few details are available on the other 45 ovarian tumors in hybrid toads (Nishioka & Ueda, 1987).

Teratoma. These neoplasms are a mixture of normal and neoplastic tissue derived from at least two of

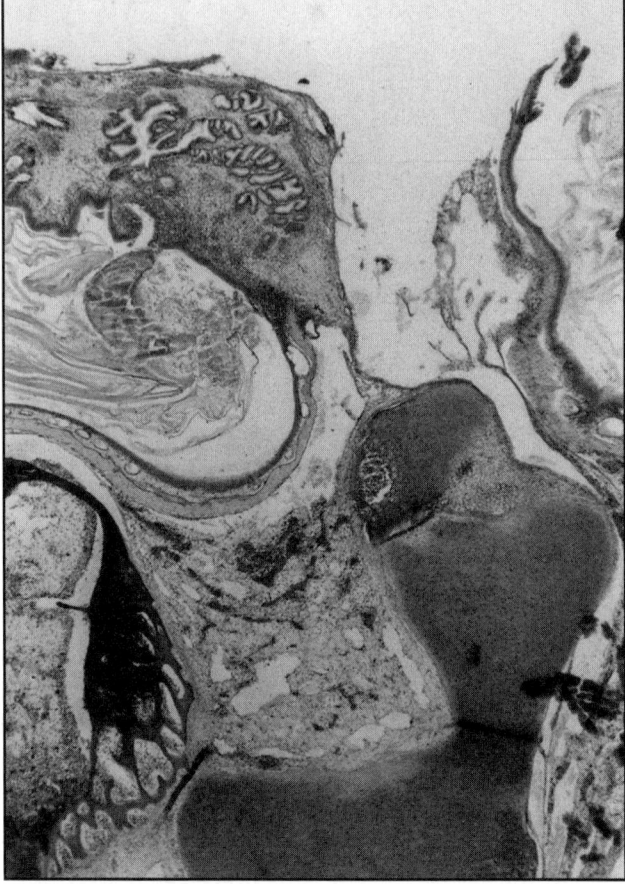

Figure 26.75. Ovarian teratoma in a northern leopard frog, *Rana pipiens*. This highly variable neoplasm has tissues of three germ layers: endoderm (intestine-like epithelial glands at top), ectoderm (keratinized skin at left), and mesoderm (bone with hematopoietic cells and cartilage at bottom and right). (J.C. Streett, RTLA 436)

26.8.3 Neoplasms of the Female Nongonadal Reproductive Organs

No primary neoplasms of the oviduct have been reported in amphibians.

26.9 NEOPLASMS OF THE ENDOCRINE ORGANS

26.9.1 Thyroid Neoplasms

No neoplasms of the thyroids have been reported in amphibians. However, massive goiters have been documented as spontaneous and experimental diseases of amphibians, and could be mistaken for neoplasms.

26.9.2 Interrenal Neoplasms

A neoplasm of possible interrenal cell origin was described in an adult female edible frog, *Rana esculenta* (Carl, 1913). The neoplasm was considered distinct from the herpesviral renal carcinomata observed in the northern leopard frog, *Rana pipiens* (Lucke, 1934). The neoplasm was diagnosed as a hypernephroma (Carl, 1923), but using more modern terminology would now be referred to as an interrenal adenoma (a malignant neoplasm would be called an interrenal carcinoma). Grossly, the tumor was 1–2 cm, firm, round, had a slightly uneven surface, was the same color as normal renal tissue, and projected ventrally from the left mesonephros. Histologically, neoplastic cells formed cords and regions of solid patternless cellularity. Cells were pleomorphic and had large nuclei resembling interrenal cell nuclei more than renal tubular nuclei. No vacuoles, glycogen, chromaffin-positive cytoplasmic granules, or metastases were evident.

26.9.3 Neoplasms of the Islets of Langerhans (Endocrine Pancreas)

Spontaneous neoplasms of islet cells have been reported only in experimentally produced, captive hybrid anurans in one laboratory in Japan. A variety of other spontaneous neoplasms of the kidneys, ovaries, exocrine pancreas, and liver were also found in these hybrid anurans (Masahito et al., 1995; Nishioka & Kondo, 1987; Nishioka & Ueda, 1987). Islet cell neoplasms are described in Section 26.6.3, Pancreatic Neoplasms.

26.9.4 Pituitary and Pineal Neoplasms

No pineal, adenohypophyseal, or neurohypophyseal neoplasms have been reported from amphibians.

26.10 NEOPLASMS OF THE RESPIRATORY SYSTEM

Very few hyperplasias and neoplasms of the respiratory system have been described in amphibians. Most reports are over 30 years old, descriptions are poor or lacking, and subsequent re-evaluations are not possible. The axolotl, *Ambystoma mexicanum*, may be prone to developing neoplasms of the nasal cavity that are first evident in the palate. It is not clear whether these naso-oral neoplasms are adenocarcinomata of mucosal epithelial origin, or neuroepitheliomata of neurosensory cell origin. Neuroepitheliomata resemble tumors of lateral line (neuromast cell) origin. Tracheobronchial neoplasms have not been reported in amphibians. One gill papilloma of epithelial origin was experimentally induced in a neotenic barred tiger salamander, *Ambystoma tigrinum mavortium* (RTLA #2541), following injection of the chemical perylene (Rose, 1981).

Only one neoplasm of the lung has been described (Elkan, 1960). The tumor was considered a multicentric adenocarcinoma, but was described histologically only at the subgross level. No cellular details were given. The neoplasm occurred in a captive adult female natterjack toad, *Bufo calamita,* that slowly became lethargic, anorectic and emaciated. Grossly, both lungs had numerous, 1–2 mm diameter, firm white nodules. Subgrossly, the nodules consisted of papillary projections that appeared to fill small air spaces. The multifocal or miliary nature of the neoplasm suggests it was either multicentric in origin or, more likely, was metastatic from some other primary focus, such as a kidney. This neoplasm is provisionally accepted as a multicentric pulmonary adenocarcinoma pending reports of additional pulmonary neoplasms in amphibians to determine if there is indeed a propensity for multicentricity.

Approximately five specimens of the northern leopard frog, *Rana pipiens,* had microscopic nodules of hypertrophied or metaplastic pulmonary epithelial cells (Duryee, 1965) that were misinterpreted as carcinomata (Balls & Clothier, 1974; Duryee, 1965). Each nodule was a tuftlike projection of tall columnar cells within the grasp of suckers of lung flukes. Although neoplasia has been associated with various helminthic parasites in a few species of endothermic animals, it is doubtful these minute nodules in leopard frog lungs were neoplasms. The preferred diagnosis is verminous hyperplasia.

26.11 NEOPLASMS OF THE CENTRAL AND PERIPHERAL NERVOUS SYSTEMS

Intracranial neoplasms of amphibians have not been reported, and those that were purported to be intracranial meningeal tumors were nodules of verminous granulomatous meningitis (Lautenschlager, 1959) or xanthomatous granulomas (Carpenter et al., 1986). Two extra-cranial neoplasms of possible nerve cell and nerve sheath origin have been reported in a red-spotted newt, *Notophthalmus viridescens*, and a bullfrog, *Rana catesbeiana* (Counts, 1980; Schlumberger & Lucke, 1948). The bullfrog neoplasm was briefly described as a "mass ... composed of interlacing bundles and whorls which resembled neoplastic connective tissue. In general appearence the tumor was similar to ... nerve sheath tumors of man" (Schlumberger & Lucke, 1948). The newt neoplasm reported as a neuroblastoma (Counts, 1980), has been reexamined with an appropriate special stain, and has been reclassified as a mast cell tumor (see Section 26.4.4, Mast Cell Tumors).

Malformations and proliferations of the brain occur in caudate and anuran larvae subjected to certain experimental manipulations of the egg and sperm. These include larvae derived from irradiated sperm (Hertwig, 1953), and possibly from larvae derived from so-called "overripe eggs" (Briggs, 1941; Witschi, 1922, 1930) or eggs stimulated into development with only the maternal or paternal genome. In many cases of so-called hybridism between two distinct species in the same genus, the sperm's genome is often eliminated because it is incapable of fusing with the maternal genome, resulting in embryogenesis with a haploid (maternal) genome only, a situation referred to as "false hybrids" (Hertwig, 1953). The precise nature of the proliferations of the brain and other ectodermal tissues in these manipulated larvae do not appear to have been studied since the early 1950s, hence, it is not clear whether these growths are hyperplastic, metaplastic, hamartomatous, or benign or malignant neoplasms.

26.12 NEOPLASMS OF THE EYE AND ADNEXA

No primary neoplasms of the eye have been reported in amphibians, but one neoplasm of the Harderian gland was reported in a captive African clawed frog, *Xenopus laevis* (Elkan, 1968). The adnexal neoplasm bulged into the oral cavity and markedly displaced the left eye outward. The frog survived over 6 months following detection of the neoplasm. Histologically, the neoplasm was well encapsulated, at least 18 mm in greatest dimension, and caused marked compression and displacement of the globe, but no invasion of adjacent tissues. The neoplasm was composed of tubules of various sizes and shapes with collapsed or prominent empty lumina. Many tubules were folded giving a false impression of simple papillary projections. Mild amounts of fibrovascular stroma separated each tubule. Each neoplastic tubule was lined by a single layer of columnar cells with basally oriented nuclei, leaving the apical 30–50% of each cell to consist only of pale cytoplasm. Nuclei are round to oval and dark. No mitoses were evident (Elkan, 1968). Since no features of malignancy were described, the neoplasm was most likely a benign, albeit large, adenoma of the Harderian gland.

Experimentally, a retinal tumor occurred in a 28-day-old larval smooth newt, *Triturus vulgaris*, that was the product of a normal egg that was inseminated by radium-irradiated sperm (Hertwig, 1953).

26.13 NEOPLASMS OF THE BONES, JOINTS, AND NOTOCHORD

26.13.1 Tumorlike Osteochondrous Dysplasia

Tumorlike osteochondrous dysplasia affecting the hindlimbs of wild specimens of the Inkiapo frog, *Rana chensinensis*, was found in two localities associated with effluents from a paper factory and sewage (Mizgireuv et al., 1984). At the site contaminated by paper factory effluents, 126 (11.5%) of 1095 metamorphs of the Inkiapo frog, *R. chensinensis*, had bone lesions, while the site contaminated by sewage had 202 (5.5%) affected frogs out of 3651. At a third site, none of 1614 frogs were affected. The condition is mentioned in this section on neoplasia, because the authors characterized some lesions as "tumorlike dysplasia," or resembling "medullary chondroma," "chondromatosis," "osteochondroma," and "chondrosarcoma" (Mizgireuv et al., 1984). Numerous other developmental anomalies were detected in the frogs near the paper factory, including microcephaly, unilateral anophthalmia, tail abnormalities, and failure of hindlimb digits or metatarsals to develop. Interestingly, two other anurans in the region, the Chusan Island toad, *Bufo gargarizans*, and the Khabarovsk frog, *Rana amurensis*, did not have developmental anomalies or chondrodysplastic lesions.

Grossly, chondrodysplastic lesions were detected in froglets as early as 2–3 weeks after metamorphosis. The diaphyses of the tibia, fibula, and distal femur were affected with one or two dense, elastic to firm, light yellow nodules that were 1×1 mm in froglets, and up to 5×7 mm in adult frogs.

Histologically, the dysplastic nodules were of two types. The first type, or chondroma-like dysplasia, consisted of nodules of mature medullary chondrocytes with a periosteum. The cells were monomorphic and spherical with weakly basophilic cytoplasm and an oval hyperchromatic nucleus. Subperiosteal and peripheral cells were smaller while central cells were larger. In some lesions, the central chondrocytes degenerated and were replaced by bone, or became centrally cystic. These lesions were considered to resemble osteochondromas and osteal (bone) cysts, respectively. The second type of chondrodysplasia was characterized by larger nodules composed of atypical pleomorphic chondroblast-like cells with vacuolated basophilic cytoplasm and large pleomorphic nuclei. This type was considered to resemble a chondrosarcoma. However, none of the cartilagenous nodules penetrated the periosteum and no metastases were detected. The authors concluded that all lesions were a form of chemically induced chondrodysplasia but the precise chemical agent was not determined.

26.13.2 Chondromyxoma (Myxochondroma, Fibromyxochondroma)

Characterization of chondromyxomas is imprecise. It is not clear whether tumors of this type are truly neoplasms or various forms of reactive exuberant chronic inflammation, hyperplasia, metaplasia, or even callous formation at the site of an unrecognized bone fracture. Tumors of this group have been encountered in two specimens of the Pacific chorus frog, *Pseudacris regilla* (Figure 26.76), and "*Rana fusca*" (Pirlot & Welsch, 1934). These tumors appear associated with or adjacent to skeletal structures of the head or limb. Histologically, the fibrous and chrondromatous portions of these tumors are solidly cellular, while the myxomatous component may be composed mostly of myxedematous extracellular material that is strikingly hypocellular. In domestic animals (farm animals) and man, many neoplasms may have a myxoid component, and it is generally accepted that this component is ignored and the diagnosis is based on the other cell components (Lattes, 1982). The amounts of myxomatous and fibrous tissue varies from region to region and between tumors. Myxomatous cells are usually found peripherally, and, moving centrally into the tumor, are progressively replaced by denser regions of fibrocyte-like cells, which in turn become chondrocyte-like cells. In the Pacific chorus frog, *P. regilla*, the chondrocytes were associated with fragments of bone that may have been preexisting, but necrotic, bones of the skull. All three cell types are well differentiated, and mitotic figures are few and normal-appearing. Until the full range of normal callus development in the flat bones of the skull and long bones of the limbs are studied and fully characterized in amphibians, it is considered prudent to consider the above lesions only as suspected neoplasms.

26.13.3 Osteosarcoma (Osteogenic Sarcoma)

Only one spontaneous osteosarcoma has been reported (Ohlmacher, 1898), however, subsequent authors

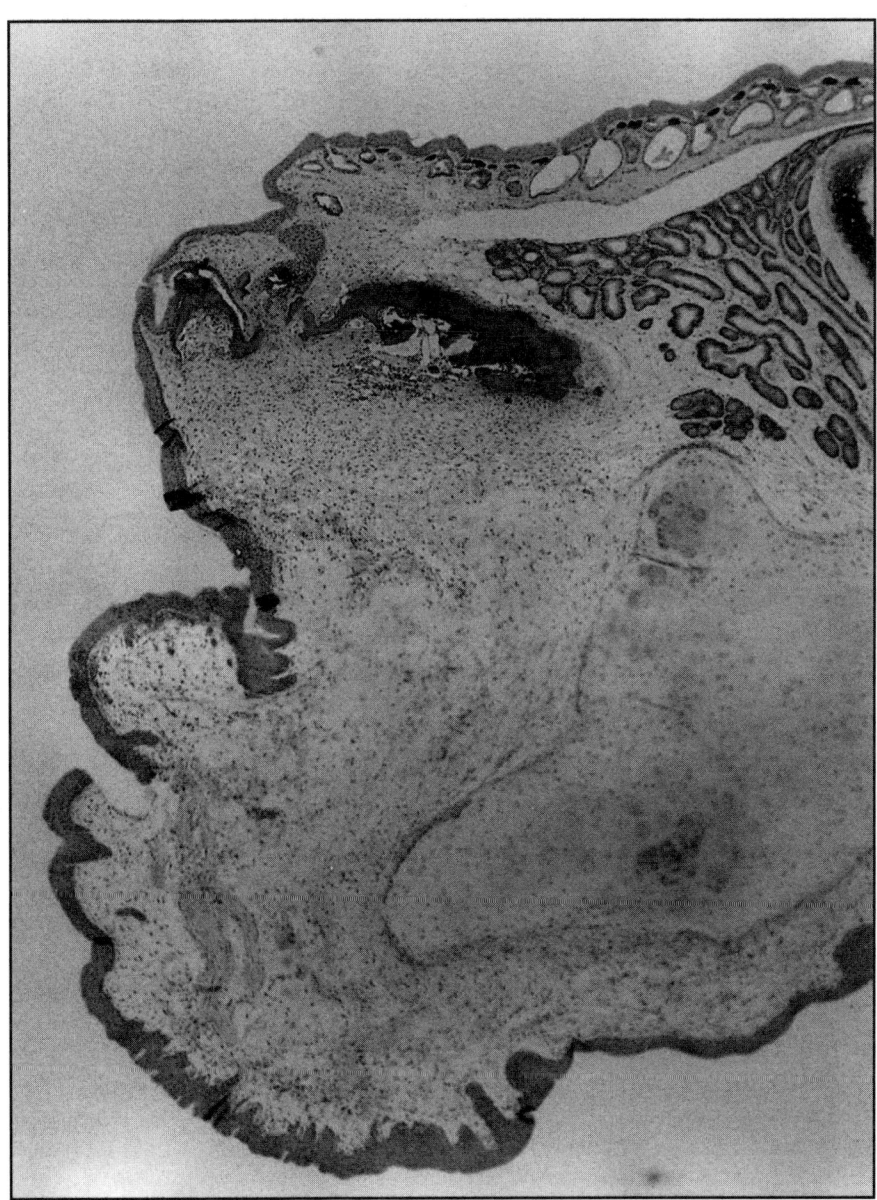

Figure 26.76. "Myxochondroma" or callus formation or chronic inflammation of maxillary (snout) region in a Pacific treefrog, *Pseudacris regilla*. This proliferation of mesenchymal tissue has been called a neoplasm, a hyperplastic lesion, and an exuberant reparative process (callus) in skull bones. (Compare to Figure 27.4.) Near top center are frayed necrotic (preexisting) bones with proliferation of fibrocytes ventrally. At right center, proliferating cartilage is incompletely surrounded by fibrocytes, and considerable myxedematous (myxoid) tissue is located peripherally. Normal glandular skin at top and oral mucous membrane at bottom. (F.L. Frye, RTLA 1080)

have suggested the tumor was not neoplastic but a physiologic callus after a bone fracture (Schlumberger & Lucke, 1948). The purported neoplasm occurred in the femur of a frog "*Rana virescens*," and was a spindle-shaped swelling up to 8 mm in diameter that enclosed most of the diaphysis of the femur. Histologically, the tumor was composed of cartilage and bony trabeculae surrounded by large spaces containing proliferating mononuclear cells suggestive of bone marrow (Schlumberger & Lucke, 1948). Since no features of malignancy were mentioned, it is unlikely this early report was a true bone neoplasm. Excluding this one uncertain case, malignant bone tumors have not been reported in amphibians.

26.13.4 Chordoma

No neoplasms of the notochord have been reported in wild or wild-caught amphibians, however, there are multiple reports of chordomas arising spontaneously in laboratory-produced, hybrid toads (Flindt et al., 1968; Hertwig, 1953; Schipp, 1969; Schipp et al., 1968), and the neoplasm may have been induced in salamanders by experimental lathyrism (intoxication by the sweet pea, *Lathyrus odorata*) (Levy & Godman, 1955). All chordomas have occurred in hybrid tadpoles or larvae, and mostly in individuals that fail to metamorphose, suggesting significant endocrinological abnormalities are also present. In hybrid tadpoles ("bastardlarven") of European bufonids, "The malformations manifest themselves primarily in a disturbed longitudinal growth of the notochord, secondarily in the appearance of tumors in the sacral region which infiltrate the neighboured tissues and destroy them" (Schipp et al., 1968). However, malformations and proliferation of the notochord also occur over much of its length, resulting in a marked increased cross-sectional diameter of the notochord. Dorsal proliferations rupture the sheath of the notochord (or, alternatively, the sheath weakens and allows herniation of chordocytes) and may progress "to a nearly complete displacing of the spinal tube" (Flindt et al., 1968). The proliferations into the spinal canal were called "neoplasma-like swellings" (Flindt et al., 1968).

Chordomas are composed of rather characteristic, large cells with abundant vesicular cytoplasm and distinct cell borders. Some purported neoplastic notochord cells are significantly larger than normal mature chordocytes. Immature notochord cells, chordoblasts, are smaller cells with proportionately larger nuclei that are found at the periphery (subsheath region) of the normal notochord, but in suspected notochord tumors may be found throughout the mass, often as nests of cells. The mitotic rate may be minimal or marked. Fibrovascular stroma is absent or minimal, although PAS-positive notochord sheathlike material may be scattered irregularly through the mass resembling septae and dividing the mass into irregular nodules.

Etiologically, it must be noted that chordomas have been observed only in hybrid toad tadpoles that have either a markedly delayed metamorphosis or an inability to undergo metamorphosis. The hybrid toad tadpole with a suspected cranial chordoma reported was 9 months old (Hertwig, 1953), while normal tadpoles of the parents undergo metamorphosis within 3–4 months. Significant endocrinological abnormalities (e.g., absence of hypophysis and gonads) have been noted in other hybrid toad tadpoles, suggesting this proliferation of the notochord may be in response to hormonal deficiencies. Alternatively, as experiments with lathyrus factor (the toxic component of sweet peas) suggest, defects in the notochordal sheath may allow herniation of chordocytes. Such herniated cells are known to proliferate (Levy & Godwin, 1955). Whether these herniated and proliferating chordocytes represent true neoplasms (chordomas) or forms of hyperplasia is unclear.

26.14 MISCELLANEOUS NEOPLASMS

26.14.1 Mesothelioma

This neoplasm of the epithelial lining (mesothelium) of the body cavity has not been well documented in amphibians. One papillomatous tumor of the mesentery that was mentioned may have been a mesothelioma, but it was not described histologically (Pawlowski, 1912).

26.14.2 Teratoma

Teratomas are most often associated with a gonad in vertebrates, and were previously discussed. However, the occurrence of one exceptionally well-documented case of teratoma in the paracloacal muscles of an axolotl, *Ambystoma mexicanum*, suggests that amphibian teratomas may not conform to this general vertebrate tropism (Brunst & Roque, 1969). The neoplasm was a domed mass caudal to the left hindlimb in a 2.5-year-old animal, whose sex was not stated. The mass was 20 × 20 × 8 mm, and the cut surface showed areas of solid cellularity with interspersed multiple cavities containing mucoid material and separated by thin septae. Histologically, cells and tissues derived from all three germ layers were evident: glands composed of various cell types (endoderm), cartilage and isolated striated muscle cells (mesoderm), epidermal cells (ectoderm), and neuroepithelial cells with cytoplasmic fibroglia (neuroectoderm). Notochord tissue was not evident.

26.14.3 Hamartoma

Two vascular hamartomata have been reported in the African clawed frog, *Xenopus laevis* (Balls, 1962). No further details or descriptions were given.

Table 26.1. Spontaneous neoplasms of amphibians.						
Key: TNTC = too numerous to count ~ = approximately * = experimentally induced tumors AFIP = Armed Forces Institute of Pathology RTLA = Registry of Tumors in Lower Animals						
Neoplasm, Revised Diagnosis	Neoplasm, Published Diagnosis	Site of Origin	N =	Host Species	Reference or RTLA Contributor	RTLA Number
Integument epidermal tumors						
Hyperplasia, pseudo-epitheliomatous (PEH)	papilloma	skin	TNTC	Ambystoma tigrinum	Harshbarger & Snyder, 1989	702
Hyperplasia, pseudo-epitheliomatous (PEH)	papilloma	skin of elbow	1	Rana pipiens	Duryee, 1965	491B
Papilloma, squamous cell	papilloma/ epithelioma	skin of head, body, limbs, tail	TNTC	Cynops pyrrhogaster	Bryant, 1973; Asashima et al., 1982; Pfeiffer et al., 1989	513 539 540
Papilloma, squamous cell	papilloma/ epithelioma	skin of head, body, limbs	7	Hynobius lichenatus	Asashima & Meyer-Rochow, 1988	
Papilloma, squamous cell	papilloma	skin of head, body, tail	TNTC	Ambystoma tigrinum	Rose & Harshbarger, 1977	704 910 912
Papilloma, squamous cell		skin	2	Ambystoma mexicanum	Fox (RTLA)	3304
Papilloma, squamous cell	papilloma	skin of tail	1	Taricha rivularis	Frye (RTLA)	4227
Papilloma, squamous cell		skin of body	1	Cryptobranchus alleganiensus bishopi	Trauth (RTLA)	6035
Papilloma, squamous cell	papilloma	skin	~6	Rana pipiens	Van Der Steen et al., 1972	656
Papilloma, squamous cell	papillomatosis	skin of body	1	Andria japonicus	Frye et al., 1989b	3765
Papilloma, squamous cell	epidermal papilloma	skin around tympanum	1	Rana nigromaculata	Kabisch et al., 1991	
Papilloma, squamous cell	adenopapilloma	skin of back	1	Rana ridibunda	Khudoley (RTLA)	5372
Fibropapilloma	fibroma, dermal	dermis	>2	Ambystoma tigrinum	Rose & Harshbarger, 1977	705 909
Intracutaneous cornifying epithelioma (ICE)	epidermal hyperplasia	skin	~2	Rana pipiens	Van Der Steen et al., 1972	658

Table 26.1. Spontaneous neoplasms of amphibians. (Continued)

Key: TNTC = too numerous to count
~ = approximately
* = experimentally induced tumors
AFIP = Armed Forces Institute of Pathology
RTLA = Registry of Tumors in Lower Animals

Neoplasm, Revised Diagnosis	Neoplasm, Published Diagnosis	Site of Origin	N =	Host Species	Reference or RTLA Contributor	RTLA Number
Integument epidermal tumors (*Continued*)						
Epithelioma, unclassified	epithelioma	snout/maxilla	1	*Ambystoma mexicanum*	Sheremetieva-Brunst, 1953	
Epithelioma, unclassified	facial epithelioma	head	>1	*Xenopus laevis*	Elkan, 1976	
Epithelioma, carcinoma type	transmissible epithelioma	skin of flank	6	*Triturus alpestris*	Champy & Champy, 1935 *fide* Lucke & Schlumberger, 1949	
Carcinoma, squamous cell	adeno-carcinoma	skin of leg	2	*Rana* sp.	Murray, 1908	
Carcinoma, squamous cell	carcinoma	skin of head	1	*Triturus cristatus*	Murray, 1908	
Carcinoma, squamous cell	carcinoma	skin of head	1	*Triturus alpestris*	Richenbacher, 1950	
Carcinoma, squamous cell	squamous cell carcinoma	skin of sternum, abdomen, back, and legs	6	*Rana pipiens*	Van Der Steen et al., 1972	657 658
Carcinoma, squamous cell	ulcus rodens	skin of head	1	*Rana temporaria*	Elkan, 1963	
Carcinoma, squamous cell	epithelioma epidermique	skin of body	1	*Triturus alpestris*	Matz, 1982	70
Integument adnexal (dermal gland) tumors						
Adenoma (?)	adenoma	skin	2	*Rana* sp.	Pawlowski, 1912 *fide* Balls, 1962	
Adenoma	adenoma	skin	17	"*Rana fusca*"	Pirlot & Welsch, 1934	
Cystadenoma	cystadenoma	skin of leg	1	*Rana esculenta*	Secher, 1919 *fide* Schlumberger & Lucke, 1948	
Cystadenoma	cystadenoma	skin	>1	*Rana temporaria*	Khudoley (RTLA)	2127
Adenoma, papillary	multiple adenome	60 skin nodules	1	*Rana* sp.	Eberth, 1868 *fide* Lucke, 1934	
Adenoma, papillary	adenopapilloma	skin of body	1	*Rana ridibunda*	Khudoley & Mizgireuv, 1980	5372

Table 26.1. Spontaneous neoplasms of amphibians. (*Continued*)						
Key: TNTC = too numerous to count ~ = approximately * = experimentally induced tumors AFIP = Armed Forces Institute of Pathology RTLA = Registry of Tumors in Lower Animals						
Neoplasm, Revised Diagnosis	**Neoplasm, Published Diagnosis**	**Site of Origin**	**N =**	**Host Species**	**Reference or RTLA Contributor**	**RTLA Number**
Integument adnexal (dermal gland) tumors (*Continued*)						
Cystadenoma, papillary	adenoma, multiple	24 skin nodules	1	*Rana* sp.	Pentimalli, 1914	
Cystadenoma, papillary	cystadenoma	skin of abdomen and legs	1–15	*Rana ridibunda*	Khudoley & Mizgireuv, 1980	2127
Cystadenoma, papillary	cystadeno-papillomata	skin	3	*Rana temporaria*	Khudoley, 1977	
Cystadenoma, papillary	cystadenoma	skin	1–6	*Rana temporaria*	Khudoley & Mizgireuv, 1980	2127
Myoepithelioma (myoepithelial adenoma)	chondroms	skin of head, body, and leg	1	*Triturus vulgaris*	Broz, 1947	
Myoepithelioma	myxofibro-chondroma	skin of leg	1	"*Rana fusca*"	Pirlot & Welsch, 1934	
Mixed cell adenoma	basal cell tumor	skin of neck	1	*Ambystoma opacum*	Counts et al., 1975	820
Adenocarcinoma		skin	1	*Hyla* sp.	Teutschlaender, 1920 *fide* Balls, 1962	
Adenocarcinoma	epithelioma cutane	skin of body and leg	1	*Rana esculenta*	Masson & Schwartz, 1923 *fide* Lucke, 1934	
Adenocarcinoma	malignant adenoma	skin	1	*Rana* sp.	Pawlowski, 1912 *fide* Schlumberger & Lucke, 1948	
Adenocarcinoma	epitelioma glandular	skin of head	1	*Rana catesbeiana*	Duany, 1929	
Adenocarcinoma	adenocarcinoma	skin of leg	1	*Rana pipiens*	Van Der Steen et al., 1972	659
Adenocarcinoma	adenocarcinoma	skin of abdomen	1	*Rana temporaria*	Khudoley (RTLA)	5373
Adenocarcinoma	pseudo-adenomatous carcinoma	skin of head	1	*Triturus alpestris*	Richenbacher, 1950 *fide* Balls, 1962	
Cystadenocar-cinoma	cystadeno-carcinoma	skin of abdomen and legs	1–16	*Rana ridibunda*	Khudoley & Mizgireuv, 1980	
Cystadenocar-cinoma	cystadeno-carcinoma	skin of abdomen and legs	1–6	*Rana temporaria*	Khudoley & Mizgireuv, 1980	

Table 26.1. Spontaneous neoplasms of amphibians. (*Continued*)						

Key: TNTC = too numerous to count
~ = approximately
* = experimentally induced tumors
AFIP = Armed Forces Institute of Pathology
RTLA = Registry of Tumors in Lower Animals

Neoplasm, Revised Diagnosis	Neoplasm, Published Diagnosis	Site of Origin	N =	Host Species	Reference or RTLA Contributor	RTLA Number
Integument pigment cell (chromatophore) tumors						
Melanophoroma	melanoma	skin	1–7	*Ambystoma mexicanum*	Sheremetieva-Brunst & Brunst, 1948	
Melanophoroma	melanoma	skin of tail	7	*Ambystoma mexicanum*	Sheremetieva, 1965	
Melanophoroma	melanophoroma	skin of tail, head and legs	2	*Ambystoma mexicanum*	Khudoley & Mizgireuv, 1980	1886
Melanophoroma	melanophoroma	skin of body	1	*Ambystoma mexicanum*	Delanney (RTLA)	3482
Melanophoroma	melanoma, intradermal	skin	TNTC	*Ambystoma tigrinum*	Rose & Harshbarger, 1977	707 791 905 906 916 et al.
Melanophoroma	melanoma, dermal	skin of snout	1	*Xenopus laevis*	Elkan, 1963	
Melanophoroma	melanoma-like lesions	skin	1–3	*Triturus carnifex*	Zavanella, 1995	
Melanophoroma	melanophoma	skin of leg	3	*Xenopus laevis*	Asashima et al., 1989	
Melanophoroma	melanic tumor	vent region	1	*Rana temporaria*	Rostand, 1958 fide Balls, 1962	
Malignant melanophoroma	melanophoroma malignum	skin	1	*Ambystoma mexicanum*	Krontovsky, 1916 fide Balls, 1962	
Malignant melanophoroma	melanosarcoma	skin	1	*Ambystoma mexicanum*	Teutschlaender, 1920 fide Balls, 1962	
Malignant melanophoroma	invasive melanoma	skin	>5	*Ambystoma tigrinum*	Rose & Harshbarger, 1977	950 954 957 969 et al.
Malignant melanophoroma		skin of head	1	*Ambystoma tigrinum*	Smith (RTLA)	3286
Malignant melanophoroma	malignant melanoma	skin of back	1	*Phrynohyas venulosa*	University of Tennessee	AFIP # 1761009

Table 26.1. Spontaneous neoplasms of amphibians. (*Continued*)

Key: TNTC = too numerous to count
~ = approximately
* = experimentally induced tumors
AFIP = Armed Forces Institute of Pathology
RTLA = Registry of Tumors in Lower Animals

Neoplasm, Revised Diagnosis	Neoplasm, Published Diagnosis	Site of Origin	N =	Host Species	Reference or RTLA Contributor	RTLA Number
Integument pigment cell (chromatophore) tumors (*Continued*)						
Malignant melanophoroma	melanoma, epithelioma	skin	>2	Triturus cristatus	Leone & Zavanella, 1969	
Malignant melanophoroma	melanoma-like tumor	skin of back	1	Triturus cristatus	Zilakos et al., 1991	5558
Malignant melanophoroma	melanophoma	skin of back	5	Xenopus laevis	Asashima et al., 1989	
Erythrophoroma	none		0			
Xanthophoroma	none		0			
Iridophoroma	none		0			
Laminophoroma	none		0			
Integument neurosensory cell (lateral line and ampullary organ) tumors						
Neuromastoma	epithelioma	head	1?	Triturus alpestris	Champy & Champy, 1935	
Neuromastoma	neuro-epithelioma	head	2	Triturus alpestris	Matz, 1982	70 2890
Neuromastoma	neuro-epithelioma	mouth	2	Ambystoma mexicanum	Humphrey, 1969	
Neuromastoma	adenocarcinoma	mouth	3	Ambystoma mexicanum	Sheremetieva-Brunst, 1961	
Neuromastoma		body	1	Ambystoma mexicanum	Delanney (RTLA)	1674
Neuromastoma	neuro-epithelioma	mouth	2	Ambystoma mexicanum	Brunst & Roque, 1967	
Soft (mesenchymal) tissue tumors						
Fibroma	intradermal fibroma	dermis	>10	Ambystoma tigrinum	Rose & Harshbarger, 1977	705 706
Fibroma	fibroma	subcutis	1	Andrias japonicus	Schwarz, 1923 fide Balls, 1962	
Fibroma	fibroma	footpad	1	Andrias japonicus	Vaillant & Pettit, 1902 fide Balls & Clothier, 1974	
Fibroma	fibroma	mouth	1	Rana esculenta	Vaillant & Pettit, 1902 fide Balls, 1962	

Table 26.1. Spontaneous neoplasms of amphibians. (Continued)

Key: TNTC = too numerous to count
~ = approximately
* = experimentally induced tumors
AFIP = Armed Forces Institute of Pathology
RTLA = Registry of Tumors in Lower Animals

Neoplasm, Revised Diagnosis	Neoplasm, Published Diagnosis	Site of Origin	N =	Host Species	Reference or RTLA Contributor	RTLA Number
Soft (mesenchymal) tissue tumors (Continued)						
Fibroma	polypoid fibroma	pelvic coelom	1	Xenopus laevis	Elkan, 1960	
Fibroma	facial tumors	head near nares	1	Xenopus laevis	Elkan, 1960	
Fibrosarcoma	fibrosarcoma	head and body	many	Ambystoma tigrinum	Rose & Harshbarger, 1977	1133
Fibrosarcoma	fibrosarcoma	leg and liver	1	Ceratophrys ornata	Volterra, 1928 fide Lucke, 1934	
Fibrosarcoma	fibrosarcoma	skin	1	Conraua goliath	Frye et al., 1991	
Fibromyxoma	myxofibroma	dermis	many	Ambystoma tigrinum	Rose & Harshbarger, 1977	792
Myxosarcoma	myxosarcoma	tail	1	Rana clamitans (tadpole)	Lucke, 1937	
Lipoma	lipoma	fat body	1	Xenopus laevis	Balls, 1962	
Lipoma	lipoma	fat body/ urinary bladder	1	Xenopus laevis	Reichenbach-Klinke & Elkan, 1965	
Liposarcoma	liposarcoma	spleen	1	Rana pipiens	Duryee, 1965	
Granular cell tumor*	granular cell tumor	head	1	Xenopus laevis	Janisch & Schmidt, 1980	2219
Rhabdomyoma	none		0			
Rhabdomyosarcoma	embryonal rhabdomyosarcoma	leg	1	Rana pipiens	Mizell et al., 1966a, b	
Rhabdomyosarcoma	rhabdomyosarcoma	"retrocoelom"	1	hybrid Chinese ranid	Masahito et al., 1995	
Mesenchymal cell tumor, unclassified	unclassified mesenchymal cell tumor	footpad	1	hybrid Chinese ranid	Masahito et al., 1995	
Hematolymphatic tumors						
Nodular hematopoiesis		liver	1	Ambystoma tigrinum	Anderson (RTLA)	2468
Nodular lymphatic hyperplasia		kidney	1	Necturus maculosus	Nauman (RTLA)	97

Table 26.1. Spontaneous neoplasms of amphibians. (*Continued*)						
Key: TNTC = too numerous to count ~ = approximately * = experimentally induced tumors AFIP = Armed Forces Institute of Pathology RTLA = Registry of Tumors in Lower Animals						
Neoplasm, Revised Diagnosis	**Neoplasm, Published Diagnosis**	**Site of Origin**	**N =**	**Host Species**	**Reference or RTLA Contributor**	**RTLA Number**
Hematolymphatic tumors (*Continued*)						
Lymphosarcoma		liver & mesonephroi	1	*Xenopus laevis*	Snyder (RTLA)	3577
Lymphosarcoma		liver & spleen	1	*Xenopus laevis*	Cosgrove (RTLA)	1665
Lymphosarcoma	renal cell carcinoma	mesonephroi & viscera	1	*Xenopus laevis*	Elkan, 1968	238
Lymphosarcoma (?)	lymphosarcoma	viscera	2	*Rana pipiens*	Duryee, 1965	
Lymphosarcoma		spleen & viscera	3	*Xenopus laevis*	Verhoeff-DeFremery (RTLA)	1769 1996 2325
Lymphosarcoma		intestine	1	*Ambystoma mexicanum*	Graham (RTLA)	4920
Lymphosarcoma	lymphosarcoma	skin	1	*Ambystoma mexicanum*	Delanney & Blackler, 1969	506
Lymphosarcoma	leukemic lymphosarcoma		1	"Treefrog"	Griner, 1983	
Lymphosarcoma	lymphosarcoma, T-cell	thymus	5	*Xenopus laevis*	Robert & DuPasquier, 1995	
Plasmacytoma/myeloma	plasmacytoma	muscles of leg	1	*Rana pipiens*	Schochet & Lampert, 1969	
Monocytoid leukosis	monocytoid leukemia	blood	15	*Bufo regularis*	El-Mofty et al., 1995	
Myeloid leukemia		liver	1	*Xenopus laevis*	Hoover & Dworkin (RTLA)	2318
Myeloid leukemia		liver & mesonephroi	1	*Bufo marinus*	Hruban et al., 1989	4156
Myeloid leukemia		spleen	1	African *Bufo* sp.	Snyder (RTLA)	1030
Mast cell tumor	mast cell tumor	skin	18	*Ambystoma mexicanum*	Delanney et al., 1981	1675 to 1690+
Mast cell tumor	dermal fibroma, fibrosarcoma, and myxosarcoma	skin	>3	*Ambystoma tigrinum*	Rose (RTLA)	990 991 999
Mast cell tumor	neuroblastoma	skin of neck	1	*Notophthalmus viridescens*	Counts, 1980	1135

Table 26.1. Spontaneous neoplasms of amphibians. (*Continued*)

Key: TNTC = too numerous to count
~ = approximately
* = experimentally induced tumors
AFIP = Armed Forces Institute of Pathology
RTLA = Registry of Tumors in Lower Animals

Neoplasm, Revised Diagnosis	Neoplasm, Published Diagnosis	Site of Origin	N =	Host Species	Reference or RTLA Contributor	RTLA Number
Hematolymphatic tumors (*Continued*)						
Mast cell tumor	mesenchymal cell tumor	skin of neck	1	*Notophthalmus viridescens*	Burns & White, 1971	
Unclassified hematopoietic neoplasm	unclassified round cell neoplasm	hindlimb	1	hybrid Chinese ranid	Masahito et al., 1995	
Neoplasia of the mesonephroi (kidney) and urinary system						
Nephroblastoma*	nephroblastoma	mesonephros	2	*Pleurodeles waltl*	Janisch & Schmidt, 1980	2182
Nephroblastoma	nephroblastoma	mesonephros	1	*Xenopus laevis*	Elkan, 1963	32
Nephroblastoma	nephroblastoma	mesonephros	1	*Cynops pyrrhogaster*	Zwart, 1970	214
Nephroblastoma	carcinosarcoma	mesonephros	1	*Rana pipiens*	Mizell et al., 1966a	
Lucke renal carcinoma	hypernephroma	mesonephros	1	*Rana pipiens*	Smallwood, 1905 *fide* Schlumberger & Lucke, 1948	
Lucke renal carcinoma	epithelial tumor of the intestine	"abdomen"	1	*Rana pipiens*	Downs, 1932; Balls, 1962	
Lucke renal carcinoma	adenocarcinoma	mesonephroi	>600	*Rana pipiens*	Lucke, 1938	577 (donated by Duryee in 1971)
Lucke renal carcinoma	Lucke renal tumors	mesonephroi	8.9%	*Rana pipiens*	McKinnell, 1965	
Lucke renal carcinoma	Lucke renal carcinoma	mesonephroi	6.8%	*Rana pipiens* "burnsi"	Zambernard et al., 1966	
Lucke renal carcinoma	Lucke renal carcinoma	mesonephroi	24%	*Rana pipiens*	McKinnell & John, 1995	
Renal cell carcinoma		mesonephros	1	*Ceratophrys ornata*	Frye et al., 1989a	3982
Renal cell carcinoma	adenocarcinoma	mesonephros	1	*Necturus maculosus*	Schlumberger, 1958	
Renal cell carcinoma	tubular renal tumors	mesonephroi	>22	hybrid Japanese ranids	Nishioka & Kondo, 1987	

Table 26.1. Spontaneous neoplasms of amphibians. (*Continued*)

Key: TNTC = too numerous to count
~ = approximately
* = experimentally induced tumors
AFIP = Armed Forces Institute of Pathology
RTLA = Registry of Tumors in Lower Animals

Neoplasm, Revised Diagnosis	Neoplasm, Published Diagnosis	Site of Origin	N =	Host Species	Reference or RTLA Contributor	RTLA Number
Neoplasia of the mesonephroi (kidney) and urinary system (*Continued*)						
Renal cell carcinoma	renal carcinoma	mesonephros	1	*Xenopus laevis*	Reichenbach-Klinke & Elkan, 1965	
Transitional cell carcinoma		paracloaca	1	*Ambystoma tigrinum*	Miller (RTLA)	3238
Unclassified neoplasms	kidney tumors	mesonephroi	2	hybrid ranids	Masahito et al., 1995	
Reproductive organ tumors						
Teratoma	teratoma	ovary	1	*Rana pipiens*	Streett, 1964	465
Teratoma	teratoma	paracloaca	1	*Ambystoma mexicanum*	Brunst & Roque, 1969	
Paraovarian cyst	paraovarian cyst	ovary	1	*Ambystoma tigrinum*	Rose (RTLA)	947
Granulosa cell tumor	granulosa cell tumor	ovary	1	*Ceratophrys ornata*	Snyder (RTLA)	3575
Carcinoma	carcinoma	ovary	1	*Rana k. esculenta*	Plehn, 1906 *fide* Schlumberger & Lucke, 1948	
Cystadenocarcinoma	cystadenocarcinoma	ovary	1	*Rana pipiens*	Abrams, 1969	
Ovarian neoplasms	ovarian neoplasms	ovary	47	hybrid toads	Nishioka & Ueda, 1987	
Sertoli cell tumor	carcinoma	testis	1	*Andrias japonicus*	Pick & Poll, 1903 *fide* Schlumberger & Lucke, 1948	
Sertoli cell tumor	teratocarcinoma	testis	1	hybrid *Rana* sp.	Hardy & Gillespie, 1976	
Sertoli cell tumor	adenoma of seminiferous epithelium	testis	1	*Cryptobranchus alleganiensis*	Cosgrove & Harshbarger, 1971	272
Sertoli cell tumor	tumors	testis	16	*Ambystoma mexicanum*	Humphrey, 1969	
Bidder's organ tumor, unclassified	tumor	Bidder's organ	~8	hybrid toads	Nishioka & Ueda, 1987	

Table 26.1. Spontaneous neoplasms of amphibians. (Continued)

Key: TNTC = too numerous to count
~ = approximately
* = experimentally induced tumors
AFIP = Armed Forces Institute of Pathology
RTLA = Registry of Tumors in Lower Animals

Neoplasm, Revised Diagnosis	Neoplasm, Published Diagnosis	Site of Origin	N =	Host Species	Reference or RTLA Contributor	RTLA Number
Reproductive organ tumors (*Continued*)						
Bidder's organ tumor, unclassified	tumor	Bidder's organ	~2	hybrid toads	Nishioka & Kondo, 1987	
Liver and pancreas tumors						
Hepatoma (hepatocellular adenoma)	hepatoma	liver	1	*Rana esculenta*	Willis, 1964	
Hepatoma	hepatoma	liver	2	*Rana pipiens*	Abrams, 1969	
Hepatoma	hepatocellular carcinoma	liver	1	*Hyla gratiosa*	Harshbarger & Snyder, 1989	3579
Hepatoma		liver	1	*Leptodactylus pentadactylus*	National Zoo/AFIP	AFIP# 1403734
Hepatoma	hepatocellular adenoma	liver	1	Chinese hybrid ranid	Masahito et al., 1995	
Hepatoma	hepatocellular adenoma	liver	1	*Phrynohyas venulosa*	National Zoo/AFIP	AFIP# 1403734
Carcinoma, hepatocellular*	hepatocarcinoma	liver	1	*Ambystoma mexicanum*	Harshbarger & Snyder, 1989	2543
Hepatoblastoma	hepatoblastoma	liver	1	*Xenopus laevis*	Harshbarger & Snyder, 1989	3577
Bile duct adenoma	poorly differentiated adenoma	liver	1	*Xenopus laevis*	Reichenbach-Klinke & Elkan, 1965	
Bile duct adenoma	bile duct adenoma	liver	1	Chinese hybrid ranid	Masahito et al., 1995	
Cholangiocarcinoma	cholangiocarcinoma	liver	4	*Xenopus borealis*	Khudoley (RTLA)	2123 2124 2125 2126
Cholangiocarcinoma	cholangiocarcinoma	liver	1	*Ambystoma tigrinum*	Rose (RTLA)	2604
Alimentary system tumors						
Fibroma	fibroma	oral cavity	1	*Rana k. esculenta*	Vaillant & Pettit, 1902 *fide* Balls, 1962	

Table 26.1. Spontaneous neoplasms of amphibians. (*Continued*)

Key: TNTC = too numerous to count
~ = approximately
* = experimentally induced tumors
AFIP = Armed Forces Institute of Pathology
RTLA = Registry of Tumors in Lower Animals

Neoplasm, Revised Diagnosis	Neoplasm, Published Diagnosis	Site of Origin	N =	Host Species	Reference or RTLA Contributor	RTLA Number
Alimentary system tumors (*Continued*)						
Carcinoma, squamous cell		colon	1	Bombina orientalis	Green (RTLA)	5850
Adenocarcinoma	anaplastic intestinal carcinoma	intestine	1	Xenopus laevis	Elkan, 1970	
Adenocarcinoma		cloacal gland	1	Ambystoma mexicanum	Verhoeff-deFremery (RTLA)	2847
Adenocarcinoma		colon	1	Bufo marinus	Herron (RTLA)	1921
Miscellaneous alimentary "tumors"						
Granulomata	leiomyoma	stomach	19	Cynops pyrrhogaster	Pfeiffer & Asashima, 1990	
Callus of fracture	chrondromyxoma	mouth	2	Pseudacris regilla	Frye (RTLA)	1010 1080
Respiratory and cardiovascular tumors						
Papilloma, epidermal*	papilloma	gill	1	Ambystoma tigrinum	Rose (RTLA)	2541
Carcinoma	multicentric adenocarcinoma	lung	1	Bufo calamita	Elkan, 1960	
Hyperplasia, verminous epithelial	carcinoma in situ	lung	5	Rana pipiens	Duryee, 1965	
Tumors of the brain, spinal cord and nerves						
Neurofibrosarcoma	neurosarcoma	sacral plexus	1	Rana catesbeiana	Schlumberger & Lucke, 1948	
Tumors of the eye, eyelid, ear, and special sensory organs						
Neuroepithelioma	neuroepithelioma	mouth/nasal cavity/ Jacobson's organ (?)	2	Ambystoma mexicanum	Brunst & Roque, 1967	
Carcinoma, squamous cell	squamous cell carcinoma	eyelid	1	Rana temporaria	Reichenbach-Klinke & Elkan, 1965	

Table 26.1. Spontaneous neoplasms of amphibians. (Continued)						
Key: TNTC = too numerous to count ~ = approximately * = experimentally induced tumors AFIP = Armed Forces Institute of Pathology RTLA = Registry of Tumors in Lower Animals						
Neoplasm, Revised Diagnosis	**Neoplasm, Published Diagnosis**	**Site of Origin**	**N =**	**Host Species**	**Reference or RTLA Contributor**	**RTLA Number**
Tumors of the eye, eyelid, ear, and special sensory organs (Continued)						
Adenoma, papillary	malignant adenocarcinoma	Harderian gland	1	Xenopus laevis	Elkan, 1968	
Skeletal tissue and notochord tumors						
Dysplasia, osteochondrous	dysplasia, osteochondrous	leg bones	328	Rana chinsenensis	Mizgireuv et al., 1984	
Chondroma			0			
Chondrosarcoma			0			
Callus after fracture	osteosarcoma, medullary	leg (femur)	1	Rana virescens	Ohlmacher, 1898 fide Schlumberger & Lucke, 1948	
Osteoma			0			
Osteosarcoma			0			
Notochord hypertrophy or hyperplasia	chordoma	sacral notochord	many	hybrid European toad tadpoles	Schipp et al., 1968	
Notochord hypertrophy or hyperplasia	neoplasma-like swellings	spinal column	many	hybrid European toad tadpoles	Flindt et al., 1968	
Notochord hypertrophy or hyperplasia	chordoma	cranial notochord	1	hybrid European toad tadpoles	Hertwig, 1953	

ACKNOWLEDGMENTS

The authors thank Phyllis Spero, Kathy Price, Marilyn Slatick, and Norman Wolcott for clerical, computer, and histotechnologic support. This chapter is designated Maryland Department of Agriculture contribution number 101–97.

REFERENCES

Abrams, G.D. 1969. Diseases in an amphibian colony, in Mizell, M. (Ed): Biology of Amphibian Tumors. Springer-Verlag, New York, pp. 419–428.

Afifi, A., A. Dalcq, and J.J. Picard. 1991. Pathologic lesions induced in Xenopus by sequential administration of N-nitrosodi-methylamine, 2-acetylaminofluorene and phenobarbital. Herpetopathologia 2:11–21.

Anver, R.A. and C.L. Pond. 1984. Biology and diseases of Amphibians, in Fox, J.G., B.J. Cohen, and F.M. Loew (Eds.): Laboratory Animal Medicine. Academic Press, Orlando, FL, pp. 427–447.

Asashima, M. and S. Komazaki. 1980. Spontaneous progressive skin papilloma in newts (Cynops pyrrhogaster). Proceedings of Japan Academy, Series B 56B:638–642.

Asashima, M. and V.B. Meyer-Rochow. 1988. Papilloma in Hynobius lichenatus Boulenger 1883 (Amphibia, Urodela). Z. Mikrosk. Anat. Forsch. 102:756–759.

Asashima, M. and V.B. Meyer-Rochow. 1989. Neoplasia in the stomach in wild Japanese newts, Cynops pyrrhogaster. Amphibia-Reptilia 10:189–192.

Asashima, M., T. Oinuma, and S. Komazaki. 1989. Electron microscopical and histochemical studies of the spontaneous tumors of Xenopus laevis. Zoological Science 6:899–905.

Asashima, M., T. Oinuma, and V.B. Meyer-Rochow. 1987. Tumors in Amphibia. Zoological Science 4:411–425.

Asashima, M., S. Komazaki, C. Satou, and T. Oinuma. 1982. Seasonal and geographical changes of spontaneous skin papillomas in the Japanese newt, Cynops pyrrhogaster. Cancer Research 42:3741–3746.

Asashima, M., T. Oinuma, H. Matsuyama, and M. Nagano. 1985. Effects of temperature on papilloma growth in the newt, *Cynops pyrrhogaster*. Cancer Research 45:1198–1205.

Asashima, M., M. Seki, H. Kanno, and H. Koyama. 1986. Morphological changes in newt epitheliomas caused by controlled temperature. Proceedings of the Japan Academy, Series B 62B:83–86.

Asfari, M. 1988. *Mycobacterium*-induced infectious granuloma in *Xenopus*: Histopathology and transmissibility. Cancer Research 48:958–963.

Asfari, M. and C.H. Thiebaud. 1988. Transplantation studies of a putative lymphosarcoma of *Xenopus*. Cancer Research 48:954–957.

Balls, M. 1962. Spontaneous neoplasms in Amphibia: A review and descriptions of six new cases. Cancer Research 22:1142–1154.

Balls, M. 1965. Lymphosarcoma in the South African clawed toad, *Xenopus laevis*: A virus tumor. Annals of the New York Academy of Sciences 126:256–273.

Balls, M. and R.H. Clothier. 1974. Spontaneous tumours in Amphibia. Oncology 29:501–519.

Balls, M. and R.H. Clothier. 1989. Neoplasia in reptiles and amphibians: Terminology and criteria. Herpetopathologia 1:5–6.

Balls, M. and L.N. Ruben. 1964. A review of the chemical induction of tumours in Amphibia. Experientia 20:241–247.

Balls, M. and L.N. Ruben. 1968. Lymphoid tumors in amphibia: A review. Progress in Experimental Tumor Research 10:238–260.

Balls, M., R.H. Clothier, and K.R. Knowles. 1983. Tumour incidence in NMU-treated *Xenopus laevis*. Proceedings of 1st International Colloquium on Pathology of Reptiles and Amphibians, pp. 163–172.

Balls, M., R.H. Clothier, L.N. Ruben, and J.C. Harshbarger. 1989. The incidence and significance of malignant neoplasia in amphibians. Herpetopathologia 1:97–104.

Barch, S.H., J.R. Shaver, and G.B. Wilson. 1965. Some aspects of the ultrastructure of cells of the Lucke renal adenocarcinoma. Annals of the New York Academy of Sciences 126:188–203.

Bouchard, P.R., C.H. Fortna, P.H. Rowland, and R.M. Lewis. 1995. An immunohistochemical study of three equine pulmonary granular cell tumors. Veterinary Pathology 32:730–734.

Breedis, C. 1952. Induction of accessory limbs and of sarcoma in the newt (*Triturus viridescens*) with carcinogenic substances. Cancer Research 12:861–966.

Briggs, R.W. 1941. The development of abnormal growths in *Rana pipiens* embryos following delayed fertilization. Anatomical Record 81:121–135.

Broz, O. 1947. Mnohocetne "chondromy" v kuzi *Triton taeniatus*—Multiple "chondroms" in the skin of *Triton taeniatus*. Vestnik Ceskoslovenske Spolecnosti Zoologicke 11:89–91.

Brunst, V.V. and A.L. Roque. 1967. Tumors in amphibians. I. Histology of a neuroepithelioma in *Siredon mexicanum*. Journal of the National Cancer Institute 38:193–204.

Brunst, V.V. and A.L. Roque. 1969. A spontaneous teratoma in an axolotl (*Siredon mexicanum*). Cancer Research 29:223–229.

Bryant, S.V. 1973. Spontaneous epidermal tumor in an adult newt, *Cynops pyrrhogaster*. Cancer Research 33:623–625.

Burns, E.R. and H.J. White. 1971. A spontaneous mesenchymal cell neoplasm in the adult newt, *Diemictylus viridescens*. Cancer Research 31:826–829.

Carl, W. 1913. Ein Hypernephrom beim Frosch. Zentr. Allg. Path. Path. Anat. 24:436–438.

Carpenter, J.L., A. Bachrach, D.M. Albert, S.J. Vainisi, and M.A. Goldstein. 1986. Xanthomatous keratitis, disseminated xanthomatosis, and atherosclerosis in Cuban treefrogs. Veterinary Pathology 23:337–339.

Carter, D.B. 1979. Structure and function of the subcutaneous lymph sacs in the anura (Amphibia). Journal of Herpetology 13:321–327.

Champy, C. and M. Champy. 1935. Epithelioma transmissible du triton. Bulletin de l'Association Francaise pour l'Etude du Cancer 24:206–220.

Clothier, R.H. 1983. Chemical carcinogenesis in amphibians. Proceedings of 1st International Colloquium on Pathology of Reptiles and Amphibians, pp. 185–186.

Clothier, R.H. and M. Balls. 1973. Mycobacteria and lymphoreticular tumours in *Xenopus laevis*, the South African clawed toad. Oncology 28:445–457.

Clothier, R.H., S.W. Wilson, K.R. Knowles, and M. Balls. 1989. A transmissible lymphoblastic lymphoma in *Xenopus laevis*, the South African clawed toad. Herpetopathologia 1:7–11.

Cosgrove, G.E. and J.C. Harshbarger. 1971. Testicular tumor in a salamander. Journal of the American Veterinary Medical Association 159:582.

Counts, C.L. III. 1980. A neural neoplasm in the eastern newt, *Notophthalmus viridescens*. Herpetologica 36:46–50.

Counts, C.L. III., C.T. Wilson, and R.W. Taylor. 1975. Occurrence of a basal cell neoplasm in *Ambystoma opacum* (Amphibia: Caudata). Herpetologica 31:422–424.

Darquenne, J. 1972. Cancerologie experimentale: Actions de substances cancerigenes sur le regenerat de la queue de *Triturus alpestris* Laur. (Amphibiens, Salamandrides). Comptes Rendus de l'Academie des Sciences, Paris 273D:1460–1462.

Dawe, C.J. 1969a. Neoplasms of blood cell origin in poikilothermic animals. A status summary, in Dutcher, R.M. (Ed.): Comparative Leukemia Research, No. 36. Karger, Basel, Switzerland, 1970, pp. 634–637.

Dawe, C.J. 1969b. Neoplasms of blood cell origin in poikilothermic animals—A review. National Cancer Institute Monograph 32: Comparative Morphology of Hematopoietic Neoplasms. U.S. Department of Health, Education and Welfare, Bethesda, MD, pp. 7–28.

Dawe, C.J. 1969c. Some comparative morphological aspects of renal neoplasms in *Rana pipiens* and of lymphosarcomas in Amphibia, in Mizell, M. (Ed.): Biology of Amphibian Tumors. Springer-Verlag, New York, pp. 429–440.

Delanney, L.E. 1969. Lymphosarcoma in the Mexican axolotl, *Ambystoma mexicanum*, in Dutcher, R.M. (Ed.): Comparative Leukemia Reasearch, No. 36. Karger, Basel, Switzerland 1970. p. 642.

Delanney, L.E. 1974. Genetic analysis of a strain-specific lymphosarcoma grown in crosses of allogeneic strains of axolotls (Urodela) [Abstr]. Amercian Zoologist 16:261.

Delanney, L.E. and K. Blackler. 1969. Acceptance and regression of a strain-specific lymphosarcoma in Mexican axolotls, in Mizell, M. (Ed.): Biology of Amphibian Tumors. Springer-Verlag, New York, pp. 399–408.

Delanney, L.E., K.V. Prahlad, and A.H. Meier. 1964. A malignant tumor in the Mexican axolotl [Abstr]. American Zoologist 4:279.

Delanney, L.E., K. Blackler, and K.V. Prahlad. 1967. The relationship of age to allograft and tumor rejection in Mexican axolotls [Abstr]. American Zoologist 7:763.

Delanney, L.E., S.C. Chang, J. Harshbarger, and C. Dawe. 1981. Mast cell tumors in the caudate amphibian, *Ambystoma mexicanum*, in Yohn, D.S., B.A. Lapin, and J.R. Blakeslee (Eds.): Advances in Comparative Leukemia Research. Elsevier North Holland. pp. 221–222.

Downs, A.W. 1932. An epithelial tumour of the intestine of a frog. Nature 130:778.

Duany, P. 1929. Un epitelioma glandular en una *Rana* bullfrog. Archivos de la Sociedad de Estudios Clinicos de la Habana 19:186–195.

DuPasquier, L. and J. Robert. 1992. In vitro growth of thymic tumor cell lines from *Xenopus*. Developmental Immunology 2:295–307.

Duryee, W.R. 1965. Factors influencing development of tumors in frogs. Annals of the New York Academy of Sciences 126:59–84.

Eberth, C.J. 1868. Multiple Adenome der Froschhaut. Virchows Archiv 44:12–22.

Elkan, E. 1960. Some interesting pathological cases in amphibians. Proceedings of the Zoological Society, London 134:275–296.

Elkan, E. 1963. Three different types of tumors in Salientia. Cancer Research 23:1641–1645.

Elkan, E. 1968. Two cases of epithelial malignancy in salientia. Journal of Pathology and Bacteriology 96:496–499.

Elkan, E. 1970. A spontaneous anaplastic intestinal metastasizing carcinoma in a South African clawed toad (*Xenopus laevis* Daudin). Journal of Pathology and Bacteriology 100:205–207.

Elkan, E. 1976. Pathology in the Amphibia, Chapter 6, in Lofts, B. (Ed.): Physiology of the Amphibia, Volume 3. Academic Press, New York, pp. 273–312.

Elkan, E. 1983. Random samples from herpetopathology. Proceedings of the 1st International Colloquium on Pathology of Reptiles and Amphibians (Angers, France). pp. 1–8.

El-Mofty, M.M. and S.A. Sakr. 1988. The induction of neoplastic lesions by aflatoxin-B1 in the Egyptian toad (*Bufo regularis*). Nutrition and Cancer 11:55–59.

El-Mofty, M.M., N.E. Abdel Meguid, and A.E. Essaway. 1995. Pathological changes of the blood cells in griseofulvin-treated toads. Oncology Reports 2:167–170.

El-Mofty, M.M., V.V. Khudoley, S.A. Sakr, S.I. Osman, and B.A. Toulan. 1991a. Adriamycin-induced neoplastic lesions in the Egyptian toad, *Bufo regularis*. Oncology 48:171–174.

El-Mofty, M.M., V.V. Khudoley, and M.H. Shwaireb. 1991b. Carcinogenic effect of force-feeding an extract of black pepper (*Piper nigrum*) in Egyptian toads (*Bufo regularis*). Oncology 48:347–350.

El-Mofty, M.M., I.A. Sadek, and S. Bayoumi. 1980. Improvement in detecting the carcinogenicity of bracken fern using an Egyptian toad. Oncology 37:424–425.

El-Mofty, M.M., R. Galal, A. El Sebae, and A.E. Essawy. 1983. Liver neoplasms in toads (*Bufo regularis*) enforced fed with chlordime-form. Proceedings of 1st International Colloquium on Pathology of Reptiles and Amphibians, pp. 173–176.

El-Mofty, M.M., V.V. Khudoley, A.E. Essawy, and H.M. Abdel-Kerim. 1993. Induction of hepatocellular carcinomas in the Egyptian toad, *Bufo regularis*, by an antifungal drug (griseofulvin). Oncology 50:267–269.

El-Mofty, M.M., V.V. Khudoley, S.A. Sakr, and N.F. Ganem. 1992. Induction of neoplasma in Egyptian toads, *Bufo regularis*, by oil of chenopodium. Oncology 49:253–255.

Flindt, V.R., H. Hemmer, and R. Schipp. 1968. Zur morphogenese von Missbildungen bei Bastardlarven *Bufo calamita* X *Bufo viridis*: Stoerungen in der ausbildung des axialskelettes. Zoologische Jahrbucher Abteilung fur Anatomie und Ontogenie der Tiere 85:51–71.

Frye, F.L., S.L. Barten, and J.C. Harshbarger. 1989a. Renal carcinoma with pulmonary metastasis in an Argentine horned frog, *Ceratophrys ornata*. 3rd International Colloquium on Pathology of Reptiles & Amphibians, 13–15 January 1989, Orlando, FL, pp. 106–107.

Frye, F.L., D.S. Gillespie, and J.C. Harshbarger. 1989b. Squamous cell papillomatosis in a Japanese giant salamander. 3rd International Colloquium on Pathology of Reptiles & Amphibians, 13–15 January 1989, Orlando, FL, p. 112.

Frye, F.L., D.S. Gillespie, and E. Maruska. 1991. Multifocal fibrosarcoma in a goliath frog (*Gigantorana goliath*). 4th International Colloquium on Pathology and Medicine of Reptiles and Amphibians. German Veterinary Association, pp. 177–178.

Gatalica, Z., S. Grujic, A. Kovatich, and R.O. Peterson. 1996. Metanephric adenoma: histology, immunophenotype, cytogenetics, ultrastructure. Modern Pathology 9:329–333.

Gheorghiu, I. 1930. Contribution a l'etude du cancer de la grenouille. Comptes Rendus de Societe de Biologie (Roumaine) 103:280–281.

Griner, L.A. 1983. Pathology of Zoo Animals. Zoological Society of San Diego, CA, pp. 7–17.

Hadji-Azimi, I. 1970. Transmission of the "lymphoid tumour" of *Xenopus laevis* in injection of cell-free extracts. Experientia 26:894–897.

Hardy, J.D.Jr. and J.H. Gillespie. 1976. Hybridization between *Rana pipiens* and *Rana palustris* in a modified natural environment. Bulletin of the Maryland Herpetological Society 12:41–53.

Harshbarger, J.C. and R.L. Snyder. 1989. Selected cases of neoplasia in amphibians and reptiles from the Registry of Tumors in Lower Animals. 3rd International Colloquium on Pathology of Reptiles & Amphibians, 13–15 January 1989, Orlando, FL, pp. 67–68.

Helmboldt, C.F. and D.S. Wyand. 1971. Nephroblastoma in a striped bass. Journal of Wildlife Diseases 7:162–165.

Hertwig, G. 1953. Das Auftreten einer Chordoms bei einer Kroeten-bastardlarve und die moeglichen Ursachen seiner Entstehung. Zentralblatt fur Allgemeine Pathologie und Pathologische Anatomie 91:56–64.

Hruban, Z., W.E. Carter, T. Meehan, F.L. Frye, and J.C. Harshbarger. 1989. Neoplasia in reptiles and amphibians in the Lincoln Park Zoological Garden. 3rd International Colloquium on Pathology of Reptiles & Amphibians, 13–15 January 1989, Orlando, FL, pp. 76–77.

Humphrey, R.R. 1969. Tumors of the testis in the Mexican axolotl (*Siredon mexicanum*), in Mizell, M. (Ed.): Biology of Amphibian Tumors. Springer-Verlag, New York, pp. 220–228.

Ingram, A.J. 1972. The lethal and hepatocarcinogenic effects of dimethylnitrosamine injection in the newt, *Triturus helveticus*. British Journal of Cancer 26:206–215.

Inoue, S. and M. Singer. 1970. Lymphosarcomatous disease in the newt, *Triturus pyrrhogaster, in:* Dutcher, R.M. (Ed.): 4th International Symposium on Comparative Leukemia Research. S. Karger, Basel, Switzerland, pp. 640–641.

Inoue, S., M. Singer, and J. Hutchinson. 1965. Causative agent of a spontaneously originating visceral tumor in the newt, *Triturus*. Nature 205:408–409.

Janisch, W. and T. Schmidt. 1980. Tumorinduktion bei spanischen Rippenmolchen (*Pleurodeles waltl*) durch Alkylnitrosoharnstoffe. Archiv fur Geschwulstforschung 50:253–265.

Jarrett, W.F.H. and L.J. Mackey. 1974. International classification of tumors of domestic animals. II. Neoplastic diseases of the haematopoietic and lymphoid tissues. Bulletin of the World Health Organization 50:21–34.

Kabisch, K., K. Brauer, J. Seeger, and H-J Herrmann. 1991. A case of epidermal papilloma of *Rana nigromaculata*. Herpetopathologia 2:51–57.

Kapa, E., M. Szigeti, A. Juhasz, and G. Csaba. 1970. Phylogenesis of mast cells. I. Mast cells of the frog, *Rana esculenta*. Acta Biologica Academiae Scientiarum Hungaricae 21:141–147.

Khudoley, V.V. 1977. Tumor induction by carcinogenic agents in anuran amphibian, *Rana temporaria*. Archive fur Geschwulstforschung 47:385–395.

Khudoley, V.V. and V.V. Eliseiv. 1979. Multiple melanomas in the axolotl, *Ambystoma mexicanum*. Journal of the National Cancer Institute 63:101–104.

Khudoley, V.V. and I.V. Mizgireuv, 1980. On spontaneous skin tumors in Amphibia. Neoplasma 27:289–293.

Khudoley, V.V. and J.J. Picard. 1980. Liver and kidney tumors induced by N-nitroso-dimethylamine in *Xenopus borealis* (Parker). International Journal of Cancer 25:679–683.

Koyama, H., M. Asashima, and V.B. Meyer-Rochow. 1989. Carcinoma in the axolotl, *Siredon = Ambystoma mexicanum* (Amphibia: Urodela). Zoologischer Anzeiger 223:26–32.

Krontovsky, A.A. 1916. On comparative and experimental pathology of tumors [in Russian]. Bacteriological Institute, Kiev. [*fide* Brunst & Roque, 1967].

Lattes, R. 1982. Tumors of the Soft Tissues. Atlas of Tumor Pathology, 2nd Series, Fascicle 1. Armed Forces Institute of Pathology, Washington DC, 264 pp.

Lautenschlager, E.W. 1959. Meningeal tumors of the newt associated with trematode infection of the brain. Proceedings of the Helminthological Society of Washington 26:11–14.

Leone, V.G. and T. Zavanella. 1969. Some morphological and biological characteristics of a tumor of the newt, *Triturus cristatus* Laur, *in* Mizell. M. (Ed.): Biology of Amphibian Tumors. Springer-Verlag, New York, pp. 184–194.

Levy, B.M. and G.C. Godman. 1955. Tumors of the notochord of the salamander, *Ambystoma punctatum,* produced by crystalline lathyrus factor. Cancer Research 15:184–187.

Lucke, B. 1934. A neoplastic disease of the kidney of the frog, *Rana pipiens*. American Journal of Cancer 20:352–379.

Lucke, B. 1937. Tumor in a tadpole. Archives of Pathology 23:292.

Lucke, B. 1938. Carcinoma in the leopard frog: Its probable causation by a virus. Journal of Experimental Medicine 68:457–468.

Lucke, B. 1952. Kidney carcinoma in the leopard frog: A virus tumor. Annals of the New York Academy of Sciences 54:1093–1109.

Lucke, B. and H.G. Schlumberger. 1949. Neoplasia in cold-blooded vertebrates. Physiological Reviews 29:91–126.

Marlow, P.B. and S. Mizell. 1972. Incidence of Lucke renal adenocarcinoma in *Rana pipiens* as determined by histological examination. Journal of the National Cancer Institute 48:823–829.

Masahito, P., M. Nishioka, H. Ueda, Y. Kato, I. Yamazaki, K. Nomura, H. Sugano, and T. Kitagawa. 1995. Frequent development of pancreatic carcinomas in the *Rana nigromaculata* group. Cancer Research 55:3781–3784.

Masson, P. and E. Schwartz. 1923. Un cas d'epithelioma cutane chez la grenouille verte (A case of cutaneous epithelioma in the green frog). Bulletin de L'Association Francaise pour L'Etude du Cancer 12:719–725.

Matz, G. 1966. Un cas d'epithelioma epidermique chez *Triturus alpestris* Laur. (Amphibien, Salamandride). Bulletin de la Societe Zoologique de France 91:707–708.

Matz, G. 1982. Tumeurs spontanees et experimentales observees chez *Triturus alpestris* (Laurent) (Salamandridae). Proceedings of 1st International Colloquium on Pathology of Reptiles and Amphibians, pp. 129–133.

McKinnell, R.G. 1965. Incidence and histology of renal tumors of leopard frogs from the North Central States. Annals of the New York Academy of Sciences 126:85–98.

McKinnell, R.G. 1969. Lucke renal adenocarcinoma: Epidemiological aspects, *in* Mizell, M. (Ed.), Biology of Amphibian Tumors. Springer-Verlag, New York, pp. 254–260.

McKinnell, R.G. and D.P. DuPlantier. 1970. Are there renal adenocarcinoma-free populations of leopard frogs? Cancer Research 30:2730–2735.

McKinnell, R.G. and J.C. John. 1995. An unexpectedly high prevalence of spontaneous renal carcinoma found in *Rana pipiens* obtained from northern Vermont, U.S.A. Proceeding of 5th International Colloquium on the Pathology of Reptiles and Amphibians. Herpetopathologia 1995:279–280.

McKinnell, R.G. and B.K. McKinnell. 1968. Seasonal fluctuation of frog renal adenocarcinoma prevalence in natural populations. Cancer Research 28:440–444.

McKinnell, R.G., E. Gorhan, and F.B. Martin. 1979. A major reduction in the prevalence of the Lucke renal adenocarcinoma associated with greatly diminished frog populations. Journal of the National Cancer Institute 63:821–824.

McKinnell, R.G., E.D. Seppanen, J.M. Lust, D.K. Carlson, and B.R. Hunter. 1989. Lucke renal adenocarcinoma: Cell of origin, characterization of malignancy, and genomic potential. Proceedings of 3rd International Colloquium on the Pathology of Reptiles and Amphibians, Orlando, FL, pp. 72–73.

Mizell, M., S.S. Schochet, Jr, and J. Isaacs. 1966a. Two new tumors in *Rana pipiens* [Abstr. #253]. American Zoologist 6:356.

Mizell, M., S.S. Schochet, Jr., J. Weichert, and C. Stackpole. 1966b. Ultrastructural observations on a frog embryonal rhabdomyosarcoma [Abstr. #254]. American Zoologist 6:356.

Mizgireuv, I.V., N.L. Flax, L.J. Borkin, and V.V. Khudoley. 1984. Dysplastic lesions and abnormalities in amphibians associated with environmental conditions. Neoplasma 31:175–181.

Mori, H. 1954. Observation of the liver sarcoma in the newt, *Triturus pyrrhogaster*. Science Reports of the Research Institute of Tohoku University, Series 4 (Biology) 20:187–188.

Mulcare, D.J. 1969. Non-specific transmission of the Lucke tumor, in Mizell, M. (Ed.): Biology of Amphibian Tumors. Springer-Verlag, New York, pp. 240–253.

Murray, J.A. 1908. The zoological distribution of cancer. Third Scientific Report, Imperial Cancer Research Fund, pp. 41–60.

Nielsen, S.W. and D.H. Lein. 1974. International histological classification of tumours of domestic animals. VI. Tumours of the testis. Bulletin of World Health Organization 50:71–78.

Nielsen, S.W., L.J. Mackey, and W. Misdorp. 1976. International classification of tumors of domestic animals, XVIII. Tumors of the kidney. Bulletin of the World Health Organization 53:237–245.

Nishioka, M. and Y. Kondo. 1987. Frequent occurrence of renal tumors in the hybrids between *Bufo japonicus* and *B. raddei* [Abstr]. Zoological Science (Japan) 4:1069.

Nishioka, M. and H. Ueda. 1987. Abundant tumors which recently occurred in the Laboratory for Amphibian Biology [Abstr]. Zoological Science (Japan) 4:1069.

Nishioka, M., H. Ueda, Y. Kondo, P. Masahito, Y. Kato, and T. Kitagawa. 1994. Pancreas carcinomas and renal cell carcinomas respectively developed in Japanese-Chinese pond frog and bufo hybrids (Abstr). 8th International Conference of the International Society of Differentiation (ISD), 22–26 October 1994.

Oinuma, T., M. Seki, and M. Asashima. 1984. Histological and electron microscopical studies on neoplasia subcutaneously occurring in *Xenopus laevis*. Proceedings of Japan Academy Series B. 60B:265–268.

Oka, K., K. Kishi, T. Shiroya, M. Asashima, and C.J. Pfeiffer. 1992. Reduction of papilloma size by ultraviolet irradiation in the Japanese newt, *Cynops pyrrhogaster*. Journal of Comparative Pathology 106:1–8.

Olmacher, H.P. 1898. Several examples illustrating the comparative pathology of tumours. Bulletin, Ohio Hospital for Epileptics 1:223–236.

Pawlowski, E.N. 1912. Zur Kasuistik der Tumoren beim Frosch (On the occurrence of tumors in frogs.) [Abstr. #94]. Zentralblatt fur Allgemeine Pathologie und Pathologische Anatomie 23:94.

Pentimalli, F. 1914. Ueber die Geschwulste bei Amphibien. Zeitschrift fur Krebsforschung 14:623–632.

Pfeiffer, C.J. and M. Asashima. 1990. Gastric leiomyomas in the Japanese newt, *Cynops pyrrhogaster*: ultrastructural observations. Journal of Comparative Pathology 102:79–80.

Pfeiffer, C.J., M. Asashima, and K. Hirayasu. 1989. Ultrastructural characterization of the spontaneous papilloma of Japanese newts. Journal of Submicroscopic and Cytologic Pathology. 21:659–668.

Pfeiffer, C.J., T. Jagai, M. Fujimura, and T. Tobe. 1979. Spontaneous regressive epitheliomas in the Japanese newt, *Cynops pyrrhogaster*. Cancer Research 39:1904–1910.

Pick, L. and H. Poll. 1903. Uber einige bemerkenswerte Tumorbildungen aus der Tierpathologie, insbesondere uber gutartige und krebsige Neubildungen bei Kaltblutern. Berliner Klinische Wochenschrifte 40:572–574.

Pirlot, J.M. and M. Welsch. 1934. Etude anatomique et experimentale de quelques tumeurs chez la grenouille rousse (*Rana fusca* L.). Archives Internationales de Medicine Experimentale 9:341–365.

Plehn, M. 1906. Uber Geschwulste bei Kaltblutern. Zeitschrift fur Krebsforschung. 4:525–564.

Ponomarkov V. and L.J. Mackey. 1976. International histological classification of tumours of domestic animals. XIII. Tumours of the liver and biliary system. Bulletin of World Health Organization 53:187–195.

Rafferty, K.A., Jr. 1964. Kidney tumors of the leopard frog: A review. Cancer Research 24:169–185.

Reichenbach-Klinke, H. and E. Elkan. 1965. Diseases of Amphibians. TFH Publications, Inc., Neptune City, NJ, pp. 321–353.

Richenbacher, J. 1950. Uber ein spontan enstandenes Carcinom bei *Triton alpestris*. Revue Suisse de Pathologie et de Bacteriologie 13:497–503.

Robert, J. and L. Du Pasquier. 1995. The immune system of *Xenopus* and metamorphosis. Madoqua 19:49–55.

Robert, J. and L. Du Pasquier. 1996. *Xenopus* lymphoid tumor cell lines (Chapter 33.5), in Lefkovits, I. (Ed.): Immunology Methods Manual. Academic Press, San Diego, CA, pp. 1–11.

Robert, J., C. Guiet, and L. Du Pasquier. 1994. Lymphoid tumor of *Xenopus laevis* with different capacities of growth in larvae and adults. Developmental Immunology 3:297–307.

Robert, J., C. Guiet, and L. Du Pasquier. 1995. Ontogeny of the alloimmune response against a transplanted tumor in *Xenopus laevis*. Differentiation 59:135–144.

Rose, F.L. 1976. Tumorous growths of the tiger salamander, *Ambystoma tigrinum*, associated with treated sewage effluent. Progress in Experimental Tumor Research 20:251–262.

Rose, F.L. 1981. The tiger salamander (*Ambystoma tigrinum*): A decade of sewage-associated neoplasia, in Dawe, C.J., J.C. Harshbarger, S. Kondo, T. Sugimura, and S. Takayama (Eds): Phyletic Approaches to Cancer. Japan Science Society Press, Tokyo, pp. 91–100.

Rose, F.L. and J.C. Harshbarger. 1977. Neoplastic and possibly related skin lesions in neotenic tiger salamanders from a sewage lagoon. Science 196:315–317.

Rostand, J. 1958. Anomalies des amphibiens anoures. S.E.D.E.S. Paris.

Ruben, L.N. and J.M. Stevens. 1970. A comparison between granulomatosis and lymphoreticular neoplasia in *Diemictylus viridescens* and *Xenopus laevis*. Cancer Research 30:2613–2619.

Sanford, S.E., D.M. Hoover, and R.B. Miller. 1984. Primary cardiac granular cell tumor in a dog. Veterinary Pathology 21:489–494.

Schipp, R. 1969. Die Bedeutung quergestreifter Faserstrukturen fur die Fibrillogenese in der Scheide von Chordomen bei Amphibien-bastardlarven. Protoplasma 67:345–360.

Schipp, R., H. Hemmer, and R. Flindt. 1968. Vergleichende licht- und elektronenmikroskopische Untersuchungen an Chordomen von Krotenbastardlarven. Beitrage zur Pathologischen Anatomie und zur Allgemeinen Pathologie 138:109–133.

Schlumberger, H.G. 1958. Krankheiten der Fische, Amphibien, und Reptile, in Cohrs, P., R. Jaffe, and H. Meesen (Eds.): Pathologie der Laboratoriumstiere, Vol. 1. Springer, Heidelberg, pp. 733–746.

Schlumberger, H.G. and B. Lucke. 1948. Tumors of fishes, amphibians, and reptiles. Cancer Research 8:657–753.

Schochet, S.S. and C.J. Lampert. 1969. Plasmacytoma in a *Rana pipiens*, in Mizell, M. (Ed.): Biology of Amphibian Tumors. Springer-Verlag, New York, pp. 204–214.

Schwarz, E. 1923. Uber zwei Geschwulste bei Kaltblutern. Zeitschrift fur Krebsforschung 20:353–357.

Secher, K. 1919. Kasuistische beitraege zur kenntnis der geschwuelste bei tieren. Zeitschrift fur Krebsforschung 16:297–313.

Sheremetieva, E.A. 1965. Spontaneous melanoma in regenerating tails of axolotls. Journal of Experimental Zoology 158:101–122.

Sheremetieva-Brunst, E.A. 1953. An epithelioma in the axolotl [Abstr]. Proceedings of the American Association for Cancer Research 1:51.

Sheremetieva-Brunst, E.A. 1961. Melanoma and adenocarcinoma in the regenerating organs of the axolotl, in Proceedings of the Frog Kidney Adenocarcinoma Conference (16 September 1961, National Institutes of Health, National Cancer Institute, Bethesda, MD, USA), pp. 115–135.

Sheremetieva-Brunst, E.A. and V.V. Brunst. 1948. Origin and transplantation of a melanotic tumor in the axolotl, in Gordon, M. (Ed.): The Biology of Melanomas. New York Academy of Sciences Special Publication 4:269–287.

Smallwood, W.M. 1905. Adrenal tumors in the kidney of the frog. Anatomischer Anzeiger 26:652–658.

Streett, J.C. 1964. A note on a teratoma occurring in the leopard frog. Texas Journal of Science 16:493.

Teutschlaender, O. 1920. Beitrage zur vergleichenden Onkologie mit Berucksichtigung der Identitatsfrage. Zeitschrift fur Krebsforschung 17:285–407.

Vaillant, L. and A. Pettit. 1902. Fibrome observe sur un *Megalobatrachus maximus,* Schlegel, a la menageri du museum. Bulletin du Museum d'Histoire Naturelle, Paris 8:301–304.

Van Der Steen, A.B.M., B.J. Cohen, D.H. Ringler, G.D. Abrams, and C.M. Richards. 1972. Cutaneous neoplasms in the leopard frog (*Rana pipiens*). Laboratory Animal Science 22:216–222.

Volterra, M. 1928. Uber eine seltene bosartige Geschwulst bei einem exotischen Frosch (*Ceratophrys ornata*). Zeitschrift fur Krebsforschung 27:457.

Walder, E.J. and T.L. Gross. 1992. Neoplastic diseases of the skin: Epithelial tumors, *in* Gross, T.L., P.J. Ihrke, and E.J. Walder (Eds.): Veterinary Dermatopathology. Mosby Year Book, Saint Louis, MO, pp. 343–373.

Weiss, E. 1974. International histological classification of tumours of domestic animals. VII. Tumours of the soft (mesenchymal) tissues. Bulletin of the World Health Organization 50:101–110.

Weiss, E. and K. Frese. 1974. International histological classification of tumours of domestic animals. VII. Tumours of the skin. Bulletin of the World Health Organization 50:79–100.

Willis, R.A. 1964. Pathology of Tumours, 4th Ed. Butterworths, London, p. 433.

Witschi, E. 1922. Uberreife der Eier als kausaler Faktor bei Entstchung von Mehrfachbildungen und Teratomen. Verhandlungen der Naturforschenden Gesellschaft in Basel 34:33.

Witschi, E. 1930. Experimentally produced neoplasms in the frog. Proceedings of the Society for Experimental Biology and Medicine 27:475–477.

Wood, D.A. 1967. Tumors of the Intestines, Series VI, Fascicle 22. Armed Forces Institute of Pathology, Washington, DC, 261 pp.

Zambernard, J., A.E. Vatter, and R.G. McKinnell. 1966. The fine structure of nuclear and cytoplasmic inclusions in primary renal tumors of mutant leopard frogs. Cancer Research 26:1688–1700.

Zavanella, T. 1974. Il melanoma del tritone crestato: Stato attuale delle ricerche. Atti Della Accademia Nazionale dei Lincei 56:1031–1042.

Zavanella, T. 1975. Epidemiologia del melanoma del tritone crestato [Abstr]. Tumori 61:123.

Zavanella, T. 1995. Spontaneous tumors in the crested newt, *Triturus carnifex*. Herpetopathologia 1995:287.

Zilakos, N.P., P.A. Tsonis, K. Del Rio-Tsonis, and R.E. Parchment. 1992. Newt squamous carcinoma proves phylogenetic conservation of tumors as caricatures of tissue renewal. Cancer Research 52:4858–4865.

Zwart, P. 1970. A nephroblastoma in a fire-bellied newt, *Cynops pyrrhogaster*. Cancer Research 30:2691–2694.

CHAPTER 27
PATHOLOGY OF AMPHIBIA

D. Earle Green, DVM, Diplomate ACVP

27.1 DISEASES AND PATHOLOGY OF EGGS AND EMBRYOS

The diagnostic approach to amphibian eggs should parallel that of fish egg examinations (Thoesen, 1994).

27.1.1 Genetically Based Egg Pathology

The Haploid Syndrome. Eggs of many amphibians may be stimulated to commense development by a variety of methods in the absence of fertilization by sperm. The maternal genome may also be microsurgically removed to allow only the sperm's genome to initiate development. Typically, haploid embryos develop abnormally with a group of characteristic features (Porter, 1939), referred to as the haploid syndrome (Browder, 1975). Haploid blastulas and embryos show delayed cell division, retarded differentiation, specific defects of eyes, brain, and other organs, hydrops, and about 90–99% mortality at days 8–12. Gastrulation in haploid eggs of the Northern leopard frog, *Rana pipiens,* is delayed 1 hour over diploid eggs. The neural tube normally forms on the third day, and in haploid embryos the neural plate remains about 33% shorter and the neural groove is shallower. Also on day 3 of development, the tail bud is shorter, the abdomen is abnormally large and rounded, and the head is shortened and smaller. On day 4, the haploid embryo has temporary lordosis of the tail, a shortened abnormally rounded abdomen, and the head is bent dorsally. On day 6, the tail and spine straighten, but the overall length remains subnormal. About 50% of haploid embryos have a beating heart whereas in diploid embryos the heartbeat begins at day 5. On day 7, edema of the dermis and abdomen begins and progressively worsens for 1–5 more days until death. On day 8, the operculum develops normally in both haploid and diploid embryos. Only those haploid embryos that develop cardiovascular circulation survive beyond 10–12 days, and show more successful differentiation of organs. Haploid embryos that successfully hatch remain inactive, often lying on the bottom on their sides. Haploid tadpoles often fail to react to physical stimulation, but when sufficiently provoked, they respond by swimming in erratic circles. Approximately 65% of embryos die between days 8 and 12 of development, and less than 5% survive beyond 24 days (Porter, 1939). Haploid embryos rarely survive to sexual maturity (Miyada, 1960).

Haploid anuran embryos may develop anomalous eyes, brain, ventricles, ears, and intestines (Porter, 1939). Grossly, the intestine does not coil, but remains almost a straight tube through the body cavity. The intestinal wall in cross section appears moderately thickened, and the cells remain packed with cytoplasmic yolk droplets. The pronephroi appear to develop normally and have patent tubules, nephrostomes, and ducts to the cloaca which suggests that abnormal renal function may not be the cause of the hydrops. Until haploid and diploid embryos are 4–5 days old, the yolk content of the cells in all regions is so great that microscopic comparisons are without value. After that time the eyes of haploid embryos are smaller than normals and development lags. The ventrolateral margins of the optic cups fail to fuse, leaving a wide choroid fissure. The lens shows initial development until about day 5, then lags. Lenses are absent or smaller than normal. The spinal cord appears to develop normally but the brain does not. In most haploids, the ventricles are prominently reduced by a marked proliferation of cells of the "brain wall." Neurons are more numerous than in diploid embryos, and if the haploid survives beyond 10 days, the neuropil becomes vacuolated and pyknotic nuclei increase in number. Insipient white matter is poorly delineated, and usually contains excessive numbers of cells. Many ectodermal structures, such as the oral suckers, olfactory pits, operculum, and mouth parts appear normal in haploids. The epidermis prior to day 7 appears thicker and more wrinkled than normal, but as dermal edema begins and progresses, the epidermis becomes thinner. It has been reported that "tumorlike proliferations of the ectoderm occasionally appear, and are not unlike those shown by frog embryos treated with weak solutions of 2,4-dinitrophenol, or with high temperatures, or developed from over-ripe eggs" (Porter, 1939).

"Over-ripe Egg" Syndrome. Myriad abnormalities have been attributed to frog eggs that were "over-ripe" at the time of fertilization (Witschi, 1930). Normally, the frog egg passes into a brief ("a few hours") resting period following the second polar spindle-metaphase awaiting fertilization. Fertilization may be delayed about 3 days with no perceptible impairment of egg vigor, but by the fifth day the eggs are dead. Unfertilized eggs between the third and fifth days are considered "over-ripe," and if fertilization occurs, numerous abnormalities become evident in the eggs and subsequent developing embryos. Many of the abnormalities in developing embryos that are attributed to "over-ripe" eggs, are remarkably similar to the anomalies observed in the haploid syndrome.

Over-ripe eggs are prone to polyspermy, which may progress to multiple segmentation of the zygote. Monosperm over-ripe eggs develop animal blastomeres that are reduced in size. Later development of over-ripe eggs results in a high percentage of embryos that have axial duplications and supernumerary limbs. Embryos have have an abundance of light brown pigment granules. Numerous anomalies of internal organs are also detected. Hypophyseal atresia, lack of ocular lenses, poorly differentiated ocular vesicles, numerous brain abnormalities, a poorly differentiated spinal cord that lacks a central canal, and poorly developed spinal ganglia and peripheral nerves are seen. Most embryos that develop from over-ripe eggs are dead by about 2 weeks of age (Witschi, 1930).

Another unusual feature of embryogenesis of over-ripe eggs is the formation of hyperplastic, neoplastic or hamartomatous growths. Similar growths were described in developing haploid eggs (Porter, 1939). Nodular cellular growths may occur in the skin and intestinal wall of embryos and larvae hatched from over-ripe eggs. These epidermal nodules were characterized as a "wild growth" of cells and were classified as epitheliomas (Witschi, 1930). The epidermal growths were also characterized as three distinct types of hyperplasia (Briggs, 1941). Transplantation of one growth from an embryo into normal tadpoles resulted either in rejection of the cells or their proliferation and invasion of local tissues and the circulatory system (Witschi, 1930). The transplanted invading cells were spindle-shaped or round, and usually contained considerable pigment. Neoplastic-like cells were transplanted intraperitoneally into a froglet. Fifty days later the froglet developed a massively swollen firm abdomen and survived to 62 days post-transplantation at which time a large tumor was found attached to the peritoneum, mesentery, and urinary bladder. Cells were also infiltrating the intestine and liver. The precise nature of these growths was not fully investigated (Witschi, 1930). Further characterization of the growths in embryos from haploid and over-ripe eggs is needed.

Pigment Mutations. Pigment mutations have been studied and characterized in five genera of amphibians: *Ambystoma*, *Pleurodeles*, *Bombina*, *Rana*, and *Xenopus*. Of these, only two pigment mutations are evident in the eggs and embryos of *Xenopus* spp.: pale eggs (Droin & Fischberg, 1984) and periodic albinism (Hoperskaya, 1975). True albinism has been reported in many amphibians, and affected females, if fertile, consistently lay unpigmented eggs (Humphrey, 1975). The pigment in all amphibian eggs is maternal, hence all true albino females lay unpigmented eggs, but unpigmented eggs may also be produced by apparently normally pigmented females. On the other hand, maternally derived egg pigments may mask inherited pigment defects of the offspring during the cleavage, gastrula, and embryonic stages (Briggs, 1972). Some defects may be noted in embryos before hatching, but others may not become evident until the free-swimming tadpole stage (Briggs & Briggs, 1984).

27.1.2 Egg—Toxicological Etiologies

Ultraviolet Radiation. Anthropogenic degradation of atmospheric ozone has been attributed to transport exhausts and halocarbons. The rapidly proliferating and differentiating embryonic tissues of surface and shallow water amphibians may be particularily radiosensitive (Blaustein et al., 1994a; Williams & Smith, 1984; Worrest & Kimeldorf, 1976). Evidence of ultraviolet-B (radiation with a wavelength from 290–315 nm) radiosensitivity in amphibian embryos comes from studies conducted in the western U.S.A. (Blaustein et al., 1994a; Blaustein et al., 1995a; Worrest & Kimeldorf, 1975, 1976), but recent studies have generated controversy (Blaustein et al., 1995b).

When eggs and tadpoles of the western toad, *Bufo boreas*, were exposed to increased levels of ultraviolet-B radiation, no significant gross effects were found on eggs, embryos, and young tadpoles until after stage 30, the stage immediately preceeding development of digits on the hindlimbs. Between stages 30 and 35, when hindlimbs are nearly fully formed, mortality rises dramatically to over 90%. Affected tadpoles showed lordosis and ocular lesions. Ocular changes were confined to the cornea, and consisted of abnormal retention of melanin pigment in the epidermal layer. Retained melanin was distinctly more prominent in the dorsal half of the cornea and this pigment persisted in those tadpoles surviving to metamorphosis (Worrest & Kimeldorf, 1976).

Experimental irradiation of embryos of the northern leopard frog, *Rana pipiens*, with unspecified wavelengths of ultraviolet light may produce abnormalities of the primordial germ cells (PGC) and gonads. When ultraviolet light is directed to the vegetal pole (ventral hemisphere) of eggs in the two-cell stage, a fate which may not occur naturally, developmental defects in the gonads are detected much later in tadpole and recent metamorph stages. Following ultraviolet exposure of eggs, tadpoles at stage 25 lack PGC in their genital ridges, but a few days later, only 33% were sterile, suggesting a delay in migration of PGC. Of the 67% of tadpoles having PGC, cell numbers were markedly reduced to between 2–13 cells. At stage V, the gonads of irradiated tadpoles are one-sixth the size of controls. Shortly after metamorphosis is complete, gonads contain nearly normal numbers of PGC, but testes and ovaries are less than half the size of nonirradiated frogs (Williams & Smith, 1984). These developmental lesions have not been documented as a natural disease in wild amphibians.

Histologically, tadpoles of the western toad, *Bufo boreas*, irradiated with ultraviolet-B develop epidermal hyperplasia in the putative cornea and epidermis of the dorsal head and body. The histologic changes in the skin are described as increased epidermal thickness (4–5 cells thick), abnormal arrangement of epidermal cells, and hyperpigmentation. Ultraviolet-B irradiation of the dorsal epidermis of a tadpole also causes severe desquamation of cells (Worrest & Kimeldorf, 1976). Ultrastructural changes have been reported (Williams & Smith 1984).

Toad embryos and tadpoles seem to be provided some protection from high levels of ultraviolet-B radiation if they are previously or subsequently exposed to visible and ultraviolet-A radiation (Blaustein et al., 1994a; Worrest & Kimeldorf, 1976).

Acid Precipitation. Amphibian eggs, embryos and larvae vary in their susceptibility to acidification of their aquatic environment depending on species and stage of development (Pierce, 1985). The effects of acidified waters on amphibians and fish are not purely a function of hydrion (H+) concentration because acidity affects a number of other water quality factors, such as oxygen concentrations, and concentrations and bioavailability of elements such as aluminum and calcium (Freda, 1991). Naturally acidic waters of the Pine Barrens of New Jersey limit amphibian distributions (Gosner & Black, 1957).

Acidification of surface waters (i.e., breeding ponds) is due principally to sulfur dioxide (SO_2) and oxides of nitrogen from coal and liquid petroleum exhausts. Consequently, acidification of surface water is principally a problem in regions of heavy human activity and industrialization, such as northern Europe and eastern Canada and the USA, but there is conflicting evidence that acidification is a factor in population declines in western USA and tropical regions (Bradford et al., 1992, 1994; Corn & Vertucci, 1992; Harte & Hoffman, 1989). In surface waters with less than pH 5, aluminum rises in concentration, its speciation shifts, and calcium concentrations decline (Freda, 1991). The combination of acidity, elevated trivalent aluminum, and declining calcium have been considered by some to be the cause of the yolk-plug defects in amphibian embryos (Beattie & Tyler-Jones, 1992); however, the same yolk lesions are reproduced experimentally at pH 4.5 in the absence of aluminum. At low pH, cellular sodium retention is adversely affected (Freda & Dawson, 1984), suggesting that low pH affects calcium, sodium, and aluminum metabolism.

In the spotted salamander, *Ambystoma maculatum*, the gross lesions in embryos affected by acidification are similar in experimental and natural situations (Pough, 1976). At pH 4.5 the mortality of eggs and embryos remains under 1.3% during early embryonic development. Mortalities begin during stages of neurulation, and again at later stages of gill development and hatching. A pH of 5–6 results in edema of the ventral thoracic region overlying the heart, and stunting and asymmetry of the gills. Severe stress occurs at pH 4.5–5, causing the following additional lesions: failure to internalize the yolk into the coelomic cavity and deformation of the posterior body. At or below pH 4 the egg membranes shrink, the egg appears dessicated, and embryos become tightly coiled (Pough, 1976). Curled embryos that are incapable of hatching have also been reported in the wood frog, *Rana sylvatica*, the American toad, *Bufo americanus*, and the northern leopard frog, *Rana pipiens*, kept at pH 4.2. Affected embryos often have a wrinkled appearance (Karns, 1992). Hatching failure in fully developed embryos is a significant cause of mortality, and also occurs in embryos without the curling defect (Freda, 1991). However, ambystomid embryos at the center of an egg mass may survive while those at the periphery suffer the greatest morbidity and mortality. Salamander embryos are more susceptible to low pH than their larvae and tadpoles, but the measured difference is only 0.3–0.4 pH units (Bradford et al., 1992). Histological examinations have not been reported on amphibian embryos affected by acid precipitation.

Embryos of frogs and toads also develop gross lesions when stressed or fatally affected by low pH or low pH in combination with elevated aluminum concentrations. Reduced snout-to-tail-tip length of recently hatched tadpoles was the principal defect reported in the Yosemite toad, *Bufo canorus*, and the mountain yellow-legged frog, *Rana muscosa* (Bradford et al., 1992), and many other frogs and toads (Freda, 1990). "Fluid-filled blebs" in the skin may occur in newly hatched tadpoles of the northern leopard frog, *Rana pipiens*. This edema may be linked to a major loss of sodium and chloride ions in high acid waters (Freda, 1991; Freda & McDonald, 1990). The

European common frog, *Rana temporaria,* shows both stunting and failure to internalize the yolk (Beattie & Tyler-Jones, 1992); however the yolk defect has not been observed consistently in other anurans (Bradford et al., 1992).

Combined Low pH and Ultraviolet Radiation. A synergistic lethal effect of combined ultraviolet-B radiation and acid water was observed under experimental conditions in embryos of the northern leopard frog, *Rana pipiens* (Long et al., 1995). Embryos in water at pH 4.5 were exposed to approximately double the natural level of ultraviolet-B and experienced a 50% mortality rate, while those exposed to similar levels of ultraviolet-B at pH 6 had a 1–3% mortality rate. Lethally affected embryos showed defects typical of low pH, namely, failure of embryonic membranes to expand, curling of the embryos, and failure to hatch. Hence, elevated levels of ultraviolet-B radiation, that were equivalent to an estimated 30% reduction in the protective atmospheric ozone shield, greatly elevates the prevalence and severity of the acidic water-associated curling defect (Long et al., 1995).

Heavy Metals and Metalloids. A variety of cations have been demonstrated to cause deformities, developmental failures, and death in aquatic amphibian eggs and embryos. Cases of metal poisoning in wild amphibians are rarely documented, and must be gleaned from reports that were principally concerned with mass mortalities among waterfowl or fish. Copper and selenium intoxications are documented or strongly suspected in wild amphibians in Great Britain and California, respectively. Most metal intoxications are documented in adult amphibians, hence aspects of these metals on reproductive success, incorporation of the metals into eggs, and embryonic development are infrequently examined. Since water hardness, pH, dissolved organics, and temperature have large effects on metal toxicity, published results of experimental studies on metal toxicity in amphibians must be compared cautiously (Freda, 1991).

Aluminum. The toxicity of aluminum is an extremely complex phenomenon that is influenced by water hardness (calcium concentration), pH, oxygen content, and the species and developmental stage of the amphibian. In natural situations, it is extremely difficult to separate the effects of low pH from rising aluminum concentrations, because the two occur concurrently (Freda, 1991). Because toxic concentrations of aluminum are likely to be found only in association with acidic water, the lesions generally are considered the same.

Copper. Pertinent studies on copper toxicity in amphibians were concisely reviewed (Freda, 1991; Power et al., 1989). It appears that eggs and embryos are resistent to copper, possibly being afforded protection from many cations by the vitelline membrane. However, larvae may die of intoxication quickly after hatching in the same copper concentrations in which the embryo developed fully (Birge & Black, 1979; Dilling & Healey, 1925; Kaplan & Yoh, 1961). Concentrations of 0.31–1.56 μg/L are lethal to hatchlings of the northern leopard frog, *Rana pipiens,* but in another study, the 72-h LC_{50} was 150 μg/L and growth was inhibited in tadpoles by 60 μg/L (Lande & Guttman, 1973). In tadpoles of the African clawed frog, *Xenopus laevis,* the 96-h LC_{50} was 157 μg/L and the 7-day LC_{50} for copper, cadmium, and zinc were 40, 40, and 10 μg/L, respectively (Birge, 1978; Freda, 1991). In tadpoles of the western toad, *Bufo boreas,* the lethal limits of copper, zinc, and iron (common ions in mine tailings) were 20–44, 100–500, and 20,000–30,000 μg/L, respectively (Porter & Hakanson, 1976).

Lead. Lead is highly toxic and teratogenic to amphibian eggs and embryos, but adult anurans are much less sensitive (Power et al., 1989). Lead salts severely inhibit growth of tadpoles. Eggs of ranids that are exposed to lead produce tadpoles that, later in development, have fewer primordial germ cells. Effects of lead on the eggs of the eastern narrowmouth toad, *Gastrophryne carolinensis,* African clawed frog, *Xenopus laevis,* and black-spotted frog, *Rana nigromaculata,* have been reported (reviewed by Power et al., 1989). In static water assays containing 0.001 mg/L lead, 18% of clawed frog eggs were killed and 82% of embryos had deformities. Levels of 10 mg/L lead resulted in 100% mortality of clawed frog eggs. The presence of other metals in the solution, such as magnesium, may ameliorate the effects of lead (Miller & Landesman, 1978).

Lithium. When cleavage-stage embryos of the African clawed frog, *Xenopus laevis,* are exposed to lithium, the entire mesoderm becomes dorsalized, leading to radial embryos that lack all organs ventral to the vertebral column. Later in embryonic development, one ventral organ does form, a beating heart (Drysdale et al., 1994; Kao & Elinson, 1988).

Mercury. Mercury is one of the most toxic elements to embryos and larvae of most aquatic invertebrates and ectothermic aquatic vertebrates (Birge et al., 1979), however, there are no analytical or histological studies of mercury (and lead) on nervous tissue of larval and adult amphibians (Power et al., 1989). Mercury is neurotoxic and gametotoxic to adult vertebrates, lethal to amphibian larvae, and teratogenic to nearly all vertebrate embryos (Birge et al., 1979). The mechanisms of action of mercury include binding of sulfhydryl groups in proteins, potent inhibition of mitotic cell division, and production of chromosomal aberrations such as induction of polyploidy and somatic mutations (Birge et al., 1979). Mercury readily bioaccumulates so that concentrations in tissues greatly increase with passage in the food chain. Females pass inorganic mercury into forming eggs, especially concentrating it in the yolk.

The African clawed frog, *Xenopus laevis*, accumulated residues of 0.49 μg mercury/g of gonadal tissue when experimentally exposed to 0.2 μg inorganic mercury/l for 11 months. When eggs from these mercury-laden clawed frogs were allowed to develop in mercury-free water, survival was over 80% suggesting that accumulation and deposition of inorganic mercury in vitellogenic eggs is not efficient in this species. However, if eggs from the *X. laevis* are allowed to develop in mercury solutions, 50% are killed in 7 days at a mercury concentration of 0.16 μg/L (Birge et al., 1979). When the eggs and larvae of 12 anuran species native to southeastern United States were exposed to inorganic mercury, the LC_{50} varied by a factor of 50. The eastern narrowmouth toad, *Gastrophryne carolinensis*, was most sensitive, having an LC_{50} of 1.3 μg/L. The gray treefrog complex, *H. chrysoscelis*, and *H. versicolor*, the barking treefrog, *H. gratiosa*, squirrel treefrog, *H. squirella*, and the spring peeper, *Pseudacris crucifer* had LC_{50}s of 2.4–2.8 μg/L. The northern leopard frog, *Rana pipiens*, and the Blanchard's cricket frog, *Acris crepitans blanchardi*, had LC_{50}s of 7.3 and 10.4 μg/L, respectively. The LC_{50}s for three bufonids (the Fowler's toad, *Bufo woodhousei fowleri*, the red-spotted toad, *B. punctatus*, and the Eastern green toad, *B. debilis debilis*) and two ranids (the river frog, *Rana heckscheri*, and the pig frog, *R. grylio*) were 37–67 μg/L. In the marbled salamander, *Ambystoma opacum*, the LC_{50} was 107.5 μg/L, but it is not clear if this high tolerance to mercury is characteristic of other salamanders.

Teratogenic effects of organic mercury were demonstrated in the northern leopard frog, *Rana pipiens* (Dial, 1976). Anomalies included impaired gastrulation, and various defects in the tail and vertebral column, including lordosis, abrupt kinks or bends, curling, and scoliosis (Dial, 1976). The same lesions were observed in tadpoles of the ornate rice frog, *Microhyla ornata*, and, in addition, there were vesicles on the body (Ghate & Mulherkar, 1980). Methylmercuric chloride at 30 ppb caused 100% mortality in embryos of the northern leopard frog, *Rana pipiens* (Dial, 1976).

Selenium. Selenium is toxic at concentrations above 1 ppm in water to embryos and tadpoles of the African clawed frog, *Xenopus laevis* (Browne & Dumont, 1979). When fertilized eggs are allowed to develop in water with concentrations of 2–20 ppm selenium, there is reduced hatching, and deformities in those embryos that successfully hatch. Deformities include flattened, irregularly shaped heads, lordosis of the tail or lateral flexure of the tail up to 90°, large epidermal, fluid-filled blisters, and reduction in melanin pigmentation on head and abdomen. These gross lesions have not been studied histologically (Browne & Dumont, 1979).

There are suggestions in the literature that spontaneous selenosis may occur in amphibians and reptiles, as it does in waterfowl in specific regions in California and neighboring Nevada (Ohlendorf et al., 1988), but definitive evidence is lacking. At Kesterson National Wildlife Refuge in central California waterfowl show infertility, teratologic effects in developing embryos, and specific gross lesions in adult birds. No gross or histological abnormalities have been observed in the sympatric populations of the bullfrog, *Rana catesbeiana*, even though selenium concentrations in their livers were exceptionally high and in ranges where infertility and teratologic effects would be expected in birds. The concentration of hepatic selenium in normal bullfrogs was 6.2 μg/g, while bullfrogs at Kesterson National Wildlife Refuge had concentrations of 45 μg/g (dry weight analyses) (Ohlendorf et al., 1988).

Silver. Silver is as toxic as mercury to amphibian embryos and larvae (Birge, 1978).

Zinc. Zinc is teratogenic to amphibian and fish embryos, but teratogenicity in mammals is inconclusive since zinc may protect against some mammalian teratogens (Eisler, 1993). Zinc is also a component of some carbamate insecticides such as Zineb® and Ziram®. At concentrations of 0.01 and 2.4 ppm zinc, 50% of the embryos of the eastern narrowmouth toad, *Gastrophryne carolinensis*, and the marbled salamander, *Ambystoma opacum*, respectively, were dead or deformed in a 7–8 day exposure (EPA, 1987). Low-level exposure of tadpoles to zinc initially stimulates multiplication of primordial germ cells, but chronic treatment has a toxic effect on germ cells of the developing ovary (Gipouloux et al., 1986). In the Frog Embryo Teratogenesis Assay *Xenopus* (FETAX), embryos of the African clawed frog, *Xenopus laevis*, developed anomalies characterized as severe edema of the eye and pericardium, abnormal coiling of the intestine, microphthalmia, micrencephaly, and severe kinking of the vertebral column when exposed to levels greater than 4 ppm zinc (Fort et al., 1989).

Petroleum. Major sources of oil in the environment are run-offs from roads, use of oils for dust control on roads, illicit dumping, accidental spills, and, increasingly, seepage from underground storage tanks.

In an experimental study on eggs, embryos and tadpoles of the green treefrog, *Hyla cinerea*, hatching success was minimally affected by up to 100 mg/L of used crankcase oil, but tadpole growth and successful metamorphosis were significantly decreased. At levels of 55 and 100 mg/L, tadpoles were stunted, but growth rebounded following dilution of oil concentrations. At the highest studied concentration (100 mg/L), no tadpoles successfully metamorphosed (Mahoney, 1994).

Retinoic Acid. Retinoic acid induces multiple anomalies in embryos of the African clawed frog, *Xenopus laevis*, and has been studied especially for its effects on the developing heart (Drysdale et al., 1994). Retinoic acid and other metabolites of provitamin-A compounds probably have multiple metabolic pathways in amphibians because amphibians incorporate these pigmentary vitamins into vesicles in the pigment cells, xanthophores (Frost-Mason et al., 1994).

If retinoic acid is applied to embryoes of *X. laevis* prior to heart determination, the amount of formed cardiac tissue is sharply reduced (Sive et al., 1990) while cement glands, hatching glands, olfactory pits, and eyes fail to form or are reduced in size. The lymph hearts located dorsocaudally to the eyes of embryos and tadpoles of *X. laevis* are not affected by retinoic acid and commense contractions normally, but show compensatory hypertrophy in the absence of the heart (Drysdale et al., 1994).

Teratogenesis. The more prolific a species, the more likely spontaneous malformed offspring will be found (Elkan, 1983). A large volume of literature exists on experimental teratogenesis in amphibians. Significant data has resulted from Frog Embryo Teratogenesis Assays on *Xenopus laevis* (FETAX) (American Society for Testing and Materials, 1991). *An Atlas of Abnormalities* (Bantle et al., undated) details many induced anomalies in embryos of the African clawed frog, *Xenopus laevis,* and serves as a starting point for investigation of spontaneously occurring defects in anurans. Over 60 defects of eyes, skeleton, heart, intestine, and head were illustrated.

27.1.3 Infectious Diseases of Eggs

The egg and embryo cannot generate an inflammatory cell reaction in response to pathogens.

Virus Infections. There are no reports of spontaneous virus infections in amphibian eggs or embryos, however, frog virus-3 (FV3, a ranavirus) when injected into embryos of the northern leopard frog, *Rana pipiens* (the host animal from which the virus was originally isolated), causes exceptionally high mortality rates (Came et al., 1968; Tweedell & Granoff, 1968). These studies have been overlooked for decades, but suggest a need for greater virological studies in wild amphibian eggs, and especially in those species involved in population declines. Frog virus-3 is discussed in greater detail in the section on Infectious Etiologies—Viral infections of Section 27.2.2, Integumentary System.

Saprolegniasis. Saprolegniasis is a disease caused by multiple genera of Oomycete watermolds that are ubiquitous in nature. The main pathogenic watermold of fish is the species group *Saprolegnia diclina-parasitica* (Noga, 1993a). In the Pacific Northwest of the USA, *Saprolegnia ferax* has been implicated in mass destruction of eggs of the western toad, *Bufo boreas* (Blaustein et al., 1994b; Kiesecker & Blaustein, 1995). Most reported watermold infections in amphibians are not fully identified, nor is it certain that the isolates that are pathogenic to fish are equally pathogenic to amphibians.

Watermold infestations of eggs in the wild and captivity are common in anurans and salamanders. Saprolegniasis occurs as both a normal decompositional process in infertile or dead eggs, and as an opportunistic disease. Watermolds colonize dead eggs more readily than viable eggs (Noga, 1993a). Infertile and dead amphibian eggs decay and disappear in a period of days (Pough, 1976). Often, a few eggs or a low percentage of eggs in a cluster will be affected, but occasionally whole egg masses are infected (Blaustein et al., 1994b). Watermolds have been implicated in serious population declines and local extinctions of amphibians due to infections of eggs and tadpoles (Blaustein et al., 1994b; Bragg, 1958; Kiesecker & Blaustein, 1995).

Factors predisposing eggs to saprolegniasis include decomposition of infertile eggs, early embryonic death, and trauma (physical or chemical) to the protective egg membranes and capsule(s). When whole clusters of eggs in the wild or captivity are affected, consideration should be given to poor water quality (low dissolved oxygen, high concentrations of organic wastes), water-borne chemicals or pollutants, infectious or toxic diseases of the reproductive tract of one or both parents, improper incubation temperatures, and an imbalance of bacterial flora on the eggs. Some bacteria (e.g., *Alteromonas* sp.) associated with the eggs of shrimp, *Palaemon* sp., produce potent antifungal chemicals (e.g., 2,3-indolinedione or isatin). Shrimp eggs that are experimentally deprived of bacteria are infected and destroyed by watermolds (Gil-Turnes et al., 1989; Noga, 1993a). The normal bacterial flora of wild amphibian eggs appears unstudied, making it difficult to document watermolds as a primary pathogen. When dead eggs of multiple taxa are found in the wild, then attention should be directed to toxicologic and water quality studies, as is necessary in the investigation of fish kills (Meyer & Barclay, 1990). Deficiencies or mutations of antifungal enzymes and disruption of the oviduct (e.g., by endocrine-modulating chemicals in the environment) which produces the membranes and capsules of amphibian eggs are unstudied factors in amphibian watermold infections.

Affected eggs have a roughened surface, and the capsule loses its typical transparency. The capsule may become so white and opaque as to obscure the yolk. Hyphae project from the surface and penetrate the capsule. With close examination or use of a hand lens, cottony tangles of filaments (hyphae) are usually evident. Histologically, hyphae are most abundant in the capsule. Hyphae are usually 2–40 μm in diameter, nonseptate, and irregularly branching (Figures 27.1, 27.2). Hyphae may invade and perforate the vitelline membrane to infect the yolk or embryo. However, recent descriptions suggest watermold infections of western toad, *Bufo boreas*, eggs and embryos by *Saprolegnia ferax* may begin within the vitelline space. At stage 13 (neural plate stage), hyphae were first clearly found on the embryos and in the vitelline space. "Within 24 h[ours], the fungus attached to the embryo and formed a stalk that branched outward toward the [vitelline] membrane. The stalk eventually erupted through the vitelline membrane and formed a branchwork of hyphae." (Kiesecker & Blaustein, 1995). In some eggs, only the capsule will be infected, possibly because the fertilization membrane of live eggs is a rather effective enzyme-rich barrier. Hyphae and zoospores may stain weakly or not at all in periodic acid-Schiff (PAS) and hematoxylin and eosin

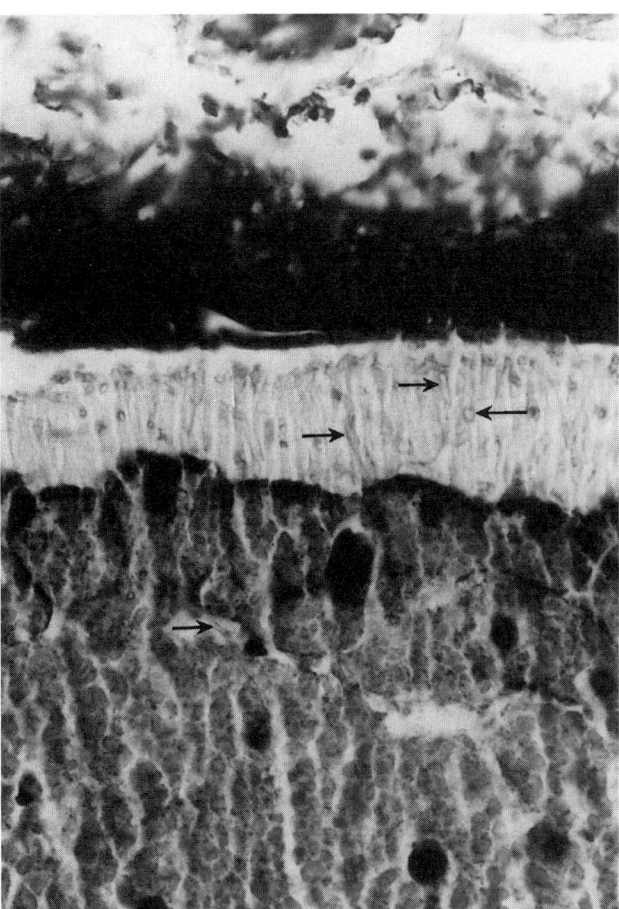

Figure 27.2. Saprolegniasis in eggs of the red-legged frog, *Rana aurora* (see Figure 27.1). Massive numbers of hyphae have invaded the vitelline space (central pale zone) and lesser numbers are present in the yolk material. Hyphae (arrows) of the watermolds may be 2–40 μm in diameter, show sparing septae, and infrequent branching. (D.E. Green)

stain. The capsule and fertilization membrane are strongly PAS-positive so other stains (e.g., Giemsa stain) are more helpful in demonstrating watermolds.

Fungal Infections of Terrestrial Eggs. An unidentified fungal infection was noted in terrestrial eggs deposited in caves by the Jamaican frog, *Eleutherodactylus cundalli* (Diesel et al., 1995).

27.1.4 Metamorphosis

Metamorphosis is a period when glucocorticoid and thyroxine levels rise, and dramatic morphological and physiological changes occur that result in the expression of new adult antigens, and, necessarily, dramatic shifts in lymphocyte populations so that new major histocompatibility complex antigens are recognized as self (tolerance) (Ruben et al., 1994). The changes in the immunologic system, evident grossly by loss of larval lymphomyeloid organs and appearance (in anurans) of new lymphoid organs, also appears to result in a temporary immunologic deficiency

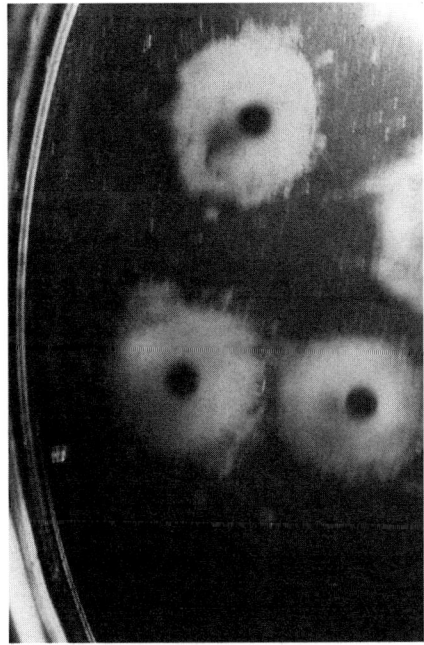

Figure 27.1. Saprolegniasis in eggs of the red-legged frog, *Rana aurora*. Note the whitish cottony growths in the capsules and projecting from the surface. Several genera of Oomycete watermolds may cause the disease, saprolegniasis, in aquatic organisms but watermolds are also common postmortem invaders. The precise identity of this watermold infection was not determined, but in regions of the Pacific Northwest in the USA the most common cause of anuran egg infections is *Saprolegnia ferax*. (D.E. Green)

(Marx et al., 1987; Ruben et al., 1992). The clinical importance of this immunological impairment to wild amphibian populations has been neglected.

Postmetamorphic Death Syndrome. Metamorphs may experience exceptionally high mortality rates, but rarely are the precise etiologies or pathogeneses determined. Many mortalities in metamorphs are attributed to red leg syndrome. "Postmetamorphic death syndrome" (PDS) occurs among ranids, and possibly bufonids, in the western United States (Scott, 1993). The syndrome has been noted especially in the Tarahumara leopard frog, *Rana tarahumarae,* and the Chiricahua leopard frog, *R. chiricahuensis,* in Arizona and New Mexico, and may be similar to die-offs involving anurans in the Colorado Rocky Mountains, and California Sierra Nevada. In the latter locations, populations of the western toad, *Bufo boreas,* the Yosemite toad, *B. canorus,* and the Wyoming toad, *B. hemiophrys baxteri,* have a lower postmetamorphic death rate than ranids, but mortalities as high as 80% have been noted. Six epidemiological features of postmetamorphic death syndrome have been noted: 1) mortality of most or all postmetamorphic individuals occurs in a short period, 2) a pattern of local synchrony occurs but does not involve all regions of a taxon's population, 3) a "ripple effect" may be detected in which mortalities progress in a gradually expanding perimeter through a watershed, 4) dead and moribund anurans are most often encountered during or immediately after winter or cold periods, 5) all species of a genus in the same locality are not afflicted equally, and 6) in the spring, breeding adults may first experience a high mortality, then tadpoles experience very high mortality during or shortly after metamorphosis. These epidemiological features, especially the lack of synchrony of die-offs in a region, the sparing of closely related taxons, and the "ripple effect," suggest that a novel pathogen, such as chytridiomycosis, may be present. Also it remains to be determined whether PDS is one syndrome, or consists of multiple disease entities.

27.2 DISEASES AND PATHOLOGY OF LARVAE, METAMORPHS, AND ADULTS

27.2.1 Musculoskeletal System

The notochord is prominent in larval stages of anurans and salamanders. The embryologic formation of the notochord in salamanders and the clawed frog, *Xenopus* spp., has been reviewed (Brun & Garson, 1984; Novoselov, 1995). The notochord of the tail and body undergoes marked degeneration and has essentially disappeared from the body at the completion of metamorphosis. Degeneration involves a fibrous transformation of notochord cells, formation of intracytoplasmic phagolysosomes, and nuclear pyknosis. Degenerate regions are infiltrated by macrophages which phagocytose debris. Ultrastructural and biochemical changes during the degenerative process have been studied (Fox, 1981). Portions of the notochord persist in metamorphosed amphibians as the intervertebral discs.

Abnormalities of the Notochord. The spontaneous abnormalities of the notochord that have been reported in tadpoles resulted from a trematode infection and a bizarre neoplastic-like proliferation in hybrid (experimental and natural) tadpoles that fail to undergo metamorphosis (Flindt et al., 1968; Schipp et al., 1968). Experimental diseases of the notochord have been observed in microgravity (space flight) and in lathyrism (intoxication by sweat peas) (Levy & Godman, 1955). The encysted immature trematode, *Cercaria elodes,* was found in the notochord of tadpoles of the northern leopard frog, *Rana pipiens* (Walton, 1964). Tadpoles of the African clawed frog, *Xenopus laevis,* were launched into space as tail-bud-stage embryos. After 12 days of microgravity these tadpoles developed lordosis (dorsal curling of the tail) and a deformed notochord. The notochord was mildly increased in diameter when compared to age-matched controls, and showed marked irregularities in shape in cross-sections. The notochord's dorsal and ventral midline notches, normally present for the spinal cord and aorta, were abnormal and markedly asymmetrical. Other differences were evident in the length of the tail, size of the body, head, and lungs, and underdevelopment of the thymus, branchial baskets, and gills. However, tadpoles that developed from eggs that were fertilized in microgravity did not develop dorsal curling (lordosis) of the tail which suggests that features of the launch (high acceleration and vibration) or an abrupt change in gravity may be a major factor in the observed musculoskeletal deformities (Snetkova et al., 1995).

Congenital Anomalies—Limb Deformities. In an apparently healthy population of the northern crested newt, *Triturus cristatus carnifex,* in Italy, a wide variety of deformities were detected (Zaffaroni et al., 1989). All defects occurred distal to the humeri and femurs. The percentage of affected animals was high: 35.5% of males and 20.5% of females. Missing digits constituted less than half of these defects and may have been due to trauma. Other defects included supernumerary phalanges and digits, fused carpal bones, atrophied and distorted phalanges, and a "bent" radius and ulna in one newt (which was insufficiently described to determine whether it was a varus or valgus deformity).

In a study of more than 13,000 wild specimens of the Japanese firebelly newt, *Cynops pyrrhogaster,* 2.26%

had limb abnormalities (Meyer-Rochow and Asashima, 1988). Supernumerary limbs, digits, or tails were found in 1.04% of newts, and missing limbs or digits were present in 1.22%. Three newts (0.02%) had exuberant webbing between digits.

Among one population of the terrestrial Western slimy salamander, *Plethodon albagula,* in Texas, 60% (6 of 10) had abnormalities of the limbs. Nearby populations in the same county and other counties lacked comparable abnormalities, except for missing digits that were attributed to trauma. As in the Italian population of the northern crested newt, *Triturus cristatus carnifex,* all anomalies occurred distal to the humeri and femurs. Illustrated anomalies consisted of syndactyly, a forked digit, and a duplication of the carpus with all digits (Lazell, 1995).

Numerous musculoskeletal deformities have been detected in both wild and captive larvae (Bantle et al., undated; Worrest & Kimeldorf, 1976; Zwart et al., 1991). Some defects have been attributed to elevated water temperature (Muto, 1969; Zwart et al., 1991), but investigators should be aware of the specific defects associated with acidic water, deionized water, and ultraviolet-B radiation, as well as limb anomalies associated with vitamin B deficiency. The Frog Embryo Teratogenesis Assay-*Xenopus* (FETAX) demonstrates that tadpoles may develop innumerable defects, which are not limited to the musculoskeletal system, in response to a wide variety of chemicals and mixed-pollutant environments (American Society for Testing and Materials, 1991; Bantle et al., undated).

Congenital Anomalies—Supernumerary Limbs. In anurans extra limbs may develop during the tadpole stage and are retained through metamorphosis (Ludicke, 1971). Recent detailed examinations of populations of amphibians with high prevalences of supernumerary limbs have demonstrated that the most likely etiology of this disorder is dermal penetration and encystment by metacercaria (Sessions & Ruth, 1990). Supernumerary limbs have been produced experimentally by various methods (Bryant & Iten, 1976; Sessions & Ruth, 1990). There is evidence that irradiation of egg or sperm of ranid frogs causes anomalous numbers of limbs, and this abnormality is passed to at least the second generation (Kawamura & Nishioka, 1978 as cited by Meyer-Rochow & Koebke, 1986). Scientific and popular press reports of supernumerary limbs in amphibians have been reviewed (Maden, 1982; Van Vallen, 1974).

Over 90% of the cases of supernumary limbs noted in North American anurans involve the hindlimbs while extra forelimbs are rare (Meyer-Rochow & Koebke, 1986). In European anurans, extra forelimbs are not uncommon (Flindt et al., 1968). In one population of the long-toed salamander, *Ambystoma macrodactylum,* in California, extra digits on the forelimbs were as common as on the hindlimbs (Sessions & Ruth, 1990). The extra appendages may be digits with or without metatarsals, a portion of a hindlimb, an entire hindlimb, as many as ten extra hindlimbs, and may involve duplication of the pelvis (Lopez & Maxson, 1990; Reynolds & Stephens, 1984; Sessions & Ruth, 1990). Duplication of the tail, however, has not been reported. Most affected individuals have a single extra hindlimb located posterior to the normal limb. It is uncommon for an extra whole limb to be positioned dorsally or ventrally to the normal limb.

Although only single affected adult individuals may be found (Van Vallen, 1974), the problem of supernumerary limbs often begins with larval amphibians in a natal pond. All larvae of the long-toed salamander, *Ambystoma macrodactylum,* with supernumerary limbs had trematode cysts in the skin and subcutis, however all sympatric tadpoles of the Pacific treefrog, *Pseudacris regilla,* had trematode cysts, including normal-appearing individuals. Hence, mere skin damage during penetration by the metacercariae is insufficient to cause supernumerary limbs; concurrent nerve damage may also be necessary. The encysted immature trematodes were identified as *Manodistomum syntomentera,* a digenic trematode, the final host of which is the garter snake, *Thamnophis* spp. Most encysted trematodes were found in the region of the vent, hindlimbs, and tail base of the amphibians (Sessions & Ruth, 1990).

The pathogenesis of supernumerary limbs was examined experimentally (Sessions & Ruth, 1990). Resin beads were implanted in the subcutis of tadpoles of the clawed frog, *Xenopus* spp., and larvae of the axolotl, *Ambystoma mexicanum.* These beads were approximately the same size as the metacercarial cysts found in wild tadpoles and larvae with naturally occurring supernumerary limbs. Nine (20%) of 44 experimental amphibians developed limb abnormalities including duplicate limbs and digits, at sites in "close physical association" with the resin beads. In natural cases of supernumerary limbs, dermal trematode cysts were found in close proximity to the base of the extra appendage.

One captive European common frog, *Rana temporaria,* had a well developed extra forelimb when captured, but over a period of 5 years the extra limb gradually atrophied and became so emaciated that it was expected to slough (Meyer-Rochow & Koebke, 1986).

Genetic Etiologies. Several recessive and dominant traits affecting the musculoskeletal system have been identified in laboratory colonies of the African clawed frog, *Xenopus laevis,* and the axolotl, *Ambystoma mexicanum* (Graveson & Armstrong, 1994; Gurdon & Woodland, 1975; Humphrey, 1967; Lipsett, 1941; Malacinski & Brothers, 1974; Uelhinger, 1966; Washabaugh et al., 1993).

Nutritional Etiologies—Forelimb Anomalies in Tadpoles. A high percentage of forelimb defects were induced in tadpoles of the African clawed frog, *Xenopus laevis*, by feeding only yeast, by placing tadpoles in deionized water, or both (Pollack & Leibig, 1989). Additionally, larvae fed yeast had defects in the number and arrangement of motor neurons in the lateral spinal column. All tadpoles raised in deionized water and fed yeast only developed limb defects. Hindlimbs were much less affected than forelimbs. Return of tadpoles to normal water and feed failed to promote healing or generation of normal limbs. Dendrobatid tadpoles raised in water enriched with vitamin B-complex often do not develop spindly legs (see Section 18.1, Spindly Leg). The occurrence of limb defects among tadpoles raised in deionized water suggests deficiency of calcium, and other essential trace minerals (e.g., magnesium) may also contribute to the anomalies.

Nutritional Etiologies—Spindly Leg. Spindly leg is a syndrome of multiple etiologies including nutritional deficiencies. A more accurate term for this condition is skeletal and muscular underdevelopment (SMUD) (Hakvoort et al., 1995; Reichenbach-Klinke, 1983; Zwart et al., 1991), but it is unlikely this will supplant the use of lay terms such as "spindly leg" (English), "match(-stick) legs" (from "Steichholzbeinchen," German), and "luciferpootjes" (Dutch). Spindly leg syndrome has been reported in dendrobatids, the oriental firebelly toad, *Bombina orientalis*, the orange-legged leaf frog, *Phyllomedusa hypocondrialis*, and the painted frog, *Discoglossus pictus*, and a variety of other anurans. Abnormal development of the forelimbs, and to a lesser extent, the hindlimbs, is variably expressed. Mild spindly leg syndrome may present with weakness or thinness of otherwise normal-appearing forelimbs, to complete absence of the forelimbs with deformities of the hindlimbs. Forelimb deformities are often asymmetrical and include atrophy of muscles (a subtle to pronounced thinness of the forelimbs), poor joint development, absence of bones distal to the humeri, and maldevelopment of the humeral and carpal-metacarpal joints (Hakvoort et al., 1995).

Histologically, myocytes show a significant variation in their diameters and may be greatly reduced in numbers. The forelimb joints demonstrate great variation in development as some may be normal and others may consist only of a mass of cartilage without a synovial cavity. Intergradations of joint development were evident as a distorted synovial cavity with interrupted bridges of cartilage. Although seemingly normal in cortical thickness, the humeri had reduced diameters. Integument, blood vessels, inflammatory cells, and amounts of lipocytes and fibrous tissue appear normal (Hakvoort et al., 1995; Reichenbach-Klinke, 1983). The etiology is unknown. Theories on the etiology of spindly leg syndrome include B vitamin deficiency, calcium deficiency, abnormal water temperature, water acidity, and combinations of several factors (Hakvoort et al., 1995) (see also Sections 7.9, Spindly Leg, and 18.1, Spindly Leg). Spindly leg appears similar to the abnormalities induced experimentally in tadpoles of the clawed frog, *Xenopus* spp., that are maintained in deionized water or fed only vitamin B-deficient yeast (Pollack & Liebig, 1989).

Nutritional Etiologies—Malnutrition and Elevated Temperatures. Various reports suggest that nutritional deficiencies and elevated water temperatures affect the development of the limbs of the axolotl, *Ambystoma mexicanum* (Brunst, 1955; Muto, 1969; Schmalhausen, 1925). Many reports are anecdotal and others fail to report the specific missing nutrients. Additional factors such as water pH, calcium concentration, aluminum concentration, and other trace elements that are known to affect myoskeletal development are seldom reported. Further research is needed to verify the effects of single factors in developmental anomalies of amphibians.

Nutritional Etiologies—Starvation. Long-term starvation in the clawed frog, *Xenopus* spp., has two distinct phases that are characterized as phase I, lasting for the first 4–6 months, and phase II, commencing when the fat body has completely atrophied (Merkle, 1990). Phase I has little impact on the musculoskeletal system as the energy reserves of the fat body and gonads are catabolyzed, but during phase II catabolism of tissue proteins accelerates. Onset of protein catabolism marks the end of lipid and carbohydrate reserves and the onset of marked skeletal muscle atrophy. In starved specimens of the edible frog, *Rana esculenta*, their skeletal muscle loss was 45% (Grably & Piery, 1981).

Nutritional Etiologies—Para-articular Xanthomatosis. Accumulation of lipid-laden foamy macrophages (xanthoma cells) in soft tissues adjacent to limb joints is one of several abnormalities associated with corneal lipidosis of captive female anurans. Xanthomas also involve the nerves of the limbs and often there is atherosclerosis of major arteries, but involvement of the articular surfaces and synovial membranes has not been reported. Grossly, the lesion consists of discrete pale plaques overlying the joints of the stifle and hock. The plaques remain superficially attached to the joint capsule following removal of the skin. The plaques consist of large lipid-laden foamy macrophages, with variable amounts of fibroplasia, lymphocytes, occasional multinucleated giant cells, and other inflammatory cells (Carpenter et al., 1986).

Nutritional Etiologies—Metabolic Bone Disease, Rickets, and Osteoporosis. Calcium and vitamin D deficiency may be encountered in aquatic and terrestrial postmetamorphic amphibians. Hypervitaminosis A also may induce osteoporosis-like disease (Bruce & Parkes, 1950). Calcium deficiency is difficult to detect in larval amphibians because the skeletal system consists principally of unmineralized cartilage and the notochord. During metamorphosis, calcium reserves in the endolymphatic sacs are mobilized for calcification of bones. When larvae of the African clawed frog, *Xenopus laevis*, are fed low calcium or high phosporus diets, such as horse liver or skeletal muscle, they develop into frogs with protrusion of the mandible, humpbacks, and paresis of the hindlimbs. Close inspection may also reveal bending and other deformities of the long bones and pelvis in both young and adult frogs. Radiographs may show obvious inadequate calcification of the vertebrae and major limb bones, absence of calcification of the phalanges and multiple greenstick or complete fractures of the femurs and tibiofibulae (Bruce & Parkes, 1950).

Toxicological Etiologies—Hypervitaminosis A. Overdosing with vitamin A may occur in captive amphibians. Horse liver contains 3–10 times as much vitamin A as rabbit and bovine liver, and was the source of excess vitamin A in one colony of the African clawed frog, *Xenopus laevis*. Hypervitaminosis A resembles osteoporosis since the cortices of long bones become thin, multiple fractures may occur, and the mandible may project beyond the maxilla. Histologic examinations of affected frogs were not attempted (Bruce & Parkes, 1950).

Toxicological Etiologies—X-Radiation-Induced Limb Atrophy. Experimental X-irradiation of the limbs of the adult red-spotted newt, *Notophthalmus viridescens*, resulted in atrophy, degeneration and sloughing of the limb at doses of 700–2000 rads. Doses of 1500–2000 rads caused limb sloughing in all newts. No obvious gross changes occur in irradiated forelimbs for 3–4 weeks and 4–6 weeks for hindlimbs. The first sign of radiation injury is multifocal hemorrhage and swelling near a joint. Tissue degeneration and necrosis then occur distal to the hemorrhages and include the swollen region(s). Sloughing of digits occurs, and progresses proximally to include all irradiated regions. Even if the entire limb was irradiated, a short stump usually remains. The stump heals with a fibrous scar, and no further degeneration or regeneration occurs in newts observed for over one year postirradiation. Similarly, X-irradiation of limb stumps following amputation inhibits limb regeneration (Rose & Rose, 1965).

Toxicological Etiologies—Fertilizer (Nitrate) Toxicity. Acute and chronic toxicity caused by ammonium nitrate (an agricultural fertilizer) in numerous species of North American amphibians has been documented (Hecnar, 1995; Huey & Beitinger, 1980). Chronic exposure to nitrate at 5–10 mg/L produced nonspecific clinical disease and gross lesions in tadpoles of the American toad, *Bufo americanus*, the Western chorus frog, *Pseudacris triseriata*, and the northern leopard frog, *Rana pipiens*. Gross lesions include bent tails (which caused affected tadpoles to swim in circles), loss of pigmentation, hydrocoelom, and reduced body weight at completion of metamorphosis (Hecnar, 1995). Reduced feeding and weight loss have been reported in tadpoles of the common European toad, *Bufo bufo*, and White's treefrog, *Pelodryas caerulea* exposed to 40 and 100 mg/L of sodium nitrate (Baker & Waights, 1993, 1994). Tadpoles of the green frog, *Rana clamitans melanota*, were not affected by chronic exposure to 10 mg/L nitrate (Hecnar, 1995). As in birds and mammals, ingested nitrate is reduced to nitrite, which is absorbed into the blood. Nitrite complexes with hemoglobin and forms methemoglobin. Blood containing methemoglobin has a very reduced capacity to carry oxygen. Formation of methemoglobin in tadpoles of the bullfrog, *Rana catesbeiana*, exposed to nitrate has been demonstrated (Huey & Beitinger, 1980). The histological changes associated with nitrate poisoning in larval amphibians have not been reported.

Traumatic Etiologies—Limb Regeneration. Regeneration of amputated tadpole and salamander limbs has been studied for centuries (Bryant et al., 1981; Iten & Bryant, 1973; Morgan, 1906; Smith, 1978; Spallanzani, 1768; Stocum, 1991; Tassava et al., 1993; Tsonis, 1991; Van Stone, 1964). The three basic stages of regeneration—wound healing, blastema formation and growth, and differentiation—have been well described (Bodemer, 1960; Goss & Holt, 1992; Maden & Holder, 1984; Stocum & Dearlove, 1972). Early larval stages of anurans have limb regenerative capabilities, but the capacity for regeneration of segments of the limbs is lost in a progressive proximal-to-distal sequence (Fry, 1966). Tadpoles gradually lose their regenerative ability as they approach metamorphosis (Pollack & Maheras-Rarick, 1990). Adult anurans have abbreviated limb regenerative capabilities, and may only be able to regenerate cartilage spikes. Successful complete regeneration of limbs and tails occurs primarily in young tadpoles, and larval and adult salamanders.

Regenerative capabilities of salamanders are not limited to limb and tail appendages, but include spinal cord, cardiac tissue, lens, retina, mandible, and intestine (Stocum, 1991).

In experimental amputations on salamanders, it has been noted that certain chemicals may have dramatic effects on the morphology of the regenerated limb. (Maden, 1993; Mohanty-Hejmadi et al., 1992; Scadding, 1990; Scadding & Maden, 1994; Zavanella et al., 1984).

Traumatic Etiologies—Fractures. Fracture repair in the European common frog, *Rana temporaria,* the viviparous lizard, *Lacerta vivipara,* and the laboratory rat were compared histologically (Pritchard & Ruzicka, 1950). There are significant differences in rate and method of anuran fracture repair compared to the reptile and mammal. Formation of the callus begins with fibroblastic proliferation (blastema formation) encircling the hemorrhagic region (hematoma). In the European common frog, *R. temporaria,* the blastema cells originate mostly from the periosteum and medulla. As the blastema invades and replaces the hematoma it transforms almost exclusively into cartilage. Endochondral ossification of the cartilagenous callus, if it occurs, is extremely slow in the frog. By 70 days postfracture (when the study was terminated), the majority of the callus was still cartilage but union of the fracture ends by cartilage was evident (Figure 27.3). The cartilagenous callus erodes very slowly in the frog, and occurs chiefly from "within" by enlargement of vascular channels. Replacement of cartilage by bone and calcification of cartilage in the frog is extremely slow, with only very thin rims of calcification evident around blood vessels within the erosion cavities. It was concluded that cartilage was transformed into bone rather than replaced by typical mammalian-type endochondral bone but observations were not made beyond 70 days postfracture to verify how cartilage was finally replaced by bone. The rate of fracture repair in the frog was markedly influenced by environmental temperature. Rate of fracture repair at 26°C (79°F) was approximately twice that at 18°C (64°F), but it should be noted that frogs died at temperatures over 28°C (82°F).

Infectious Etiologies—Fungal Infections. An *Ichthyophonus*-like myositis has been detected in adults of the red-spotted newt, *Notophthalmus viridescens,* from West Virginia (Herman, 1984) and Vermont (Green et al., 1995b). Clinical and subclinical infections occur. Affected newts are lethargic, and may tend to float just below the water's surface. Mild to moderate asymmetrical, plaquelike swellings occur dorsolaterally on the caudal half of the body, over the rump, and on the proximal half of the tail. The proximal hindlimbs may also be swollen. The overlying skin is usually intact and normal in color, but appears subtly roughened. The underlying skeletal muscles are grayish or black. No lesions of internal organs are present.

Unstained, crushed, wet mounts of the affected skeletal muscles show numerous cylindral, cigar-shaped, thin-walled fungal elements which are light brown and average 75×175 μm (Figures 27.4, 27.5, 27.6, 27.7). Acute, chronic, and resolving stages of infection may be found in histologic preparations. Acute infections are characterized by intramyocytic fungal elements which greatly distend the cross-sectional diameter of the host cell, and markedly compress sarcoplasm and nuclei peripherally or eccentrically. Fungal elements have a thin wall, inapparent nuclei, and homogenously flocculated cytoplasm which is palely eosinophilic or basophilic. No internal structures, such as septae, daughter sphaerules, spores, hyphae, or germinations are observed. Initially, inflammatory cell reaction tends to be minimal or absent. Fungal elements are intensely periodic

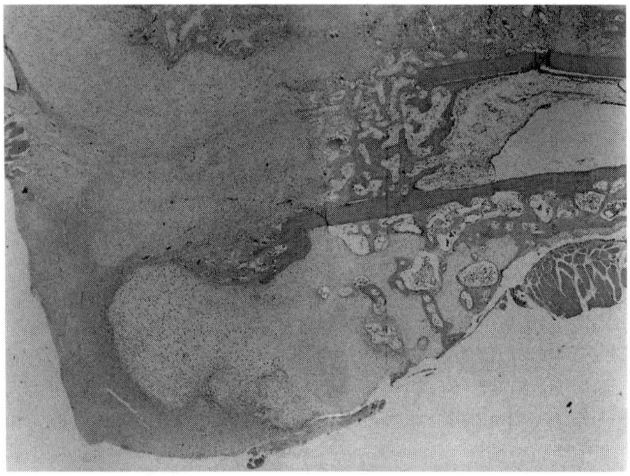

Figure 27.3. Callus of fractured femur in a northern leopard frog, *Rana pipiens.* Note the prominence of cartilage around the end of the fractured femoral shaft and from the periosteum. The apparently exuberant cartilage formation is normal in amphibians, although it has been mistaken for neoplasia. (A. Klembau, RTLA 2191)

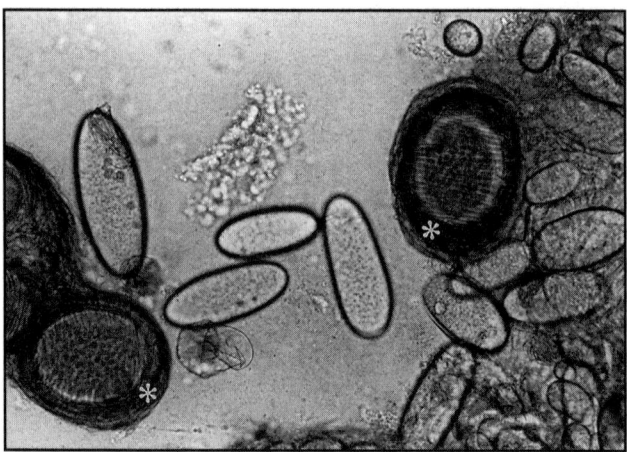

Figure 27.4. *Ichthyophonus*-like myositis in a red-spotted newt, *Notophthalmus viridescens viridescens.* This wet mount, unstained, crush smear of proximal tail muscle shows the typical elongate, thin-walled, fungal element. The thick dark walls (asterisks) around ovoid organisms are actually flattened concentric layers of epithelioid macrophages (see Figure 27.6.). Note the absence of budding, septae, and daughter spherules within the organisms. (D.E. Green)

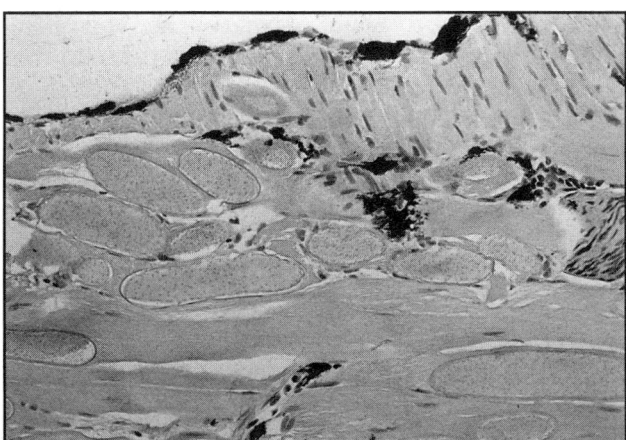

Figure 27.5. *Ichthyophonus*-like myositis in a red-spotted newt, *Notophthalmus viridescens viridescens*. In acute stages of infection, the fungal organisms are elongate, intramyocytic, and evoke little or no inflammatory reaction from the host. The organism may appear spherical in cross-section (see Figure 27.7.). (D.E. Green)

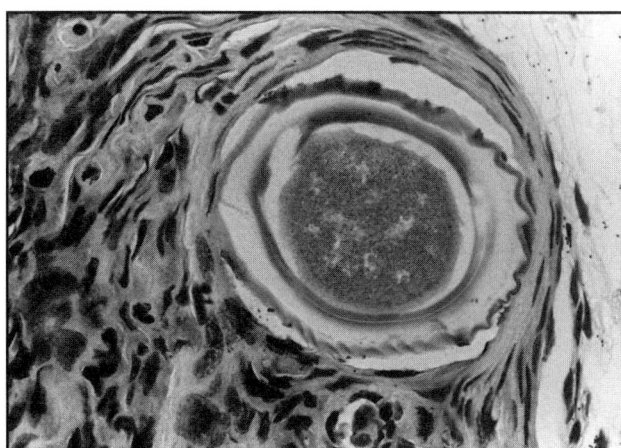

Figure 27.7. *Ichthyophonus*-like myositis in a red-spotted newt, *Notophthalmus viridescens viridescens*. A single organism in cross-section showing artifactual shrinkage and a clear space separating the fungal wall from the flattened epithelioid macrophages. (D.E. Green)

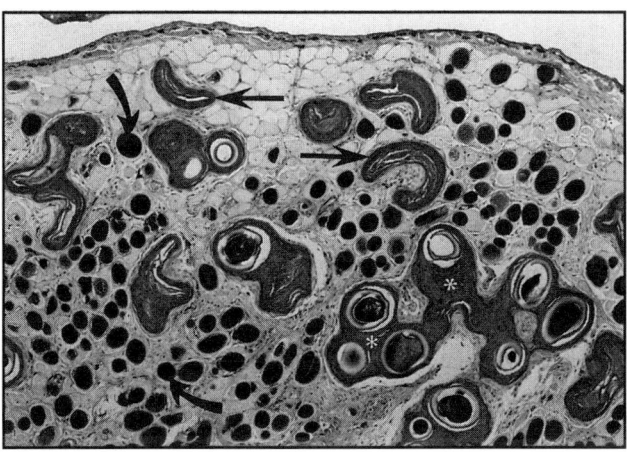

Figure 27.6. *Ichthyophonus*-like myositis in a red-spotted newt, *Notophthalmus viridescens viridescens*. Recent infections (curved arrows) lack inflammatory cells around the organisms. Chronic infections develop granulomatous inflammation composed mostly of flattened epithelioid macrophages (asterisks). Some fungal elements may collapse into C, V, or S shapes (straight arrows). (D.E. Green)

acid-Schiff-positive and stain well with silver stains. Chronic infections, sometimes in the same muscle mass as acutely infected myocytes, present with intense foci of granulomatous inflammation which may coalesce. Large numbers of flattened epithelioid macrophages surround fungal elements. Lesser numbers of lymphocytes, neutrophils and eosinophils are present. Fungal elements usually appear shrunken, leaving clear spaces or haloes separating them from the epithelioid macrophages. Again, no internal structures are evident, although the fungi lose their elongated structure and become ovoid. In histologic sections, the fungi are 36–149 μm in diameter (mean diameter: 97 μm) and 135–351 μm in length (mean length: 232 μm). Healing infections are characterized by collapsed granulomas which have C, V, or S shapes in cross-sections, and lack central fungal debris. Muscular infections are most intense in the proximal tail, rump, and distal half of the body, with decreasing numbers of fungal elements in muscles of the limbs, proximal half of the body, neck, and head. No fungi were detected in any other organs or tissues.

In the early 1950s a similar muscular infection was decribed in five recent metamorphs of the bullfrog, *Rana catesbeiana*, from Massachusettes. Each metamorph had a conspicuously swollen "rump" and was listless. The swellings were purplish red, 16–26 mm across, and in some animals extended to the muscles of the proximal hindlimbs (Goodchild, 1953). The etiological agent was named *Histocystidium ranae*, but it is likely it was *Ichthyophonus*.

Ichthyophonus sp., is a recognized pleomorphic organism with unsettled taxonomy (Lauckner, 1984; McVicar, 1982; Neish & Hughes, 1980; Rand, 1994). Clarification of the status of *Ichthyophonus* is not likely until multiple isolates are analyzed biochemically and DNA homologies are determined. *Ichthyophonus* spp. are considered fungi, while *Ichthyosporidium* is a microsporidian protozoa. *Ichthyophonus* fungal infections have been mistakenly identified as *Ichthyosporidium* (Elkan, 1976b; Reichenback-Klinke & Elkan, 1965; Thoen & Schliesser, 1984), however *Ichthyosporidium* is, at present, strictly an infection of fish (Canning & Lom, 1986).

Infectious Etiologies—Protozoal Diseases. Infection by *Sarcocystis* spp. has not been detected in amphibians (Frank, 1984; Munday et al., 1979).

A chronic wasting disease attributed to the microsporidian, *Pleistophora myotropica,* caused high mortality in a captive group of the common European toad, *Bufo bufo.* Grossly, distinct pale fusiform streaks were evident in all muscle groups including the tongue, but were most readily evident in pectoral and abdominal muscles. The streaks of pallor are infected myocytes. Ligaments, tendons, heart, and smooth muscles were not affected. Histologically, myriad small (3–4.5 μm) ovoid intramyocytic organisms with refractile walls occurred within rhabdomyocytes (Canning et al., 1964). Infected myocytes may have only frayed fragments of myofibrils among the scores or hundreds of spores. Macrophages and lymphocytes infiltrate the muscles, but exceptionally few granulocytes are found. Macrophages may contain phagocytosed spores. In chronic infections, myocytic regeneration is evidenced by rows of myocytic nuclei, but regeneration may not keep pace with myocytic destruction (Canning et al., 1964; Canning & Lom, 1986). *Pleistophora* spp. stain Gram-positive (see Section 15.8, Microsporidia), and mature spores are acid-fast-positive and have a periodic acid-Schiff-positive polar granule (Gardiner et al., 1988).

It has been suggested that *Pleistophora myotropica* and *P. danilewski* are the same organism (Canning & Lom, 1986). Precedence exists for the name *P. danilewski* which was reported previously in the skeletal muscles of frogs, lizards, turtles, and snakes in Europe. Natural infection was described in the Western chorus frog, *Pseudacris triseriata,* from Ontario, Canada, and was successfully transmitted to the common European toad, *Bufo bufo,* and the American toad, *B. americanus* (Canning & Lom, 1986).

Infectious Etiologies—Helminth-associated Diseases. Considerable literature exists on the helminthic fauna of amphibians, but seldom are gross and histological lesions reported. Over 20 genera of trematodes were tabulated which might be found in the skeletal muscles of amphibian larvae and adults (Flynn, 1973). All muscular trematodes are encysted immature stages and many may be found in extramuscular tissues as well. The inflammatory reaction to encysted trematodes is similar regardless of the host or parasite. All such "cysts" should more properly be considered verminous granulomata. Grossly the granulomata appear spherical, 0.5–2 mm in diameter, and may be whitish or black. Histologically, each trematode is surrounded by a thin (one to several cells) layer of epithelioid macrophages, which, depending on the duration of the granuloma, usually has a thin outermost rim of collagen and fibrocytes. Melanin may be present in the wall of the granuloma, reflecting the grossly observed black color. There is disagreement on whether the immature trematode produces its own "wall" or membrane. Some encysted metacercaria may produce a thin membrane that is about one micron thick, and clear or eosinophilic. Other metacercarial cysts may lack a distinct thin membrane, but may produce abundant homogenous periodic acid-Schiff-positive material that is more appropriately considered a gelatinous capsule which nearly fills the cyst and surrounds the metacercaria. Many "cysts" may appear empty, but occasional fortuitous sections will reveal fragments of the trematode. Some granulomas may collapse, apparently following death of the trematode, to become smaller, denser clusters of cells composed mostly of fibrocytes and epithelioid macrophages. Larvae of the nematode *Spiroxys* spp. also have been reported in the skeletal muscles of the red-spotted newt, *Notophthalmus viridescens,* but no gross or histological descriptions of the infection were provided (Muzzall, 1991).

Idiopathic Etiologies—Articular Gout. A case of periarticular gout in a captive pixie frog, *Pixicephalus delalandii,* was characterized as a painful swelling of one forelimb digit. The digit was amputated and fresh impression smears made from the incised digit showed birefringent microcrystals. The digit was appropriately fixed in absolute alcohol and histologically demonstrated a chronic granulomatous inflammation of periarticular regions with uratelike, birefringent microcrystals. The disease appeared to have involved only one digit, and the postsurgical survival time was over 2.5 years (Frye, 1989b), so correlation of this condition with renal disease was not established. Pedunculated digital nodules caused by uric acid gout have been observed "in other anuran species" (Stetter, 1995).

Idiopathic Etiologies—Wasting Syndromes in Wild Anurans. The giant toad, *Bufo marinus,* has been introduced to many tropical and subtropical regions of the world from its original habitat in Central America and northern South America (Easteal, 1981).

Introductions of the giant toad, *B. marinus,* are usually characterized by an initial population explosion (1000+ toads/hectare) followed by a period of relative stability for 10–40 years. Afterward, there is a gradual population decline to a low density (10–80 toads/hectare). Established low density populations of the giant toad, *B. marinus,* contain significant numbers of emaciated specimens (Freeland et al., 1986; Green et al., 1995a; Zug & Zug, 1979) (Figure 27.8). Histological examinations of more than 25 wasted specimens of the giant toad, *Bufo marinus,* from Hawaii failed to detect significant infectious diseases which could have induced cachexia (Green et al., 1995a).

In a 15-year study of wild populations of the Puerto

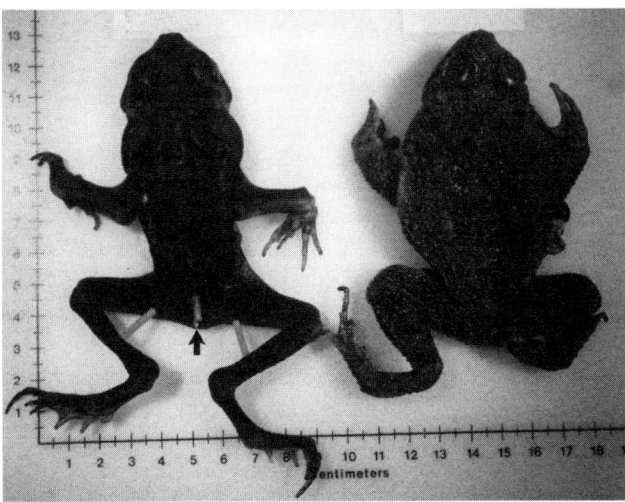

Figure 27.8. Wasting syndrome (simple starvation) in wild specimens of the giant toad, *Bufo marinus*. These toads, from Kauai Island, Hawaii, became emaciated during the winter. Note the gaunt appearance of the abdomen and thinness of the limbs. The toad on the left was so emaciated that the urostyle perforated the overlying skin. (Formalin-fixed carcasses.) (D.E. Green)

Rican coqui, *Eleutherodactylus coqui*, dead emaciated frogs with empty stomachs were found during droughts of 10–30 days' duration (Stewart, 1995). Combined desiccation and hyperthermia associated with El Niño (Southern Oscillation) were considered principal factors in the disappearance of the Alajuela golden toad, *Bufo periglenes*, and sympatric populations of the Veragoa stubfoot toad, *Atelopus varius* (Pounds & Crump, 1994). None of the involved amphibians were submitted for diagnostic evaluation.

27.2.2 Integumentary System

The microanatomy and physiology of the amphibian skin have been well studied in all three Orders (Heatwole & Barthalmus, 1994; Fox, 1994), yet many basic physiologic processes are poorly understood, such as carbon dioxide exchange and transport of water.

The skin increases in complexity throughout larval life and its reorganization climaxes during metamorphosis. Two key distinctions between larval and adult skin are the presence of many dermal glands in adults, and the formation of a superficial cornified (keratin) layer in the epidermis, features that first appear during metamorphosis.

The epidermis of amphibians is thin. Plethodontids have the thinnest epidermis (12–18 μm), ranids have variable skin depths but usually around 40 μm, while other anurans (e.g., firebelly toads, *Bombina* spp., and true toads, *Bufo* spp.) have skin thicknesses greater than 55 μm (Czopeck, 1965). The epidermis is thicker during hibernation and estivation and thinner during breeding seasons.

The epidermis of terrestrial amphibians consists of three or four strata. The single layer of cuboidal to columnar cells attached to the basement membrane is called the *stratum germinativum* or *stratum basale*. The *stratum spinosum* is 1–3 cells thick and lies adjacent to the *stratum basale*. Cells of the *stratum granulosum* lie subjacent to the cornified surface and have cytoplasmic granules akin to mammalian keratohyaline granules. Some authors lump the *stratum spinosum* and *stratum granulosum* into a single layer, the *stratum intermedium* (Elkan, 1976a). The superficial *stratum corneum* is 1–2 cells thick and is cornified; it is molted at regular intervals and is avidly consumed by most amphibians. The epidermis and dermis of larval and adult amphibians contain a variety of specialized cells (Fox, 1981; 1992; 1994; Fox & Whitear, 1990; Frost-Mason et al., 1994; Heatwole & Barthalmus, 1994; Nishikawa et al., 1992; Robinson & Heintzelman, 1987; Ruibal & Shoemaker, 1984; Warburg et al., 1994; Whitear, 1976).

The Eberth-Kastchenko layer is a striking, basophilic (in H&E-stained sections), calcium-rich layer between the *stratum spongiosum* and *stratum compactum* in many species (Elkan, 1968). To the novice histologist, this layer might be mistaken for dystrophic calcification of the dermis.

The ventral dermis of the caudal abdomen and adjacent proximal hindlimbs of many anurans is highly vascularized compared to other body regions. This region constitutes a skin organ specialized for uptake of water which has been popularly called the drinking patch or the pelvic patch. Most amphibians do not drink water but absorb it through the skin. The pelvic patch is approximately ten times more efficient at water absorption than other segments of skin (Czopeck 1965; Parsons, 1994).

Skin glands are generally very numerous in terrestrial amphibians. The secretions of skin glands enhance cutaneous respiration, slightly reduce or greatly inhibit evaporative water loss, have bacteriostatic (or antibacterial) and fungistatic components, may produce noxious or highly toxic defensive chemicals, and probably are involved in pheromone production, conspecific sexual recognition, and other functions. In addition to multicellular mucous and serous (granular) dermal glands throughout the skin, specialized defensive and secondary sexual glands are present in many amphibians. The parotid glands of bufonids secrete noxious and toxic chemicals. Some male microhylids possess dermal glands that secrete specialized adhesive or gluelike substances that cause them to adhere to the female during amplexus (Conaway & Metter, 1967). Sexually mature male salamanders may develop prominent mental (chin) glands, nuptial pads, genial (cheek) glands, or caudal glands (Houck & Sever, 1994).

Scores of bioactive chemicals have been identified in the skin of amphibians (Erspamer, 1994). The consequences of disrupted secretory functions on the pathogenesis of bacterial and fungal infections of amphibian skin have not been addressed but warrant investigation.

Genetic Etiologies—Pigment Mutations. Several mutations of pigment cells have been described in amphibians, and most occur in those taxa bred in captivity for experimental studies. Defects of pigmentation may affect only one type of chromatophore (e.g., melanophores), or all types of chromatophores (e.g., xanthophores and iridophores). Mutations of pigmentation have been reviewed (Bagnara, 1958; Bagnara et al., 1978; Bechtel, 1995; Browder, 1975; Droin, 1992; Epp, 1972; Frost et al., 1982, 1984; Humphrey, 1967, 1975; Smith-Gill et al., 1972; Tompkins, 1977; Underhill, 1967)

Although many taxa of amphibians may produce albino individuals, rarely is the trait documented as a specific homozygous recessive defect of melanin production (Bechtel, 1995). Albinism includes a spectrum of biochemical abnormalities with variable phenotypic expression from amelanosis (complete absence of melanin), to hypomelanosis (decrease in melanin), and other graded pigmentary dilutions (Droin, 1992; Frost et al., 1982, 1984; Hoperskaya, 1975; Humphrey, 1975; Smith-Gill et al., 1972; Tompkins, 1977).

Blue variants have been detected rarely among the green frog, *Rana clamitans,* the bullfrog, *R. catesbeiana,* and the northern leopard frog, *R. pipiens,* but have not been reported in the axolotl, *Ambystoma mexicanum,* and clawed frogs, *Xenopus* spp. The blue coloration is attributed to physical effects of light diffraction on abnormal iridophores and the absence of xanthophore pigments (pteridines). Ultrastructurally, the blue skin contains atrophied xanthophores with abnormal pterinosomes (Bagnara et al., 1978; Bechtel, 1995).

The Burnsi mutation is a dominant trait in the wild adult northern leopard frog, *Rana pipiens,* that was originally described as a new ranid species, *R. burnsi.* The phenotype is expressed as a reduction in the number of leg stripes and spots on the back and a great variation in the spotting pattern (Browder, 1975; Smith-Gill, 1974).

The Kandiyohi mutation is a dominant trait found in the wild northern leopard frog, *Rana pipiens,* that was described as a new species, *R. kandiyohi.* The phenotype is characterized in adults by increased black mottling of the interspot areas of the dorsal and lateral body. Up to 10% of a population of the northern leopard frog, *Rana pipiens,* show this trait in northeastern South Dakota. Tadpoles that are heterozygous for this mutation develop more quickly and successfully undergo metamorphosis more rapidly than wild-types (Browder, 1975).

The speckle mutation is attributed to an incompletely dominant gene that is variably expressed among wild specimens of the northern leopard frog, *Rana pipiens,* in the region of Lake Manitoba, Canada. Homozygous individuals are diffusely olive gray on the dorsal and lateral body skin, and have pink venters. Heterozygous frogs have normal dorsal skin patterns that are "broken up by numerous olive gray speckled markings" (Browder, 1975). Phenotypically, this trait is similar to the melanoid trait of northern leopard frogs, except that xanthophores are normal and only iridophores are greatly reduced in numbers (Browder, 1975).

Genetic Etiologies—Averusa. One Houston toad, *Bufo houstonensis,* that had been raised from wild eggs and successfully metamorphosed was observed to have abnormally smooth skin and lacked parotid glands and other epidermal [sic] glands. Out of 800 eggs that were raised at the facility, only two additional toadlets had smooth, hypoglandular skin. The additional two toadlets had parotid glands. The toad without parotid glands also had pinkish translucent ventral skin through which the visceral organs were visible. Histologic features of the disease were not reported. The disease in the glandless toad was called averusa, meaning lack of warts (Peterson & Mays, 1989).

Toxicological Etiologies—Acidity. Acid soils limit populations of terrestrial salamanders (Wyman, 1988; Wyman & Hawksley-Lescault, 1987). At soil pH lower than 4.0, disrupted sodium balance was suggested as the lethal mechanism in the redback salamander, *Plethodon cinereus,* and as the cause of reduced populations of the two-lined salamander, *Eurycea bislineata,* the mountain dusky salamander, *Desmognathus ochrophaeus,* and the American toad, *Bufo americanus.* On experimental soils with pH 3 and 4, growth, survival, and respiration were significantly depressed in redback salamanders. Juveniles and young-of-the-year were not observed on soils with a pH less than 3.7, suggesting reproductive failure or 100% mortality of eggs, embryos, or juveniles. Gross and histologic lesions were not studied (Wyman & Hawksley-Lescault, 1987).

Toxicological Etiologies—Experimental Toxic Depigmentation. In the African clawed frog, *Xenopus laevis,* various chemical toxicants have been associated with abnormal or reduced pigmentation in developing embryos and early larvae. Chemicals include the insecticide, malathion (and its more toxic metabolite, malaoxon), nabam, monosulphides and disulphides of tetraethylthiuram, and others. The mechanism of action of the latter chemicals is by chelation of copper, thus preventing its incorporation into the melanin-forming, copper-dependent enzyme, tyrosinase. The mechanism of action of the organophosphates in depigmentation is not understood (Snawder & Chambers, 1990).

Toxicological Etiologies—Gas Bubble Disease. Accidental and experimental exposure of the African clawed frog, *Xenopus laevis,* to gas-supersaturated water may result in the disease known among fish aquaculturists as gas bubble disease, and in human medicine as "the bends" (or air embolism). Gas bubble disease occurs when the total dissolved gas pressure is greater than barometric pressure (Colt et al., 1984). In 24–70 hours in supersaturated water, specimens of the African clawed frog, *X. laevis,* developed numerous minute air bubbles in the skin, most easily detected in the webbing between the toes. Mucus production by the body skin declines, epidermis sloughs, anorexia develops, and toads float at the surface. Dermal bubbles may coalesce such that the diameter of the hindlimbs doubles. Following appearance of gas bubbles in the skin, hyperemia begins at the digits and progressively ascends the limbs while petechiae and ecchymoses may develop on the limbs and abdomen. In severe cases with marked gaseous swelling of the dermis, gas bubbles may be found in the vessels of the stomach, mesonephroi, and heart. Inhibited or obstructed blood circulation in the dermis results in devitalized foci or segments that are prone to opportunistic infections by bacteria (e.g., *Aeromonas hydrophila*). This bacterium and others may be isolated from multiple internal organs of animals with gas bubble disease.

Toxicological Etiologies—Ultraviolet Radiation. Ultraviolet-B radiation (wavelengths ranging from 290–315 nm) is considered a major factor in the development of several forms of skin cancer in mammals and hybrids between the swordtail and platyfish (Setlow et al., 1989; Vander Leun & De Gruijl, 1993), but a direct relationship to skin cancer of amphibians has not been established experimentally (Zavanella & Losa, 1981). However, the northern crested newt, *Triturus cristatus carnifex,* developed epidermal hyperplasia, erosions, and ulcerations following experimental exposure to ultraviolet-B radiation. At repeated dosages of ultraviolet-B radiation (1570 J/m^2) epidermal hyperplasia was evident 6–14 days postexposure. About 75% of the irradiated newts developed slightly raised epidermal plaques or nodules. Epidermal cells showed increased intercellular space, occasional subtle whorled patterns, and mitotic figures in nonbasal cells. Inflammatory cell infiltrates were minimal to mild and consisted mostly of lymphocytes and neutrophils, with occasional eosinophils. About 15% of newts demonstrated mild fibroplasia of the upper dermis. No changes in dermal chromatophores or glands were reported.

Newts that received higher doses of ultraviolet-B radiation (4710 J/m^2) were examined 10–11 weeks after the last exposure, and about 35% of these animals developed epidermal erosions and ulcers from 3–12 mm in diameter. There was an increased rate of ecdysis within 1 week of initiating exposures. Histologically the epidermis is alternately atrophied and hyperplastic. Basal cells often are flattened, almost fibroblastic in appearance, and have pleomorphic nuclei. Ulcerated segments of skin lack epithelium. The basement membrane is irregularly thickened and occasionally disrupted. Dermal fibrosis may be prominent. Material resembling basophilic ground substance (Eberth-Kastchenko layer) became prominent in the dermis, especially on the head. Dermal elastosis was not noted. Dermal glands and chromatophores were greatly reduced in numbers or absent in many segments. Reduction in numbers of dermal melanophores persisted at least 5 months. Inflammatory cells in the ulcerated segments consisted mostly of neutrophils, while lymphocytes predominated in other segments (Zavanella & Losa, 1981).

Toxicological Etiologies—Lead. Although it has been reported that adult anurans are less sensitive to lead intoxication than their eggs and embryos, there is a lack of histological and ultrastructural studies of grossly observed lesions and the neuromuscular and integumentary systems (Power et al., 1989). The 96 h LC_{50} of lead nitrate solutions in the northern leopard frog, *Rana pipiens,* was 105 mg/L (Kaplan et al., 1967). Clinical signs and gross lesions in the leopard frogs were a permanent loss of semierect posture, sloughing of the epidermis, muscular twitching, increased salivation, lethargy, pale liver, and death. Amphibians may accumulate lead and pass it into the food chain (reviewed by Power et al., 1989).

Traumatic Etiologies—Rostral Abrasions. Despite the delicate nature of the amphibian integument, localized bacterial infections are rarely reported.

Several captive specimens of Darwin's frog, *Rhinoderma darwini,* in one collection developed a localized atrophic dermatitis of the dorsorostral-projecting skin fold. Both sexes were affected. Initial clinical signs were grayish discoloration of the snout, ulceration, or necrosis with complete atrophy of the dorsorostral fold. In some frogs, remnants of the fold were red and swollen. Internal lesions were absent, except in one frog which had severe pneumonia. Histologically, the skin fold showed disrupted and damaged epithelium, but often with partially intact overlying keratinized cells. Dermal glands contained cellular debris and the dermis was markedly edematous. Although inflammatory cell reaction was absent, masses of Gram-negative cocci and bacilli were present, usually associated with necrotic epidermal cells and adnexa. From one affected euthanized frog, *Aeromonas liquefaciens, Citrobacter freundii,* and *Acinetobacter* spp., were isolated. *Acinetobacter* was considered to be the Gram-negative cocci in the histological sections. Physical injury to the projecting rostral fold was considered a probable predisposing factor in this condition (Cooper et al., 1978).

One bullfrog, *Rana catesbeiana*, developed severe focal ulceration of the skin of the nose and upper lip that resulted in exposure of underlying bone. Necrotic debris with extensive infiltrates of macrophages, lymphocytes, and "heterophils" was evident in the ulcerated area on histological section. Bacteria were evident histologically in the cellular debris, and four bacteria were isolated, *Aeromonas hydrophila*, *Citrobacter freundii*, *Pseudomonas* spp., and a group D *Streptococcus*. Since this frog was euthanized, and *A. hydrophila* also was isolated from the heart blood, it is likely the extensive and chronic skin wound progressed to septicemia shortly before euthanasia (Li & Lipman, 1995).

Traumatic Etiologies—Atrophic Mandibular Stomatitis. In a colony of wild-caught specimens of the redback salamander, *Plethodon cinereus*, from southwestern Virginia, several developed severe ulceration of the chin which progressed to exposure of the mandibles. Dermal swelling and erythema were not detected clinically or at necropsy. In one salamander, the mandibular symphysis was lost and the exposed rami overlapped (Figure 27.9). Histologically, the integument overlying the mandible at the point of regression showed subtle disorganization of cell layers, mild necrosis of scattered epidermal cells, and mild infiltrates of neutrophils and macrophages into the epidermis and dermis. (see Figure 27.9) There was osteosis of the denuded mandibular rami, and in the unexposed segment of mandible the periosteum was elevated and degenerate. Numerous Gram-negative bacilli were evident on the exposed rami and were infiltrating viable tissue in the area between the periosteum and bone. A mixture of bacteria were isolated from the mandible of one affected euthanized salamander, including *Aeromonas caviae*, *Ochrobactrum (Achromobacter) anthropi*, and *Flavobacterium* spp. Clinically normal salamanders from the same colony had the following oral bacteria: *Flavobacterium indologenes*, *Pseudomonas fluorescens*, *Serratia liquefaciens*, *Xanthomonas maltophila*, and *Enterobacter* spp. It was presumed the condition was due to efforts to burrow into the plastic petri dish (Green & Wise, unpublished data).

Infectious Etiologies—Viral Infections. Ranaviruses and erythrocytic iridoviruses are the two groups of Iridoviridae commonly identified in amphibians. Erythrocytic iridoviruses are icosohedral and are exceptionally large (up to 450 nm in diameter) (Gruia-Gray et al., 1989a, b) compared to the ranaviruses which are usually 160–200 nm in diameter (Goorha & Granoff, 1994).

Tadpole edema virus (TEV, Ranavirus type III) is the first acutely fatal viral infection of wild tadpoles to be described (Wolf et al., 1968, 1969). Because affected tadpoles present with redleglike signs including ventral subcutaneous edema and hemorrhages of the caudal body and, especially, the proximal hindlimbs, discussion of this infection is included under integumentary diseases, even though there are no adequate histological descriptions of skin lesions. TEV is an acute, highly pathogenic, cytolytic virus infection of tadpoles of the bullfrog, *Rana catesbeiana*, bufonids (*Bufo americanus*, *Bufo woodhousei fowleri*), and a pelobatid (*Spea [Scaphiopus] intermontana*) (Wolf et al., 1968, 1969). Gross lesions were similar in all species and include marked edema, erythema and hemorrhages of the skin and subcutis of the body and proximal hindlimbs, hydrocoelom, and petechial hemorrhages in the stomach, intestines, skeletal muscles. No gross renal lesions were detected in the bullfrog tadpoles, but the *Bufo* spp. and *Spea* sp. showed pale mesonephros with miliary, spherical petechiae typical of glomerular hemorrhages (Clark et al., 1969; Wolf et al., 1968, 1969).

The glomeruli of the affected bufonid and pelobatid anurans show endothelial necrosis with extensive hemorrhages, and pyknotic nuclei in Bowman's capsule and among interstitial cells. Only mild multifocal

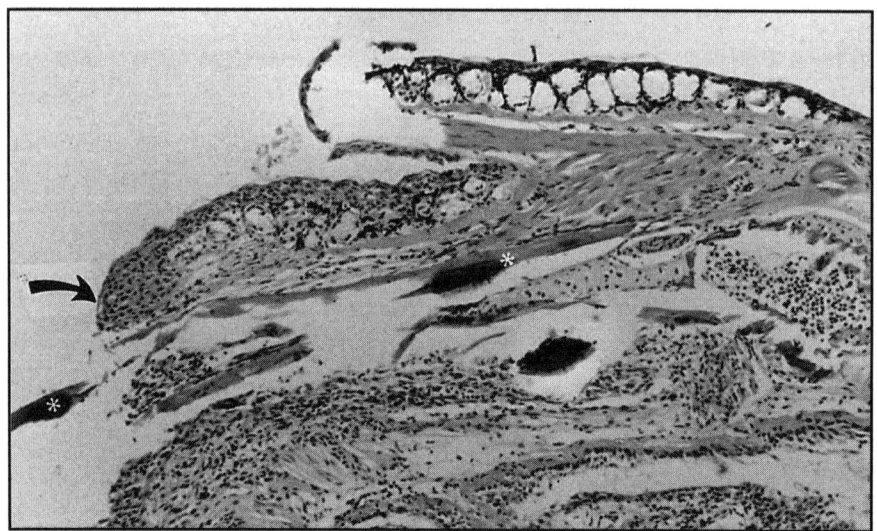

Figure 27.9. Atrophic mandibular stomatitis in a captive redback salamander, *Plethodon cinereus*. The skin (arrow) atrophies from the mandible exposing the rami (asterisks). The epidermis adjacent to the exposed bone shows subtle parakeratosis and infiltrates of acute inflammatory cells (arrow). Bacilli are present on the surface of the exposed necrotic bone, and on the epidermal and oral surfaces, and infiltrate the mandibular periosteum (see Figure 27.10). (D.E. Green)

tubular necrosis is evident (Figure 27.10). Reexamination of the histologic slides from the original studies of Wolf et al. (1968) revealed a mild hemoglobin nephrosis in some anurans. In addition, some tadpoles had intense amounts of black gritty material in the glomeruli and Bowman's spaces suggestive of free melanosomes. The source of this melanin debris was not investigated, but necrosis of one or two types of melanin-laden cells was considered probable: melanophores in the skin (and elsewhere in the body) or macrophages of melanomacrophage aggregates in the liver and other organs. In all species, the stomach had extensive hemorrhagic foci with vascular necrosis in the muscular and submucosal tunics, which supports observations by others (Clark et al., 1969) that the stomach often has the highest viral titers. Reexamination of the histologic slides by this author revealed blue intracytoplasmic inclusion bodies and massive necrosis of the glandular cells in the stomach (Figures 27.11, 27.12); the inclusion bodies suggest that not all of gastric hemorrhage and necrosis can be attributed to ischemia. Petechial hemorrhages also were detected in the lungs, fat bodies, urinary bladders, and skeletal muscles. Livers showed acute multifocal periportal necrosis as early as 48 h after virus exposure in bullfrog tadpoles (Figures 27.13, 27.14). Liver lesions advanced to a severe stage (lobar necrosis) by 8 days. Reexamination of the slides of the liver showed prominent basophilic intracytoplasmic inclusions in hepatocytes, similar to those recently described in a ranaviruslike infection in the European common frog, *Rana temporaria* (see below). Necrosis of macrophages (Kupffer cells and cells of the melanomacrophage aggregates) was marked and appeared to precede hepatocellular necrosis. In those amphibians with prominent numbers of pre-existing melanomacrophage aggregates, large numbers of free melanosomes are evident in the hepatic sinusoids and other vessels. Necrosis in the spleen and renal interstitial hematopoietic cells was present. Possible lesions in the skin and nervous tissues, which have been observed in other ranavirus infections, have not been characterized in TEV infections.

The gross lesions of TEV infection in four species of anurans are similar to lesions associated with Gram-negative bacillary septicemias (i.e., "red leg"). Viral lesions in the skin, intestines, and blood vessels may allow rapid secondary, opportunistic invasion by many Gram-negative bacilli thus obscuring the underlying viral etiology.

Frog virus-3 (FV3, Ranavirus type I) is the type-species of ranavirus in the family Iridoviridae. It was isolated from cells of a Lucke adenocarcinoma from an adult northern leopard frog, *Rana pipiens*, and for several years was assumed to be a herpesvirus (Granoff et al., 1965). Frog virus-3 and tadpole edema virus represent different strains of ranaviruses (Essani & Granoff, 1989; Granoff, 1989). Although FV3 is the best studied member of the iridovirus group (Goorha & Granoff, 1994; Granoff, 1989), little has been published on the lesions of this virus infection in amphibians. Experimentally, FV3 is rapidly fatal to embryos and tadpoles of the northern leopard frog, *R. pipiens*, and recent metamorphs of the Fowler's toad, *Bufo woodhousei fowleri* (Came et al., 1968; Tweedell & Granoff, 1968), and present a similar but milder histopathological profile than the lesions of TEV-infected toads. Histologically, lesions are "compatible with a generalized virus infection with multiple focal or confluent necrosis and hemorrhage in the tissues" of the toads (Granoff, 1989). In experimentally inoculated metamorphs of the Fowler's toad, *Bufo woodhousei fowleri*, there were ". . . hemorrhagic foci in the skeletal musculature on the ventral surface of the hind legs. Localized hemorrhagic foci were found in the stomach and

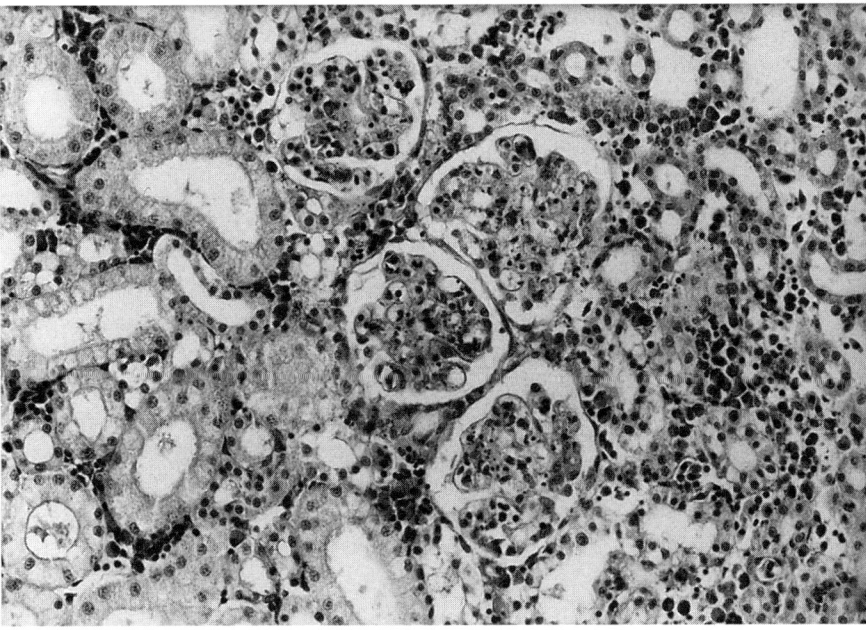

Figure 27.10. Glomerular and interstitial necrosis in experimental tadpole edema virus infection of a bullfrog tadpole, *Rana catesbeiana*. Note the mild dilation of Bowman's capsules, and the pyknotic and karyorrhectic nuclei among the glomerular and interstital cells. (K. Wolf and R.L. Herman, National Fish Health Research Laboratory, West Virginia)

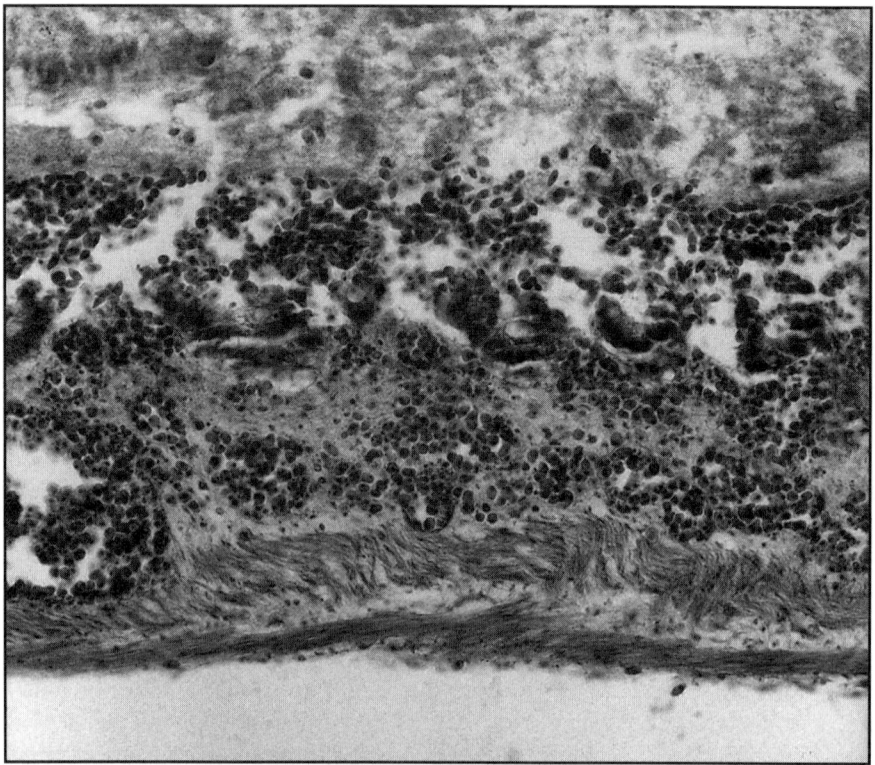

Figure 27.11. Necrohemorrhagic gastritis in experimental tadpole edema virus infection of a Great Basin spadefoot toad, *Spea intermontana*. Note the total necrosis of the gastric glands. (K. Wolf and R.L. Herman, National Fish Health Research Laboratory, West Virginia)

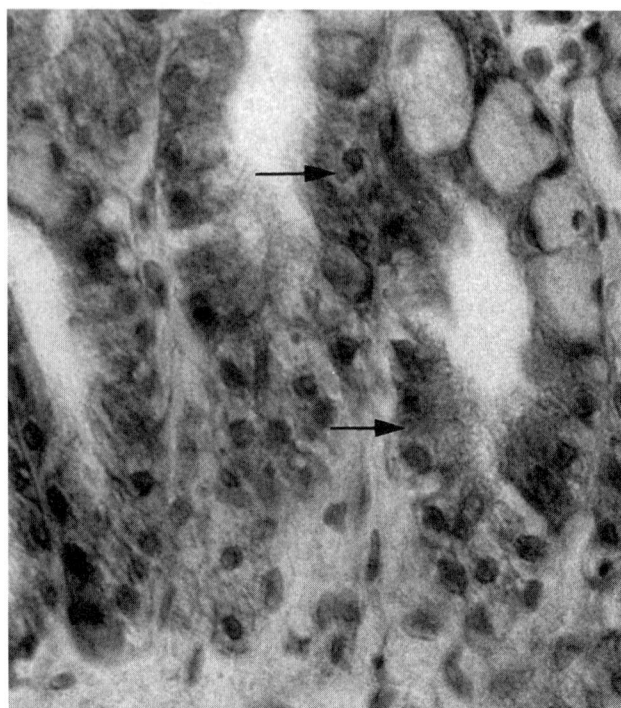

Figure 27.12. Inclusion body gastritis in experimental tadpole edema virus (TEV) infection of a Great Basin spadefoot toad, *Spea intermontana*. TEV, like other ranaviruses, produces basophilic intracytoplasmic inclusion bodies (arrows). (K. Wolf and R.L. Herman, National Fish Health Research Laboratory, West Virginia)

intestine, and massive edema was observed in many animals" (Came et al., 1968). Embryos of the northern leopard frog, *R. pipiens*, that died 3–12 days postinoculation showed depigmentation, epidermal sloughing, and lordosis. Embryos near hatching stage and tadpoles that died within 10 days showed ventral dermal hemorrhages, and abdominal edema, but 40–70% of the tadpoles survived the challenge (Tweedell & Granoff, 1968). In cell cultures, this virus, like most iridoviruses, produces basophilic intracytoplasmic inclusions; however, such inclusions have not been described histologically in FV3-infected amphibians, but are worthy of reexaminations and additional studies.

Bohle iridovirus (BIV) was isolated from metamorphs of the ornate burrowing frog, *Limnodynastes ornatus*, in Australia (Speare & Smith, 1992). Bohle iridovirus and FV3 were found to be closely related (Hengstberger et al., 1993). Experimentally, Bohle iridovirus is highly pathogenic to tadpoles and metamorphs of the ornate burrowing frog, *L. ornatus*, and to tadpoles, metamorphs and adults of the giant toad, *Bufo marinus*. Lesions produced by BIV were briefly summarized as multifocal necroses of the liver, mesonephroi, and lungs (Moody & Owens, 1994). Bohle iridovirus also causes mortality in tadpoles of the White's treefrog, *Pelodryas caerulea* (Moody & Owens, 1994), and tadpoles and recent metamorphs of the northern banjo frog, *Limnodynastes terraereginae*, and Australian variable treefrog, *Litoria latopalmata*. The relationship of BIV to a sudden and serious amphibian population decline involving at least 14 taxa of rainforest anurans in Queensland has been inferred from epidemiologic data (Anderson, 1995; Laurance et al., 1996; Speare et al., 1994a). Histologic lesions in the rainforest frogs were briefly reported

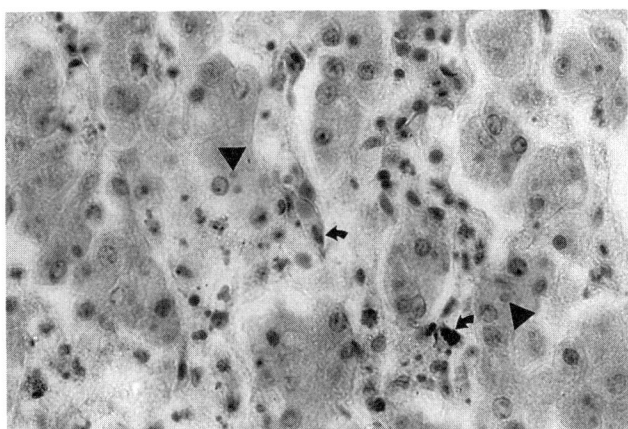

Figure 27.13. Necrosis of macrophages and inclusion body hepatitis in experimental tadpole edema virus infection of a young Fowler's toad, *Bufo woodhousei fowleri*. Macrophages in the melanomacrophage aggregates and sinusoids are necrotic (arrows), there is degeneration and necrosis of hepatocytes, and occasional hepatocytes have round blue intracytoplasmic inclusion bodies (arrowheads). (K. Wolf and R.L. Herman, National Fish Health Research Laboratory, West Virginia)

as foci of necrosis in the liver, mesonephros, spleen, and occasionally in intestinal mucosa and skin.

In experimental BIV infections of the northern banjo frog, *Limnodynastes terraereginae,* and the Australian variable treefrog, *Litoria latopalmata,* there is histological evidence of systemic infection. Necrosis is evident in the mesonephroi, livers, spleens, lungs, and stomachs. In the mesonephroi, the tubules show miliary necroses characterized by open-faced nuclei, karyolysis, and pyknosis; glomeruli show shrinkage of the tuft, nuclear pyknosis, and occasionally prominent amounts of black gritty material consistent with free melanosomes. Renal interstitial hematopoietic cells are also necrotic, and congestion and hemorrhage in the interstitial spaces may be present. The livers prominent melanomacrophage aggregates and a diffuse melanization (possibly due to many free melanosomes). Hepatocytes show apoptosis and foci of necrosis. The spleens show extensive lymphorrhexis with necrosis of hematopoietic cells. The lungs show lymphocytic ("nonsuppurative") pneumonitis with foci of necrosis and dystrophic calcification of the septae. In the brain and spinal cord, some neurons and gliocytes have open-faced or pyknotic nuclei. The stomachs have open-faced nuclei and pyknosis of the mucosal and glandular cells which may involve the underlying tunica muscularis. In many organs, erythrocytes have pyknotic nuclei. Immunohistochemistry demonstrates ranavirus antigen in the necrotic regions of the liver, lung, and renal tubules, glomeruli, and interstitial hematopoietic cells, but not in the brain or spinal cord. Skin lesions were not reported but the epidermis was not studied histologically. There has been no mention of inclusion bodies in Bohle virus-infected Australian frogs as has been reported in systemic iridovirus (ranavirus-like) infections of the European common frog, *Rana temporaria* (see below, Cunningham et al., 1996b), and experimental TEV infections of anurans.

An iridovirus-associated ulcerative dermatitis was reported in three anuran species in Queensland, Australia (Speare et al., 1994a). The three species, the sharp snout torrent frog, *Taudactylus acutirostris,* the torrent treefrog, *Litoria nannotis,* and Atherton Tableland treefrog, *L. rheocola,* were involved in a sudden severe population decline. Although minute skin ulcers and hemorrhages were noted, the clinical disease presented principally as a neurologic condition. *Aeromonas hydrophila* was isolated from 11 of 14 frogs which were submitted for bacterial cultures. Acute multifocal necroses were detected histologically in the livers, spleens, mesonephroi, intestinal mucosa, and skin. The tissue tropism and character of the histologic lesions was similar to that of tadpole edema ranavirus and Bohle iridovirus. Inflammatory cell response is generally minor. Central nervous system lesions

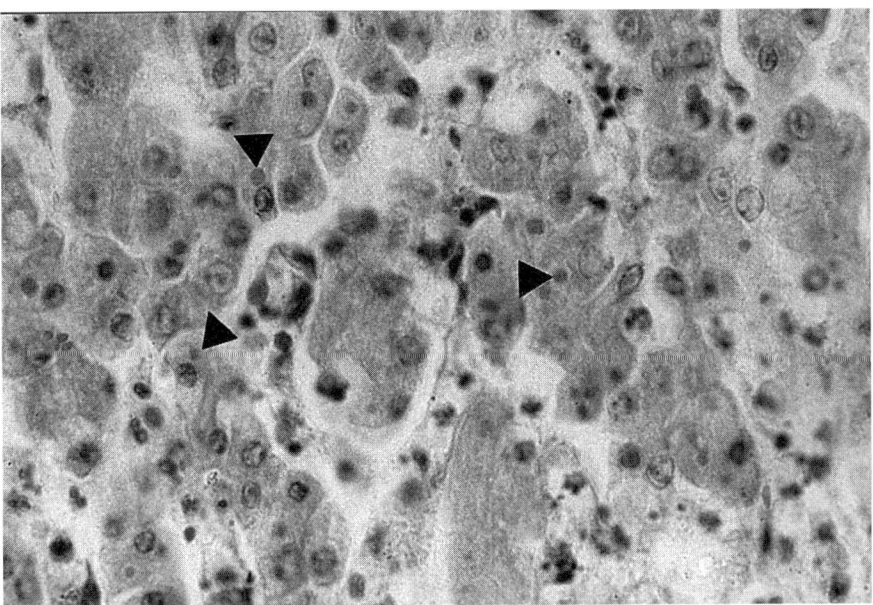

Figure 27.14. Same as Figure 27.13. Additional basophilic intracytoplasmic inclusion bodies (arrowheads) in hepatocytes. (K. Wolf and R.L. Herman, National Fish Health Research Laboratory, West Virginia)

were evident. Immunohistochemical stains utilizing a polyclonal antisera against epizootic haematopoietic necrosis iridovirus (EHNV is closely related to frog Bohle iridovirus [Moody & Owens, 1994]) demonstrated iridoviral antigen in the necrotic foci.

There are two reports of viral infections in the edible frog, *Rana kl. esculenta* from the former Yugoslavia (Fijan et al., 1991; Kunst & Valpotic, 1968). Both groups of researchers isolated viruses from clinically sick frogs, but the disease was experimentally reproduced by only one group (Kunst & Valpotic, 1968). Initial deaths and viral isolations were obtained from captive frogs in crowded conditions. Clinical signs were lethargy and tetany. The disease was called "viral hemorrhagic septicemia of frogs" (VHSF) as gross lesions included skin necrosis, edema and petechiation of the third eyelid, hemorrhagic gastroenteritis, hemorrhages in the hindlimb musculature, and skin hemorrhages at the sites of experimental scarification. Histological examinations were not attempted (Kunst & Valpotic, 1968). Subsequent studies of 16 frogs which died in captivity between 1970 and 1981 (Fijan et al., 1991) showed petechial hemorrhages of the skin, oral mucosa, tongue, limb muscles, liver, stomach, intestine, gonads, and coelomic cavity. Epidermal necrosis with inflamed edges and palbebra tertia blepharitis also were found in most frogs. The disease was reproduced in experimentally inoculated frogs (Kunst & Valpotic, 1968), but others were unable to induce clinical disease in specimens of the edible frog, *R. kl. esculenta*, that were inoculated with one of several isolates (Fijan et al., 1991). The latter authors considered the clinical and gross lesions in their frogs to be identical to VHSF (Kunst & Valpotic, 1968), but admitted that there was a "need for the inclusion of bacteriological studies in . . . further cases." The virus that was associated with VHSF has been lost (Fijan et al., 1991). Another isolate has been named *Rana esculenta* iridovirus (REIR) (Ahne et al., 1995). REIR has been shown to have common antigenic epitopes with Australian epizootic haematopoietic necrosis virus (EHNV) of fish, and a related catfish iridovirus from Italy (Ahne et al., 1995). Furthermore, Bohle iridovirus, Australian EHNV from fish, and the type Ranavirus (frog virus-3, FV3) are similar ultrastructurally, antigenically, and genomically (Hengstberger et al., 1993).

Reports of severe edema and very high mortality rates in captive-raised tadpoles of the fire-bellied toad, *Bombina orientalis*, and the European common frog, *Rana temporaria*, have been attributed to a tadpole edema viruslike infection (Fischer, 1976; Verhoeff-DeFremery, 1983). In neither report was a virus isolated.

Numerous ranavirus isolates were obtained from specimens of the red-spotted newt, *Notophthalmus viridescens viridescens*, that had been injected with Lucke carcinoma cells or normal-appearing mesonephroi cells from the northern leopard frog, *Rana pipiens*, or were received as normal uninoculated animals from one animal broker (Clark et al., 1968, 1969). These viruses were designated LT viruses (for Lucke-*Triturus*) or T viruses (for *Triturus*, the former genus name for the red-spotted newt). Fifteen isolates of ranaviruses (T-6 through T-20), that were obtained from uninoculated newts (*Notophthalmus v. viridescens* or *N. v. dorsalis*), came from one lot of animals. Repeated attempts to isolate viruses from additional lots of newts were unsuccessful (Clark et al., 1968, 1969). Due to the lack of clinical signs or lesions and their isolation in only one lot of animals, these "T" viruses are not considered a virus disease nor a spontaneous infection of wild salamanders.

Intracoelomic injection of six different ranalike viruses (Lucke-*Triturus*-1, frog virus-1, TEV, T-6, T-8, and T-15) into efts of the red-spotted newt *Notophthalmus viridescens* resulted in infection in all efts, with recovery of the viruses from the liver, spleen, mesonephroi, and testis. No gross lesions were found in experimentally infected efts and newts; histological examinations were not attempted. When groups of metamorphs of the Fowler's toad, *Bufo woodhousei fowleri*, were injected with six ranaviruses (TEV, FV1, L5, LT1, LT2, and T6), 50–67% mortality rates occurred with TEV, FV1, and LT1 at 7–20 days postinoculation. Gross lesions in the toads were described briefly as edema with visceral and skeletal muscle hemorrhages. Histological examinations of the toads were not attempted. The viruses were considered a single antigenic type and all isolates were representative of the same virus (i.e., ranavirus) (Clark et al., 1969).

An iridovirus-like dermatitis was noted in one adult bullfrog, *Rana catesbeiana*, reportedly from Mexico, which was purchased from a supplier in Wisconsin and studied in Kansas. The frog developed small whitish skin ulcers and became lethargic (Briggs & Burton, 1973). The length of time the frog had been in captivity was unknown. The described skin lesions apparently were not investigated further, so the etiology of this skin disease was not determined. However, leukocytes from this frog were ultrastructurally found to contain numerous polyhedral cytoplasmic deoxyriboviruses (PCDV) which were probably iridovirus, and possibly ranavirus.

A detailed diagnostic examination of recurring unusual mortalies in English populations of the European common frog, *Rana temporaria*, described four distinct clinical syndromes associated with ranavirus-like particles (Cunningham et al., 1996b). The syndromes, called "ulcerative syndrome" (US), "haemorrhagic syndrome" (HS), "ulcerative and haemorrhagic syndrome" (UHS), and "reddened skin syndrome" (RSS), had evidence of a ranavirus-like infection sometimes associated with mixed Gram-negative bacteria. Although the syndromes appear distinctive grossly (Plate 27.1), histologically, and ultrastructurally, the syndromes appear to be a continuum which may be due to one or more unnamed ranalike viruses (Drury et al., 1995) or a ranavirus-like infection with secondary (opportunistic) bacterial infections. The commonly isolated bacteria were *Aeromonas hydrophila* and *Acinetobacter* sp.

Grossly, live frogs with "ulcerative syndrome" (US) have two prominent abnormalities: dermal ulcerations and necrosis of distal limbs. Ulceration prominently and principally affects the femoral skin, but may involve the skin of the forelimbs and body. Ulcers may be small (1–4 mm in diameter) or much larger and cause extensive exposure of underlying musculature. Ulcers usually have a red center, and, infrequently, may have a slightly elevated grayish margin about 2–3 mm wide. About 50% of frogs with US have necrosis of distal limbs in which one to all digits may be missing or protruding denuded bones. Necrosis may be to the level of the tarsus and was once observed to the level of the distal femur. Frogs with US lacked hemorrhages in the muscles and viscera. "Haemorrhagic syndrome" (HS) was strikingly similar to previous descriptions of red leg syndrome as affected frogs had systemic petechiae and ecchymoses in myoskeletal, alimentary, and reproductive tracts. Frogs with skin ulcers and hemorrhages were classified as having "ulcerative and haemorrhagic syndrome" (UHS). Frogs with either US, HS, or UHS were often thin and 58% had no fat bodies, suggestive of cachexia due to a prolonged infection. Frogs with "reddened skin syndrome" (RSS) were thin, lethargic, and had skin erythema without hemorrhages or ulcers. Bacteriologically, 40% of frogs with RSS and 74% of frogs with US had isolates of *Aeromonas hydrophila* from at least one body site (usually skin, exposed muscle or intestine), while 90% of frogs with HS had this bacterium, and 100% of four control frogs had it. *Acinetobacter* was isolated from skin ulcers or internal organs of about 50% of frogs (Cunningham et al., 1996b).

Histologically, epidermal ulcers consist of a mixture of hyperplasia, basal cell necrosis, and segments of complete epidermal sloughing. The normal epidermis is 5–7 cells thick, while the hyperplastic regions are 10–30 cells thick, and occasionally form plaques or small papillary projections. Necrosis is generally confined to deeper cell layers, especially the stratum basale. Cell necrosis may be so extensive that the epidermis sloughs. Bacterial invasion of the exposed dermis, muscles, and bone is evident with infiltrates of granulocytes and lymphocytes; edema, congestion, and hemorrhages are also present. In several frogs with HS or UHS two types of hepatocellular intracytoplasmic inclusion bodies are evident. (Figures 27.16, 27.17, 27.18) Basophilic inclusions were round and lack clear haloes. Larger acidophilic hepatocellular inclusions with clear haloes are found in 10% of all frogs. Ultrastructurally, the basophilic inclusions are aggregates of iridovirus-like particles (mean diameter: 129 nm) surrounded by layers of rough endoplasmic reticulum (rER), while the eosinophilic inclusions consist of whorls of rER around ill-defined central cores, but without virus particles. Ultrastructurally, the skin ulcers have degenerate, shrunken, rounded cells containing intracytoplasmic iridovirus-like particles (mean diameter: 142 nm), while regions of normal skin had no detectable virus particles (Figure 27.15).

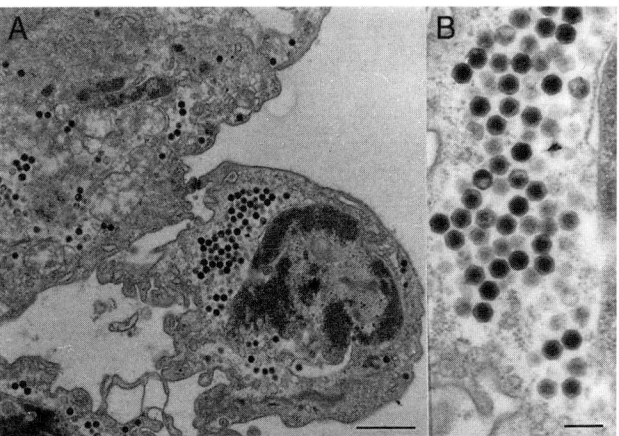

Figure 27.15. Transmission electron micrograph of skin from a wild European common frog, *Rana temporaria*, with ulcerative skin syndrome. **A.** A rounded surface epidermal cell that contains numerous iridovirus-like particles only in the cytoplasm (scale bar = 1 μm). **B.** Higher magnification of intracytoplasmic icosohedral iridovirus-like particles (scale bar = 250 μm). (A.A. Cunningham, The Zoological Society of London, taken from Cunningham et al., 1996b, with permission)

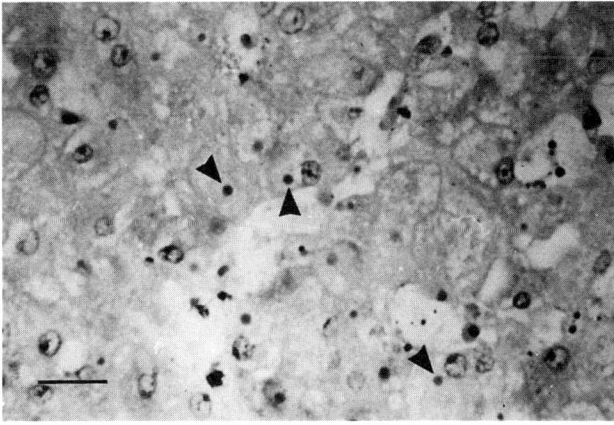

Figure 27.16. Liver from a wild European common frog, *Rana temporaria*, with ulcerative and hemorrhagic syndrome. Note the prominent round, basophilic, intracytoplasmic inclusion bodies (arrowheads) associated with iridovirus-like particles (scale bar = 25 μm). (See Figure 27.18.) (A.A. Cunningham, The Zoological Society of London, taken from Cunningham et al., 1996b, with permission)

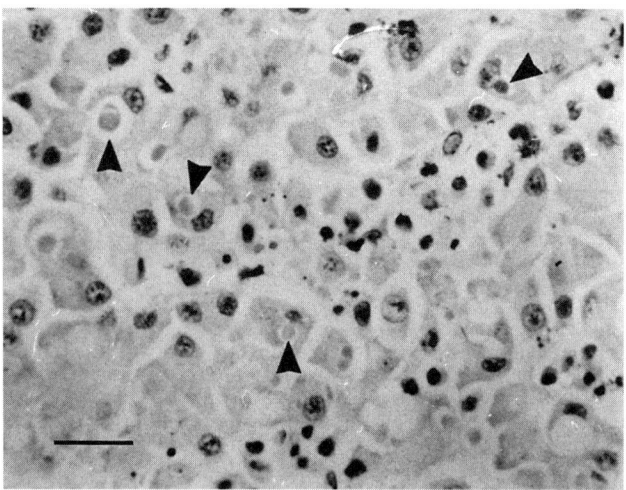

Figure 27.17. Liver from a wild European common frog, *Rana temporaria*, with hemorrhagic syndrome. Note the larger intracytoplasmic inclusion bodies with prominent clear haloes (arrowheads). This second form of intracytoplasmic inclusion (see also Figure 27.18) is eosinophilic (scale bar = 25 μm). (A.A. Cunningham, The Zoological Society of London, taken from Cunningham et al., 1996b, with permission)

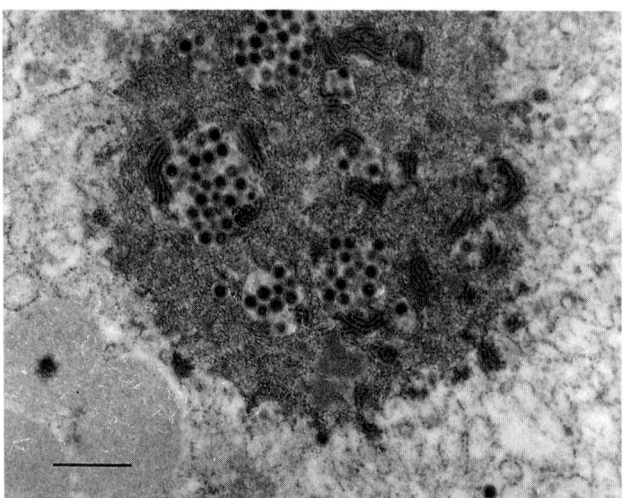

Figure 27.18. Transmission electron micrograph of a basophilic intracytoplasmic inclusion from the liver of a European common frog, *Rana temporaria*, with hemorrhagic syndrome. Note the electron-dense icosohedral virus particles, some of which have gray membranelike capsules. The electron-dense stacks of curving membranes are rough endoplasmic reticulum (scale bar = 500 nm). (A.A. Cunningham, The Zoological Society of London, taken from Cunningham et al., 1996b, with permission)

Numerous histological lesions are present in other organs. Necrosis of the renal interstitial myeloid cells occurs consistently in frogs with HS and UHS, but in few or no frogs with US and RSS. Glomerular and tubular necroses are present in less than 50% of the frogs with each syndrome. Basophilic intracytoplasmic inclusions are rarely present in tubular cells. Spleens of frogs with HS and UHS have foci of lymphorrhexis histologically; these foci of necrosis are observed grossly as white foci in some frogs. Pulmonary lesions are inconsistent but lungs may show congestion, hemorrhages, or acute focal necroses. Most frogs with HS or UHS have marked congestion or transmural hemorrhages in the gastrointestinal tract, occasionally with submucosal edema and foci of mucosal necrosis. Congestion or hemorrhages may be observed grossly or histologically in the fat bodies, pancreases, testes, ovaries, and oviducts of frogs with HS and UHS, but infrequently in frogs with US and RSS (Cunningham et al., 1996b).

Some of these described syndromes in the European common frog, *Rana temporaria*, from England have a striking resemblance to descriptions of red leg syndrome. The authors (Cunningham et al., 1996b) propose some reports of red leg syndrome are principally and primarily ranavirus-like infections and that isolated bacteria are merely secondary (opportunistic) or postmortem invaders.

Raised white skin lesions found on a common European toad, *Bufo bufo*, had eosinophilic intracytoplasmic inclusions in the epidermal cells consistent with viral particles (Scullion et al., 1989).

A herpesvirus-like dermatitis was noted in specimens of the spring frog, *Rana dalmatina*, from a region of northern Italy near Brescia. Numerous dorsal and lateral epidermal vesicles were detected in 35% and 80% of two breeding populations. The cutaneous vesicles were whitish to dark gray, 1–3 mm in diameter, and irregular in outline. No lesions were detected in internal organs. Histologically, epidermal hyperplasia, basal cell epidermolysis, and karyomegaly are evident. Epidermal cell karyomegaly consists of enlarged translucent nuclei filled with pink to purple intranuclear bodies. Negative-staining electron microscopy of skin vesicles demonstrates many herpesvirus-like particles. However, it is important to note the ultrastructural similarity of herpesviruses and iridoviruses. Sympatric amphibian species, including the smooth newt, *Triturus vulgaris*, the northern crested newt, *T. carnifex*, and the edible frog, *Rana kl. esculenta*, which shared the same breeding ponds, were not affected. Unpublished observations were cited of similar cutaneous lesions in specimens of the spring frog, *Rana dalmatina* in Switzerland (Bennati et al., 1994).

Poxviruslike particles from epidermal ulcers of specimens of the European common frog, *Rana temporaria* (Cunningham et al., 1993), were later shown by transmission electron microscopy to be typical of melanosomes (Cunningham et al., 1996b).

Infectious Etiologies—Bacteria—Red Leg Syndrome. The vast majority of reported bacterial infections of the amphibian integument seem to rapidly progress to bacteremias with widespread involvement of multiple organ systems. Bacterial infections which are truly limited to the integument are uncommon and poorly documented. Because bacterial skin infections and septicemias commonly coexist, most amphibian bacterial infections may be considered dermatosepticemias.

Red leg syndrome has been known from cultural studies since the late nineteenth century (Russell, 1898), and is most often attributed to bacterial infection by *Aeromonas hydrophila* (Boyer et al., 1971; Hubbard, 1981). Other species of *Aeromonas* and Gram-negative bacilli, mostly Enterobacteriaceae, also have been implicated in red leglike morbidities and mortalities of anurans and salamanders. Red leglike illnesses have occurred principally in anurans in captivity, but have occasionally been implicated in mass mortalities of wild amphibians (Bradford, 1991; Burton et al., 1995; Dusi, 1949; Hine et al., 1975 as cited by Hird et al., 1981; Hunsaker & Potter, 1960; Nyman, 1986; Worthylake & Hovingh, 1989). However, aeromonads such as *Aeromonas hydrophila* are commonly isolated from clinically normal, apparently healthy fish and aquatic and terrestrial amphibians (Austin & Austin, 1987; Gibbs et al., 1966; Green, unpublished data; Hird et al., 1981; Kulp & Borden, 1942). Caution is necessary when assigning etiologic diagnoses to bacteria isolated from any dead amphibians or from amphibian epidermis, gills, intestines, and feces. Dead amphibians are invaded rapidly by environmental or decompositional microorganisms, and bacterial isolates from the epidermis and the alimentary tract merely reflect the flora of the environment and diet (Vander Waaij et al., 1974). *Aeromonas hydrophila* was readily isolated from fecal samples of adult *Rana pipiens* in captivity, all of which remained healthy for over 5 months (Gibbs et al., 1966). The ease with which most suspected pathogenic bacteria (e.g., *Aeromonas* spp., *Flavobacterium* spp., *Citrobacter* spp., etc.) are isolated from the skin and alimentary tracts of normal, healthy appearing, wild populations (Green, unpublished data; Hird et al., 1981) necessitates additional proof of pathogenicity of most bacterial isolates. Confirmed diagnoses should be restricted to those cases in which internal tissues (subcutis, heart blood, spleen, liver, mesonephroi, etc.) of live or euthanized amphibians yield isolates, those cases in which Koch's postulates are fulfilled, or those cases in which virulence factors of the bacterial isolates are detected. Diagnoses of red leg syndrome that are based only on clinical signs, external lesions, skin or alimentary tract cultures, and cultures from amphibians that were found dead, are suspect.

Grossly, the redness of the skin in red leg syndrome may consist of four distinct lesions: generalized but usually ventral and digital erythema due to dilation of dermal vessels is a common presentation. (Plates 27.2, 27.3, 27.4, 27.5); sunken multiple foci of necrosis or ulceration of the epidermis; subtly raised hemorrhagic epidermal papules; and petechial or ecchymotic hemorrhages in the dermis (Cunningham et al., 1996b; Emerson & Norris, 1905; Gibbs et al., 1966; Glorioso et al., 1974; Hubbard, 1981; Kulp & Borden, 1942). Other lesions associated with bacterial dermatosepticemias in most taxa of adult amphibians include edematous, fibrinocellular or sanguinous fluids in the subcutis of the upper limbs and abdominal ventrum, hemorrhagic ulceration of the tips of digital skin sometimes progressing to exposed phalangeal bones or sloughed digits (Figure 27.19), ulcerated jaws, pale yellowish or sanguinous coelomic transudates or effusions, and hemoptysis (Emerson & Norris, 1905; Gibbs et al., 1966; Kaplan & Glaczenski, 1965; Kulp & Borden, 1942; Taylor et al., 1994, 1995). Subcutaneous edema may be so marked that it causes the appearance of generalized cutaneous pallor, a lack of erythema or hemorrhage within dermal ulcers, and a bloated appearance (sometimes termed edema syndrome) (Glorioso et al., 1974). Petechial and ecchymotic hemorrhages in adult amphibians also may be detected in skeletal muscles, mesonephroi, spleen, coelomic mesothelial surfaces, and nearly any other organ in which vascular thrombi and bacillary emboli occur (Cunningham et al., 1995; Frye, 1989a; Kulp & Borden, 1942; Olson et al., 1992). Mild weight loss to obvious emaciation may be evident in adult amphibians as atrophy of muscles and moderate to complete atrophy of fat bodies. Many amphibians succumbing peracutely or acutely to bacterial dermatosepticemias may have minimal or no gross lesions (Abrams, 1969; Boyer et al., 1971; Frye, 1989a; Gibbs et al., 1966; Kulp & Borden, 1942). Some lesions that are commonly attributed to red leg may be separate distinct virus infections (Cunningham et al., 1996b).

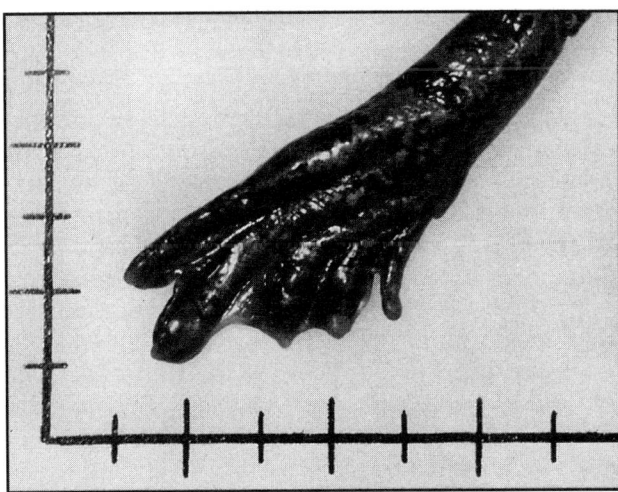

Figure 27.19. Necrosis of the tips of the hindlimb digits in a wild spotted frog, *Rana pretiosa*. Necrosis of the digits has been associated with bacteria, fungi, and viruses (5 mm between crossbars). (D.E. Green)

In tadpoles and salamander larvae, erythema and petechia are reported on ventral and lateral body skin, the tail, and legs. Hemorrhages may be present over the eyes in tadpoles of the bullfrog, *Rana catesbeiana*. Immature amphibians also may have minimal to moderate subcutaneous edema composed of clear, cloudy, or sanguinous fluids, but others in the same group may appear emaciated (Glorioso et al., 1974; Nyman, 1986).

Septicemia is a common consequence of infection by *Aeromonas* spp. and other Gram-negative bacilli. Gross manifestations of bacillary septicemias may vary depending on several factors such as the environmental temperature, immunological status of the host, virulence of the bacteria, presence of concurrent viral, fungal and parasitic infections, and duration of infection in the host. Ocular lesions of corneal edema, hypopyon, fibrinocellular endophthalmitis, and exophthalmos are observed in adult terrestrial anurans (Brooks et al., 1983; Olson et al., 1992; Taylor et al., 1993) but have not been reported in salamanders, tadpoles, and clawed frogs, *Xenopus* spp. (Frye, 1989a; Hubbard, 1981; Nyman, 1986). The blood-filled blisters over the eyes of tadpoles of the bullfrog, *Rana catesbeiana* (Glorioso et al., 1974) may refer to hemorrhages into the skin dorsal to the eyes, or hyphema. Hosts with compromised immune systems or those which are overwhelmed by bacteria, may show widespread visceral lesions including fibrinocellular or sanguinous coelomic exudates, miliary petechial or ecchymotic hemorrhages on natural and cut surfaces of organs, muscles, joints and periostea, splenomegaly, nephritis, and dilatative gastroenteritis (Emerson & Norris, 1905; Frye, 1989a; Olson et al., 1992; Russell, 1898). Some investigators have observed absence of lesions consistently in one or more organs, such as mesonephroi (Kulp & Borden, 1942), lungs, heart, or liver (Elkan, 1976b). Others report liver lesions of hepatomegaly, pale foci of necrosis, diffuse pallor, and friability (Glorioso et al., 1974; Olson et al., 1992; Russell, 1898; Zwart et al., 1991). "Dark" livers have been considered a lesion associated with dermatosepticemias (Shotts, 1984), but gray to black livers are common in clinically normal, apparently healthy amphibians and, therefore, have little significance (Zwart et al., 1991). Yellowish bile was associated with *Aeromonas* bacteria in the gall bladder of the northern leopard frog, *R. pipiens*, while dark green bile was considered normal and was consistently found to be sterile (Kulp & Borden, 1942). Myocarditis was noted in three anurans from the San Diego Zoo (Griner, 1983), and epicarditis has been found in others (Cunningham et al., 1996b; Olson et al., 1992), but valvular endocarditis has not been reported, grossly or histologically, in amphibians with septicemia.

Histologic descriptions of red leg syndrome generally confirm the gross observations. Integumentary lesions vary tremendously. Epidermal necrosis, erosions, and deep ulcerations into the subcutis and skeletal muscles may be found. Inflammation may consist solely of edema of the subcutis and dermis with dilation of lymphatic sacs, or may include an inflammatory cell component. Infiltrating integumentary leukocytes consist mostly of granulocytes (neutrophil-like cells) with lesser numbers of macrophages and lymphocytes. Dermal glands may be necrotic and have granulocytic infiltrates. Blood vessels are dilated, congested, and may have perivascular hemorrhages and contain thrombi or bacillary emboli. Air embolisms in blood vessels caused by gas bubble disease may cause miliary ischemia and infarcts in the dermis that are secondarily invaded by bacteria (Colt et al., 1984). Histologic detection of air emboli is very difficult. Bacteria are detected in the epidermis, vessels, and lymphatic sacs, but in amphibians which were not euthanized, nor promptly necropsied, nor promptly preserved in fixatives, special attention must be directed to the detection of intracellular bacteria (in phagocytic cells) to be sure that the organisms were present before death and do not represent decompositional invaders (Abrams, 1969).

Histological lesions described in visceral organs are variable and consistent with the first published description (Russell, 1898). Some authors report essentially no lesions in the mesonephroi, spleen, and liver, even when bacterial cultures of these organs are productive (Brooks et al., 1983; Taylor et al., 1993). In the spleen, congestion of sinusoids, necrosis of scattered phagocytic cells, or discrete foci of coagulative necrosis may be found (Olson et al., 1992; Russell, 1898). Hemorrhage into necrotic foci may be present (Russell, 1898). Uncharacterized splenitis is reported (Frye, 1989a). Fatty vacuolation of hepatocytes may be evident (Hubbard, 1981) depending on the degree of inanition or catabolic state prior to death. Sinusoidal congestion, hepatocellular hydropic degeneration, apoptosis (Olson et al., 1992; Russell, 1898; Zwart et al., 1991), and hepatitis occur (Frye, 1989a). Necrotic foci in the liver and spleen have been reported in association with visible bacteria (Abrams, 1969) (Figures 27.20, 27.21). Striking cardiac and pericardial lesions may present as marked fibrinopurulent epicarditis with masses of bacilli (Olson et al., 1992) or nonsuppurative myocarditis (Frye, 1989a). Lesions in the mesonephroi are inconsistent for there may be no detectable changes, acute necrosis, or tubular and glomerular mesonephritis (Frye, 1989a). The absence of glomerular thrombi and emboli in published reports is inconsistent with vascular lesions elsewhere in the body. Finally, skeletal muscles, mostly of the limbs, show interstitial edema, congestion, and hemorrhage, with myocytic degeneration and rhabdomyolysis. The inflammatory cell component is

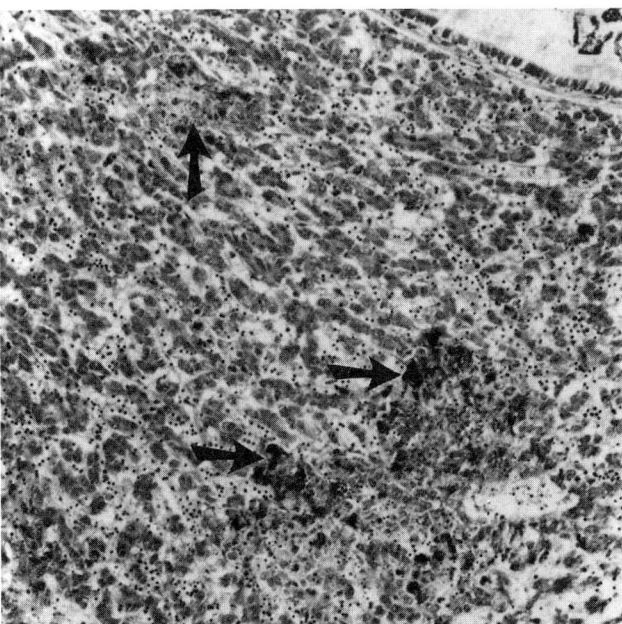

Figure 27.20. Necrotizing bacillary hepatitis in a tadpole of the wood frog, *Rana sylvatica*. Degeneration and necrosis of hepatocytes is evident with prominent clusters of bacilli centrally (arrows). Large clusters of bacilli, which appear to be spilling out of ruptured cells, generally may be attributed to continued bacterial growth after the death of the animal. (D.E. Green)

variable but usually suppurative, although mild granulomatous myositis has been reported in the clawed frog, *Xenopus* spp., (Hubbard, 1981). The presence or number of bacilli in the above lesions is highly variable, but it is always necessary to search for evidence of antemortem bacteria.

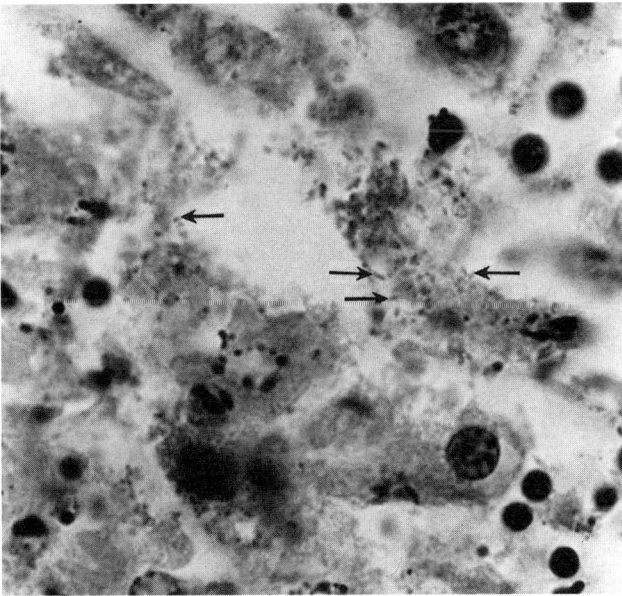

Figure 27.21. Higher magnification of Figure 27.20. Numerous bacilli are present within hepatocytes and spilling from necrotic cells (arrows). (D.E. Green)

Aeromonas salmonicida is the only major nonmotile aeromonad that is foremost a pathogen of fish. One report (Frye, 1985) documents this fish pathogen in a colony of the African clawed frog, *Xenopus laevis*. The frogs were accidentally exposed to the aeromonad when fresh Pacific salmon was included in their food. Gross findings included reddened skin, dermal hemorrhages, and extensive dermal ulcerations, especially involving the digits and stifles. Necrosis and loss of digits, exposure of patellae, hepatitis, mesonephritis, and gastroenteritis occur. *Aeromonas salmonicida* was isolated from tank water and internal organs of the affected frogs.

Infectious Etiologies—Bacteria—Para-Orbital Pustular Dermatitis. A clinical syndrome characterized by cutaneous vesicles and pustules in the skin around the eyes and ears was noted in captive specimens of the northern leopard frog, *Rana pipiens* (Abrams, 1969). It was implied the cause was not any of the bacteria associated with red leg syndrome, but the precise etiology was not reported. The syndrome occasionally causes a high mortality rate in groups of the northern leopard frog, *R. pipiens*. Vesicles and pustules are evident in the dermis and subcutis, and consist of edema, fibrin, occasionally numerous neutrophils, and degenerate and necrotic dermal structures. The overlying epidermis remains intact.

Infectious Etiologies—Mycobacteria—Mycobacteriosis. Acid-fast bacillary infections of amphibians should be referred to as mycobacterial infections or mycobacterioses. The term tuberculosis is inaccurate and should not be used when referring to mycobacteria other than tubercle (MOTT) bacilli in ectothermic animals (Thoen & Schliesser, 1984). It would be difficult to improve on the descriptions of mycobacteriosis (Elkan, 1976b), so readers are referred to this reference for a more thorough description and excellent illustrations.

In amphibians, mycobacteriosis often presents as a disease of the integument, the pathogenesis of which is widely assumed to be contamination of wounds. Cutaneous mycobacteriosis in the African clawed frog, *Xenopus laevis*, may present in one of four forms: 1) granulomas of the digital tips and webs; 2) granulomas of the lips and mouth; 3) miliary ("disseminated") dermoepidermal granulomas of the body and proximal hindlimbs; or 4) large, solitary, subcutaneous granuloma in nearly any region (Elkan, 1976b; Schwabacher, 1959). The nodules are usually pale, and free of melanin. Large cutaneous nodules may be ulcerated centrally. Cutaneous mycobacteriosis may be limited to the skin (Schwabacher, 1959) or it may spread via the lymphatic drainage. Hindlimb infections often spread to the mesonephroi, and cephalic infections often affect the respiratory system (Elkan, 1976b). Viscera may have miliary nodules, but large, solitary, sessile or pedunculated granulomas which are grossly indistinguishable from neoplasia, may be found in nearly any organ or site. Cachexia in affected animals is evident by mild to moderate muscular atrophy and severe atrophy or absence of the fat bodies.

Histologically, early granulomas are composed of mostly epithelioid macrophages and a few lymphocytes with little or no caseous necrosis. More chronic lesions present with dry caseous cores and with thick walls of viable epithelioid cells. Mineralization does not occur. Giant cells were mentioned as a component of infection in the clawed frog, *Xenopus laevis* (Schwabacher, 1959), and multiple species of toads (Elkan, 1976b; Machicao & LaPlaca, 1954; Shively et al., 1981). Acid-fast stains readily demonstrate myriad intracellular acid-fast bacilli. The bacilli may be curved, granular, beaded, or coccuslike (Aronson, 1957; Elkan, 1976b; Schwabacher, 1959; Thoen & Schliesser, 1984), but within an individual the bacterial morphology is uniform. Mycobacteria also are Gram-positive (Aronson, 1957).

Amphibians were frequently injected with isolates of mycobacteria obtained from fish, reptiles, and other amphibians (Aronson, 1957; Vogel, 1958). As a general rule, amphibians develop disease and granulomas when injected with mycobacteria isolated from ectotherms, but not mammalian mycobacteria.

Experimentally, granulomatous inflammation and lymphoreticular neoplasms in amphibians have often been confused in the literature. In reading and evaluating the published literature and future publications, the following three statements must be carefully considered: 1) granulomatous inflammation and mycobacterial granulomas of amphibians have been misdiagnosed as lymphoreticular neoplastic disease; 2) cases of suspected granulomatous and lymphoreticular diseases in amphibians must be carefully examined by use of acid-fast stains; and 3) reports of lymphoreticular disease in amphibians in which the neoplastic cells are not described in detail or adequately illustrated, and in which results of acid-fast stains are not given, should be viewed with caution (Asfari, 1988; Asfari & Thiebaud, 1988; Clothier & Balls, 1973a, b).

Experimental mycobacteriosis in amphibians usually involves inoculation of material into the dorsal lymph sac, body cavity or axillary subcutis. In the clawed frog, *Xenopus* spp., and the northern leopard frog, *Rana pipiens,* gross lesions usually appear in the liver, spleen and ventral skin at 14–21 days postinoculation (Clothier & Balls, 1973a; Joiner & Abrams, 1967). In the Japanese firebelly newt, *Cynops pyrrhogaster,* and the red-spotted newt, *Notophthalmus viridescens,* inoculated intracoelomically, the initial response in 3 days is the formation of numerous gray mealy patches on the mesothelial surfaces of many organs, especially the liver and spleen. Within 2 weeks, extensive nodules (granulomata) form in liver and spleen, with fewer smaller white granulomata in the pancreas, mesonephros, stomach, ovary, fat body, mesentery, and body wall (Inoue & Singer, 1970a). Splenomegaly is common at necropsy of mycobacteria-infected specimens of the clawed frog, *Xenopus* spp., but is not consistently found (Asfari, 1988; Clothier & Balls, 1973a). The liver and spleen consistently have granulomata in spontaneous and experimental mycobacterioses.

The first attempts at histological comparisons of lymphoid neoplasia and granulomatous mycobacteriosis in amphibians failed to recognize the non-neoplastic nature of the granulomata (Inoue & Singer, 1970a, b; Ruben & Stevens, 1970a). Experimentally inoculated amphibians develop nodules of inflammation in the liver and spleen by 16 days postinoculation. These nodules consist of about equal numbers of granulocytes and macrophages, and could be considered abscesses. Beginning at 20 days postinoculation, macrophages with abundant pale eosinophilic cytoplasm are the major cell in the cores of nodules, and could be considered acute granulomas. Beginning at about 28 days postinoculation, nodules clearly are enlarging, compressing surrounding parenchyma, forming thin fibrocytic capsules, and have small clusters or diffuse thin rims of lymphocytes at the periphery. These are considered granulomata. Clusters of granulomata with rims of lymphocytes may, at low magnifications, resemble mammalian germinal centers, and hence, may be the basis of some mistaken diagnoses of lymphosarcoma. Occasional mitotic macrophages may be present, usually at the periphery of the granulomata. Intracellular acid-fast bacilli peak in numbers within the granulomata at about 24 days postinoculation, although some granulomas contain very few or no detectable mycobacteria. Intrasinusoidal macrophages (probably Kupffer cells) also may be laden with acid-fast bacilli. Caseous necrosis within the granulomata is first detected at 31 days postinoculation, although many granulomata fail to demonstrate necrosis of central macrophages through 45 days postinoculation. Multinucleated giant cells were detected in granulomata of only one newt, and many northern leopard frogs, *Rana pipiens,* although the giant cells may be responsive to embolic oil droplets used in the inoculum (Joiner & Abrams, 1967). In clawed frogs, *Xenopus* spp., caseous necrosis and multinucleated giant cells are rarely found, even in thymectomized specimens, through 50 days postinoculation (Ruben & Stevens, 1970). The number of dead mycobacteria, the dose of bacteria, and the growth phase of the mycobacteria in the inoculum exert marked influences on the inflammatory reaction and disease progression in clawed frogs, *Xenopus* spp., (Asfari, 1988). The development of *Mycobacterium marinum*-induced granulomata in clawed frogs, *Xenopus* spp., has been summarized: "Histological studies of the different experimental animals represent a histological spectrum ranging from a mere accumulation of lymphoid cells . . . to an advanced necrotic granuloma . . . This spectrum reflects the progressive histopathological changes which occur as the disease develops: a) Soon after bacterial infection some foci of lymphoid cells appear . . . In the liver, these lymphoid cell foci are often associated with melanocytes [melanomacrophage aggregates]. b) Later on, histiocytes appear in the center of these lymphoid clumps and develop concentrically . . . c) At a later stage, these granuloma foci are surrounded by a halo of lymphoid cells . . . d) as the number of histiocytes in a granuloma . . . increases a sheath of fibroblasts is formed around the focus. e) At the final stage, necrosis appears in the center of the granuloma and develops concentrically . . . In some cases, granulomatous lesions of similar histological features display a great variation in bacterial content. . . . [A]s few as 52 colony-forming bacteria were sufficient to induce granulomas . . ." (Asfari, 1988).

Infectious Etiologies—Mycobacteria—Lepralike Mycobacteriosis. A Bolivian population of wild leptodactylids and bufonids were infected by uncultureable mycobacteria (Machicao & LaPlaca, 1954). The anurans included the Juliaca four-eyed frog, *Pleurodema cinerea,* the marbled four-eyed frog, *Pleurodema marmorata,* and the warty toad, *Bufo s. spinulosum.* Nearly all affected frogs and toads had mycobacterial granulomata in the liver and, in some, integumentary lesions were found. The location of integumentary granulomata was variable but grossly evident nodules were found at the oral commissures, lips, ventral neck, axilla, and forelimbs. Occasional granulomata were detected on the abdomen, back, and proximal hindlimbs. Raised nodules were up to 4 mm in diameter, and the overlying skin was slightly depigmented or ulcerated centrally. Granulomata were found near the brachial and sacral nerve trunks. Histologically, the dermal nodules were composed of pleomorphic foamy histiocytes, with very few lymphocytes and granulocytes. Toads had rare multinucleated giant cells, while the frogs had none. Intracellular bacteria were both Gram-positive and acid-fast-positive. The authors suggested a diagnosis of "batrachian leprosy" based on the globuslike histiocytes, slight nerve involvement, and their failure to isolate the mycobacteria in cultures. However, the authors met only one of the five principal criteria (Walsh et al., 1978) now used for identifying acid-fast bacilli as leprosy-like (i.e., noncultivability on mycobacterial media). Because all frogs with lepralike skin lesions also had massive granulomata in the visceral organs, it is equally likely the skin lesions were near-terminal dissemination of the mycobacteria. Later authors have suggested the infections in these Bolivian anurans were *Mycobacterium marinum*-like (Shively et al., 1981).

Infectious Etiologies—Fungal—Saprolegniasis. White cottony growths on the skin and gills are usually due to one of several genera of watermolds, including *Saprolegnia, Achyla, Aphanomyces, Leptolegnia,* and others. These opportunistic pathogens belong to the subdivision Diplomastigomycotina and the Class Oomycetes. Watermolds have a complex life cycle that includes multiple propagative stages (for additional information on the life cycle of Oomycetes, see Neish & Hughes, 1980, and Noga, 1993a). Although the disease saprolegniasis is considered common, cultural isolation and identification of the infecting organisms in amphibians is rarely reported. Cases are reported as consistent with *Saprolegnia* or as *Saprolegnia* spp., (Cooper, 1984; Frye & Gillespie, 1989; Jacobson, 1989). *Saprolegnia parasitica* is reported from newts and frogs, and *S. ferax, Achyla flagellata,* and *Dictyuchus monosporus* have been reported from newts (Tiffany, 1939 as cited by Reichenbach-Klinke & Elkan, 1965).

In salamanders, the clinical signs of saprolegniasis are multisystemic and include lethargy, anorexia, vomiting, respiratory distress (gaping), weight loss, and death (Frye & Gillespie, 1989). This author has observed saprolegniasis in tadpoles of the foothills yellow-legged frog, *Rana boylii,* from a mass mortality event of undetermined etiology in northern California. Affected tadpoles had discrete, multifocal grayish white, translucent tufts of tangled hyphae about the mouth and projecting from the spiracle (Figures 27.22, 27.23, 27.24). In aquatic amphibians,

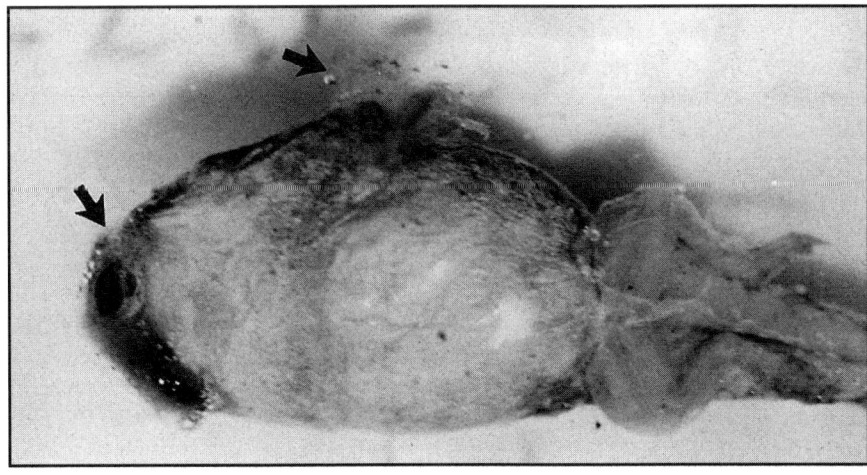

Figure 27.22. Saprolegniasis affecting the snout and spiracle of a tadpole of the foothills yellow-legged frog, *Rana boylii.* Para-oral, spiracle (arrows) and gill chamber infections were associated with a mass mortality event in these tadpoles. (D.E. Green)

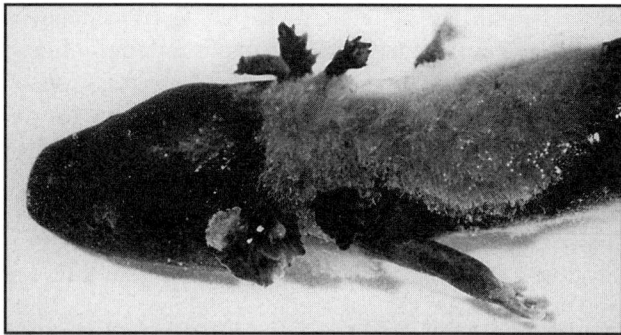

Figure 27.23. Saprolegniasis of the gills and dorsal skin of a captive mudpuppy, *Necturus maculosus*. (D.E. Green)

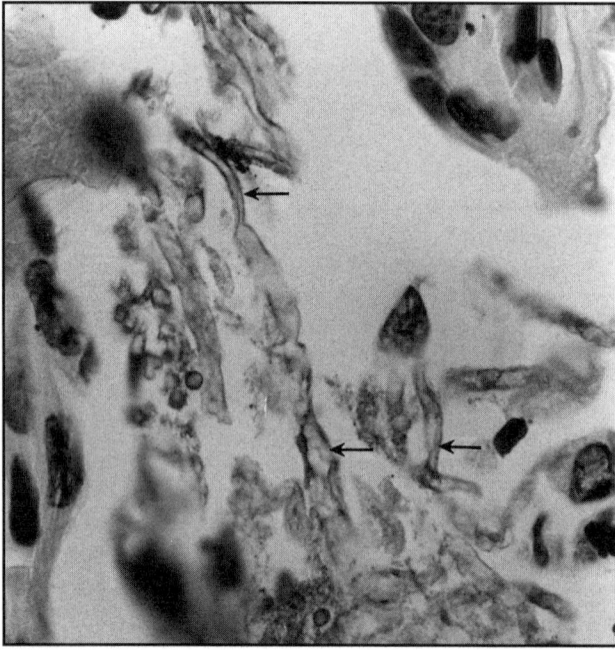

Figure 27.24. Saprolegniasis of the gills of a captive mudpuppy, *Necturus maculosus* (same as Figure 27.23). The hyphae (arrows) are variable in diameter, sparingly septate, and elicit minimal or no inflammatory response. (D.E. Green)

the white or grayish white, cottony, hyphal tangles may be present anywhere on the body or external gills (Jacobson, 1989). Skin wounds are the site of most watermold infections (Cooper, 1984; Crawshaw, 1993). The anterior snout, gills, and tail tip are common sites of infection, but infections may occur anywhere on the body and limbs. The underlying skin is discolored, necrotic or ulcerated, and inconsistently reddened. Advanced deep ulcerations which expose underlying musculature or bone (Reichenbach-Klinke & Elkan, 1965) are inconsistently hemorrhagic. The delicate cottony tangles collapse when the animal is removed from water.

Histologically, the infection is noteworthy for the paucity of inflammatory cells, extensive ulceration of skin with necrosis of underlying soft tissues, and frequent poor staining of the hyphae. Vesicles or blisters may be detected acutely in the epidermis but with minimal or no inflammatory cell response. Subacute and chronic lesions may show epithelial cell necrosis, erosions, and ulcerations in the epidermis. Necrosis may affect dermal glands, subcutis, and muscles with variable amounts of sloughed, lost tissue. Although the hyphae rarely become septicemic, extensive involvement of bone, muscle, spinal cord, and other organs may occur by direct extension from primary epithelial lesions (Bly et al., 1992; Frye & Gillespie, 1989). Tissue edema is variable but it is not clear whether it is a true host inflammatory response, or due to osmosis of water through the devitalized skin. Deep hyphal invasion of underlying soft tissues may be detected despite absence of tissue degeneration and inflammatory cells. Deep invasion of soft tissues by hyphae may be due, in part, to postmortem growth of the fungi. As in fish, dead aquatic amphibians decompose rapidly, and watermolds rapidly flourish as part of the decompositional process.

Concurrent bacterial infections are common at sites of watermold infection. Bacteremias may be the proximate cause of death in many cases, and change otherwise bland lesions into those with extensive tissue necrosis and inflammatory cell response (Bly et al., 1992; Frye & Gillespie, 1989).

Zoospores and hyphae are present in the dermal lesions. Zoospores are thin-walled, roughly spherical, 10–14 μm in diameter, and may contain 1–4 internal spores (Frye & Gillespie, 1989; Noga, 1993a). Hyphae are aseptate, occasionally branching, quite variable in stain affinity in periodic acid-Schiff and hemotoxylin and eosin preparations, have parallel walls, and are highly variable in diameter (2–40 μm) (Noga, 1993b). It is not clear whether these variable hyphal diameters represent different growth stages of one species, or mixed watermold infections.

Infectious Etiologies—Fungal—Basidiobolus sp. *Basidiobolus* is a genus of saprophytic fungus which is ubiquitous in the environment, and has been found regularly in feces of clinically normal amphibians and reptiles (Gugnani & Okafor, 1980; Okafor et al., 1984). In amphibians, this fungal infection is intraepidermal, elicits minimal inflammation, and organisms are ovoid-to-globose conidia (Groff et al., 1991). At present, the disease has been reported only in anurans in captivity (Burton et al., 1995; Groff et al., 1991; Taylor et al., 1994, 1995).

Basidiobolus is a Zygomycete with several suspected species, but only *B. microsporus* can be unequivocally identified in cultures based on formation of microspores. All other isolates are relegated to the taxon *B. ranarum*. Generally, the fungus is an opportunistic pathogen. Although it may be transmitted between anurans (Groff et al., 1991), it has not been transmitted by exposure of anurans to pure colonies of *Basidiobolus*. The fungus also has proved difficult to control in captive bufonids (Taylor et al., 1994, 1995; Burton et al., 1995).

Gross lesions of cutaneous zygomycosis by *Basidiobolus* are minimal and nonspecific. In specimens of the western dwarf clawed frog, *Hymenochirus curtipes*, subtle skin pallor and crawling out of the water were reported (Groff et al., 1991). The Wyoming toad, *Bufo hemiophrys baxteri*, had changes that were briefly described as dermatitis, most notable at the tips of digits and ventral skin, and hepatopathy. Digital dermatitis was characterized as reddening of the extremities, with occasional progression to ulceration and exposure of the distal phalanges, but these latter, more extensive lesions may have been complicated by concurrent bacterial infections (Burton et al., 1995; Taylor et al., 1994). In bufonids, infection of ventral abdominal skin in the region of the pelvic patch was detected histologically, but gross changes were inapparent or minimal.

Histologically, epidermal changes are mild and could be easily overlooked. Epidermal changes consist of mild hyperkeratosis and acanthosis with a mild (or absent) inflammatory cell infiltrate. Principal inflammatory cell types have not been described. Fungal elements in the epidermis only are spherical to ovoid conidia, 10–15 μm in diameter, and often show dense, darkly staining, clustered, internal structures. These internal structures are presumed to be formed by cleavage and are called sporangiospores (or meristospores) (Groff et al., 1991).

The very mild nature of the gross and histologic lesions of *Basidiobolus* spp. infection in anurans was totally disproportionate to the high mortality rates in the western dwarf clawed frog, *Hymenochirus curtipes* (Groff et al., 1991). Such mild lesions suggest the importance of intact epidermis for the survival of amphibians. When aquatic amphibians attempt to escape their environment, hypoxia or osmoregulatory difficulties secondary to epidermal disease are implied. In terrestrial anurans, *Basidiobolus* spp. infection of the drinking patch may sufficiently disrupt transepidermal water absorption to cause fatal dehydration. The absence of obvious lesions internally, and the subtle nature of epidermal changes in *Basidiobolus* infections, necessitate careful histological and cultural examinations of the ventral body skin, and especially the skin of the pelvic patch, in all anurans.

Infectious Etiologies—Fungal—Chromomycosis. Integumentary and systemic infections by pigmented fungi are the most frequently reported mycotic infections of terrestrial amphibians. Chromomycosis in amphibians has been thoroughly reviewed (Schmidt, 1984). Recent case reports offer little new pathological and etiological information, but epidemiologically serve to expand the list of documented host species (Ackermann & Miller, 1992; Bube et al., 1992; Miller et al., 1992; Tell et al., 1994). Most infections are detected in amphibians in captivity, although many cases are reported in free-ranging South American and Southeast Asian anurans (Correa et al., 1968; Dhaliwal & Griffiths, 1964). In addition, several pigmented fungi have been isolated from internal organs of asymptomatic and histologically normal anurans in South America (Mok et al., 1983).

Taxonomy of the fungi and terminology of the disease(s) are in a continual state of flux (Yager & Scott, 1993). The infectious agents are multiple genera of dematiaceous (pigmented) fungi, that can not be identified to species or genus level by gross or histological examinations. Specific identification of pigmented fungi requires culture. Names that have been applied to the lesions produced by pigmented fungi include chromomycosis, chromoblastomycosis, chromohyphomycosis, subcutaneous phaeohyphomycosis, and mycetoma (Ackermann & Miller, 1992; Frank & Roester, 1970; Fraser et al., 1991; Yager & Scott, 1993). The term chromomycoses is usually preceeded by the word superficial, implying an infection limited to the epidermal stratum corneum, which has not been reported in amphibians. Chromoblastomycosis refers to an infection in any organ in which the fungi are bulbous or spherical in shape (muriform cells or chlamydospores). Chromohyphomycoses are infections containing pigmented hyphae. Phaeohyphomycosis is a broad term inclusive of the previous three "chromo-" terms. Rarely, a mycetoma may occur in vertebrates. If the fungi form macroscopic granules (or grains) within a subcutaneous nodule with a draining tract, it is a mycetoma. Most mycetomas are caused by nonpigmented fungi (Yager & Scott, 1993). Usually, only one fungal form predominates, although all three forms may occur in one animal, suggesting the terms chromoblastomycosis and chromohyphomycosis are vague and unnecessary. Chromomycosis is most widely used and accepted in amphibian medicine for all infections by pigmented fungi, regardless of the fungal morphology and tissue tropism.

Unlike endotherms, amphibian chromomycosis may progress into an overwhelming systemic disease. Infections appear to originate in skin wounds or the intestinal tract (Schmidt, 1984). The author has observed masses of uncultured pigmented fungi within crickets used as prey items, paralleling bacterial studies that the intestinal flora of the northern leopard frog, *Rana pipiens*, is derived mostly from prey (Vander Waaij et al., 1974). Most chromomycotic infections have been dermal and subcutaneous. It is widely accepted that the principal sites, the head and limbs, are locations most prone to injury in captive amphibians (Schmidt, 1984), but others suggest not all infections are at sites of possible trauma (Ackermann & Miller, 1992).

Gross findings in chromomycosis are varied. Captive and wild anurans present with raised dermal nodules, up to 20 mm in diameter, on the head, body, and proximal limbs, many of which are extensively ulcerated. Smaller raised nodules, 2–4 mm in diameter, may show little discoloration but may have a central gray area. Swelling may not accompany ulcerations of the digits and distal limbs (Elkan & Philpot, 1973). Occasional ulcers may expose musculature and bone. Ulcers of the digits, snout, and ventral body are most common (Dhaliwal & Griffiths, 1963). Spread of the infection via subcutaneous lymph sacs (Carter, 1979) probably explains many secondary dermal nodules (Ackerman & Miller, 1992). Infections may spread from dermal lesions by direct extension to underlying muscle and bone and via lymphatics to internal organs, especially the mesonephros, liver, spleen, lung, heart, mesentery, intestines, and brain (in approximate descending order of involvement) (Figures 27.25, 27.26). The nodules that are evident in many internal organs are mycotic granulomata. In the northern leopard frog, *Rana pipiens*, granulomata tend to be grayish black or very black, but in other anurans, nodules are grayish white, yellowish tan, or gray; hepatic granulomata tend to be darker. Granulomata may be single or multiple, coalescing, and from barely visible grossly to 3 cm in diameter. Most granulomata are described as about 3–10 mm. Mesonephric nodules may be the largest, up to three times the size of the organ, and occasionally may fuse the mesonephroi. Liver granulomata may be equally large. Some granulomata have caseous cores, and some of these may show concentric laminations. In one captive giant toad, *Bufo marinus*, with neurologic signs, there was severe compression of the brain by a large intracranial granuloma.

Histological examinations reveal intense granulomatous inflammatory reaction or multiple organized granulomata. Within the granulomata the fungi are easily detected as golden brown, dark brown or black hyphae, sclerotic bodies or chlamydospores. Nodules are composed predominantly of macrophages and epithelioid macrophages, with variable numbers of multinucleated giant cells, lymphocytes, plasmacytes, and eosinophils. Some granulomata have numerous multinucleated giant cells and a caseous core. Fungi are extracellular and within multinucleated giant cells. Hyphae have undulating walls, septae, and irregular branching. Hyphae are highly variable in diameter, possibly depending on the fungal species, but most are 2–10 μm in diameter. Hyphae may appear constricted at the septations, and slightly to markedly bulging between septations. When hyphae are the predominant form, chromohyphomycosis may be used as a diagnosis in lieu of chromomycosis. Chlamydospores

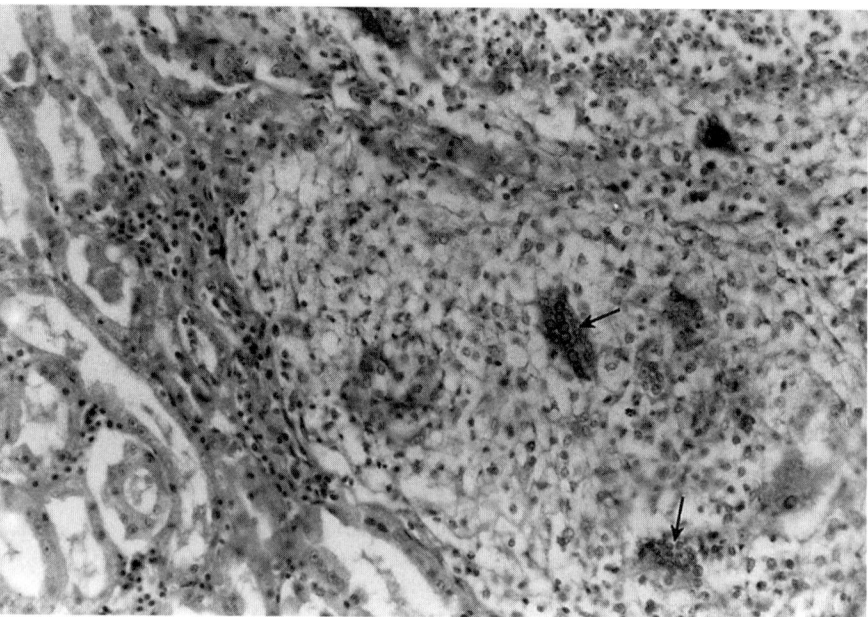

Figure 27.25. Chromomycosis in the mesonephros of a captive specimen of White's treefrog, *Pelodryas caerulea*. This fungal infection spread from an initial skin infection via the subcutaneous lymphatics to the inguinal lymph hearts, to the mesonephroi and other organs. The mesonephros has numerous discrete granulomata composed of epithelioid macrophages, multinucleated giant cells (arrows), and lesser numbers of lymphocytes, neutrophils, and eosinophils. The fungal hyphae are prominently brownish black; many are evident within multinucleated giant cells. (E. Elkan, RTLA 410)

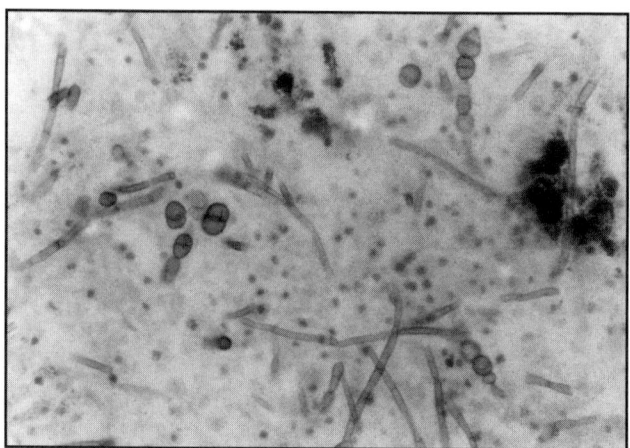

Figure 27.26. Chromomycosis in the liver of a captive northern leopard frog, *Rana pipiens*. In this acute to subacute generalized mycotic infection, brown hyphae were evident in many organs. The liver has many brown hyphae and bulbous fungal elements in a large focus of hepatocellular necrosis. (E. Elkan, RTLA 408)

form terminally and subterminally from the hyphae as spherical or elliptical structures, singly or in chains of up to 10, and are 6–17 μm in diameter. Sclerotic bodies may be found in some lesions. These are round to oval, 10–12 μm in diameter, and have septations in one or two perpendicular planes (equatorial and vertical septations). The presence of sclerotic bodies is the basis of the term, chromoblastomycosis.

Numerous special stains may be employed to better demonstrate fungal hyphae, but this usually is not necessary in cases of chromomycosis. Pigmented fungi are most readily detected in unstained paraffin sections (Migaki & Frye, 1975). Various silver impregnation stains and the periodic acid-Schiff reaction will stain hyphae black or red, respectively.

One case of chromomycosis has been reported in a captive barred tiger salamander, *Ambystoma tigrinum mavortium* (Migaki & Frye, 1975). The fungi were not cultured, but histologically, the organisms were hyphae and chlamydospores. The lesion was solitary, contained numerous multinucleated giant cells, epithelioid macrophages, and eosinophils, and was located in the left prefemoral musculature.

Infectious Etiologies—Protozoan-like Fungi—Dermocystidium spp., Dermosporidium spp., and Dermomycoides spp. As these genus names imply, these organisms cause infections of the skin in amphibians, as well as in fish and molluscs. The taxonomic status of these organisms is uncertain for some authors consider them to be fungi (Goldstein & Moriber, 1966), while others consider them protozoa (see also Section 15.9, *Dermocystidium*, the Protozoan-like Fungi).

Three different genus names have apparently been used for this group of parasites in amphibians, *Dermocystidium*, *Dermosporidium*, and *Dermomycoides* (Broz & Privora, 1952; Green et al., 1995b; Poisson, 1937; Reichenbach-Klinke & Elkan, 1965). For purposes of this discussion, the genera will be treated as one group of fungal organisms. All three genera are described principally in European amphibians, but some, or similar, organisms have been found in the Americas (Jay & Pohley, 1981). *Dermocystidium* contains two species: *Dermocystidium ranae* is described from the European common frog, *Rana temporaria*, and the edible frog, *R. kl. esculenta*, and *Dermocystidium pusula* in European newts (Broz & Privora, 1952; Flynn, 1973; Guyenot & Naville, 1922; Remy, 1931). Four species of *Dermosporidium* have been described: *D. granulosum* in the European common frog, *R. temporaria*, *D. hylarum* in a Brazilian frog, *Hyla rubra* (sic), and *D. multigranulosum* in the edible frog, *R. kl. esculenta*, and *D. penneri* in the American toad, *Bufo americanus* (Broz & Privora, 1952; Carini, 1940; Flynn, 1973; Jay & Pohley, 1981).

Dermocystidium ranae causes discrete, intensely inflammatory dermal nodules (Figures 27.27, 27.28,

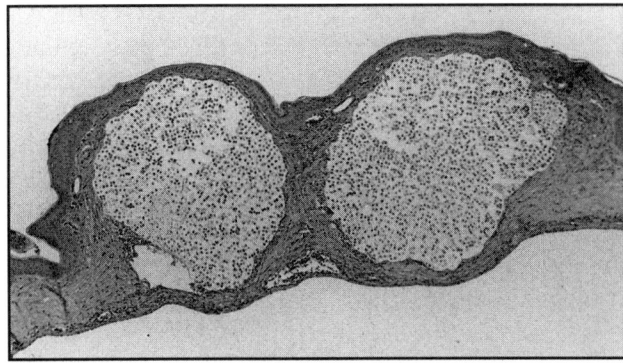

Figure 27.27. Infection of the dermis by a *Dermocystidium*-like organism in an American toad, *Bufo americanus*. This dermal infection produces 0.5–8.0 mm diameter nodules that are filled with "spores." A granulomatous inflammatory reaction to the cyst may be mild to intense. (R. Clapp, RTLA 2417)

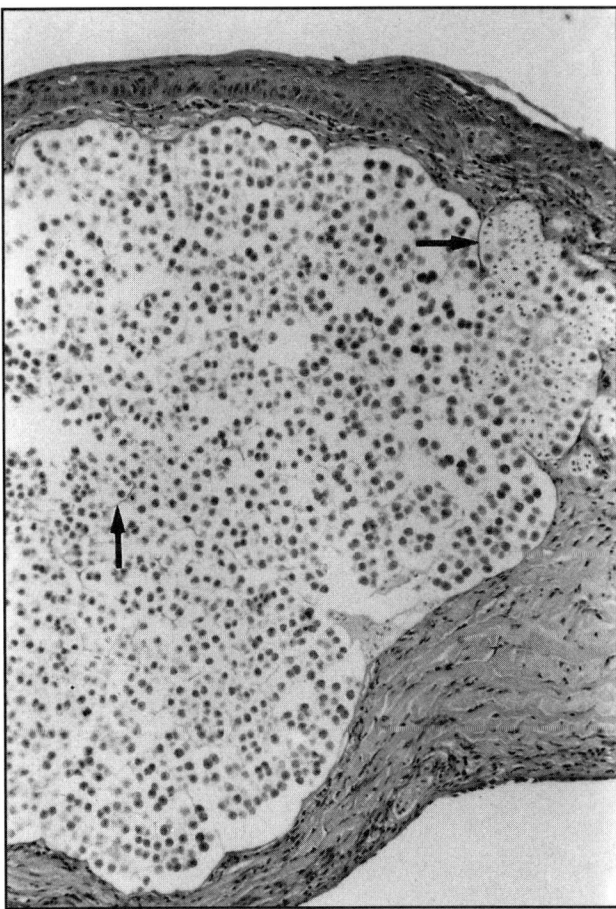

Figure 27.28. Higher magnification of Figure 27.27. A key feature of *Dermosporidium penneri* infections is the presence of thin, barely discernible septal membranes (arrows) that divide the entire "cyst" into multiple chambers. Each chamber contains four or more spores in the same stage of development. Larger spore chambers are found centrally in the "cyst," but septal membranes may break down or become indistinct. (R. Clapp, RTLA 2417)

27.29, 27.30). Some nodules are not visible at necropsy, while others may be up to 10 mm in diameter. Nodules may occur anywhere on the body and head. A prevalence of 5% in a population of the European common frog, *R. temporaria*, near Prague has been reported (Broz & Privora, 1952). The nodule consists of a cyst that is filled with sporelike organisms. Initially, the cyst is about 90 μm long, cylindrical with rounded ends, and only slightly curved. As the cyst enlarges over a period of several months, it becomes progressively more curved until at maximum development it is 1 mm long and distinctly "U" shaped. This large mature cyst is found only in adult breeding frogs in April. The wall of the cyst is 2–3 μm thick, and is filled with spherical spores, 3–12 μm in diameter. Spores have a large central or slightly eccentric clear vacuole. The single nucleus is marginated. The dermal and subcutaneous inflammatory reaction is intense. Early smaller cysts elicit intense infiltrates of macrophages, epithelioid macrophages, and fewer lymphocytes while granulocytes are rare. Epithelioid macrophages initially appear to radiate perpendicularly from the cyst wall, but as the cyst enlarges, inflammatory cells apparently are compressed and lie concentrically around it (Broz & Privora, 1952). The life cycle and method of transmission are unknown (Flynn, 1973).

Other *Dermocystidium* spp., *Dermosporidium* spp., and *Dermomycoides* spp. form spherical or irregularly spherical dermal and epidermal cysts. Grossly, in specimens of the European common frog, *Rana temporaria*, infected by *Dermosporidium granulosum*, one to three raised, dome-shaped and umbilicated nodules may be found that are 4–8 mm in diameter. The sunken central pit is considered an ulcer through which spores are released (Broz & Privora, 1952). Histologically, the cyst is about 1 mm in diameter, is located in the dermis between skin glands, and is surrounded by intense edema, macrophages, lymphocytes, and neutrophils. The cyst wall is very thin and barely discernable. The core of the cyst is divided into numerous small chambers by very thin septal membranes. Within each chamber are four or more spores, generally at the same stage of development. Those organisms in central chambers are usually more mature and spherical (spores), while those at the periphery are immature and contain smaller polygonal organisms (sporoblasts). The latter are about 7 μm in diameter, and mature spores are 10 μm. Mature spores have a central dark round nucleus, and numerous 2 μm diameter vacuoles in the cytoplasm. Prevalence of infection was highly variable. In 1947, 30% of a breeding group of the European common frog, *R. temporaria*, were infected, while in 1949, only two infected frogs could be found (Broz & Privora, 1952).

Dermosporidium multigranulare produces cylindrical cysts that are 0.4–2.0 mm long, and contain spores that are 18 μm in diameter. The parasite has been reported only from the edible frog *Rana kl. esculenta* (Broz & Kulda, 1954).

Dermosporidium hylarum of Brazilian frogs produces spherical-shaped dermal cysts that are 400–500 μm in diameter and contain spores measuring 8–10 μm (Carini, 1940). *Dermosporidium granulosum* has been considered similar to *D. hylarum* (Broz & Privora, 1952), however the spores of *D. hylarum* contain black granules of various sizes.

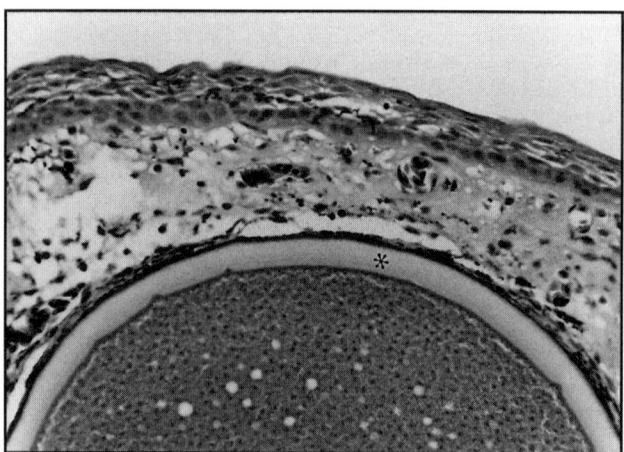

Figure 27.29. *Dermocystidium*-like dermal cyst in a leopard frog from Mexico (possibly *Rana berlandieri*). This organism (bottom) is different from the organisms in Figures 27.27 and 27.28. Note the prominent thick homogenous wall (asterisk) and nonseptate core that is packed with developing spores. (B.J. Cohen, Armed Forces Institute of Pathology 1773295)

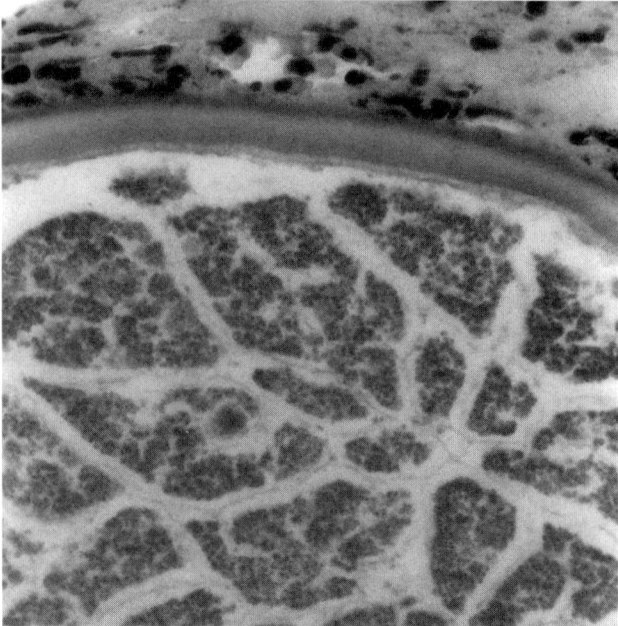

Figure 27.30. *Dermocystidium*-like dermal cyst in a leopard frog, *Rana* sp. The cyst has a thick homogenous wall and the core is divided into irregular packets of spores separated by thin septae. (B.J. Cohen, Armed Forces Institute of Pathology 1773295)

Dermosporidium penneri in the American toad, *Bufo americanus*, produces solitary or multiple 2–6 mm diameter umbilicated nodules or multifocally coalescing nodules principally in the skin of the ventral body. Histologically, spores within the nodules are 10–20 μm in diameter, lack vacuoles but contain about 70 dark, 1.2-μm granules which have been called "inclusion bodies" (Jay & Pohley, 1981).

Dermomycoides armoriacus and *D. beccari* were originally placed in the genus *Dermocystidium* (Broz & Privora, 1952). *Dermomycoides armoriacus* was described from the skin of a palmate newt, *Triturus helveticus* (Poisson, 1937). The cysts of this organism are spherical, and the spores have flagella but lack vacuoles (Broz & Privora, 1952; Reichenbach-Klinke & Elkan, 1965). The second species, *D. beccari*, was described from French specimens of the palmate newt, *T. helveticus*. Grossly, both produce miliary, distinctly raised, spherical nodules in the skin. Some authors consider both species to be indistinguishable histologically from *Dermocystidium* spp. and *Dermosporidium* spp., (Reichenbach-Klinke & Elkan, 1965).

Infectious Etiologies—Protozoal Infections—Microsporidium tritoni. A smooth newt, *Triturus vulgaris*, from Czechoslovakia had a single, ovoid, whitish elevation just anterior to the vent in the dermis. Microsporidia were described from the nodule, however, in the absence of ultrastructural studies, the precise identity, even to the genus level, remains uncertain. It was named *Microsporidum tritoni* (Canning & Lom, 1986).

Various ectoparasitic protozoa may be found in association with epidermal lesions on amphibians, but it may be uncertain whether the protozoa are primary pathogens or opportunistic invaders (Figures 27.31, 27.32, 27.33, 27.34).

Infectious Etiologies—Helminths—Visceral Larval Migrans by Rhabdias sphaerocephala. Juveniles of the giant toad, *Bufo marinus*, were experimentally exposed to large numbers of infective larvae of *Rhabdias sphaerocephala* (Williams, 1960). The larvae were hatched from eggs passed in the feces of local specimens of the giant toad. Two of three juveniles

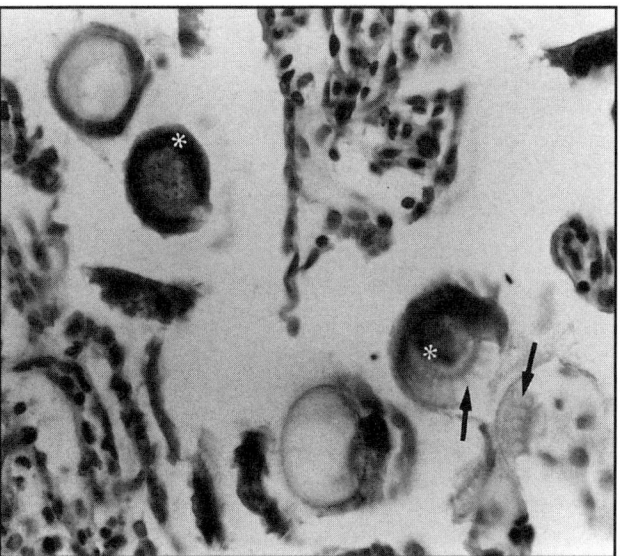

Figure 27.32. *Trichodina*-like ectoparasites in the gill chamber of a wild tadpole of the Pacific treefrog, *Pseudacris regilla*. Note the large horseshoe-shaped macronucleus (asterisks) and the denticles (arrows). Organisms in cross and tangential sections appear as slightly curved discs. (D.E. Green)

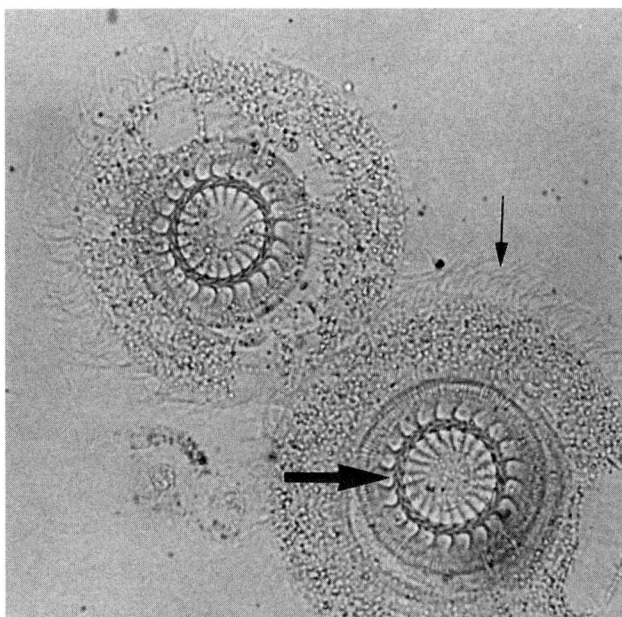

Figure 27.31. *Trichodina*-like ectoparasites from a skin scraping of a wild tadpole of the American toad, *Bufo americanus*. Identifying features of this protozoa include shape, cilia around the oral disc and elsewhere (thin arrow), and shape of the ring denticle (thick arrow). (D.E. Green)

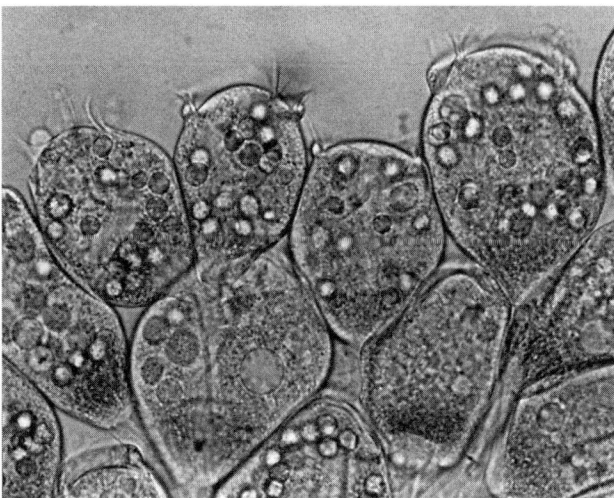

Figure 27.33. Cluster of *Epistylis*-like ectoparasites from a skin scraping of a wild tadpole of the Pacific treefrog, *Pseudacris regilla*. These sessile protozoa are often found around the eyes, spiracle, cloaca, proximal tail, and developing hindlimbs of tadpoles. (D.E. Green)

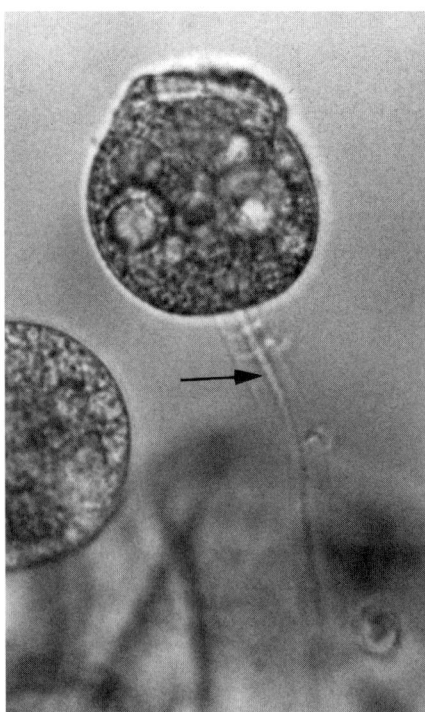

Figure 27.34. *Epistylis*-like ectoparasites from a skin scraping of a wild tadpole of the Pacific treefrog, *Pseudacris regilla*; higher magnification of Figure 27.33. Note the stalk (arrow). (D.E. Green)

died within 24 hours of exposure. Massive numbers of live active larval *Rhabdias sphaerocephala* were observed on the skin surface, on the corneas, and actively burrowing in the subcutis, skeletal muscles and internal organs. Nonencysted, nonencapsulated larvae may be observed in nearly any organ in routine histological examinations of wild and captive anurans. *Rhabdias* and *Strongyloides* are in the same family and have similar life cycles including the capacity for transcutaneous infection by larvae. Histologically, it may be impossible to determine much of the nematodes' morphologic structure in sections because of their small size (Chitwood & Lichtenfels, 1972).

Infectious Etiologies—Helminths—Foleyella spp. and Icosiella spp. Most adult filarid worms inhabit the body cavity, however, *Icosiella neglecta* and *Foleyella duboisi* are found in the dermis or subcutaneous lymph sacs of the European common frog, *Rana temporaria*, the edible frog, *Rana kl. esculenta*, and the marsh frog, *R. ridibunda* (Flynn, 1973; Witenberg & Gerichter, 1944). Microfilaria in the subcutis may cause dermal nodules (Reichenbach-Klinke & Elkan, 1965), but the lesions have not been characterized grossly or histologically. In histological sections, the microfilaria might be mistaken for *Rhabdias* spp. It has been reported that these amphibian filarids have lateral alae while *Rhabdias* spp. does not (Reichenbach-Klinke & Elkan, 1965) but it is more precise to state that the filarids have large lateral chords (Chitwood & Lichtenfels, 1972). Microfilaria are produced by mature female filarids and may be found in histologic sections of lymph and blood vessels in nearly any organ. The microfilaria of *F. brachyoptera* are 120–168 μm long with a hooked tail; those of *F. ranae* are 114–163 μm, and *F. dolichoptera* are 263–295 μm long (Flynn, 1973). In most cases it is not possible to identify microfilaria to genus or species in histologic sections.

Infectious Etiologies—Helminths—Capillarid Dermatitis. *Pseudocapillaroides xenopi* (syn = *Capillaria xenopodis*) may cause significant morbidity and mortality in captive colonies of the African clawed frog, *Xenopus laevis*. Most mortality may be attributed to secondary bacterial skin infections that progress to septicemia. The parasite inhabits the epidermis, principally on the dorsum of the body. The life cycle is direct, hence, heavy infections may develop within 6–18 months in frogs that share an enclosure. The normal smooth skin of the back becomes roughened, pitted, ulcerated, hyperemic or grayish over a period of 2–4 months. As the infection progresses, frogs become lethargic, anorectic, thin, and patches of skin may slough. It is possible to see the white nematodes occasionally beneath the mucus on the skin surface with magnification provided by a dissecting microscope. Female nematodes are 2–4 mm in length. Parasites and ova may be detected more readily in skin scrapings and in the sediment of the aquarium. Flakes of skin may contain parasites, larvated eggs, and elongate tunnels (Cunningham et al., 1996a; Stephens et al., 1987).

Histologically, the skin of the back is affected. The parasites are confined to the epidermis, although degenerative and inflammatory changes also occur in the dermis. The epidermis shows a variety of inflammatory, degenerative, and proliferative changes. Segments of the epidermis may show erosions or ulcerations, alternating with regions of acanthosis, parakeratosis, and dyskeratosis (Cunningham et al., 1996a). Vacuolization of epidermal cells, and separation of the epidermis from the basement membrane also may be present. Empty tunnels and tunnels containing nematodes or larvated eggs are evident in the epidermis (Figures 27.35, 27.36). Some tunnels become more dilated or cystic, and may contain degenerate epithelial cells, granulocytes, dead parasites or their ova, bacteria, fungi, protozoa, and proteinaceous debris. Granulocytes predominate in the epidermis, while lymphocytes are the major inflammatory cell in the dermis. Fluid accumulation may be evident in the dermis. Histological descriptions of the nematodes have not been given (Stephens et al., 1987), but they have the standard features of the nematode group, *Trichinellina* (Chitwood & Lichtenfels, 1972). The ova are different from most ova of the genus *Capillaria* in that they are thin-walled and lar-

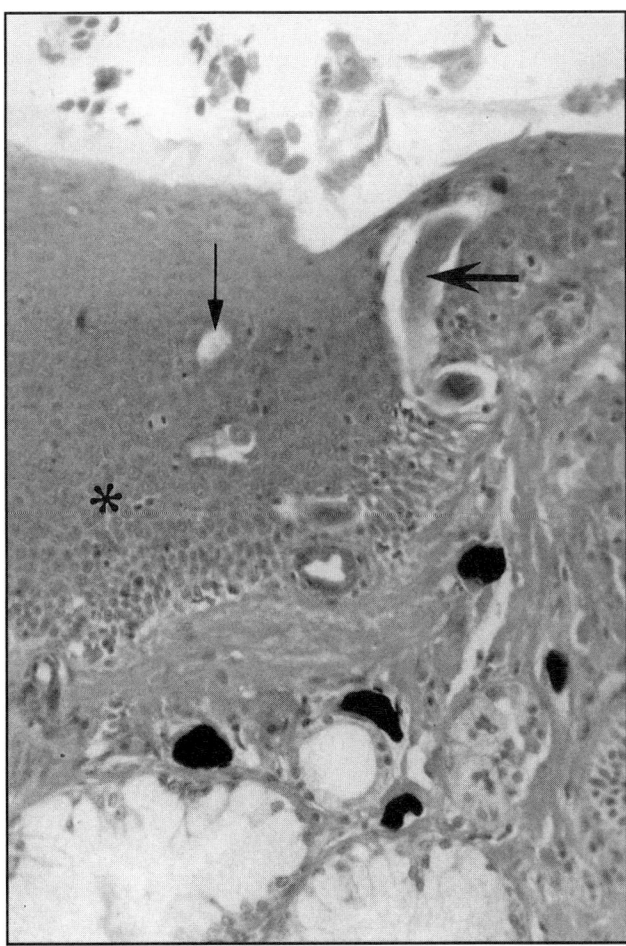

Figure 27.35. Capillarid epidermitis in a captive African clawed frog, *Xenopus laevis*. In this mild infection of the dorsal skin, *Pseudocapillaroides xenopi* (large arrow) is found only in the epidermis. There is marked epidermal hyperplasia (asterisk). Burrow holes are evident (thin arrow). (G.E. Cosgrove, RTLA 1669)

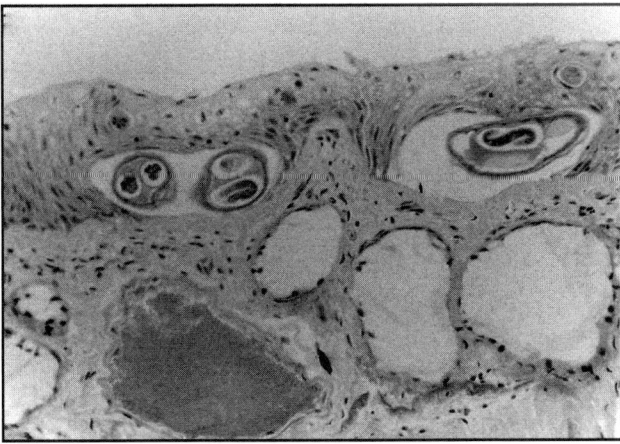

Figure 27.36. Capillarid epidermitis in a captive African clawed frog, *Xenopus laevis*. Note the larvated eggs within the oviducts of two female *Pseudocapillaroides xenopi*. (C.S. Patton, Armed Forces Institute of Pathology 2132692)

vated. The ova retain the standard features of being bioperculate (bipolar plugs) and barrel-shaped. These parasites were not found in the dermis nor any internal organs (Stephens et al., 1987).

An unidentified nematode has been found associated with similar lesions in the Cayenne caecilian, *Typhlonectes compressicauda*, at the Philadelphia Zoological Garden (personal communication, K. Wright, 1997).

Infectious Etiologies—Helminths—Epidermal Trematodes. As adults, *Glypthelmins* spp. and *Haplometra* spp., infect the intestines of multiple species of North American ranids. The cercariae (xiphidiocercariae) of these trematodes begin the infection by penetrating and "encysting" in the epidermis of the tadpole and adult frog. During ecdysis in metamorphosed frogs, the "encysted" cercariae are shed with the skin, and the skin is eaten by the frog, thus finishing the life cycle (Olsen, 1937; Rannala, 1990). The histological features of the epidermal and enteric infections have not been described.

Infectious Etiologies—Arthropods—Ticks. Larger species of toads may be host to a variety of ticks. Ticks are most often found attached to the head or neck, including the parotid glands of anurans (Zug & Zug, 1979). Up to 100% of the giant toad, *Bufo marinus*, may have ticks during certain seasons. In an extensive study of a wild population of the giant toad, *B. marinus*, secondary infections of bite wounds by ticks were not observed (Zug & Zug, 1979).

Infectious Etiologies—Arthropods—Mites and Chiggers. Larval trombiculid mites, commonly called chiggers, are often found embedded in the dermis of anurans and salamanders. Amphibian trombiculid mites remain embedded in the dermis for a prolonged time. Five genera have been described in amphibians. The genera, *Anouracarus* and *Vercannenia*, are found in Asian and Pacific amphibians, while *Endotrombicula* and *Schongastia* are found in amphibians in Africa. The fifth genus, *Hannemania*, is widespread in the Western Hemisphere. Among chiggers, only the larval stage actively feeds on vertebrates. Later stages are free-living and not parasitic. Some species of *Hannemania* may persist in the dermis for more than 9 months (Welbourn & Loomis, 1970, 1975). Several species of *Hannemania* are found in North American amphibians. The most commonly encountered taxa in the eastern United States are *H. dunni* and *H. penetrans* (Flynn, 1973). Grossly, infected amphibians have bright red nodules, 0.25–1 mm in diameter, on the skin. The most common site of infection in salamanders is the distal limbs, especially the webbing between digits (Duncan & Highton, 1979). In anurans, the most common location is the ventral and caudal skin of the hindlimbs and abdomen (Worms, 1967). However, nodules may be found anywhere on the head, body, and tail of terrestrial amphibians (Plates 27.6, 27.7, 27.8). Histologically, the larvae are present in the dermis in a roughly spherical cystlike granuloma (Hyland, 1961) (Figure 27.37). The host reaction in subacute and chronic infections is mild; there is a thin layer of flattened epithelioid macrophages adjacent to the larvum, with varying amounts of fibrocytes and collagen deposition. The larvum has a thin chitinous exoskeleton that is eosinophilic and periodic acid-Schiff-negative; other histological features of the larvum are typical of arthropoda (Chitwood & Lichtenfels, 1972).

Because the trombiculid mites feed only in the larval stage, skin mite infections in amphibians are limited to recently captured animals (less than 12 months in captivity) or ones exposed to contaminated soil or cage furnishings. In certain populations of amphibians, the prevalence may be 60–99% (Duncan & Highton, 1979; Welbourn & Loomis, 1970, 1975), while in other sympatric anurans and salamanders, prevalence may be 0–33% (Murphy, 1965; Rankin, 1937). In Arkansas, the Rich Mountain salamander, *Plethodon ouachitae,* may have a prevalence of greater than 90%, but western slimy salamanders, *P. albagula,* are rarely infested, even when they are found together under the same log (Duncan & Highton, 1979). In central East Africa, heavy infections by the trombiculid, *Schongastia rana,* were reported in the Angola frog, *Rana angolensis* (Ball, 1967). Mites have not been encountered in wild European amphibians (Worms, 1967).

Amphibians may occasionally be infected by species of chiggers that principally infect reptiles, such as *Eutrombicula alfreddugesi* and *E. splendens. Eutrombicula alfreddugesi* has been found on North American bufonids, and *E. splendens* has been reported on hylid treefrogs in the southeastern United States (Flynn, 1973).

Infectious Etiologies—Arthropods—Myiasis. Larvae (maggots) of several taxa of Diptera (flies) may infect the subcutis and nasal cavity of amphibians. Subcutaneous myiasis is not uncommon among wild Australian anurans, and also occurs in India and Europe. Different genera of flies infest the nasal cavities and subcutis. Infestations of the nasal cavity usually are by massive numbers of maggots, while subcutaneous infections generally consist of 1–10 maggots. In Australia, ten *Batrachomyia* spp., have been detected

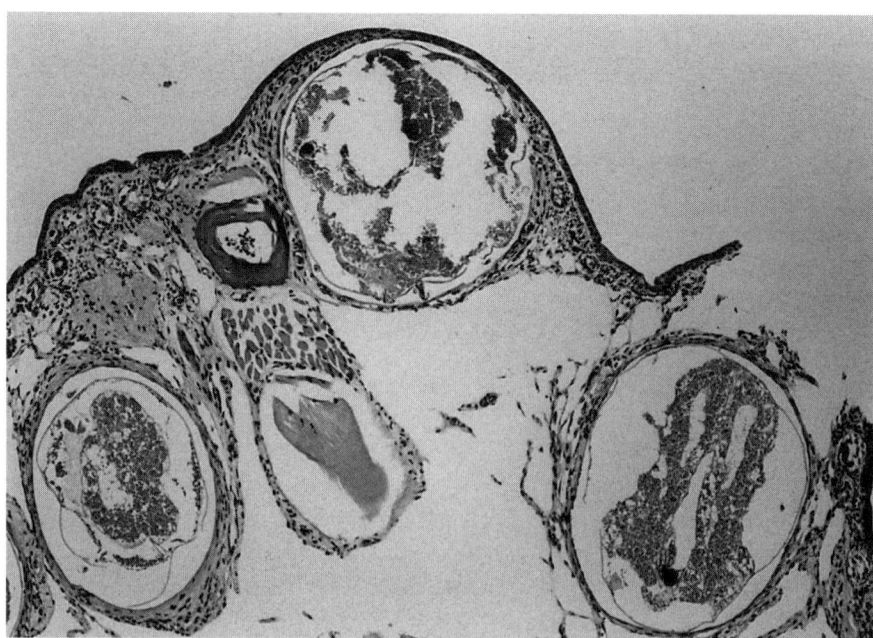

Figure 27.37. Nymphal chigger infection (*Hannemania dunni*) in a wild Fourche Mountain salamander, *Plethodon fourchensis*. (Same animal as Plates 27.7 and 27.8.) Three nymphs are embedded in the dermis of the toe webs. Although these chiggers were present for over 3 months, there is minimal inflammatory cell response. (D.E. Green)

in over 11 species of frogs and toads (Elkan, 1965; McAlpine, 1955 *fide* Vogelnest, 1994; Zumpt, 1965). In one case, a maggot lying in the dorsal lymph sac had perforated the fascia and muscular body wall to lie partially within the coelomic cavity in contact with abdominal viscera. Histologically, the fascia surrounding the maggot was thickened but otherwise free of cellular reaction (Elkan, 1965). About 10% of infected frogs may die when the maggot(s) emerge (McAlpine, 1955, as cited by Vogelnest, 1994).

However, mortality rates approach 10% in Central and South American anurans infected by *Notochaeta bufonivora*. During the dry season in Costa Rica, 1–12 maggots may be found per Veragoa stubfoot toad, *Atelopus varius*. The prevalence of infection was found to be 5.3% in one season. The early stage of infection is characterized by a "single small wound on the posterior surface on one thigh, which was noticeably swollen" (Crump & Pounds, 1985). Breathing spiracles of one or more maggots are evident in the skin ulcer. The maggots first consume the thigh musculature and then the visceral organs. Once maggots are grossly evident in the leg, death of the host invariably occurs within 4 days (Crump & Pounds, 1985). Histological features of infected anurans have not been reported.

27.2.3 Alimentary Tract

Histological examinations of the livers of amphibians are complicated by the presence of extra-medullary hematolymphopoiesis (EMH) in the subcapsular regions and sinuses, and by variable numbers of melanin-laden melanomacrophage aggregates (MMA). EMH may be mistaken for hepatitis or serositis of the liver, while MMA may constitute 50% of the hepatic section. When MMA are extensive, use of the melanin-bleach technique prior to application of standard or special stains should be considered.

Clusters of melanin-laden macrophages within the liver are known as melanomacrophage centers (MMC) or melanomacrophage aggregates. These are well known and best studied in fish (Aguis, 1980), but similar structures in amphibians have received scant attention (Barrutia et al., 1983; Manning & Horton, 1982; Saad & El Masri, 1995). MMAs are present in many organs, including liver, spleen, lymphomyeloid organs, thymus, and others. In some amphibians, the liver has large numbers of MMAs, imparting a black color at necropsy. Ultrastructurally, MMAs are composed of macrophage-like phagocytic cells; their cytoplasm is filled with melanin granules and traces of lipids, neutral mucopolysaccharides, basic proteins, membranous vacuoles, and cell debris (Saad & El Masri, 1995).

The pancreas of adult amphibians consists of exocrine and endocrine (islets of Langerhans) cells. Most amphibians have at least three distinct pancreatic lobes (or processes), the hepatic, splenic, and duodenal lobes. During metamorphosis, the larval pancreas undergoes considerable degeneration, structural change, and subsequent regeneration (Fox, 1981). Volume reduction of the pancreas between larval and postmetamorphic stages is about 70–80%. Necrotic exocrine cells are described as sloughing into sinudoidal cavities and pancreatic ducts, and being phagocytosed in situ. After metamorphosis is complete, the pancreas regenerates and increases in size. Histologically, the pancreatic acini are similar to most other vertebrates, and have been described ultrastructurally (Fox, 1981).

Herbivorous tadpoles have long, coiled intestinal tracts, which, during metamorphosis, become shorter, consistent with a change from herbivory to carnivory. Algae-eating tadpoles may depend on bacterial hydrolysis in the gut to obtain nutrition from their feed, because experimental bacteria-free tadpoles do not survive much beyond the exhaustion of yolk reserves (Timmons et al., 1977).

Nutritional Etiologies—Hypocalcemia-related Cloacal Prolapse. Cloacal prolapse occurred in bullfrogs, *Rana catesbeiana*, that developed hypocalcemic tremors following feeding trials with crickets only (Modzelewski & Culley, 1974).

Toxicological Etiologies—Petroleum Intoxication in Tadpoles. The effects of crankcase oil and fuel oil on tadpoles has been examined (Mahaney, 1994; McGrath & Alexander, 1979). At levels of 55 and 100 mg/L of used crankcase oil, tadpoles of the green treefrog, *Hyla cinerea*, show stunted growth. At the higher level, no tadpoles successfully metamophosed and most failed to develop hindlimbs (Mahaney, 1994). No attempt was made to study histological changes in the treefrog tadpoles. Many tadpoles are filter feeders, and they have been observed attacking and gulping suspended oil droplets from the water column. Tadpoles of the bullfrog, *Rana catesbeiana,* that ingest oil droplets have oil in their stomach and intestines, and have hepatomegaly and distended gall bladders. Tadpoles may appear bloated, abnormally buoyant, and have difficulty returning to the bottom of the tank (Mahaney, 1994; McGrath & Alexander, 1979). Small concentrations of fuel oil may kill late stage bullfrog tadpoles, and the abnormal buoyancy in others makes them more susceptible to predation (McGrath & Alexander, 1979). The lethal concentration for 50% (LC50) of larvae of the wood frog, *Rana sylvatica,* and the spotted salamander, *Ambystoma maculatum,* to four types of oils was lower than that for fish (Hedtke & Puglisi, 1982). Illegal dumping of waste oil in a stream caused the deaths of 46 specimens of the endangered Japanese giant salamander, *Andrias japonicus,* while other salamanders developed "severe skin damage" that was not further characterized (Matsui & Hayashi, 1992).

Toxicological Etiologies—Benzene Hexachloride. Gastric prolapse (eversion of the stomach through the mouth) and cloacal prolapse occur in experimental intoxication of the northern leopard frog, *Rana pipiens,* with the insecticide, benzene hexachloride (Kaplan & Overpeck, 1964) (Figure 27.38). No additional gross or histological details were given.

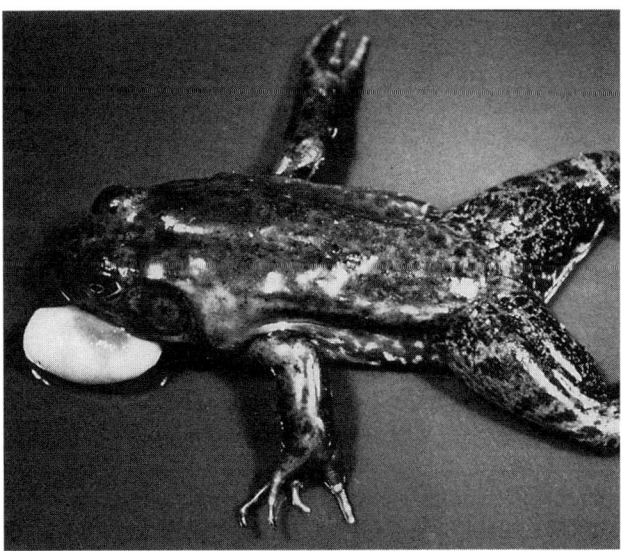

Figure 27.38. Gastric prolapse in a green frog, *Rana clamitans*. This condition is most often associated with hypocalcemia, hypoglycemia, or insecticide intoxication. (D.E. Green)

Toxicological Etiologies—Aflatoxicosis. Aflatoxin B_1 was studied experimentally for its potential carcinogenicity in the square-marked toad, *Bufo regularis* (El-Mofty & Sakr, 1988), but descriptions of acute or subacute lesions in the liver cells and bile ducts were not reported. Although the experimental exposure of toads to aflatoxin resulted in development of tumors in the livers, spleens, and mesonephroi, these tumors resembled infectious granulomata rather than neoplastic disease (Figures 27.39, 27.40).

Toxicological Etiologies—Copper. Exceptionally high levels of copper have been detected in the livers of British specimens of the European common frog, *Rana temporaria*, involved in repeated mass mortality events. However, the significance of cuprosis in the mortalities was not established, and gross and histological examinations were inconclusive due to the concurrence of Gram-negative bacillary septicemias and multiple viral agents (Cunningham et al., 1995). Hepatic copper levels in dead and euthanized frogs ranged from 291–9361 mg/kg (dry weight). The source of copper in these frogs was not investigated.

Infectious Etiologies—Viral. No enteric viral pathogens have been reported in aquatic amphibians, however, the intestine and stomach may develop lesions as part of systemic viral infections such as ranaviral infections of anurans.

Several rana- and ranalike viruses (in the family Iridoviridae) produce an inclusion body hepatitis or necrotizing hepatitis. The ranaviruses or suspected ranaviruses that have been associated with hepatitis include tadpole edema virus (TEV), Bohle iridovirus (BIV), VHSF-REIR (viral hemorrhagic septicemia of frogs, *Rana esculenta* iridovirus), and an as yet unnamed iridovirus associated with several syndromes in European common frogs, *Rana temporaria*, from southeastern England (Cullen et al., 1995; Cunningham et al., 1996b; Fijan et al., 1991; Kunst & Valpotic, 1968; Miscalencu et al., 1981; Wolf et al., 1968). Grossly, hepatic lesions are seldom observed. Histologically, TEV and BIV produce multifocal to panlobular hepatocellular necrosis (Cullen et al., 1995; Wolf et al., 1968). Initially, there is nuclear pyknosis of hepatocytes and macrophages in the melanomacrophage aggregates; this progresses to karyorrhexis and the lesions expand to involve larger and larger foci. In some experimental anurans, the entire liver may be necrotic. Experimentally, TEV causes

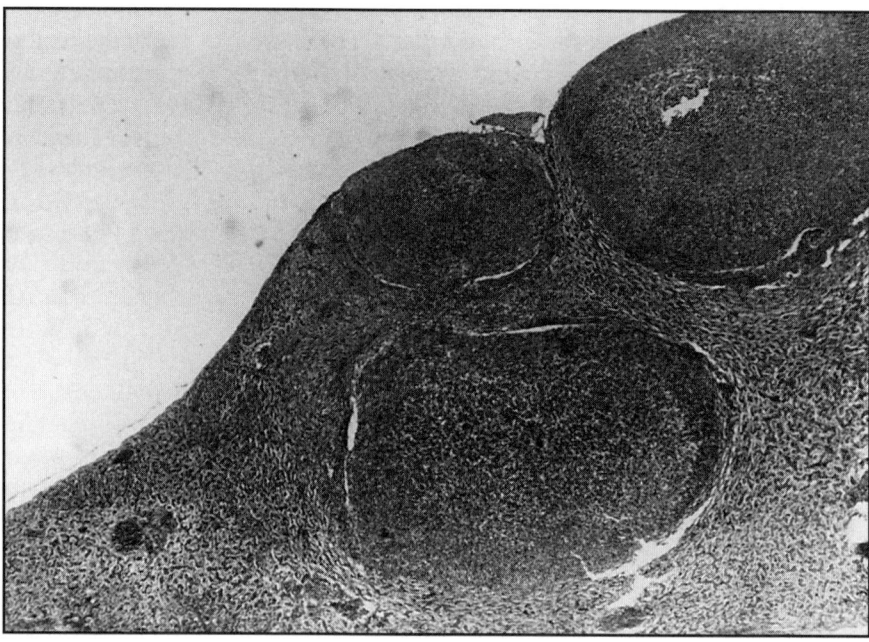

Figure 27.39. Granulomata in the liver of a captive square-marked toad, *Bufo regularis*. Note the discrete noninfiltrative nature with compression of adjacent normal tissue. Although etiology was not confirmed in this case, it is typical of mycobacterial granulomata. (M.M. El-Mofty, RTLA 2363)

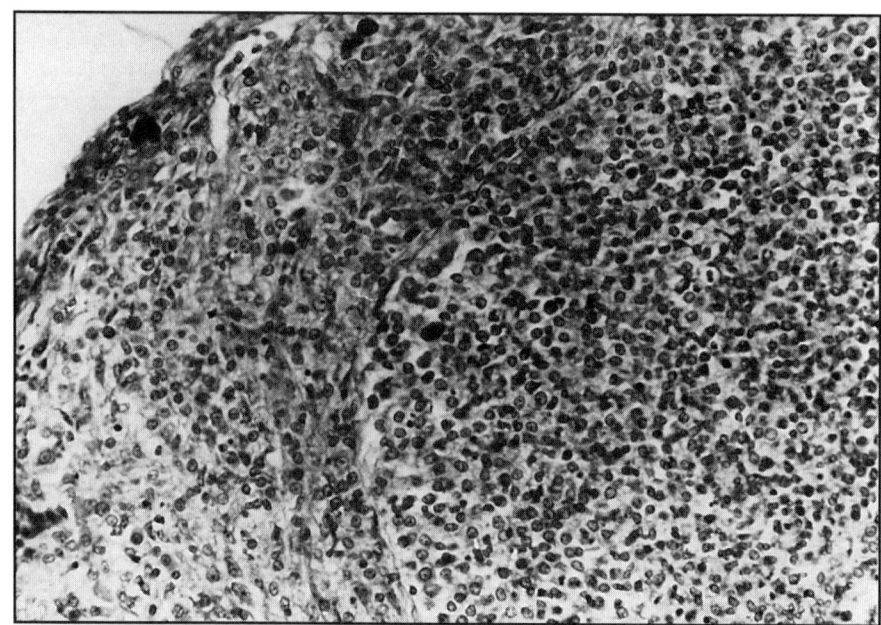

Figure 27.40. Higher magnification of Figure 27.39. The macrophages that compose this granuloma have pleomorphic nuclei, and indistinct lightly eosinophilic cytoplasm. Far fewer granulocytes and lymphocytes are present. (M.M. El-Mofty, RTLA 2363)

hepatocellular necrosis in tadpoles of the bullfrog, *Rana catesbeiana,* and metamorphs of Fowler's toad, *Bufo woodhousei fowleri,* but not metamorphs and adults of the bullfrog, *R. catesbeiana* (Wolf et al., 1968, 1969). Experimental BIV infections in Australian anurans cause hepatic necrosis with hemorrhages in tadpoles and recent metamorphs of the ornate burrowing frog, *Limnodynastes ornatus,* northern banjo frog, *Limnodynastes terraereginae,* and giant toad, *Bufo marinus,* and in adult giant toads and recent metamorphs of the Australian variable treefrog, *Litoria latopalmata* (Cullen et al., 1995; Moody & Owens, 1994). Bohle iridovirus is also lethal to tadpoles of White's treefrog, *Pelodryas (Litoria) caerulea,* but specific lesions have not been described (Moody & Owens, 1994). Inclusion bodies have not been reported in infections with BIV.

Inclusion body hepatitis, consisting of basophilic and eosinophilic intracytoplasmic inclusions, has been observed in European common frogs, *Rana temporaria,* infected by an unnamed iridovirus(es). The basophilic inclusions are dense, dark, round and about one-third the diameter of the hepatocyte's nucleus; they could be mistaken for karyorrhectic debris, except that the nucleus of the hepatocyte appears essentially normal. The eosinophilic inclusions are round, pale, have a clear halo, and are about the diameter of the nucleus. This inclusion body hepatitis was not associated with overt hepatocellular necrosis. Ultrastructurally, the basophilic inclusions consist of a core of icosohedral virus particles surrounded by rough endoplasmic reticulum (rER), while the eosinophilic inclusions are composed of whorls of rER with ill-defined central debris (Cunningham et al., 1996).

One ultrastructural study of the livers of Romanian specimens of the edible frog, *Rana kl. esculenta,* reported intracytoplasmic icosahedral viruses about 100 nm in size. No clinical signs, gross lesions, or histological findings were reported (Miscalencu et al., 1981). Morphology of the virus particles was consistent with a ranavirus or herpesvirus, although the absence of virions in hepatic nuclei makes ranavirus more likely. It is likely the observed virus was "viral hemorrhagic septicemia of frogs," which has been isolated from the same species of frog in neighboring Yugoslavia (Fijan et al., 1991; Kunst & Valpotic, 1968).

Infectious Etiologies—Chlamydial. Spontaneous chlamydiosis has been reported in the African clawed frog, *Xenopus laevis* (Howerth, 1984; Newcomer et al., 1982). Chlamydial infection causes striking hepatomegaly and hepatitis in addition to its effects on other organ systems.

Spontaneously and experimentally infected frogs show lethargy, a tendency to surface more frequently to breathe, disequilibrium, patchy depigmentation and petechiation of the skin, skin ulcers, and bloating (subcutaneous edema). Spontaneous mortality in a 2–3 month period in a group of 40,000 frogs was approximately 50%. The source of the infection was not confirmed, but was implicated as being raw chopped beef liver which had been condemned for human consumption.

At necropsy, lesions are hepatosplenomegaly, subcutaneous edema, coelomic effusion, cutaneous petechiation, and epidermal ulceration. Lesions are similar in spontaneously and experimentally infected frogs.

Histological findings in spontaneously and experimentally infected frogs are similar and consist of pyogranulomatous inflammation of the liver, spleen, mesonephros, lung, and heart. Livers are diffusely affected. There is increased cellularity in the sinusoids composed of macrophages (including swollen Kupffer cells), lymphocytes, and neutrophils, in varying mixtures. Some regions may be principally suppurative. Hepatocellular necrosis was not described but was implied by hepatic regeneration and bile duct proliferation. Basophilic intracytoplasmic inclusion bodies are readily detected in sinusoidal cells (endothelium and Kupffer cells). Inclusions are polymorphic but principally ellipsoidal or crescentric, and may fill the cytoplasm sufficiently to obscure the nucleus. The inclusions may have a central vacuole and contain numerous small coccoid elements. Splenic lesions are varied and consist of diffuse histiocytosis, foci of congestion, suppuration, and necrosis. Large subcapsular nodules of fibrinopurulent inflammation may be present. Basophilic cytoplasmic inclusions are present in cells in the splenic sinusoids (Howerth, 1984).

Glomerular and interstitial lesions developed in the mesonephroi. Glomeruli show increased eosinophilic matrix, hypercellularity, pyknotic nuclei, and intracytoplasmic inclusions. Purulent exudate may fill Bowman's space, and obliterate glomerular tufts or result in adhesions of the tuft. The inflammatory reaction involving some glomeruli extends into surounding interstitium. Hyaline casts are present in some tubules.

Lung lesions are marked and interstitial. Septae are more than five times thicker than normal, edematous and hypercellular. Interstitial cells consist of small macrophages and neutrophils in varying mixtures. Lining pneumocytes show segmental to disseminated epithelialization. Air spaces and bronchi have multiple foci of acute suppuration. Intravascular emboli may be present. Inclusions are present in interstitial macrophages, but are much fewer in number than in the liver, spleen, and mesonephros. The heart lesions consist of valvular, mural, and subendocardial inflammation. Vegetative endocarditis of the valves and atria is multifocal, composed of fibrin and neutrophils, and occurred in 100% of spontaneously infected frogs but in only 22% of experimentally infected frogs. Granulomatous and pyogranulomatous endomyocarditis may be diffuse in the ventricles, but myofiber necrosis and inclusions are mild (Howerth, 1984; Newcomer et al., 1982).

Ultrastructurally, hepatic inclusions consist of two populations of double membrane-bound organisms within a single membrane-bound space in the host cytoplasm. Smaller particles (elementary bodies) are 250–400 nm and have a central or eccentric denser core. Larger particles (initial bodies) are 400–1000 nm with a internal structure composed primarily of small granules, some of which resemble ribosomes. Intermediate stages of development with characteristics of both elementary and initial bodies may be found.

Infectious Etiologies—Bacterial. The gastrointestinal tract may develop lesions with other visceral organs in Gram-negative bacillary dermatosepticemias. *Salmonella* and *Yersinia* have been isolated from asymptomatic adult frogs and toads but there appear to be no reports of enteropathogens in larvae. *Salmonella* isolates have not been reported in aquatic adult amphibians but *Yersinia intermedia, Y. enterocolitica,* and other *Yersinia* spp. have been obtained from the intestines of asymptomatic specimens of the red-spotted newt, *Notophthalmus viridescens* (Green, unpublished data). No gross or histologic lesions were found in the intestines. The distribution of this pathogen in extraintestinal organs remains unknown. Over 24 species of *Salmonella* have been isolated from the feces and intestines of wild specimens of the giant toad, *Bufo marinus* (Bool & Kampelmacher, 1958; O'Shea et al., 1990). *Salmonella*-associated disease in amphibians has not been documented conclusively (Anver & Pond, 1984), but one report describes a frog with paralysis and ecchymotic hemorrhages on the ventral skin (Urbain, 1944 as cited by Reichenbach-Klinke & Elkan, 1965). *Salmonella paratyphi-B* was recovered from the frog but there is no evidence that this was the cause of the clinical signs. In one *Salmonella* survey of wildlife on two Caribbean islands, 25 (40%) of 60 specimens of the giant toad, *Bufo marinus,* and one of two specimens of the lesser treefrog, *Hyla minuta,* carried one or more species of *Salmonella* (Everard et al., 1979). In other areas *Salmonella* recovery rates may be low. In the laboratory of the author, over 250 wild amphibians have been cultured specifically for *Salmonella* with no isolates to date. *Salmonella* has also been isolated from frogs' legs intended for human consumption (Mayrick, 1976) and from captive pet frogs that were implicated in human infections (Bartlett et al., 1977; Trust et al., 1981). *Salmonella*-infected wild amphibians may reflect environmental contamination by sewage, and isolations may be more common from amphibians in developing countries (Anver & Pond, 1984), while in captivity the bacteria isolated from the intestines of anurans most likely originates from the invertebrates that are fed as live food (Vander Waaij et al., 1974).

Long segmented filamentous bacteria have been observed in cytological smears of the intestine from captive adults of the clawed frog, *Xenopus* spp. (Klaasen et al., 1993). Spiral bacteria have been detected in the intestines of many anurans, but their significance is unknown (Figures 27.41, 27.42).

High levels of unspeciated *Clostridium* bacteria

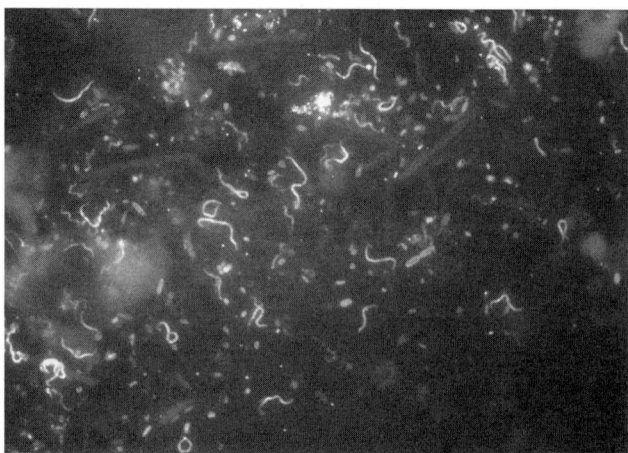

Figure 27.41. Spiral bacteria in the intestine of a wild spotted frog, *Rana pretiosa,* revealed by direct fluorescent antibody test. Massive numbers of spiral bacteria and a few short thick bacilli are fluorescing (white). The antibody is not specific for leptospires. The significance of spiral bacteria in amphibians is unknown. (D.E. Green)

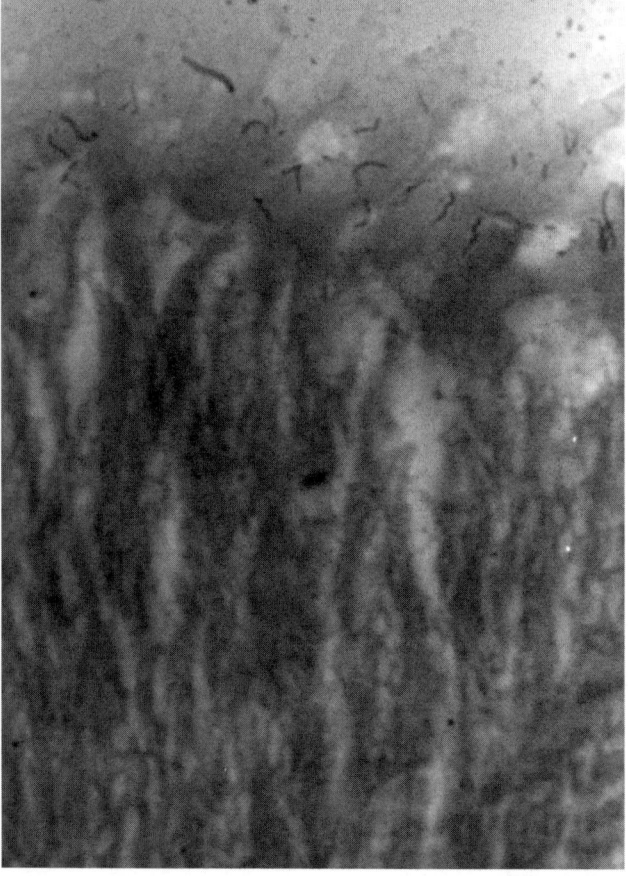

Figure 27.42. Spiral bacteria on the colonic mucosa of a wild giant toad, *Bufo marinus* (Warthin-Starry stain). These unidentified spiral bacteria (top) were not associated with any lesions. (D.E. Green)

were detected in the livers of ill larvae of the tiger salamander, *Ambystoma tigrinum nebulosum,* in Arizona, but no gross or histologic lesions in the liver were reported. The affected larvae were "diseased," prone to cannibalism, prone to late summer mass mortalities, inhabited lakes frequented by livestock, and, probably as a consequence of the livestock, were from lakes with Gram-negative bacterial counts over four times that of lakes not frequented by livestock. The clinical signs in affected larvae were lethargy with a tendency to float at the surface of the pond, reddening of the skin around the vent and proximal limbs, and death within one week of onset (Pfennig et al., 1991).

Cloacal prolapse occurred in specimens of the northern leopard frog, *Rana pipiens,* that died with tremors and convulsions due to advanced red leg syndrome (Emerson & Norris, 1905).

Infectious Etiologies—Mycobacterium. Mycobacteriosis due to *Mycobacterium marinum* begins as an infection of the intestines in experimental infections of young tadpoles (probably *Rana pipiens*) (Nonidez & Kahn, 1937). Nearly all cases of amphibian mycobacteriosis have been reported in adult anurans. Although liver granulomata are most likely to be observed at necropsy, the first cells to be infected in tadpoles that ingest the bacteria are intestinal goblet cells (Nonidez & Kahn, 1937).

Mycobacteriosis in clawed frogs, *Xenopus* spp., may present as a solitary massive granuloma in nearly any organ or tissue (Elkan, 1976b), but this appears to be uncommon in terrestrial adult amphibians. Usually, the amphibian is presented in an advanced stage in which the disease is generalized. Miliary granulomas may be observed in many organs (Asfari, 1988; Darzins, 1952; Jara, 1972; Machicao & LaPlaca, 1954), but in the subclinical or early stages of mycobacteriosis, the intestines, spleen, and liver are most consistently affected. Weight loss and emaciation are not constant findings in mycobacteriosis. In a study of wild specimens of the Juliaca four-eyed frog, *Pleurodema cinerea,* the marbled four-eyed frog, *Pleurodema marmoratus,* and the warty toad, *Bufo spinulosus,* in Bolivia, 129 (19.6%) of 663 frogs, and 3 (0.5%) of 600 toads had mycobacteriosis (Machicao & LaPlaca, 1954). In a study of Brazilian South American bullfrogs (gias), *Leptodactylus pentadactylus,* from an urban area, 100% (n = 60) had mycobacteriosis, while only 20% from "remote" regions of the same state were infected (Darzins, 1952). The livers consistently had granulomas. In a study of 234 toads and frogs from the Amazon region of Brazil, no animals had gross lesions of mycobacteriosis, but *Mycobacterium cheloni abscessus* was isolated from the liver or spleen or 4 (6%) of 66 wild specimens of the giant toad, *Bufo marinus,* and from the mesonephros or coelomic fluid of 2 (2%) of 86 wild specimens of the common lesser toad, *Bufo granulosus* (Mok & Carvalho, 1984). Granulomata have been described as highly variable in size, spherical, firm to fibrous, and consistently pale (unpigmented). Larger granulomata have a whitish to yellowish caseous core. Mineralization and cavitation have not been reported in amphibian mycobacteriosis.

Detailed gross and histological observations of the acute stages of experimental mycobacteriosis by *M. marinum* in tadpoles have been reported (Nonidez & Kahn, 1937). Following ingestion of cultured mycobacteria, massive numbers of acid-fast bacilli persist in the intestinal lumen, despite frequent changes of sterile water, suggesting that the mycobacteria proliferate intraluminally. The first cells to be infected, within 48 hours of ingestion, were goblet cells which had recently discharged their mucous vacuoles. The process by which the intraluminal mycobacteria entered only these cells was not determined. Within hours, infected goblet cells degenerate and become necrotic. Macrophages phagocytose the cellular debris and mycobacteria, but were not observed to contain acid-fast bacilli until 6–7 days after exposure. Macrophages migrate back to the submucosa, and those containing mycobacteria may degenerate, attracting more macrophages. The precise route of movement of the mycobacteria-laden macrophages to other organs was not determined but did not appear to be via the blood circulation because no mycobacteria were found in serial sections of the heart and major blood vessels. The authors theorized that migrating mycobacteria-laden macrophages enter lymphatics or the coelomic cavity to reach the liver and developing lungs. Granulomata develop in the submucosa of the intestines (but not in the stomach) and in the liver near portal regions. Large numbers of mycobacteria, both extracellular and within macrophages, were detected in the lumen of the lungs, even though the lungs lack a patent airway to the pharynx (the larynx is undeveloped and lacks a lumen). Older tadpoles with a patent larynx appear to efficiently clear intraluminal mycobacteria by the mucociliary escalator. Granulomas in the intestinal submucosa and other organs, especially the liver, develop as mycobacteria-laden macrophages degenerate and attract more and more macrophages.

Some intracoelomically injected amphibians developed granulomata in nearly all coelomic organs, with the spleen and liver most prominently affected and death occuring within 60–90 days. In other studies distinct gross lesions were not evident 60 days postinoculation (Inoue et al., 1965; Inoue & Singer, 1963, 1970a; Mok & Carvalho, 1984). Histologically, the grossly evident granulomata have been mistakenly diagnosed (and published) as various lymphoproliferative diseases (e.g., lymphosarcoma). In some experimentally challenged toads lacking grossly evident granulomata, acid-fast bacilli are readily found in scattered single macrophages of many organs. The number of mycobacteria-laden macrophages steadily increases with time (Mok & Carvalho, 1984).

Mycobacterial granulomas consist predominantly of epithelioid macrophages. Small granulomas are solidly cellular, while larger granulomas may have a caseonecrotic core with a thick cortex of viable epithelioid macrophages. Larger and chronic granulomas usually have a distinct fibrocytic and collagenous capsule (Darzins, 1952; Rowlatt & Roe, 1966). Mineralization has never been reported in amphibian mycobacterial granulomas, and multinucleated giant cells are rare or absent. It has been suggested that if multinucleated giant cells are common in a granuloma, the etiology is most likely mycotic or a foreign body (Elkan, 1976b). Although these fibrous capsules appear more slowly in ectotherms than endotherms, the thickness of the fibrous capsule may become more pronounced (Ippen, 1964). Acid-fast stains demonstrate myriad acid-fast bacilli within epithelioid macrophages in deeper locations of the granuloma. Acid-fast bacilli are also present in the cellular debris of the caseous core. The mycobacteria are also Gram-positive, and morphologically are usually described as beaded, but may be curved, thick rods, long and thin, or tangled masses.

Infectious Etiologies—Fungal. Mycotic infections by the fungus *Mucor amphibiorum* have been reported in captive anurans in Europe and wild toads in Australia (Frank et al., 1974; Speare et al., 1994b) Mucormycosis is a systemic infection.

Gross lesions in the giant toad, *Bufo marinus,* occur as small yellow granulomata, less than 5 mm in diameter, in many organs, especially the liver, urinary bladder, mesonephros, spleen, heart, and lung, and occasionally in the subcutaneous lymph sacs, skeletal muscles, stomach, intestines, brain, and skin (Speare et al., 1989).

Histologic features of mucormycosis are characteristic: presence of unpigmented spherical organisms called sphaerules within inflammatory nodules. Organisms are found almost exclusively within inflammatory nodules of two types. Acute inflammatory nodules consist of neutrophils, lymphocytes, and macrophages with mostly centrally placed fungi. The more common nodule, a granuloma, consists of macrophages, multinucleated giant cells, and lesser numbers of lymphocytes and eosinophils. Fibrocytes and collagen occur peripherally (Speare et al., 1989). Coalescence of granulomata may occur. The fungal sphaerules have three major sizes and shapes: 1) simple, nearly spherical sphaerules with no internal structures and are 5–14.5 μm in diameter; 2) larger ("mother") sphaerules, that contain 2–11 daughter sphaerules, and are 14.5–37 μm in diameter; and 3) collapsed oval and crescentric fungi. Daughter sphaerules and simple sphaerules are similar morphologically. Daughter sphaerules are also variable in size with a mean diameter of 5.3 μm (range: 2.4–10.5 μm). Sphaerules stain well with hematoxylin and eosin and many special stains (Speare et al., 1994b).

Differential diagnoses of systemic mycotic infections, including several fungi that have yet to be detected in amphibians, have been reviewed (Green et al., 1995b; Speare et al., 1994b).

A colorless spherical algae was implicated in retarded growth of captive tadpoles of the northern leopard frog, *Rana pipiens.* The organisms were 5–19 μm in diameter and were associated with impaired growth in situations of crowding and coprophagy. The identity of the colorless algae was not determined, but it was *Prototheca*-like. Elimination of crowding and coprophagy appeared to allow tadpoles to eliminate the algae from their gastrointestinal tracts. No histological studies were attempted (Richards, 1958).

Infectious Etiologies—Protozoal. Tadpoles and salamander larvae have a rich diversity of enteric protozoa. Most ciliates, opalinids, and flagellates are widely assumed to be innocuous or commensals. A high density of intestinal protozoa is not evidence of disease (Poynton & Whitaker, 1994). No gross or histologic lesions have been associated with the presence of enteric opalinids. The intestinal protozoa of amphibians have been reviewed (Flynn, 1973; Frank, 1984; Upton & McAllister, 1988; Upton et al., 1993) (see also Chapter 15, Protozoa and Metazoa Infecting Amphibians).

Loss of diversity of intestinal protozoa has been reported in wild-caught anurans that were held in captivity for many months and remained healthy. However, examination of voided feces may not result in detection of all intestinal protozoa due to desiccation and encystment of some organisms. Some protozoa which are commonly assumed to be pathogenic, such as coccidia, may not be detected by fecal examinations (Poynton & Whitaker, 1994).

Infectious Etiologies—Protozoal—Coccidia. Clinical disease associated with heavy infections by intestinal coccidia has been seen in captive anurans, especially dendrobatids (see Section 15.7.2, Apicomplexa in the Tissues). However, in wild populations of anurans the prevalence of infection is low (Upton et al., 1993). Clinical signs in captive frogs may include depression, weight loss, anorexia, dehydration, and loose, off-colored feces (Poynton & Whitaker, 1994). Histologically, infected dendrobatids may have mild disseminated to severe diffuse intestinal epithelial inflammation with typical intra-epithelial macrogamete, microgamete, and oocyst stages (personal communication, B. Whitaker, 1996).

Intestinal coccidiosis of ranid tadpoles has been reported twice in Europe. *Isospora* spp., and *Eimeria* spp., have been reported in adults worldwide, and each species of coccidia is probably species-specific in anurans (reviewed by Upton & McAllister, 1988).

Clinical disease associated with intestinal coccidiosis in captive salamanders has been reported in Austria in the alpine salamander, *Salamandra atra* (Frank, 1984). Infections by *Eimeria grobbeni* were considered massive in the intestines. Infected salamanders developed conspicuous depigmentation of the skin over the head, neck, and abdominal regions. Histologically, intestinal epithelial necrosis and desquamation were found with inflammatory cell infiltrates in the mucosa and submucosa.

Reports of coccidia in wild salamanders are uncommon but this most likely reflects the lack of attention given to salamanders rather than the actual prevalence of infection. Two species of *Isospora* and numerous *Eimeria* spp. have been detected and identified in the stools of wild salamanders worldwide (reviewed by Upton et al., 1993).

One captive giant toad, *Bufo marinus*, was found dead with lesions of dehydration and hemorrhagic gastroenteritis. Coccidia oocysts, Gram-negative bacteria, and an unidentified amoeba were found in this toad, so the gross and histologic lesions cannot be attributed solely to the coccidia (Valentine & Stoskopf, 1984).

Oocysts of *Eimeria bufomarini* in the intestinal epithelium of the giant toad, *Bufo marinus*, often rupture and release their sporocysts (Paperna & Lainson, 1995a). Wet mount smears of fresh feces are best for examinations of anurans for coccidian oocysts and sporocysts (Upton & McAllister, 1988).

Infectious Etiologies—Protozoal—Amoeba. Numerous genera and species of amoeba have been identified in amphibians, however, only two species are potentially pathogenic, *Entamoeba ranarum* and *E. ilowaiskii* (Frank, 1984). *Entamoeba ilowaiskii* is reported to be pathogenic in the European common frog, *Rana temporaria*, but details of the lesions are lacking (Ghosh, 1977). *Entamoeba ranarum* was isolated from a liver abscess of an axolotl, *Ambystoma mexicanum*, but intestinal lesions, considered a prerequisite of amoebic liver disease, were not described (Frank, 1984).

Infectious Etiologies—Protozoal—Hepatosphaera molgarum. Fatal liver infections by *Hepatosphaera molgarum* in the northern crested newt, *Triturus cristatus*, were reported in wild and captive animals (Gambier, 1924). Wild newts were sluggish and easily captured. Once captured, infected newts often died within 2 days. *Hepatosphaera molgarum* infection of newts causes hepatic necrosis with the presence of massive numbers of spherical, uninucleate, 6–10 μm in diameters, organisms. The hepatic organisms were illustrated by camera lucida drawings only, so the taxonomy of this protozoan organism is uncertain.

Infectious Etiologies—Protozoal—Hepatozoon sipedon. The northern leopard frog, *Rana pipiens*, is an obligate intermediate host of *Hepatozoon sipedon* infection in anurophagus snakes. The mosquito is the definitive host since sexual reproduction of the parasite occurs only in the invertebrate. The frog becomes infected by ingesting an infected mosquito. The mosquito is incapable of transmitting the parasite to frogs or snakes by merely taking a blood meal. *Hepatozoon* spp. infections of terrestrial anurans are consistently hepatocellular, and, sometimes, concurrently erythrocytic. In the liver, small ovoid cysts measure 22 × 18.4 μm; each cyst contains two cystozoites, each of which contains a nucleus and a larger homogenous paranuclear crystalloid inclusion. An inflammatory reaction to these cysts has not been reported, and the cysts often stain poorly with standard histological and cytological stains. Phase contrast microscopy is most helpful in detecting the dizoic cysts (Smith, 1996; Smith et al., 1994).

Infectious Etiologies—Protozoal—Tritrichomonas augusta. One northern leopard frog, *Rana pipiens*, was observed to have hepatic lesions from which the flagellated protozoan *Tritrichomonas augusta* was identified. Experimental reproduction of the disease in frogs was attempted but failed (Walton, 1964), hence, the pathogenicity of this protozoan is uncertain (Frank, 1984).

Infectious Etiologies—Protozoal—Hexamita intestinalis. *Hexamita intestinalis* is a small flagellated protozoan principally inhabiting the intestines, but in heavy intestinal infections in captive anurans, it may invade the gall bladder. No specific lesions have been attributed to the presence of this protozoan (Reichenbach-Klinke & Elkan, 1965).

Infectious Etiologies—Protozoal—Alloglugea bufonis. A new genus and species of microsporidium that infects the intestines and other viscera of wild tadpoles of the giant toad, *Bufo marinus*, in Brazil was described (Paperna & Lainson, 1995b). The microsporidium is named *Alloglugea bufonis*. Infected tadpoles have about 5–50 white nodules on the serosa of the intestine and in the spleen and mesonephroi. The nodules are roughly spherical, and 0.25 mm in diameter. The nodules are called xenomas, and contain masses of developing or mature spores that are up to 10 μm in length in the immature (plasmodial, meront or sporont) stage, and 1.5 × 0.7 μm in the mature (spore) stage. Smaller xenomas are observed histologically within the submucosal and muscular tunics. Xenomas are a massively enlarged host cell, probably a macrophage, filled with immature and mature organisms. The host nucleus is greatly enlarged, and the xenoma may be partially surrounded by a thin layer of fibrocyte-like cells. Organisms are usually concentrated near the host cell's cytoplasmic membrane.

Xenomas may rupture and release spores into the body to form additional xenomas in other organs, principally the spleen and mesonephroi. Heavy infections may result in splenomegaly. Most heavily infected tadpoles successfully metamorphose, and the xenomas rapidly disappear as the toadlet matures (Paperna & Lainson, 1995b). Microsporidia have characteristic special staining features: all stages are Gram-positive, and the mature spores are acid-fast and have a periodic acid-Schiff-positive polar granule (Gardiner et al., 1988).

Infectious Etiologies—Myxozoans (Myxosporeans). (Note: This author prefers to use the term myxozoan for this group of organisms rather than the term myxosporeans (see also Section 15.10, Myxosporea). The myxozoans, *Myxidium immersum, M. serotinum,* and *M. haldari* occur in the lumen of the gall bladder in numerous adult anurans in South America and Australia, North America, and India, respectively. The host records of *Myxidium* spp. in amphibians were reviewed (Delvinquier, 1986). The distribution of the parasite in amphibians is irregular (Clark & Shoemaker, 1973; Kudo, 1922a, b). It appears that *Myxidium immersum* was introduced into Australia with the giant toad, *Bufo marinus,* in 1935 (Delvinquier, 1986). It now occurs in 19 species of native frogs in Queensland and northeastern New South Wales, but not in indigenous frogs in those Australian states that lack the giant toad, *B. marinus*. In North America, adults and larvae of the two-lined salamander, *Eurycea bislineata,* are also infected by *M. serotinum*. Spores of unidentified species of *Myxidium* and *Henneguya* were found in the gall bladder of one recently imported Surinam toad, *Pipa pipa,* but the only described lesion was that the bile was gelatinous (Frank, 1984).

Other than gelatinous bile (Frank, 1984), no gross or histologic lesions have been associated with myxozoan infections of the amphibian gall bladder. The organisms are best detected in fresh, wet mount smears of the contents of the gall bladder. Cytologically, the organism may be present only as trophozoites in tadpoles and larvae, while in adult amphibians, both trophozoites and spores may be found. Infections are usually light, with only 3–12 trophozoites per animal (Delvinquier, 1986). The life cycles of all amphibian myxozoans are unknown, but direct transmission between amphibians does not occur (Clark & Shoemaker, 1973). It is unknown how myxozoans gain entry to the gall bladder, metanephroi or gonads, nor what as-yet-undetected intermediate stages may be necessary to establish infections of the internal organs (Siddall et al., 1995).

Infectious Etiologies—Helminths. Tadpoles, larval and neotenic salamanders, and other aquatic amphibians are intermediate and definitive hosts for nematodes, trematodes, cestodes, and acanthocephalids. Even in cases of heavy gastrointestinal infections, clinical signs, gross lesions, and histologic changes are seldom found. However, acanthocephalids and some cestodes have "thorny heads" and spiney scolices which may penetrate or perforate the gastrointestinal wall. Such parasitic attachment sites may provide entry into the intestinal tissues and circulatory system for opportunistic bacteria, fungi, and other microorganisms. As in higher vertebrates, verminous perforations usually result in bacterial coelomitis and death. Heavy infections by helminths, in particular the cestode, *Nematotaenia dispar,* may cause mechanical obstruction with fatal gangrenous enteritis in toads in captivity (Canning et al., 1964; Elkan, 1960a, b; Reichenbach-Klinke & Elkan, 1965). Numerous studies and reviews of gastrointestinal parasites have been published (Brooks, 1984; Flynn, 1973; Lees, 1962; Prokopic & Krivanec, 1975; Reichenbach-Klinke & Elkan, 1965; Walton, 1964).

Numerous cestodes, trematodes, nematodes, and pentastomids may be encountered in the liver, pancreas, and associated ducts (Flynn, 1973) (Figure 27.43).

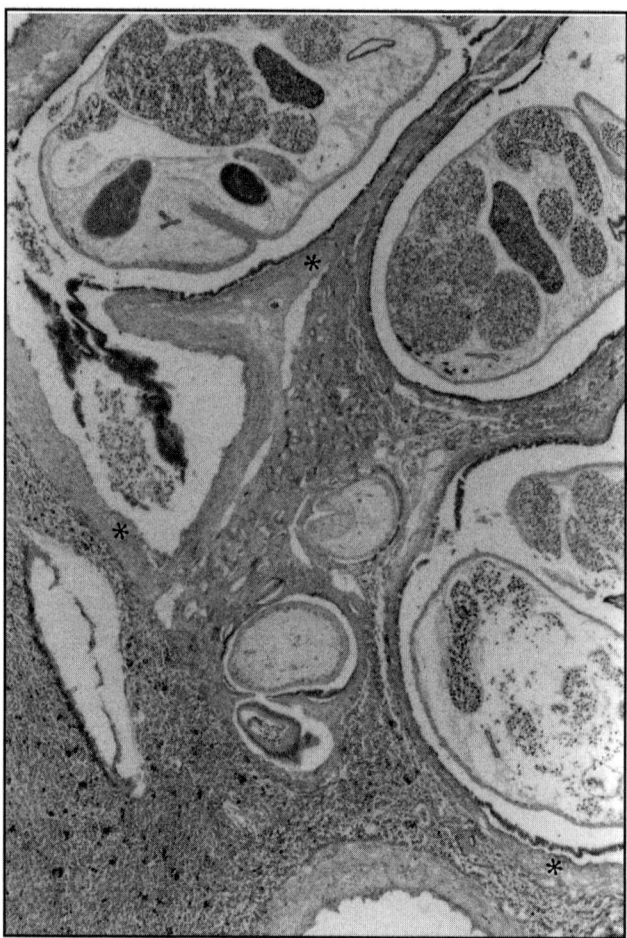

Figure 27.43. Biliary trematodiasis in a wild giant toad, *Bufo marinus*. Adult trematodes are intraductal. There is dilation of biliary ducts, compression atrophy of hepatocytes, and moderate fibrosis around infected ducts (asterisks). (G.R. Zug, RTLA 1523)

Trematodes and nematodes may be immature or mature worms, while most of the other taxa occur as immature worms that are migrating, encysted, or encased in granulomata, and utilize amphibians as an intermediate or paratenic host. Cysts of immature trematodes may occupy as much as 50% of the liver (Green, unpublished; Zug & Zug, 1979).

Tetrathyridia (immature forms of *Mesocestoides* spp.) utilize a variety of ectothermic and endothermic intermediate hosts, and have been reported from eight species of wild adult anurans in North America (McAllister & Conn, 1990). Although the prevalence of infection in an anuran population is usually less than 5%, the intensity of infection in an individual may be severe. Tetrathyridia may be detected in the liver, the mesentery, intestinal wall, and free in the body cavity and muscle fascia. In the liver, the cysts generally lack intraluminal and capsular inflammatory cells. Compression of surrounding hepatocytes usually is minimal. The tetrathyridium has a thin syncytial tegument, pale loose cellular body, no body cavity, and characteristic blue mineralized bodies called calcareous corpuscles. In fortuitous sections an invaginated tunnel (or canal) in the head, a densely cellular hind-body, and a tetra-acetabulate scolex may be found (Chitwood & Lichtenfels, 1972; McAllister & Conn, 1990).

Infectious Etiologies—Pentastomids. Amphibians function as intermediate and paratenic hosts for multiple genera of pentastomids (Flynn, 1973). Immature pentastomids are called nymphs, and as few as 20 nymphs can be fatal to an adult ranid. Histologically, acute hemorrhagic tracts may be found in many organs, especially the stomach and liver (Boyce & Kazacos, 1991).

Idiopathic Etiologies—Cholelithiasis. A gallstone was reported in an adult female red-eyed treefrog, *Agalychnis callidyras* (Stetter, 1994). At necropsy, the treefrog had a full, firmly distended gall bladder that could not be expressed by palpation. One hard greenish stone, measuring $2 \times 1 \times 1$ mm, was determined to consist of calcium carbonate. The cholelith was detected in a whole body radiograph, but results of histologic examination of the gall bladder were not reported (Stetter, 1994). Choleliths must be carefully distinguished from inspissated, concentrated bile.

Idiopathic Etiologies—Hepatic Hydropic Degeneration and Steotosis. Swelling of hepatocytes, loss of glycogen, and accumulation of excessive lipid (steotosis) occurred in surgically splenectomized specimens of the Vienna newt, *Triturus carnifax.* Newts had been spleenless for over 10 months and the steotosis was attributed to chronic hypoxia (Frangioni & Borgioli, 1993). Hepatocellular hydropic degeneration and loss of glycogen granules occurred in experimental African clawed frogs, *Xenopus laevis,* that were administered the radioactive isotope Ca^{45}. At 7–10 days postinoculation, other assumed parameters of hepatic function were abnormal (elevated AST, ALT, and GGT, and hypoalbuminemia) and, grossly, massive hydrocoelom and ovarian edema were found (Giannetti et al., 1990).

27.2.4 Urinary System

Amphibians have separate kidneys in the larval and adult life stages. Larvae have primitive aglomerular pronephric kidneys located anterior to the later-developing mesonephric kidneys (Fox, 1963). Amphibians do not have true metanephric kidneys as do mammals, birds, and reptiles. The paired pronephroi are initially the sole excretory and osmoregulatory organ of larval amphibians. There is evidence that their growth, differentiation, and eventual complete degeneration are controlled mainly by thyroid hormones (Fox, 1981). The mesonephric kidneys begin developing in amphibian larvae well before metamorphic climax.

Genetic Etiologies. Three inherited traits affecting the mesonephroi of axolotls, *Ambystoma mexicanum,* have been described: short toes, lethal renal insufficiency, and ascites (Egar & Jarial, 1991; Humphrey, 1964, 1975; Washabaugh et al., 1993).

Toxicological Etiologies—Tricaine methanesulfonate. Tricaine methanesulfonate caused severe edma in the mesonephroi of the northern leopard frog, *Rana pipiens* (Clark et al., 1968). No other reports of this suspected adverse drug reaction have been found.

Toxicological Etiologies—Oxalates. Oxalate nephosis has been noted in captive-raised tadpoles that are fed certain oxalate-containing plants such as spinach and kale. Oxalate crystals may form in the mesonephroi. Gross and histologic lesions have not been described (Stetter, 1995). A few oxalate crystals may form in the mesonephroi in active, healthy amphibians without apparent deleterious effect.

Infectious Etiologies—Viral. Lucke's renal carcinoma is a herpesvirus-induced neoplasm of the mesonephroi of the northern leopard frog, *Rana pipiens* (see Section 26.5, Neoplasms of the Urinary System).

In addition to iridoviruses, at least three other taxa of viruses have been isolated from normal mesonephroi and Lucke's tumor cells of adult specimens of the northern leopard frog, *Rana pipiens*: adenoviruses, papovalike viruses, and a calicivirus (reviewed by Granoff, 1989). The adeno-like and papova-like viruses were incidental findings in early studies on the etiology of Lucke's tumor, and no clinical illness or lesions have been associated with these viruses (Clark et al., 1973; Granoff, 1989).

The calicivirus was isolated from multiple organs, including one mesonephros, of two specimens of the ornate horned frog, *Ceratophrys ornata,* and several taxa of snakes in a zoological park (Smith et al., 1986).

Infectious Etiologies—Bacterial—Leptospirosis. Serotypes of *Leptospira interregans* have been detected in anurans serologically and by cultural isolation (Babudieri et al., 1973; Diesch et al., 1967; Everard et al., 1983, 1988; Minette, 1983). However, gross and histological lesions of leptospiral infections have not been detected or reported in amphibians.

Infectious Etiologies—Protozoal—Trichodina spp. Trichodinids may parasitize the skin, urinary bladder, mouth, and gill chamber of amphibians. Urinary bladder infections by *Trichodina urinicola* are reported principally from adult aquatic European anurans and salamanders (Lom, 1958). No pathologic effects have been described (Flynn, 1973).

Infectious Etiologies—Protozoal—Coccidia. *Isospora lieberkuehni* (formerly *Diplospora lieberkuhni*, *Hyaloklossia lieberkuhni*, and *Klossia lieberkuhni*) infects the renal tubular epithelium of adult ranids in Europe and North America, and the firebelly toad *Bombina variegata* in Europe. Other reports of the parasite in the common European toad, *Bufo bufo*, the Gulf Coast toad, *B. valliceps*, and the Common Eurasian spadefoot toad, *Pelobates fuscus*, have been discounted (Upton & McAllister, 1988). In view of the theory that *Isospora* spp., and *Eimeria* spp., are species-specific in anurans (Upton & McAllister, 1988), this renal protozoan is either an exception, or further species of renal coccidia await description. In the northern leopard frog, *Rana pipiens*, the only documented ranid host in North America, 1–12 merozoites are present in the cytoplasm of a tubule cell. Merozoites are elongate, slightly curved, about 7 µm long, and have a central spherical or slightly squarish 1 µm diameter nucleus. Merozoites lie loosely in the host cell cytoplasm and may completely destroy the cytoplasm. The host cell nucleus is basal and may appear normal or pyknotic, but no host inflammatory cell reponse has been reported (Levine & Nye, 1977).

Infectious Etiologies—Protozoal Amoeba. Amoebic nephritis was reported in a captive giant toad, *Bufo marinus* (Valentine & Stoskopf, 1984). Marked lymphohistiocytic nephritis was found and extracellular amoebae, 11–32 µm in diameter, were evident. Each amoeba was circular to ovoid, and most had a single nucleus, but a few had as many as four nuclei, each 3–4 µm in diameter. Karyosomes were either not found or were single, small, and central. The precise identity of the amoeba was not determined, but the size of the trophozoites was considered suggestive of *Entamoeba ranarum*. In the absence of lesions in the intestines, it was suggested the amoeba had ascended from the cloaca to the mesonephroi (Valentine & Stoskopf, 1984). Trophozoites of *Entamoeba ranarum* have a single nucleus (Kudo, 1922b), while cysts usually have four, but sometimes as many as 16 nuclei (Flynn, 1973).

Infectious Etiologies—Myxozoans (Myxosporeans). The myxozoan parasite, *Leptotheca ohlmacheri*, is a common infection of the renal tubules of the northern leopard frog, *Rana pipiens*, and the green frog, *R. clamitans*, in North America (Kudo, 1922a, b). The parasite has been recorded in the mesonephroi of many other species of ranids and bufonids in Europe and North America. In the 1960s, during extensive studies of the Lucke renal carcinoma, the parasite was regularly detected and illustrated (Duryee, 1965; McKinnell, 1965).

No specific disease has been attributed to this myxozoan. The parasite is considered an extracellular organism that lies within the tubular lumina and the glomerular space, but the infective stage and prerenal stages have not been detected or reported (Siddall et al., 1995). Histologically, there is minimal change in the affected renal tubules. When large numbers of organisms are present, the tubule will appear dilated and the epithelial cells flattened. Intraluminal organisms stain variably with hematoxylin and eosin, and may be mistaken for sloughed degenerate epithelial cells. The Giemsa stain demonstrates myxozoans well.

Infectious Etiologies—Helminths. Reports of trematodes in the mesonephroi of tadpoles often do not specify whether the pronephroi, mesonephroi, or both, are involved. "Kidney" flukes of amphibians may be found in the urinary bladder, mesonephric ducts, body cavity, and, possibly, the pronephroi.

Immature and mature trematodes of several genera may be found in the mesonephroi of aquatic and terrestrial amphibians. Some trematodes (e.g., *Alaria* spp. and *Echinostoma* spp.) use amphibians as an intermediate host, and for others (e.g., *Gorgodera amplicava*), the amphibian is the final host. The metacercariae of *Alaria* spp. are called mesocercariae (Dunn, 1969). Most renal trematodes are acquired during the aquatic larval periods in sympatry with snails. Snails release cercariae which infect aquatic amphibians. Grossly, multiple, subcapsular and parenchymal, somewhat varicose, white nodules are found. *Gorgodera amplicava* may use the mesonephroi temporarily for development and maturation. Some may mature in the mesonephroi and others return to the urinary bladder where they attain sexual maturity; within the mesonephroi, these flukes are also detected as firm whitish nodules (Goodchild, 1950). *Echinostoma* also form cysts that are whitish if the metacercariae are alive but cysts containing dead immature flukes are dark brown (Martin & Conn, 1990).

Histological changes associated with the renal trematodes consist of two distinct sets of lesions, corresponding to whether the amphibian is an intermediate or final host. The lesions associated with encysted metacercariae and mesocercariae are more destructive, and may cause renal dysfunction and debilitation of the host (Martin & Conn, 1990). Most histological studies have concentrated on the "cyst" formed by metacercariae and mesocercariae. Encysted mesocercaria and metacercaria are found in the renal interstitium, capsule, glomerular space, and tubules. The renal lesion produced by immature encysted trematodes consists of two parts, the "cyst" that is the parasite and its wall, and the host's inflammatory cell reaction. The host reaction to the trematode cysts has been variously described as encapsulation, fibrous capsules, or, rarely, granulomata. Initial inflammatory reactions to metacercariae are not commonly reported because most studies are conducted on postmetamorphic amphibians, and it is principally in the tadpole stage that flukes invade the amphibian. The least mature granulomas often contain granulocytes. Epithelioid macrophages later replace granulocytes. Fibroblastic cell reaction appears to quickly surround the cyst, and, occasionally, mononuclear cells are mentioned. In granulomata that contain live echinostomatids, the peripheral fibroplasia is mild, while in those nodules with dead trematodes, the fibrous layer is thicker. Heavy metacercarial infections may be common in some ponds or populations, and coalescence of granulomata may result in reduction of functional renal tissue (Martin & Conn, 1990).

Gorgodera spp., *Gorgoderina* spp., and *Phyllodistomum* spp. are common in the urinary bladder of amphibians (Flynn, 1973). The first two genera occur in anurans and salamanders in Europe, Africa, and North and South America, and all are reported to cause listlessness, anorexia, uremia, and death in heavy infections (Flynn, 1973). The latter genus occurs commonly in mole salamanders, *Ambystoma* spp., and dusky salamanders, *Desmognathus* spp. *Gorgodera amplicava* has a prevalence of up to 35% in wild populations of the bullfrog, *Rana catesbeiana*, in the southern United States. *Gorgodera amplicava* and *Gorgoderina attenuata* also may be found in the ureters and mesonephroi. Heavy infections may cause obstruction of renal tubules or ureters, postrenal uremia, and death (Flynn, 1973; Goodchild, 1950). There is a well delineated, focal hyperplasia of the host urothelium within the fluke's sucker which has been variously described as hyperplasia, metaplasia, carcinoma in situ, and a precursor lesion of Lucke renal carcinomata (Duryee, 1965). Mild histological lesions associated with *Gorgodera amplicava* infection in a bullfrog, *R. catesbeiana*, from Missouri, were described as multifocal erosions of the transitional epithelium with a mild mixed leukocytic infiltrate in the underlying mucosa which occasionally extended into the muscular tunic (Li & Lipman, 1995). In the same bullfrog, 20–24 mature *Gorgodera amplicava* were found free in the body cavity yet the urinary bladder was intact. These trematodes were 3–4.5 mm long and had a large ventral sucker that was about 2 mm in diameter. Other infectious and parasitic diseases were also present in this bullfrog, *R. catesbeiana*, including trematodes, allegedly *Gorogdera amplicava*, encysted in the wall of the stomach and free in the lumina of the lungs but it is likely the frog was infected by multiple taxa of trematodes (i.e., *Haematoloechus* spp.).

Two possible routes of infection of the coelomic cavity in adult anurans by adult bladder flukes, *Gorgodera* spp., apparently have not been considered (Li & Lipman, 1995): 1) long-lived tadpoles (1–3 years in the larval stage) may develop trematode infections of the pronephroi and pronephric ducts, and then during metamorphic degeneration of the pronephroi, the trematodes would be released into the body cavity; or 2) immature trematodes may migrate up the pronephric duct, into the pronephric tubules, and could simply fall into the coelomic cavity from the aglomerular nephrostome. Such lengthy migration in tubules is not unprecedented since metaceracariae have been detected in the glomerular space of the mesonephroi in the northern leopard frog, *Rana pipiens*, and the green frog, *R. clamitans* (Narajian, 1953, 1954; Martin & Conn, 1990).

Idiopathic Etiologies. Occasional reports of mesonephric disease of unknown etiology may be found associated with seemingly unrelated conditions (Stephens et al., 1987). In mature clawed frogs, *Xenopus* spp., interstitial lymphocytic mesonephritis, mesonephrocalcinosis, suppurative mesonephritis, and mesonephrosis have been reported. The etiologies of these lesions were not determined, although the suppurative mesonephritis may have been associated with bacterial dermatitis that progressed to bacterial septicemia (Stephens et al., 1987).

27.2.5 Respiratory System

Introduction. The principal respiratory organ in aquatic amphibians is the skin. About 70% of the total oxygen uptake, and over 85% of carbon dioxide elimination in tadpoles of the bullfrog, *Rana catesbeiana*, is via the skin (Burggren & West, 1982). Gills, lungs and the buccopharyngeal cavity account for the balance of gas exchange in larval and neotenic aquatic amphibians. Nonrespiratory functions of amphibian gills include ion exchange, water balance, and feeding. In tadpoles, external and internal sets of gills develop, while larval and neotenic salamanders have external gills only. The internal location of the gills in tadpoles makes external, noninvasive examinations difficult. Despite its ubiquitous nature in embryonic and larval stages of all three orders, the amphibian gill is one of the least studied of vertebrate respiratory organs (Malvin, 1989).

Adaptive branchial hypertrophy by tadpoles and salamanders in hypoxic waters has been recognized for almost a century (Burggren & Mwalukoma, 1983).

Metamorphic Degeneration of Gills. In anuran metamorphosis, the gills and tail normally undergo complete degeneration. These degenerative processes are normal physiological and ontological changes but could be mistaken for pathological processes. Three discrete phases of cellular activity have been described in the regression of the internal gills and tail. First, there is a selective decrease in the rate of protein synthesis within branchial cells. The second and dramatic phase is that of histolysis, followed by the final phase of elimination of cellular debris (Duellman & Trueb, 1986; Fox, 1981). Degeneration of the anuran external gills has been studied ultrastructurally (Michaels et al., 1971). To avoid confusing normal involution of the the gills and tail with true disease processes, it is essential to determine the developmental stage of the larval amphibian, perferrably during gross examination.

Genetic Etiologies. At least four autosomal recessive traits, expressed phenotypically as defective gills, have been reported in the axolotl, *Ambystoma mexicanum*. These traits are gill lethal, fragile gills, twisted gills, and slow growth with abnormal gills (Humphrey, 1959, 1975; Malacinski, 1978). In addition, gill abnormalities may develop in conjunction with other congenital anomalies (Humphrey, 1975).

Experimental Etiologies—Nonaerated Lungs in Larval Amphibians. Experimental studies of various amphibian taxa show that larvae denied access to air are unable to inflate their lungs, develop more slowly, are more lethargic, develop cardiomegaly, and have atrophied (or hypoplastic) lungs and other developmental anomalies. Noninflated lungs were about 33–50% of the size of age-matched controls, and lumina were partially or completely filled with undifferentiated mesenchyme in 26% of tadpoles denied access to air. Other anomalies were forked lungs (consisting of more than one sac), invagination of the posterior region, and abnormal spherical or triangular shapes (Pronych & Wassersug, 1994).

Infectious Etiologies—Viral. Two specimens of the ornate horned frog, *Ceratophrys ornata*, died in a zoo during an epizootic of calicivirus infection in reptiles and amphibians (Smith et al., 1986). Although the authors were reluctant to attribute death or any observed lesions to the isolated calicivirus, both frogs had lung lesions characterized as necrotic interstitial pneumonia.

Infectious Etiologies—Bacterial. The lungs of anurans begin development well before metamorphosis and with careful dissection may be observed grossly. Pneumococcal pneumonia was found in tapdoles of the mission golden-eyed treefrog, *Phrynohyas resinifictrix* (Zwart et al., 1991). The movement of affected tadpoles was hampered by an emphysematous overfilling of the lungs with gas bubbles. Histologically, the lungs had infiltrates of phagocytic cells which were laden with bacteria. The specific identity of the pneumococci was not reported.

Infectious Etiologies—Helminths. Nematodes (*Rhabdias* spp.) and trematodes (*Haematoloechus* spp. = *Pneumonoeces* spp., and *Haplometra* spp.) are lungworms of adult amphibians (Brooks, 1984; Flynn, 1973; Lees, 1962; Rees, 1964) (Figure 27.44). Although, 15 species of the North American genera *Haematoloechus* have been described, these were revised and consolidated into six species (Kennedy, 1981). In addition, numerous other immature stages of cestodes, trematodes, and nematodes may be detected in pulmonary tissues in encysted, nonencysted (actively migrating) stages, or in granulomata. The larval stages of amphibians may have gill infections by monogenic trematodes such as *Polystoma* spp. Some

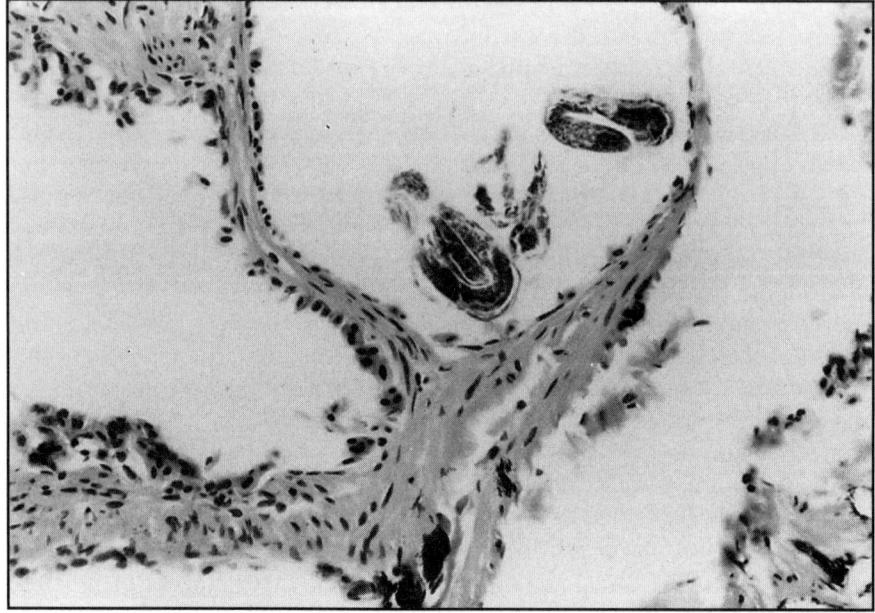

Figure 27.44. *Rhabdias* lungworms in a northern leopard frog, *Rana pipiens*. Rhabditida typically are of small diameter, have prominent dark-staining ova, and occur in the lungs. *Rhabdias* typically have a smooth cuticle, platymyarian muscles on cross-section, low cuboidal intestinal cells with a single nucleus and low microvillus border, and large basophilic ova. (J. Carney, RTLA 1926)

species of these trematodes mature and migrate to the urinary bladder during anuran metamorphosis, while others mature on the gills and are eliminated during metamorphosis.

Descriptions of gross and histological features of *Haematoloechus longiplexus* infections in the bullfrog, *Rana catesbeiana*, were attempted (Shields, 1987). Larger mature trematodes, which may be up to 9 mm long, are generally found free in the lumen of the lung or main bronchi. Minimal changes are associated with intraluminal trematodes, such as loss of cilia on adjacent epithelium, increased mucus production with possible increased numbers of goblet cells, rarely squamous metaplasia, and poorly delineated nodules of lymphocytes and macrophages in the submucosa. Smaller trematodes may partially burrow into cavae, and may produce nodules containing 1–4 trematodes. These nodules consist of compression capsules with minimal inflammation. The nodules are often visible grossly from the serosal surface. Segments of the nodule, especially nearest the pleura, may appear thin, hypocellular, compressed, and fibrous, while other segments may show edematous fibroplasia, and atrophy of smooth muscle cells. Leukocytic infiltrates are usually slight, but may consist of macrophages, lymphocytes, and granulocytes. Trematode ova, mucus, and degenerate pulmonary epithelial cells and leukocytes may be present in the nodule's lumen (Rees, 1964).

Since lung trematodes are hematophagous, erythrocytes may be found in the nodules and free in the lumina of the airways (Rees, 1964; Shields, 1987). The histological features of the pulmonary tissue entrapped by the suckers of the trematodes have been interpreted erroneously as pulmonary adenocarcinomata in situ (Duryee, 1965). The plugs of pulmonary epithelium within the suckers often have a compressed stalk with a fungiform hemispherical mass of hypertrophied columnar epithelial cells in the lumen of the oral sucker. Detachment of the fluke from the lung may leave behind the same peculiar nodule of hyperplastic cells, that actually has some resemblance to a minute carcinoma in situ (illustrated by Duryee, 1965). Metastatic foci in the lungs from Lucke renal carcinomata might be mistaken for such hyperplastic epithelial nodules, but metastatic carcinomata should have a clear intravascular association.

Dead lung trematodes elicit a greater inflammatory response in the lungs by the production of parenchymal granulomata and polypoid pleural granulomata, that have been inaccurately characterized as fibrous cysts (Shields, 1987). Parenchymal and polypoid granulomata have a core of amorphous decomposed trematodes, degenerating eggs and leukocytes, and granular detritus and crystals. Variable numbers of epithelioid macrophages surround the central debris, and a prominent fibrous capsule is present peripherally. Lung flukes may become life-threatening infections by occlusion of bronchial lumina by their sheer numbers, and by allowing secondary bacterial or fungal infections at the site of attachment by oral suckers (Brooks, 1984).

Polystomatids are an unusual taxon of monogeans which parasitize the gills and urinary bladders of tetrapods (Combes et al., 1995). Anuran polystomatids are oioxenous (each species of fluke parasitizes only one host) (Vaucher, 1990), hence detection of the parasite in the gills or bladder, grossly or histologically, allows for identification to genus and species. No reports of specific lesions associated with infection of anurans were found.

Infectious Etiologies—Arthropods. Several taxa of dipteran flies deposit their eggs on the skin of anurans. These eggs hatch into larvae which either directly penetrate the skin to cause subcutaneous infections, or migrate to the nostrils and into the nasal cavity. Old World anurans and salamanders are infested by the toad fly, *Bufolucilia bufonivora* (Sandner, 1955). *Bufolucilia bufonivora* is considered an obligate parasite of amphibians. Infestations (myiasis) of the nasal cavity may be massive and fatal to the host. Larvae are white and reach a maximum length of 10–18 mm. Larvae cause severe ulceration of nasal mucosa and extensive loss of bone around the nostrils and septum. Larvae may penetrate the skull, invade the brain, and may infest the conjunctiva, orbit, and tympanic region. In North America, *Bufolucilia silvarum* occasionally infects adult anurans (Bleakney, 1963; Flynn, 1973; Zumpt, 1965).

27.2.6 Cardiovascular System

Fluid accumulation in the body cavity of amphibians is referred to as hydrocoelom. Ascites is the accumulation of serous fluid in the abdominal cavity. Since amphibians do not have separate thoracic and abdominal cavities, the term is inappropriate in amphibian medicine. Hydrops is the preferred term for combined fluids in the subcutis, tissues, and coelomic cavity in larval amphibians (Figure 27.45). Anasarca

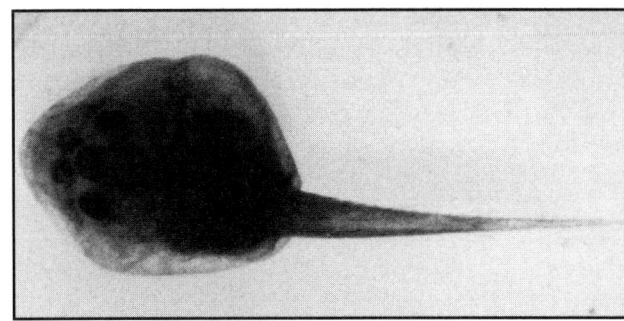

Figure 27.45. Hydrops in a tadpole of the western toad, *Bufo boreas*. The etiology of hydrops in tadpoles is rarely determined. (D.E. Green)

may be considered synonymous with hydrops, but is most often applied to postneonatal terrestrial animals. Hydrops and hydrocoelom have been reported as separate entities in larval amphibians. Occlusion of the lymphatic vessels and lymphatic hearts in amphibians does not consistently induce hydrops, although it has been implicated in some cases (Elkan, 1983; Verhoeff-DeFremery, 1989).

The hearts of adult amphibians are three-chambered, consisting of left and right atria and a single ventricle. Anuran and salamander hearts are markedly different anatomically (Boutilier et al., 1992). There is little literature on the cardiac anatomy of Gymnophiona.

The extent or even presence of lymphatics in amphibians is variable depending on life stage and species (Baculi & Cooper, 1967; Carter, 1979; Conklin 1930; Ecker, 1881; Elkan, 1957). Among anurans, the lymph fluid does not "filter" through lymphomyeloid organs ("lymph nodes") but is transported to the lymph hearts, then to the venous circulation. The subcutis of amphibians, especially anurans, is considered a series of lymph sacs. Skeletal movement greatly facilitates movement of fluids in the lymph sacs, from one sac to another, and to the lymph hearts (Carter, 1979).

Lymph hearts are located in the dorsal subcutis; one pair, the anterior lymph hearts, lies beneath the scapula, while the posterior lymph hearts, which vary in number from 1–5 pairs, lie on each side of the urostyle (Carter, 1979). Anterior lymph hearts receive lymph from the head, neck and, usually, the forelimbs, and pump lymph fluid into the vertebral veins, while posterior hearts receive lymph from the coelom, hindlimbs, and tail, and pump into renal portal veins. Lymph hearts have three histological layers: an endothelium, a tunica media of muscle cells, and an indistinct adventitia that blurs with the surrounding tissue.

Genetic Etiologies. The cardiac lethal mutation of the axolotl, *Ambystoma mexicanum*, is a recessive lethal trait that causes hydrops (Erginel-Unaltuna & Lemanski, 1994; Humphrey, 1972; Lemanski, 1978; Shen & Lemanski, 1989; Smith & Armstrong, 1990). The caudal edema trait of the Spanish ribbed newt, *Pleorodeles waltl*, is a lethal recessive autosomal mutation of the larval tail. (Beetschen & Jaylet, 1966; Gallien, 1969). Postmetamorphic subcutaneous edema of the African clawed frog, *Xenopus laevis*, has been described (Uehlinger & Beauchemin, 1968).

Congenital Anomalies. Few spontaneous defects of the heart have been described. A captive-bred African clawed frog, *Xenopus laevis*, had a ventral thoracic lump due to herniation of the heart through a defective pectoral girdle (Elkan, 1976b). The precise pectoral defect was not explained, nor were any abnormalities of the heart described, other than its ectopic location. Numerous cardiac anomalies have been detected and illustrated during standardized toxicological and teratological tests in the Frog Embryo Teratogenesis Assay-*Xenopus* (FETAX) (Bantle et al., undated).

Experimental Etiologies. Tadpoles of the clawed frog, *Xenopus* spp., normally inflate their lungs within hours of hatching by gulping air at the air/water interface. These tadpoles have gills as well as functional trachea, bronchi, and lungs at the time of hatching. When tadpoles are denied access to air, the lungs remain uninflated. If tadpoles are unable to inflate their lungs for over 2 weeks, cardiomegaly develops. The hearts of tadpoles with uninflated lungs are approximately twice the size of age-matched controls with aerated lungs (Pronych & Wassersug, 1994). The precise hypertrophied regions of the heart have not been described.

Curare causes cessation of contractions of lymph hearts. If a northern leopard frog, *Rana pipiens*, is curarized and immersed in water, it will increase its body weight by 10–30% within 6 hours due to marked swelling of the lymph sacs (Conklin, 1930).

Infectious Etiologies. Carditis is reported rarely in amphibians, despite the presumed widespread prevalence of Gram-negative bacillary septicemias. Systemic chlamydial infections of clawed frogs, *Xenopus* spp., frequently produce a granulomatous endomyocarditis with characteristic intracytoplasmic inclusions. A rather high prevalence of 3–26% of captive crested newts, *Triturus cristatus*, developed pericarditis principally around the conus arteriosus. The cause was not determined, but enteritis was also common in these newts (Zavanella et al., 1989) suggesting an undetected infectious agent.

The heart may be involved in septicemic bacterial infections with lesions of epicarditis and myocarditis, but there are no bacterial diseases specific to the heart, and endocardial and valvular diseases have not been described in association with bacteremias.

Helminths, especially trematodes, may be found encysted in the myocardium and free in the pericardial sac. Wild-caught specimens of the African clawed frog, *Xenopus laevis*, may harbor dozens of immature nonencysted larvae of *Tylodelphys xenopi* flukes in the pericardial sac (King & Van As, 1997). Large numbers of these strigeid flukes may produce a slight pericarditis, occasional adhesions between the epicardium and pericardium, and massive hydropericardium with decreased cardiac output, respiratory embarrassment, hypoxia, and death. The larvae may live 2 years or longer in the host (Flynn, 1973; Nigrelli & Maraventano, 1944). The wild clawed frogs are intermediate hosts for this parasite; the final host is a fish-eating bird, *Anhinga melanogaster*, but the fluke does not develop in gulls and ducks (King & Van As, 1997).

Idiopathic Etiologies. Abnormalities of the posterior lymph hearts are assumed to be a cause of hydrops and subcutaneous edema in anuran tadpoles and adults, yet there are few descriptions of lymph heart lesions. Hydropic specimens of the clawed frog, *Xenopus* spp., have thrombosed, nonfunctional lymph hearts and become immensely bloated due to an excess of fluid in the lymph sacs, but no further gross, histologic, or etiologic details were given (Carter, 1979).

Aortic and arterial atherosclerosis have been reported in captive tree frogs affected with corneal lipidosis and xanthomatosis (Carpenter et al., 1986; Russell et al., 1990; Zwart & Vander Linde-Sipman, 1989).

27.2.7 Hematolymphopoietic System

The anatomy and histomorphology of the hematolymphopoietic system of immature caecilians, tadpoles, and salamander larvae have been reviewed (Zapata & Cooper, 1990). Information on the anatomy and physiology of the larval amphibian immune system is extensive, but is limited principally to ranids, bufonids, pipids (e.g., *Xenopus* spp.), and the axolotl, *Ambystoma mexicanum*. Lymphoid, myeloid, and erythroid tissue may occur in many organs of the body. There is very little information regarding gross and histological responses of the organs of the immune system to pathogens (Haynes et al., 1992).

Adult terrestrial amphibians retain some hematolymphopoietic organs from their larval stages, but there are significant developmental changes during metamorphosis. Most terrestrial amphibians (except caecilians) have functional bone marrow which they lacked as tadpoles and larvae, and the thymus does not involute with onset of sexual maturity as it does in some higher endotherms. Amphibians do not have an organ equivalent to the bursa of Fabricius in birds. Only the thymus, spleen, and, possibly, gut-associated lymphoid tissue exist as discrete hematolymphopoietic organs in all amphibians.

As a general rule, bone marrow is found in terrestrial stages of amphibians and is absent from aquatic forms and caecilians. Bone marrow equivalents in aquatic amphibians (larvae, tadpoles, neotenic adults) are found principally in the liver and kidneys (pronephros and mesonephros). In primitive salamanders, such as the Japanese giant salamander, *Andrias japonicus*, the ventral meninges has bone marrowlike tissue. Hematolymphopoietic tissue has also been described in gonads and intestines of other taxa.

Larval and adult amphibians have paired thymuses, usually situated posteroventral to the ears. In some amphibians the thymus is a single pair of organs derived from the second pharyngeal pouch (DuPasquier et al., 1989), but in others there may be three pairs that are derived from three branchial pouches. During metamorphosis, there is extensive turnover of the lymphocytic population in the thymus (Robert & Du Pasquier, 1995). Since metamorphosis results in the expression of new major histocompatability complex antigens, old T-lymphocytes are lost and new tolerant T-lymphocytes are necessary which will not reject tissues expressing new antigens of the adult major histocompatability complex (Rollins-Smith et al., 1993; Ruben et al., 1994).

Seasonal variation in the size and cellularity of the ranid thymus is striking. Hibernating and spring-breeding amphibians usually have much reduced thymic lobes with greatly reduced numbers of small lymphocytes, and blurred corticomedullary zones. The cortical region may also have multiple small cysts. By mid-summer and early autumn, the thymuses are large, heavy, and have prominent lymphocyte-rich cortices (Zapata et al., 1992). Thymuses undergo marked involution and atrophy in amphibians stressed by recent captivity or malnutrition (Plytycz et al., 1995).

Red pulp and white pulp are found in the spleen. The white pulp contains lymphopoietic cells and the subcapsular red pulp is the principal site of erythropoiesis (Manning & Horton, 1969). Distinct B-lymphocyte and T-lymphocyte regions are not evident in the spleen or lymphomyeloid organs. Seasonal changes in the spleen are much less than in the thymus, but a distinct involution occurs in wild anurans held in captivity (Plytycz et al., 1995). It is not clear whether this captivity-induced splenic atrophy is due to stress or a more favorable, bacteria-free environment (Mika et al., 1995).

The number of "lymph nodes" in tadpoles varies greatly from genus to genus and from species to species. Although the term "lymph node" is often used, based on anatomy, circulation, and function, the term lymphomyeloid organ is more appropriate.

Larval and adult anuran lymphomyeloid organs are not related. Larval organs undergo modification and retrogression until they disappear during metamorphosis (Cooper, 1967; Horton, 1971).

Functionally, anuran lymphomyeloid organs trap and process antigens, and produce strong humoral immune responses in a manner resembling the "true" lymph nodes of mammals (Zapata & Cooper, 1990).

Histologically, normal lymphomyeloid organs have a thin collagenous capsule, indistinct or absent trabeculae, and relatively homogenous masses of lymphocytes throughout, with no distinct cortical, paracortical, and medullary regions (Baculi et al., 1970).

Gut-associated lymphoid tissue (GALT) has been described in salamanders and anurans from the esophagus to cloaca (Ardavin et al., 1982; Jurd et al., 1995; Wong, 1972). These lymphoid aggregates are composed of small and medium sized lymphocytes, which, in the intestine, are consistently located amesenterically in the tunicas mucosa and submucosa. The lymphocytes readily infiltrate between mucosal epithelial cells. Discrete aggregates of lymphoid cells in the gut have not been found in some aquatic salamanders (Plytycz et al., 1995). The GALT also shows striking seasonal changes in cellularity and size: it is atrophied in hibernating anurans and well developed by mid-summer.

Genetic Etiologies. Stasis mutation in the axolotl, *Ambystoma mexicanum,* is a lethal trait in which nearly all erythrocytes in the body become lodged in the liver and circulation fails (Humphrey, 1975).

Anemic mutation is a nonlethal trait that occurs in the white trait axolotl, *Ambystoma mexicanum.* Affected homozygous larvae suffer a temporary severe anemia that results in a marked generalized pallor and mild reduction in growth. Hematopoiesis and coloration are eventually regained (Humphrey, 1975; Malacinski & Brothers, 1974).

Infectious Etiologies—Viral. The effects of viral infections on the amphibian immune system are unstudied. Despite a number of histological studies of tadpole edema virus, Bohle iridovirus, other ranaviruses, and Lucke herpesvirus, no specific lesions of the thymus, lymphomyeloid organs, bone marrow, or GALT have been reported. "Lymphoid hyperplasia" was reported in an ornate horned frog, *Ceratophrys ornata,* infected with a reptilian calicivirus, but the affected tissue or organ was not mentioned (Smith et al., 1986). Viral inclusions were detected histologically and ultrastructurally, in the spleen of one wild giant toad, *Bufo marinus* (Speare et al., 1991).

Intraerythrocytic inclusion body disease has been recognized in fish, amphibians, and reptiles for over a century (Gruia-Grey et al., 1989a, b). Literature prior to 1980 is confusing because these viral infections were misidentified and misnamed as artifacts and protozoan parasites. The protozoan names applied to these viral infections were *Pirhemocyton* spp. and *Toddia* spp. When infected erythrocytes were examined by electron microscopy, their viral nature was obvious (Bernard et al., 1968; Gruia-Grey et al., 1989a; Sousa & Weigl, 1976). Attempts to isolate frog erythrocytic virus (FEV) in cultures have failed, but numerous biochemical and biophysical properties of FEV have been reported (Gruia-Grey et al., 1989a, b).

Cytological examination of Giemsa-stained blood smears demonstrates a red or sometimes blue intracytoplasmic inclusion, often surrounded by several smaller inclusions (Desser & Barta, 1984a; Gruia-Grey & Desser, 1992; Speare et al., 1991). These dense inclusions are usually spherical, occasionally ovoid or pleomorphic, and 1–3 μm in diameter. Often, the cytoplasm also contains a larger pale or clear albuminoid vacuole. A third, bizarre inclusion, called an elongate (or crystalloid) body, is infrequently found. The elongate body is membrane-bound, dense, large (10–20 μm long), distinctly rectagular or trapezoidal, and often distorts the erythrocyte (Gruia-Grey et al., 1989a). The elongate body's rectangular inclusions are both intranuclear and intracytoplasmic, and are best demonstrated by differential interference contrast microscopy or in Heinz body (e.g., new methylene blue) stains. However, intranuclear crystalloid inclusions have not been detected in FEV of Canadian specimens of the bullfrog, *Rana catesbeiana* (Gruia-Grey et al., 1989b). Up to 90% of erythrocytes may contain the former smaller inclusions, but typically, 20–50% of erythrocytes are infected (Alves De Matos & Paperna, 1993; Gruia-Grey & Desser, 1992; Speare et al., 1991).

Infected erythrocytes are usually slightly or distinctly spheroidal. The nucleus is slightly to markedly eccentric and also appears mildly condensed. Anemia is minimal to moderate, with the red blood cell count being 28% lower than uninfected frogs in the same wild population. Mean corpuscular volume (MCV), mean corpuscular hemoglobin (MCH), and mean corpuscular hemoglobin concentration (MCHC) were usually similar to uninfected frogs, although in frogs with high intensity of infected erythrocytes, a 20% increase in MCV was found (Gruia-Grey & Desser, 1992). Peripheral blood smears also demonstrate a mild to moderate increase in circulating immature erythrocytes. Immature erythrocytes may comprise 17–30% of erythrocytes in the smear (Alves De Matos & Paperna, 1993; Gruia-Grey & Desser, 1992). Immature erythrocytes are more intensely infected by the iridovirus. The infected bullfrog, *Rana catesbeiana,* may have a spherocytic anemia (Gruia-Grey et al., 1989a).

Ultrastructurally, the smaller dense cytoplasmic inclusions of FEV consist of paracrystalline arrays of hexagonal (icosahedral) virus particles. Virus particles of FEV are found only in the cytoplasm, as is typical of all iridoviruses. Virus particles bud from cytoplasmic membranes or acquire envelopes from intracytoplasmic lamellar membranes; envelopes may be single or double. Size of the virus particles varies considerably from amphibian to amphibian but is usually consistent within the individual and species. Diameters (vertex to vertex) of the viral cores have been reported as 175–198 nm in the Banguella grassland frog, *Ptychadena anchietae* (Alves De Matos & Paperna, 1993), 200–300 nm in the northern leopard frog, *Rana pipiens* (Bernard et al., 1968), 293–312 nm in one wild Costa Rican giant toad, *Bufo marinus* (Speare et al., 1991), and 300–370 nm in Canadian specimens of the bullfrog, *Rana catesbeiana* (Gruia-Grey et al.,

1989a). The enveloped virus particles are large, measuring up to 450 nm in diameter. The albuminoid vacuoles are, ultrastructurally, stacks of lamellar membranes. The elongate crystalloid bodies consist of proteinaceous material forming distinct striations which run parallel to the long axis. The large size of intraerythrocytic iridoviruses and repeated failures at isolation, distinguish FEV viruses from the smaller, readily cultured ranaviruses (tadpole edema virus, Bohle virus, frog virus 3, and others).

Gross and histological lesions associated with FEV infections have not been described.

Epidemiological aspects of FEV in wild and captive Canadian anurans have been reported. The vector is suspected to be a mosquito, *Culex territans,* or a midge, *Forcipomyia fairfaxensis,* which feeds on terrestrial anurans. In recapture studies of the bullfrog, *R. catesbeiana,* 9% of uninfected and 4% of infected frogs were recaptured, suggesting that viral infection may contribute to the mortality of juveniles (Gruia-Grey & Desser, 1992).

One adult bullfrog, *Rana catesbeiana,* with lethargy had small ulcers on the skin of the body. The skin lesions were not studied, but ultrastructurally, leukocytes were found to contain polyhedral (icosahedral) cytoplasmic deoxyriboviruses (PCDV). Nonenveloped virions were 160 nm in diameter (vertex to vertex), strictly intracytoplasmic, and were observed budding from cell membranes. Lymphocytes, monocytes, and heterophils were infected. Heterophils were most heavily infected (Briggs & Burton, 1973). The morphology of the virus is consistent with a ranavirus, but the possibility remains that the virus was an FEV-like iridovirus.

Infectious Etiologies—Bacterial—Rickettsia (Aegyptianella spp.). The intraerythrocytic inclusions of amphibians caused by rickettsial organisms were initially misidentified and misnamed as the protozoan *Cytamoeba.* The intraerythrocytic rickettsia of North American anurans have been named *Aegyptianella ranarum,* and the similar organism in anurans from Europe is *A. bacterifera* (Desser, 1987; Desser & Barta, 1989). The older literature, which used the mistaken protozoan name, *Cytamoeba bacterifera* or *Cytamoeba* spp., has been summarized (Johnston, 1975), yielding reports from five anurans and five salamanders in North America, seven anurans from South America, and three anurans from Japan and the Phillipines. More recently, *Aegyptianella ranarum* was clearly identified and described from the bullfrog, *Rana catesbeiana,* the green frog, *R. clamitans,* and the mink frog, *R. septentrionalis* (Desser, 1987). The prevalence of infection in these three species varied considerably from year to year, from location to location, and from species to species.

Clinical signs and gross and histological lesions have not been described or associated with *Aegyptianella* spp. In Giemsa-stained blood smears, the organisms form distinct round or elliptical translucent vacuoles with dark encircling rims which are 3–11 μm in diameter. Smaller inclusions contain densely packed, dark-staining rods, arranged in parallel. Larger inclusions contain pink filamentous material (Desser, 1987). The organisms are Gram-negative. By electron microscopy, *A. ranarum* is rod-shaped, 1–1.7 μm long by 0.2–0.3 μm in diameter, while *A. bacterifera* is up to 5 μm long by 0.5 μm in diameter. *Aegyptianella bacterifera* is present at 1–12 organisms per vacuole, while vacuoles of *A. ranarum* contain 90–120 organisms.

Infectious Etiologies—Epidemic Splenomegaly. Beginning in March 1990, an uncultured intracellular coccoid organism has been found in many groups of clawed frogs, *Xenopus* spp. (Haynes et al., 1992). The coccobacilloid organism is approximately 1 μm in diameter, is found in macrophages and peripheral blood monocytes, exhibits motility when extracellular, and cannot be isolated in multiple standard bacterial media. One to many organisms may be found in "nonlymphoid leukocytes." The organism appears highly contagious as it has spread in one laboratory to infect all frogs, and has been detected in newly purchased frogs from four different vendors in the United States and Republic of South Africa. The organism may belong to the family Rickettsiaceae, and is possibly *Coxiella* or *Ehrlichia.* Infection in the clawed frog, *Xenopus* spp., is clinically silent and has not been associated with increased mortalities.

The only gross lesion is splenomegaly, a condition which may be difficult to assess when all colony animals are infected, as was the case at one research facility. The infection has not been studied histologically, nor are special stain characteristics reported. However, the immunological stimulation of infected toads is profound and involves activation of T-lymphocytes, production of T-cell growth factor (TCGF), expression of TCGF receptors on splenic lymphocytes (a trait exhibited exclusively by activated lymphocytes), and production of antibodies (IgM and IgY) (Haynes et al., 1992).

Infectious Etiologies—Streptococcal Bacteria. Streptococcal septicemia was described in an outdoor colony of 100,000 specimens of the bullfrog, *Rana catesbeiana,* in Brazil (Amborski et al., 1983). Mortality rate in 2 months was about 75% of the colony. Ten sick and ten normal-appearing frogs were cultured. Nonhemolytic group B streptococcal bacteria were isolated from sick frogs, but also were isolated from spleens of some apparently healthy frogs.

Grossly, sick specimens of the bullfrog, *R. catesbeiana,* had spleens that were twice normal size. No other gross lesions were reported, but clinically, affected frogs floated and had difficulty submerging (Amborski et al., 1983).

Gram-positive cocci were observed in the blood smears and were demonstrated intracellularly in histological sections of sick frogs. Histologically, the spleen, liver, and mesonephroi showed necrosis and phagocytosed cocci. Splenic lesions were striking and consisted of acute cellular necrosis, increased number of reticuloendothelial cells, and depletion of small lymphocytes. Livers showed acute multifocal coagulative necrosis with hemorrhage. Other hepatocytes appeared atrophied, and hepatic cords were disorganized. Within hepatic sinusoids, Kuppfer cells were increased in number and often contained phagocytosed cocci. Melanomacrophage aggregates were hyperplastic. Mesonephroi of three frogs had three changes: marked interstitial hemorrhage, segmental necrosis of glomerular tufts, and numerous cocci with minimal cellular change. Cocci were observed in blood vessels of other organs (Amborski et al., 1983).

Streptococcal bacteria were also isolated from 73–80% of tadpoles and adults of the bullfrog, *R. catesbeiana* (Glorioso et al., 1974), but were considered to be nonpathogenic.

Infectious Etiologies—Thrombocytozoons spp. The precise identity of this organism as a prokaryote or eukaryote is unclear. Originally, *Thrombocytozoons ranarum* was thought to be a protozoan infection of the marsh frog, *Rana ridibunda,* in Bulgaria (Tchacarof, 1963, as cited by Barta & Desser, 1984), however, recent ultrastructural studies suggest the organism is a Gram-positive-like bacterium (Desser & Barta, 1984b). The organism was detected in 3 (4%) of 75 specimens of the mink frog, *R. septentrionalis,* in Ontario, Canada (Barta & Desser, 1984), and 5.4% of the Bulgarian frogs. The organism is intrathrombocytic, forms a clearly defined cytoplasmic vacuole containing, usually, one bacillus-shaped to elongate organism with two or more pale spherical intraorganismal vacuoles. Rarely, two bacilli may be found in one thrombocyte. The organism is 9.5×2.6 μm (range: $7.8–11.5 \times 1.6–3.3$ μm), and has rounded or club-shaped ends. Because cytoplasm is sparse in ranid thrombocytes, the bacillus-shaped organism is usually adjacent to the nucleus and seems to fill the cytoplasm. No clinical signs, gross lesions, or histological features were reported in infected frogs.

Infectious Etiologies—Protozoal. Among wild-caught amphibians, protozoan parasitemias are commonly encountered. These protozoa may be extracellular (e.g., *Trypanosoma* spp.) or intraerythrocytic (e.g., *Hepatozoon* spp., *Lankesterella* spp.). The taxomomy of intraerythrocytic haemogregarines of amphibians is not precise (Desser, 1993). In addition, the literature is confused with protozoan names for viral and rickettsial infections. Recently, it has been suggested that all amphibian and reptilian blood parasites that were named *Haemogregarina* should be reclassified as the genus *Hepatozoon* (Siddall, 1995), with the possible exceptions of an obscure protozoan of toads called *Hemolivia* and two erythrocytic protozoans of crocodilians. Based on morphology alone in blood smear slides, it is not possible to distinguish the intraerythrocytic gamonts of *Hepatozoon* from *Haemogregarina,* nor is it possible to distinguish the two in histological sections of the hepatic meronts. The identity, even to the genus level, of nearly all reported frog haemogregarines is questionable, except the newly described *Hepatozoon catesbeianae* (Desser et al., 1995).

All described blood protozoan infections of amphibians have been considered asymptomatic, and some are host-specific (Desser, et al., 1995). However, some blood protozoa are capable of infecting multiple taxa of amphibians (e.g., *Trypanosoma ranarum, Babesiosoma stableri,* and *Lankesterella minima*).

Many amphibian protozoal infections of the blood are transmitted by leeches, but some are transmitted by hematophagous insects such as mosquitoes and midges. Mosquitoes may transmit protozoan parasites while taking a blood meal from an amphibian, or, as in the case of *Hepatozoon* spp., when they are eaten by anurans (Desser et al., 1995).

All *Hepatozoon* spp. infections of terrestrial anurans are consistently hepatocellular, and, sometimes, concurrently erythrocytic.

Hepatozoon catesbeianae is a recently described erythrohepatocytic infection of the bullfrog, *Rana catesbeiana*. The parasite cycles between the mosquito, *Culex territans,* and the frog. The mosquito is infected when it feeds on a frog that has circulating intraerythrocytic gamonts. The frog becomes infected only by ingesting an infected mosquito. Following ingestion of the mosquito, the sporozoites are released and reach the liver to form meronts. Each intrahepatocellular meront produces numerous merozoites, which are eventually released to infect erythrocytes. Merozoites enlarge and mature within the erythrocyte to become gamonts (Desser et al., 1995).

Clinical disease and gross lesions of *Hepatozoon catesbeianae* infection of the bullfrog, *Rana catesbeiana,* have not been reported. Mature gamonts within erythrocytes measure 22×5 μm, and are halteridial with pale-staining cytoplasm and a central compact nucleus. The mature gamonts markedly displace the erythrocyte's nucleus laterally (Desser et al., 1995).

Grossly, the only reported lesion of *Hepatozoon* spp. (formerly *Haemogregarina* spp.) infections is splenomegaly, reported in infections of the square-marked toad, *Bufo regularis,* by *H. boueti* in Egypt (Saad & El Masri, 1995).

Babesiosoma spp. and *Dactylosoma* spp. are intraerythrocytic protozoa of adult anurans that are probably transmitted by leeches but can be transmitted experimentally by injected blood (Barta et al., 1987; Schmittner & McGhee, 1961). The life cycles of these two genera are unknown and presently they are considered members of the order Eucoccidia (Barta et al., 1987). Two principal species are of concern among anurans: the North American *B. stableri* and the European *D. ranarum*. Both protozoa appear to infect only erythrocytes since no organisms have been detected in other organs or cells by cytological examinations (Schmittner & McGhee, 1961). No gross or histological lesions have been described. Cytologically, intraerythrocytic gamonts of *Dactylosoma* are blue in Giemsa's stain, 7.0 × 3.4 μm, and have a "tail" that folds back about 80% of the length of the gamont (Barta et al., 1987). Secondary merozoites of *Babesiosoma stableri* often have a distinct cruciform shape in erythrocytes (Barta & Desser, 1984) while the gamonts lack the recurved tail and usually lie fully extended within the erythrocytic cytoplasm.

Multiple genera of Lankesterellidae have been described from ectothermic vertebrates, but until life cycles are elucidated and cross-species transmission studies are performed, many proposed genera and species remain uncertain (Desser, 1993). The best studied of these amphibian parasites are *Lankesterella minima* and *Schellackia balli*. The prevalence of *L. minima* in the bullfrog, *Rana catesbeiana*, in Ontario, Canada, was 55% in tadpoles and 29% in metamorphosed frogs (Desser et al., 1990). The site of development of infective sporozoites in the amphibia host corresponds to the route of infection: *Lankesterella* spp. sporozoites infect endothelial cells throughout the body and cells of the reticuloendothelial system (Lainson & Paperna, 1995) while ingestion of vector mites harboring *Schellackia* spp. results in initial infection of the amphibian's intestinal mucosal epithelium. *Schellackia* spp. initially form microgamounts in the intestinal mucosa, then secondarily invade cells of the lamina propria to form sporozoite-laden oocysts. In the case of *S. balli* in the giant toad, *Bufo marinus*, the respiratory epithelium may be infected. *Schellackia* spp. produce only eight sporozoites per oocyst, while *L. minima* in the bullfrog, *R. catesbeiana*, produces about 70 sporozoites per infected endothelial cell (Desser, 1993; Desser et al., 1990). In the edible frog, *Rana kl. esculenta*, oocysts of *L. minima* produce 16–50 sporozoites (Noller, 1912 *fide*, Desser et al., 1990). *Lankesterella hylae* of White's treefrog, *Pelodryas caerulea*, produces only eight sporozoites per oocyst (Stehbens, 1966). Sporozoites released by oocysts infect erythrocytes, and cytologically, intraerythrocytic sporozoites in wild Canadian ranids measure 12.7 × 2.1 μm, and have a characteristic mild concavity of the organism adjacent to the erythrocyte's nucleus (Barta & Desser, 1984).

Trypanosomes of amphibians are transmitted principally or entirely by leeches. Cytological and ultrastructural descriptions of trypanosomes have been reported, and excellent epidemiological studies also exist, but no gross or histologic lesions have been described in infected amphibians (Gill & Mock, 1985; Jones & Woo, 1994; Martin & Desser, 1990, 1991; Martin et al., 1992; Mock, 1987; Mock & Gill, 1984; Siddall & Desser, 1992; Werner et al., 1988).

Infectious Etiologies—Helminths. Filarid worm infections are common in ranid frogs in North America and Europe, and have been reported on other continents. Infections have been noted in ranids and amphiumas, *Amphiuma* spp. (Flynn, 1973), by *Foleyella* spp. and *Icosiella* spp. Several proposed species of amphibian filaria are based on observations of the microfilaria only, and are therefore considered incomplete identifications (Witenberg & Gerichter, 1944). All adults of *Foleyella* spp. occur in the coelomic cavity, subvertebral lymphatics or mesentery as does *Icosiella quadrituberculata*, while adults of *Icosiella neglecta* of Old World ranids occurs in the dermis and subcutis. When both male and female filarids infect the frog, the female releases ensheathed microfilaria which enter the circulatory system and may survive 2 years awaiting ingestion by a mosquito intermediate host. In the mosquito, the microfilaria develop into an infective larva, which is passed to the host when the mosquite again takes a blood meal from the amphibian (Flynn, 1973). Most infected anurans are asymptomatic, but heavy infections by the filarids may cause listlessness and eventual death. Microfilaria may cause dermal nodules, but the nodules have not been characterized histologically (Reichenbach-Klinke & Elkan, 1965).

Miscellaneous Etiologies—Glucocorticosteroid-Induced Changes. Tadpoles of the bullfrog, *Rana catesbeiana*, adults of the Eastern newt, *Notophthalmus viridescens*, and adults of the axolotl, *Ambystoma mexicanum*, show a marked peripheral blood lymphopenia and neutrophilia when injected with corticosteroids. In the axolotl, *A. mexicanum*, the thymus undergoes severe lymphorrhexis with atrophy of both the cortex and medulla (Tournefier, 1982), however lymphocytes in the spleen appear to increase in number.

The effects of exogenous corticosteroids on adult amphibians is much the same as in aquatic larval amphibians. Marked thymic lymphorrhexis, lymphopenia, and neutrophilia occur (Garrido et al., 1987). In some amphibians the spleen shows lymphorrhexis and atrophy of white pulp while lymphocytes appear to increase in numbers in the bone marrow of adult anurans (Zapata et al., 1992).

27.2.8 Endocrine System

The endocrine organs of aquatic amphibians are basically similar to those of higher vertebrates, with some important exceptions. The principal endocrine organs are the pituitary, pineal, thryroid, parathyroids, ultimobranchial bodies, interrrenals ("adrenals"), islets of Langerhans, and gonads. In the skin, gastrointestinal tract, and elsewhere, amphibians also have scattered neuroendocrine cells (Chester-Jones et al., 1987a), sometimes referred to as APUD cells (amine precursor uptake, decarboxylation cells), which embryologically originate from neural crest cells. As with many other amphibian organs, endocrine glands may vary seasonally in size, functional activity, and cellular morphology (Dodd & Callan, 1955).

The thyroid consists of two lobes with a common embryological origin in the ventral midline of the oropharynx. In most amphibians the thyroid has no obvious capsule, and in tadpoles it tends to be loosely aggregated in the wall of the gill chamber, somewhat similar to the distribution in fish. In salamanders the thyroid usually forms two discrete lobes. In experimentally thyroidectomized specimens of the Eastern newt, *Notophthalmus viridescens,* accessory thyroid follicles were evident histologically in 30% of animals (Schmidt, 1958). Calcitonin cells (C-cells) are not present in the amphibian thyroid, but instead cluster as the paired ultimobranchial bodies. One pair of parathyroids are present in anurans, but many taxa of salamander larvae appear to lack parathyroids (Stiffler, 1993; Waggener, 1930).

Thyroidal histology changes during metamorphosis (Coleman et al., 1967, 1968a). As metamorphosis begins the tadpole's thyroid is stimulated by thyroid-stimulating hormone (TSH), causing follicular cells to hypertrophy and colloid to accumulate in the follicles. Nuclei are usually round and central in the cell. Droplets of colloid within the cell cytoplasm are rare. At the completion of metamorphosis, the thyroid is a discrete bilobed organ. Thyroid follicles are lined by low cuboidal cells, and PAS-positive colloid is present in the lumina.

The adult pituitary of anurans, salamanders, and caecilians differ morphologically. The pituitary of permanently neotenous salamanders resembles that of dipnoan fish. The amphibian hypophysis consists of glandular (adenohypophysis) and neural (neurohypophysis) parts. Two acidophilic and three basophilic (mucoid) cell types occur in the amphibian adenohypophysis. The special staining features and secretions of these cells have been reviewed (Chester-Jones et al., 1987c).

In aquatic larval amphibians, the pineal is a saccular organ originating from the roof of the diencephalon and is composed of two cell types, photoreceptor cells and supportive cells. In anurans, there is evidence the pineal photoreceptor cells are similar to photoreceptors of the retina. During metamorphosis the pineal is markedly reorganized and loses its central lumen. The pineal becomes flattened and solidly cellular. Over half the cells in the adult pineal are produced following metamorphosis. In both the larvae and adult, 14–18% of cells in the pineal are photoreceptors (Hendrickson & Kelly, 1969; Kelly, 1965; Kelly & Smith, 1964).

The term adrenal is used when the organ is near, but separate from the kidney, as is characteristic of mammals, birds, and reptiles. When adrenocortical cells mingle, to varying degrees, with the renal tissue, as in amphibians and fish, the more appropriate term is interrenal gland. Possibly because amphibians have a mesonephric kidney, rather than metanephroi as in mammals, and because the endoderm gives rise to both interrenal and mesonephric tissue, the two organs remain intermingled (Accordi & Milano, 1990). The interrenal of amphibians is not a discrete encapsulated gland, but lies ventrally in the mesonephroi and intermingles with renal tubules in the renal interstitium. In anurans, interrenal cells are present superficially in the ventral region of the mesonephroi (Accordi & Cianfoni, 1981; Accordi et al., 1981; Chester-Jones, 1987). In salamanders, the interrenal tissue may consist of interrupted segments or islands of cells, located mostly in the ventral midline of each mesonephros.

Three cell types have been described in the interrenals of amphibians: interrenal (cortical), Stilling, and chromaffin (medullary) cells. Cortical cells are rich with lipid droplets (cytoplasmic vacuoles) and have round nuclei. Chromaffin cells (medullary cells of neural crest origin) occur singly and in small groups in the mesonephric interstitium and among interrenocortical cells. Chromaffin cells tend to be larger than cortical cells, are polygonal to elongate, and have an ovoid eccentric nucleus. Their cytoplasm is finely granular; these cytoplasmic granules stain positively in most silver stains. A third cell type, Stilling cells, occur in ranids only and are clearly evident by their prominent eosinophilic, periodic acid-Schiff-positive, cytoplasmic granules (Accordi & Cianfoni, 1981). The function and possible homology of Stilling cells to higher vertebrates are unresolved (Chester-Jones, 1987).

The islets of Langerhans, or endocrine pancreas, occur as discrete clusters of cells in the lobes (or processes) of the adult exocrine pancreas. Islet cells may occur singly or in clusters. Clusters may be small or large, depending on the species of amphibian. No clear pattern of distribution, organization, or cluster size occurs, despite numerous studies (Gorbman,

1964). Four islet hormones (glucagon, insulin, pancreatic polypeptide, and somatostatin) have been demonstrated in amphibian pancreases (Chester-Jones et al., 1987b).

In tadpoles, the islets are embryonic and minimally functional. Larval islets have slight secretory capacity. Maturation and function of the insulin-secreting beta cells does not become important in blood glucose regulation until mid-metamorphosis (Frye, 1964).

Scattered single cells in many organs, especially in the epithelium of the gastrointestinal tract (GIT), secrete a variety of polypeptide hormones. Various names have been proposed for these cells including the "diffuse endocrine system," but the name amine precursor uptake and decarboxylation (APUD) cells is probably most widely accepted. In addition to cells of the GIT, APUD cells include interrenal medullary cells, and some cells of the adenohypophysis.

Genetic Etiologies—Goiters. Goiter mutation in tadpoles of the African clawed frog, *Xenopus laevis*, inhibits metamorphosis (Fischberg et al., 1963; Gurdon & Woodland, 1975).

Congenital Etiologies—Absence of the Pituitary in Tadpoles. In a group of 28 cross-bred tadpoles of the northern leopard frog, *Rana pipiens*, six were silvery due to an expansion of iridophores and contraction of melanophores, which suggested a deficiency of the hormone intermedin. Histological examinations revealed absence of the pituitary (Underhill, 1967). It has been suggested the trait was recessive (Browder, 1975).

Congenital Etiologies—Giantism in Tadpoles. Very large wild tadpoles which fail to metamorphose have been reported since 1905 (Elkan, 1976b; Reichenbach-Klinke & Elkan, 1965). Affected animals may be 2–3 times larger than normal, and all tadpoles in a pond may be affected. Affected giant tadpoles fail to metamorphose, fail to extrude their forelimbs, retain weak poorly developed hindlimbs, and have misshapen mouths. Giant tadpoles have histologically abnormal thyroids, pituitaries, and thymuses (Elkan, 1976b). The thyroid consists of large, thin-walled cysts which lack colloid while the pituitary is markedly hyperplastic and in some individuals had one or more large cysts containing a periodic acid-Schiff-positive material. Thymuses have normal cortices but in the medulla there are multiple thin-walled cysts also containing a periodic acid-Schiff-positive material. Rising levels of thyroid hormones are a major factor in initiating metamorphosis in tadpoles, hence any process which interferes with iodine metabolism or thyroid function may be expressed as defective metamorphosis in amphibians.

Idiopathic Etiologies. In some neotenic newts, clinically and grossly obvious goiters may be found (Dodd & Callan, 1955). Goiters may cause marked, bilobed, ventral swellings of the neck and intermandibular region with extensive compression and displacement of structures.

Toxicological Etiologies—Experimental Goiters. Several chemicals have goitrogenic properties including thiourea, propyl-thiouracil, potassium thiocyanate, and potassium perchlorate. Goiters and a hypothyroid state may be induced in tadpole and adult clawed frogs, *Xenopus* spp., by chronic immersion (3–20 months) in aqueous solutions of any of these four chemicals (Coleman et al., 1968a, b; Rollins-Smith et al., 1993). Terrestrial anurans have similar histological changes in the thyroids following treatment with thiourea (Hussain & Saidapur, 1982). The known goitrogen thiourea fails to induce clinical goiters in newts (Adams, 1946) although histologically the thyroid follicles are much smaller, lined by columnar epithelium, and have very little colloid.

27.2.9 Reproductive System

Gonads of all amphibians lie within the body cavity. Among temperate zone amphibians and those from climatic zones having distinct wet and dry seasons, there is marked seasonal fluctuation of gametogenesis and size of gonads and accessory sex organs. In continuously moist tropical climates, gametogenesis may occur year-round. In female amphibians from temperate zones that are held in captivity, failure to provide cold seasons may result in continued development of ova. Ova that are twice the size of normal wild amphibians have been reported in captive amphibians. However, adverse effects of oversized ova have not been reported.

In ranids, sex determination is a notoriously labile phenotypic characteristic. The larval gonad consists of indifferent cortex and medulla. The ovary is derived from the cortex, and the testis from the medulla (Browder, 1975). In anurans, the female is heterogametic, and the male is homogametic. Genetic determination of sex can be experimentally reversed by temperature or hormone treatments. Matings of sex-reversed females with normal females result in all offspring being female (Browder, 1975). In the Spanish ribbed newt, *Pleurodeles waltl*, the male is homogametic (ZZ) while the female is heterogametic (ZW). When larvae of this newt are raised at elevated temperature, 30°C (86°F) rather than a normal 18–22°C (64–72°F), the percentage of phenotypic males greatly increases, and intersexes and hermaphrodites develop. Sexually reversed females (phenotypic males) are capable of breeding as males (Dournon, 1983).

In the African clawed frog, *Xenopus laevis*, genetic males are easily and efficiently converted to females by treatment of the developing embryos with estradiol. Genetic females may be converted to males by transplantation of testes (Gurdon & Woodland, 1975).

Temperate zone salamanders have annual cycles of spermatogenesis, and their testes are considered zonal, and consist of locules (germinal cysts). Each locule contains clones of gametes in the same stage of development, such that each testis shows a marked gradation of maturing locules with the most mature gametes located rostrally (Callard, 1992; Dawley & Crowder, 1995).

Bidder's organ is a structure that is a remnant of the ovary in bufonid males only. It is located ventral and anterior to each testis, and may be a lateral band, roundish nodule, or an anterior caplike structure. Bidder's organs are remnants of the cortical region of the embryonic germinal ridge. Immature ova are evident histologically in Bidder's organs (Duellman & Trueb, 1986). The presence of ovarian tissue in male bufonids should not be mistaken for evidence of hermaphroditism.

Amphibians have symmetrical, paired ovaries and oviducts (urogenital ducts). The ovaries are suspended by the mesovarium, and surrounded by a very thin sheath of connective tissue, the ovisac. Rupture of the ovisac releases mature ova into the body cavity. The coelomic mesothelium is ciliated, and ciliary action moves the ova anteriad and into the infundibulum of the oviduct. Oviducts form from the embryonic Mullerian ducts, and course parallel and ventrolateral to the mesonephroi. Oviducts are are straight in caecilians, slightly convoluted in salamanders, and very convoluted in anurans. Segments of the oviduct nearest the cloaca in oviparous amphibians are lined by mucus-secreting epithelial cells that produce the capsules on eggs (Duellman & Trueb, 1986).

Retention of developing embryos with provision of nutrition within the oviduct (viviparity) occurs in all three living orders of amphibians. In anurans and salamanders, less than 1% of species evidence viviparity, while in caecilians the majority of the known 170 species are viviparous. The taxa of amphibians that are viviparous and ovoviviparous have been reviewed (Wake, 1993).

Neoteny is the condition in which salamander larvae fail to undergo metamorphosis into terrestrial adult amphibians, and instead become sexually mature in an aquatic form, usually with retention of external gills and other larval features. Grossly and histologically, the endocrine organs of neotenes appear normal (Pierce & Smith, 1979).

Congenital Etiologies. Hermaphroditism was reported in a captive tomato frog, *Dyscophus antongilii* (Frye & Miller, 1994). At necropsy, the animal had well developed ovaries containing deeply pigmented and yolked ova. The testes were not observed grossly because they were not suspected and were dorsal to the ovaries. Histologically, the testes were active. The ovaries were distinctly separate from and were not attached to the testes as occurs with Bidder's organs. The presence of separate, functionally active, male and female gonads in this animal was diagnostic of true hermaphroditism.

Toxicological Etiologies. It is becoming increasingly clear that multiple widely used household, industrial, and agricultural chemicals are estrogenic to fish and reptiles (Gross et al., 1994; Jobling et al., 1996; Palmer & Selcer, 1996).

Based on one experimental study of injected diethylstilbesterol and the pesticide DDT (o, p' -DDT: 1-chloro-2- [2,2,2,-trichloro-1-(4-chlorophenyl)ethyl] benzene) in adults of the African clawed frog, *Xenopus laevis,* it is evident that these xenobiotic estrogenic chemicals induce hepatic production and release of measurable levels of the yolk lipoprotein, vitellogenin, into the blood of male amphibians (Palmer & Palmer, 1995). Furthermore, the production of vitellogenin in response to DDT in males *X. laevis* (which normally do not produce it) can be used as a specific (qualitative) as well as quantifiable biomarker of estrogenic exposure. However, the effects on wild amphibians of environmental estrogen-mimicking xenobiotics, the duration of vitellogenin in the serum of estrogen-stimulated males, and adverse physiological and reproductive effects of such exposures have yet to be documented, although it has been suggested that estrogen-mimicking xenobiotics may contribute to reproductive impairment and population declines in wild amphibians (Palmer & Palmer, 1995).

Mercury is embryotoxic and gametotoxic in amphibians. Mercury is toxic to germ cells and may inhibit proliferation of primordial germ cells, resulting in smaller gonads and partial sterility (Power et al., 1989). In mature male Cyan five-fingered frogs, *Euphlyctis (Rana) cyanophlyctis,* which have continuous spermatogenesis, mercuric chloride caused reduction in the number of spermatocytes in each testicular lobule, but increased numbers of spermatogonia, suggesting maturation of spermatogonia into spermatocytes was inhibited (Kanamadi & Saidapur, 1992).

Infectious Etiologies—Protozoal. Two microsporidian infections are reported in the gonads of anurans, *Microsporidium schuetzi* in the ova of the northern leopard frog, *Rana pipiens,* and *Pleistophora bufonis* in Bidder's organ of bufonids in Switzerland and the United States (Canning & Lom, 1986; Guyenot & Ponse, 1926; King, 1907). In the common European toad, *B. bufo,* the organism essentially destroys both Bidder's organs. The organisms measure 2.4–5.2 μm. Within Bidder's organs, the microsporidia are located within ova. Although not specifically demonstrated or reported for this organism, all microsporidia are considered Gram-positive, have a periodic acid-Schiff-positive polar cap, and mature sporonts are acid-fast (Gardiner et al., 1988).

Microsporidiosis of the ova of the northern leopard frog, *Rana pipiens*, may be fairly common, and often overlooked. It has been encountered in many females from Vermont (Schuetz et al., 1978), with the assigned name, *Microsporidium schuetzi* (Canning & Lom, 1986). The infection was obvious grossly by the marked abnormal enlargement and discoloration of ova. Affected ova were about 50% greater in volume, and instead of having discrete melanosis of the animal pole and a yellowish ventral vegetal hemisphere, the infected ova are homogenously pale brown to whitish gray. The prevalence in wild frogs was not reported, but affected female frogs had 8 to about 120 infected ova, which was a small fraction of the total number of normal, fully developed oocytes (Schuetz et al., 1978).

Infectious Etiologies—Myxozoans (Myxosporeans). Myxozoan (Myxosporean) infections of the the male reproductive tract have been reported in anurans for more than 100 years (reviewed by Upton et al., 1992) (Figure 27.46). *Myxobolus* spp., have been recorded from frogs and toads in Australia, New Guinea, Africa, and Europe. *Myxobolus hylae* was common in the green and golden bell frog, *Litoria aurea*, in the region near Sydney. It infects the testes, vas deferens, oviduct, and urinary bladder, and may be host-specific since it was not detected in any sympatric anurans. The recent description of *M. bufonis* in Hallowell's toad, *Bufo maculatus*, from Cameroon, Africa, is instructive of the infections in general.

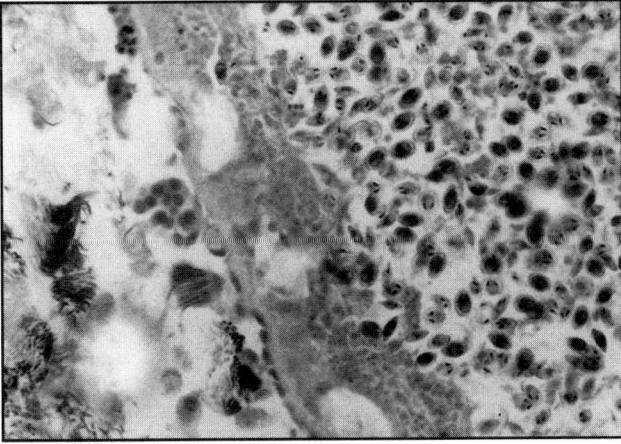

Figure 27.46. Myxosporidiosis in the testis of a sandy big-eyed frog, *Nyctimystes kubori*. Normal testicular tissue on the left, massive numbers of myxozoan spores on the right. Note the ovoid to spindle shape of these small multicellular parasites. Dark-staining paired piriform nucleus-like structures in each spore are actually separate cells called polar capsules or cnidocysts. (E. Elkan, RTLA 412)

Grossly, white, oval nodules, about 0.5–0.9 mm in diameter, are evident on at least one but usually both testes. Histologically, each cyst contains hundreds or thousands of trophozoites and spores. There is compression atrophy of adjacent locules, a thin fibrous capsule and minimal inflammatory cell reaction. Spores are disc-shaped and measure about 9 μm in diameter and 4 μm thick. No striations are evident on the valvelike cells of the spore. Polar capsules are paired, symmetrical, piriform, and measure 4.1 × 3.2 μm (Upton et al., 1992).

27.2.10 Central, Peripheral, and Autonomic Nervous Systems

The brain develops and changes during metamorphosis as nuclear regions for special sensory organs change from an aquatic emphasis on olfactory and lateral line systems to an emphasis on the ocular and auditory systems in terrestrial adults. Topography and histomorphology of the adult amphibian nervous system has been the subject of several reviews and monographs (Herrick, 1948; Kemali & Braitenberg, 1969; Kuhlenbeck, 1973; Oksche & Ueck, 1976).

The sympathetic nervous system of amphibians has been reviewed (Smith, 1994).

Metamorphic Transitions in the Nervous System. The brains of tadpoles and salamander larvae have been considered a mosaic of regions that respond differently to thyroid hormones during metamorphosis. Some regions of the central nervous system grow and differentiate in response to rising levels of thyroid hormones. Other areas atrophy, necrose, and disappear, and some neurons (e.g., Mauthner neurons) atrophy after metamorphic climax when thyroid levels decline (Kollros, 1981).

The neurons of the mesencephalic nucleus of the trigeminal nerve (Vth) increase steadily in larval stages but increase markedly during metamorphosis as proprioceptors of the remodeling mandible. The medulla oblongata of larvae is substantially smaller in cross-sectional diameter compared to animals in metamorphosis. In the lumbar spinal cord, tadpoles of the clawed frogs, *Xenopus* spp., and the northern leopard frog, *Rana pipiens*, have over 10,000 neurons per hemisphere in the lateral motor column (LMC) during early larval stages. Numbers of LMC neurons decline markedly during metamorphosis, resulting in about 2000 neurons at completion of metamorphosis. The cerebellum of tadpoles is relatively simple and primitive until early stages of metamorphosis. The cerebellum develops rapidly as the hindlimbs form, and then very rapidly as the tail begins resorption. The maturation of the cerebellum includes loss of the external granular cell layer by cell migration to the internal granular cell layer, and growth and differentiation of

Purkinje cells from small, immature forms into large mature neurons.

In contrast to the selective degeneration of some neural components of the brain and body spinal cord at metamorphosis, the tail cord degenerates completely. Degeneration begins distally and progresses proximally. The tail neural tube reduces its luminal diameter, neural cells accumulate lipid and pigment, degenerate, and necrotic cellular debris accumulates in the lumen. Ultrastructurally, neural cells develop autophagic vacuoles, large cytolysosomes, and many membrane-bound bodies. Macrophages and granulocytes infiltrate the tube and phagocytose necrotic neural cells (Fox, 1981).

Genetic Etiologies. Several mutations have been described and partially characterized in common laboratory amphibians (Droin & Beauchemin, 1975; Gurdon & Woodland, 1975; Humphrey, 1975; Ide, 1978; Ide et al., 1977; Reinschmidt & Tompkins, 1984).

Nutritional Etiologies. Cholesterol granulomata have been reported in the cranial cavity of mature female frogs with corneal lipidosis/disseminated xanthomatosis syndrome (Carpenter et al., 1986; Russell et al., 1990; Zwart & Vander Linde-Sipman, 1989). The granulomata consist of swollen foamy macrophages laden with lipids, fibrocytes, and lesser numbers of lymphocytes, granulocytes, and occasional multinucleated giant cells. The foamy macrophages contain neutral fats which are positive by various special stains for fat (e.g., oil-red-O). Cholesterol crystals (or clefts) may also be present. Some granulomata cause severe compression of the brain due to their size. The precise site of origin of these masses has not been determined or discussed.

Toxicological Etiologies—Insecticides. No specific or diagnostically useful lesions are detectable grossly or histologically in cases of insecticide poisoning in most adult vertebrates. However, several pronounced defects or malformations occur in embryonic and larval amphibians that are exposed to a variety of insecticides (Honrubia et al., 1993; Osborn et al., 1981; Snawder & Chambers, 1989). Insecticide intoxications are discussed in this section on the nervous system because the mode of action of organophosphate, carbamate, and pyrethroid insecticides occurs at the biochemical level involving inhibition of acteylcholinesterase and sodium channels. Although pesticide-associated fatalities are commonly reported in conjunction with mass mortalities of fish, birds, or mammals, rarely are levels of insecticides determined in mass amphibian casualties. Insecticide poisoning and persistence in the environment has been implicated in local extinctions of amphibians (Russell et al., 1995). The effects of pesticides may be species-specific (Honrubia et al., 1993), with variations in response depending on the life stage of the amphibian.

Toxicological Etiologies—Insecticides—Organochlorines. Use of organochlorine pesticides in North America and Europe has decreased since the 1970s, but they continue to pose threats to many vertebrate taxa because of environmental persistence, localized regions of massive spills, and tendency to accumulate in food chains. Manufacture of organochlorines for export to developing countries continues in industrialized countries, hence toxic spills remain a threat, even in those countries where their use is banned. Local extinctions of three species of amphibians has been attributed to repeated applications of dichlorodiphenyltrichlorethane (DDT) for mosquito control in the 1960s and 1970s in a Canadian national park. In the same national park, specimens of the spring peeper, *Pseudacris crucifer,* were assayed for organochlorines 26 years after the last application of DDT and were found to have levels of DDT and its metabolites of 1188 µg/kg. Levels of 1,000 µg/kg in fish may be toxic to fish-eating birds (Russell et al., 1995).

Limited data are available on the toxicity of dieldrin and DDT and its metabolites to amphibians. The DDT metabolite, DDD, is 3–8 times more toxic to bufonid tadpoles than DDT. Dieldrin is approximately four times more toxic to bufonid tadpoles than DDD, and is eight times more toxic than DDT (Sanders, 1970). Clinical signs of DDT intoxication in bufonid tadpoles are incoordination, hyperactivity, loss of equilibrium, weight loss, and death (Cooke, 1972; Russell et al., 1995; Sanders, 1970). The toxicity of seven organochlorine insectides was assessed in adults of the northern leopard frog, *Rana pipiens* (Kaplan & Overpeck, 1964). Frogs exposed cutaneously by immersion in various concentrations of aldrin, benzene hexachloride (BHC), chlordane, dieldrin, endrin, methoxychlor, and toxaphene, showed clinical signs of skin discoloration (grayish or blackish green), decreased cardiac and respiratory rates, hyperactivity, hyperreaction to stimuli, occasional course tremors, hindlimb extensor rigidity, poor righting reflex, and repeated convulsions. Excessive mucus secretion of the skin and hyperptyalism also occurred. Frogs immersed in benzene hexachloride reacted differently. These frogs were lethargic, failed to respond to stimuli, and made weak or no efforts to escape capture or handling. Prolonged immersion in 17 ppm BHC caused vomiting, gastric prolapse, and cloacal prolapse. Gross lesions were nonspecific and included occasional petechiation of the intestines and myocardial pallor in all organochlorines except benzene hexachloride. Frogs intoxicated with benzene hexachloride had enlarged congested hearts and enlarged livers that were "olive to yellowish" (Kaplan & Overpeck, 1964). Hemograms were also studied and reported in experimental intoxications of the northern leopard frog, *R. pipiens,* by organochlorine insecticides (Kaplan & Overpeck, 1964). Toxaphene has been used in deliberate attempts to kill aquatic salamanders, so that fish could be stocked in a pond (Rose, 1977).

Dieldrin and DDT are associated with deformities of the snout or maxillary region of growing tadpoles (Cooke, 1972, 1979; Osborn et al., 1981).

Toxicological Etiologies—Insecticides—Carbamates. The mode of action of carbamate and organophosphate insecticides in vertebrates is inhibition of acetylcholinesterase in synapses (Fikes, 1990). However, these insecticides also have potent teratologic effects in amphibian embryos and larvae that are not usually recognized in endotherms. Exposure of tadpoles of the tiger frog, *Rana tigrina,* and the Coruna frog, *R. perezi,* to carbaryl and pirimicarb, respectively, results in numerous developmental anomalies (Honrubia et al., 1993; Marian et al., 1983). Tadpoles of the tiger frog, *R. tigrina,* that were exposed to carbaryl were examined grossly only showed changes in dermal pigmentation, greatly reduced intestinal coiling, deformation of the notochord, and an increased volume of the heart and blood vessels (Marian et al., 1983). Similar gross defects were induced in tadpoles of the Coruna frog, *R. perezi,* and the defects were studied histologically (Honrubia et al., 1993). Acute miliary degeneration and necrosis of gill epithelium occurs within 24 hours of exposure to primicarb, and in those tadpoles that survive acute intoxication, repair is completed in a few days. The gall bladder also shows transient change. The epithelium of the gall bladder is simple cuboidal, but for about 14 days following exposure, the epithelium is distinctly flattened as if recovering from loss of epithelial cells. The liver develops slowly in exposed tadpoles. The hepatic cords remain thin and the hepatocytes small for about 14 days. Hepatocytes also contain many clear vacuoles suggestive of lipid accumulation. The atria of the heart was mildly dilated. The notochord, which normally is circular in cross-section, is pleomorphic, and the perinotochordal sheath of fibrocytes is irregularly thickened or hypoplastic. As in studies of organophosphate exposures in bird embryos (Wyttenbach & Thompson, 1985), it was suggested that anomalies of the heart and notochord in tadpoles are due to carbamate-induced defects in collagen synthesis (Honrubia et al., 1993).

Toxicological Etiologies—Insecticides—Organophosphates. Organophosphates act on the central and peripheral nervous systems by inhibiting acetylcholinesterase. Some organophosphates are reversible while others are nonreversible inhibitors (Berrill et al., 1995; Fikes, 1990). Use of agricultural organophosphates such as fenitrothion has been cited as an example of a commonly used forest pesticide that may contribute to amphibian population declines (Vial & Saylor, 1993). Clinically, most organophosphate insecticides cause paralysis, inability to respond to stimuli, and sometimes death in amphibian larvae, but minimally affect embryos (Berrill et al., 1994, 1995). Each species of amphibian varies in sensitivity to organophosphates depending on the insecticide, its concentration, and the life stage at exposure (Berrill et al., 1995).

Fenitrothion and malathion are the better studied organophosphates in amphibian taxa (e.g., Berrill et al., 1994, 1995; Elliott-Feeley & Armstrong, 1982; Snawder & Chambers, 1990). Concentrations as low as 1–4 ppm fenitrothion in water may cause temporary or permanent paralysis of larvae. Concentrations of 2.5 ppm have been detected in vernal forest ponds used by breeding amphibians following aerial spraying of fenitrothion (Berrill et al., 1995). Paralysis and death are the only described clinical signs of intoxication by fenitrothion; no gross or histological lesions have been reported. However, developmental anomalies caused by the organophosphate malathion have been reported in experimentally exposed specimens of the African clawed frog, *Xenopus laevis* (Snawder & Chambers, 1989, 1990). Many of the embryological anomalies are attributable to defects in formation of connective tissues and epithelia (Honrubia et al., 1993; Snawder & Chambers, 1989).

Toxicological Etiologies—Insecticides—Pyrethroids. Synthetic pyrethroids are increasingly popular for control of insects in agricultural, veterinary, aquatic, and household environments. While synthetic pyrethroids have low toxicity to birds and mammals, they are extremely toxic to aquatic organisms (Materna et al., 1995). In experimental studies with the African clawed frog, *Xenopus laevis,* allethrin caused clinical signs of hyperexcitation and convulsions within 10 min of exposure to 5000 µg/L, while 1000 µg/L caused excitability in 30 min (Vanden Bercken et al., 1973). Three species of tadpoles (northern leopard frog, *Rana pipiens,* southern leopard frog, *R. sphenocephala,* and the plains leopard frog, *R. blairi*) were exposed to esfenvalerate, and all species developed lethargy and inactivity in the first 24 h, followed quickly by spasmodic, convulsive twisting and twitching movements of the body and tail (Materna et al., 1995). Stimulated tadpoles of the green frog, *R. clamitans,* and the American toad, *Bufo americanus,* that had been exposed to permethrin or fenvalerate (0.1–2.0 ppm) also reacted by twisting and jerking in an incoordinated manner, and often curled into twisting balls. Exposure of embryos of the green frog, *R. clamitans,* to permethrin (1.0–2.0 ppm) for 96 h also resulted in 92% not forming an operculum by 15 days of age while in normal tadpoles, 93% had fully formed opercula (Berrill et al., 1993). Mortalities occurred within 96 h of exposure to concentrations over 7 μg/L, while concentrations of 3–7 μg caused convulsive behavior. Mortalities are greatly enhanced at temperatures over 20°C (68°F). Embryos and recently hatched tadpoles of multiple species of ranids and bufonids also develop a characteristic kinked tail or bent back within 96 h of exposure (Berrill et al., 1993; Materna et al., 1995). Newly hatched tadpoles are considerably more sensitive to esfenvalerate than embryos, and tadpoles of the green frog, *R. clamitans,* are more sensitive than tadpoles of the northern leopard frog, *R. pipiens* (Berrill et al., 1993).

Pyrethrins are derivatives of the flowers of chrysanthemums, and the mechanism of action of both naturally purified pyrethrins and synthetically produced pyrethroids is blockage of sodium, and possibly calcium, channels in cell membranes of nerves and muscles (Berrill et al., 1995; Whittem, 1995). In mammals some pyrethroids also may bind to gamma-aminobutyric acid (GABA) receptors in the brain (Whittem, 1995). The precise mode of action of pyrethroids in amphibians appears unstudied.

Toxicological Etiologies—Organotin. A variety of organotin compounds have uses as agricultural fungicides, paint additives to inhibit barnacle growth, molluscicides, anthelminthics, and more recently as antitumor agents (Socaciu et al., 1994). The most toxic forms of organotins are the triorganotins, but their toxicity differs markedly among animal taxa (Fleming et al., 1991; Semlitsch et al., 1995). Likewise, organ tropisms for the triorganotins varies. Triethyltin and trimethyltin are neurotoxic, inducing pronounced spongiform encephalopathy or neuronal degeneration in the brainstem, respectively, in various experimental animals (Chang et al., 1982; Fleming et al., 1991). Tributyltins and triphenyltins have effects on many organ systems but are considered principally immunotoxic (Socaciu et al., 1994). Triphenyltins are used worldwide as agricultural fungicides and are highly toxic to fish and many aquatic invertebrates, but the toxicities of most triorganotins to amphibians are unstudied.

Toxicological Etiologies—Herbicides. There are many herbicides in use in many regions of the world, each having distinct modes of action, and each has minimal to severe adverse impact on aquatic organisms (invertebrate and vertebrate). In toxicity tests of 15 herbicides in 1980, acrolein was the most toxic to fish (Environmental Protection Agency, 1980). Yet, in trials with the African clawed frog, *Xenopus laevis,* amphibians were found to be even more susceptible to acrolein than fish (Holcombe et al., 1987). Acrolein killed frogs at doses of 7 μg/L, while the LC_{50} levels for rainbow trout, bluegill, fathead minnow, brown shrimp, and Australian freshwater snail were 29–77, 79–100, 84–150, 100, and around 3000 μg/L, respectively (Eisler, 1994). The pathological effects of fatal acrolein exposure on amphibians is unstudied. Intoxication by the herbicide, acrolein, should be suspected in any agricultural areas experiencing mass mortalities of aquatic organisms. Acrolein is used principally as an aquatic herbicide in irrigation canals and ponds. It is the only aquatic herbicide in use in Australia (Eisler, 1994).

The herbicide, 2,4-dichlorophenoxyacetic acid (2,4-D), has been used extensively worldwide. Of concern to amphibians is its use as an aquatic herbicide in rice fields. At low exposure levels of 10–50 ppm for 3 months, no gross or histological lesions were detected in the northern crested newt, *Triturus cristatus,* although there was equivocal impairment of limb regeneration (Arias et al., 1989).

Paraquat and diquat are herbicides used in agricultural and aquatic environments. Embryos and tadpoles of the northern leopard frog, *Rana pipiens,* did not develop the characteristic edematous atypical interstitial pneumonia, nephrosis and adrenal necrosis observed in poisonings of mammals with these two herbicides (Dial & Bauer-Dial, 1987). The eggs of the northern leopard frog, *R. pipiens,* were resistant to diquat and paraquat. The embryos hatch normally, but then high mortalities occur in tadpoles 4–9 days posthatching on exposure doses of 0.5 mg/L of paraquat and 5 mg/L of diquat. In paraquat-treated eggs, mortality rates in tadpoles by age 16 days was 33% and 95% at doses of 0.5 mg/L and 2 mg/L, respectively. Suggested concentrations for aquatic application of paraquat are 0.1–2.0 mg/L, but local environmental concentrations can be significantly higher. In tadpoles of the northern leopard frog, *R. pipiens,* paraquat is more than 20 times as toxic as diquat (Dial & Bauer-Dial, 1987). Because larval mortalities may not be observed for 1–2 weeks following application of diquat or paraquat, there may be a tendency to overlook this intoxication in amphibian larval die-offs.

Paraquat, but not diquat, at prescribed application rates, is teratogenic to the northern leopard frog, *Rana pipiens.* Abnormalities include retarded growth, tail malformations, and aberrant development of the head (Dial & Bauer, 1984; Dial & Bauer-Dial, 1987).

Toxicological Etiologies—Paper Factory Effluents. Numerous developmental anomalies have been detected in wild specimens of the Inkiapo frog, *Rana chensinensis,* from South Sakhalin, Russia, associated with effluents from a paper factory (Mizgireuv et al., 1984). Microencephaly, unilateral anophthalmia, hindlimb chondrodysplasia, and absence of hindlimb digits have been reported, but the brain and ocular lesions were not further characterized grossly or histologically. The precise chemical in the effluent that was associated with these defects was not identified.

Toxicological Etiologies—Lead. Although lead is known to be neurotoxic in many classes of vertebrates, there are no neuropathologic studies or toxicological analyses of central or peripheral nervous tissue for this element in amphibians (Power et al., 1989).

Toxicological Etiologies—Chronic Zinc Intoxication. Captive specimens of the northern crested newt, Triturus cristatus, developed darkening of the skin, anorexia, and lethargy 6–12 weeks after being placed in an aquarium with a zinc-plated bottom. When newts were removed from the zinc-contaminated aquarium and hibernated by placing animals in a covered moss-lined box at 4°C (39°F) for 3 months, only 50% survived. Gross abnormalities were not reported. Histologically, the neurons of the primordial hippocampus (medial to the lateral ventricles) and mesencephalon demonstrated black granular deposits in the axonal cones. The granular deposits were not described in H&E stained sections, but were characterized as rod-shaped or V-shaped deposits in Bodia stains. Degenerative changes, glial reactions, and inflammatory changes in the brains were not described (Taban et al., 1982).

Infectious Etiologies—Viral. Two togaviruses, Western equine encephalitis (WEE) and sindbis (SIN), have been isolated from ranids. In addition, titers to WEE were detected in 12% of a population of northern leopard frogs, Rana pipiens, in Saskatchewan, Canada, but not in other sympatric amphibians such as the wood frog, Rana sylvatica, Plains spadefoot toad, Spea bombifrons, and the gray tiger salamander, Ambystoma tigrinum diaboli (Burton et al., 1966; Spalatin et al., 1964). Naturally infected frogs with virus isolates or titers have appeared clinically normal, and experimental infections of northern leopard frogs with WEE failed to induce clinical disease or lesions (Spalatin et al., 1964).

A sindbislike virus was isolated from the blood of wild specimens of the marsh frog, Rana ridibunda, but clinical disease and lesions in the amphibians were not described (Kozuch et al., 1977).

There are no detailed published descriptions of viral encephalomyelitis in amphibians, although there are hints of the condition in Australian rain forest anurans (Cullen et al, 1995; Laurence et al., 1996; Speare et al., 1994a) and a captive group of the European green toad, Bufo viridis, in Europe (personal communication, A. Cunningham, 1996). The disease in the toads was briefly characterized as a lymphocytic (nonsuppurative) myelitis and polyganglioneuritis. A virus infection was suspected.

Infectious Etiologies—Protozoal—Glaucoma spp. Protozoan infections of the brain have been reported occasionally. A ciliate Glaucoma sp. has been found in the brain and spinal cord of a larval smallmouth salamander, Ambystoma texanum (Shumway, 1940). This ciliated protozoan is closely related to Tetrahymena. The Glaucoma sp. from the brain measured 60 × 25 × 17 μm, and had 20 rows of cilia. Up to 42 ciliates were detected in a single horizontal section of brain. The invasive route to the brain was not determined. Protozoa were evident in the meninges, neuropil, and ventricles, but there was little evidence of inflammatory reaction.

Tetrahymena spp. infection of recently hatched larvae of the spotted salamander, Ambystoma maculatum (Ling & Werner, 1988), may be an acute stage of the Glaucoma spp. infection previously reported (Shumway, 1940). Infections developed in larvae hatched from eggs from two of three breeding ponds in Michigan in 1984. Among larvae that successfully hatched, 16–24% were infected fatally. All larvae that were infected usually died in 24 hours. The organism has also been reported in amphibian egg masses (Corliss, 1954). Grossly, infected larvae had marked edema of the subcutis of the head and gills, and this edematous fluid yielded large numbers of ciliated protozoa that were 47 × 27 μm. The subcutaneous swelling spread caudally in late stage infections and caused larvae to coil ventrally. Histologically, the larvae had masses of protozoa in the subcutis of the head and in nervous tissue (Ling & Werner, 1988). The short duration of the fatal infection may preclude inflammatory cell infiltrates.

Infectious Etiologies—Protozoal—Amoeba. Although Naegleria-type amoeba may cause encephalitis in reptiles (Frank, 1984), experimental infections of the European common frog, Rana temporaria, failed to induce lesions. The amoeba had the capability of invading the circulatory system following intraperitoneal injection, and were reisolated from the brains of experimental frogs. No gross brain lesions were seen in experimentally infected frogs but histological findings were not reported.

Infectious Etiologies—Protozoal—Sporozoans. Sporozoan infections of the anuran brain and spinal cord, often reported as Toxoplasma, Toxoplasma-like, Lankesterella, or Dactylosoma-like organisms, have been reported several times (DaCosta & Pereira, 1971; De Alencar, 1957; Levine & Nye, 1977; Manwell et al., 1953; Stensaas et al., 1967; Stone & Manwell, 1969). However, the precise identity of the organism(s) involved in these encephalomyelitic infections remains to be determined, even though ultrastructural studies were attempted, and species names have been proposed and revised (DaCosta & Pereira, 1971; DaCosta et al., 1975; Levine & Nye,

1976; Manwell et al., 1953; Stensaas et al., 1967; Stone & Manwell, 1969).

An intra-axonal infection by a sporozoan was described in South American amphibians, and was named *Lankesterella alencari* (DaCosta & Pereira, 1971; Stensaas et al., 1967). In a group of wild-caught specimens of the common toad, *Bufo arenarum,* from Uruguay that were held in captivity for a few weeks, 55% had spinal cord infections (Stensaas et al., 1967). Protozoa were found to infect axons mostly in submeningeal regions. Protozoal cysts were roundish, densely compacted, up to 30 μm in diameter, and consisted of a large single cell with aggregates of smaller organisms, each about 2 μm in diameter. Up to 80 smaller organisms with subterminal nuclei may be found forming a dense cluster. Organisms were unstained in the periodic acid-Schiff reaction. Organisms caused marked dilation of axons, but no obvious degenerative or necrotic changes. No protozoa were found in blood smears, dorsal or ventral spinal nerve roots, sensory ganglia, liver, spleen, intestine, or skin. This intra-axonal protozoan in the common toad, *Bufo arenarum,* was indistinguishable from an organism described in the giant toad, *B. marinus* (De Alencar, 1957).

Infectious Etiologies—Protozoal—"Toxoplasma-like" Organisms. At least three species of *Toxoplasma,* all of which caused infections of the brain of frogs and toads, have been proposed. These are *T. ranae* (Levine & Nye, 1976), *T. serpai* (Scorza et al., 1956), and *T. alencari* (DaCosta & Pereira, 1971; Levine & Nye, 1976). There remains doubt as to the correct classification and genus name for these three organisms.

Toxoplasma ranae is based on an infection of one Rio Grande frog, *Rana berlandieri* (Levine & Nye, 1976). *Toxoplasma serpai* was found in specimens of the giant toad, *Bufo marinus,* from Venezuela (Scorza et al., 1956), and *T. alencari* (synonym: *Lankesterella alencari*) was found in the brains of four specimens of the Criolla frog, *Leptodactylus ocellatus* (DaCosta & Pereira, 1971). All three proposed species of *Toxoplasma* produce pseudocysts within neurons, neuroglial cells, and, possibly, endothelial cells of the central nervous system. Pseudocysts are spherical, ovoid or ellipsoidal, thin-walled, and 45–106 μm in diameter. In about 25% of pseudocysts, a large crescentric host nucleus may be found pressed against the margin of the cell. In a section of a pseudocyst, up to 500 slightly curved, elongate zoites, each 4–7 μm long, may be found. One end of each zoite contains a periodic acid-Schiff-positive glycogen granule, about the same size as the nucleus. Zoite nuclei are 1–2 μm in diameter, and are central in *T. ranae* and subterminal in *T. alencari.* No inflammatory cells or other host reactions to the protozoa have been reported histologically or ultrastructurally.

Infectious Etiologies—Helminths. Helminths, predominantly trematode cercariae, may be encountered in brain and meninges of amphibians. *Diplostomum* spp. infection may occur elsewhere but the meninges and ventricles may be the preferred site of these immature trematodes. Within the ventricles, metacercariae of the strigeid trematode, *Tylodelphys* spp., may be encountered in European frogs (Reichenbach-Klinke & Elkan, 1965).

In the brain and eyes of the Eastern newt, *Notophthalmus viridescens,* metacercariae of the fluke, *Diplostomum scheuringi,* may be found. In some populations and in some years, prevalence may approach 100% (Etges, 1961). In a study of 40 infected newts (Lautenschlager, 1959), 5–35 active, nonencysted metacercariae were found in the meninges and ventricles. Histological changes associated with these flukes were negligible to moderate. Hydrocephalus was noted histologically with atrophy or absence of the choroid plexi of the lateral ventricles. The ependymal cells were hypertrophied and contained increased amounts of melanin. The meninges showed diffuse minimal to mild hyperplasia with possible hyperplasia of the endolymphatic ducts and paraphysis. One newt had a nodular mass of cells within the meninges dorsal to the paraphysis that was poorly characterized. The route of entry of the metacercariae into the calvarium has not been determined, and it is not clear whether the newt is an effective intermediate host, or a dead-end host.

Idiopathic Etiologies—Myelomalacia. In 1994, myelomalacia was detected in one paralyzed and one dead specimen of the wild mountain yellow-legged frog, *Rana muscosa,* found in a national park in California during amphibian surveys (Figures 27.47,

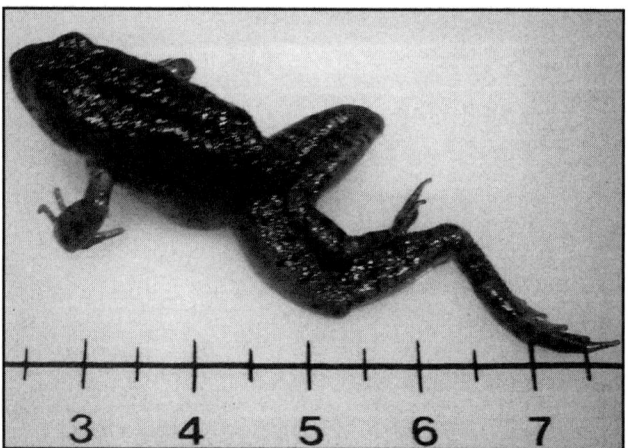

Figure 27.47. Hindlimb paralysis in a wild mountain yellow-legged frog, *Rana mucosa*. The right hindlimb was paretic while the left hindlimb was paralyzed. Segmental myelomalacia was detected in the thoraco-lumbar spinal cord (see Figure 27.48). (D.E. Green)

27.48). Upon capture, the live frog convulsed and had extensor rigidity of the hindlimbs. Within 72 hours, the rigid hindlimbs became flaccid. Macroscopic lesions in the euthanized frog included an atrophied spleen, and a recent laceration of the skin overlying the left tarsus. Histologically, the thoracic spinal cord had a large segment of acute malacia with loss of neurons, pyknotic neuroglia, and edema. Ependyma of the central canal was necrotic with cellular debris in the lumen. Hemorrhage was present in the malacic focus, but the surrounding meninges and vertebrae were normal. No microorganisms were detected histologically or in bacterial cultures of internal organs, but a few neurons appeared to have karyomegaly or karyolysis. The etiology of the myelomalacia was not determined.

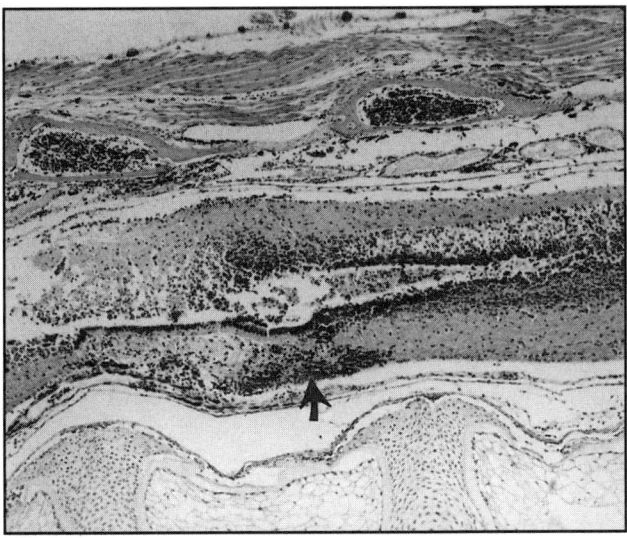

Figure 27.48. Spinal cord from frog in Figure 27.47. Extensive segmental meyelomalacia of unknown etiology. Necrotic ependymal cells have sloughed into dilated central canal, neurons and astrocytes are necrotic around the central canal, and there is a focus of marked submeningeal hemorrhage (arrow). There is no evidence of associated trauma. (D.E. Green)

Idiopathic Etiologies—Paralysis. Captive specimens of the African clawed frog, *Xenopus laevis*, may develop paralysis of the hindlimbs which prevents surfacing to breathe and subsequent drowning. No abnormalities of the brain or spinal cord were detected in several affected frogs, so the etiology remains unknown although a neurotoxic factor was suggested (Elkan, 1960a).

A syndrome involving hindlimb extensor rigidity, ventral dermal abrasions, and death has been observed in several captive adult Veragoa stubfoot toads, *Atelopus varius*, which had been raised from eggs obtained in the wild in Panama. Affected animals have fully extended hindlimbs which, when moved into a "normal" resting position, promptly return to full extension. There also is a slight arching of the back, but the toad is generally alert and willing to feed (Whitaker, unpublished).

A progressive, often ascending, flaccid paralysis of poison dart frogs has been observed by two large public aquaria, and many individual cases by veterinarians and amphibian hobbyists in the USA. Approximately 3% of captive anurans were affected at one facility, but five out of six specimens of the yellow-banded poison dart frog, *Dendrobates leucomelas*, at the second facility died. Affected species include the harlequin poison dart frog, *Dendrobates histrionicus*, the yellow-banded poison dart frog, *D. leucomelas*, the blue poison dart frog, *D. azureus*, the dyeing poison frog, *D. tinctorius*, the pleasing poison dart frog, *Epipedobates bassleri*, the three-striped poison dart frog, *E. trivittatus*, and the black-legged poison dart frog, *Phyllobates bicolor*. The disease presents as ataxia, general weakness, or hindlimb flaccid paralysis, which may progress over a period of days or weeks to forelimb paralysis, tremors, head tilt, and death. Affected frogs generally remain alert and willing and able to feed if prey is provided (Whitaker, unpublished).

Grossly, no specific lesions have been observed, except for the expected ventral skin abrasions and secondary dermatosepticemias in frogs that crawl using only their forelimbs. Four distinct histologic changes have been observed in the central nervous system: hydrocephalus of the IVth ventricle, demyelination of the spinal cord, axonal swelling, and neuronal vacuolation (Figures 27.49, 27.50, 27.51, 27.52). All lesions are mild and free of inflammatory cell infiltrates. Ultrastructurally, the demyelination appears bland and free of virus particles. Degeneration of myelin presents as dense myelin whorls, and there are unidentified smaller intraneuronal cytoplasmic discoid structures with moderately electron-lucent cores (Whitaker, unpublished). Ataxia, flaccid paralysis, and neuronal vacuolation have also been reported in wild Australian tropical anurans associated with a ranavirus-like infection (Cullen et al., 1995; Speare et al., 1994a). Because the duration of the clinical disease often is not known and because each affected frog shows only one of the main lesions, it is not clear if the lesions represent a continuum of one disease, or multiple disease entities (Whitaker, unpublished data).

27.2.11 Eyes, Ears, and Special Sensory Organs

The anatomy of the amphibian eye and metamorphic changes have been reviewed (Kaltenbach, 1953; Millichamp, 1991; Muntz, 1977; Reyer, 1977; Williams & Whitaker, 1994).

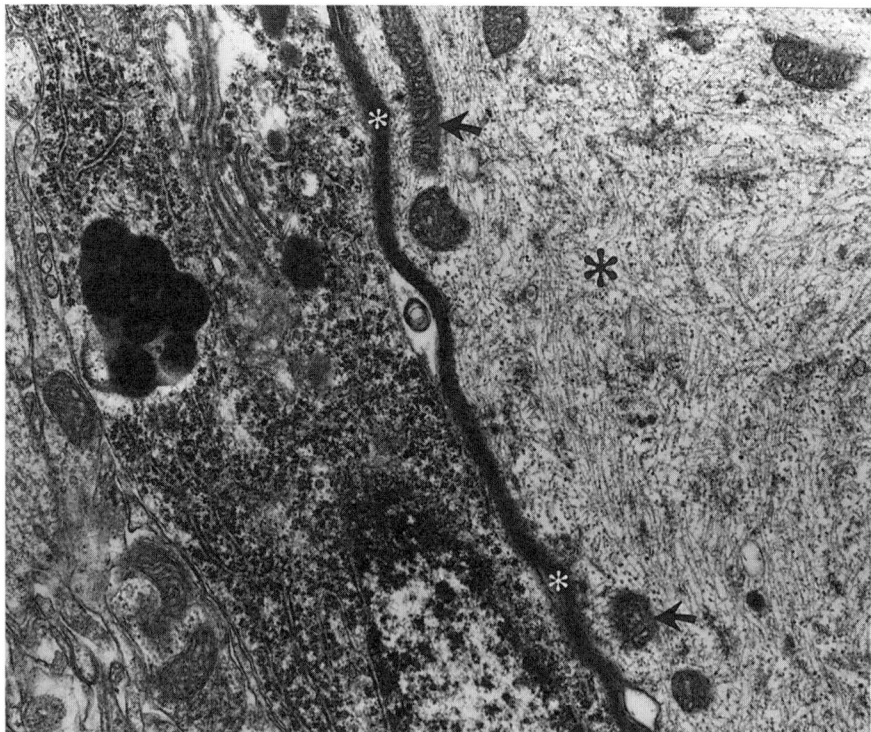

Figure 27.49. Transmission electron micrograph of the brain of a harlequin poison frog, *Dendrobates histrionicus,* with flaccid paralysis. Shown is a portion of a swollen axon (black asterisk) with mitochondria (arrows) and an intact myelin sheath (white asterisks). The cluster of electron-dense granules on the left in an adjacent cell is considered nonviral. No organisms have been observed in this condition. (Brent Whitaker)

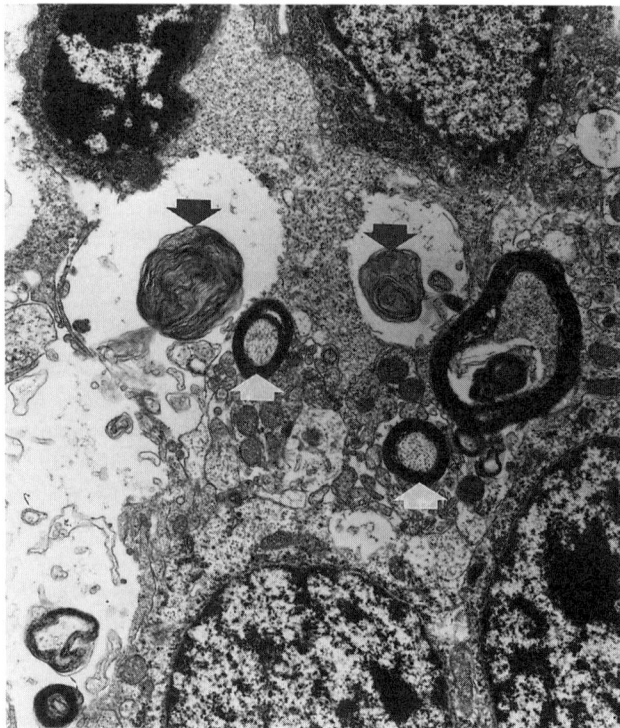

Figure 27.50. Same frog as Figure 27.49. Transmission electron micrograph of the brain. Myelin figures (black arrows) and normal myelin sheaths (white arrows). (Brent Whitaker)

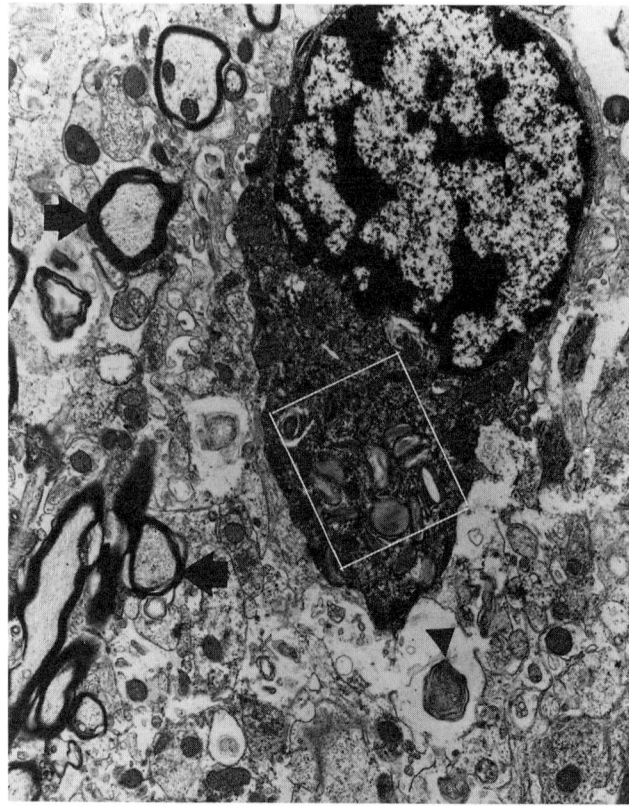

Figure 27.51. Same frog as Figure 27.49. Transmission electron micrograph of the brain. Myelin figure (arrowhead) and normal myelin sheaths (arrows), and unidentified cytoplasmic structures (in box, see Figure 27.52). (Brent Whitaker)

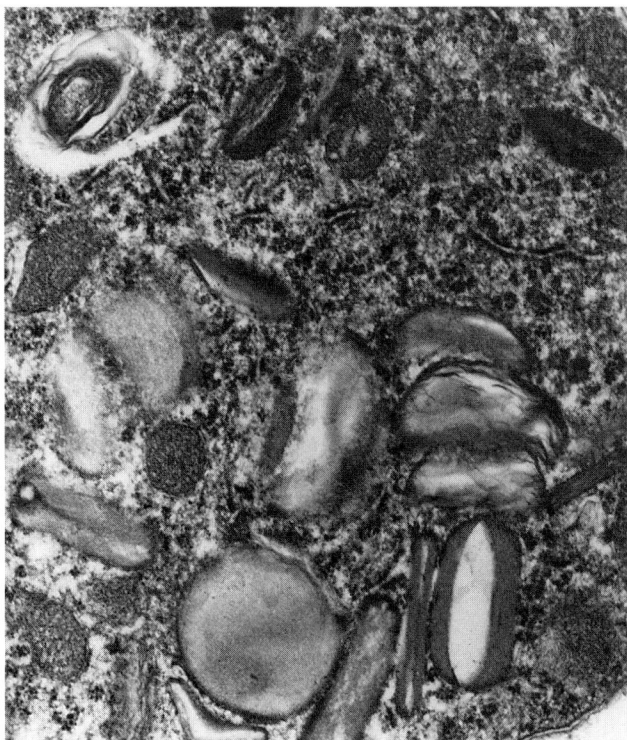

Figure 27.52. Same frog as Figure 27.49. Transmission electron micrograph of the brain. Unidentified, probably degenerate, cytoplasmic structures. (Brent Whitaker)

The anatomy and development of the inner ear in amphibians has been reviewed (Hertwig & Hentschel, 1990; Wever, 1985). Although the inner ear and labyrinths are well formed by the time amphibian embryos hatch into free-swimming tadpoles and larvae, the full development of the auditory apparatus is delayed until metamorphosis.

The three-dimensional shape, and ultrastructure of the sensory epithelia and otoconia ("otoliths") of the labyrinths (semicircular canals) have been described in various aquatic, terrestrial, and cave-dwelling amphibians (Bulog, 1989a, b; Lewis et al., 1985).

Although no special sensory function has been attributed to the paravertebral endolymphatic sacs, their embryological origin and function are related to the inner ear and otoliths. The endolymphatic sacs arise as endolymphatic ducts from between the sacculus and utriculus of the ear (Pilkington & Simkiss, 1966). The ducts expand into the cranium to encircle the myelencephalon (hindbrain) and are intimately associated with the choroids of the fourth ventricle. From the hindbrain the ducts project bilaterally in the arachnoid through the entire length of the spinal canal. At each intervertebral foramina, bilateral diverticuli accompany the spinal nerve roots, envelope the spinal ganglia, and expand to form small discoid cysts called "lime sacs." The diverticulae are not simple sacs as their name implies, but are multiloculated glandlike structures with prominent central cavities. These endolymphatic sacs are lined by low cuboidal epithelium which secretes orthorhombic doubly refractile crystals of calcium carbonate. The composition of the material secreted by the endolymphatic sacs is similar to that of the otoliths (Schlumberger & Burk, 1953), while the calcium in bones and in lesions of dystrophic mineralization is 85–90% calcium phosphate. It has been suggested that larval amphibians accumulate calcium in the endolymphatic sacs for later use in bone mineralization during metamorphosis (Guardabassi, 1960). When the skeleton begins to mineralize during metamorphosis, calcium carbonate is mobilized in a gradient from the posterior to anterior sacs (Pilkington & Simkiss, 1966).

The lateral line system, ampullary organs, and pit organs are present in the tadpoles of some anurans (e.g., clawed frogs, *Xenopus* spp.), most salamander larvae, and most neotenic salamanders. The lateral line and pit organs are mechanoreceptors, while the ampullary organs are electroreceptors. The mechanoreceptive cells of the lateral lines and pit organs are called neuromast cells and are arrayed as oval-shaped organs in rows on the surface of the head and trunk. Ampullary and pit organs are located on the head only, while the lateral lines, as in fish, usually extend from the head to the tail on each side of the body. The axolotl, *Ambystoma mexicanum*, has three pairs of lines on the body, but only the middle pair project on the tail almost to the tip. Tadpoles of the northern leopard frog, *Rana pipiens*, have three pairs of lateral lines on the body, two of which extend onto the tail. The three pairs of lateral lines on the body have been named the dorsal, middle and ventral body lines. On the head, neuromasts are arrayed in irregular, usually curved, lines which may intersect. Two pairs of lines are oriented tangential to the orbits, and another pair occurs in the mandibular skin (Smith et al., 1988). Ampullary organs are recessed below the epidermis, and open to the surface by a short canal (Northcutt & Bleckmann, 1993). The embryological migration and ultrastructural morphology of neuromast cells and pit organs have been studied (Northcutt & Bleckman, 1993; Northcutt et al., 1994, 1995; Smith et al., 1988).

The amphibian vomeronasal organ (Jacobson's organ) is a lateral diverticulum of each nasal cavity in salamanders and a medial diverticulum in anurans (Dawley & Bass, 1989). The vomeronasal organs are considered a chemical sensory system similar to but autonomous from the main olfactory system. It has been suggested that the nerves coursing from the vomeronasal organ to the brain could be considered a separate cranial nerve. Three cell types have been described: receptor (sensory) cells, supporting cells, and basal cells. Basal cells may be a reservoir of undifferentiated sensory cells. Plethodontid salamanders have a nasolabial groove extending from each upper lip to the lateral opening of the nostril. The "nose-tapping" behavior of these salamanders enhances the movement of nonvolatile chemicals by a sort of capillary action up the nasolabial groove to the vomeronasal organ (Dawley & Bass, 1989). Subtle seasonal changes and sexual dimorphism in the size of the vomeronasal organ have been reported (Dawley & Crowder, 1995).

The gustatory chemoreceptor organs are rosettes of fusiform cells localized principally on the tongue. The embryologic origin of taste bud receptor cells in vertebrates was recently demonstrated in the axolotl, *Ambystoma mexicanum*, to be endodermal cells of the mouth, and not the neural crest or epibranchial placodes as had been theorized for many years (Barlow & Northcutt, 1995). The taste cells of amphibians are large, directly sample the external environment, consist of 50–100 cells, and, at least in some salamanders, consist of multiple distinct cell types: elongate light and dark cells, and two types of smaller basal cells, undifferentiated cells and Merkel-like neuroendocrine cells (Delay et al., 1993; Nagai, 1993). Taste buds are innervated by the glossopharyngeal (IX) cranial nerve, and the Merkel-like cells have synapses with taste bud cells and the innervating cranial nerves fibers (Delay et al., 1993). No spontaneous diseases specific to taste buds have been described in amphibians.

Genetic Etiologies. At least four distinct recessive traits affecting the eyes have been described in the axolotl, *Ambystoma mexicanum* (Brun, 1990, 1993; Epp, 1978; Malaciniski, 1978). Additional traits having multiorgan involvement also may express ocular anomalies, and many studies of toxic chemicals in developing embryos may express ocular malformations.

One mutation of otoliths has been described in the African clawed frog, *Xenopus laevis* (Droin, 1967, as cited by Gurdon & Woodland, 1975).

Nutritional Etiologies—Corneal Lipidosis. There are multiple reports of corneal lipidosis (lipid keratopathy) in captive ranid, hylid, and leptodactylid frogs. When the sex is reported, the vast majority are female. Affected anurans are usually over 3 years old. Affected taxa in published reports include the Cuban treefrog, *Osteopilus septentrionalis,* the European treefrog, *Hyla arborea,* White's treefrog, *Pelodryas caerulea,* the Mexican leaf frog, *Pachymedusa dacnicolor,* the veined treefrog, *Phrynohyas venulosa,* and the Sabinal frog, *Leptodactylus melanonotus* (Carpenter et al., 1986; Dziezyc & Millichamp, 1989; Russell et al., 1990; Zwart & Vander Linde-Sipman, 1989). Hazy white to gray opacities of the superficial corneal stroma usually begin at the nasal or temporal limbus and may progress into white, globular or plaquelike dense opacities in the stroma that cause marked corneal thickening and irregularities in the surface epithelium (Millichamp, 1991). Over the course of 8–20 months, 60–100% of the cornea may be affected. Corneal melanosis and pannus may occur in chronic severe cases (Zwart & Vander Linde-Sipman, 1989). Blindness and weight loss may also occur (Russell et al., 1990). Many affected frogs also have systemic gross lesions of cutaneous and periarticular xanthomatosis, intracranial granulomata, atherosclerosis, and mesothelial lipid granulomata.

As suggested by the widespread gross lesions, corneal lipidosis is usually a sign of serious systemic disease. Histological examinations reveal lipidotic, xanthomatous, and atherosclerotic changes in many organs and tissues. Affected organs include, but are not limited to, brain, pituitary, choroid plexuses, meninges, peripheral nerves, aorta, liver, mesonephros, ovary, joints, and mesothelial surfaces (Carpenter et al., 1986; Russell et al., 1990; Zwart & Vander Linde-Sipman, 1989). The histological lesions in the corneas consist of discrete nodules or diffuse infiltrates of large, foamy, lipid-laden macrophages within the stroma and, occasionally, the ciliary body. Smaller macrophages may be present adjacent to clear cholesterol clefts (lenticular clefts, cholesterol crystals), and lakes of amorphous, weakly stained material may dissect the corneal stroma parallel to Descemet's membrane. A mix of other inflammatory cells may be present, including fibroblasts, lymphocytes, granulocytes, multinucleated giant cells, and mast cells. In some cases, fibrosis of the corneal stroma is prominent. Descemet's membrane shows minimal deformation, but Bowman's membrane and the corneal epithelium are often markedly undulating or bulging due to nodular accumulations of foamy macrophages. Infiltrating melanocytes and blood vessels may be found peripherally in the corneal stroma. Mineralization may be present, usually subjacent to Bowman's membrane. The iris, choroid, retina, and vitreous are usually normal. Cholesterol and fats within macrophages are lost during routine histological processing, but frozen sections examined under polarized light show birefringent crystals in the clefts. Fat stains (e.g., oil-red-O) applied to frozen sections of cornea or other systemic xanothomatous and atherosclerotic lesions demonstrate the neutral lipids as large globules and intracytoplasmic droplets within macrophages.

Nutritional Etiologies—Glucose-associated Transient Cataracts. Transient cataracts developed in sick dendrobatids that were administered 5% glucose solutions. Cataracts may occur in conjunction with numerous other ocular diseases such as malnutrition, infections, and intoxications (Williams & Whitaker, 1994).

Toxicological Etiologies—Hypervitaminosis-D. Doses of 30,000–50,000 units of vitamin D$_2$ result in increased production of calcium carbonate by the epithelial cells of the endolymphatic sacs, with marked expansion of the diverticulae (sacs) and increased radiodensity (Schlumberger & Burk, 1953). In the absence of calcium in the feed or water, calcium is mobilized from the bones and appears to be secreted into the sacs as calcium carbonate. As the sacs expand with calcium carbonate crystals, the epithelium becomes flattened (squamous). Following dosing with vitamin D$_2$, peak accumulation of calcium carbonate occurs 3–5 weeks later, but becomes radiographically evident in about 2 weeks. The otoliths are not affected as determined radiographically by hypervitaminosis-D (Schlumberger & Burk, 1953). Prominent endolymphatic sacs may be detected at necropsy of many anurans, and should not be mistaken for vertebral ankylosis, gout, or pseudogout (calcium pyrophosphate deposition disease). The post metamorphic function of the endolymphatic sacs and their calcium carbonate secretions apparently have not been studied.

A case of exuberant calcium deposition in the endolymphatic sacs was reported in a captive adult male giant monkey frog, *Phyllomedusa bicolor*. Grossly, the nodules were asymmetrical and up to 3 mm in diameter. Histologically, basophilic and yellow anisotropic granules were present in the ducts and sacs, and there were infiltrates of macrophages and proliferation of fibrocytes with compression of one spinal nerve root (Stetter & Nichols, 1994).

Metastatic calcification may be induced in frogs by hypervitaminosis-D. The most frequent site of metastatic calcification is the tubules of the mesonephroi. This mesonephrocalcinosis is predominantly intraluminal. Calcium deposits are infreqently detected in tubular epithelial cells, and calcification of the tubular basement membranes has not been described. Intraluminal calcium deposits are present in all regions of the nephron, but are most abundant in the proximal convoluted tubules. Epithelial cells surrounding large intraluminal desposits of calcium are often flattened but it is not clear whether this is a mechanical change or degenerative. Metastatic calcification of the heart, lungs, and gastric mucosa, as reported in mammals, was not detected in experimental hypervitaminosis-D of frogs (Schlumberger & Burk, 1953).

Toxicological Etiologies—Ultraviolet-B Radiation. In naturally dark, melanotic tadpoles of many toads, *Bufo* spp., pigment within the cornea normally dissipates completely by stage 23, leaving a transparent cornea. However, experimentally enhanced ultraviolet-B radiation causes retention of melanin pigment in the dorsal hemisphere of the cornea, and generalized increased melanosis of the skin in the western toad, *Bufo boreas*. This corneal melanosis persists into metamorphosis (Worrest & Kimeldorf, 1976), but it is not clear how long it persists in metamorphosed toads with developed eyelids. Neither is it clear whether amphibians develop corneal melanosis if exposed to elevated ultraviolet-B after metamorphosis is complete. Histologically, tadpoles have mild dorsal corneal epithelial hyperplasia and melanin within corneal epithelial cells.

Infectious Etiologies—Bacterial. Bacterial ophthalmitis has been reported in anurans only, namely in the northern leopard frog, *Rana pipiens,* and the firebelly toad, *Bombina orientalis*. Single or mixed bacteria have been isolated. Most infections are caused by Gram-negative bacilli, and many are the sequelae of bacterial septicemias (e.g., red leg syndrome). It appears that any bacterium that causes bacteremia or septicemia may cause ophthalmitis. Careful examinations of anurans with bacterial ophthalmitis usually reveals concurrent involvement of other special sensory organs (e.g., middle and inner ears, and labyrinths), and productive bacterial cultures from many internal organs such as liver, spleen, heart, and mesonephroi. All reports have been in captive anurans, and usually in specimens that were recently subjected to stress, such as crowding or transport. The bacteria that have been implicated by cultural isolations include *Aeromonas hydrophila, Citrobacter freundii, Providencia alcalifaciens,* an unnamed Gram-negative bacillus in group IV E, *Flavobacterium indologenes,* and *F. meningosepticum* (Brooks et al., 1983; Olson et al., 1992; Taylor et al., 1993).

Bacterial ophthalmitis appears in acute and subacute forms. In the acute form, generalized active lesions of septicemia may be present, resembling red leg syndrome. Subcutaneous edema, pericarditis, serosanguinous coelomic exudates, muscular hemorrhages, and hepatosplenomegaly may be present (Olson et al., 1992). In the subacute stage, the visceral lesions may be absent; lesions appear confined to the eyes, ears, and meninges (Brooks et al., 1983; Taylor et al., 1993).

Clinical and gross lesions in the eyes include corneal edema, hyphema, hypopyon, and fibrin in the anterior chamber (Brooks et al., 1983). Clinical signs relating to involvement of the ears and brain include opisthotonus, circling, torticollis, and deficient righting reflexes.

Histologically, the ocular lesions are a purulent or fibrinopurulent panophthalmitis. Specifically there is corneal edema with mild stromal infiltrates of inflammatory cells with purulent iridocyclitis and chorioretinitis. Inflammatory cell infiltrates in the choroid may cause detachment of the retina. The anterior and posterior chambers and vitreous may be mildly to severely infiltrated by granulocytes, fibrin, and bacteria. Granulocytes within the chambers are often degenerate. The lens may show proliferation of the anterior epithelium with subcapsular cataractous change (Brooks et al., 1983; Olson et al., 1992; Taylor et al., 1993).

Otitis and meningitis frequently accompany bacterial ophthalmitis in anurans. Meningeal lesions involve the outermost layer and may cause separation of the meninges and periosteum from the bones of the skull. The neuropil and ventricles are often spared, while involvement of the choroids, paraphysis, and endolymphatic ducts have not been specifically addressed. Purulent otitis of the inner and middle ears may fill the chambers with neutrophils and fibrin, and may result in erosion of osseous structures. Although the same bacteria which were isolated from the eyes may be isolated from internal organs such as heart, liver, and mesonephroi, usually, the internal organs in the subacute stage of ophthalmitis, are reported as lacking abnormalities histologically (Brooks et al., 1983; Taylor et al., 1993).

Ocular (and generalized) mycobacteriosis has been described in a captive South American bullfrog, *Leptodactylus pentadactylus* (Rowlatt & Roe, 1966).

Infectious Etiologies—Protozoal. The lateral lines, and ampullary and pit organs may be infected by various protozoan ectoparasites as part of a generalized dermatitis or branchitis.

Infectious Etiologies—Helminths—Rhabdias spp. Experimentally, massive numbers of recently hatched *Rhabdias sphaerocephala* larvae and three recently metamorphosed specimens of the giant toad, *Bufo marinus*, were placed in petri dishes. Within 2–24 hours, two toads were dead or prostrate. Large numbers of live larvae of *R. sphaerocephala* were found on the epidermis, in the subcutis, in skeletal muscles, on the cornea, and in the vitreous body. Histological examinations were not attempted (Williams, 1960).

Infectious Etiologies—Helminths—Trematodes. Three species of trematodes have been reported as infecting the eyes of tadpoles, adult anurans, newts, and a siren, *Siren lacertina*. The trematodes are *Diplostomum scheuringi*, *D. flexicaudum,* and *Clinostomum attenuatum.* The former trematode also infects the meninges of the brain in newts and fish, and all flukes occur as immature stages in eyes or brains of amphibians (Etges, 1991). The definitive hosts of the *Diplostomum* spp. were not determined (Etges, 1961), but probably are various piscivorous birds. Experimental exposure of larvae of the Eastern newt, *Notophthalmus viridescens,* to massive numbers of infective cercariae in water resulted in 100% mortality of the newts within 2 hours. The infective cercariae are capable of penetrating the cornea of larvae, efts and adult newts and are capable of penetrating the skin of larvae. Cercariae avoid penetration of the skin of efts and adult newts. Adults of the red salamanders, *Pseudotriton* spp., and tadpoles and adults of the northern leopard frog, *Rana pipiens,* and the pickerel frog, *R. palustris,* are resistent to the cercariae of *D. scheuringi.* Studies on newt larvae show that cercariae penetrate the skin and cornea at any point, cause small subcutaneous hemorrhages, migrate via the circulation, and accumulate in the brain. The route the cercariae may take from the eyes to the brains of efts and adult newts is not known, but is suspected to be along the optic nerves (Etges, 1961). Within the vitreous of the eyes and the brain, cercariae of *Diplostomum* spp. remain active and do not encyst, although *Clinostumum* spp. may form a thin-walled cyst on the retina. The lens is not affected and no specific histological lesions in the eye have been reported.

The trematode *Halipegus eccentricus* infests the eustachian tubes of wild specimens of the green frog, *Rana clamitans,* the northern leopard frog, *R. pipiens,* the bullfrog, *R. catebesbeiana,* and other frogs of North America. Tadpoles become infected when they consume the second intermediate hosts, copepods and ostracods. The trematode is retained during metamorphosis, and may be found in the middle ears, but clinical disease, and gross and histological lesions have not been reported (Flynn, 1973; Goater et al., 1990; Thomas, 1937). Other species of *Halipegus,* such as *H. occidualis* and *H. amhertensis,* occur principally in the mouth of the same species of frogs, but may invade the eustachian tubes.

Trematode infection of the lateral line sensory organs has been reported. The infection occurred in captive specimens of the clawed frog, *Xenopus* spp., and was caused by strigeids of the trematode *Neascus* spp. (Elkan & Murray, 1952). Normally, the integument of the clawed frog is dark, and the lateral line system is subtly evident as rows of small pale rods. In infected frogs, the lateral line segments become dark (melanotic) and the skin becomes pale (grayish). Heavy infections result in detailed melanotic delineation of the lateral line system of the frogs. Histologically, the trematodes form thick-walled, pigmented granulomata in the dermis subjacent to the neuromast organ (Elkan, 1960a; Elkan & Murray, 1952).

Idiopathic Etiologies—Vascularizing Keratitis (Pannus). Invasion of the avascular cornea by vessels from the sclera has been reported in a captive ornate horned frog, *Ceratophrys ornatus* (Williams & Whitaker, 1994) and is known in other species. Corneal neovascularization may have been in response to corneal stromal opacities or crystalline epithelial deposits. As the corneal lesion progresses, the corneal epithelium may retain a smooth contour or become roughened. Vascularizations may eventually affect vision. Such anurans then fail to feed on their own and become emaciated. Histological changes were briefly described as corneal infiltrates of macrophages and lymphocytes. In more severe cases, additional sequellae have been reported in the form of corneal melting (stromal collagenolysis) and descemetocoeles. No consistent etiology has been detected. Occasionally, Gram-negative bacteria have been isolated from affected amphibians as well as clinically normal frogs. Most affected frogs had been maintained under near continuous ultraviolet-B lighting (Williams & Whitaker, 1994).

Idiopathic Etiologies—Glaucoma. Only one case of glaucoma appears to have been reported in amphibians. The affected captive animal was a common European toad, *Bufo bufo*, with clinical buphthalmos (Williams & Whitaker, 1994). The toad was not necropsied, nor was the globe examined histologically.

Idiopathic Etiologies—Spontaneous Lens Anomalies. Gross examinations of wild specimens of the northern leopard frog, *Rana pipiens*, detected a prevalence of 0.4% with cataracts (Peltz & Pezella, 1976). Lenticular disorders in 48 specimens of the northern leopard frog, *R. pipiens*, were studied histologically (Peltz et al., 1978). A high incidence of abnormalities was observed in frogs from Vermont, Wisconsin, and Minnesota. The histological changes included disruption of fibers (87%), irregularly distributed epithelial cells (60%), and abnormal cell nuclei (63%). Nuclear cataracts were observed in two frogs (4%). The northern leopard frog, *R. pipiens*, has such a high incidence of lenticular irregularities that their usefulness in experimental investigations is limited (Peltz et al., 1978).

ACKNOWLEDGMENTS

The author thanks the staff of the College Park Animal Health Diagnostic Laboratory and Fish Diagnostic Laboratory, Maryland Department of Agriculture, for their support, and Andrew A. Cunningham for useful comments on this chapter. This chapter is designated Maryland Department of Agriculture Number 98–97.

REFERENCES

Abrams, G.D. 1969. Diseases in an amphibian colony, *in* Mizell, M. (Ed.): Biology of Amphibian Tumors. Springer-Verlag, New York, pp. 419–428.

Accordi, F. and P. Cianfoni. 1981. Histology and ultrastructure of the adrenal gland of *Rhacophorus leucomystax* (Amphibia, Anura). Bollettino di Zoologia. 48:277–288.

Accordi, F. and E.G. Milano. 1990. Evolution and development of the adrenal gland in amphibians. Fortschritte der Zoologie 38:257–268.

Accordi, F., V.P. Gallo, and E.G. Milano. 1981. The adrenal gland of *Xenopus laevis* (Daudin) (Anura, Pipidae): Histological and ultrastructural observations. Monitore Zoologico Italiano 15:163–174.

Ackermann, J. and E. Miller. 1992. Chromomycosis in an African bullfrog, *Pyxicephalus adspersus*. Bulletin of the Association of Reptilian and Amphibian Veterinarians 2:8–9.

Adams, A.E. 1946. The effect of thiourea on the thyroids of *Triturus viridescens* [Abstr]. Anatomical Record 94:532.

Aguis, C. 1980. Phylogenetic development of melanomacrophage centres in fish. Journal of Zoology 191:11–31.

Ahne, W., Z. Matasin, and G. Bovo. 1995. Antigenic relationship of epizootic haematopoietic necrosis virus (EHNV) and iridovirus-like isolates from European green frogs (*Rana esculenta*). Bulletin of the European Association of Fish Pathologists 15:142–144.

Alves de Matos, A.P. and I. Paperna. 1993. Ultrastructure of erythrocytic virus of the South African anuran *Ptychadena anchietae*. Diseases of Aquatic Organisms 16:105–109.

Amborski, R.L., T.G. Snider, R.L. Thune, and D.D. Culley, Jr. 1983. A non-hemolytic, group B *Streptococcus* infection of cultured bullfrogs, *Rana catesbeiana*, in Brazil. Journal of Wildlife Diseases 19:180–184.

American Society for Testing and Materials. 1991. Standard guide for conducting the frog embryo teratogenesis assay-Xenopus (FETAX), Designation E-1439–91. *in* Annual Book of ASTM Standards, Philadelphia, PA, 11 pp.

Anderson, I. 1995. Is a virus wiping out frogs? New Scientist 145:7.

Anver, M.R. and C.L. Pond. 1984. Biology and diseases of amphibians, Chapter 14, *in* Fox, J.G., B.J. Cohen, and F.M. Loew (Eds.): Laboratory Animal Medicine. Academic Press, Orlando, FL, pp. 427–447.

Ardavin, C.F., A. Zapata, A. Villena, and M.T. Solas. 1982. Gut-associated lymphoid tissues (GALT) in the amphibian Urodele, *Pleurodeles waltl*. Journal of Morphology 173:35–41.

Arias, E., T. Zavanella, and N.P. Zaffaroni. 1989. Teratogenic effects of 2,4-D on the regenerating limb of the crested newt. Herpetopathologica 1:1–4.

Aronson, J.D. 1957. Tuberculosis of cold-blooded animals, a review. Leprosy Briefs 8:21–32.

Asfari, M. 1988. Mycobacterium-induced infectious granuloma in *Xenopus*: Histopathology and transmissibility. Cancer Research 48:958–963.

Asfari, M. and C.H. Thiebaud. 1988. Transplantation studies of a putative lymphosarcoma of *Xenopus*. Cancer Research 48:954–957.

Austin, B. and D.A. Austin. 1987. Bacterial fish pathogens, *in* Disease in Farmed and Wild Fish. Ellis Horwood Limited, Chichester, UK, and John Wiley & Sons, New York, 384 pp.

Babudieri, B., E.R. Carlos, and E.T. Carlos. 1973. Pathogenic leptospira isolated from toad kidneys. Tropical and Geographical Medicine 25:297–299.

Baculi, B.S. and E.L. Cooper. 1967. Lymphomyeloid organs of amphibia. II. Vasculature in larval and adult *Rana catesbeiana*. Journal of Morphology 123:463–480.

Baculi, B.S., E.L. Cooper, and B.A. Brown. 1970. Lymphomyeloid organs of amphibia. V. Comparative histology in diverse anuran species. Journal of Morphology 131:315–328.

Bagnara, J.T. 1958. Hypophyseal control of guanophores in anuran larvae. Journal of Experimental Zoology 137:265–284.

Bagnara, J.T., S.K. Frost, and J. Matsumoto. 1978. On the development of pigment patterns in amphibians. American Zoologist 18:301–312.

Baker, J. and V. Waights. 1993. The effect of sodium nitrate on the growth and survival of toad tadpoles (*Bufo bufo*) in the laboratory. Herpetology Journal 3:147–148.

Baker, J. and V. Waights. 1994. The effects of nitrate on tadpoles of the tree frog (*Litoria caerulea*). Herpetology Journal 4:106–108.

Ball, G.H. 1967. Blood sporozoans from East African amphibia. Journal of Protozoology 14:521–527.

Bantle, J.A., J.N. Dumont, R.A. Finch, and G. Linder. Undated. Atlas of Abnormalities: A guide for the Performance of FETAX. [Available from J.A. Bantle, Department of Zoology, 430 LSW, Oklahoma State University, Stillwater, OK 74078.]

Barlow, L.A. and R.G. Northcutt. 1995. Embryonic origin of amphibian taste buds. Developmental Biology 169:273–285.

Barrutia, M., J. Leleta, J. Foneria, E. Garrido, and A. Zapata. 1983. Non-lymphoid cells of the anuran spleen: An ultrastructural study in the natterjack, *Bufo calamita*. American Journal of Anatomy 167:83–94.

Barta, J.R. and S.S. Desser. 1984. Blood parasites of amphibians from Algonquin Park, Ontario. Journal of Wildlife Diseases 20:180–189.

Barta, J.R., Y. Boulard, and S.S. Desser. 1987. Ultrastructural observations on secondary merogony and gametogony of *Dactylosoma ranarum* Labbe, 1894 (Eucoccidiida: Apicomplexa). Journal of Parasitology 73:1019–1029.

Bartlett, K.H., T.J. Trust, and H. Lior. 1977. Small pet aquarium frogs as a source of *Salmonella*. Applied and Environmental Microbiology 33:1026–1029.

Beattie, R.C. and R. Tyler-Jones 1992. The effects of low pH and aluminum on breeding success in the frog *Rana temporaria*. Journal of Herpetology 26:353–360.

Bechtel, H.B. 1995. Reptile and Amphibian Variants: Colors, Patterns, and Scales. Krieger Publishing Co., Malabar, FL, 224 pp.

Beetschen, J.C. and A. Jaylet. 1966. Sur un facteur recessif semi-lethal determinant l'apparition d'ascite caudale (*ac*) chez le Triton, *Pleurodeles waltlii*. Compte Rendu Hebdomadeire des Seances de l'Academie des Sciences, D: Sciences Natural 261D:5675–5678.

Bennati, R., M. Bonetti, A. Lavazza, and D. Gelmetti. 1994. Skin lesions associated with herpesvirus-like particles in frogs (*Rana dalmatina*). Veterinary Record 135:625–626.

Bernard, G.W., E.L. Cooper, and M.L. Mandell. 1968. Lamellar membrane encircled viruses in the erythrocytes of *Rana pipiens*. Journal of Ultrastructural Research 26:8–16.

Berrill, M., S. Bertram, A. Wilson, S. Louis, D. Brigham, and C. Stromberg. 1993. Lethal and sublethal impacts of pyrethroid insecticides on amphibian embryos and tadpoles. Environmental Toxicology and Chemistry 12:525–539.

Berrill, M., S. Bertram, L. McGillivray, M. Kolohon, and B. Pauli. 1994. Effects of low concentrations of forest-use pesticides on frog embryos and tadpoles. Environmental Toxicology and Chemistry 13:657–664.

Berrill, M., S. Bertram, B. Pauli, D. Coulson, M. Kolohon, and D. Ostrander. 1995. Comparative sensitivity of amphibian tadpoles to single and pulsed exposures of the forest-use insecticide, fenitrothion. Environmental Toxicology and Chemistry 14:1011–1018.

Birge, W.J. 1978. Aquatic toxicology of trace elements of coal and fly ash, *in* Thorp, J.H. and J.W. Gibbons (Eds.): Energy and Environmental Stress in Aquatic Systems. US Department of Energy Symposium Series (CONF-771114), Washington, DC, pp. 219–240.

Birge, W.J. and J.A. Black. 1979. Effects of copper on embryonic and juvenile stages of aquatic animals, *in* Nriagu, J.O. (Ed.): Copper in the Environment, Part II. John Wiley & Sons, New York, pp. 590–631.

Birge, W.J., J.A. Black, A.G. Westerman, and J.E. Hudson. 1979. The effects of mercury on reproduction of fish and amphibians, *in* Nriagu, J.O. (Ed.): The Biogeochemistry of Mercury in the Environment. Elsevier, Amsterdam and New York, pp. 629–655.

Blaustein, A.R., P.D. Hoffman, D.G. Hokit, J.M. Kiesecker, S.C. Walls, and J.B. Hayes. 1994a. UV repair and resistance to solar UV-B in amphibian eggs: A link to population declines? Proceedings of National Academy of Sciences, USA 91:1791–1795.

Blaustein, A.R., D.G. Hokit, R.K. O'Hara, and R.A. Holt. 1994b. Pathogenic fungus contributes to amphibian losses in the Pacific Northwest. Biological Conservation 67:251–254.

Blaustein, A.R., B. Edmond, J.M. Kiesecker, J.J. Beatty, and D.G. Hokit. 1995a. Ambient ultraviolet radiation causes mortality in salamander eggs. Ecological Applications 5:740–743.

Blaustein, A.R., D. Reznick, T. Halliday, and D.R. Formanowicz. 1995b. Ecological research [4 Letters]. Science 269:1201–1205.

Bleakney, J.S. 1963. First North American record of *Bufolucilia silvarum* (Meigen) (Diptera:Calliphoridae) parasitizing *Bufo terrestris americanus* Holbrook. Canadian Entomologist 95:107.

Bly, J.E., L.A. Lawson, D.J. Dale, A.J. Szalai, R.M. Durborow, and L.W. Clem. 1992. Winter saprolegniasis in channel catfish. Diseases of Aquatic Organisms 13:155–164.

Bodemer, C.W. 1960. The importance of quantity of nerve fibres in development of nerve-induced limbs in *Triturus*, and enhancement of the nervous influence by tissue implants. Journal of Morphology 107:47–59.

Bool, P.H. and E.H. Kampelmacher. 1958. Some data on the occurrence of *Salmonella* in animals in Suriman. Antonie van Leeuwenhoek 24:76–80.

Boutilier, R.G., D.F. Stiffler, and D.P. Toews. 1992. Exchange of respiratory gases, ions, and water in amphibious and aquatic amphibians, *in* Feder, M.E. and W.W. Burggren (Eds.): Environmental Physiology of the Amphibians. University of Chicago Press, Chicago, pp. 81–124.

Boyce, W.M. and E.A. Kazacos. 1991. Histopathology of nymphal pentastomid infections (*Sebekia mississippiensis*) in paratenic hosts. Journal of Parasitology 77:105–110.

Boyer, C.I., K. Blackler, and L.E. Delanney. 1971. *Aeromonas hydrophila* infection in the Mexican axolotl, *Siredon mexicanum*. Laboratory Animal Science 21:372–375.

Bradford, D.F. 1991. Mass mortality and extinction in a high-elevation population of *Rana muscosa*. Journal of Herpetology 25:174–177.

Bradford, D.F., C. Swanson, and M.S. Gordon. 1992. Effects of low pH and aluminum on two declining species of amphibians in the Sierra Nevada, California. Journal of Herpetology 26:369–377.

Bradford, D.F., C. Swanson, and M.S. Gordon. 1994. Effects of low pH and aluminum on amphibians at high elevation in the Sierra Nevada, California. Canadian Journal of Zoology 72:1272–1279.

Bragg, A.N. 1958. Parasitism of spadefoot tadpoles by *Saprolegnia*. Herpetologica 14:34.

Briggs, R.W. 1941. The development of abnormal growths in *Rana pipiens* embryos following delayed fertilization. Anatomical Record 81:121–135.

Briggs, R.T. 1972. Further studies on the maternal effect of the *o* gene in the Mexican axolotl. Journal of Experimental Zoology 181:271–280.

Briggs, R.T. and F. Briggs. 1984. Discovery and initial characterization of a new conditional (temperature-sensitive) maternal effect mutation in the axolotl. Differentiation 26:176–181.

Briggs, R.T. and P.R. Burton. 1973. Fine structure of an amphibian leukocyte virus. Journal of Submicroscopic Cytology 5:71–78.

Brooks, D.R. 1984. Platyhelminths, *in* Hoff, G.L., F.L. Frye, and E.R. Jacobson (Eds.): Diseases of Amphibians and Reptiles. Plenum Press, New York, pp. 247–258.

Brooks, D.E., E.R. Jacobson, E.D. Wolf, S. Clubb, and J.M. Gaskin. 1983. Panophthalmitis and otitis interna in fire-bellied toads. Journal of American Veterinary Medical Association 183:1198–1201.

Browder, L.W. 1975. Frogs of the genus *Rana*, *in* King, R.C. (Ed.): Handbook of Genetics, Vol 4, Vertebrates of Genetic Interest. Plenum Press, New York, pp. 19–33.

Browne, C.L. and J.N. Dumont. 1979. Toxicity of selenium to developing *Xenopus laevis* embryos. Journal of Toxicology and Environmental Health 5:699–709.

Broz, O. and J. Kulda. 1954. *Dermosporidium multigranulare* n. sp. parasit z kuze *Rana esculenta*. Vestnik Ceskoslovensk Zoologick Spolenosti 18:91–97.

Broz, O. and M. Privora. 1952. Two skin parasites of *Rana temporaria*: *Dermocystidium ranae* Guyenot and Naville and *Dermosporidium granulosum* n. sp. Parasitology 42:65–69.

Bruce, H.M. and A.S. Parkes. 1950. Rickets and osteoporosis in *Xenopus laevis*. Journal of Endocrinology 7:64–81.

Brun, R.B. 1990. In the Mexican salamander (*Ambystoma mexicanum*) homozygous for the gene eyeless, unilateral neural fold rearrangements stimulate bilateral eye formation. Journal of Experimental Zoology 254:107–113.

Brun, R.B. 1993. Bilateral eye formation in the eyeless mutant Mexican salamander following unilateral, partial excision of neural fold tissues: A quantitative study. Journal of Experimental Zoology 265:542–548.

Brun, R.B. and J.A. Garson. 1984. Notochord formation in the Mexican salamander (*Ambystoma mexicanum*) is different from notochord formation in *Xenopus laevis*. Journal of Experimental Zoology 229:235–240.

Brunst, V.V. 1955. The axolotl. II. Morphology and pathology. Laboratory Investigation 4:429–449.

Bryant, S.V. and L.E. Iten. 1976. Supernumerary limbs in amphibians: Experimental production in *Notophthalmus viridescens* and a new interpretation of their formation. Developmental Biology 50:212–234.

Bryant, S.V., V. French, and P.J. Bryant. 1981. Distal regeneration and symmetry. Science 212:993–1002.

Bube, A., E. Burkhardt, and R. Weiss. 1992. Spontaneous chromomycosis in the marine toad (*Bufo marinus*). Journal of Comparative Pathology 106:73–77.

Bulog, B. 1989a. Tectorial structures on the inner ear sensory epithelial of *Proteus anguinus* (Amphibia, Caudata). Journal of Morphology 201:59–68.

Bulog, B. 1989b. Differentiation of the inner ear sensory epithelial of *Proteus anguinus* (Urodela, Amphibia). Journal of Morphology 202:325–338.

Burggren, W.W. and M. Mwalukoma. 1983. Respiration during chronic hypoxia and hyperoxia in larval and adult bullfrogs (*Rana catesbeiana*). I. Morphological responses of lungs, skin, and gills. Journal of Experimental Biology 105:191–203.

Burggren, W.W. and N.H. West. 1982. Changing respiratory importance of gills, lungs and skin during metamorphosis in the bullfrog, *Rana catesbeiana*. Respiration Physiology 47:151–164.

Burton, A.N., J. McLintock, and J.G. Rempel. 1966. Western equine encephalitis virus in Saskatchewan garter snakes and leopard frogs. Science 154:1029–1031.

Burton, M.S., E.T. Thorne, A. Anderson, D.R. Kwiatkowski. 1995. Captive management of the endangered Wyoming toad at the Cheyenne Mountain Zoo. Bulletin of the Association of Reptilian and Amphibian Veterinarians 5:6–8.

Callard, G.V. 1992. Autocrine and paracrine role of steroids during spermatogenesis: Studies in *Squalus acanthias* and *Necturus maculosus*. Journal of Experimental Zoology 261:132–142.

Came, P.E., G. Geerling, L.J. Old, and E.A. Boyse. 1968. A serological study of polyhedral cytoplasmic viruses isolated from amphibia. Virology 36:392–400.

Canning, E.U., and J. Lom. 1986. The microsporidia of amphibia and reptiles, in The Microsporidia of Vertebrates. Academic Press, London, pp. 173–187.

Canning, E.U., E. Elkan, and P.I. Trigg. 1964. *Plistophora myotrophica* spec. nov., causing high mortality in the common toad, *Bufo bufo*, with notes on the maintenance of *Bufo* and *Xenopus* in the laboratory. Journal of Protozoology 11:157–166.

Carini, A. 1940. Sobre um parasito semelhante ao "*Rhinosporidium*," encontrado em quistos da pele de uma "*Hyla*." Arquivos do Instituto Biologico, Sao Paolo 11:93–98.

Carpenter, J.L., A. Bachrach, D.M. Albert, S.J. Vainski, and M.A. Goldstein. 1986. Xanthomatous keratitis, disseminated xanthomatosis, and atherosclerosis in Cuban tree frogs. Veterinary Pathology 23:337–339.

Carter, D.B. 1979. Structure and function of the subcutaneous lymph sacs in the anura (Amphibia). Journal of Herpetology 13:321–327.

Chang, L.W., T.M. Tiemeyer, G.R. Wenger, D.E. McMillan, and K.R. Reubl. 1982. Neuropathology of trimethyltin intoxication. I. Light microscopy study. Environmental Research 29:435–444.

Chester-Jones, I. 1987. Structure of the adrenal and interrenal glands, in Chester-Jones, I., P.M. Ingleton, and J.G. Phillips (Eds.): Fundamentals of Comparative Vertebrate Endocrinology. Plenum Press, New York, pp. 95–120.

Chester-Jones, I., P.M. Ingleton, and J.G. Phillips. 1987a. The gastrointestinal endocrine system, in Fundamentals of Comparative Vertebrate Endocrinology. Plenum Press, New York, pp. 541–577.

Chester-Jones, I., P.M. Ingleton, and J.G. Phillips. 1987b. The endocrine pancreas, in Fundamentals of Comparative Vertebrate Endocrinology. Plenum Press, New York, pp. 579–620.

Chester-Jones, I., P.M. Ingleton, and J.G. Phillips. 1987c. The structure and function of the hypothalamus and pituitary gland, in Fundamentals of Comparative Vertebrate Endocrinology. Plenum Press, New York, pp. 285–409.

Chitwood, M. and J.R. Lichtenfels. 1972. Identification of parasitic metazoa in tissue sections. Experimental Parasitology 32:407–519.

Clark, J.G. and J.P. Shoemaker. 1973. *Eurycea bislineata* (Green), the two-lined salamander, a new host of *Myxidium serotinum* Kudo and Sprague, 1940 (Myxosporida, Myxidiidae). Journal of Protozoology 20:365–366.

Clark, H.F., J.C. Brennan, R.F. Zeigel, and D.T. Karzon. 1968. Isolation and characterization of viruses from the kidneys of *Rana pipiens* with renal adenocarcinoma before and after passage in the red eft (*Triturus viridescens*). Journal of Virology 2:629–640.

Clark, H.F., C. Gray, F. Fabian, R. Zeigel, and D.T. Karzon. 1969. Comparative studies of amphibian cytoplasmic virus strains isolated from the leopard frog, bullfrog, and newt, in Mizell, M. (Ed.): Biology of Amphibian Tumors. Springer-Verlag, New York, pp. 310–326.

Clark, H.F., F. Michalski, K.S. Tweedell, D. Yohn, and R.F. Zeigel. 1973. An adenovirus, FAV-1, isolated from the kidney of a frog (*Rana pipiens*). Virology 51:392–400.

Clothier, R.H. and M. Balls. 1973a. Mycobacteria and lymphoreticular tumours in *Xenopus laevis*, the South African toad. I. Isolation, characterization and pathogenicity for *Xenopus* of *M. marinum* isolated from lymphoreticular tumour cells. Oncology 28(5):445–457.

Clothier, R.H. and M. Balls. 1973b. Mycobacteria and lymphoreticular tumours in *Xenopus laevis*, the South African Toad II. Have mycobacteria a role in tumour initiation and development? Oncology 28(5):458–480.

Coleman, R., P.J. Evennett, and J.M. Dodd. 1967. The ultrastructural localization of acid phosphatase, alkaline phosphatase and adenosine triphosphatase in induced goitres of *Xenopus laevis* Daudin tadpoles. Histochemie 10:33–43.

Coleman, R., P.J. Evennett, and J.M. Dodd. 1968a. Ultrastructural observations on the droplets of experimentally-induced goitres in *Xenopus laevis* with special reference to the development of Uhlenhuth colloid cells. Zeitschrift fur Zellforschung 84:490–496.

Coleman, R., P.J. Evennett, and J.M. Dodd. 1968b. Ultrastructural observations on some membranous cytoplasmic inclusion bodies in follicular cells of experimentally-induced goitres in tadpoles and toads of *Xenopus laevis* Daudin. Zeitschrift fur Zellforschung 84:497–505.

Colt, J., K. Orwicz, and D. Brooks. 1984. Gas bubble disease in the African clawed frog, *Xenopus laevis*. Journal of Herpetology 18:131–137.

Combes, C., G. Barchvarov, A. Fournier, and N.D. Sinnappah. 1995. Polystomatids (Monogenea). Arguments for a long-lasting coevolution with their amphibian and reptilian hosts. Herpetopathologia (Proceedings of 5th International Colloquium on Pathology of Reptiles and Amphibians) 1995:73–76.

Conaway, C.H. and D.E. Metter. 1967. Skin glands associated with breeding in *Microhyla carolinensis*. Copeia 1967:672–673.

Conklin, R.E. 1930. The formation and circulation of lymph in the frog. American Journal of Physiology 95:79–109.

Cooke, A.S. 1972. The effects of DDT, dieldrin, and 2,4-D on amphibian spawn and tadpoles. Environmental Pollution 1:51–68.

Cooke, A.S. 1979. The influence of rearing density on the subsequent response to DDT dosing for tadpoles of the frog *Rana temporaria*. Bulletin of Environmental Contamination & Toxicology 21:837–841.

Cooper, E.L. 1967. Lymphomyeloid organs of Amphibia. I. Normal appearance during larval and adult stages of *Rana catesbeiana*. Journal of Morphology 122:381–398.

Cooper, J.E. 1984. Physical influences, in Hoff, G.L., F.L. Frye, and E.R. Jacobson (Eds.): Diseases of Amphibians and Reptiles, Plenum Press, New York, pp. 607–624.

Cooper, J.E., J.R. Needham, and J. Griffin. 1978. A bacterial disease of the Darwin's frog (*Rhinoderma darwini*). Laboratory Animals 12:91–93.

Corliss, J.O. 1954. The literature on Tetrahymena: Its history, growth, and recent trends. Protozoology 1:156–169.

Corn, P.S. and F.A. Vertucci. 1992. Descriptive risk assessment of the effects of acidic deposition on Rocky Mountain amphibians. Journal of Herpetology 26:361–369.

Correa, R., I. Correa, G. Garces, D. Mendez, L.F. Morales, and A. Restrep. 1968. Lesiones micoticas (cromomicosis?) observadas en sapos (*Bufo* spp.). Antioquia Medica 18:175–184.

Crawshaw, G.J. 1993. Amphibian medicine. in Fowler, M.E. (Ed.): Zoo & Wild Animal Medicine, Current Therapy 3. W.B. Saunders Co., Philadelphia, PA, pp. 131–139.

Crump, M.L. and J.A. Pounds. 1985. Lethal parasitism of an aposematic anuran (*Atelopus varius*) by *Notochaeta bufonivora* (Diptera: Sarcophagidae). Journal of Parasitology 71:588–591.

Cullen, B.R., L. Owens, and R.J. Whittington. 1995. Experimental infection of Australian anurans (*Limnodynastes terraereginae* and *Litoria latopalmata*) with Bohle iridovirus. Diseases of Aquatic Organisms 23:83–92.

Cunningham, A.A., T.E.S. Langton, P.M. Bennett, S.E.N. Drury, R.E. Gough, and J.K. Kirkwood. 1993. Unusual mortality associated with poxvirus-like particles in frogs (*Rana temporaria*). Veterinary Record 133:141–142.

Cunningham, A.A., T.E.S Langton, and P.M. Bennett. 1995. Investigations into unusual mortalities of the common frog (*Rana temporaria*) in the United Kingdom. Herpetopathologia (Proceedings of the 5th International Symposium on Pathology of Reptiles & Amphibians) 1995:19–27.

Cunningham, A.A., A.W. Sainsbury, and J.E. Cooper. 1996a. Diagnosis and treatment of a parasitic dermatitis in a laboratory colony of African clawed frogs (*Xenopus laevis*). Veterinary Record 138:640–642.

Cunningham, A.A., T.E.S. Langton, P.M. Bennett, J.F Lewin, S.E.N. Drury, R.E. Gough, and S.K. MacGregor. 1996b. Pathological and microbiological findings from incidents of unusual mortality of the common frog (*Rana temporaria*). Philosophical Transactions of the Royal Society of London (Biological Sciences) 351B:1539–1557.

Czopek, J. 1965. Quantitative studies on the morphology of respiratory surfaces in amphibians. Acta Anatomica 62:296–323.

DaCosta, S.C.G. and N.M. Pereira. 1971. *Lankesterella alencari* n. sp., a *Toxoplasma*-like organism in the central nervous system of *Amphibia* (Protozoa, Sporozoa). Memorias do Instituto Oswaldo Cruz 69:397–424.

DaCosta, S.C.G., M.A. DeSousa, and D.R. Weigl. 1975. The ultrastructure of *Lankesterella alencari* [Abstr]. Journal of Protozoology 22:36A.

Darzins, E. 1952. The epizootic of tuberculosis among the gias in Bahia. Acta Tuberculosea Scandinavica 26:170–174.

Dawley, E.M. and A.H. Bass. 1989. Chemical access to the vomeronasal organs of a plethodontid salamander. Journal of Morphology 200:163–174.

Dawley, E.M. and J. Crowder. 1995. Sexual and seasonal differences in the vomeronasal epithelium of the red-back salamander (*Ambystoma cinereus*). Journal of Comparative Neurology 359:382–390.

De Alencar, A.A. 1957. Toxoplasmose espontanea e inaparente em anfibios dos generos *Leptodactylus* e *Bufo*. Jornal Brasileiro de Neurologia 9:137–146.

Delay, R.J., R. Taylor, and S.D. Roper. 1993. Merkel-like basal cells in *Necturus* taste buds contain serotonin. Journal of Comparative Neurology 335:606–613.

Delvinquier, B.L.J. 1986. *Myxidium immersum* (Protozoa: Myxosporea) of the cane toad, *Bufo marinus*, in Australian anura, with a synopsis of the genus in amphibians. Australian Journal of Zoology 34:843–853.

Desser, S.S. 1987. *Aegyptianella ranarum sp. n.* (Rickettsiales, Anaplasmataceae): Ultrastructure and prevalence in frogs from Ontario. Journal of Wildlife Diseases 23:52–59.

Desser, S.S. 1993. The Haemogregarinidae and Lankesterellidae, in Kreier, J.P. (Ed.): Parasitic Protozoa, Volume 4, 2nd Edition. Academic Press, San Diego, CA, pp. 247–272.

Desser, S.S. and J.R. Barta. 1984a. An intraerythrocytic virus and rickettsia of frogs from Algonquin Park, Ontario. Canadian Journal of Zoology 62:1521–1524.

Desser, S.S. and J.R. Barta. 1984b. *Thrombocytozoons ranarum* Tchacarof 1963, a prokaryotic parasite in thrombocytes of the mink frog, *Rana septentrionalis*, in Ontario. Journal of Parasitology 70:454–456.

Desser, S.S. and J.R. Barta. 1989. The morphological features of *Aegyptianella bacterifera*: An intraerythrocytic rickettsia of frogs from Corsica. Journal of Wildlife Diseases 25:313–318.

Desser, S.S., H. Hong, and D.S. Martin. 1995. Life history, ultrastructure, and experimental transmission of *Hepatozoon catesbeianae n. comb.*, an apicomplexan parasite of the bullfrog, *Rana catesbeiana* and the mosquito, *Culex territans* in Algonquin Park, Ontario. Journal of Parasitology 81:212–222.

Desser, S.S., M.E. Siddall, and J.R. Barta. 1990. Ultrastructural observation on the developmental stages of *Lankesterella minima* (Apicomplexa) in experimentally infected *Rana catesbeiana* tadpoles. Journal of Parasitology 76:97–103.

Dhaliwal, S.S. and D.A. Griffiths. 1963. Fungal disease in Malayan toads: An acute lethal inflammatory reaction. Nature 1963 (No. 4866):467–469.

Dhaliwal, S.S. and D.A. Griffiths. 1964. Fungal disease of Malayan toads (*Bufo melanostictus*). Sabouraudia 3:279–287.

Dial, N.A. 1976. Methylmercury: teratogenic and lethal effects in frog [*Rana pipiens*] embryos. Teratology 13:327–334.

Dial, N.A. and C.A. Bauer. 1984. Teratogenic and lethal effects of paraquat on developing frog embryos. Bulletin of Environmental Contamination & Toxicology 33:592–597.

Dial, N.A. and C.A. Bauer-Dial. 1987. Lethal effects of diquat and paraquat on developing frog embryos and 15-day-old tadpoles, *Rana pipiens*. Bulletin of Environmental Contamination & Toxicology 38:1006–1011.

Diesch, S.L., W.F. McCulloch, and J.L. Braun. 1967. Experimental leptospirosis in frogs. Nature (London) 214:1139–1140.

Diesel, R., G. Baurle, and P. Vogel. 1995. Cave breeding and froglet transport: A novel pattern of anuran brood care in the Jamaican frog, *Eleutherodactylus cundalli*. Copeia 1995:354–360.

Dilling, W.J. and D.W. Healey. 1925. Influence of lead and the metallic ions copper, zinc, thorium, beryllium, and thallium on the germination of frogs' spawn and on the growth of tadpoles. Annals of Applied Biology 13:177–188.

Dodd, J.M. and H.G. Callan. 1955. Neotony with goiter in *Triturus helveticus*. Quarterly Journal of Microscopic Science 96:121–128.

Dournon, C. 1983. Development somatique et inversion sexuelle sous l'action de la temperature chez les amphibiens. Proceedings of 1st International Colloquium on Pathology of Reptiles & Amphibians. pp. 227–231.

Droin, A. 1967. Une mutation letale recessive, otolithless chez *Xenopus laevis* Daudin. Revue Suisse de Zoologie 74:628–636.

Droin, A. 1992. Genetic and experimental studies on a new pigment mutant in *Xenopus laevis*. Journal of Experimental Zoology 264:196–205.

Droin, A. and M.L. Beauchemin. 1975. 'Immobile' (*im*), a recessive lethal mutation of *Xenopus laevis* tadpoles. Journal of Embryology & Experimental Morphology 34:435–449.

Droin, A. and M. Fischberg. 1984. Two recessive mutations with maternal effect upon colour and cleavage of *Xenopus l. laevis* eggs. Roux's Archives of Developmental Biology 193:86–89.

Drury, S.E.N., R.E. Gough, and A.A. Cunningham. 1995. Isolation of an iridovirus-like agent from common frogs (*Rana temporaria*). Veterinary Record 137:72–73.

Drysdale, T.A., K.F. Tonissen, K.D. Patterson, M.J. Crawford, and P.A. Krieg. 1994. Cardiac troponin I is a heart-specfic marker in the *Xenopus* embryo: Expression during abnormal heart morphogenesis. Developmental Biology 165:432–441.

Duellman, W.E. and L. Trueb. 1986. Biology of Amphibians. McGraw-Hill Book Company, New York. 670 pp.

Duncan, R. and R. Highton. 1979. Genetic relationships of the Eastern large *Plethodon* of the Ouachita Mountains. Copeia 1979:95–110.

Dunn, A.M. 1969. Veterinary Helminthology. Lea & Febiger, Philadelphia, PA, 302 pp.

Du Pasquier, L., J. Schwager, and M.F. Flajnik. 1989. The immune system of *Xenopus*. Annual Review of Immunology 7:251–275.

Duryee, W.R. 1965. Factors influencing development of tumors in frogs. Annals of the New York Academy of Sciences 126:59–84.

Dusi, J.L. 1949. The natural occurrence of "redleg," *Pseudomonas hydrophila*, in a population of American toads, *Bufo americanus*. Ohio Journal of Science 49:70–71.

Dziezyc, J., and N.J. Millichamp. 1989. Lipid keratopathy of frogs. 3rd International Colloquium on the Pathology of Reptiles & Amphibians, Orlando, FL, pp. 95–96.

Easteal, S. 1981. The history of introductions of *Bufo marinus* (Amphibia: Anura): A natural experiment in evolution. Biological Journal of the Linnean Society 16:93–113.

Ecker, A. 1881. Die Anatomie des Frosches. Ein Handbuch fur Physiologen, Arzle und Studirende. Friedrich Vieweg & Sohn, Braunschweig.

Egar, M.W. and M.S. Jarial. 1991. Structural changes in the proximal tubule of the short-toes axolotl mutant. Tissue & Cell 23:631–639.

Eisler, R. 1993. Zinc hazards to fish, wildlife, and invertebrates: A synoptic review. Contaminant Hazard Reviews Report 26, US Fish and Wildlife Service, Technical Report Series, 106 pp.

Eisler, R. 1994. Acrolein hazards to fish, wildlife, and inverte-brates: A synoptic review. Contaminant Hazard Reviews Report 28, National Biological Survey, US Department of the Interior, 29 pp.

Elkan, E. 1957. Observations on the lymphatic system of the South African claw-footed toad (*Xenopus laevis* Daudin). British Journal of Herpetology 2:37–53.

Elkan, E. 1960a. Some interesting pathological cases in amphibians. Proceedings of the Zoological Society, London 134:275–296.

Elkan, E. 1960b. The common toad (*Bufo bufo* L.) in the laboratory. British Journal of Herpetology 2:177–181.

Elkan, E. 1965. Myiasis in Australian frogs. Annals of Tropical Medicine & Parasitology 59:51–54.

Elkan, E. 1968. Mucopolysaccharides in the anuran defense against desiccation. Journal of Zoology, London 155:19–53.

Elkan, E. 1976a. Ground substance: An anuran defense against desiccation, Chapter 3, in Lofts, B. (Ed.): Physiology of the Amphibia, Volume 3. Academic Press, New York, pp. 101–110.

Elkan, E. 1976b. Pathology in the Amphibia, Chapter 6, in Lofts, B. (Ed.): Physiology of the Amphibia, Volume 3. Academic Press, New York, pp. 273–312.

Elkan, E. 1983. Random samples from herpetopathology. Proceedings of 1st International Colloquium on Pathology of Reptiles & Amphibians. pp. 1–8.

Elkan, E. and R.W. Murray. 1952. A larval trematode infection of the lateral line system of the toad, *Xenopus laevis*. Proceedings of the Zoological Society of London 122:121–126.

Elkan, E. and C.M. Philpot. 1973. Mycotic infections in frogs due to a *Phialophora*-like fungus. Sabouraudia 11:99–105.

Elliott-Feeley, E. and J.B. Armstrong. 1982. Effects of fenitrothion and carbaryl on *Xenopus laevis*. Toxicology 22:319–335.

El-Mofty, M.M. and S.A. Sakr. 1988. The induction of neoplastic lesions by aflatoxin-B1 in the Egyptian toad (*Bufo regularis*). Nutrition & Cancer 11:55–59.

Emerson, H. and C. Norris. 1905. "Red leg," an infectious disease of frogs. Journal of Experimental Medicine 7:32–58.

Environmental Protection Agency (US EPA). 1980. Ambient water quality criteria for acrolein. EPA Report 440/5-80-016. 94 pp.

Environmental Protection Agency (US EPA). 1987. Ambient water quality criteria for zinc. EPA Report 440/5-87-003. 207 pp.

Epp, L.G. 1972. Development of pigmentation in the eyeless mutant of the Mexican axolotl, *Ambystoma mexicanum*, Shaw. Journal of Experimental Zoology 181:169–180.

Epp, L.G. 1978. A review of the eyeless mutant in the Mexican axolotl. American Zoologist 18:267–272.

Erginel-Unaltuna, N. and L.F. Lemanski. 1994. Immunofluorescent studies on titin and myosin in developing hearts of normal and cardiac mutant axolotls. Journal of Morphology 222:19–32.

Erspamer, V. 1994. Bioactive secretions of the amphibian integument. *in* Heatwole, H. and G.T. Barthalmus (Eds.): Amphibian Biology, Volume 1, The Integument. Surrey Beatty & Sons, Chipping Norton, New South Wales, Australia, pp. 178–350.

Essani, K. and A. Granoff. 1989. Amphibian and piscine iridoviruses proposal for nomenclature and taxonomy based on molecular and biologic properties. Intervirology 30:187–193.

Etges, F.J. 1961. Contributions to the life history of the brain fluke of newts and fish, *Diplostomulum scheuringi* Hughes, 1929 (Trematoda: Diplostomatidae). Journal of Parasitology 47:453–458.

Etges, F.J. 1991. *Clinostomum attenuatum* (Digenea) from the eye of *Bufo marinus*. Journal of Parasitology 77:634–635.

Everard, C.O.R., B. Tota, D. Bassett, and C. Ali. 1979. *Salmonella* in wildlife from Trinidad and Grenada, West Indies. Journal of Wildlife Diseases 15:213–219.

Everard, C.O.R., G.M. Fraser-Chanpong, L.J. Bhagwandin, M.W. Race, and A.C. James. 1983. Leptospires in wildlife from Trinidad and Grenada. Journal of Wildlife Diseases 19:192–199.

Everard, C.O.R., D. Carrington, J. Korver, and J.D. Everard. 1988. Leptospires in the marine toad (*Bufo marinus*) on Barbados. Journal of Wildlife Diseases 24:334–338.

Fijan, N., Z. Matasin, Z. Petrinec, I. Valpotic, and L.O. Zwillenberg. 1991. Isolation of an iridovirus-like agent from the green frog (*Rana esculenta* L.). Veterinarski Arhiv 61:151–158.

Fikes, J.D. 1990. Organophosphorous and carbamate insecticides. Veterinary Clinics of North America Small Animal Practice 20:353–367.

Fischberg, M., A.W. Blackler, V. Uehlinger, J. Reynaud, A. Droin, and J. Stock. 1963. Nucleo-cytoplasmic control of development. *in* Geerts, S.J. (Ed): Genetics Today, Volume 2. Pergamon Press, Oxford, pp. 187–198.

Fischer, J.L. 1976. L'oedeme generalise chez la grenouille rousse. Bulletin de la Societe Linnaeus, Lyon 45:43–46.

Fleming, W.J., E.F. Hill, and J.J. Momot. 1991. Toxicity of trimethyltin and triethyltin to mallard ducklings. Environmental Toxicology & Chemistry 10:255–260.

Flindt, V.R., H. Hemmer, and R. Schipp. 1968. Zur morphogenese von Missbildungen bei Bastardlarven *Bufo calamita* X *Bufo viridis*: Stoerungen in der ausbildung des axialskeletts. Zoologische Jahrbucher Abteilung fur Anatomie & Ontogenie der Tiere 85:51–71.

Flynn, R.J. 1973. Parasites of laboratory reptiles and amphibians. *in* Parasites of Laboratory Animals. Iowa State University Press, Ames, IA, pp. 507–642.

Fort, D.J., B.L. James, and J.A. Bantle. 1989. Evaluation of the developmental toxicity of five compounds with the frog embryo teratogenesis assay: *Xenopus* (FETAX) and a metabolic activation system. Journal of Applied Toxicology 9:377–388.

Fox, H. 1963. The amphibian pronephros. Quarterly Review of Biology 38:1–25.

Fox, H. 1981. Cytological and morphological changes during amphibian metamorphosis, *in* Gilbert, L.I. and E. Frieden (Eds.): Metamorphosis, A Problem in Developmental Biology, 2nd Ed. Plenum Press, New York, pp. 327–362.

Fox, H. 1992. Figures of Eberth in the amphibian larval epidermis. Journal of Morphology 212:87–97.

Fox, H. 1994. The structure of the integument, *in* Heatwole, H. and G.T. Barthalmus (Eds.): Amphibian Biology, Volume 1, The Integument. Surrey Beatty & Sons, Chipping Norton, New South Wales, Australia. pp. 1–32.

Fox, H. and M. Whitear. 1990. Cellular elements of the dermis and collagen remodelling during larval life of anurans. Archives of Histology & Cytology 53:381–391.

Frangioni, G. and F. Borgioli. 1993. Consequences of splenectomy on the conpensatory mechanism of cutaneous respiration in the newt. Journal of Experimental Zoology 267:1301–136.

Frank, W. 1984. Non-hemoparasitic protozoans. *in* Hoff, G.L., F.L. Frye, and E.R. Jacobson (Eds.). Diseases of Amphibians and Reptiles. Plenum Press, New York, pp. 259–284.

Frank, W. and U. Roester. 1970. Amphibian als trager van *Hormiscium* (*Hormodendrum*) dermatitis (Kano, 1937) einen Erreger der Chromoblastomykose (Chromomykose) des Menschen. Zeitschrift fur Tropenmedizin und Parasitologie 21:93–108.

Frank, W., U. Roester, and H.J. Scholer. 1974. Sphaerulenbildung bei einer *Mucor*-spezies in inneren Organen von Amphibien. Vorlaufige mitteilung. Zentralblatt fur Bakteriologie und Hygiene, Abteilung Originale A226:405–417.

Fraser, C.M., J.A. Bergeron, A. Mays, and S.E. Aiello. 1991. Fungal infections (mycoses), *in* The Merck Veterinary Manual, 7th Ed. Merck & Company, Rahway, NJ, pp. 340–344.

Freda, J. 1990. Effects of acidification on amphibians, *in* Baker, J.P., D.P. Bernard, S.W. Christensen, and M.J. Sale (Eds.): Biological Effects of Changes in Surface Water Acid-Base Chemistry. State-of-Science Technology Report 13. National Acid Precipitation Assessment Program, Washington, DC, pp. 114–129.

Freda, J. 1991. The effects of aluminum and other metals on amphibians. Environmental Pollution 71:305–328.

Freda, J. and W.A. Dawson. 1984. Sodium balance of amphibian larvae exposed to low environmental pH. Physiological Zoology 57:435–443.

Freda, J. and D.G. McDonald. 1990. The effects of aluminum on the leopard frog, *Rana pipiens*: Life stage comparisons and aluminum uptake. Canadian Journal of Fisheries & Aquatic Science 47:210–216.

Freeland, W.J., B.L.J. Delvinquier, and B. Bonnin. 1986. Decline of cane toad, *Bufo marinus*, populations: Status of urban toads. Australian Wildlife Research 13:597–601.

Frost, S.K., M.S. Ellinger, and J.A. Murphy. 1982. The pale mutation in *Bombina orientalis*: Effects on melanophores and xanthophores. Journal of Experimental Zoology 221:125–129.

Frost, S.K., F. Briggs, and G.M. Malacinski. 1984. A color atlas of pigment genes in the Mexican axolotl (*Ambystoma mexicanum*). Differentiation 26:182–188.

Frost-Mason, S.K., R. Morrison, and K. Mason. 1994. Pigmentation, *in* Heatwole, H. and G.T. Barthalmus (Eds.): Amphibian Biology, Volume 1, The Integument. Surrey Beatty & Sons, Chipping Norton, New South Wales, Australia, pp. 64–97.

Fry, A.E. 1966. Hind limb regeneration in *Rana pipiens* larvae. Copeia 1966:530–534.

Frye, B.E. 1964. Metamorphic changes in the blood sugar and the pancreatic islets of the frog, *Rana clamitans*. Journal of Experimental Zoology 155:215–224.

Frye, F.L. 1985. An unusual epizootic of anuran aeromoniasis. Journal of the American Veterinary Medical Association 187:1223–1224.

Frye, F.L. 1989a. *Aeromonas* and *Citrobacter* epizootics in an institutional amphibian collection [Abstr.]. 3rd International Colloquium on Pathology of Reptiles & Amphibians, 13–15 January 1989, Orlando, FL, pp. 31–32.

Frye, F.L. 1989b. Periarticular gout in a pixie frog (*Pixicephalus delalandii*). 3rd International Colloquium on Pathology of Reptiles & Amphibians, 13–15 January 1989, Orlando, FL, p. 108.

Frye, F.L. and D.S. Gillespie. 1989. Saprolegniasis in a zoo collection of aquatic amphibians. Proceedings of the 3rd International Colloquium on the Pathology of Reptiles and Amphibians, 13–15 Jan 1989, Orlando, FL, p. 43.

Frye, F.L. and H. Miller. 1994. Hermaphroditism in a tomato frog (*Dyscophus antongilii*). Journal of Zoo & Wildlife Medicine 25:154–157.

Gallien, L. 1969. Spontaneous and experimental mutations in the newt, *Pleurodeles waltlii* Michah, *in* Mizell, M. (Ed.): Biology of Amphibian Tumors. Springer-Verlag, New York, pp. 35–42.

Gambier, H. 1924. Sur un protiste parasite et pathogene des tritons: *Hepatosphaera molgarum* n.g., n. sp. Comptes Rendus des Seances de la Societe de Biologie & de ses Filiales 90:439–441.

Gardiner, C.H., R. Fayer, and J.P. Dubey. 1988. An Atlas of Protozoan Parasites in Animal Tissues. U.S. Department of Agriculture, Agriculture Handbook Number 651. 83 pp.

Garrido, E., R.P. Gomariz, J. Leceta, and A. Zapata. 1987. Effects of dexamethasone on the lymphoid organs of *Rana perezi*. Developmental & Comparative Immunology 11:375–384.

Ghate, H.V. and L. Mulherkar. 1980. Effect of mercuric chloride on embryonic development of the frog *Microhyla ornata*. Indian Journal of Experimental Biology 18:1094–1096.

Ghosh, T.N. 1977. Studies on the genus *Entamoeba*. III. *Entamoeba* from amphibians [Abstr. 131]. Journal of Protozoology (Supplement 2) 24:21A.

Giannetti, M., A. Trux, B. Gianetti, and Z. Zubrzycki. 1990. *Xenopus laevis* South African clawed toad—A potential indicator for radioactive contamination in ecological systems? Fortschritte der Zoologie 38:279–285.

Gibbs, E.L., T.J. Gibbs, and P.C. Van Dyck. 1966. *Rana pipiens*: Health and disease. Laboratory Animal Care 16:142–160.

Gill, D.E. and B.A. Mock. 1985. Ecological and evolutionary dynamics of parasites: The case of *Trypanosoma diemyctyli* in the red-spotted newt *Notophthalmus viridescens*, in Rollinson, D. and R.M. Anderson (Eds.): Ecology and Genetics of Host-Parasite Interactions. Academic Press, London and Orlando, pp. 157–183.

Gil-Turnes, M.A., M.E. Hay, and W. Fenical. 1989. Symbiotic marine bacteria chemically defend crustacean embryos from a pathogenic fungus. Science 246:116–118.

Gipouloux, J.D., C. Girard, and S. Gipouloux. 1986. Number of somatic and germ cells during early stage of gonadal development in frog larvae treated with zinc sulphate. Roux's Archives of Developmental Biology 195:193–196.

Glorioso, J.C., R.L. Amborski, G.F. Amborksi, and D.D. Culley. 1974. Microbiological studies on septicemic bullfrogs (*Rana catesbeiana*). American Journal of Veterinary Research 35:1241–1245.

Goater, T.M., M. Mulvey, and G.W. Esch. 1990. Electrophoretic differentiation of two *Halipegus* (Trematoda: Hemiuridae) congeners in an amphibian population. Journal of Parasitology 76:431–434.

Goldstein, S. and L. Moriber. 1966. Biology of a problematic marine fungus, *Dermocystidium* sp. I. Development and cytology. Archiv fur Mikrobiologie 53:1–11.

Goodchild, C.G. 1950. Establishment and pathology of gorgoderid infections in anuran kidneys. Journal of Parasitology 36:439–446.

Goodchild, C.G. 1953. A subcutaneous, cyst-parasite of bullfrogs: *Histocystidium ranae*, n. g., n. sp. Journal of Parasitology 39:395–405.

Goorha, R.M. and A. Granoff. 1994. Frog virus 3, in Webster, R.G. and A. Granoff (Eds.): Encyclopedia of Virology. Academic Press, London, pp. 503–508.

Gorbman, A. 1964. Endocrinology of the Amphibia. V. Islets of Langerhans, in Moore, J.A. (Ed.): Physiology of the Amphibia, Academic Press, New York, pp. 393–398.

Gosner, K. and I.H. Black. 1957. The effects of acidity on the development and hatching of New Jersey frogs. Ecology 38:256–262.

Goss, R.J. and R. Holt. 1992. Epimorphic vs. tissue regeneration in *Xenopus* forelimbs. Journal of Experimental Zoology 261:451–457.

Grably, S. and Y. Piery. 1981. Weight and tissues changes in long term starved frogs, *Rana esculenta*. Comparative Biochemistry & Physiology 69A:683–688.

Granoff, A. 1989. Viruses of amphibians: An historical perspective, in Ahne, W. and E. Kurstak (Eds.): Viruses of Lower Vertebrates. Springer-Verlag, Berlin, pp. 1–12.

Granoff, A., P.E. Came, and K.A. Rafferty. 1965. The isolation and properties of viruses from *Rana pipiens*: Their possible relationship to the renal adenocarcinoma of the leopard frog. Annals of New York Academy of Sciences 126:237–255.

Graveson, A.C. and J.B. Armstrong. 1994. In vivo evidence that the premature death (*p*) mutation of *Ambystoma mexicanum* affects an early segregating subpopulation of neural crest cells. Journal of Experimental Zoology 269:327–335.

Green, D.E., et al. 1995a. Mass morbidity and mortality of wild cane toads (*Bufo marinus*) on Kaua'i Island, Hawai'i (USA) in 1992 and 1994. Herpetopathologia (Proceedings of 5th International Colloquium on the Pathology of Reptiles & Amphibians) 1995:201–214.

Green, D.E., J. Andrews, and J. Abell. 1995b. Preliminary investigations on a mycotic myositis in red-spotted newts (*Notophthalmus viridescens*) from Vermont. Herpetopathologia (Proceedings of 5th International Colloquium on the Pathology of Reptiles & Amphibians) 1995:51–62.

Griner, L.A. 1983. Pathology of Zoo Animals. Zoological Society of San Diego, pp. 3–17.

Groff, J.M., A. Mughannam, T.S. McDowell, A. Wong, M.J. Dykstra, F.L. Frye, and R.P. Hedrick. 1991. An epizootic of cutaneous zygomycosis in cultured dwarf African clawed frogs (*Hymenochirus curtipes*) due to *Basidiobolus ranarum*. Journal of Medical & Veterinary Mycology 29:215–223.

Gross, T.S., L.J. Guillette, H.F. Percival, G.R. Masson, J.M. Matter, and A.R. Woodward. 1994. Contaminant-induced reproductive anomalies in Florida. Comparative Pathology Bulletin 26:1–8.

Gruia-Gray, J. and S.S. Desser. 1992. Cytopathological observations and epizootiology of frog erythrocytic virus in bullfrogs (*Rana catesbeiana*). Journal of Wildlife Diseases 28:34–41.

Gruia-Gray, J., M. Petric, and S.S. Desser. 1989a. Ultrastructural, biochemical, and biologic properties of an erythrocytic virus of frogs from Ontario, Canada, in Ahne, W. and E. Kurstak (Eds.): Viruses of Lower Vertebrates. Springer-Verlag, Berlin, pp. 69–78.

Gruia-Gray, J., M. Petric, and S.S. Desser. 1989b. Ultrastructural, biochemical, and biophysical properties of an erythrocytic virus of frogs from Ontario, Canada. Journal of Wildlife Disease 25:497–506.

Guardabassi, A. 1960. The utilization of the calcareous deposits of the endolymphatic sacs of *Bufo bufo* in the mineralization of the skeleton. Investigations by means of Ca^{45}. Zeitschrift fur Zellforschung 51:278–282.

Gugnani, H.C. & J.I. Okafor. 1980. Mycotic flora of the intestine and other internal organs of certain reptiles and amphibians with special reference to characterization of *Basidiobolus* isolates. Mykosen 23:260–268.

Gurdon, J.B. and H.R. Woodland. 1975. *Xenopus*, in: King, R.C. (Ed.): Handbook of Genetics, Vol 4, Vertebrates of Genetic Interest. Plenum, New York, pp. 35–50.

Guyenot, E. and A. Naville. 1922. Un nouveau Protiste, due genre *Dermocystidium*, parasite de la grenouille. *Dermocystidium ranae* nov. spec. Revue Suisse de Zoologie 29:133–145.

Guyenot, E. and K. Ponse. 1926. Une microsporidie, *Plistophora bufonis*, parasite d'organe de Bidder du Crapaud. Revue Suisse de Zoologie 33:213–250.

Hakvoort, J.H.M., E.J. Gouda, and P. Zwart. 1995. Skeletal and muscular underdevelopment (SMUD) in Dendrobatidae. Herpetopathologia (Proceedings of the 5th International Colloquium on Pathology of Reptiles & Amphibians) 1995:271–275.

Harte, J. and E. Hoffman. 1989. Possible effects of acidic deposition on a Rocky Mountain population of the tiger salamander *Ambystoma tigrinum*. Conservation Biology 3:149–158.

Haynes, L., F.A. Harding, A.D. Koniski, and N. Cohen. 1992. Immune system activation associated with a naturally occurring infection in *Xenopus laevis*. Developmental & Comparative Immunology 16:453–462.

Heatwole, H. and G.T. Barthalmus. 1994. Amphibian Biology, Volume 1, The Integument. Surrey Beatty & Sons, Chipping Norton, New South Wales, Australia, 418 pp.

Hecnar, S.J. 1995. Acute and chronic toxicity of ammonium nitrate fertilizer to amphibians from southern Ontario. Environmental Toxicology & Chemistry 14:2131–2137.

Hedtke, S.F. and F.A. Puglisi. 1982. Short-term toxicity of five oils to four freshwater species. Archives of Environmental Contamination & Toxicology 11:425–430.

Hendrickson, A.E. and D.E. Kelly. 1969. Development of the amphibian pineal organ: Cell proliferation and migration. Anatomical Record 165:221–228.

Hengstberger, S.G., A.D. Hyatt, R. Speare, and B.E.H. Coupar. 1993. Comparison of epizootic haematopoietic necrosis and Bohle iridoviruses, recently isolated Australian iridoviruses. Diseases of Aquatic Organisms 15:93–107.

Herman, R.L. 1984. *Ichthyphonus*-like infection in newts (*Notophthalmus viridescens* Rafinesque). Journal of Wildlife Diseases 20:55–56.

Herrick, C.J. 1948. The Brain of the Tiger Salamander, *Ambystoma tigrinum*. University of Chicago Press, Chicago, 407 pp.

Hertwig, I. and J. Hentschel. 1990. Anatomy and development of the inner ear in amphibians. Fortschritte der Zoologie 38:177–186.

Hine, R.L., B.L. Les, B.F. Hellmich, et al. 1975. Preliminary report on leopard frog (*Rana pipiens*) populations in Wisconsin. Wisconsin Department of Natural Resources Research Report 81.

Hird, D.W., S.L. Diesch, R.G. McKinnell, E. Gorham, F.B. Martin, S.W. Kurtz, and C. Dubrovolny. 1981. *Aeromonas hydrophila* in wild caught frogs and tadpoles (*Rana pipiens*) in Minnesota. Laboratory Animal Science 31:166–169.

Holcombe, G.W., G.L. Phipps, A.H. Sulaiman, and A.D. Hoffman. 1987. Simultaneous multiple species testing: Acute toxicity of 13 chemicals to 12 diverse freshwater amphibian, fish, and invertebrate families. Archives of Environmental Contamination & Toxicology 16:697–710.

Honrubia, M.P., M.P. Herraez, and R. Alvarez. 1993. The carbamate insecticide ZZ-Aphox® induced structural changes of gills, liver, gall-bladder, heart, and notochord of *Rana perezi* tadpoles. Archives of Environmental Contamination & Toxicology 25:184–191.

Hoperskaya, O.A. 1975. The development of animals homozygous for a mutation causing periodic albinism (*a*ᵖ) in *Xenopus laevis*. Journal of Embryology & Developmental Biology 34:253–264.

Horton, J.D. 1971. Histogenesis of the lymphomyeloid complex in the larval leopard frog, *Rana pipiens*. Journal of Morphology 134:1–20.

Houck, L.D. and D.M. Sever. 1994. Role of the skin in reproduction and behavior, *in* Heatwole, H. and G.T. Barthalmus (Eds.): Amphibian Biology, Volume 1, The Integument. Surrey Beatty & Sons, Chipping Norton, New South Wales, Australia, pp. 351–381.

Howerth, E.W. 1984. Pathology of naturally occurring chlamydiosis in African clawed frogs (*Xenopus laevis*). Veterinary Pathology 21:28–32.

Hubbard, G.B. 1981. *Aeromonas hydrophila* infection in *Xenopus laevis*. Laboratory Animal Science 31:297–300.

Huey, D.W. and T.L. Beitinger. 1980. Toxicity of nitrate to larvae of the salamander, *Ambystoma texanum*. Bulletin of Envirnomental Contamination & Toxicology 25:909–912.

Humphrey, R.R. 1959. A linked gene determining the lethality usually accompanying a hereditary fluid imbalance in the Mexican axolotl. Journal of Heredity 50:279–286.

Humphrey, R.R. 1964. Genetic and experimental studies on a lethal factor (*r*) in the axolotl which induces abnormalities in the renal system and other organs. Journal of Experimental Zoology 155:139–150.

Humphrey, R.R. 1967. Albino axolotls from an albino tiger salamander through hybridization. Journal of Heredity 58:95–101.

Humphrey, R.R. 1972. Genetic and experimental studies on a mutant gene (*c*) determining absence of heart action in embryos of the Mexican axolotl, *Ambystoma mexicanum*. Developmental Biology 27:365–375.

Humphrey, R.R. 1975. The axolotl, *Ambystoma mexicanum*, *in* King, R.C. (Ed.): Handbook of Genetics, Vol 4, Vertebrates of Genetic Interest. Plenum Press, New York, pp. 3–17.

Hunsaker, D. and F.E. Potter. 1960. "Red leg" in a natural population of amphibians. Herpetologica 16:285–286.

Hussain, M.M. and S.K. Saidapur. 1982. Effect of thiourea on the pituitary and thyroid gland of the toad, *Bufo melanostictus*. Journal of Animal Morphology and Physiology 29:64–70.

Hyland, K.E. 1961. Parasitic phase of chigger mite, *Hannemania hegeneri* on experimentally infested amphibians. Experimental Parasitology 11:212–225.

Ide, C. 1978. Genetic dissection of cerebellar development: Mutations affecting cell position. American Zoologist 18:281–287.

Ide, C.F., R. Tompkins, and N. Miszkowski. 1977. Neuroanatomy of spastic, a behavior mutant of the Mexican axolotl: Purkinje cell distribution in the adult cerebellum. Journal of Comparative Neurology 176:373–386.

Inoue, S. and M. Singer. 1963. Transmissibility and some histopathology of a spontaneously originated visceral tumor in the newt, *Triturus pyrrhogaster*. Cancer Research 23:1679–1684.

Inoue, S. and M. Singer. 1970a. Experiments on a spontaneously originated visceral tumor in the newt, *Triturus pyrrhogaster*. Annals of the New York Academy of Science 174:729–764.

Inoue, S. and M. Singer. 1970b. Lymphosarcomatous disease of the newt, *Triturus pyrrhogaster*. Bibl Haematol 36:640–641.

Inoue, S., M. Singer, and J. Hutchinson. 1965. Causative agent of a spontaneously originating visceral tumour in the newt, *Triturus*. Nature 205:408–409.

Ippen, R. 1964. Vergleichende pathologische Untersuchungen uber die spontane und experimentelle Tuberkulose der Kaltbluter. Abhand. Deutsch Akad die Wissenschaft. Springer-Verlag, Berlin.

Iten, L.E. and S.W. Bryant. 1973. Forelimb regeneration from different levels of amputation in the newt, *Notophthalmus viridescens*: Length, rate, and stages. Wilhelm Roux's Archives 173: 263–282.

Jacobson, E. 1989. Mycotic diseases of amphibians and reptiles: A review. Proceedings of the 3rd International Colloquium on the Pathology of Reptiles and Amphibians, pp. 41–42.

Jara, Z. 1972. Gruzlica ryb i innych kregowcow zmiennocieplnych (Tuberculosis of fish and other homeothermic vertebrates). Medycyna Weterynaryjna 28:705–710.

Jay, J.M. and W.J. Pohley. 1981. *Dermosporidium penneri* sp. n. from the skin of the American toad, *Bufo americanus* (Amphibian: Bufonidae). Journal of Parasitology 67:108–110.

Jobling, S., D. Sheahan, J.A. Osborne, P. Matthiessen, and J.P. Sumpter. 1996. Inhibition of testicular growth in rainbow trout (*Oncorhynchus mykiss*) exposed to estrogenic alkylphenolic chemicals. Environmental Toxicology & Chemistry 15:194–202.

Johnston, M.R.L. 1975. Distribution of *Pirhemocyton* Chatton & Blanc and other, possibly related, infections of poikilotherms. Journal of Protozoology 22:529–535.

Joiner, G.N. and G.D. Abrams. 1967. Experimental tuberculosis in the leopard frog. Journal of the American Veterinary Medical Association 151:942–949.

Jones, S.R.M. and P.T.K. Woo. 1994. Morphology and infectivity of cultivated *Trypanosoma ambystomae*. Journal of Parasitology 80:521–525.

Jurd, R.D., L.D.S. Gainey, and I.R. John. 1995. Gut-associated lymphoid tissue in Urodela. Herpetopathologia 2:151–155.

Kaltenbach, J.C. 1953. Local action of thyroxin on amphibian metamorphosis. II. Development of the eyelids, nictitating membrane, cornea, and extrinsic ocular muscles in *Rana pipiens* larvae affected by thyroxin-cholesterol implants. Journal of Experimental Zoology 122:41–51.

Kanamadi, R.D. and S.K. Saidapur. 1992. Effects of exposure to sublethal mercuric chloride on the testis and fat body of the frog *Rana cyanophlyctis*. Journal of Herpetology 26:499–501.

Kao, K.R. and R.P. Elinson. 1988. The entire mesodermal mantle behaves as Speman's organizer in dorsoanterior enhanced *Xenopus laevis* embryos. Developmental Biology 127:64–77.

Kaplan, H.M. and S.S. Glaczenski. 1965. Salamanders as laboratory animals: *Necturus*. Laboratory Animal Care 15:151–155.

Kaplan, H.M. and J.G. Overpeck. 1964. Toxicity of halogenated hydrocarbon insecticides for the frog, *Rana pipiens*. Herpetologica 20:163–169.

Kaplan, H.M. and L. Yoh. 1961. Toxicity of copper for frogs. Herpetologica 17:131–135.

Kaplan, H.M., T.J. Arnolt, and J.E. Payne. 1967. Toxicity of lead nitrate solutions for frogs (*Rana pipiens*). Laboratory Animal Care 17:240–246.

Karns, D.R. 1992. Effects of acidic bog habitats on amphibian reproduction in a northern Minnesota peatland. Journal of Herpetology 26:401–412.

Kawamura, T. and M. Nishioka. 1978. Abnormalities in the descendants of *Rana nigromaculata* produced from irradiated eggs or sperm. Science Report of the Laboratory of Amphibian Biolology, Hiroshima University 3:1–187.

Kelly, D.E. 1965. Ultrastructure and development of amphibian pineal organs. Progress in Brain Research 10:270–287.

Kelly, D.E. and S.W. Smith. 1964. Fine structure of the pineal organs of the adult frog, *Rana pipiens*. Journal of Cell Biology 22:653–674.

Kemali, M. and V. Braitenberg. 1969. Atlas of the Frog's Brain. Springer-Verlag, Berlin, 74 pp.

Kennedy, M.J. 1981. A revision of the species of the genus *Haematoloechus* Looss, 1899 (Trematoda: Haematoloechidae) from Canada and the United States. Canadian Journal of Zoology 59:1836–1846.

Kiesecker, J.M. and A.R. Blaustein. 1995. Synergism between UV-B and a pathogen magnifies amphibian embryo mortality in nature. Proceedings of National Academy of Sciences USA 92:11049–11052.

King, H.D. 1907. *Bertramia bufonis*, a new parasite of *Bufo lentiginosus*. Proceedings of the Academy of Natural Science (Philadelphia) 59:273–278.

King, P.H. and J.G. Van As. 1997. Description of the adult and larval stages of *Tylodelphys xenopi* (Trematoda: Diplostomidae) from southern Africa. Journal of Parasitology 83:287–295.

Klaasen, H.L.B.M., J.P. Koopman, M.E. Vanden Brink, M.H. Bakker, F.G.J. Poelma, and A.C. Beynen. 1993. Intestinal, segmented, filamentous bacteria in a wide range of vertebrate species. Laboratory Animals 27:141–150.

Kollros, J.J. 1981. Transitions in the nervous system during amphibian metamorphosis, *in* Gilbert, L.I. and E. Frieden (Eds.): Metamorphosis, A Problem in Developmental Biology, 2nd Ed. Plenum Press, New York, pp. 445–459.

Kozuch, O., M. Labuda, and J. Nosek. 1977. Isolation of sindbis virus from the frog, *Rana ridibunda*. [Abstr.] Acta Virologica 22:78.

Kudo, R.R. 1922a. On the morphology and life history of a myxosporidian, *Leptotheca ohlmacheri*, parasitic in *Rana clamitans* and *R. pipiens*. Parasitology 14:221–224.

Kudo, R.R. 1922b. On the protozoa parasitic in frogs. Transactions of the Amercian Microscopical Society 41:59–76.

Kuhlenbeck, H. 1973. The Central Nervous System of Vertebrates, Vol III, Part 2. S. Karger, Basel.

Kulp, W.L. and D.G. Borden. 1942. Further studies on *Proteus hy-*

drophilus, the etiological agent in "red leg" disease of frogs. Journal of Bacteriology 44:673–685.

Kunst, L. and I. Valpotic. 1968. Nova zarazna bolest zaba uzrokovana virusom. Veterinarski Archiv (Zagreb) 38:108–113.

Lainson, R. and I. Paperna. 1995. Light and electron microscope study of a *Lankesterella petiti* n. sp. (Apicomplexa: Lankesterellidae) infecting *Bufo marinus* (Amphibia: Anura) in Para, north Brazil. Parasite 2:307–313.

Lande, S.P. and S.I. Guttman. 1973. The effects of copper sulfate on the growth and mortality rate of *Rana pipiens* tadpoles. Herpetologica 29:22–27.

Lauckner, G. 1984. Agents: Fungi, *in* Kinne, O. (Ed.): Diseases of Marine Animals, Part 1, Volume IV. Biologische Anstalt Helgoland, Hamburg, Germany, pp. 89–113.

Laurance, W.F., K.R. McDonald, and R. Speare. 1996. Epidemic disease and the catastrophic decline of Australian rain forest frogs. Conservation Biology 10:406–413.

Lautenschlager, E.W. 1959. Meningeal tumors of the newt associated with trematode infection of the brain. Proceedings of the Helminthological Society of Washington 26:11–14.

Lazell, J. 1995. *Plethodon albagula* (western slimy salamander). Foot anomalies. Herpetological Review 26:198.

Lees, E. 1962. The incidence of helminth parasites in a particular frog population. Parasitology 52:95–102.

Lemanski, L.F. 1978. Morphological, biochemical and immunohisto-chemical studies on heart development in cardiac mutant axolotls, *Ambystoma mexicanum*. American Zoologist 18:327–348.

Levine, N.D. and R.R. Nye. 1976. *Toxoplasma ranae* sp. n. from the leopard frog *Rana pipiens* Linnaeus. Journal of Protozoology 23:488–490.

Levine, N.D. and R.R. Nye. 1977. A survey of blood and other tissue parasites of leopard frogs, *Rana pipiens*, in the United States. Journal of Wildlife Diseases 13:17–23.

Levy, B.M. and G.C. Godman. 1955. Tumors of the notochord of the salamander, *Ambystoma punctatum*, produced by crystalline lathyrus factor. Cancer Research 15:184–187.

Lewis, E.R., E.L. Levernez, and W.S. Bialek. 1985. The Vertebrate Inner Ear. CRC Press, Boca Raton, FL.

Li, X. and N.S. Lipman. 1995. Peritoneal gorgoderiasis in a bullfrog (*Rana catesbeiana*). Laboratory Animal Science 45:309–311.

Ling, R.L. and J.K. Werner. 1988. Mortality in *Ambystoma maculatum* larvae due to *Tetrahymena* infection. Herpetological Review 19:26.

Lipsett, J.C. 1941. Disproportionate dwarfism in amblystoma. Journal of Experimental Zoology 86:441–445.

Lom, J. 1958. A contribution to the systematics and morphology of endoparasitic trichodinids from amphibians, with a proposal of uniform specific characteristics. Journal of Protozoology 5:251–263.

Long, L.E., L.S. Saylor, and M.E. Soule. 1995. A pH/UV-B synergism in amphibians. Conservation Biology 9:1301–1303.

Lopez, T.J. and L.R. Maxson. 1990. *Rana catesbeiana* (bullfrog) polymely. Herpetological Review 21:90.

Ludicke, M. 1971. Ein funfbeiniger Grasfrosch (*Rana temporaria* L.). Zoologische Anzeiger 186:188–197.

Machicao, N., and E. LaPlaca. 1954. Lepra-like granulomas in frogs. Laboratory Investigation 3:219–227.

Maden, M. 1982. Supernumerary limbs in amphibians. American Zoologist 22:131–142.

Maden, M. 1993. The homeotic transformation of tails into limbs in *Rana temporaria* by retinoids. Developmental Biology 159:379–391.

Maden, M. and N. Holder. 1984. Axial characteristics of nerve induced supernumerary limbs in the axolotl. Roux's Archives of Developmental Biology 193:394–401.

Mahaney, P.A. 1994. Effects of freshwater petroleum contamination on amphibian hatching and metamorphosis. Environmental Toxicology & Chemistry 13:259–265.

Malacinski, G.M. 1978. The Mexican axolotl, *Ambystoma mexicanum*: Its biology and developmental genetics, and its autonomous cell-lethal genes. American Zoologist 18:195–206.

Malacinski, G.M. and A.J. Brothers. 1974. Mutant genes in the Mexican axolotl. Science 184:1142–1147.

Malvin, G.M. 1989. Gill structure and function: Amphibian larvae, *in* Wood, S.C. (Ed.), Comparative Pulmonary Physiology, Current Concepts, Vol 39, Lung Biology in Health and Disease. Marcel Dekker, New York, pp. 121–151.

Manning, M.J. and J.D. Horton. 1969. Histogenesis of lymphoid organs in larvae of the South African clawed toad, *Xenopus laevis* (Daudin). Journal of Embryology & Experimental Morphology 22:265–277.

Manning, M.J. and J.D. Horton. 1982. RES structure and function of the Amphibia, *in* Cohen, N. and M. Sigel (Eds.): The Reticuloendothelial System: A Comprehensive Treatise, Phylogeny and Ontogeny. Plenum Press, New York, pp. 423–459.

Manwell, R.D., E. Bernstein, and R. Dillon. 1953. Toxoplasma in frogs. Journal of Parasitology 39:406–407.

Marian, M.P., V. Arul, and T.J. Pandian. 1983. Acute and chronic effects of carbaryl on survival, growth and metamorphosis in the bullfrog, *Rana tigrina*. Archives of Environmental Contamination & Toxicology 12:271–275.

Martin, T.R. and D.B. Conn. 1990. The pathogenicity, localization, and cyst structure of echinostomatid metacercariae (Trematoda) infecting the kidneys of the frogs *Rana clamitans* and *Rana pipiens*. Journal of Parasitology 76:414–419.

Martin, D.S. and S.S. Desser. 1990. A light and electron microscopic study of *Trypanosoma fallisi* n. sp. in toads (*Bufo americanus*) from Algonquin Park, Ontario. Journal of Protozoology 37:199–206.

Martin, D.S. and S.S. Desser. 1991. Infectivity of cultured *Trypanosoma fallisi* (Kinetoplastida) to various anuran species and its evolutionary implications. Journal of Parasitology 77:498–500.

Martin, D.S., S.S. Desser, and J.K. Werner. 1992. Allozyme comparison and infectivity of cultured stages of *Trypanosoma fallisi* from southern Ontario and a trypanosome of toads from northern Michigan. Journal of Parasitology 78:1083–1086.

Marx, M., L.N. Ruben, C. Nobis, and D. Duffy. 1987. Compromised T-cell regulatory functions during anuran metamorphosis: The role of corticosteroids. Developmental & Comparative Immunology 11:129–140.

Materna, E.J., D.F. Rabeni, and R.W. LaPoint. 1995. Effects of the synthetic pyrethroid insecticide, esfenvalerate, on larval leopard frogs (*Rana* spp.). Environmental Toxicology & Chemistry 14:613–622.

Matsui, M. and T. Hayashi. 1992. Genetic uniformity in the Japanese salamander, *Andrias japonicus*. Copeia 1992:232–235.

Mayrick, E.A. 1976. *Salmonella* in frogs' legs. Medical Journal of Australia 2:700.

McAllister, C.T. and D.B. Conn. 1990. Occurrence of tetrathyridia of *Mesocestoides* sp. (Cestoidea: Cyclophyllidea) in North American anurans (Amphibia). Journal of Wildlife Diseases 26:540–543.

McAlpine, D.K. 1955. Entomology honours thesis. Australian Museum, Sydney.

McGrath, E.A. and M.M. Alexander. 1979. Observations on the exposure of larval bullfrogs to fuel oil. Transactions of the Northeastern Fish & Wildlife Conference 80:45–51.

McKinnell, R.G. 1965. Incidence and histology of renal tumors of leopard frogs from the north central states. Annals of the New York Academy of Sciences 126:85–98.

McVicar, A.H. 1982. *Ichthyophonus* infection of fish, *in* Roberts, R.J. (Ed): Microbial Diseases of Fish. Academic Press, London, pp. 243–269.

Merkle, S. 1990. Effects of starvation in *Xenopus*. Fortschritte der Zoologie 38:311–320.

Meyer, F.P. and L.A. Barclay. 1990. Field manual for the investigation of fish kills. US Government Printing Office, Washington, DC 20401 (stock number 024-010-00685-4), 120 pp.

Meyer-Rochow, V.B. and M. Asashima. 1988. Naturally occurring morphological abnormalities in wild populations of the Japanese newt, *Cynops pyrrhogaster* (Salamandridae; Urodela; Amphibia). Zoologische Anzeiger 221:70–80.

Meyer-Rochow, V.B. and J. Koebke. 1986. A study of the extra extremity in a five-legged *Rana temporaria* frog. Zoologische Anzeiger 217:1–13.

Michaels, J.E., J.T. Albright, and D.I. Patt. 1971. Fine structural observations on cell death in the epidermis of the external gills of the larval frog, *Rana pipiens*. American Journal of Anatomy 132:301–318.

Migaki, G. and F.L. Frye. 1975. Mycotic granuloma in a tiger salamander. Journal of Wildlife Diseases 11:525–528.

Mika, J., M. Chadzinska, M. Stosik, and B. Plytycz. 1995. Bacterial survival in spleens of *Bombina variegata, B. bombina,* and *Rana esculenta*. Herpetopathologia (Proceedings of 5th International Colloquium on the Pathology of Reptiles & Amphibians) 1995:129–133.

Miller, J.C. and R. Landesman. 1978. Reduction of heavy metal toxicity to embryos by magnesium ions. Bulletin of Environmental Contamination & Toxicology 20:93–95.

Miller, E.A., R.J. Montali, E.C. Ramsay, and B.A. Rideout. 1992. Disseminated chromoblastomycosis in a colony of ornate-horned frogs (*Ceratophrys ornata*). Journal of Zoo & Wildlife Medicine 23:433–438.

Millichamp, N.J. 1991. Exotic animal ophthamology, *in* Gelatt, K.N. (Ed.): Veterinary Ophthalmology, 2nd Ed., Lea & Febiger, Philadelphia, PA, pp. 685–686.

Minette, H.P. 1983. Leptospirosis in poikilothermic vertebrates. A review. International Journal of Zoonoses 10:111–121.

Miscalencu, D., M.E. Alfy, F. Mailat, and G.R. Mihaescu. 1981. Viral particles in the hepatocytes of *Rana esculenta* (L.). Revue Roumaine de Medecine: Virologie 32:123–125.

Miyada, S. 1960. Studies on haploid frogs. Journal of Science of Hiroshima University, Series B Division 1, 19:1–57.

Mizgireuv, I.V., N.L. Flax, L.J. Borkin, and V.V. Khudoley. 1984. Dysplastic lesions and abnormalities in amphibians associated with environmental conditions. Neoplasma 31:175–181.

Mock, B.A. 1987. Longitudinal patterns of trypanosome infections in red-spotted newts. Journal of Parasitology 73:730–737.

Mock, B.A. and D.E. Gill. 1984. The infrapopulation dynamics of trypanosomes in red-spotted newts. Parasitology 88:267–282.

Modzelewski, E.H. and D.D. Culley. 1974. Growth responses of the bullfrog, *Rana catesbeiana*, fed various live foods. Herpetologica 30:396–405.

Mohanty-Hejmadi, P., S.K. Dutta, and P. Mahapatra. 1992. Limbs generated at site of tail amputation in marbled balloon frog after vitamin A treatment. Nature 355:352–353.

Mok, W.Y. and C.M. Carvalho. 1984. Occurrence and experimental infection of toads (*Bufo marinus* and *B. granulosus*) with *Mycobacterium cheloni* subsp. *abscessus*. Journal of Medical Microbiology 18:327–333.

Mok, W.Y., C.M. Carvalho, L.C. Ferreira, and J.W.S. Meirelles. 1983. Natural mycotic infections in Amazonian anurans. Proceedings of 1st International Colloquium on Pathology of Reptiles & Amphibians, pp. 59–65.

Moody, N.J.G. and L. Owens. 1994. Experimental demonstration of the pathogenicity of a frog virus, Bohle iridovirus, for a fish species, barramundi *Lates calcarifer*. Diseases of Aquatic Organisms 18:95–102.

Morgan, T.H. 1906. The physiology of regeneration. Journal of Experimental Zoology 3:457–500.

Munday, R.L., W.J. Hartley, K.E. Harrigan, P.J.A. Presidente, and D.L. Obendorf. 1979. *Sarcocystis* and related organisms in Australian wildlife. II. Survey findings in birds, reptiles, amphibians, and fish. Journal of Wildlife Diseases 15:57–73.

Muntz, W.R.A. 1977. The visual world of the Amphibia, *in* Crescitelli, F. (Ed.): The Visual System in Vertebrates (Handbook of Sensory Physiology, Vol VII/5). Springer-Verlag, New York, pp. 309–390.

Murphy, T.D. 1965. High incidence of two parasitic infestations and two morphological abnormalities in a population of the frog, *Rana palustris* Le Conte. American Midland Naturalist 74:233–239.

Muto, Y. 1969. Anomalies in the hindlimb skeletons of the toad larvae reared at a high temperature. Congenital Anomalies (Senten Ijo) 9:61–73.

Muzzall, P.M. 1991. Helminth infracommunities of the newt, *Notophthalmus viridescens*, from Turkey Marsh, Michigan. Journal of Parasitology 77:87–91.

Nagai, T. 1993. Transcellular labeling by DiI demonstrates the glossopharyngeal innervation of taste buds in the lingual epithelium of the axolotl. Journal of Comparative Neurology 331:122–133.

Narajian, H.H. 1953. The life history of *Echinoparyphium flexum* (Linton, 1892) (Dietz, 1910) (Trematoda: Echinostomatidae). Science 117:564–565.

Narajian, H.H. 1954. Developmental stages in the life cycle of *Echinoparyphium flexum* (Linton, 1892) (Dietz, 1910) (Trematoda: Echinostomatidae). Journal of Morphology 94:165–198.

Neish, G.A. and G.C. Hughes. 1980. Fungal diseases of fishes, Book 6, *in* Sniesko, S.F. and H.R. Axelrod (Eds.): Diseases of Fishes. TFH Publications, Neptune City, NJ.

Newcomer, C.E., M.R. Anver, J.L. Simmons, B.W. Wilcke, and G.W. Nace. 1982. Spontaneous and experimental infections of *Xenopus laevis* with *Chlamydia psittaci*. Laboratory Animal Science 32:680–686.

Nigrelli, R.F. and L.W. Maraventano. 1944. Pericarditis in *Xenopus laevis* caused by *Diplostomulum xenopi* sp. nov., a larval strigeid. Journal of Parasitology 30:184–190.

Nishikawa, S., J. Hirata, and F. Sasaki. 1992. Fate of ciliated epidermal cells during early development of *Xenopus laevis* using whole-mount immunostaining with antibody against chondroitin 6-sulphate proteoglycan and anti-tubulin: Transdifferentiation of metaplasia of amphibian epidermis. Histochemistry 98:355–358.

Noga, E.J. 1993a. Watermold infections of freshwater fish: Recent advances. Annual Review of Fish Diseases 3:291–304.

Noga, E.J. 1993b. Fungal and algal diseases of temperate freshwater and estuarine fishes, *in* Stoskopf, M.K. (Ed.): Fish Medicine, W.B. Saunders Co., Philadelphia, PA, pp. 278–283.

Noller, W. 1912. Uber eine neue Schizogonie von *Lankesterella minima* Chaussat. Archiv fur Protisten Kunde 24:201–208.

Nonidez, J.F. and M.C. Kahn. 1937. Experimental tuberculosis infection in the tadpole and the mechanism of its spread. American Review of Tuberculosis 36:191–211.

Northcutt, R.G. and H. Bleckmann. 1993. Pit organs in axolotls: A second class of lateral line neuromasts. Journal of Comparative Physiology A172:439–446.

Northcutt, R.G., K.C. Catania, and B.B. Criley. 1994. Development of lateral line organs in the axolotl. Journal of Comparative Neurology 340:480–514.

Northcutt, R.G., K. Brandle, and B. Fritzsch. 1995. Electroreceptors and mechanosensory lateral line organs arise from single placodes in axolotls. Developmental Biology 168:358–373.

Novoselov, V.V. 1995. Notochord formation in amphibians: Two directions and two ways. Journal of Experimental Zoology 271:296–306.

Nyman, S. 1986. Mass mortality in larval *Rana sylvatica* attributable to the bacterium, *Aeromonas hydrophila*. Journal of Herpetology 20:196–201.

Ohlendorf, H.M., R.L. Hothem, and T.W. Aldrich. 1988. Bioaccumulation of selenium by snakes and frogs in the San Joaquin Valley, California. Copeia 1988:704–710.

Okafor, J.I., D. Testrake, H.R. Mushinsky, and B.G. Yangco. 1984. *Basidiobolus* sp. and its association with reptiles and amphibians in Southern Florida. Sabouraudia 22:47–51.

Oksche, A. and M. Ueck. 1976. The nervous system, *in* Lofts, B. (Ed): Physiology of the Amphibia, Volume III. Academic Press, New York, pp. 313–419.

Olsen, O.W. 1937. Description and life history of the trematode, *Haplometrana utanensis* sp. nov. (Plagiorchiidae) from *Rana pretiosa*. Journal of Parasitology 23:13–28.

Olson, M.E., S. Gard, M. Brown, R. Hampton, and D.W. Morck. 1992. *Flavobacterium indologenes* infection in leopard frogs. Journal of the American Veterinary Medical Association 201:1766–1770.

Osborn, D., A.S. Cooke, and S. Freestone. 1981. Histology of a teratogenic effect of DDT on *Rana temporaria* tadpoles. Environmental Pollution 25A:305–319.

O'Shea, P., R. Speare, and A.D. Thomas. 1990. Salmonellas from the cane toad, *Bufo marinus*. Australian Veterinary Journal 67:310.

Palmer, B.D. and S.K. Palmer. 1995. Vitellogenin induction by xenobiotic estrogens in the red-eared turtle and African clawed frog. Environmental Health Perspectives 103:19–25.

Palmer, B.D. and K.W. Selcer. 1996. Vitellogenin as a biomarker for xenobiotic estrogens: A review, *in* Bengtson, D.A. and D.S. Henshel (Eds.): Environmental Toxicology and Risk Assessment: Biomarkers and Risk Assessment, Vol. 5, ASTM STP 1306, American Society for Testing and Materials, pp. 3–22.

Paperna, I. and R. Lainson. 1995a. Life history and ultrastructure of *Eimeria bufomarini* n. sp. (Apicomplexa: Eimeriidae) of the giant toad, *Bufo marinus* (Amphibia: Anura) from Amazonian Brazil. Parasite 2:141–148.

Paperna, I. and R. Lainson. 1995b. *Alloglugea bufonis* nov. gen., nov. sp. (Microsporea: Glugeidae), a microsporidian of *Bufo marinus* tadpoles and metamorphosing toads (Amphibia: Anura) from Amazonia Brazil. Diseases of Aquatic Organisms 23:7–16.

Parsons, R.H. 1994. Effects of skin circulation on water exchange, *in* Heatwole, H. and G.T. Barthalmus (Eds.): Amphibian Biology, Volume 1, The Integument. Surrey Beatty & Sons, Chipping Norton, New South Wales, Australia, pp. 132–146.

Peltz, R. and K. Pezzella. 1976. Cellular alterations accompany opacification in the cultured lens. Cytobios 16:203–210.

Peltz, R., K. Pezzella, and A. Wilson. 1978. Lens structural disorders in the leopard frog (*Rana pipiens*) supplied to the laboratory from wild populations. Laboratory Animal Science 28:190–192.

Peterson, K.H. and S.R. Mays. 1989. Abnormal epidermis in the Houston toad (*Bufo houstonensis*). Herpetopathologia 1:49–51.

Pfennig, D.W., M.L.G. Loeb, and J.P. Collins. 1991. Pathogens as a factor limiting the spread of cannibalism in tiger salamanders. Oecologia 88:161–166.

Pierce, B.A. 1985. Acid tolerance in amphibians. BioScience 35:239–243.

Pierce, B.A. and H.M. Smith. 1979. Neotony or paedogenesis? Journal of Herpetology 13:119–121.

Pilkington, J.B. and H.M. Simkiss. 1966. The mobilization of the calcium carbonate deposits in the endolymphatic sacs of metamorphosing frogs. Journal of Experimental Biology 45:329–341.

Plytycz, B., J. Bigaj, and A. Miodonski. 1995. Amphibian lymphoid organs and immunocompetent cells. Herpetopathologia (Proceedings of 5th International Colloquium on the Pathology of Reptiles & Amphibians) 1995:115–127.

Poisson, R. 1937. Sur une nouvelle espece du genre *Dermomycoides* Granata 1919: *Dermomycoides armoriacus* Poisson 1936, parasite cutane de *Triturus palmatus* Schneider. Bulletin Biologique de la France & de la Belgique 71:81–116.

Pollack, E.D. and V. Liebig. 1989. An induced developmental disorder of limbs and motor neurons in *Xenopus*. American Zoologist 29:163A.

Pollack, E.D. and J.M. Maheras-Rarick. 1990. Differential limb regeneration in diploid and triploid *Rana pipiens* larvae with reference to spinal motor neuron development. Journal of Experimental Zoology 254:276–285.

Porter, K.R 1939. Androgenetic development of the egg of *Rana pipiens*. Biological Bulletin 77:233–257.

Porter, K.R. and D.E. Hakanson. 1976. Toxicity of mine drainage to embryonic and larval boreal toads. Copeia 1976:237–331.

Pough, F.H. 1976. Acid precipitation and embryonic mortality of spotted salamanders, *Ambystoma maculatum*. Science 192:68–70.

Pounds, J.A. and M.L. Crump. 1994. Amphibian declines and climate disturbance: The case of the golden toad and the harlequin frog. Conservation Biology 8:72–85.

Power, T., K.L. Clark, A. Harfenist, and D.B. Peakall. 1989. A review and evaluation of the amphibian toxicological literature. Canadian Wildlife Service Technical Report 61:4–47.

Poynton, S.L. and B.R. Whitaker. 1994. Protozoa in poison-dart frogs (Dendrobatidae): Clinical assessment and identification. Journal of Zoo & Wildlife Medicine 25:29–39.

Pritchard, J.J. and A.J. Ruzicka. 1950. Comparison of fracture repair in the frog, lizard, and rat. Journal of Anatomy 84:236–261.

Prokopic, J. and K. Krivanec. 1975. Helminths of amphibians, their interaction and host-parasite relationships. Acta Scientiarum Naturalium Academie Scientarium Bohemoslovacae Brno 9:1–48.

Pronych, S. and R. Wassersug. 1994. Lung use and development in *Xenopus laevis* tadpoles. Canadian Journal of Zoology 72:738–743.

Rand, T.G. 1994. An unusual form of *Ichthyophonus hoferi* (Ichthyophonales: Ichthyophonaceae) from yellowtail flounder *Limanda ferruginea* from the Nova Scotia shelf. Diseases of Aquatic Organisms 18:21–28.

Rankin, J.S. 1937. An ecological study of parasites of some North Carolina salamanders. Ecological Monographs 7:169–269.

Rannala, B.H. 1990. Electrophoretic evidence concerning the relationship between *Haplometrana* and *Glypthelmins* (Digenea: Plagiorchiiformes). Journal of Parasitology 76:746–748.

Rees, G. 1964. Two new species of the genus *Haematoloechus* (Digenea: Plagiorchiidae) from *Rana occipitalis* (Gunther) in Ghana. Parasitology 54:345–368.

Reichenbach-Klinke, H. 1983. Streichholzbeine bei Amphibien als zeichen einer Mangelerkrankung. Proceedings of 1st International Colloquium on Pathology of Reptiles & Amphibians, pp. 23–24.

Reichenbach-Klinke, H. and E.E. Elkan. 1965. The principal diseases of lower vertebrates: Diseases of Amphibians. TFH Publications, Inc., Neptune City, NJ, 240 pp.

Reinschmidt, D.C. and R. Tompkins. 1984. *Unresponsive*, a new behavioral mutant in *Xenopus laevis*. Differentiation 26:189–193.

Remy, P. 1931. Presence de *Dermocystidium ranae* Guyenot and Naville, chez une *Rana esculenta* L. de Lorraine. Annales de Parasitologie 9:1–13.

Reyer, R.W. 1977. The amphibian eye: Development and regeneration, *in* Crescitelli, F. (Ed.): The Visual System in Vertebrates (Handbook of Sensory Physiology, Vol VII/5). Springer, New York, pp. 309–390.

Reynolds, T.D. and T.D. Stephens. 1984. Multiple ectopic limbs in a wild population of *Hyla regilla*. Great Basin Naturalist 44:166–169.

Richards, C.M. 1958. The control of tadpole growth by alga-like cells. Physiological Zoology 35:285–296.

Robert, J. and L. DuPasquier. 1995. The immune system of *Xenopus* and metamorphosis. Madoqua 19:49–55.

Robinson, D.H. and M.B. Heintzelman. 1987. Morphology of ventral epidermis of *Rana catesbeiana* during metamorphosis. Anatomical Record 217:305–317.

Rollins-Smith, L.A., T. Davis, and P.J. Blair. 1993. Effects of thyroid hormone deprivation on immunity in postmetamorphic frogs. Developmental & Comparative Immunology 17:157–164.

Rose, F.L. 1977. Tissue lesions of tiger salamanders (*Ambystoma tigrinum*): Relationship to sewage effluents. Annals of the New York Academy of Sciences 298:270–279.

Rose, F.C. and S.M. Rose. 1965. The role of normal epidermis in recovery of regenerative ability in X-rayed limbs of *Triturus*. Growth 29:361–393.

Rowlatt, U.F. and F.J. Roe. 1966. Generalized tuberculosis in a South American frog, *Leptodactylus pentadactylus*. Pathologica Veterinarius 3:451–460.

Ruben, L.N. and J.M. Stevens. 1970. A comparison between granulomatosis and lymphoreticular neoplasia in *Diemictylus viridescens* and *Xenopus laevis*. Cancer Research 30:2613–2619.

Ruben, L.N., M.A. Scheinman, R.O. Johnson, S. Shiigi, R.H. Clothier, and M. Balls. 1992. Impaired T-cell functions during amphibian metamorphosis: IL-2 receptor expression and endogenous ligand production. Mechanisms in Development 37:167–172.

Ruben, L.N., P. Ahmadi, R.O. Johnson, D.R. Buchholz, R.H. Clothier, and S. Shiigi. 1994. Apoptosis in the thymus of developing *Xenopus laevis*. Developmental & Comparative Immunology 18:343–352.

Ruibal, R. and V. Shoemaker. 1984. Osteoderms in anurans. Journal of Herpetology 18:313–328.

Russell, F.H. 1898. An epidemic, septicemic disease among frogs due to the *Bacillus hydrophilus fuscus*. Journal of the American Medical Association 80:1442–1449.

Russell, R.W., S.J. Hecnar, and G.D. Haffner. 1995. Organochlorine pesticide residues in southern Ontario spring peepers. Environmental Toxicology & Chemistry 14:815–817.

Russell, W.C., D.L. Edwards, E.L. Stair, and D.C. Hubner. 1990. Corneal lipidosis, disseminated xanthomatosis, and hypercholesterolemia in Cuban tree frogs (*Osteopilus septentrionalis*). Journal of Zoo & Wildlife Medicine 21:99–104.

Saad, A.H. and M. El Masri. 1995. Histopathology of amphibian lymphoid organs. Herpetopathologia (Proceedings of 5th International Colloquium on the Pathology of Reptiles & Amphibians) 1995:135–153.

Sanders, H.O. 1970. Pesticide toxicities to tadpoles of the western chorus frog, *Pseudacris triseriata*, and Fowler's toad, *Bufo woodhousei fowleri*. Copeia 1970:246–251.

Sandner, H. 1955. *Lucilia bufonivora* Moniez, 1876 (Diptera) in Poland. Acta Parasitologica Polonica 2:319–329.

Scadding, S.R. 1990. Histological effects of vitamin A on limb regeneration in the larval axolotl, *Ambystoma mexicanum*. Canadian Journal of Zoology 68:159–167.

Scadding, S.R. and M. Maden. 1994. Retinoic acid gradients during limb regeneration. Developmental Biology 162:608–617.

Schipp, R., H. Hemmer, and R. Flindt. 1968. Vergleichende licht- und elektronenmikroskopische Untersuchungen an Chordomen von Krotenbastardlarven. Beitrage zur Pathologischen Anatomie & zur Allgeneimen Pathologie 138:109–133.

Schlumberger, H.G. and D.H. Burk. 1953. Comparative study of the reaction to injury. II. Hypervitaminosis D in the frog with special reference to the lime sacs. AMA Archives of Pathology 56:103–124.

Schmalhausen, I. 1925. Uber die Beeinflussung der Morphogenese der Extremitaten der Axolotl durch vershiedene Faktoren. Wilhelm Roux's Archiv fur Entwicklungsmechanik der Organismen 105:483–500.

Schmidt, A.J. 1958. Forelimb regeneration of thyroidectomized adult newts. Journal of Experimental Zoology 139:95–134.

Schmidt, R.E. 1984. Amphibian chromomycosis, *in* Hoff, G.L., F.L. Frye, and E.R. Jacobson (Eds.): Diseases of Amphibians and Reptiles. Plenum Press, New York, pp. 169–181.

Schmittner, S.M. and R.B. McGhee. 1961. The intra-erythrocytic development of *Babesiosoma stableri nov. sp.* in *Rana pipiens pipiens*. Journal of Protozoology 8:381–386.

Schuetz, A.W., K. Selman, and D. Samson. 1978. Alterations in growth, function and composition of *Rana pipiens* oocytes and follicles associated with microsporidian parasites. Journal of Experimental Zoology 204:81–94.

Schwabacher, H. 1959. A strain of mycobacterium isolated from skin lesions of a cold-blooded animal, *Xenopus laevis*, and its relation to typical acid-fast bacilli occuring in man. Journal of Hygiene 57:57–67.

Scorza, J.V., C. Dagert, and L.I. Arocha. 1956. Estudo sobre hemoparasitos de *Bufo marinus* L. da Venezuela. 1. Hemogregarinas. 2. Uma nova especie de *Toxoplasma*. Memorias do Instituto Oswaldo Cruz 54:373–392.

Scott, N.J. 1993. Postmetamorphic death syndrome. FrogLog #7:1–2.

Scullion, F.T., J.E. Cooper, and A. Skuse. 1989. Virus-like particles associated with skin lesions in a toad (*Bufo bufo*)[Abstr.]. 3rd International Colloquium on the Pathology of Reptiles and Amphibians. 13–15 January 1989, Orlando, FL, p. 90.

Semlitsch, R.D., M. Foglia, A. Mueller, I. Steiner, E. Fioramonti, and K. Fent. 1995. Short-term exposure to triphenyltin affects the swimming and feeding behavior of tadpoles. Environmental Toxicology & Chemistry 14:1419–1423.

Sessions, S.K. and S.B. Ruth. 1990. Explanation for naturally occurring supernumerary limbs in amphibians. Journal of Experimental Zoology 254:38–47.

Setlow, R.B., A.D. Woodhead, and E. Grist. 1989. Animal model for ultraviolet radiation-induced malignant melanoma: Platyfish-swordtail hybrid. Proceedings of the National Academy of Science USA 86:8922–8926.

Shen, P-S. and L.F. Lemanski. 1989. Immunofluorescent, immunogold, and electrophoretic studies for desmin in embryonic hearts of normal and cardiac mutant Mexican axolotls, *Ambystoma mexicanum*. Journal of Morphology 201:243–252.

Shields, J.D. 1987. Pathology and mortality of the lung fluke *Haematoloechus longiplexus* (Trematoda) in *Rana catesbeiana*. Journal of Parasitology 73:1005–1013.

Shively, J.N., J.G. Songer, S. Prchal, M.S. Keasey III, and C.O. Thoen. 1981. *Mycobacterium marinum* infection in Bufonidae. Journal of Wildlife Diseases 17:3–7.

Shotts, E.B. 1984. *Aeromonas, in* Hoff, G.L., F.L. Frye, and E.R. Jacobson: Diseases of Amphibians and Reptiles. Plenum Press, New York, pp. 49–57.

Shumway, W. 1940. A ciliate protozoan parasitic in the central nervous system of larval *Ambystoma*. Biological Bulletin 78:283–288.

Siddall, M.E. 1995. Phylogeny of adeleid blood parasites with a partial systematic revision of the *Haemogregarine* complex. Journal of Eukaryotic Microbiology 42:116–125.

Siddall, M.E. and S.S. Desser. 1992. Alternative leech vectors for frog and turtle trypanosomes. Journal of Parasitology 78:562–563.

Siddall, M.E., D.S. Martin, D. Bridge, S.S. Desser, and D.K. Cone. 1995. The demise of a phylum of protists: Phylogeny of Myxozoa and other parasitic Cnidaria. Journal of Parasitology 81:961–967.

Sive, H.L., B.W. Draper, R. Harland, and H. Weintraub. 1990. Identification of a retinoic acid-sensitive period during axis formation in *Xenopus laevis*. Genes & Development 4:932–942.

Smith, A.R. 1978. Digit regeneration in the amphibian, *Triturus cristatus*. Journal of Embryology & Experimental Morphology 44:105–112.

Smith, A.W., M.P. Anderson, D.E. Skilling, J.E. Barlough, and P.K. Ensley. 1986. First isolation of calicivirus from reptiles and amphibians. American Journal of Veterinary Research 47:1718–1721.

Smith, P.A. 1994. Amphibian sympathetic ganglia: An owner's and operator's manual. Progress in Neurobiology 43:439–510.

Smith, S.C. and J.B. Armstrong. 1990. Heart induction in wild-type and cardiac mutant axolotls (*Ambystoma mexicanum*). Journal of Experimental Zoology 254:48–54.

Smith, S.C., M.J. Lannoo, and J.B. Armstrong. 1988. Lateral-line neuromast development in *Ambystoma mexicanum* and a comparison with *Rana pipiens*. Journal of Morphology 198:367–379.

Smith, T.G. 1996. The genus *Hepatozoon* (Apicomplexa: Adeleina). Journal of Parasitology 82:565–585.

Smith, T.G., S.S. Desser, and D.S. Martin. 1994. The development of *Hepatozoon sipedon* sp. nov. (Apicomplexa: Adeleina: Hepatozoidae) in its natural host, the Northern water snake (*Nerodia sipedon sipedon*), in the culicine vectors *Culex pipiens* and *Culex territans*, and in an intermediate host, the Northern leopard frog (*Rana pipiens*). Parasitology Research 80:559–568.

Smith-Gill, S.J. 1974. Morphogenesis of the dorsal pigmentary pattern in wild-type and mutant [burnsi] *Rana pipiens*. Developmental Biology 37:153–170.

Smith-Gill, S.J., C.M. Richards, and G.W. Nace. 1972. Genetic and metabolic bases of two "albino" phenotypes in the leopard frog, *Rana pipiens*. Journal of Experimental Zoology 180:157–168.

Snawder, J.E. and J.E. Chambers. 1989. Toxic and developmental effects of organophosphorus insecticides in embryos of the South African clawed frog. Journal of Environmental Science & Health B24:205–218.

Snawder, J.E. and J.E. Chambers. 1990. Critical time periods and the effect of tryptophan in malathion-induced developmental defects in *Xenopus laevis*. Life Sciences 46:1635–1642.

Snetkova, E., N. Chelnaya, L. Serova, S. Saveliev, E. Cherdanzova, S. Pronych, and R. Wassersug. 1995. Effects of space flight on *Xenopus laevis* larval development. Journal of Experimental Zoology 273:21–32.

Socaciu, C., A.I. Baba, and O. Rotaru. 1994. Histopathologic investigations of acute and subchronic toxicities of some organotin compounds in chickens. Veterinary & Human Toxicology 36:535–539.

Sousa, M.A. and D.R. Weigl. 1976. The viral nature of *Toddia* Franca, 1912. Memorias do Instituto Oswaldo Cruz 74:213–230.

Spalatin, J., R. Connell, A.N. Burton, and B.J. Gollop. 1964. Western equine encephalitis in Saskatchewan reptiles and amphibians, 1961–1963. Canadian Journal of Comparative Medicine & Veterinary Science 28:131–142.

Spallanzani, L. 1768. Prodromo da un Opera da Imprimersi Sopra le Riproduzioni Animali [An essay on animal reproductions]. Modena.

Speare, R. and J.R. Smith. 1992. An iridovirus-like agent isolated from the ornate burrowing frog *Limnodynastes ornatus* in northern Australia. Diseases of Aquatic Organisms 14:51–57.

Speare, R., W.J. Freeland, and S.J. Bolton. 1991. A possible iridovirus in erythrocytes of *Bufo marinus* in Costa Rica. Journal of Wildlife Diseases 27:457–462.

Speare, R., P. O'Shea, P.W. Ladds, and A.D. Thomas. 1989. The pathology of mucormyosis of free-ranging cane toads, *Bufo marinus*, in Australia. Proceedings of 3rd International Colloquium on the Pathology of Reptiles & Amphibians, Orlando, FL, p. 45.

Speare, R., K. Field, J. Koehler, and K. McDonald. 1994a. Disappearing Australian rainforest frogs: Have we found the answer? [Abstr.] FrogLog #9:2.

Speare, R., A.D. Thomas, P. O'Shea, and W.A. Shipton. 1994b. *Mucor amphibiorum* in the toad, *Bufo marinus*, in Australia. Journal of Wildlife Diseases 30:399–407.

Stehbens, W.E. 1966. Observations on *Lankesterella hylae*. Journal of Protozoology 13:59–62.

Stensaas, L.J., S.S. Stensaas, and J.R. Sotelo. 1967. An intra-axonal protozoon in the spinal cord of the toad, *Bufo arenarum* (Hensel). Journal of Protozoology 14:585–595.

Stephens, L.C., D.M. Cromeens, V.W. Robbins, P.C. Stromberg, and J.H. Jardine. 1987. Epidermal capillariasis in South African clawed frogs (*Xenopus laevis*). Laboratory Animal Science 37:341–344.

Stetter, M.D. 1994. Clinical challenge case 2. Journal of Zoo & Wildlife Medicine 25:177–178.

Stetter, M.D. 1995. Noninfectious medical disorders of amphibians. Seminars in Avian & Exotic Pet Medicine 4:49–55.

Stetter, M.D. and D. Nichols. 1994. Clinical challenge case 3. Journal of Zoo & Wildlife Medicine 25:179–180.

Stewart, M.M. 1995. Climate driven population fluctuations in rain forest frogs. Journal of Herpetology 29:437–446.

Stiffler, D.F. 1993. Amphibian calcium metabolism. Journal of Experimental Biology 184:47–61.

Stocum, D.L. 1991. Limb regeneration: A call to arms (and legs). Cell 67:5–8.

Stocum, D.L. and G.E. Dearlove. 1972. Epidermal-mesodermal interaction during morphogenesis of the limb regeneration blastema in larval salamanders. Journal of Experimental Zoology 181:49–62.

Stone, W.B. and R.D. Manwell. 1969. Toxoplasmosis in cold-blooded hosts. Journal of Protozoology 16:99–102.

Taban, C.H., M. Cathieni, and P. Borkard. 1982. Changes in newt brain caused by zinc water-pollution. Experientia 38:683–685.

Tassava, R.A., M Castilla, J-P. Arsanto, and Y. Thouveny. 1993. The wound epithelium of regenerating limbs of *Pleurodeles waltl* and *Notophthalmus viridescens*: Studies with mAbs WE3 and WE4, phalloidin, and DNase 1. Journal of Experimental Zoology 267:180–187.

Taylor, F.R., R.C. Simmonds, and D.G. Loeffler. 1993. Isolation of *Flavobacterium meningosepticum* in a colony of leopard frogs (*Rana pipiens*). Laboratory Animal Science 43:105.

Taylor, S.K., E.S. Williams, K. Mils, A. Boerger-fields, E.T. Thorne, D.R. Kwiatkowski, S.L. Anderson, and M.S. Burton. 1994. The Wyoming toad (*Bufo hemiophrys baxteri*): A review of causes of mortality in the captive population. Proceedings of the Association of Reptilian and Amphibian Veterinarians & American Association of Zoo Veterinarians, pp. 73–75.

Taylor, S.K., E.S. Williams, K.W. Mills, A. Boerger-fields, C.J. Lynn, C.E. Hearn, E.T. Thorne, and S.L. Pistono. 1995. A review of causes of mortality and the diagnostic investigation for pathogens of the Wyoming toad (*Bufo hemiophrys baxteri*). [Reported to:] U.S. Fish & Wildlife Division, Laramie, WY, 36 pp.

Tchacarof, W.E. 1963. Parasitose elective intrathrombocytaire chez la *Rana ridibunda*. Comptes Rendus de l'Acadmie Bulgare des Sciences 16:845–848.

Tell, L., D.K. Nichols, and M. Bush. 1994. Clinical challenge case 1 [chromoblastomycosis]. Journal of Zoo & Wildlife Medicine 25:173–175.

Thoen, C.O. and T. Schliesser. 1984. Mycobacterial infection in cold-blooded animals, *in* Kubica, G.P. and L.G. Wayne: The *Mycobacteria*: A Sourcebook. Dekker-Marcel, New York, pp. 1297–1311.

Thoesen, J.C. (Ed.). 1994. Suggested procedures for the detection and identification of certain finfish and shellfish pathogens. 4th ed., Version I, Fish Health Section, American Fisheries Society, Bethesda, MD, 326 pp.

Thomas, L.J. 1937. Life cycle of a fluke, *Halipegus eccentricus n. sp.*, found in the ears of frogs. Journal of Parasitology 23:207–221.

Tiffany, W.N. 1939. The identity of certain species of the Saprolegniaceae parasitic in fish. Journal of the Elisha Mitchell Scientific Society 55:134–151.

Timmons, E.H., G.M. Olmstead, and J.M. Kaplan. 1977. The germfree leopard frog (*Rana pipiens*): Preliminary report. Laboratory Animal Science 27:518–521.

Tompkins, R. 1977. Grafting analysis of the periodic albino mutant of *Xenopus laevis*. Developmental Biology 57:460–464.

Tournefier, A. 1982. Corticosteroid action on lymphocyte subpopulations and humoral immune response of axolotl urodele amphibian. Immunology 46:145

Trust, T.J. K.H. Bartlett, and H. Lior. 1981. Importation of salmonellae with aquarium species. Canadian Journal of Microbiology 27:500–504.

Tsonis, P.A. 1991. Amphibian limb regeneration. In Vivo 5:541–550.

Tweedell, K. and A. Granoff. 1968. Viruses and renal carcinoma of *Rana pipiens*. V. Effect of frog virus 3 on developing frog embryos and larvae. Journal of the National Cancer Institute 40:407–410.

Uehlinger, V. 1966. Description chez *Xenopus laevis* D. d'une mutation dominante 'Screwy' (*S*), letale a l'etat homozygote. Revue Suisse de Zoologie 73:527–534.

Uehlinger, V. and M-L. Beauchemin. 1968. L'oedeme subcutane, une maladie hereditaire de la pre- et post-metamorphose chez *Xenopus laevis*. Revue Suisse de Zoologie 75:697–706.

Underhill, D.K. 1967. Spontaneous silver color and pituitary abnormality in tadpoles from a laboratory cross of *Rana pipiens*. Copeia 1967:673–674.

Upton, S.J. and C.T. McAllister. 1988. The coccidia (Apicomplexa: Eimeriidae) of Anura, with descriptions of four new species. Canadian Journal of Zoology 66:1822–1830.

Upton, S.J., P.S. Freed, D.A. Freed, C.T. McAllister, and S.R. Goldberg. 1992. Testicular myxosporidiasis in the flat-backed toad, *Bufo maculatus* (Amphibia: Bufonidae), from Cameroon, Africa. Journal of Wildlife Diseases 28:326–329.

Upton, S.J., C.T. McAllister, and S.E. Trauth. 1993. The coccidia (Apicomplexa: Eimeriidae) of Caudata (Amphibia), with descriptions of two new species. Canadian Journal of Zoology 71:2410–2418.

Urbain, A. 1944. La paratyphose des grenouilles, *Rana esculenta*. Comptes Rendus de les Societe Biologie Paris 183:458–459.

Valentine, B.A. and M.K. Stoskopf. 1984. Amebiasis in a neotropical toad. Journal of the American Veterinary Medical Association 185:1418–1419.

Vanden Bercken, J., L.M. Akkermans, and J.M. Vander Zalm. 1973. DDT-like action of allethrin in the sensory nervous system of *Xenopus laevis*. European Journal of Pharmacology 21:95–106.

Vander Leun, J.C. and F.R. De Gruijl. 1993. Influences of ozone depletion on human and animal health, *in* Tevini, M. (Ed.), UV-B Radiation and Ozone Depletion: Effects on Humans, Animals, Plants, Microorganisms, and Materials. Lewis Publishers, Boca Raton, FL, pp. 95–123.

Vander Waaij, D., B.J. Cohen, and G.W. Nace. 1974. Colonization patterns of aerobic Gram-negative bacteria in the cloaca of *Rana pipiens*. Laboratory Animal Science 24:307–317.

Van Stone, J.M. 1964. The relationship of nerve number to regenerative capacity in the developing hind limb of *Rana sylvatica*. Journal of Experimental Zoology 155:293–302.

Van Vallen, L. 1974. A natural model for the origin of some higher taxa. Journal of Herpetology 8:109–121.

Vaucher, C. 1990. *Polystoma cuvieri* n. sp. (Monogenea: Polystomatidae), a parasite of the urinary bladder of the leptodactylid frog *Physalaemus cuvieri* in Paraguay. Journal of Parasitology 76:501–504.

Verhoeff-DeFremery, R. 1983. Disease in the amphibian facility of the Hubrecht Laboratory (*Ambystoma mexicanum*, *Xenopus laevis*, *Discoglossus pictus*, *Rana pipiens*, *Rana lessonae*, *Bombina orientalis*). Proceedings of 1st International Colloquium on Pathology of Reptiles & Amphibians, pp. 9–10.

Verhoeff-DeFremery, R. 1989. Abnormalities occurring during early development of *Ambystoma mexicanum* and *Xenopus laevis*. Herpetopathologia 1:35–39.

Vial, J.L. and L. Saylor. 1993. Status of amphibian populations. Working Document of Declining Amphibian Populations Task Force, IUCN/SSC. The Open University, Milton Keynes, UK.

Vogel, H. 1958. Mycobacteria from cold-blooded animals. American Review of Tuberculosis & Pulmonary Disease 77:823–838.

Vogelnest, L. 1994. Myiasis in a green tree frog, *Litoria caerulea*. Bulletin of Association of Reptilian & Amphibian Veterinarians 4:4.

Waggener, R.A. 1930. An experimental study of the parathyroids in the anura. Journal of Experimental Zoology 57:13–55.

Wake, M.H. 1993. Evolution of oviductal gestation in amphibians. Journal of Experimental Zoology 266:394–413.

Walsh, G.P., C.H. Binford, and W.M. Meyers. 1978. Leprosy in the nine-banded armadillo (*Dasypus novemcinctus*), *in* Montali, R.J. (Ed.): Mycobacterial Infections of Zoo Animals. Smithsonian Institution Press, Washington, DC, pp. 253–257.

Walton, A.C. 1964. The parasites of amphibia. Journal of Wildlife Diseases, Microfiche No. 40.

Warburg, M.R., D. Lewinson, and M. Rosenberg. 1994. Ontogenesis of amphibian epidermis, *in* Heatwole, H. and G.T. Barthalmus (Eds.): Amphibian Biology, Volume 1, The Integument. Surrey Beatty & Sons, Chipping Norton, New South Wales, Australia, pp. 33–63.

Washabaugh, C.H., K. Del Rio-Tsonis, and P.A. Tsonis. 1993. Variable manifestations in the short toes (*s*) mutation of the axolotl. Journal of Morphology 218:107–114.

Welbourn, W.C. and R.B. Loomis. 1970. Three new species of *Hannemania* (Acarina, Trombiculidae) from amphibians of western Mexico. Bulletin of the Southern California Academy of Sciences 69:65–73.

Welbourn, W.C. and R.B. Loomis. 1975. *Hannemania* (Acarina: Trombiculidae) and their anuran hosts at Fortynine Palms Oasis, Joshua Tree National Monument, California. Bulletin of the Southern California Academy of Sciences 74:15–19.

Werner, J.K., J.S. Davis, and K.S. Slaght. 1988. Trypanosomes of *Bufo americanus* from northern Michigan. Journal of Wildlife Diseases 24:647–649.

Wever, E.G. 1985. The Amphibian Ear. Princeton University Press, Princeton, NJ, 405 pp.

Whitear, M. 1976. Identification of the epidermal "Stiftchenzellen" of frog tadpoles by electron microscopy. Cell Tissue Research 175:391–402.

Whittem, T. 1995. Pyrethrin and pyrethroid insecticide intoxication in cats. Compendium on Continuing Education for the Practicing Veterinarian 17:489–493.

Williams, R.W. 1960. Observations on the life history of *Rhabdias sphaerocephala* Goodey 1924 from *Bufo marinus* L., in the Bermuda Islands. Journal of Helminthology 34:93–98.

Williams, M.A. and L.D. Smith. 1984. Ultraviolet irradiation of *Rana pipiens* embryos delays the migration of primordial germ cells into the genital ridges. Differentiation 26:220–226.

Williams, D.L. and B.R. Whitaker. 1994. The amphibian eye—A clinical review. Journal of Zoo & Wildlife Medicine 25:18–28.

Witenberg, G. and C. Gerichter. 1944. The morphology and life history of *Foleyella duboisi* with remarks on allied filarids of Amphibia. Journal of Parasitology 30:245–256.

Witschi, E. 1930. Experimentally produced neoplasms in the frog. Proceedings of the Society for Experimental Biology & Medicine 27:475–477.

Wolf, K., G.L. Bullock, C.E. Dunbar, and M.C. Quimby. 1968. Tadpole edema virus: A viscerotropic pathogen for anuran amphibians. Journal of Infectious Disease 118:253–262.

Wolf, K., G.L. Bullock, C.E. Dunbar, and M.C. Quimby. 1969. Tadpole edema virus: Pathogenesis and growth studies and additional studies of virus-infected bullfrog tadpoles. *in* Mizell, M. (Ed.): Biology of Amphibian Tumors. Springer-Verlag, New York, pp. 327–336.

Wong, W.C. 1972. Lymphoid aggregations in the oesophagus of the toad (*Bufo melanostictus*). Acta Anatomica 83:481–487.

Worms, M.J. 1967. Parasites in newly imported animals. Journal of the Institute of Animal Technicians 18:39–47.

Worrest, R.C. and D.J. Kimeldorf. 1975. Photoreactivation of potentially lethal, UV-induced damage to boreal toad (*Bufo boreas*) tadpoles. Life Sciences 17:1545–1550.

Worrest, R.C. and D.J. Kimeldorf. 1976. Distortions in amphibian development induced by ultraviolet-B enhancement (290–315 nm) of a simulated solar spectrum. Photochemistry & Photobiology 24:377–382.

Worthylake, K.M. and P. Hovingh. 1989. Mass mortality of salamanders (*Ambystoma tigrinum*) by bacteria (*Acinetobacter*) in an oligotrophic seepage mountain lake. Great Basin Naturalist 49:364–372.

Wyman, R.L. 1988. Soil acidity and moisture and the distribution of amphibians in five forests of south-central New York. Copeia 1988:394–399.

Wyman, R.L. and D.S. Hawksley-Lescault. 1987. Soil acidity affects distribution, behavior and physiology of the salamander, *Plethodon cinereus*. Ecology 68:1819–1827.

Wyttenbach, C.R. and S.C. Thompson. 1985. The effects of the organophosphate insecticide, malathion, on very young chick embryos: Malformations detected by histological examination. American Journal of Anatomy 174:187–202.

Yager, J.A. and D.W. Scott. 1993. The skin and appendages, *in* Jubb, K.V.F., P.C. Kennedy, and N. Palmer (Eds.): Pathology of Domestic Animals, 4th Ed., Vol. 1. Academic Press, San Diego, CA, pp. 532–738.

Zaffaroni, N.P., T. Zavanella, and E. Arias. 1989. Spontaneous skeletal malformations of the forelimbs in the adult crested newt. Herpetopathologia 1:49–50.

Zapata, A.G. and E.L. Cooper. 1990. The Immune System: Comparative Histophysiology. John Wiley & Sons, Chichester and New York, 335 pp.

Zapata, A.G., A. Varas, and M. Torroba. 1992. Seasonal variations in the immune system of lower vertebrates. Immunology Today 13:142–147.

Zavanella, T. and M. Losa. 1981. Skin damage in adult amphibians after chronic exposure to ultraviolet radiation. Photochemistry & Photobiology 34:487–492.

Zavanella, T., N.P. Zaffaroni, and E. Arias. 1984. Abnormal limb regeneration in adult newts exposed to the fungicide, Maneb-80. A histological study. Journal of Toxicological & Environmental Health 13:735–745.

Zavanella, T., N.P. Zaffaroni, and E. Arias. 1989. Evaluation of the carcinogenic risk of 2-methyl-4-chlorophenoxy acetic acid (MCPA) in the adult crested newt. Herpetopathologia 1:51–56.

Zug, G.R. and P.B. Zug. 1979. The marine toad, *Bufo marinus*: A natural history resume of native populations. Smithsonian Contributions to Zoology 284:1–58.

Zumpt, F. 1965. Myiasis in Man and Animals in the Old World: A Textbook for Physicians, Veterinarians, and Zoologists. Butterworth, London, 267 pp.

Zwart, P. and J.S. Vander Linde-Sipman. 1989. Lipid keratopathy in a European tree frog (*Hyla arborea*). Herpetopathologia 1(2):91–95.

Zwart, P., H. Claessen, M.J.L. Kik, and L. Lambrechts. 1991. Survey of amphibian diseases, *in* Gabrisch, K., B. Schildger, and P. Zwart (Eds.): 4th International Colloquium on Pathology and Medicine of Reptiles and Amphibians. Deutsche Veterinarmedizinische Gesellschaft, pp. 323–327.

APPENDIX

TABLES

2.1.	Common names of amphibians	4–5
3.1.	Examples of sexually dimorphic characters in some anuran species	18
5.1.	Addresses and publications of scientific herpetological organizations	36
7.1.	Equations for calculating resting metabolism of anurans	78
7.2.	Equations for calculating resting metabolism of salamanders	78
7.3.	Equations for calculating resting metabolism of caecilians	78
7.4.	Standard Metabolic Rate of anurans by body mass and temperature	78
7.5.	Standard Metabolic Rate of salamanders by body mass and temperature	84
7.6.	Standard Metabolic Rate of caecilians by body mass and temperature	84
7.7.	Estimated caloric content of some prey items fed to amphibians	84
8.1.	Commercially available products for amphibian veterinary care	89–90
8.2.	Suggested supplies for the examination room	96
8.3.	Electrocardiogram information on four anurans under sodium pentobarbital	104
10.1.	Representative microbial isolates recovered from ill anurans	127
11.1.	Natt-Herrick's solution	133
11.2.	Average values for hematocrit, hemoglobin, erythrocyte count, volume, and dimensions for some amphibians	135
11.3A.	Hemograms and plasma chemistries of a captive bullfrog with metabolic bone disease	141
11.3B.	Hemograms and plasma chemistries of a captive bullfrog with metabolic bone disease supplemented with calcium glubionate/vitamin D after diagnosis	141
11.3C.	Hemograms and plasma chemistries of a free-ranging bullfrog	141
11.3D.	Average values for hemograms of anesthetized captive bullfrogs	142
11.3E.	Average values for serum chemistries of anesthetized captive bullfrogs	142
11.3F.	Hemograms and plasma chemistries of two Japanese giant salamanders	142
11.3G.	Hemograms and plasma chemistries of an adult male South American bullfrog with metabolic bone disease	143
11.3H.	Hemograms and plasma chemistries of an adult female South American bullfrog with corneal lipidosis	143
11.3I.	Hemograms and plasma chemistries of an adult female axolotl with ovarian neoplasia	144
12.1.	Suggested water quality parameters for most adult and larval amphibians	148
12.2.	Water quality log	149
12.3.	Percent of total ammonia in un-ionized form for 5–30°C and pH 6 to 9	153
13.1.	Some bacteria associated with red leg syndrome	163
13.2.	Species of *Aeromonas* isolated from amphibians	165
13.3.	Species known to be susceptible to mycobacterioses	168
13.4.	Bacteria generally considered nonpathogenic in amphibians	172
14.1.	Amphibians known as asymptomatic carriers of *Basidiobolus ranarum*	182
14.2.	Species of amphibians reported with chromomycosis	187
15.1.	Common distribution of protozoa and metazoa in the organ systems of amphibians	195
15.2.	Identification of protozoa	203
15.3.	Features used to distinguish the different flagellate groups living in the digestive tracts of amphibians	218
15.4.	Identification of metazoa from amphibians	219
22.1.	Hormonal manipulation for artificial reproduction of select amphibian species	290–292
22.2.	Physiological solutions used for diluting sperm or maintaining eggs	295–296
24.1	Antibacterial and antifungal agents used in amphibians	320–323
24.2.	Antiparasitic agents used in amphibians	323–325

24.3	Two formulas for the production of water suitable for amphibian husbandry	325
24.4.	Holtfreter's and modified Holtfreter's solutions	326
24.5.	Steinberg's solutions	326
24.6A.	Amphibian Ringer's solution	326
24.6B.	Hypertonic amphibian Ringer's solution	326
24.7.	Whitaker-Wright solution	327
24.8.	Measured osmolality and pH of various solutions used in managing amphibians	327
24.9.	Miscellaneous drugs and other products used in amphibians	328–329
25.1.	Amphibian pathology questionnaire	332
25.2.	Gross necropsy worksheet	333
25.3.	Necropsy tissue checklist	334
26.1.	Spontaneous neoplasms of amphibians	385–396

INDEX

Abah river flying frog, 13
Abdominal distention. *See also* coelomic distension; hydrocoelom; hydrops.
　ultrasonography and, 261
Abdominal palpation, 77, 101. *See also* palpation.
Abrasions, 233–234
Acanthocephala, 212, 446
　diagnosis of, 212
　treatment of, 212
Acclimation and maladaptation syndrome, 304–306
Accommodation, 247
Achyla flagellata, 184
Achroia grisella. See wax worms.
Acid-base metabolism, 33
Acidosis, carbon dioxide and, 150
Acid precipitation, 403–404
Acid soils, salamanders and, 416
Acinetobacter haemolyticus (calcoaceticus), 166
Acrolein, 464
Activated carbon, water conditioning and, 156
Acyclovir, 309
Adenocarcinoma, cloacal, 376
　intestinal, 375–376
　tubular type, 345–347
Adenoviruses, 447
Adrenal gland. *See* interrenal gland.
Adrenocorticotropin (ACTH), 28
Aegyptianella ranarum, 455
Aerobic scope, 33
Aerolysin, 165
Aeromonas hydrophila, 164–165, 423
　red leg syndrome and, 161–164, 425
Aeromonas salmonicida, 165–166, 427
Aeromonas septicemia, 426
Aflatoxicosis, 440
African clawed frog, 8, 9
African clawed toad, 8
African mouse-eating bullfrog, 4t
African reed frogs. *See* Hyperolidae.
Agalychnis callidryas, 11
Albinism, 416
Alloglugea bufonis, 206, 445
Alpine newts, 7
Aluminum toxicity, eggs and, 404
Alvarobufotoxin. *See* skin secretions.
Alytes spp., 8
Ambystoma andersoni, 7
Ambystoma maculatum, 7
Ambystoma mexicanum, 7
Ambystoma opacum, 7
Ambystomatidae, 7
Ambystoma tigrinum, 4t, 7
American brook salamanders, 8
American giant salamanders. *See* Dicamptodontidae.
American toad, 10–11
Amikacin, 311, 315
Ammonia, excretion of, 32, 151
　test kits for, 151
　toxicity of, 151, 230–231
　un-ionized vs. ionized, 151, 153t, 230

Amoebae, 203–204, 445, 448
　Acanthamoeba, 203
　diagnosis of, 203–204
　Entamoeba, 203, 448
　infection of brain with, 465
　Naegleria, 203
　treatment of, 204, 312, 315
　Vahlkampfia, 203
Amphibian Ringer's solution, diluting sperm or maintaining eggs, 294, 296t
　formula for, 296t, 326t
Amphiuma, 6, 350–351, 469
Amphiuma spp., 4t, 6
Amphiumidae, 6
Amphotericin-B, 314
Ampullary organ, 350–351, 469
Amputation
　affect on hematology, 139
　for blood collection, 132
　surgical, 277–278
　traumatic, 234–235
Anaerobiasis, 33
Anaerobic infections. *See also* specific bacterial agents.
　treatment of, 312, 315
Analgesia, postoperative, 282
Anamnesis, diagnostic examination and, 91–96
　postmortem examination and, 331
Anasarca. *See* hydrocoelom; hydrops.
Anatomy, 15–29
　adult amphibians, 16–29
　cardiovascular system, 27–28, 452
　endocrine system, 28
　epidermis, 415
　hematolymphopoietic system, 28
　integumentary system, 19–21
　larval amphibians, 15–16
　musculoskeletal system, 17–19
　nervous system, 19
　ocular, 245–247
　ovary and oviduct, 460
　respiratory system, 24–26
　urinary system, 23–24
Anderson's axolotl, 7
Andrias davidianus, 6
Andrias japonicus, 6
Anemia, erythrocyte inclusions and, 132
　iodine toxicity and, 227
　nematode infection and, 211
　nodular hyperplasia of hematopoietic tissue and, 360
　pentastome infection and, 214
　radiation poisoning and, 238
　spherocytic, 454
　viral infection and, 454–455
Anemic mutation, 454
Anesthesia,
　fasting and, 115
　induction chambers and, 117, 119
　monitoring of, 115
　preparation for, 114–115
Anesthetics. *See also* individual anesthetic agents.
　inhalant, 119–120

Anesthetics (*Continued*)
　injectable, 118, 120
　intubation and, 26, 119
　topical, 115–119
Anorexia. *See* cachexia.
Anthelmintics. *See* pharmacotherapeutics.
Antibacterial agents, administration of, 311
　availability of pharmacokinetic data, 309–310
　combination therapies, 313, 315
　saline baths and, 312
　temperature and, 310, 314
Antidiuretic hormone (ADH), 28
Antifungal agents. *See* pharmacotherapeutics.
Antiprotozoal agents. *See* pharmacotherapeutics.
Antiviral agents. *See* pharmacotherapeutics.
Anura, 3, 8–13. *See also* specific organisms or families.
Anurans, 8
Apicomplexa, 203t, 204–205. *See also* specific organisms and diseases.
　in blood, 204
　　Babesiosoma, 204, 456–457
　　Dactylosoma, 204, 457
　　diagnosis of, 204
　　Hemogregarina, 204, 456
　　Hepatozoon, 204, 445, 456
　　Lankesterella, 204, 457, 465–466
　　Schellackia, 204
　　treatment of, 205
　in tissues, 205
　　diagnosis of, 205
　　Eimeria, 205, 445
　　Isospora, 205, 445, 448
　　treatment of, 205
Apoda. *See* Gymnophiona.
APUD cells. *See* neuroendocrine cells.
Aquatic caecilian, 4t
Aquatic caecilians. *See* Typhlonectidae.
Aquatic toads, 9
Aqueous humor, drainage of, 247
Arboreal salamander, 4t
Argentine horned frog, 4t
Arginine vasotocin, 28
Argulus, 213
Artemia salina. See brine shrimp.
Artificial fertilization, 294–296
Artificial pond water, diluting sperm or maintaining eggs, 295t
　formula for, 295t, 325t
Artificial slime, 236, 238, 319
Ascaphis truei, 8
Ascites. *See* hydrocoelom; hydrops.
Asian horned frog, 4t
Asian salamander. *See* Hynobiidae.
Asian spadefoot toad, 9
Asian tree toads, 10–11
Assist-feeding, 82–83
Atelopus spp., 5t, 10–11
Atherosclerosis, 453
Atmospheric pressure, reproduction and, 288
Atrophic mandibular stomatitis, 234, 418
Auscultation, 99

Australian froglets. See Myobatrachidae.
Australian green treefrog, 4t
Averusa, 416
Axolotl, 7

Babesiosoma stableri, 456–457
Bacterial disease, 159–179, 442–443, 448, 450, 455–456, 471–472. See also specific bacterial agents.
Barbiturates, anesthetic, 120
  euthanasia and, 121
Barth's solution (modified), diluting sperm or maintaining eggs, 295t
Basal cell tumor, 341
Basidiobolus microsporus, 430
Basidiobolus ranarum, 182–183
  chytridiomycosis and, 185
  red leg syndrome and, 162, 182–183, 430
Basidiobolus spp., 430–431
  gross lesions of, 431
  histology of, 431
Basking, 56
Basophil, 137–138
Batrachochytrium dendrobatidis, 185
Batrachomyia mertensi. See frog fly.
Batrachoseps spp., 4t
Beaked caecilians. See Rhinatrematidae.
Behavioral fever, 31, 39, 310
Bell's horned frog, 4t
Benzalkonium chloride, surgical preparation and, 274
  treatment of fungi and, 313–314
Benzene hexachloride, 439, 462–463
Benzocaine, 118–119
  anesthesia with, 119
  dosage for, 119
  stability of, 119
Bidder's organ, 460
  microsporidian infections of, 205, 297, 460
  neoplasms of, 379
Bile duct hyperplasia vs. neoplasia, 372
Biopsy, 276–277
Biting amphibians, 114
Black worms, 65
Bladder, 23
Bladder flukes, 449
Bloodworms, 65
Blue plasma, 129, 142t
Bohle iridovirus (BIV), 420, 440–441
Bolitoglossa spp., 4t, 8
Bombina spp. 8
Bone cysts, 382
Bone marrow, 453
Boophis spp., 5t, 13
Brachycephalidae, 11
  lack of Bidder's organ, 11
Brachycephalus ehippium, 11
Brain, changes in metamorphosis and, 461
  over-ripe syndrome and, 402
Branchiurans, 213. See also specific organisms and diseases.
  diagnosis of, 213
  treatment of, 213
Brine shrimp, 65
Brown blood disease, 153. See also nitrite toxicity.
Buccopharyngeal respiration, 24–26
Budgett's frog, 4t
Bufo americanus, 10–11
Bufo guttatus, 5t, 10
Bufo hemiophrys baxteri, 10
Bufo houstonensis, 10

Bufolucilla spp. See toad fly.
Bufo marinus, 4t, 5t, 10
Bufonidae, 10–11
  Bidder's organ and, 10
Bufo periglenes, 10
Bufo viridis, 10
Bullfrog, 12
Bullous keratopathy, 249
Burnsi mutation, 416
Burns, treatment of, 236

Cachexia, 81–82
Cadmium, 228, 404
Caecilia thompsoni, 4
Caecilidae, 3–4
Calcitonin, 28, 34, 458
Calcium absorption, 156
Calcium carbonate, endolymphatic sacs and, 469. See also cholelithiasis; hypervitaminosis D.
  mineral supplement and, 69
  tube-feeding formula and, 85
Calcium oxalate, in plants, 64
Calcium phosphate, dystrophic mineralization and, 469
Calculi, cystic. See cystic calculi.
Calculi, urate. See urate calculi.
Calicivirus, 447–448, 450, 454
Calling, hormonal influence of, 286
Candida guilliermondii, 189
Candidiasis, 188–189
Cane toad, 4t
Cannibalism, 16, 241
Capillaria infection, 210, 436–437
Carbamate toxicosis, 224–226, 463
  treatment of, 225–226
Carbaryl toxicity, 463
Carcinogenesis, experimental, 335–336
Carcinosarcoma, 365
Cardiocentesis, 102, 131
Cardiomegaly, 452
Cardiomyopathy, 451–453
Cardiovascular circulation, haploid syndrome and, 401
Cardiovascular flukes, 452
Carditis, 452
Cataract, 250, 470, 473
Caudata, 3, 5–8. See also specific organisms or families.
Caudates. See Caudata. See also newt; salamander.
Cayenne caecilian. See Typhlonectes compressicauda.
Celiocentesis, 101–102
Celioscopy. See laparoscopy.
Celiotomy, 279–281
Centrolene spp., 11
Centrolenella spp., 11
Centrolenidae, 11
Cepedietta. See ciliates.
Ceratobatrachus guentheri, 5t, 12
Ceratophrynae, 10
Ceratophrys cornuta, 10
Ceratophrys cranwelli, 10
Ceratophrys ornata, 4t, 5t, 10
Ceratophrys spp., 5t
Cestodes, 209–210
  Bothricephalus, 209
  Cephalochlamys, 209
  diagnosis of, 210
  Diphyllobothrium, 209
  Mesocestoides, 447

Cestodes (Continued)
  Nematotaenia, 210, 446
  treatment of, 210
Ceylon sticky caecilian. See Ichthyophis glutinosus.
Chiggers. See mites.
Chinese giant salamander, 6
Chiromantis spp., 4t
Chironomidae. See bloodworms.
Chlamydia psittaci. See also Chlamydiosis.
  red leg syndrome and, 162
Chlamydiosis, 162, 441–442
  endocarditis and, 452
  granulocytic leukemia and, 360
  treatment of, 170, 315
Chloramine, 41, 94, 156
Chloramphenicol, 312, 315
Chlorine, 41, 94, 156, 227
Chloroquine, treatment of hemoflagellates and, 200
Cholangiocarcinoma, 372–373
Cholangioma, 372–373
Cholelithiasis, 447
Cholesterol, dietary requirement for, 81
Chondroblasts, 383
Chondroma, 382
Chondromata, 345
Chondromyxoma, 383
Chondrosarcoma, 382
Chordoma, 384
Chorus frogs, 11
Chromoblastomycosis, 431. See also chromomycosis.
Chromohyphomycosis, 431–432. See also chromomycosis.
Chromomycosis, 187–188, 431–433
  gross lesions of, 432
  histology of, 432
Chytridiomycosis, 184–185
  Basidiobolus ranarum and, 185
  postmetamorphic death syndrome and, 241, 408
  treatment of, 185
Ciliates, 196–198
  external and in urinary bladder, 197–198
    Carchesium, 197
    diagnosis of, 197
    sessile peritrichs, 197
    treatment of, 198
    trichodinids, 197
    Vorticella, 197
  in brain, 465
    Glaucoma, 465
    Tetrahymena, 465
  in gastrointestinal tract, 196–197
    Balantidium, 196
    Cepedietta, 196
    diagnosis of, 197
    Haptophyra. See Cepedietta.
    Nyctotheroides, 196
    Sicuophora, 196
    Tetrahymena, 196
    treatment of, 197
Ciprofloxacin, 311, 315
Cladosporium spp., 186–187
Clawed frogs. See Pipidae.
Clawed salamanders, 6
Cleaning and disinfection, 95, 97, 306–307
  disinfection vs. sterilization, 306
  parasitic infections and, 317
  recommendations for the established collection, 306–307
  recommendations for the quarantined collection, 307

Cleaning and disinfection (*Continued*)
  surgical scrubs and, 274
  tools and, 302
Climbing salamander, 4t
Clinical techniques, 89–109. *See also* specific techniques.
  weighing amphibians, 97
Clinostomum attenuatum, 209, 250, 472
Cloacal prolapse, 243, 281, 439, 443
Cloacal wash, 102–103
Clostridium, 442–443
Clotrimazole, treatment of fungi with, 314
Coccidiosis, 205, 444–445
  diagnosis of, 105–106, 205, 444–445
  treatment of, 205, 312, 316
Cochranella. *See Centrolenella* spp.
Coelocanth, 1
Coelomic distension, 261. *See also* hydrocoelom; hydrops.
Colestethus spp., 12
Collembolla. *See* springtails.
Coloration, 286
  acclimation and maladaptation syndrome and, 306
  bacterial dermatitis and, 160
  chemically altered, 416–417
  ivermectin toxicity and, 317
  organophosphates and, 416–417
Common caecilians. *See* Caeciliidae.
Common reed frog, 12.
Computerized axial tomography (CT), 253, 263
Conger eels, 6
Conraua goliath, 12
Copepods, treatment of, 318
Copper, 156, 228, 316, 440
  immunosuppression and, 316
  pH and, 156
  toxicity to embryos and larvae, 404
Copper sulfate, treatment of ciliates and, 200
  treatment of flagellates and, 198
Corneal lipidosis, 81, 249, 410, 462, 470
Corneal ulcer (ulcerative keratitis), 249–250
  treatment of, 251
Cornea, UV radiation and, 402–403
Corticosteroids, 28, 457
  treatment of drowning and, 237
  treatment of shock and, 235, 238
  treatment of spinal cord injury and, 235
Costia. *See Ichthyobodo*.
Cranial nerves, 19
Cranwell's horned frog, 10
Crayfish, 65
Crickets, 65
  gut-loading diet, 67–68
Crocodile newt, 7
Cross-banded treefrogs, 11
Cryosurgery, 277
Cryptobranchidae, 6
Cryptobranchiids, 6
Cryptobranchus alleganiensis, 6
Cryptosporidiosis, 302–303
  disinfectants and, 302
  treatment of, 316
Cryptosporidium. *See* cryptosporidiosis.
C-type retrovirus particles, 373
Cuban treefrog, 11
Cutaneous respiration, 24–26
Cyclops spp. *See* water fleas.
Cynops pyrrhoghaster, 4t, 7
Cystadenocarcinoma, 345
Cystadenoma, 345, 367
  papillary, 343

Cystic calculi, 280–281. *See also* dehydration; oxalate nephrosis; oxalates; oxalate toxicity, urate calculi, gout.
Cystotomy, 280–281
Cytamoeba spp., 455

Dactylosoma-like organisms, 465
Dactylostomatids. *See* Apicomplexa.
Daphnia spp. *See* water fleas.
Dart-poison frog. *See* Dendrobatidae. *See also* Mantellinae.
Darwin's frogs. *See* Rhinodermatidae.
DDT (diphenyltrichlorethane), toxicity of, 462
De Boer's solution, diluting sperm or maintaining eggs, 296t
Dehydration, 236–237, 318
  gout and bladder stones and, 33, 241
  treatment of, 319
Dendrobates auratus, 12
Dendrobates spp. 12
Dendrobates tinctorius, 4t
Dendrobatidae, 12
Dermatitis, bacterial, 427
  mycotic, 181–185
  ulcerative, 427
Dermatophagy, 21, 69
Dermatosepticemia, bacterial, 161–166. *See also* red leg syndrome.
  culture of, 126
Dermocystidium, 206, 433–435
  diagnosis of, 206
  lesions of, 433–435
  treatment of, 206
Dermocystidium pusula, 206
Dermomycoides. *See Dermocystidium*.
Dermophis mexicanus, 3, 5
Dermosporidium. *See Dermocystidium*.
Descemetocele, 250
Desmognathus spp., 8
Dexamethasone, 303, 309
Diagnostic equipment and supplies, 89–90t, 96t, 96–98
Dicamptodon ensatus, 6
Dicamptodontidae, 6
Dictyuchus monosporus, 184
Digenea, 208–209. *See also* specific organisms and diseases.
  Alaria, 448
  Clinostomum, 209, 250, 472
  diagnosis of, 209
  Diplostomum, 209, 466, 472
  Echinostoma, 448
  Glypthelmins, 437
  Gorgodera, 209, 448–449
  Gorgoderina, 209, 449
  Haematoloechus, 209, 450–451
  Halipegus, 472
  Haplometra, 437, 450
  Neascus, 472
  Phyllodistomum, 449
  treatment of, 209
  Tylodelphys, 452, 466
Dinoflagellates, 199
  Oodinium, 199
  Piscinoodinium, 199
Diplomonads, 200–203. *See also* specific species and diseases.
  Brugerolleia, 200
  Enteromonas, 218t
  Giardia, 200, 218t
  Hexamita, 200, 218t, 445

Diplomonads (*Continued*)
  Octomitus, 218t
  Spironucleus, 218t
  Trimitus, 218t
Diplostomum flexicaudum, 250, 472
Diplostomum scheuringi, 209, 250, 466, 472
Diquat, toxicity of, 464
Discoglossidae, 8
Discoglossus spp., 5t
Disinfection. *See* cleaning and disinfection.
Doppler, 98, 99
  monitoring anesthesia with, 115, 118
Doxapram hydrochloride, drowning and, 237
Drinking patch, 32
  Basidiobolus infection, 431
Drosophila, 65
  heidii, 71
  melanogaster, 71
Drowning, 237
Dumpy treefrog, 4t
Dusky salamanders, 8
Dusting, 68–69
Dwarf clawed frogs, 9
Dwarf siren, 5
Dyeing poison frog, 4t
Dyscophus antongilli, 13
Dyscophus guineti, 4t, 13

Earthworms, 65, 66, 67. *See also* red worms.
Edema, hypocalcemia and, 242
  in haploid embryos, 401
  mast cell tumors and, 362
  saprolegniasis and, 430
  tadpole edema virus and, 418
  treatment of, 318–319
Edema syndrome, 164, 242–243, 425
Edwardsiella spp., 171
Egg retention, 297
Eggs, mycotic infection of, 186–187
  over-ripe, 402
  pigments of, 402
  toxicants and, 223, 226
Eimeria bufomarini, 445
Eimeria grobbeni, 445
Ekatin, 225
Electrical shock, 237
Electrocardiography (ECG), 103–105, 104t, 115
Electrolytes, loss of, 318
Electrolyte solutions, treatment of external fungi and, 313–314
  treatment of leeches and, 318
  treatment of protozoans and, 319
Eleuthrodactylus spp., 10
Embryo, effect of low pH on, 403–404
Emesis, 91, 115
Enchytraeus spp. *See* white worms.
Endocrine organs, 28, 458. *See also* specific organs.
Endolymphatic sacs, 34, 469
  hypervitaminosis D and, 471
Endorphins, 282
Endoscopy, 105, 278–279
Enrofloxacin, 311, 315
Entamoeba ilowaiskii, 445
Entamoeba ranarum, 445, 448
Enteritis, treatment of, 312
Enucleation, 281–282
Eosinophil Unopette® method, for a total leukocyte count, 133–134

Epidemic splenomegaly, 455
Epidermal hyperplasia, 337
Epidermal papillomata, 335
Epidermis, thickness of, 415
Epinephrine, 28
　treatment of drowning and, 237
Epipedobates spp., 5t, 12
Epipedobates tricolor, 12
Epithelioma, over-ripe egg syndrome and, 402
Erythema, restraint and, 113, 117
　tadpole edema virus and, 418–420
Erythrocyte, 134–136, 135t
Erythrocytic iridoviruses, 418
Erythropoiesis, 28, 135–136, 453
Escapes, 45
Estivation, 53, 55, 79. See also hibernation.
　epidermal thickness and, 415
　obesity and, 77
Estrogen, 28
Estrogenic chemicals, 460
Ethanol, use as an anesthetic, 120
　euthanasia and, 121
Ethylenediamine-tetra-acetic acid (EDTA), 130
Ethyl *m*-amino benzoate. See tricaine methanesulfonate.
European edible frog, 12
European fire salamander, 7
European green toad, 10
European newt, 4t
European olm, 6
Eurycea spp., 8
Euthanasia, 121
　carbon dioxide and, 121
　chemical use and, 121
　freezing and, 121
　pithing and, 121
　traumatic, 121
Evolution of Amphibia, 1
Exogenous hormones, use of. See hormones.
Extra-medullary hematolymphopoiesis (EMH), 438
Eye. See also specific diseases.
　anatomy of, 245–247
　examination of, 247–248
　neoplasia of, 250
　parasites of, 250
　treatment of, 250–251
Eyelids, 245

Facial tumors, 352
Fatigue, 33
Fat neoplasms, 353
Fecal collection and evaluation, 105–106
Feeder fish, 65
Femoral vein, 102
Fenbendazole, 211, 303, 317
　prophylaxis during quarantine and, 303
Fenitrothion, 225, 463
Fenvalerate, 226, 463
FETAX (Frog Embryo Teratogenesis, Assay of *Xenopus*), 231, 405–406, 452
Fibroma, 352
Fibromyxoma, 352–353
Fibropapilloma, 340, 352
Fibrosarcoma, 353
Filarial worms, 211–212, 436, 457
　granulomata and, 356
Filtration, 154–155
　biological, 151–154
　box filter, 154

Filtration (*Continued*)
　canister filters, 154–155
　sponge or foam filters, 154
　trickle or wet-dry filters, 155
　undergravel filters, 154
Finquel®. See tricaine methanesulfonate.
Firebelly toads, 8
Fish caecilians. See Ichthyophiidae.
Flagellates, 199–203, 201t. See also specific organisms and diseases.
　ectoparasitic flagellates, 199–200
　　diagnosis of, 199
　　Ichthyobodo, 199
　　Oodinium, 199
　　Picinoodinium, 199
　　treatment of, 200
　hemoflagellates, 200
　　diagnosis of, 200
　　diplomonads, 200
　　trypanosomes, 200
　intestinal flagellates, 200–203
　　diagnosis of, 202–203
　　treatment of, 203
Flat-tailed caecilian, 4t
Flavobacterium spp., 166
　bacterial meningitis and, 160
　edema syndrome and, 164
Flies, as food, 65
Flour beetles, 65, 70
Fluconazole, treatment of fungi with, 314
Fluid therapy, 318–319
Flunixin meglumine, 282
Fluorescein stain, use in the diagnosis of ocular disease, 248
Flying frogs. See Rhacophoridae.
Fly larvae. See myiasis.
Foam-nest frog, 4t
Foam-nest treefrog, 4t
Foleyella brachyoptera, 436
Foleyella dolichoptera, 436
Foleyella duboisi, 436
Foleyella ranae, 436
Follicle-stimulating hormone (FSH), 28, 290–292t, 294
Fonsecaea spp., 187
Formalin, 316,
　carcinogenicity of, 198
　treatment of ciliates with, 198
　treatment of flagellates with, 200
　treatment of trematodes with, 317
Fractures, 235–236, 412
Freezer burn, 236
Freshwater mussel, 215
Frog, 8
Frog erythrocytic virus (FEV), 454–455
Frog fly, 215. See also myiasis.
Frog virus-3 (FV3, Ranavirus type I), 406, 419. See also ranaviruses.
Fruit flies, culturing, 71
Fungal dermatitis, treatment of, 314
Fungal infection. See mycosis.
Fungi, pigmented, 431

Gallstones. See *Cholelithiasis*.
Gambusia affinis. See mosquito fish.
Gardiner's Seychelles frog, 9
Gas bubble disease, 98, 150, 228–229, 417
　secondary infections and, 417, 426
Gastric-brooding frog, 9
Gastric impaction, 79,
Gastric overload, 79, 280–281
Gastric prolapse, 100, 243, 439

Gastric wash, 108
Gastrotheca spp., 11
Gastrotomy, 280
Gentamicin, 311–313
Germ-free strains of amphibians, 171
Ghost frogs. See Heleophrynidae.
Giant glass frogs, 11
Giant leaf frog, 4t
Giant salamanders. See Cryptobranchidae.
Giant toad, 10
Giardia sp., 200
Gill, 449–451
　degeneration of, 450
　function of, 449
　genetic and congenital abnormalities, 450
　retention of, 297
Glands, cloacal, 343
　skin, 343
Glass frogs, 11
Glassworms, 65
Glaucoma, 250, 473
Glottis, 25
Glucocorticoids, affect on hematology, 139, 457
　metamorphosis and, 407
Glucosuria, 109
Glues and sealants, toxicity of, 229–230
　use of, 41
Glycolysis, 33
Goitrogenic chemicals, 459
Golden Alajuela toad, 10
Golden frog, 5t
Golden mantella, 12
Golden shiner, 66
Golden tomato frog, 4t
Goliath frog, 12
Gonadal biopsy, 281
Gonadal tumor, imaging of, 264
Gonadectomy, 281
Gonadotropin-releasing hormone (Gn-RH), 293–294
Gout, 33, 241–242, 414
Granular cell tumor, 354
Granulosa cell tumor, 379
Grass shrimp, 65
Greater siren, 5–6
Green and black poison frog, 12
Griseofulvin, monocytic leukemia and, 361
Growth inhibition, algae and, 444
Gunther's triangle frog, 12
Gut-associated lymphoid tissue (GALT), 28, 453
Gymnophiona, 3–5. See also specific organisms and families.
Gymnopis multiplicata, 4, 5

Halipegus amhertensis, 472
Halipegus eccentricus, 472
Halipegus occidualis, 472
Halloween newt, 4t
Halogens, 227
Halothane, 114, 120
Hamartoma, 384
Hand-feeding. See assist-feeding.
Handling amphibians, 112
Haploid syndrome, 401–402
Harderian gland, 245
　adenoma of, 382
Harlequin frogs. See Pseudidae.
Heleophrynidae, 9
Hellbender, 6

Hemangioma, 355
Hemangiosarcoma, 355
Hematology, 129–144
  anticoagulants, 130
  blood volume, 129
  complete blood count, 133–134, 139–140, 141–144t
  cytology, 134–139
  plasma chemistries, 134, 140, 141–144t
  sample processing, 129–130
  stains and, 132–133
Hematopoieitic cells, 360, 372
Hemiphractys spp., 11
Hemogregarines. *See* apicomplexa.
Hemolivia, 456
Hemorrhagic syndrome, 422–424
Hemostasis, 274
Hepatic hydropic degeneration, 447
Hepatitis, mycotic, 186
  viral, 440
Hepatoblastoma, 372
Hepatocellular carcinoma, 370–372
Hepatoma, 370, 371
Hepatosphaera molgarum, 445
Hepatotoxic chemicals, 370, 372
Hepatozoon catesbeianae, 456
Hepatozoon sipedon, 445
Herbicides, 226
Hermaphroditism, 460
Herpesvirus, Lucke's renal carcinoma and, 365, 447
Herpesvirus-like dermatitis, 424
Heterophil, 137
Hexamita intestinalis, 445
Hibernation, 236. *See also* estivation.
  epidermal thickness and, 415
  gastrointestinal flora and, 159
Holtfreter's solution, 326t
  diluting sperm or maintaining eggs and, 295t
  formula for, 295t, 326t
  treatment of mites and, 214
  treatment of protozoa and, 198, 319
Hormones. *See also* individual hormones.
  exogenous use of, 285, 289–294
  reproduction and, 288–294
  sexual dimorphism and, 286
Horned treefrogs, 11
Horn frog, 5t
Housing. *See* husbandry and housing.
Houston toad, 10
Human chorionic gonadotropin (HCG), 290–292t, 293–294
Humidity, measuring, 56, 94
  providing, 57, 301
Husbandry and housing, 35–61
  environmental control, 55–59
    macro vs. microenvironment, 39
    thermal and moisture gradients, 38–39, 49
    water quality, 41
  handling and transportation, 36–37
  housing, 38–55
    cage design, 93
    cage furnishings, 44
    enclosures, 38–55
      aquatic pond, 45–47
      arboreal, 53–55
      basic amphibian, 39–41
      cliffside arboreal, 53, 55
      stream, 47–49
      stream-side, 49–50
      terrestrial forest floor, 50–51
      terrestrial fossorial, 51–53

housing (*Continued*)
    enclosure set-up and maintenance, 41–45
    ground cover, 42–43
    location of enclosure, 45
    retreats, 44–45
    spartan vs. enriched enclosures, 38
    substrates, 41–42
  information sources, 35, 36t
  nutrition, 59–60
  social structure, 93
Hydrocoelom, 98–99, 101–102
  edema syndrome and, 242–243
  gonadal tumors and, 264
  protein deficiency and, 66
  ranaviruses and, 243
  tadpoles and, 243
  treatment of, 243, 318–319
Hydrops, 451–452. *See also* hydrocoelom.
  cardiac lethal mutation and, 452
Hyla andersoni, 11
Hyla spp., 11
Hylidae, 11
Hymenochirus spp., 9
Hynobiidae, 6
Hyoid bones, 18–19
Hypercalcemia, 34
Hyperglycemia, 140
Hyperolidae, 12–13
Hyperolius marmoratus, 13
Hyperolius spp., 13
Hyperolius viridiflavus, 12
Hyperthermia, 236
Hypertonic electrolyte solutions, treatment of mites and, 214
Hypervitaminosis A, 67, 74, 411
Hypervitaminosis D, 76, 471
Hypocalcemia, 34, 74–75
  cloacal prolapse and, 439
  edema and, 242
Hypothermia, 236

Ichthyobodo, 199
Ichthyophiidae, 4
Ichthyophis glutinosus, 4
Ichthyophis kohtaoensis, 4t, 4–5
Ichthyophonus spp., 185–186, 412
Icosiella neglecta, 436
Identification guides, 13–14
Identification techniques, 275–276
Idiopathic syndromes, 239–243
Immunoglobulin production, 138
Immunosuppression, ammonia exposure and, 151–153
  copper and, 316
  estivation and, 159
  metamorphosis and, 107
  temperature and, 31, 148, 236
Inclusion body hepatitis, 441
Indian caecilians. *See* Uraeotyphlidae.
Infectious wart, 337–340
Inner ear, development of, 469
Insulin, 28, 459
Interrenal gland, 458
Intestinal mycoses, 186
Intracutaneous cornifying epithelioma, 340–341
Intranuclear inclusion bodies, 367
Intraocular fluid, collection of, 248
Intromittent organ, 17, 29
Intubation, 26, 119
Intussusception, intestinal, 280
Iodine toxicosis, 227, 274

Iridoviridae, 418
Iridovirus infection, erythrocyte parameters and, 140
  ulcerative dermatitis and, 421
Iris, iridescence of, 247
Iron, toxicity to tadpoles and, 404
Islets of Langerhans, 458–459
Isoflurane, 114, 119–120
Isospora lieberkuehni, 448
Itraconazole, 313–314
  treatment of *Dermocystidium* and, 206
Ivermectin, 317, 318
  prophylaxis during quarantine and, 303
  toxicity of, 317
  treatment of fly larvae and, 215
  treatment of mites and, 214
  treatment of pentastomes and, 214
  treatment of ticks and, 214

Jacobson's organ. *See* vomeronasal organ.
Japanese firebelly newt, 7
Japanese giant salamander, 6
  blue plasma and, 129, 142t

Kale and oxalates, 64, 447. *See also* cystic calculi; oxalate nephrosis; spinach and kidney stones.
Kaloula pulchra, 5t, 13
Kandiyohi mutation, 416
Kassina spp., 13
Keratitis, 249–250, 472–473
  diagnosis of, 250
  treatment of, 251
Keratoconjunctivitis sicca, 248
Ketamine hydrochloride, 114, 120
  administration of, 120
  dosage for, 120
Ketoconazole, 314
  treatment of *Dermocystidium* and, 206
Kidney flukes, 448
Koh Tao Island caecilian. *See* *Ichthyophis kohtaoensis*.

Labyrinthodontia, 1
Lacerations, 234
Lactate, metabolism of, 33
  and muscle fatigue, 33
Lactated Ringer's solution, 33, 319
Lactic acid, and fluid therapy, 319
Lake Titicaca frog, 10
Lampsilis cardium, 215
Lankesterella alencari, infection of brain and, 466
Lankesterellids. *See* apicomplexa.
Laparoscopy, 278–279
Lateral line system, 350–351, 469
  trematode infection and, 472
Lathyrus factor, neoplasia and, 384
Latimeria chalumnae. *See* coelocanth.
Lead, toxicity of, 404, 417, 465
Leeches, 212–213
  diagnosis of, 213
  treatment of, 213, 318
Leiomyoma, 353–354
Leiomyomata, 354
Leiomyosarcoma, 353–354
Leiopelma spp., 8
Leiopelmatidae, 8, 17

Lens, anomalies of, 473
  haploid embryo and, 401
  over-ripe eggs and, 402
Lepidobatrachus asper, 4t
Lepidobatrachus spp., 10
Lepomis spp. See sunfish.
Lepospondylia, 1
Leptodactylidae, 10
Leptodactylus pentadactylus, 5t, 10
Leptodactylus spp., 4t
Leptospira interregans, 448
Leptothea ohlmacheri, 448
Lesser siren, 5–6
Leukemia, basophilic myeloid, 361
  eosinophilic myeloid, 361
  granulocytic, 360–361
  plasmocytoma and, 359–360
Leukocytes, 137–139
Levamisole hydrochloride, toxicity of, 316
  treatment of fly larvae and, 215
  treatment of nematodes and, 211, 316–317
  treatment of pentostomids and, 214
  use in quarantine, 303
Levator bulbi muscle, 245
Leydig cell tumors, 379
Lice. See branchiurans.
Light, 58–59. See also photoperiod.
  bulb selection and replacement, 58
  growth of tadpoles and, 241
  measurement of, 58
  reproductive success and, 285
  ultraviolet-B and biogenesis of vitamin D_3, 58, 93
Limb deformities, congenital, 408–409
Limb regeneration, 277–278, 411–412
Lime sacs, 469
Lingual vein, 102, 106, 130
Lipid keratopathy. See corneal lipidosis.
Lipoma, 353
Lissamphibia, 1
Listeria monocytogenes, 170
Lithium, embryo development and, 404
Lithium heparin, 102, 130
Litoria caerulea. See *Pelodryas caerulea.*
Litoria infrafrenata, 5t, 11
Liver, reparative process, 370
Loperamide, 212
Louse. See Branchiurans.
Lowland Caribbean toad, 10
Lucke's renal adenocarcinoma, 335, 354, 365–368, 447
Lucke tumor herpesvirus (LTV), 365
Lumbriculus variegatus. See black worms.
Lumbricus spp. See earthworms.
Lung, calicivirus infection and, 450
  nonaerated lungs and development of, 450, 452
  parasitic infection of, 450
Lungless salamanders. See Plethodontidae.
Lung worms. See *Rhabdias* spp.
Luteinizing hormone (LH), 28, 288–289
Luteinizing hormone-releasing hormone (LH-RH), 289, 290–292t, 293–294
Lymphangioma, 355
Lymphatic system, 27–28
Lymph hearts, 27–28, 452
  edema and, 243
Lymphocytes, 138
Lymphocytopoiesis, 28
Lymphomyeloid organs, 453–454
Lymphopoiesis, 357
Lymphoproliferative disorders, differentiation from mycobacteriosis, 336, 357

Lymphosarcoma, 357–359
Lymphosarcomata, 357–359

Madagascan bright-eyed frogs, 13
Madagascan dart-poison frogs. See Mantellinae.
Madagascan frogs. See *Mantidactylus* spp.
Madagascan treefrog, 5t
Magnetic resonance imaging (MRI), 253, 263
Malachite green, carcinogenicity of, 198
  growth inhibition of tadpoles and, 198
  treatment of ciliates and, 198
  treatment of flagellates and, 200
  treatment of fungi and, 313–314
Maladaptation syndrome. See acclimation and maladaptation syndrome.
Malathion, toxicity of, 463
Malaysian narrowmouth toad, 13
Malignant melanophoroma, 350
Malpighian body, 23
Mandarin newt, 4t
Mandibular fracture, 278
Mantella aurantiaca, 5t, 12
Mantellas, 12
Mantella spp., 12
Mantellinae, 12
Mantidactylus spp., 5t, 12
Marbled reed frog, 13
Marbled salamander, 7
Marine toad, 5t
Marsh frog, 12
Marsupial treefrogs, 11
Mast cell, 138
Mast cell tumor, 355, 361–364, 382
Mealworms, 65, 70
  gut-loading diet, 67–68
Megophrys montana, 4t, 9
Melanomacrophage centers, 439
Melanophores, 347, 348
Melanophore-stimulating hormone (MSH), 28
Melanophoroma, dendritic type, 348
  epithelioid type, 348–350
  fibromatous type, 348
Meningitis, bacterial, 160, 472
  verminous, 381
Mental gland, 17
Mercury, toxicity of, 404–405, 460
  teratogenic effects of, 405
Mesenchymal cell neoplasm, 355–356
Mesonephritis, 449
Metabolic bone disease, 73–76, 411
Metabolism, equations for, 78t
  standard metabolic rate for anurans, 78t
  standard metabolic rate for caecilians, 84t
  standard metabolic rate for salamanders, 84t
Metals. See also specific metals.
  toxicity of, 227–228, 404
Metal screening, 227, 301, 305
Metamorphosis, 15, 285, 407–408
  CNS and, 461–462
  crowding and, 240–241
  failure to undergo, 459
  gills and, 450
  inhibition of, 406
  injuries to the tail and, 241
  inner ear and, 469
  intestinal tract and, 439

Metamorphosis (*Continued*)
  kidneys and, 447
  pancreas and, 439
  skeletal mineralization and, 469
  skin changes and, 415
  thymus and, 453
  thyroid and, 458
  transitions in the nervous system and, 461–462
Metastatic calcification, 471
Methemoglobinemia, 153. See also nitrite toxicity.
Methoxyflurane, 119
Methylene blue, furazolidone, and monofuracin treatment, 313
Metronidazole, treatment of amoebiasis with, 204, 312, 315
  treatment of anaerobic infections with, 312, 315
  treatment of ciliates with, 197
  treatment of diarrhea with, 312
  treatment of flagellates with, 203
  treatment of new arrivals with, 315
  use in quarantine, 303
Mexican burrowing toad, 8–9. See also Rhinophrynidae.
Mexican caecilian. See *Dermophis mexicanus.*
Miconozole, treatment of fungi with, 314
Microbiology, 123–128, 171–176
  bacterial culture and sensitivities, 171–176
    antibiotic sensitivities, 125–126, 175–176
    culture media for, 123–124, 172–173
    identification of isolates, 125–126, 172–174
    incubation of, 123, 331
    preservation of isolates, 174–175
    sample collection, 103, 124–125, 126–128, 172
  fungal culture, 124
    culture media for, 124, 189
    identification of isolates, 126, 189
    incubation of, 189
    preservation of isolates, 189–190
    sample collection, 103, 189
Microfilaria, 436
  detection of, 129–130
Microhylidae, 13
Microliter pipette, use of, 101, 106–107
Microsporidia, 205–206, 413–414, 435–436, 460–461. See also specific organisms and diseases.
  Alloglugea, 205
  diagnosis of, 206
  infection of oocytes and, 297
  Microsporidium, 205, 435, 460–461
  Pleistophora, 205–206, 414, 460–461
  treatment of, 206
Microsporidium schuetzi, 460–461
Microsporidium tritoni, 435
Microtags, 276
Midwife toads, 8
Mites, 214, 437–438
  Anouracarus, 437
  diagnosis of, 214, 437–438
  Endotrombicula, 437
  Eutrombicula, 214, 438
  Hannemania, 214, 437
  Neotrombicula, 214
  Schongastia, 437

Mites (*Continued*)
　treatment of, 214, 318
　trombiculid. See *Hannemania*.
　Vercannenia, 437
Mixed cell adenoma, 343–344
Modified Giemsa stain for protozoa, 216
Molchpest, 242
Mole salamanders. See Ambystomatidae.
Molliensia latispina. See molly.
Molly, 66
Monkey treefrog, 5t
Monocytes, 138–139
Monocytoid leukemia, 361
Monogenea, 207–208. See also specific organisms and diseases.
　diagnosis of, 208
　Gyrodactylus, 207
　monopisthocotylea vs. polyopisthocotylea, 207
　Polystoma spp., 450–451
　treatment of, 208, 317
Monopisthocotylea, 207
Morphine sulfate, analgesia and, 282
Mosquito fish, 66
Mott cells, 359
Mouse-eating frog, 5t
Mouth-brooding frogs, 11
MS-222. See tricaine methanesulfonate.
Mucor amphibiorum, 188, 444
Mucormycosis, 444
Mucor spp., 183, 188
Mudpuppy, 6
Musca spp. See flies.
Muscle wasting, 99–100
Musculoskeletal deformities, water temperature and, 409
Mushroom tongue salamander, 4t
Mycelia spp., 187
Mycetoma, 431
Mycobacteriosis, 167–169, 305, 427–429, 443–444, 472
　clinical findings and, 167
　definition of, 167
　diagnosis of, 167
　disinfection of, 307
　epidemiology of, 167
　experimental, 428, 443
　forms of, 427
　histology of, 428–429, 442–443
　lesions of, 167, 427–428, 443
　lymphoreticular neoplastic disease and, 428
Mycobacterium, 167–169, 427–429, 443–444
　zoonosis and, 169
Mycosis, 181–190, 412–413, 429–433, 444. See also specific organisms and diseases.
　of eggs and larvae, 186–187
Mydriasis, 248
Myelomalacia, 466
Myelopoiesis, 28
Myeloproliferative disease, unclassified, 361
Myelothrombocytopoiesis, 28
Myiasis, 214–215, 438, 451
　diagnosis of, 215
　treatment of, 215, 318
Myobatrachidae, 9
Myoblastoma, 354–355
Myocardial fibrosis, 267
Myoepithelial adenoma, 344–345

Myositis, mycotic, 185–186
Myxobolus bufonis, 461
Myxobolus hylae, 461
Myxochondroma, 353
Myxolipoma, 353
Myxoma, 352–353
Myxosarcoma, 353
Myxosporea, 207, 461
　Chloromyxum, 207
　diagnosis of, 207, 446
　Leptotheca, 207, 448
　Myxidium, 207, 446
　Myxobolus, 207, 461
　treatment of, 207

Nalidixic acid, 312
Narrowmouth toads. See Microhylidae.
Nasolacrimal duct, 245
Naso-oral neoplasms, 381
Natt-Herrick's solution, 133
Necropsy, 331–334
　anamnesis, 331
　cultures and, 126–128, 331, 334
　cytology and, 331
　equipment for, 331
　procedures for, 332–334
　sample collection for metal analysis, 228
Necturus maculosus, 6
Necturus spp., 4t, 6
Nematodes, 210–212. See also specific organisms and diseases.
　Aplectana, 210
　Cosmocerca, 210
　Cosmocercoides, 210
　diagnosis of, 211
　direct vs. indirect life cycles, 210
　Dranunculus, 210
　filarial worms, 211–212, 436
　Foleyella, 211, 436, 457
　Icosiella, 457
　infecting the lung, 210
　infecting the skin, 210–211
　Pseudocapillaroides, 210, 436–437
　Rhabdiasis, 210, 435–436
　treatment of, 211–212, 316–317
Nematotaenia dispar, 446
Neoplasia, cloacal and rectal prolapse and, 281
　reproductive disorders and, 297
　tumors vs., 335
　viruses and, 335
Neoplastic and hyperplastic lesions. See also specific diseases.
　alimentary tract, 374–377
　　adenocarcinoma of the stomach, 374
　　hyperkeratosis of the tongue, 374
　　intestinal neoplasms, 374–377
　　neuroepithelioma of the mouth, 374
　bones, joints, and notochord, 382–384
　endocrine organs, 381
　　interrenal neoplasms, 381
　　Islet of Langerhans neoplasms, 381
　　pituitary and pineal neoplasms, 381
　　thyroid neoplasms, 381
　eyes and adnexa, 382
　hematopoietic and lymphoid cells and organs, 356–364
　　granulocytic cell neoplasms, 360–361
　　histiocytic cell neoplasms, 361
　　lymphoproliferative disease, 356–360
　　mast cell neoplasms, 361–364
　　thymus neoplasms, 364

Neoplastic and hyperplastic lesions (*Continued*)
　integument, 336–352
　　chromatophore neoplasms, 347–350
　　dermal gland neoplasms, 343–347
　　epidermal neurosensory neoplasms, 350–352
　　epithelial cell neoplasms, 337–343
　kidneys and urinary bladder, 364–370
　　kidney neoplasms, 364–369
　　urinary bladder neoplasms, 369–370
　liver, biliary system, and pancreas, 370–374
　　bile duct neoplasms, 372–373
　　hepatic neoplasms, 370–372
　　pancreatic neoplasms, 373–374
　mesenchymal tissues, 352–356
　　blood and lymph vessel neoplasms, 355
　　fat tissue neoplasms, 353
　　fibrous tissue neoplasms, 352–353
　　mesenchymal cell and undifferentiated neoplasms, 355–356
　　muscle tissue neoplasms, 353–355
　miscellaneous neoplasms, 384
　nervous system, 381–382
　reproductive system, 377–381
　　female reproductive tract neoplasms, 379–381
　　male reproductive tract neoplasms, 377–379
　respiratory system, 381
Neotenic salamanders. See Proteidae.
Neoteny, 16, 460
Neotropical giant toad, 5t
Nephroblastoma, 364–365
Neuroendocrine cells, 458–459
Neuroepithelioma, 350–352
Neuromast cells, 350
Neuromastoma, 350–352
New Guinea giant treefrog, 11
Newt, 5
New tank syndrome, 153–154
New Zealand tailed frog, 8
Nicotine toxicity, 230
Nitrate toxicity, 230–231, 411
Nitrite toxicity, 153, 230, 411
Nitrofurantoin, 312
Nitrogen cycle, 151–154
Nitrogenous waste, 23–24, 32
N-nitroso-dimethylamine, cholangiocarcinomata and, 371–372
　hepatocellular carcinomas and, 371
Nodular hyperplasia, lymphoproliferative disease and, 355–356
　hematopoietic tissue and, 360
Norepinephrine, 7
North American tailed frog, 8
Northern leopard frog, 12
Notemigonus crysoleucas. See golden shiner.
Notochaeta bufonivora. See sarcophagid fly.
Notochord neoplasms, 384
Notophthalmus viridescens, 7
Nuptial pads, 17, 286
Nutrition, 63–71, 95
　diets for captive amphibians, 63–71
　　adult aquatic amphibians, 65–66
　　larval amphibians, 63–65
　　recording the diet, 69
　　terrestrial amphibians, 66
　frequency and time of feeding, 59–60, 67
　oophagous tadpoles, 63, 287
　overfeeding, 59
　paresis and, 411
　prey items, 60, 63–64, 65–67

Nutrition (*Continued*)
  caloric content of, 84t
  culturing food items, 69–71
  rodents as a food source, 67
 reproduction and, 293
 spinach and kidney stones, 60, 64, 447
 vitellogenesis and, 286
Nutritional supplementation, 67–69, 95
 for ill and anorectic amphibians, 82–87, 305
 methods of, 68–69, 73–74

Obesity, 59, 77–79
Olfaction, 36, 39
Olm, 6
Olympic salamanders, 6
Onychodactylus spp., 6
Oogenesis, 288
Oophagous tadpoles, 287
Opalinids, 198–199, 444
 Cepedea, 198
 diagnosis of, 199
 Opalina, 198
 Protoopalina, 198
 Protozelleriella, 198
 treatment of, 199
 Zelleriella, 198
Ophthalmic examination, 100
Oral cavity, examination of, 100
Organochlorine toxicity, 462–463
Organophosphate toxicosis, 224–226, 463
 treatment of, 225–226
Ornate horned frog, 10
Orthopedic procedures, 278
Osmolality, of plasma, 32, 140, 318
Osmoregulation, 39
Osteochondromas, 382
Osteomyelitis, 278
Osteopilus septentrionalis, 11
Osteoporosis, 411
Osteosarcoma, 383–384
Otitis, 472
Ovarian adenocarcinoma, 379–380
Ovariectomy, 281
Over-ripe egg syndrome, 402
Oxalate nephrosis, 447. See also calcium oxalate; cystic calculi; kale and oxalates; spinach and oxalates.
Oxalates, 447. See also calcium oxalate.
Oxalate toxicosis, 77. See also oxalate nephrosis.
Oxymonads, *Monocercomonoides*, 218t
Oxytetracycline, 311, 315

Pachytriton brevipes, 7
Pachytriton spp., 4t
Pacific giant salamander, 6
Pac-man frog, 5t
Paddle tail newt, 4t
Painted-belly monkey frog. See waxy treefrog.
Painted frog, 5t
Painted frogs. See Discoglossidae.
Painted toad, 5t
Palaemonetes spp. See grass shrimp.
Palm salamander, 4t
Palpation, abdominal, 101
 bladder, 281
 fracture and, 235
 gall bladder stone and, 447
 gastric overload and, 79
 gout and, 241

Palpation (*Continued*)
 ovarian cysts and, 297
 starvation and, 82
 steatitis and, 77
 tongue and, 374
Pancreas, endocrine 458–459
Pancreatic carcinoma, 358
Pancreatic islets, 28
Pannus, 250. See also keratitis.
Panophthalmitis, 161, 248–249
Papova-like viruses, 447
Papillary adenocarcinoma of the urinary bladder, 369–370
Para-articular xanthomatosis, 410
Paradox frog, 5t
Paraguay horned frogs, 10
Paralysis, 80–81, 467
 ivermectin toxicity and, 317
 levamisole toxicity and, 316
 pathology of, 80
 treatment of, 81
Paramesotriton spp., 4t
Para-orbital pustular dermatitis, 427
Paraquat, toxicity and teratogenic effects of, 464
Parasitic disease, 194, 413–414, 435–438, 444–447, 448–451, 455–457, 465–466, 472. See also specific organisms and classifications.
 commensal vs. parasitic, 193
 identification of protozoa and metazoa, 215–219
 life cycles of, 193
 management of protozoa and metazoa, 193, 196
Parathormone, 34
Parathyroid gland, 28
Parathyroid hormone (PTH), 28
Parental care, 285, 287
 Dendrobates pumilio and, 287
Paresis, hindlimb, 411
Paromomycin, treatment of amoebiasis with, 315
 treatment of ciliates and, 197
Parotid glands, 17
Parsley frogs, 9. See Pelodytidae.
Passive integrated transponder tags (PIT tags), 276
Pathology and diseases of. See also specific pathological or disease conditions.
 eggs and embryos, 401–407
  genetically based, 401–402
  infectious disease, 406–407
  toxicological etiologies, 402–406
 eyes, ears, and special organs, 467–473
  genetic etiologies, 470
  idiopathic etiologies, 472–473
  infectious etiologies, 472
  nutritional etiologies, 470
  toxicological etiologies, 471–472
 larvae, metamorphs, and adults, 408–473
  alimentary tract, 438–447
   idiopathic etiologies, 447
   infectious etiologies, 440–447
   nutritional etiologies, 439
   toxicological etiologies, 439–440
  cardiovascular system, 451–453
   congenital etiologies, 452
   experimental etiologies, 452
   genetic etiologies, 452
   idiopathic etiologies, 453
   infectious etiologies, 452
  endocrine system, 458–459
   congenital etiologies, 459
   genetic etiologies, 459

Pathology (*Continued*)
   idiopathic etiologies, 459
   toxicological etiologies, 459
  hematolymphopoietic system, 453–454
   genetic etiologies, 454
   infectious etiologies, 454–457
   miscellaneous etiologies, 457
  integumentary system, 415–438
   genetic etiologies, 416
   infectious etiologies, 418–438
   toxicological etiologies, 416–417
   traumatic etiologies, 417–418
  musculoskeletal system, 408–415
   abnormalities of notochord, 408
   congenital abnormalities, 408–409
   genetic etiologies, 409
   idiopathic etiologies, 414–415
   infectious etiologies, 412–414
   nutritional etiologies, 410–411
   toxicological etiologies, 411
   traumatic etiologies, 411–412
  nervous system, central, peripheral, and autonomic, 461–467
   genetic etiologies, 462
   idiopathic etiologies, 466–467
   infectious etiologies, 465–466
   metamorphic transitions in, 461–462
   nutritional etiologies, 462
   toxicological etiologies, 462–465
  reproductive system, 459–461
   congenital etiologies, 460
   infectious etiologies, 460–461
   toxicological etiologies, 460
  respiratory system, 449–451
   experimental etiologies, nonaerated lungs, 450
   genetic etiologies, 450
   infectious etiologies, 450–451
   metamorphic degeneration of the gills, 450
  urinary system, 447–449
   genetic etiologies, 447
   idiopathic etiologies, 449
   infectious etiologies, 447–449
   toxicological etiologies, 447
Pectoral girdle, defect of, 452
Pedostibes spp., 10–11
Pelobatidae, 9
Pelodryas caerulea, 4t, 11
Pelodytes spp., 9
Pelodytidae, 9
Peltophryne lemur, 5t
Pelvic patch. See drinking patch.
Pentastomids, 213–214, 447
 diagnosis of, 214
 treatment of, 214
Pentobarbital, anesthesia and, 120–121
 euthanasia and, 120–121
Pericardial effusion, 260, 264
Pericardial fluid, collection and analysis of, 131–132
Permethrin, 226, 463–464
Petroleum intoxication, 405–406, 439
Phaeohyphomycosis, 431. See also chromomycosis.
Phantasmal dart frog, 5t, 12
Pharmacotherapeutics, 309–329
 administration of, 106–107
 anthelmintics, 316–318, 323–325t
 antibacterial agents, 309–313
 antifungal agents, 313–314, 320–323t
 antiprotozoal agents, 315–316, 319, 323–325t
 antiviral agents, 309
 emergency treatment and, 314–315

Pharmacotherapeutics (*Continued*)
  failure of treatment and, 310
  thermal gradients and, 148, 310
Pharyngostomy tube, 278
Pheromones, 36, 39
Phialophora spp., 187
Phlebotomy, 102, 130–132
Photoperiod, 59, 305
  feeding behavior and, 67
  oogenesis and, 288
  reproductive success and, 285–286
Phyllobates, 12
Phyllomedusa bicolor, 4t
Phyllomedusa sauvagii, 5t
Phyllomedusa spp., 5t, 11
Physical examination, anamnesis and, 91–96
  examining the patient, 98–101
Physiology, 31–33
  calcium metabolism, 33–34
  energy metabolism, 33
  thermal homeostasis, 31
  water homeostasis, 31–33
Pigment mutations, 402, 416
Pineal body, 28, 458
Pine Barrens treefrog, 11
Pipa pipa, 9
Piperacillin, 315
Pipidae, 9
Pirhemocyton spp., 454
Pit organs, 469
Pituitary gland, 28, 458
  congenital absence of, 459
Pituitary pars distalis homogenate (PDH), 291t
Pixie frog, 5t
Plants, 43–44
  aquatic, 44
  oxalates and, 43, 94, 447
  parasites and, 44
  preparing for use, 44
  recommendations for, 43, 53–54
Plasma cell, 139
Plasmocytoma, 359–360
Pleistophora bufonis, 460–461
Pleistophora danilewski, 414
Pleistophora myotropica, 205–206, 414
Plethodon spp., 8
Plethodontidae, 7–8
Pleurodeles spp., 4t
Pleurodeles waltl, 7
Pneumonia, mycotic, 186
  pneumococcal, 450
Poison-arrow frogs. See Dendrobatidae.
Poison-dart frogs. See Dendrobatidae.
Poison frogs. See Dendrobatidae.
Polyhedral cytoplasmic deoxyriboviruses (PCDV), 422
Polyopisthocotylea, 207
Polyvinyl chloride glues, 229–230. See also Glues and sealants.
Pool frog, 12
Postmetamorphic death syndrome, 241
Potassium permanganate, treatment of external ciliates and, 198
  treatment of fungi and, 313–314
Praziquantel, prophylaxis during quarantine and, 303
  treatment of cestodes and, 210, 317
  treatment of trematodes and, 208, 317
Precipitation, stimulation of reproduction and, 57–58, 285
Preferred body temperature, 31
Pregnant mare serum gonadotropin (PMSG), 292t, 293–294
Preventive medicine, 95–96

Primicarb toxicity, 463
Progesterone, 28, 288
Prolactin (PRL), calcium metabolism and, 34
  vitellogenesis and, 288
Protargol silver protein stain, 216
Proteidae, 6
Proteromonads, *Karotomorpha,* 201, 203, 218t
  Proteromonas, 218t
Proteus anguinis, 6
Prototheca algae, growth inhibition and, 240
Protractor lentis muscle, 246, 247
Pseudacris spp., 11
Pseudidae, 11
Pseudis paradoxa, 5t, 11
Pseudobranchus axanthus, 5
Pseudobranchus spp. 5–6
Pseudobranchus striatus, 5
Pseudocapillaroides xenopi, 210, 436–437
Pseudomonas aeruginosa, 166
Pseudotriton spp., 8
Puerto Rican crested toad, 5t
Pulmonary adenocarcinoma, 381
Pulse oximetry, 115
Pupillary light reflexes, 248
Pyrethrin toxicosis, 226
Pyrethroid toxicosis, 226, 463–464
Pyxicephalus adspersus, 4t, 5t, 12
Pyxicephalus delalandii, 5t

Quarantine, 37–38, 95–96, 301–307
  cultures and, 304
  disinfection of tools and, 302
  parasite evaluation and treatment, 302–304
  protocols for, 301–304
  record keeping and, 304
  spartan vs. enriched environments, 38, 301
Quinilones, use of, 311
Quinine sulfate, treatment of hemoflagellates, 200

Radiation, 237–238
Radiography, 253–258
  barium enema, 258,
  cholecystogram, 258
  double contrast coelogram, 258
  pneumocoelogram, 258
  radiographic techniques, 254–258
Rain chambers, 57–58, 290t
Rana catesbeiana, 5t, 12
Rana esculenta, 12
  klepton concept and, 12
Rana esculenta iridovirus (REIR), 422
Rana lessonae, 12
Ranalike viruses, 422–423, 467
Rana pipiens, 12
Rana ridibunda, 12
Rana sylvatica, 12
Ranaviruses, 406, 418–420, 422. See also specific organisms.
  red leg syndrome and, 162
  tadpole edema virus (TEV), 418
Ranidae, 12
Rectal prolapse, nematodiasis and, 93, 281
  treatment of, 281
Redbelly newt, 4t
Reddened skin syndrome, 422–424
Red-eyed treefrog, 11
Red leg syndrome, 161–164, 424–427
  lesions of, 425–426
  ophthalmitis and, 471
  treatment of, 163–164

Red salamanders, 8
Red-spotted newt, 7
Red worms, 70
Reflexes, 99
Renal calculi, 77
  calcium oxalates and, 64, 77
Renal cell carcinoma, 358, 368–369
Renal portal system, 28
Reproduction, 285–297, 459–461
  atmospheric pressure and, 288
  disorders of, 296–297
  hormonal manipulation and, 285, 289–294, 290–292t
  nutrition and, 286, 293
  oogenesis, 288
  ovulation, 288, 293–294
  parental care, 287
  rainfall and, 57, 285
  reproductive cycle, 287–289
  sexual maturity and, 287
  spermatogenesis, 29, 288–289, 460
  temperature and, 147, 287
Reproductive strategies, 285–286
  internal vs. external fertilization, 285
  parental care, 285
  seasonal breeding, 285
  sperm storage, 285
  viviparous vs. oviparous, 285
Respiration, 24–26
Respiratory infection, culture of, 126
Restraint, manual, 36–37, 111–114
  chemical, 114–121
  hypothermia and, 114
  radiography and, 253
Reticulum cell sarcoma, 361
Retina, structure and nourishment of, 247
Retinoic acid, cardiac formation and, 406
Retortamonads, *Chilomastix,* 201, 218t
  Retortamonas, 201, 218t
Retractor bulbi muscle, 245
Rhabdias bufonis, 210
Rhabdiasis, 210, 435–436, 450, 472
  diagnosis of, 211
  treatment of, 211, 316–317
Rhabdias sphaerocephala, 435–436, 472
Rhabdias spp., 210, 211
Rhabdomyoma, 354
Rhabdomyosarcoma, 354
Rhacophoridae, 13
Rhacophorus nigropalmatus, 13
Rhacophorus spp., 4t, 13
Rheobatrachus spp., 9
Rhinatrematidae, 4
Rhinodermatidae, 11
Rhinophrynidae, 8–9
Rhinophynus dorsalis, 8–9
Rhyacotritonidae, 6
Rhyacotriton spp., 6
Rickets, 411
Rickettsia, 455
Rio Cauca caecilian. See *Typhlonectes natans.*
Robber frogs, 10
Rocket frogs. See *Colestethus* spp.
Rodents as a food source, 67
Rose Bengal stain, use in the diagnosis of ocular disease, 248
Rostral injuries, 38, 99, 160, 233, 304, 417–418
  histology of, 417
  preventing, 38, 304–305
  treatment of, 99, 233–234
Rotenone toxicosis, 226
Roughskin newt, 7
Rubber eel, 4t

Running frogs, 13
Russel bodies, 359

Saddleback toads, 11
Salamander, 5
Salamandra salamandra, 7
Salamandridae, 5, 6–7
Salientia. *See* Anura.
Salmonella spp., 170–171, 442
Salt bath, treatment of branchiurans and, 213
Salt toxicosis, 228
Sambava tomato frog, 13
Saprolegnia ferax, 184, 186
Saprolegnia parasitica, 184, 186
Saprolegniasis, 183–184, 186–187, 429–430
　eggs and embryos and, 406–407
　oviduct and, 297
　treatment of, 184
Sarcocystis, 413
Sarcophagid fly, 214, 438. *See also* myiasis.
Schellackia balli, 457
Scolecomorphidae, 4
Scolecosbasidium humicola, 187–188
Scoliosis, mercury toxicity and, 405
　microgravity and, 408
　prevention of, 65, 80
Selenium toxicity, 405
Seminoma, 379
Septicemia, emergency treatment of, 314–315
Serratia spp., 167
Sertoli cell tumor, 377–379
Sex determination, alteration of, 459–460
Sexual dimorphism, 286, 18t
　cloacal glands and, 286
　coloration in anurans and, 286
　mental glands and, 17
　nuptial pads and, 17, 286
　permanent vs. seasonal characteristics and, 286
　tympanic membrane and, 286
Seyechelles frog, 10
Seychelles frogs. *See* Sooglossidae.
Shock, therapy for, 234
Silver toxicity, 405
Sinbis virus, 465
Sirenidae, 5
Siren intermedia, 5–6
Siren lacertina, 5–6
Sirens. *See* Sirenidae.
Skeletal and muscular underdevelopment. *See* spindly leg.
Skin, permeability of, 33
Skin glands, 415–416
Skin scrape, performing, 107–108
Skin secretions, 93, 111, 415
　alvarobufotoxin, 111
　defensive chemicals, 415
　gluelike substances, 415
Smilisca spp., 11
Smokey jungle frog, 5t
Smooth muscle neoplasms, 353–354
Smooth-sided toad, 5t
Snails, removal from tank, 44
Sodium absorption, 156
Sodium balance, acid soils and, 416
Sodium chloride, treatment of ciliates and, 198
　treatment of flagellates and, 200
　treatment of fungi and, 313
Soft tissue sarcomas, 356
Solomon Island eyelash frog, 5t
Solomon Island leaf frog, 5t

Solutions. *See also* individual solutions.
　for diluting sperm or maintaining eggs, 295–296t
Sooglossidae, 9–10
Sooglossus gardineri, 9
Sooglossus seychellensis, 10
South American bullfrog, 10
Spadefoot toads. *See* Pelobatidae.
Spanish ribbed newt, 7
Speckle mutation, 416
Spermatogenesis, 29, 288–289
　environmental changes and, 289
　gonadotropins and, 289, 293
Spermatophore, 29
　anchoring of, 286
Spinach and kidney stones, 60
Spinal cord, haploid syndrome and, 401
　over-ripe eggs and, 402
　and oxalates, 64, 77. *See also* cystic calculi; kale and oxalates; oxalate nephrosis.
Spindly leg, 65, 80, 239–241, 410
Spiral bacteria, 442
Spix's saddleback toad, 11
Spontaneous neoplasms, 385–396t
Spotted salamander, 7
Spotted toad, 10
Springtails, 65, 70
Squamous cell carcinoma, 341–343
　of the colo-cloacal region, 376–377
Squamous cell papilloma, 337–340
Squamous metaplasia of submucosal glands, 374
Starvation, 410
Steatitis, 76–77
Steinberg's solution, diluting sperm or maintaining eggs, 294, 296t
　formula for, 296t, 326
　treatment of mites and, 214
　treatment of protozoa and, 198, 319
Steotosis, 447
Streptococcus spp., 167, 455–456
Stress, inhibition of reproduction and, 289
　physiological changes and, 309
　thymus and, 453
Stubfoot toads, 10–11
Substrate, 41–42, 93
　anchoring spermatophore and, 286
Sunburn, 238
Sunfish, 66
Supernumerary limbs and digits, 402, 408–409
　congenital, 408–409
　over-ripe egg syndrome and, 402
　trematodes cysts and, 409
Supersaturation. *See* Gas bubble disease.
Surgical instruments, 274
Surgical techniques, 273–282. *See also* specific procedures.
　patient preparation, 273–274
　postoperative analgesia, 282
　procedures, 274–275
Surinam horned frog, 10
Surinam toad, 9
Suture material, 274
Swimming frog, 11

Tadpole edema virus (TEV, Ranavirus type III), 418, 422, 440–441
　inclusion bodies and, 419
　liver necrosis and, 419
　stomach and, 419
　tubular necrosis and, 419

Tadpoles, filtration for, 154
　separating carnivorous tadpoles, 155
Tail, degeneration of, 450
Tailed frogs. *See* Leiopelmatidae.
Taricha spp., 4t, 7
Taste bud receptor cells, 470
Taxonomy, 3–13
Telmatobius culeus, 10
Temperature, air temperature, 45, 55–57
　body temperature, 31, 38, 56, 94, 305–306
　malnutrition and, 410
　measuring, 56, 94
　physiological effect of, 148
　reproduction and, 56, 285–286, 287
　transporting and, 37
　treatment of toxicosis and, 223
Tenebrio molitor. See mealworms.
Teratogenesis, 406
Teratoma, 379, 380, 384
Testicular neoplasms, 377
Testosterone and dihydrotestosterone, 286
　sexual dimorphism and, 286
Tetany, hypocalcemia and, 34
Tetracycline hydrochloride, 312
Tetraiodothyronine, 15, 28
Tetrathyridia. *See* cestodes, *Mesocestoides*.
Texas blind salamander, 8
T_4. *See* Tetraiodothyronine.
Thermal gradient, 38–39, 56–57, 95, 310
　pharmacotherapeutics and, 310
　recommendations for, 56–57, 310
Thermoregulation, 310
Thiabendazole, treatment of pentastomes and, 214
Thiamine deficiency, 76
Thompson's caecilian. *See Caecilia thompsoni*.
Thrombocyte, 136–137
Thrombocytozoons, 456
Thymoma, 364
Thymosin, 28
Thymus, 28, 453
Thyroid gland, 458
Thyroid hormones, metamorphosis and, 407, 447, 461
Thyroxine, 407
Ticks, 214, 437
　Amblyomma dissimile, 214
　diagnosis of, 214
　treatment of, 214
Tiger salamander, 7
Tiletamine HCl and zolazepam, 120
Tissue regeneration, 411–412. *See also* limb regeneration.
Toad, 8
Toad fly, 214–215, 451. *See also* myiasis.
Toad-licking, 111
Toddia spp., 454
Toe-clipping, 275–276
Togaviruses, 465
Tolnaftate, treatment of fungi with, 314
Tomato frog, 13
Touch preparations, 108
Toxicity, skin secretions and, 111
Toxicology, 223–231. *See also* specific agents.
　halogens and, 227
　herbicides and, 226, 464
　metals and, 227–228
　organophosphorous and carbamate insecticides and, 224–226, 462–464
　organotin, 464
　paper factory effluents, 464–465
　polyvinyl chloride glues and, 229–230
　pyrethrin and pyrethroid insecticides and, 226, 462–464

Toxicology (*Continued*)
  rotenone, 226
  salt, 228
Toxicosis, diagnosis of, 223–224
  treatment of, 224
Toxoplasma, infection of brain and spinal cord, 465–466
Toxoplasma alencari. See *Lankesterella alencari*.
Toxoplasma ranae, 466
Toxoplasma serpai, 466
Trachea, 25
Tracheal lung, 25
Tracheal wash, 109
Tracheobronchial neoplasms, 381
Transillumination, 113
Transitional cell carcinoma, 369
Transporting amphibians, 36–37, 90–91
Treefrogs. See Hylidae.
Tree salamander, 4t
Treetoads, 8
Trematode cysts, histology of, 449
Trematodes. See also Monogenea; Digenea.
  brain and meninges and, 466
  eustachian tube and, 472
  eyes and, 472
  lateral line infection and, 472
  musculature and, 414
Triboleum confusum. See flour beetles.
Tributyltins and triphenyltins, toxicity of, 464
Tricaine methanesulfonate, 114, 115–118
  absorption and metabolism of, 118
  anesthesia and, 116–117
  buffering of, 116
  cardiac rate and, 116–117
  dosage for, 116
  euthanasia and, 121
  pH and, 116
  preparation of injectable solution, 118
  toxicity of, 447
Trichlorfon, 225
Trichodina urinicola, 197, 448
Trichodinids, 197, 448
Trichomonads, *Hexamastix*, 218t
  Monocercomonas, 218t
  Tetratrichomonas, 218t
  Trichomitus, 218t
  Tritrichomonas, 201, 218t, 445
Triethyltin, toxicity of, 464
Triiodothyronine, 15, 28
Trimethoprim and sulfamethoxazole, 303, 311–312, 315–316
Trimethyltin, toxicity of, 464
Tritrichomonas augusta, 445
Triturus spp., 4t, 7
Tropical caecilians. See Scolecomorphidae.
Tropical frogs. See Leptodactylidae.
Tropical lungless salamanders, 8
True frogs. See Ranidae.
True salamanders. See Salamandridae.
True toads. See Bufonidae.
Trypanosoma diemyctyli, 200
Trypanosoma inopinatum, 200
Trypanosoma pipientis, 200
Trypanosoma ranarum, 200
Trypanosomes, 200, 456. See also specific organisms.
  transmission of, 457
Tschudi's African bullfrog, 12
Tsitou newt, 7
T_3. See Triiodothyronine.
Tube-feeding, 83
Tubifex tubifex. See tubifex worms.

Tubifex worms, 65
Tumorlike osteochondrous dysplasia, 382–383
2,4-dichlorophenoxyacetic acid, teratogenic effects of, 464
Tylodelphys xenopi, 452
Tylototriton shanjing, 4t, 7
Tylototriton verrucosus, 4t, 7. See also *Tylototriton shanjing*.
Typhlomolge rathbuni, 8
Typhlonectes compressicauda, 4t, 4–5
Typhlonectes natans, 4–5
Typhlonectes spp., 4t
Typhlonectidae, 4

Ulcerative and hemorrhagic syndrome (UHS), 422–424
Ulcerative syndrome (US), 422–424
Ultimobranchial glands, 28
Ultrasonography, 258–263
Ultraviolet radiation (light), 58, 93, 237–238, 402–404, 417
  corneal melanosis and, 471
  ecdysis and, 417
  eggs and embryos and, 402–404
  epidermal erosions and ulceration, 417
  epidermal hyperplasia and, 403, 417
  keratitis and, 249
  prey recognition and, 305
Uraeotyphlidae, 4
Urate bladder stones, 33. See also cystic calculi.
Urate calculi, 280. See also cystic calculi.
Uricotelic, 32.
Urinalysis, 109
Urinary bladder, 365
  Gorgodera and, 208
  Gorgoderina and, 208
  Monogenea and, 207
  myxozoan infection of, 461
  Trichodena urinicola and, 197
  ultrasonography of, 261
Urodela. See Caudata.
Urostyle, 18
Uveitis, 161, 248–251
  fungal, treatment of, 314

Varagua caecilian. See *Gymnopis multiplicata*.
Ventilation, 301
Ventral abdominal vein (midabdominal), 102, 106, 131
Ventral caudal vein, 131
Verminous granulomata, 414
Verminous granulomatous meningitis, 381
Verminous hyperplasia, 381
Viral hemorrhagic septicemia of frogs (VHSF), 422, 440–441
Viral infections. See also specific viral agents.
  eggs and embryos and, 406
  larvae, adults, and metamorphs, 418–424, 440–441, 447–448, 450, 454–455, 465
Vitamin A deficiency, squamous metaplasia and, 374
Vitamin B, importance of, 80
Vitamin D_3, 58, 66, 73–76
  hypervitaminosis A and, 74
  hypervitaminosis D, 471
Vitellogenesis, 288
Vitreous humor, 247

Vocal sacs, 26
Vomeronasal organ, 469–470

Wangiella dermatitidis, 187
Warty newt, 4t
Wasting syndrome, 414–415
Water, buffering capacity of, 151
  calcium-deficient, 156
  conditioning of, 41, 156
  source of, 156
  supersaturation of, 150
Waterdog, 4t
Waterdogs, 6
Water filtration, 47, 154–155
  ponds and streams and, 155
  types of filters and, 154–155
Water fleas, 65
Water homeostasis, 31–33. See also dehydration; water loss.
Water loss, 236–237
  resistance to, 31–32
Water quality, 41, 94, 147–157
  alkalinity, 151
  carbon dioxide, 150
  hardness, 151
  log, 147, 149t
  nitrogen cycle and, 151–154
  oxygen, 148–150
  pH, 150–151
  recommended parameters, 148t
  record keeping and, 147, 149t
  salinity, 156, 228
  testing, 97, 147, 151
Wax worms, 65
  gut-loading diet, 68
Waxy treefrog (syn. painted-belly monkey frog), 5t
Weight loss, 305
Weight reduction, 78
Western equine encephalitis virus, 465
Whitaker-Wright solution, formula for, 318–319, 327t
White-lipped treefrog, 5t
White's treefrog, 11
White worms, 65, 69–70
Wolffian duct, 29
Wood frog, 12
Woodland salamanders, 8
Wound healing, 235
Wyoming toad, 10

Xanthomas, 249, 381
Xenobiotic estrogens, 460
Xenoma, 445–446
Xenopus laevis, 8, 9
X-radiation, induced limb atrophy and, 411

Yellow-striped caecilian, 4t
Yersinia spp., 171, 442

Zelleriella. See opalinids.
Zinc, CNS lesions and, 465
  teratogenicity of, 405
  toxicity to tadpoles, 405
Zygomycoses, 188